D1547899

ELECTROSURGERY IN DENTISTRY

Second Edition

MAURICE J. ORINGER, D.D.S., F.A.C.D., F.A.A.D.E., F.R.S.H.

Guest Instructor in Electrosurgery, Faculties of Continuing Dental Education,
at Loyola University School of Dentistry, Southern Illinois University School of
Dental Medicine, U.C.L.A. School of Dentistry, University of Pavia (Italy) School
of Dentistry, University of Washington School of Dentistry. Also Guest Instructor in
Electrosurgery, Dental Society Continuing Education Programs in Australia,
Brazil, Canada, France, Italy, Germany, Japan, Switzerland, Venezuela, and the
United States. Formerly Professorial Lecturer in Electrosurgery, Undergraduate
and Graduate, St. Louis University School of Dentistry. Formerly Guest Instructor,
Faculties of Continuing Dental Education, at Ohio State University School of
Dentistry, St. Louis University School of Dentistry, Temple University School of
Dentistry, Tufts University School of Dental Medicine, University of Bologna
(Italy) School of Dentistry, University of California School of Dentistry, University
of Detroit School of Dentistry, University of Oregon School of Dentistry, University
of Pittsburgh School of Dental Medicine, University of Zurich (Switzerland) Institute
of Stomatology, U.S. Naval Dental School, Western Reserve University School of
Dentistry, and Albert Einstein University Medical School's Dental Division.
Consultant for Electrosurgical Devices to the American Dental Association's
Council on Dental Materials and Devices. Consultant in Oral Diagnosis and
Oral Surgery and to the Oral Cancer Detection and Prevention Center, St. Francis
Hospital, Poughkeepsie, New York. Founder, American Academy of Dental
Electrosurgery. Fellow, American College of Dentists. Fellow, American
Academy of Dental Electrosurgery. Fellow, Royal Society of Health (England).
Professeur Honoraire du Centre de Perfectionnement en Odonto-Stomatologie,
Provence–Côte d'Azur, France.

1975 W. B. SAUNDERS COMPANY PHILADELPHIA LONDON TORONTO

W. B. Saunders Company: West Washington Square
Philadelphia, Pa. 19105

12 Dyott Street
London, WC1A   1DB

833 Oxford Street
Toronto, Ontario M8Z 5T9, Canada

Library of Congress Cataloging in Publication Data

Oringer, Maurice J.

Electrosurgery in Dentistry, 2nd edition

Includes bibliographies.

1. Dentistry, Operative.   2.   Electrosurgery.   I.   Title.
[DNLM: 1. Electrosurgery.   2. Surgery, Oral.   WU600
069e 1974]

RK501.5.07 1974   617.6   70–186952

ISBN 0–7216–7001–6

Electrosurgery in Dentistry   ISBN 0-7216-7001-6

Last digit is the print number: 9   8   7   6   5   4   3   2   1

TO MY WIFE
HELEN J. ORINGER
FOR HER UNFLAGGING
ENCOURAGEMENT

PREFACE TO THE SECOND EDITION

Why a Second Edition?

The first edition of this book was published more than 10 years ago, prior to which compilation of the original text took another three years. All in all, substantially more than a decade has elapsed.

Science has made incredible advances during this decade . . . from Sputnik to Apollo's men on the moon, satellite communications, weather satellites, solid-state and microwave electronics, the laser, and other marvels far too numerous to mention.

Medicine and its related basic sciences have shared in these advances—from the nuclear cardiac pacemaker and open heart surgery to heart, liver, and other organ transplants; biologic investigation and synthesis of DNA; sex and gene control, and a host of comparable developments.

Of course dentistry has shared in these advances, and so has dental electrosurgery. New, more sophisticated, clinically superior electrosurgical equipment has become available. Clinical needs have led to the development of a host of new clinical electrosurgical techniques for an ever-expanding range of clinical applications, and for revision or refinement of old techniques. Perhaps most noteworthy of all, electrosurgical experimental research by competent investigators has resulted in an impressive accumulation of valid research data, thermal and histologic, that help to explain many of the phenomena experienced with electrosurgery. These data have been especially useful to verify exactly how and why electrosurgery affects the tissues and produces the remarkable therapeutic results we enjoy when adequately potent fully rectified electrosection is properly utilized. These data as well as data regarding the effects of electrosurgery on the heart will be fully reported in a section devoted to electrosurgical research.

Like its predecessor, this edition is essentially a clinical text for the clinician. Its primary purpose is to review comprehensively all the safe, effective electrosurgical techniques that have been developed to facilitate and improve dental therapy and simplify the practice of dentistry.

Nevertheless, a section of the text is devoted to electrosurgical research for what I consider several valid reasons: First, the thermal and histologic evidence provided by heat sensors and by light and electron microscopes proves conclusively that when electrosurgery is used properly, the tissue response to it is remarkably favorable, and that it can be employed with full confidence in its safety. Second, as a direct outcome of competent research investigations a number of revisions and refinements that improve technique and produce more favorable clinical results have been perfected.

Moreover, not only is the competent clinician influenced by the research findings, but in his unceasing effort to improve old techniques and develop better ones, he is likely to become personally involved in either structuring or conducting new research studies. Thus, although this is a clinical text, I am firmly convinced that far from being incompatible with the clinical aspect of the text, the research section will augment its clinical value by reassuring the clinician that electrosurgery is a safe as well as a wonderfully useful modality, and will also help him to use it more judiciously.

In the interval since the first edition was published a number of readers have sent me letters chiding me for having failed to include in that text specific electrosurgical techniques for treatment of a wide variety of conditions ranging from the commonplace, such as bleaching discolored teeth, to the rare, such as the evulsion of the mental nerve. It was the consensus of opinion among the communicants that because of electrosurgery's unique qualities, its clinical uses should be expanded to develop new techniques to help simplify treatment or to achieve superior operative results in many areas that had not been covered in the first edition.

The electrosurgical techniques most frequently suggested as especially desirable included the following: bleaching discolored teeth; treatment of traumatic and mechanical pulp exposure; treatment of the chronically suppurating root canal; mandibular and maxillary edentulous ridge extension vestibulotomy; radectomy of totally involved maxillary molar palatal roots to preserve the teeth as functionally useful abutments; treatment of ankyloglossia, of leukoplakia, and of papillary hyperplasia. Other requests included treatment of cavernous hemangioma, ranula, traumatic cyst and evulsion of the mental nerve.

These requests challenged the author to broaden the scope of application and increase the clinical usefulness of electrosurgery in dentistry. In response to this challenge, and to increase and more fully utilize electrosurgery's remarkable advantages, I have succeeded in developing specific electrosurgical techniques that effectively treat the conditions just enumerated.

There are a few isolated instances among the cases reported in the section on clinical electrosurgical techniques of seeming similarity that may create an impression of unnecessary duplication. In each instance, however, despite the similarity, critical differences in instrumentation or treatment plan, or both, fully justify their inclusion. Moreover, since the results achieved were so spectacularly more favorable than can be achieved by other methods, these duplications may indirectly serve another useful purpose. They may help to resolve any lingering doubts in the reader's mind about whether these results were really relatively typical and predictable, or simply isolated fortuitous accidents.

In the decade since the first edition was published I have become acutely aware of the vast difference that may exist between the author's intent and the reader's interpretation thereof. Several items that have caused confusion and misinterpretation have been thoroughly clarified in this edition.

In compiling the material for the first edition I included all the dental electrosurgical techniques that had been reported in the literature—some I was personally unfamiliar with; others did not meet with my personal approval. This procedure has been dispensed with; only those techniques that have given ample proof of their efficiency and safety will be considered in this edition.

Most of the techniques that were reviewed in the first edition have withstood the test of time and have fully proved their merit. A few, however, have failed to do so. These have been deleted or thoroughly revised.

One such important area, in which clinical experience has dictated need for re-evaluation and in which extensive deletion and revision proved necessary, is the preparation of the subgingival trough for full crown restoration. A totally new technique that eliminates the postoperative hazards of gingival proliferation or recession is presented in this edition.

A related technique for preparation of the subgingival trough in very thin marginal gingiva is also presented. This technique eliminates the virtually inevitable gingival recession that has occurred, regardless of the technique used to prepare the tooth, when the maxillary cuspid is restored with a full crown that extends subgingivally.

The rapid rate and superb quality of tissue healing that is typically experienced when fully rectified current of adequate potency is properly utilized shall be seen repeatedly in case after case throughout this text.

When slow, unfavorable healing is encountered despite comparable electrosurgery, the atypical result is as unexpected as it is unwelcome. In the isolated instances when unfavorable healing occurs unexpectedly and unaccountably despite good technique, the cause invariably is neither accidental nor inexplicable. The patient who fails to heal normally from electrosurgery properly performed almost invariably is an unsuspected victim of a blood dyscrasia, severe vitamin or hormone deficiency, diabetes or other metabolic dysfunction, or a comparable systemic factor that impairs the body's ability to repair itself.

When a systemic disease is suspected preoperatively, the patient's physician is of course consulted and laboratory tests are initiated to establish a diagnosis. If the laboratory tests confirm a systemic involvement, treatment is immediately instituted to cure the systemic condition, or at least ameliorate it long enough to assure a normal postoperative response to the electrosurgery.

If, however, no systemic disease was suspected preoperatively, as is all too often the case, and the procedure results in poor healing which can be attributed to neither the technique used nor the electrosurgery, there is a subconscious tendency to axiomatically assume that in some way we must have done something wrong, or that the electrosurgery is to blame. This guilt complex is especially likely to occur when the therapist is still a relative neophyte in the use of electrosurgery and has not had the opportunity to develop the self-confidence that comes with experience.

Such mental wringing of the hands and self-blame is not only pointless, but it deprives the individual of the opportunity to render an invaluable service to the patient by discovering serious systemic disease at the preclinical stage, before the clinical medical symptoms associated with the disease have been manifested and serious, perhaps irreparable, permanent inroads have been made on the patient's health.

If, instead, we condition ourselves to think in terms of the *total patient* rather than just the dental problem, and initiate steps to uncover any systemic disease that had not been previously suspected, we shall have rendered a service that is more important by far than the dental therapy itself.

A number of such cases are included in this text to describe the nature and extent of the healing impairment and the response of the tissues to the corrective therapy.

There has been a notable increase in the number of schools that now are including some measure of electrosurgical instruction at the undergraduate level. A chapter on proper introduction of the undergraduate student to electrosurgical instrumentation is therefore also included in this edition.

Unfavorable postoperative pain and tissue destruction caused by faulty local anesthesia injection technique all too often is improperly attributed to electrosurgical procedures. A greatly expanded separate chapter devoted to techniques of local anesthesia has been included in this text in the hope that this will help to eliminate such unfavorable results that have tended to discredit electrosurgery.

Although pedodontic dentistry is essentially similar to the practice of dentistry for adults, there are problems that are unique to this discipline. A chapter dealing with the advantageous contributions electrosurgery can make toward favorably resolving some of these problems has also been included.

Finally, an Appendix of drugs, instruments, and other items mentioned in the text and their sources has been compiled to aid the reader.

In conjunction with the Rochester University School of Medicine, the author is currently conducting comprehensive laboratory investigations to compare the effects of identical wounds created in the labial gingival mucosa of six dogs with new Bard-Parker steel scalpels and with needle electrodes activated by continuous wave (surgery 1) current and modified continuous wave (surgery 2) current of the Ritter unit and the fully rectified current of the Coles Radiosurg Scalpel IV unit. The experiments have been concluded, and the results will be determined histologically by double-blind study. Thus far, the only histological specimens have been tissue removed at the initial session, 3 hours postoperatively, and all tissues appear to be in satisfactory condition. Since it is a double-blind study, identification of the specimens will not be made until all have been interpreted histologically by code number designation. The results will be valuable not only because of the specific comparative data but because they may offer a pattern for similar studies by manufacturers of electrosurgical circuits to qualify for approval by the ADA Council on Dental Materials and Devices.

PREFACE TO THE
FIRST EDITION

Persisting outmoded prejudices and fundamental misconceptions remain the principal barriers to more universal utilization of the numerous advantages electrosurgery offers dentistry. This link with the past, nurtured in the miasma of faulty, antiquated concepts, is a stumbling block to progress and a challenge that still remains to be met. To the hope of meeting that challenge this book is dedicated.

Electrosurgery has come a long way since those momentous occasions more than two centuries ago when for the first time electricity was used therapeutically for tumor surgery at the Middlesex and St. Bartholomew's hospitals in London, England.

Today, electrosurgery is, in effect, virtually indispensable for many clinical procedures in the practice of medicine and dentistry. It is used extensively in many of the medical specialties, especially in tumor surgery, neurosurgery, dermatology, rhinolaryngology, urology, proctology and gynecology. The role that this modality is playing in the present-day practice of these specialties was highlighted in a talk to a dental group by the internationally famous neurosurgeon, Dr. Juan Negrin.[*]

Describing some of the handicaps under which many Latin-American neurosurgeons must operate, he exclaimed, "Can you imagine anyone having to perform modern neurosurgery without the use of suction or electrocoagulation?"

Although it is indispensable in many medical specialties, electrosurgery can be valuable to an even greater extent in dentistry. Electrosurgery does not play a significant role in the general practice of medicine, and therefore it is of relatively little interest to the general medical practitioner. In dentistry, however, the usefulness of electrosurgery is by no means restricted to a few specialties; it is virtually universal. Properly and judiciously employed, it is a remarkably valuable adjunct to the modern practice of dentistry, equally beneficial to general practitioner and specialist alike.

---

[*]Delivered as guest speaker at the 1958 annual meeting of the Pan-American Odontological Association.

Despite infinitely more universal usefulness and applicability in dentistry, and ardent championing by a few competent pioneers such as Ogus, Strock and Saghirian, electrosurgery has received all too little attention in the dental literature. Unlike the medical literature, which has been replete with reports on use of electrosurgery for office and hospital procedures, the dental literature has rarely included authoritative articles about the advantages electrosurgery offers in treatment of inflammatory, infectious or neoplastic dental diseases, or description of the numerous special electrosurgical techniques that have been developed and perfected for specific dental procedures.

Despite the fact that it has proved its incomparable usefulness for a vast variety of clinical procedures, confusion still exists about the role and scope of electrosurgery in dentistry. Responsibility for this paradox must be attributed primarily to four factors. One is the failure of our undergraduate and postgraduate dental curricula to include adequate courses devoted to teaching the fundamentals and clinical applications of electrosurgery. Another factor is the relative dearth of electrosurgical contributions to the current literature.* Still another is the distressing lack of uniformity in electrosurgical nomenclature. And finally, the confusion has undoubtedly been most harmfully compounded by a hard core of skeptics. These men, although well informed about other phases of dentistry, are often totally unqualified by either training or personal clinical experience to be competent judges of electrosurgery; nevertheless, many persist in perpetuating the myth that this modality is inherently dangerous or that it is unsuited for dental procedures.

Despite the confusion and the definite handicaps these factors impose, electrosurgery has been proved to be practical and indispensable for so many dental procedures within the past decade that the profession has finally awakened to an appreciation of its remarkable potential usefulness.

This interest has stimulated a demand by the profession for electrosurgical training. It is regrettable that despite the ever-increasing demand, neither training facilities nor curricula have yet been adequately expanded to meet the growing need. And helpful articles relating to dental electrosurgical uses and techniques of treatment are still far too few and too widely scattered in the numerous dental journals to be readily reviewed and properly evaluated by the busy practitioner.

This book has been compiled for a dual purpose: to try to explain electrosurgery simply and clearly, and to present many practical and safe dental electrosurgical uses and techniques. To accomplish this objective, I have attempted to correlate review of the fundamentals of electrosurgery and a selective search of the available literature, with experience gained from many years of practical clinical use and postgraduate teaching of electrosurgery, in the hope that such work will help to overcome the existing confusion and provide a sound foundation for the successful incorporation of this modality into the everyday practice of dentistry.

---

*And, as was demonstrated in one instance in 1957, articles may contain inaccuracies and misconceptions.

Electrosurgery is *not* a substitute for special training in the dental disciplines. It *is* a refined method of instrumentation which facilitates and simplifies existing specialized techniques. The innumerable advantages inherent in this modality make possible invaluable additional techniques that cannot be performed efficiently by other methods of instrumentation.

Skillful proficiency in performing specialized dental techniques requires years of training and practice. It is unrealistic to assume that skillful proficiency in the use of electrosurgery can be achieved without the same requirement. Unfavorable sequelae are the inevitable result of misguided optimism.

When the necessary proficiency is achieved and electrosurgery is properly and judiciously employed, it soon becomes virtually indispensable. It can be adapted for advantageous use in all the modern dental disciplines, and can be effectively employed in areas that are relatively inaccessible to other forms of instrumentation. Its action and effects can be controlled. It can be applied so precisely that its action is limited and its effect confined exclusively to tissue that requires treatment. It is capable of producing effective hemostasis. The resultant clear operative field accelerates treatment; the ease with which it can be employed also facilitates treatment. Normal healing that is cosmetically advantageous and functionally useful is promoted by the supple soft scar repair tissue completely free of cicatricial contraction, which characterizes electrosurgical healing.

Electrosurgical techniques, with just two exceptions — desensitizing hypersensitive dentin and sterilizing root canals — are surgical procedures designed to implement therapeutic and restorative dental treatment. For the sake of order, the various electrosurgical techniques that have been designed and adapted to meet special needs of specific dental disciplines will be presented under their respective discipline headings.

In operative dentistry, electrosurgery is invaluable for a wide variety of procedures, ranging from desensitizing sensitive cervical erosions to eliminating hypertrophic granulation tissue that proliferates into, and obliterates, cavities or cavity margins and interferes with preparation or accurate seating and cementing of restorations. It is also highly effective for drying and sterilizing root canals, destroying necrotic tissue, and numerous other adjunctive operative procedures.

In crown and bridge work, electrosurgery is dramatically useful for elongating the clinical crowns of abutment teeth, for exposing the reclaiming retained roots as key abutments, and for construction of subgingival trenches around the shoulders of prepared teeth to facilitate techniques for taking impressions of multiple prepared teeth. It is also useful for reducing hypertrophic mucosa from edentulous alveolar ridges to restore harmonious contour and create sufficient space for insertion of normal-sized pontics.

In orthodontia it is useful for elongating clinical crowns of teeth for banding; for exposing permanent dentition in delayed eruptions; for frenectomy; for reducing hypertrophic gingivae.

Electrosurgery is invaluable in the treatment of periodontal disease for performing gingivoplasty — repositioning the gingivae, frenectomy, eradication of infrabony pockets; for gingivectomy—to resect detached unsupported periodontal pocket tissue and to recontour the gingival architecture rapidly and accurately without massive hemorrhage such as invariably accompanies other methods of periodontal instrumentation.

Electrosurgery can be used to great advantage in prosthetic dentistry for resecting or coagulating hypertrophic mucosa; for submucous dissections; for pushbacks to perform ridge extensions and recreate the mandibular labial sulcus; for channeling to deepen the maxillary buccal vestibule; for muscle-raising and frenectomy or frenotomy; for destruction of undesirable papillomatous tissue tabs; for alveoloplasty, and many other useful surgical aids to prosthetics.

In oral surgery, electrosurgery is invaluable for performing rapid, painless incisions for drainage; for resection of diseased pericoronal tissue; for destruction of adherent necrotic and cystic tissue shreds, and epithelial-lined fistulous tracts and their orifices; for flap incisions; for biopsy and resection of neoplastic masses, and for other uses for which cold-steel cutting is usually performed. It is also a highly effective means to provide hemostasis, and is a superb substitute for the dangerous, uncontrollable escharotics, such as trichloroacetic acid, that are used for coagulating tissue to produce hemostasis.

In brief, electronic electrosurgical equipment, basically the so-called radioknife, ranks close to the dental unit and the x-ray machine as one of the most useful and versatile instruments available to our armamentarium to assist and simplify the modern practice of dentistry.

MAURICE J. ORINGER, D.D.S.

ACKNOWLEDGMENTS

To all who have contributed directly or indirectly to the compilation of this second edition I wish to express my gratitude.

I am particularly grateful to the research investigators who, by making available to me the complete data of their experimentation, have made possible the Section on Electrosurgical Research that is featured in this edition: James D. Harrison, D.D.S., formerly Assistant Dean, Professor and Chairman, Department of Crown and Bridge Prosthodontics, and Director of Research, St. Louis University School of Dentistry, now at Southern Illinois University School of Dental Medicine; William J. Kelly, Jr., D.D.S., formerlyAssistant Professor, Department of Crown and Bridge Prosthodontics, St. Louis University School of Dentistry; William F. Malone, D.D.S., Professor and Chairman, Department of Fixed Prosthodontics, Loyola University School of Dentistry; Richard Evans, D.D.S., Director of Dentistry, Jefferson Medical College; John E. Flocken, D.M.D., Professor of Restorative Dentistry and Director of Continuing Education, U.C.L.A. School of Dentistry; and James D. Schieda, D.D.S., of Cleveland, Ohio.

I am further indebted to Drs. Harrison, Kelly and Malone for having also made available to me reports of representative cases of crown and bridge electrosurgical techniques from their case files. I am also greatly indebted to Dr. William W. Dolan (Coral Gables, Florida), Dr. Charles J. Miller (Pittsburgh, Pennsylvania), and Dr. Peter K. Thomas (Beverly Hills, California) for having made available reports of representative cases involving uses of electrosurgery for crown and bridge prosthodontics from their case files; and to Donald M. Pipko, D.M.D., Assistant Professor, and Mohammed El-Sadeek, D.D.S., Visiting Associate Professor, Department of Restorative Dentistry, University of Pittsburgh School of Dental Medicine, for their collaboration in developing the techniques of preclinical student electrosurgical instruction. I am also greatly indebted to Wallace C. Bedell, M.D., former Chief of Surgery, St. Francis Hospital, Poughkeepsie, New York; Melvin Engelman, Chief of Dental Service, St. Francis Hospital; and M. Joel Schackner, Chief of the Oral Cancer Detection and Prevention Center, St. Francis Hospital, for their thoughtful cooperation in making available to me the data on their treatment of oral cancer by electrocoagulation that enabled me to include a report of their case.

Also my deep appreciation to Dr. Charles W. Conroy, Associate Professor of Dental Research and Graduate Periodontics, Ohio State University School of Dentistry, for making available his case on comparative treatment of dilantin hypertrophy by steel scalpel and electrosurgical gingivectomy, and to Dr. Peter M. Beck of Toronto, Ontario, Canada, for his implant case reports; to Dr. William B. Trice of Erie, Pennsylvania, for his case report on bleaching discolored teeth; to Brian F. Pollack, D.M.D., of New York City, for making available the report of his case of repair of a defective veneer crown; and to Dr. Manuel Weissman of Augusta, Georgia, for his case report on rubber dam isolation of a retained fractured root for endodontic therapy.

I am also indebted to Mr. William Honig, formerly Director of Electronic Research, Cavitron Corporation, New York, now Professor of Physics, University of Western Australia, Perth, Australia, for his invaluable technical information about the constant wave and coaxial shielding circuitry reviewed in this text; and to Mr. Stephen Andrews, Mr. John Nugent, and Mr. Egon Weickgenannt of the Ritter Company's Engineering Division, and Mr. Sutherland, a Consultant to that Division, for their cooperation and invaluable information about the modified continuous wave current and self-regulating circuitry which they have developed and which are reviewed in the text.

I also wish to express my appreciation to my medical and dental colleagues whose patient referrals made available to me the clinical material without which this book could not have been written. Also my appreciation to Mrs. Dunleavy of the New York Academy of Medicine Library Staff for her assistance with the reference research, and to Mr. Carroll Cann, Mrs. Carol Cramer, Mrs. Diane Forti, Mr. Raymond Kersey, Mr. Grant Lashbrook, Mr. George Laurie, and the other members of the staff of the W. B. Saunders Company who participated in the preparation of this edition, for their cooperation and encouragement.

MAURICE J. ORINGER

CONTENTS

Section One
THE PHENOMENON CALLED ELECTROSURGERY

Part 1
HISTORICAL BACKGROUND... 3

Part 2
THE BASIC PHYSICS OF ELECTROSURGERY 10

Chapter One
The Therapeutic Electrosurgical Currents 10

Chapter Two
Dental Electrosurgical Equipment and Instrumentation Techniques ... 42

Chapter Three
Indications and Contraindications... 83

Section Two
PRECLINICAL INSTRUMENTATION EXERCISES

Chapter Four
Prelaboratory Practice for the Undergraduate Dental Student 93

Chapter Five
Experimental Practice Techniques for the Practitioner and Student..... 101

Section Three
ELECTROSURGICAL RESEARCH

Part 1
INDICATIONS AND STANDARDS FOR RESEARCH 135

Chapter Six
Relationship of Research to Clinical Electrosurgery........................... 136

Part 2
EXPERIMENTAL RESEARCH REPORTS 141

Chapter Seven
Behavioral Research 141

Chapter Eight
Laboratory Evaluation of Efficacy of Clinical Electrosurgical
Techniques 154

Chapter Nine
Clinical Research on Human Subjects 191

Section Four
INTERRELATED NONELECTROSURGICAL FACTORS

Part 1
ANESTHESIA 211

Chapter Ten
Pharmacodynamics of the Local Anesthetic Drugs 212

Part 2
MEDICATION 236

Chapter Eleven
Use of Systemic and Local Drugs 236

Section Five
CLINICAL ELECTROSURGICAL TECHNIQUES

Part 1
RESTORATIVE DENTISTRY 265

Chapter Twelve
Operative Dentistry 266

Chapter Thirteen
Uses in Pedodontics — Treatment of Deciduous Teeth and Aids to
Eruption of Permanent Dentition 309

Chapter Fourteen
Endodontic Uses of Electrosurgery 321

Chapter Fifteen
Clinical Techniques for Crown and Bridge Prosthesis........................ 378

Part 2
ORTHODONTICS 505

Chapter Sixteen
Preorthodontic Procedures... 507

Chapter Seventeen
Techniques Adjunctive to Treatment in Cleft Palate and
Comparable Abnormalities... 537

Part 3
PERIODONTICS 559

Chapter Eighteen
Electrosurgery for Definitive Conservative Modern
Periodontal Therapy.. 559

Chapter Nineteen
Clinical Techniques in Periodontal Electrosurgery........................... 581

Part 4
PREPROSTHODONTIC ELECTROSURGERY 728

Chapter Twenty
Repair of Soft Tissue Defects 731

Part 5
ORAL SURGERY... 807

Chapter Twenty-One
Minor Oral Surgery... 816

Chapter Twenty-Two
Major Oral Surgery 902

Section Six
**ELECTROSURGICAL BIOPSY FOR DIAGNOSIS OF
ORAL PATHOLOGY**

Chapter Twenty-Three
Fundamentals of Biopsy Procedure... 985

Chapter Twenty-Four
Clinical Electrosurgical Biopsy Techniques 1003

Section Seven
ADVANCED ORAL CANCER

Chapter Twenty-Five
Treatment of Advanced Oral Cancer by Electrocoagulation 1089

Chapter Twenty-Six
Medicaments and Instruments Mentioned in the Text 1102

INDEX... 1119

Section One

THE PHENOMENON CALLED ELECTROSURGERY

PART 1

HISTORICAL BACKGROUND

Ever since primitive man discovered fire, heat *in one form or another* has been used therapeutically to destroy diseased tissue or to control hemorrhage. According to Ewing, the earliest recorded surgical use of heat was when Hippocrates cauterized a malignant growth on the back of the neck of a man to destroy it.[1]

Before commercial electricity became available, surgeons used metal bars heated to red or white incandescent glow or molten pitch therapeutically to destroy diseased tissue and to seal off severed blood vessels to staunch hemorrhage by cauterization.

With the advent of commercially available electricity, tumor surgeons, in their never-ending search for more efficient methods to destroy malignant tissue, substituted electrically generated heat called electrocautery for the flame-heated metal bars. The surgical use of electrocautery was first demonstrated publicly by tumor surgeons at the Middlesex and St. Bartholomew's Hospitals in London, more than 250 years ago.

Many consider electrocautery as an electrosurgical device and procedure, since in the broadest sense electrosurgery may be defined as the application of electrically generated heat energy to alter or destroy tissue cells. Such an interpretation would, however, be unrealistic and impractical, since, according to this broad definition, a soldering iron, a laundry iron, or in fact any other electrically heated device that can burn tissue would have to be considered an electrosurgical instrument. Since such devices can scarcely qualify as surgical instruments, it becomes apparent that if a device *is* to qualify as a surgical instrument it must meet several basic essential minimal requirements beyond the mere fact that it is capable of altering or destroying tissue.

To qualify as a *surgical* instrument the device must be self-limiting in its destructiveness to at least a reasonable degree. The therapist must be able to control the instrument's destructiveness to at least a reasonable degree. Finally, the end result of the destruction must be favorable tissue repair, and not the typical repair of a third degree burn.

As shall be seen elsewhere in this text, electrocautery fails to meet any of

3

these minimal requirements, and cannot be considered an electrosurgical device or procedure. Nevertheless, it was a great improvement over the infinitely more primitive and uncontrollable flame-heated cautery or molten pitch. The electrocautery therefore was used extensively by surgeons until the spark-gap generator, the first of the high-frequency electrosurgical instruments, was developed.

The spark-gap generator developed as a result of D'Arsonval's experiments in 1891, which established that when alternating current oscillates at high frequency, meaning at more than 10,000 oscillations per second, and is applied to living tissue, it does not produce potentially lethal neuromuscular shock such as results from applications of alternating current oscillating at low frequencies to living tissues. All that happens when the high-frequency current is applied is a slight rise in the internal temperature of the tissues through which it passes.[2] This phenomenon is the basis upon which medical and surgical diathermy are predicated. The latter is commonly known as electrosurgery.

The spark-gap generator fulfills the minimal basic requirements for an electrosurgical instrument and its use soon largely replaced electrocautery as a surgical modality. Although the spark-gap generator is incapable of producing true surgical cutting energy, the tissue destruction by electrocoagulation and electrodesiccation that it provided continued to be usefully employed until DeForest's invention of the three-element radio vacuum tube power generator made possible the electronic high-frequency (RF) circuits that deliver true surgical cutting energy. This highly advanced phase in the evolutionary use of electrically generated heat energy to living tissue for therapeutic purposes has made possible modern dental electrosurgery.

The prototype electronic scalpel capable of delivering true surgical cutting energy was developed in 1924 by Dr. George A. Wyeth, a noted tumor surgeon. Wyeth called his instrument an *endotherm knife,* and referred to the technique for its use as "electrothermic endothermy."

As might be anticipated, Wyeth and his colleagues encountered some resistance to change by tumor surgeons and other medical specialists accustomed to, and more familiar with, the earlier therapeutic electrical modalities. This resistance to change was correctly attributed to confusion of the surgical cutting current made available by the electronic scalpel with the dehydrating and coagulating currents produced by the spark-gap and cautery devices.

Wyeth authored a text, *Surgery of Neoplastic Diseases by Electrothermic Methods,*[3] in an attempt to present an indisputable clear-cut picture of the vastly superior performance possible with electronic surgery as compared to what could be accomplished with the other electrosurgical modalities.

Although this text was published in 1926, many of the observations by Wyeth and his colleagues still hold true and bear repetition. Although the techniques they refer to deal only with tumor surgery, their comments about the effects of their "electrothermic" techniques are revealing.

"The idea of an electric current of cutting power . . . has been the basis of considerable experimentation for several years."

"The endotherm knife [or radioknife] is not a true knife but a current operating through the . . . needle [an electrode applied to the tissues]. . . . *It is the current which cuts, or, more properly, which causes a disintegration of the tissue. . . . The needle [electrode] is but the applicator by which the operator directs the incision.*"*

". . . Kowarschik [a colleague] discusses . . . DeForest's use of a short spark, and says if these sparks were concentrated upon a needle point, and if the needle was drawn across a tissue, the tissue fell apart as if split by a knife. . . . *If the electrode was not held too long in one place the cut was as fresh and clean as that produced by a very sharp knife.** The arc not only formed a scalpel that cut like any other knife but it also possessed the decided advantage *that it sterilized the cut.*"*4

"We took [DeForest's] three-element vacuum tube and successfully applied it to surgery (undamped oscillations), incorporating it into the endotherm."

"Our interest in . . . the endotherm knife was stimulated by the following experience:

"Operating on a case of tumor of the bladder, the usual incision was made by the scalpel. The growth was thoroughly exposed by electric light in the bladder, and treated after the technique of monopolar endothermy (electrosurgery). The bladder was sutured in the usual way, without drain.

"After three months, cystoscopic examination showed that the site of the lesion was free and clean. *So smooth had been the healing that it was difficult to be sure just where the growth had been,** but on turning the beak of the cystoscope upward the observer was amazed to see along the line of the scalpel's incision three carcinomatous nodules. There could hardly be a more graphic picture of the beneficial healing action of the high-frequency current as contrasted with the lack of protection against implantation provided by the scalpel.

"From that time forward the development of a practical (surgical) cutting current was felt to be a matter of urgency, and the endotherm knife is the result."

". . . the cutting current is developed by the three-element vacuum tube system and is of such extremely high frequency that *it produces a molecular dissolution of the tissues, sealing lymphatics as it cuts** by a thin line of coagulation. The incrustation which characterizes the cut of the 'cautery knife' does not follow the use of the endotherm's cutting current, and our records show an unbroken list of *healings by primary union, with a thinner, finer, less conspicuous scar,** which is gratifying to the operator and to the patient."

"To say that the endotherm knife is the equipment for a new surgery . . . is not to intimate that standard surgical technique is not employed in its use. *Its successful employment is founded on sound surgical training".*

This training must be combined with study of the electrosurgical currents and their waveforms, and of the special endothermy techniques which have been developed.

---

*Author's italics.

Dr. Howard A. Kelly, one of Dr. Wyeth's colleagues, and the coauthor with Dr. Ward of an excellent text on medical electrical modalities, emphasized this, stating: "These methods [of electrosurgery] are not to be learned in a week or a year. They call for careful attention to a new technique, for discriminating judgment in their application and for increasing boldness with a growing experience."[*5] Kelly also stated: "It is possible that primary union which follows incision by the endotherm knife is promoted because of sterilization of the skin edges."

"One of the the first things noted by the surgeon who seeks to employ electrosurgery in place of the scalpel is that with the former no pressure need be, or ought to be, exerted; light contact only is required, and we have a new sense of feeling the tissues separating as if of themselves before the tip of the small electrode. *The operator directs the line of incision; he does not,* by pressure, 'make' it."[*6]

Kelly goes on to say that the choice of electrode is determined by the nature of the tissues: "If the incision is to be made in delicate tissue only, a fine needle electrode is used; if working in heavier tissue, a heavier electrode is used. The amount of current required is to be determined by the size of the electrode. *With a fine needle as the active electrode, the endotherm knife is capable of cutting so fine a line as to heal almost without scar formation.*"[*]

The endotherm knife appears to be equally effective for use on skin and mucous membrane. Beck and Pollock reported on successful use of the endotherm knife in mouth lesions, describing two typical cases: one, carcinoma of the tonsil; the other, carcinoma of the tongue.[7] In the tonsil case there was no bleeding and quick recovery. In the tongue case one half of the tongue was resected and the result was good. It is noteworthy that the endotherm knife, although it seals off the lymph and smaller blood vessels as it cuts, will not protect against hemorrhage if larger vessels are traversed.

Wise, reporting a technique for treatment of leukoplakia of the tongue and buccal mucosa by electrodesiccation, stated: "... shows better results with this treatment [endothermy] than can be obtained by any other method."[8]

Grant E. Ward, in reporting a technique for treating ranula by endothermy, stated that he found the method much simpler and more efficient than the older methods of treatment. He summarized the reasons for his preference of the electrosurgical procedure thus:

Advantages

1. Dangers and discomforts of radical operations and general anesthesia avoided.
2. Operation technically simple.
3. Danger of hemorrhage avoided.
4. Rapid healing with no scar or deformity.
5. Minimal hospitalization.[9]

Dr. Lewis McArthur at the meeting of the American Medical Association in St. Louis in May of 1922 urged upon his colleagues the importance of

---

*Author's italics.

deviating from accepted surgical axioms, and even, in certain rare instances, operative procedures at variance with established surgical teaching, Dr. McArthur concluded that: ". . . otherwise surgical judgement is banished, and surgery becomes a set of formulas, the surgeon disappears, and there remains only the operator."[10]

The purpose and high aim of surgery in malignancy is to remove not only diseased tissue but also the paths by which malignant cells reach locations beyond the primary focus. The metastases which follow surgical operations and the frequent implantation of malignant cells along the line of the steel scalpel's incision are evidence that that ideal is not always realized.

Dr. W. J. Mayo, referring to the fact that only particles of molecular size such as sugars, amino acids and other crystalloids are absorbed directly through the vascular capillaries of the body, while colloids and large particles are picked up by the lymphatics, said: "Bacteria and malignant cells do not pass directly into the capillaries, but are carried by phagocytes into the lymphatics, which are a closed system of vessels."[11] Hence the danger of mechanical dissemination which lies in the steel scalpel's severance of lymphatics from a malignant area, and the advantage to the operator and patient inherent in the employment of the endotherm knife, which seals off these channels as it cuts.

As for usefulness of electrosurgery for biopsy, Dr. Case has stated: "We believe, in most instances, that the danger of removing a biopsy specimen is not great. It is well in all cases to use the electrical knife (radiotherm) both for removing the specimen and for sealing over the edges of the wound from which the specimen is taken. We believe that in this manner it is safe to take biopsy specimens in practically every accessible tumor encountered."[12]

Fears have been expressed that removal of a section of tissue with the endotherm knife for microscopic examination would cauterize the wound and make valueless any section for histologic examination. *Confusion will inevitably result whenever the terms electrocautery and electrosurgery are used interchangeably. To cauterize is to burn; endothermy does not burn.* By the technique of endothermy we take the tissue section with confidence and feel a safety unshared by one who employs the old surgical methods.

Dr. Harmer reported that in his experience electrosurgery is the best method for treatment of growths in the upper air passages. Excision by cold-steel scalpel yielded only 33⅓ per cent cures. Recurrences were almost invariably in the scar, suggesting that dissemination had taken place at the time of operation. He found better than 70 per cent cure with endothermy; *there was striking absence of fever or toxemia. He considers the relief from pain and the smooth and pliant scars which resulted to be remarkable.* His conclusions were that this treatment should be employed in cases of diseases of mucous membranes.[13]

Dr. Cumberbatch of St. Bartholomew's Hospital reported successful use of electrosurgery in cases of nevi, lupus and cancer of the tonsil and pharyngeal wall, and concluded that: "Even if the final results of [this treatment] were no better than those given by cutting operations, *the quickness of* *the newer method, the absence of bleeding . . . the absence of shock and the very short stay in bed with little discomfort** would render diathermy [electrosurgery] a formidable rival to the knife in the treatment of malignant diseases."[14] The *soft noncontracting scar* which results from electrothermic operation is one of the great advantages of the method. Many others have also praised the suppleness of the scar and its remarkable similarity to surrounding normal tissue.

To compare Wyeth's endotherm knife with the electrosurgical circuitry currently available is equivalent to comparing Lindbergh's "Spirit of St. Louis" to a 747 jet plane. The electrosurgical achievements of Wyeth and his colleagues have not only been equalled but greatly surpassed as more sophisticated electrosurgical equipment has been developed.

For dentistry the most significant advance in electrosurgical circuitry was the invention of a fully rectified circuit by William Coles, an engineer. Coles developed his circuit to meet specific needs of the dental profession by eliminating the coagulation that inherently accompanies cutting with partially rectified current.[15]

Coles' concept of a surgically pure cutting current, as well as the actual circuit design, was so great a departure from pre-existing electrosurgical circuitry that the U.S. Patent Office issued Patent #2-835-254 for his circuit. He also pioneered in use of solid-state circuitry for electrosurgery. His original circuit utilized mercury vapor rectifying tubes. Well over a decade ago he substituted banks of rectifiers for the tubes: first, selenium rectifiers, and when these proved inadequate, silicon rectifiers. By converting the circuit to partial solid-state he eliminated the need to heat up the mercury vapor rectifying tubes to vaporize the mercury, thereby making possible instantaneous use of the current at all times. The surgically pure cutting current this circuit provided made possible most of the dental electrosurgical techniques that have been developed, and his circuit remains the prototype for all the fully rectified and continuous wave equipment that is being produced.

In view of the superior quality of the therapeutic currents that modern electrosurgical equipment provides, and the remarkable clinical results that are being achieved with them, it is inexplicable and incomprehensible that the misconceptions, fears and resistance to the use of electrosurgery experienced in the pioneering days tend to persist in some areas of dental therapy.

---

*Author's italics.

FOOTNOTE REFERENCES

1. Ewing, J.: Neoplastic Diseases. A Treatise on Tumors. 2nd ed. Philadelphia, W. B. Suanders Co., 1922, p. 17.
2. D'Arsonval: Compt. rend. Soc. de Biol., 43:283, 1891; 45:122, 1893.
3. Wyeth, G. A.: Surgery of Neoplastic Diseases by Electrothermic Methods. New York, Paul B. Hoeber, Inc., 1926.
4. Kowarschik, J.: Die Diathermie. 3rd ed. Vienna, 1921, p. 258.
5. Kelly, H. A., in Kelly, H. A. and Ward, G. E.: The radical breast operation with the endotherm knife and without ligatures. Ann. Surg., 83:42, Jan., 1926.

6. Kelly, H. A.: Endothermy, the new surgery. M. J. & Rec., *122*, July, 1925.
7. Beck, J. C., and Pollock, H. L.: The present status of electrotherapeutic measures used in the practice of otolaryngology. Ann. Otol., Rhinol. & Laryngol., *34:*405, June, 1925.
8. Wise, F., and Eller, J.: Endothermy (electrodesiccation) in dermatology. Arch. Dermat. & Syph., *13:*344, Mar., 1926.
9. Ward, G. E.: A conservative operation for cure of ranula by endothermy. Med. Rev. of Rev., *31:*587, 1925.
10. McArthur, L. L.: Atypical operations on the jaws and mouth for malignant growths. A.M.A.J., 79:1484–1486, 1922.
11. Mayo, W. J.: The relative values of surgery and radiotherapy. Minnesota Med., 8:7, Jan., 1925.
12. Case, J. T.: Radiation therapy of malignant disease. A.M.A.J., *34:*108–111, 1925.
13. Harmer, D.: Surgical diathermy. Proc. Roy. Soc. Med., *15:*87, 1922.
14. Cumberbatch, E. P.: Diathermy: Its production and uses in medicine and surgery. London, 1921; id., Proc. Roy. Soc. Med., *15:*87, 1922.
15. Coles, W.: Personal communication.

THE BASIC PHYSICS OF ELECTROSURGERY

Chapter One

THE THERAPEUTIC ELECTROSURGICAL CURRENTS

Introduction

Responsibility for much of the general confusion still prevalent pertaining to the phenomenon of electrosurgery must be attributed to lack of uniformity in electrosurgical nomenclature. Unquestionably the most persistent factor, and in all probability the one most responsible for the nomenclatural chaos, has been the failure to unmistakably differentiate *electrocautery* from *electrosurgery.*

Theoretically, the term *electrosurgery* might be interpreted as *the application of electrically generated heat energy to living tissue to alter or destroy it for therapeutic purposes.* Any electrical device with which the heat energy can be produced and applied to the tissues theoretically might be regarded as an electrosurgical instrument.

From a practical standpoint, however, this is an unrealistic and factually inaccurate generalization. It is basic and elementary that if an electrical device is to qualify as a therapeutically useful electrosurgical instrument, it must offer much more than the mere ability to alter or destroy tissue — it must meet a number of specific minimum requirements. Its currents must be self-limiting in their destructiveness to an acceptable degree. It must permit the operator to fully control and limit the extent of tissue alteration or destruction achieved. It must permit and promote desirable tissue repair.

ELECTROCAUTERY VS. ELECTROSURGERY

The electrocautery is a low-voltage monoterminal device. It operates on commercial electric current that passes through a step-down transformer and is converted to low-voltage current. When activated, its single active or working electrode gets red or white hot, and, like its more primitive ancestor, the red-hot metal bar, it sears and destroys the tissues as it comes into contact with them. The incandescent heat generated by the hot electrode penetrates into the tissues by *convection* (searing heat radiating outward from the heated metal), penetrating unpredictable distances beyond the site of electrode tissue contact. All the tissue cells affected by the incandescent heat are destroyed by mass coagulation necrosis identical in all respects with that produced by any third degree burn.

Tissue repair likewise is identical to that from a burn, i.e., by production of contractile cicatricial bands of fibrous scar connective tissue. Such scar repair tissue is usually cosmetically disfiguring and functionally impairing. Electrocautery literally cooks the tissues, and the operator has no effective control over the extent or quality of tissue destruction produced. Electrocautery is totally unsuited for precise surgery or for biopsy, since tissue subjected to such mass coagulation necrosis cannot be histologically differentiated for diagnostic interpretation.

Electrocautery completely fails to fulfill the minimum requirements and criteria for therapeutic electrosurgery. Therefore, this primitive modality should **never** be considered as, or indiscriminately classified as, an electrosurgical instrument or an electrosurgical procedure.

Diathermy

MEDICAL DIATHERMY

When therapeutic high-frequency current is introduced into the body by applying two electrodes of equal or near-equal size on either side of the body part to be treated, the current density is evenly dispersed within the intervening tissues as the current radiates through the body. This produces a generalized rise in the internal temperature of the body tissues, with a dilatation of the blood vessels, resulting from the increased temperature. This phenomenon is called *medical* diathermy.

SURGICAL DIATHERMY ⟷ ELECTROSURGERY

If instead of using electrodes of equal size one electrode is large and the other small enough, the current radiates through the tissues from the site of contact of the small electrode with the tissues toward the larger electrode, then back to the power oscillator of the electrosurgical unit, and back again to the site of contact of the small electrode with the tissues, in a continuing radiating cycle. The current is no longer evenly dispersed but instead attains a density or concentration at the site of entry into the tissues from the small electrode that is great enough to produce actual cellular destruction — that is, *surgical* diathermy, best known as electrosurgery.[1]

In the modern meaning of the term, electrosurgery is based upon the principle, discovered by D'Arsonval, that when alternating current oscillates at sufficiently high frequency it can be passed through living tissue without shock. However, as the current radiates through the tissues, resistance to passage of the current offered by the body produces heat within the tissues.[2-12]

The type of current used and its method of application to the tissues determines the amount of heat generated. Such heat ranges in intensity from a mild awareness of warmth to total molecular dissolution of individual tissue cells.[13-16] When fully rectified true RF current is properly employed, the operator has complete control over the instrument and its therapeutic behavior. Since individual cells are affected, no generalized mass necrosis results, only dehydration, coagulation, or volatilization of individual cells. Application of heat can therefore be pinpointed and accurately confined to the tissue undergoing treatment. Tissue repair, therefore, is free from cicatricial contraction. Healing is rapid and painless, with formation of a supple scar which is soft in texture and identical in all respects to the surrounding normal tissue. Since cellular destruction is not *en masse*, but by alteration or destruction of individual cells, tissue resected by electrosection can be histopathologically differentiated for diagnostic interpretation. Electrosection is therefore ideally suited for biopsy.

ELECTROSURGICAL TERMINOLOGY

Many of the technical electrical terms relating to electrosurgery lend themselves to multiple interpretations, and thus tend to confuse most dentists. Since this is a text for dentists and not for electrical engineers, the author has taken the liberty of attempting to define and categorize some of the major offenders in nontechnical terms that can be more easily understood and differentiated by most dentists. Naturally this often can be accomplished only at the risk of deviating somewhat from purely technical accuracy of the definitions, but the author feels the need for clarification warrants this risk.

Electrode Contact Points

Monopolar and bipolar

The terms "monopolar" and "bipolar" and also "monoterminal" and "biterminal" are among the worst offenders. These terms have been applied interchangeably to the electrodes that convey the currents to the tissues and also to the manner in which the currents are delivered to the patients.

For the sake of clarity the author recommends that the terms monopolar and bipolar be applied exclusively to denote the number of tissue contacting tips at the end of the surgical electrode, and that the terms monoterminal and biterminal be reserved exclusively to describe the method of delivery of the current to the patient.

When the surgical electrode has only one tip projecting from its end, it is a monopolar electrode. If it has two tips, it is a bipolar electrode.

Monoterminal and biterminal

A terminal usually denotes the end of a line; for example, a railroad terminal. Monoterminal suggests use of only one connection or electrode from the electrosurgical device to deliver the current to the patient, whereas biterminal suggests two connections, or two electrodes, used simultaneously to deliver the current. Thus, if the patient is seated on an indifferent electrode that is plugged into the conductive socket on the instrument panel of an electrosurgical unit, the current will flow from the power output of the unit to and through the patient, into the indifferent electrode, and directly back to the unit's power generator. This is a biterminal application of the current (Fig. 1-1A). If the indifferent electrode is not employed, there is a single unit-patient contact, only that of the surgical electrode, and the current returns to the unit indirectly. This is monoterminal application of the current (Fig. 1-1B). The details and merits of these methods of application will be elaborated in the discussion of the electrosurgical electrodes.

Waveform

This term is mystifying to anyone who is unfamiliar with electrical terminology. Waveform refers to the pattern that current forms as it flows. Each variety of electrosurgical current produces its own unique wavy pattern of cur-

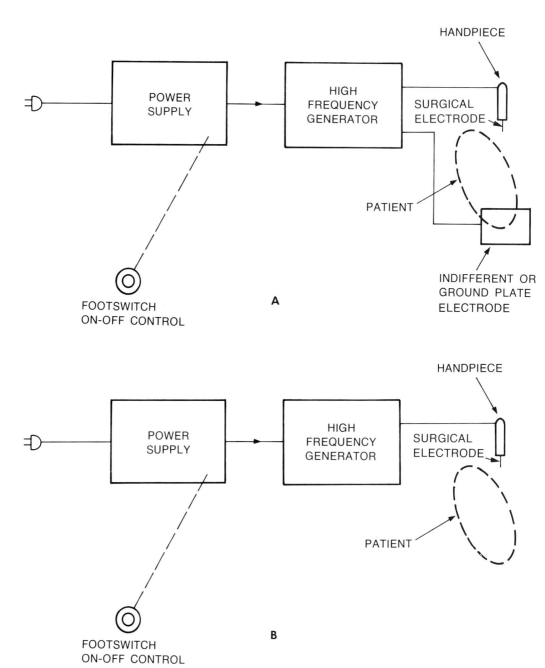

Figure 1-1.   General block diagram of electrosurgical equipment. *A,* Biterminal application of current *with* the indifferent electrode. *B,* Monoterminal application of the current *without* the indifferent electrode.

rent flow that identifies it just like a human fingerprint identifies the individual it belongs to. The waveforms created by the various currents can be visualized and photographed on the screen of an oscilloscope, or traced on an oscillograph.

When interruptions in the continuity of the flow of high-frequency current occur, such as those which characterize the flow of Oudin spark-gap current and that of a partially rectified circuit, it is referred to as a "damping" of the current. The damping effect is illustrated in Fig. 1–4A and B. Thus spark-gap current is referred to as a highly damped current; partially rectified current as a moderately damped current; and fully rectified current as an undamped current. The electrosurgical waveforms will be thoroughly reviewed later in this chapter.

Oscilloscope

This is an electronic instrument for projecting the forms of electromagnetic waves on the fluorescent screen of a cathode-ray tube. When an electrosurgical unit is attached to it and activated, the waveforms produced by the particular current being employed appear clearly visible on the oscilloscope screen.

Oscillograph

This is an instrument on which the waveforms of the current can be traced as a graph, in a manner similar to the tracings of an electrocardiogram.

Amplitude

This refers to the peak height or value attained by an alternating current during one complete cycle. If the amplitude remains constant at its maximum level, without breaks in the continuity of the current flow, it is a fully rectified current. Breaks in the continuity of current flow, or variations in the amplitude, differentiate the various current waveforms.

Current Density

This refers to how tightly the current is packed together in a given region of space or tissue. The greater the intensity of current in this region of space or tissue, the more potent is the energy it can produce. The depth of penetration is determined by the speed with which the current is applied to the tissues.

Alternating Cycle "Envelope"

A single cycle of alternating current actually consists of two half-cycles, as shall be visualized later in this chapter. The envelope is the imaginary space in which the two half-cycles are contained.

RF Current

RF current means radio-frequency sound waves generated by a high-frequency power oscillator. The electrosurgical circuit is a high-frequency power oscillator; thus, in effect, it is a radio transmitter, or radio-sending circuit. Electrosurgical circuits differ from radio broadcasting transmitters in that the latter transmit audible signals, whereas electrosurgical units transmit inaudible signals. Despite this difference, the inaudible as well as the audible signals are emissions of pure radio-frequency (RF) current.

The number of oscillations that a high-frequency oscillator can produce is regulated by each nation, since unrestricted use of RF wavebands (frequencies) would cause chaotic disrupting interference with airplane signals and other forms of communication. Since the electrosurgical unit is an RF power oscillator, its frequency, or the number of oscillations per second it may produce, is assigned and regulated in the U.S. by the F.C.C.; and in other countries by its counterparts.

Diode

A diode is either an electron tube or its solid-state substitute that permits electrons to pass in one direction only and thus acts as a rectifier.

Transistor

This is a miniature device for control and amplification of an electron current. It is made of semiconductor material and has three or more electrodes, the current between one pair of electrodes controlling the amplified current between the other pair, with one of the electrodes being common to both pairs.

When a number of these devices are incorporated into a circuit to substitute for radio vacuum tubes, it is referred to as a solid-state circuit. The latter, especially silicon wafer integrated circuitry, is a relatively recent phenomenon and is still surrounded by an aura of mystery and glamour that can be misleading.

Solid-state circuitry enjoys a number of advantages over the older vacuum tube systems. There are no tubes to break or filaments to burn out. No preheating period is required, and the circuit provides instantaneous use. It is more conducive to miniaturization of equipment, making it possible to incorporate clinically advantageous features and more refined and consistent performance without creating excessive increase in the size of the unit.

Electromagnetic Waves

All forms of radiant energy, ranging from radio and light waves to gamma and cosmic rays produced by a system of electric and magnetic fields, are varieties of electromagnetic waves. Thus the therapeutic high-frequency RF currents used in electrosurgery are included among the electromagnetic wave energies.

Watts

A watt is a measurement of heat established by a mathematical formula:
$$R_1 = R \text{ load}$$
It is defined as "the practical unit of electric power, activity, or rate of work equivalent to one joule second, or one volt-ampere." In electrosurgery this would be equated with the amount of heat energy being delivered to the tissues at the site of their contact with the activated electrode. The electrosurgical conversion of RF current into heat energy results from tissue resistance to the passage of current. Electronically this resistance is called "impedance." For household electrical appliances such as toasters, grills, or steam irons, the manufacturer's certification of the number of watts that the appliance is capable of producing is a consistent index of the amount of heat the appliance's circuit will produce, and is therefore a reliable index of its capabilities and performance.

The situation is quite different with electrosurgical devices. These are transmitters that transmit RF current to the tissues. Transmitters are affected to a much greater degree than ordinary electrical appliances by the factor inherent to electrical circuitry, "internal impedance."

Impedance

Electrically, impedance is the total opposition to alternating current created by the circuit itself. It is defined as the measure of voltage drop in the current flowing through a circuit element. The circuit element may consist of any combination of resistance, capacitance, or inductance. The latter two become more significant as the frequency increases.

This impedance, or resistance, converts the RF current into heat energy great enough to at least cook the tissue cells and coagulate their organic contents, or to disintegrate and volatilize them into atomic carbon.

If an electrosurgical circuit is to be able to transmit or deliver to the tissues all the wattage that it is capable of generating, it must maintain closely the ratio of the mathematical equation $R_1 = R$ load. If the circuit's internal impedance is high, this balance between R_1 and R load is disrupted and creates a varying degree of difference in wattage reaching the tissues. Thus the manufacturer's certification of the number of watts an electrosurgical unit can produce does not necessarily represent the number of watts it is producing at the site of electrode contact with the tissues, and is therefore an unreliable and often misleading index of the capabilities and performance of the circuit.

INTERNAL IMPEDANCE. In addition to tissue impedance, there is internal impedance. Translated into simple, nontechnical language, this refers to the internal resistance to the current flow that is created inherently in all circuitry and is somewhat comparable to the factor of friction in a mechanical model. It is unpredictably variable from one circuit to another and causes a loss of wattage being produced by its power generator in the process of transmitting the current power source to its output source. This internal impedance can be a significant factor in electrosurgery.

In an electrosurgical unit it is a factor in the transmitting or delivery of the current to the clinical end of the circuit. Specifically, internal impedance in a circuit creates a distinct difference between the amount of watts of heat the circuit develops and the amount of that heat it loses as the current flows through the wire cable and handpiece and the surgical electrode in order to reach the tissues. If the circuit has a low internal impedance factor and is capable of developing 70 watts of heat at its power source, it will deliver most of that wattage to the tissues and provide enough heat energy at the site of application to perform its cutting function efficiently under any conditions likely to be encountered in the mouth. If, however, the circuit has a high internal impedance factor, even though it develops 70 watts of heat at its power source, it can deliver only a fraction of the wattage to the tissues. Thus, just as the unit that produces an unrealistically low wattage at its power source is incapable of providing adequate cutting power except under optimal conditions and using a fine needle electrode, a circuit that produces a much higher number of watts at its power source but has a high internal impedance is likely to prove equally incapable of providing adequate cutting power except under similar optimal conditions.

It therefore becomes inescapably obvious that wattage alone is an unreliable index of the efficiency of an electrosurgical unit. In the final analysis the only infallibly reliable index of how an electrosurgical circuit will perform is when the current is applied to the tissues.

PRINCIPLES OF ELECTROSURGERY

It has already been established that electrosurgery is based upon the phenomenon that when high-frequency alternating current is introduced into the body, heat is generated within the tissues as a result of resistance offered by the body to passage of the current through them.

The Electrosurgical Electrodes

Two totally different basic types of electrodes are used in electrosurgery. Since it would be impossible to perform electrosurgery without them, the most important types are the small active, working or *surgical* electrodes. There are two varieties, and each variety comes in many sizes and shapes:

1. *Cutting Electrodes.* For dental electrosurgery these are hair-thin wire needles or loops made, as a rule, of tungsten wire. The loops may be completely closed or partially open (Fig. 1-2).

2. *Coagulating or Dehydrating Electrodes.* These are made of solid metal and are round, cylindrical or conical in shape (Fig. 1-2).

The second basic type of electrode is the large passive or dispersive electrode called the indifferent electrode, of which there are three varieties (Fig. 1-3):

1. Metallic wristbands usually placed on the patient's wrist. (One company recommends that the doctor wear the wristband and hold that hand against the patient's cheek opposite to the surgical field.)

2. Square or rectangular metal plates placed under the patient seated in the dental chair. The author has designed a modification of this variety that is flexible and can be inserted under the Naughahyde of the dental chair seat as a permanent internal installation, or fitted into a Naughahyde envelope of a color similar to that of the chair upholstery, and attached externally to the seat portion of the chair. These square- or rectangular-shaped electrodes are referred to as indifferent plates.

3. Cylindrical metal electrodes that are hand-held by the patient.

The indifferent electrode is not used when performing electrodesiccation or fulguration. Since this electrode also does not participate *directly* in the surgical effects of the cutting or coagulating currents at the surgical site, performing electrosection or electrocoagulation without using an indifferent plate is *technically* possible. This technicality has resulted in recent claims that the indifferent plate does not have to be used with certain equipment. These claims are causing much confusion and have given rise to hazardous misconceptions about the function of the indifferent electrode and its relation to the *efficiency* of the electrosurgery.

Inasmuch as this electrode *does* play a critically important role in the *consistency* and *potency* of the electrosurgical currents delivered to the tissues by the surgical electrode, the author considers it important to try to clarify this matter and bring the issue into proper focus.

A high-frequency generator (electrosurgical unit) delivers its output of RF current between leads A and B as shown in Figure 1-4. During surgery the current flows through the handpiece lead, A, through the electrode tip, through the tissues, into the indifferent electrode and back to point B at the generator. When the patient sits on the indifferent plate, the capacitance be-

COLES ELECTRODES

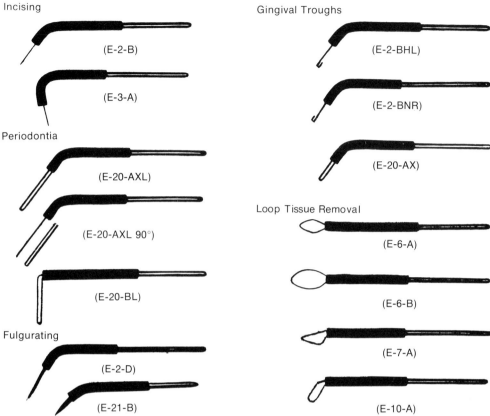

Incising

(E-2-B)

(E-3-A)

Periodontia

(E-20-AXL)

(E-20-AXL 90°)

(E-20-BL)

Fulgurating

(E-2-D)

(E-21-B)

Gingival Troughs

(E-2-BHL)

(E-2-BNR)

(E-20-AX)

Loop Tissue Removal

(E-6-A)

(E-6-B)

(E-7-A)

(E-10-A)

Figure 1-2. Types of surgical electrodes (courtesy of Clev-Dent Division, Cavitron Corp., Cleveland, Ohio, and Gebrueder Martin, Tuttlingen, Germany), author's block holder for electrode assortment, and aspirating-coagulating electrode handle (courtesy of Cameron-Miller). Each manufacturer of electrosurgical equipment provides electrodes similar to these under his own code name and number designation. To avoid confusion, electrodes used in the case reports have been described according to their physical appearance rather than code name and number.

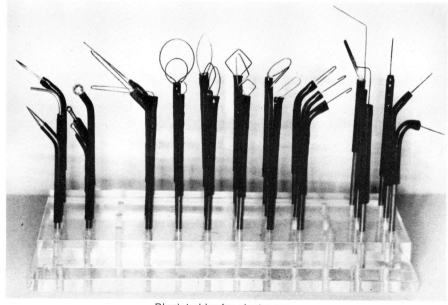

Block holder for electroges

COLES ELECTRODES (*continued*)

MARTIN ELECTRODES

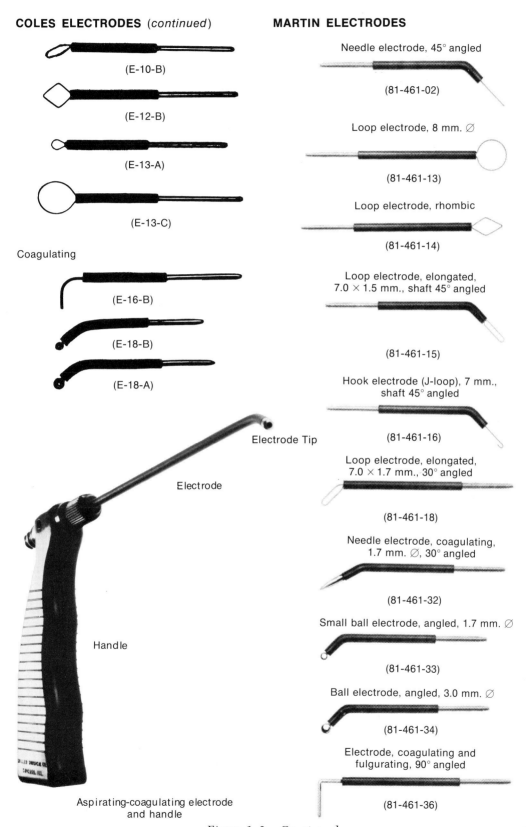

(E-10-B)

(E-12-B)

(E-13-A)

(E-13-C)

Coagulating

(E-16-B)

(E-18-B)

(E-18-A)

Electrode Tip

Electrode

Handle

Aspirating-coagulating electrode
and handle

Needle electrode, 45° angled

(81-461-02)

Loop electrode, 8 mm. ⌀

(81-461-13)

Loop electrode, rhombic

(81-461-14)

Loop electrode, elongated,
7.0 × 1.5 mm., shaft 45° angled

(81-461-15)

Hook electrode (J-loop), 7 mm.,
shaft 45° angled

(81-461-16)

Loop electrode, elongated,
7.0 × 1.7 mm., 30° angled

(81-461-18)

Needle electrode, coagulating,
1.7 mm. ⌀, 30° angled

(81-461-32)

Small ball electrode, angled, 1.7 mm. ⌀

(81-461-33)

Ball electrode, angled, 3.0 mm. ⌀

(81-461-34)

Electrode, coagulating and
fulgurating, 90° angled

(81-461-36)

Figure 1–2. Continued.

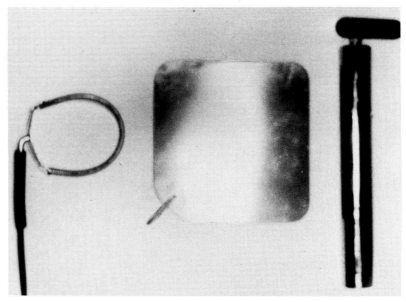

Figure 1-3. Indifferent (passive or dispersive) electrode; three types include metallic wristband, metal plate to be placed beneath patient, and metal hand-held cylinder.

tween the patient and the indifferent electrode is high enough to permit the high-frequency RF current to flow satisfactorily through the patient and into the indifferent electrode. The major impedance during the cutting occurs at the electrode tip and the tissues around it. Thus, although the current is the same throughout the entire circuit, cutting occurs because the current, owing to the high impedance, becomes tremendously concentrated at the site where the small surgical tip makes contact with the tissues.

When the current spreads over a much larger area, as in the indifferent electrode, there is no appreciable increase in impedance and therefore little or no physical or physiological effect at that site of contact.

The diagram in Figure 1–4A visualizes the direct RF current flow pathway clearly. However, as can be seen in the diagram in Figure 1–4B, the current flow can also be via an indirect connection, called the earth ground connection, instead of through the direct connection provided by the indifferent electrode.

The power available from a 60-cycle, 110-volt input power plug flows through two slots which provide the power to the electrosurgical equipment. There is a third slot or hole in the wall socket which is called the earth ground lead. This third connection does not carry voltage but is electrically connected to the physical ground of the earth. Connection to this earth ground point usually is from the case of the electrosurgical unit and the metal parts of the dental chair. In addition, almost all the metal pipes in the operatory usually are connected to this earth ground.

If, as is shown in Figure 1–4B, a connection is made between point B and the earth ground connection, this may simultaneously connect the dental chair to point B. When this occurs, one may be able to use the surgical elec-

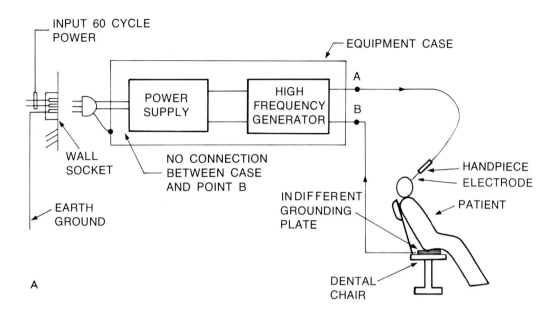

A

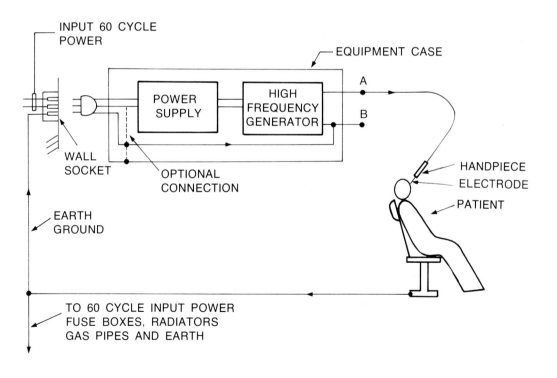

B

Figure 1-4. Path of current during operation *A*, with the indifferent plate, and *B*, without it.

trode handpiece lead A directly on a patient sitting in the chair, but without a directly connected indifferent electrode.

This admittedly is a means of eliminating the indifferent plate from the circuit. Moreover, even when there is no three-prong connection to the equipment, which contains the earth ground lead, one side of the 110-volt plug is usually close to ground potential, and the point B on the high-frequency oscillator can also be connected to this point and still be used as an input electrode, which would permit the ground or indifferent electrode to be eliminated.

Although it is possible to operate the equipment in this manner, it is clinically inadvisable to do so for many reasons. The dental operatory may or *may not* have the correct ground connection. If it does, and if the power output requirement is relatively nominal, adequate electrosurgery may be performed, because the return current to point B can flow through such ground connections from the dental chair to point B of the electrosurgical unit. However, this mode of operation is quite likely to cause these currents to flow along wires and pipes out of the room, down to the power mains in the cellar, and back again. Since many dentists lack the electronic know-how to assure a satisfactory grounding system, and the normal house electrical wiring system does not take this into account, this is a very uncertain arrangement on which to depend.

The major disadvantage of this indirect current flow is its unreliability. Two dentists using identical electrosurgical equipment may achieve markedly different degrees of electrosurgical efficiency if one, by pure chance, happens to have a good external ground and the other does not. Moreover, even when an acceptable external ground *is* present, this method of operation may become radically affected by rewiring or electrical modifications in neighboring apartments, in the cellar or in neighboring buildings, without the dentist being aware that the change has occurred.

Another important disadvantage is that the indirect method of current flow appears to reduce the power output potency. The author has demonstrated this by means of a simple experiment with a light bulb, which will be fully described in the section on research. When the socket containing the light bulb is introduced into the cutting circuit and the cutting current is activated, the light bulb gradually begins to glow. If the indifferent plate is also introduced into the conductive circuit of the unit, and the free hand is placed on it, the glow immediately intensifies greatly. As soon as the hand is removed from the indifferent plate, the bulb becomes dim again. This is visual evidence that when the indifferent plate is being used the power output potency is considerably greater than when it is omitted from the circuit, since the power output setting on the instrument panel remains constant throughout the test. The reason for the difference is due in large measure to the fact that the current return with the indirect current flow has to travel many feet before it returns to point B on the unit. The clinical significance is that when the tissue to be cut is very dense, thick, engorged or edematous, or, if it is necessary to use a fairly large loop electrode, it would be virtually impossible to perform efficient electrosurgery without using the indifferent electrode.

Dependence on indirect current return through the earth ground connection also appears to increase the hazard of untoward effects. The author recently learned from a reliable source an example of this — an accidental burn in a hospital medical procedure that could also happen in the dental operatory. A patient was undergoing surgery under general anesthesia and suffered a burn on the hand and around the nostrils when electrosurgery was used without the indifferent plate. Subsequent reconstruction of events revealed that the patient's hand had drooped limply after she was anesthetized and accidentally made contact with a metal edge on the operating table, causing the hand burn. Metallic contact of the facemask inhaler apparently accounted for the burn around the nostrils. Had a direct current flow into the unit with the indifferent plate been used, it is likely that this accidental burn would have been avoided or the damage minimized.

Indirect current flow creates still another problem. Since the return current usually has to travel many feet before it returns to point B on the high-frequency unit, it acts as a transmitting antenna and is likely to cause increased amounts of interference with other equipment.

Standard electrical practice and N.E.C. codes specify that the ground systems may not be used for indirect current return; such a prohibition may well become part of an F.C.C. requirement as in other countries. The National Fire Protection Association manual* regarding use of high-frequency electrosurgical equipment in hospitals prohibits its use without the indifferent patient electrode, the reasons for which also apply to its use in the dental operatory.

There is one other related matter that deserves comment. A device has recently been introduced as a substitute for the indifferent electrode that is attached to the dental chair instead of to the electrosurgical unit. This creates a direct current flow into the chair, but an indirect current flow back to the power generator at point B, via the earth-ground connection. Therefore it apparently does not eliminate the disadvantages and hazards that have been reviewed.

Electrode Placement

SURGICAL ELECTRODES

There is only one precaution regarding proper placement of these electrodes: the entire metal shaft of the electrode must be inserted into the handpiece, or covered with insulation, so that no bare metal is exposed beyond the handpiece chuck to assure against accidental burns to the patient's lips or tongue and to the therapist's fingers.

---

*High-frequency electrical equipment in hospitals: National Fire Protection Association International. Boston, Massachusetts, 1970. NFPA No. 76 CM: p. 5 (Glossary).

INDIFFERENT ELECTRODES

The indifferent electrode must be placed in a manner that will assure against accidental loss of contact with the electrode, or contact with only a small portion of it, such as its edge, since this would greatly increase the impedance at that point to the degree that the tissues at that site of contact could accidentally be burned.

The best place for the indifferent electrode is under the Naughahyde chair covering. To be placed there, the electrode should be of a flexible character; otherwise, the Naughahyde will wear out from frictional contact with the rigid metal edges. The electrode preferably should also involve a major portion of the seat area, to assure adequate contact under any and all conditions and to assure maximum dispersive action.

If the regulation indifferent electrode—that is, the one supplied with the unit—is used, it should be placed under the patient's thigh rather than under the buttock, since the thigh is more likely to remain in contact with the electrode if the patient should shift around in the chair, or lean forward to expectorate and inadvertently move the electrode in doing so. Should the patient be in the habit of crossing his legs, the electrode should be placed under the limb that remains in contact with the chair seat.

The indifferent plate electrode should be placed centrally under the patient's thigh to avoid having only the outer edge of the electrode make the contact, since this would create enough heat concentration to be painful or cause a mild burn. Special care must also be taken to avoid accidental contact of metallic objects in the patient's undergarments (such as metal clips of a garter belt) with the bare metal of the indifferent plate, especially if there is no cloth intervening between the two metal surfaces. Such contact would cause a severe burn due to the heat concentration at the contact site. The hazard of such accidental burns can be greatly minimized by shielding the indifferent plate electrode with a plastic veneer coating, encasing it in a protective cloth or plastic envelope, or inserting the electrode under the Naughahyde upholstery of the dental chair seat.

It is inadvisable to place the electrode behind the patient's back, even if the patient is going to be in a prone position, since the hollow in the small of the back formed by the curvature of the spine is in many instances great enough to fail to make firm contact with the electrode in that area, and thereby fails to provide the direct current return that is being sought. Moreover, if the spine does make contact with the indifferent plate, the vertebral bony projections are apt to make premature contacts that could create burn-producing heat concentrations.

Effective biterminal application of cutting and coagulating current is not dependent upon direct contact of the indifferent plate with the bare skin of the patient, but direct body contact is essential. In their desire to avoid burn hazards, some dentists are placing the indifferent plate behind the dental chair in the mistaken belief that such remote indirect use will provide the desired biterminal application without body contact. There is no basis for this assumption. Attaching the indifferent electrode to the external back of the dental chair merely provides for direct flow of the current into the *chair*, and from the chair into the earth-ground connection. As a result, the patient will fail to benefit from a direct conductive circuit. The advantage that the latter provides will be reviewed in the section on research.

If the power output of the high-frequency generator is adequately potent, the cutting current is powerful enough to cut efficiently under any clinical conditions even when the indifferent electrode has been inserted under the Naughahyde chair covering upholstery. Therefore, unless the current output of the generator is inadequate, there is no reason for bringing the indifferent electrode into direct contact with bare skin, especially if a vacuum seal has not been assured by applying a lubricating sealant to the skin at the site of contact, to guard against an accidental burn due to high impedance at the site of incomplete contact. As for placing the electrode on the therapist's wrist, and then placing that hand against the cheek on the side opposite to the surgical field, this is not only unnecessary with adequate power output, but may prove awkward and hazardous. In addition to the other factors mentioned, this method impairs the therapist's freedom of movement and tends to interfere with access to the operative field and impair visibility there, and also interfere with the patient's ability to cooperate by opening or closing the mouth and turning the head freely.

There is still another factor about this method that troubles the author. It may actually be quite safe to bring two to three megacycles of RF current that close to the braincase, but the author has an uneasy feeling that this may *not* be a very desirable situation, and if the unit can deliver current of adequate potency, there is no basis for using it. If, on the other hand, the high-frequency generator is incapable of delivering power output of adequate potency for efficient electrosurgery, it could hardly be considered the type of equipment ideally suited for dental electrosurgery.

Current Application — Monoterminal vs. Biterminal

When only the small surgical electrode is employed, without the indifferent plate, monoterminal current is produced. All the heat energy potentiated by monoterminal current is concentrated at the site of contact, producing a more intensely dehydrating effect on the tissues. When both electrodes are employed simultaneously, biterminal current is produced. Current produced thus may have either a coagulating or a volatilizing effect on tissue.

Waveform

Alternating current is an oscillating current, reversing its direction of flow from several to millions of times per second (Fig. 1–5). Alternating current may be unrectified, partially rectified or fully rectified. Each of these types of alternating current produces its own particular pattern of current flow, called its *waveform*. Waveforms are wavy lines that can be visualized on the oscilloscope or traced on the oscillograph. Differences in their waveforms are responsible for the variety of tissue responses produced by electrosurgical currents.

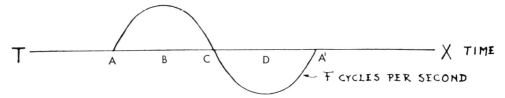

Figure 1-5.   Schematic diagram of single cycle of alternating current.

High-frequency currents may be unrectified, partially rectified or fully rectified. Unrectified current from a spark-gap generator produces a highly damped waveform (Fig. 1–6A) which has an intensely dehydrating effect on tissue. Partially rectified current has a moderately damped waveform. This current is capable of cutting effect, but it is accompanied by simultaneous inherent surface coagulating effect. Fully rectified current produces an undamped waveform (Fig. 1–9). This current produces a pure surgical cutting effect on tissue.[17] A fully filtered, fully rectified current has also recently become available. These variations and refinements of the high-frequency currents can be readily identified, and interpreted, when seen on an oscilloscope.

In order to make the proper choice of electrosurgical current for a given purpose, and to use it judiciously, it is necessary to know not only what the currents are but also their respective waveforms, since the effects the currents have on the tissues are produced by these waveforms.

UNRECTIFIED HIGHLY DAMPED
WAVEFORM

This type of current, produced by spark-gap and simulated spark-gap generators, retains the basic pattern of the cycle of alternating current but is characterized by drastic changes in the amplitude of the current. The current flow begins with an initial burst of peak amplitude that rapidly dwindles to zero, then, after a split-second pause interval or damping period, there is another burst of energy that diminishes to zero (Fig. 1–6A). Figures 1–6B and C are oscilloscopic photographs of these currents. This intermittent, make-and-break pattern of current flow produces insult to the tissues, which react by necrosis of those cells that have been the recipients of the insult (heat output). Tissue repair is slowed, and a degree of postoperative pain may result from the insult.

PARTIALLY RECTIFIED
MODERATELY DAMPED WAVEFORM

This type of current, produced by the partially rectified or "single tube" electronic circuit, is referred to technically as a "half-wave" current (Fig. 1–7A). It has been given this designation because only the first half of each individual cycle of alternating current has been converted by the power generator into high-frequency current. The second half of each cycle which

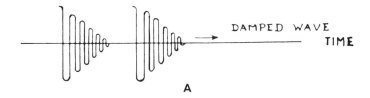

A

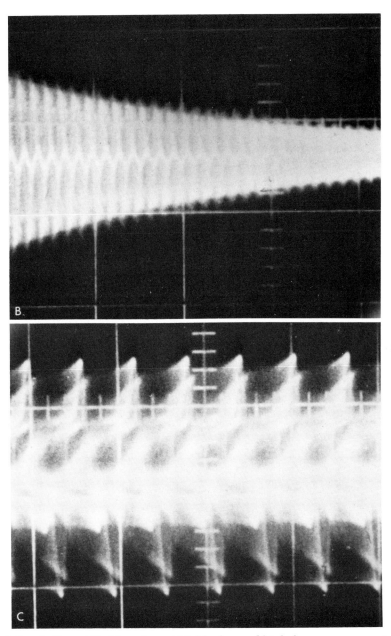

Figure 1-6. *A*, Unrectified (spark-gap) highly damped high-frequency current. *B*, A single surge of true Oudin spark-gap current. *C*, Simulated spark-gap current produced by Coles multicircuit units.

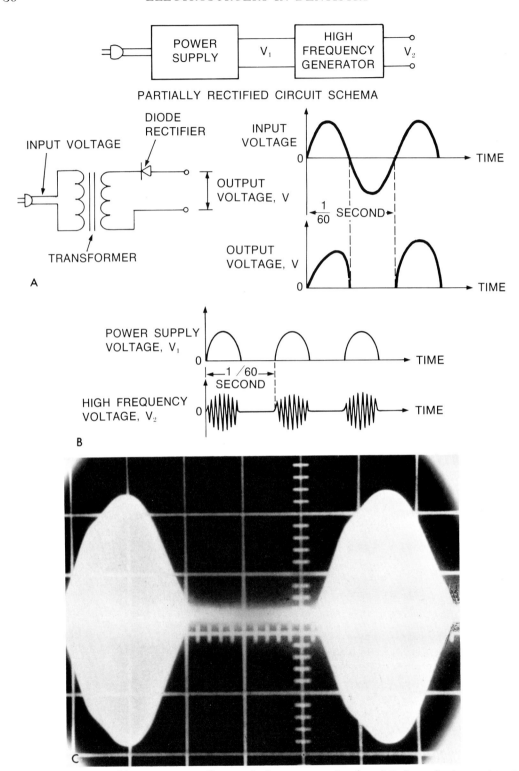

Figure 1-7. Half-wave or partially rectified power supply. *A* and *B* show the intermittent flow of the high-frequency cutting current. In *C*, the connecting bar of the waveform represents the unconverted half cycle of alternating current, while the oval areas represent the half cycles that have become converted into therapeutic high-frequency current.

is referred to as an *envelope* electronically, remains unchanged. During the second half, the high-frequency energy is at zero, or has been damped out. This produces an intermittent flow of the high-frequency cutting current (Fig. 1–7*B*). Owing to the damped period during which the cutting energy amplitude is at zero (Fig. 1–7*C*), several layers of tissue cells on the cut surfaces become coagulated as this current cuts tissue surgically, so that the cutting is automatically accompanied by an inherent degree of coagulation, even though the current is being used properly. Usually the amount of co-agulation is very minimal and not likely to interfere with primary healing of the cut tissues. However, if the electrosurgical instrumentation should fall somewhat short of perfection, this, superimposed on the inherent amount of coagulation, may impair the rate and quality of repair and prevent primary union.

FULLY RECTIFIED
UNDAMPED ELECTRONIC CURRENT

This type of current, produced by a fully rectified circuit, is known electronically as a "full-wave" current, since the entire envelope of each cycle of current is converted into high-frequency current (Figs. 1–8*A* and *B*). The continuous flow of the high-frequency current assures a continuous flow of cutting energy. Thus this current is capable of cutting tissue without any accompanying coagulation of cells on the surface of the cut tissues. However, since each individual cycle starts at zero and returns to zero (as shown in Figure 1–8*C* and *D*) there is a minute but perceptible pulsating effect which can, under special conditions, reduce the efficiency of the cutting effect a trifle. Taking this into consideration, the circuitry of the fully rectified current has been modified by electronic filtration, thereby providing us with a current that is fully rectified and also fully filtered. Thus it is now necessary to subdivide fully rectified current into full-wave and continuous-wave currents.

One additional control factor has recently been incorporated into some of the new dental electrosurgical circuits. Such units have automatic regulators, which maintain the RF output current at a constant potency, even when the input voltage changes rapidly or slowly.

FULLY RECTIFIED FULL-WAVE CURRENT. This current, as has been described, involves transformation of both halves of the cycle or envelope, so that all of each cycle is converted into high-frequency RF current that cuts tissue efficiently, without accompanying coagulation when used properly.

CONTINUOUS-WAVE FULLY RECTIFIED AND FILTERED CURRENT. The late William Coles, inventor of the fully rectified circuit, thought full rectification also provided full filtration. His diagrammatic visualization (Fig. 1–9) showed the indentations between each cycle eliminated, and a completely uniform amplitude throughout, a pattern of current flow that describes the continuous-wave current flow. He also described the fully rectified current as fully filtered, which oscilloscopic examination does not confirm.

Using his fully rectified circuit as the fountainhead, electronics engineers

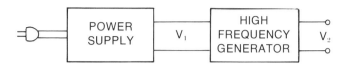

FULLY RECTIFIED CIRCUIT SCHEMA

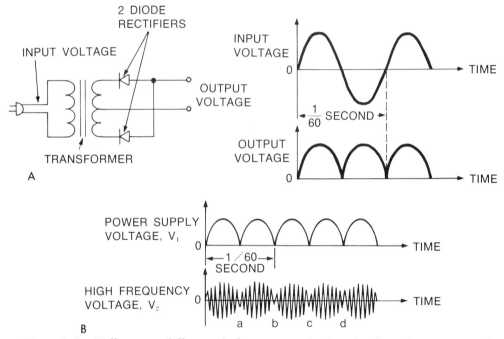

Figure 1–8.   Full-wave or fully rectified power supply. *A* and *B* show the continuous flow of high-frequency current.

Illustration continued on opposite page.

have recently introduced additional electronic components into the fully rectified circuit that filter out the constrictions seen in Figure 1–8C as each full wave begins and ends at zero (Fig. 1–10A). This filtration results in a continuous non-pulsating flow of current, which provides a smoother continuity of cutting current flow, which, under some clinical conditions, can prove most advantageous. Figures 1–10B and C illustrate this current diagrammatically. Figure 1–10D is an oscilloscopic photograph of this current. Figure 1–10E is an oscilloscopic photograph by the author of currents from a fully rectified circuit and from a continuous wave fully rectified, fully filtered circuit as they flow simultaneously through the oscilloscope.

The author also connected two fully rectified units, one of which produces higher current density than the other, to the oscilloscope. Both units were activated and a photograph was taken of their oscillations as they appeared on the oscilloscope when both were used simultaneously for electrosection (Fig. 1–10E). The unit that produced the higher current density produced more than twice as many oscillations in the same period of time and at the same power settings.

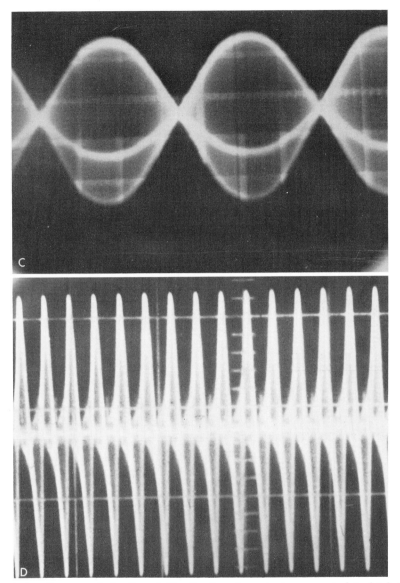

Figure 1–8. Continued. In C and D, all of each cycle is converted to high-frequency current.

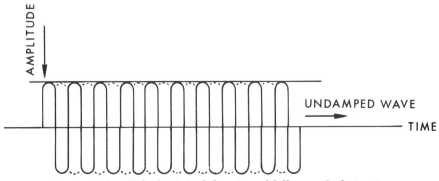

Figure 1-9. Coles' original drawing of fully rectified circuit.

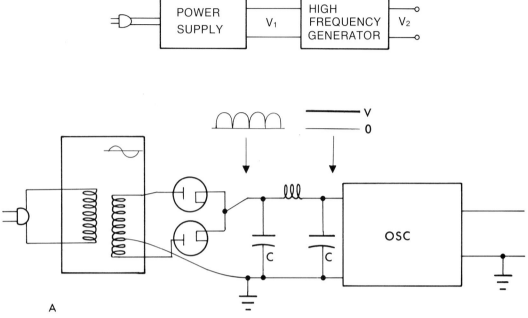

FULLY RECTIFIED CIRCUIT SCHEMA

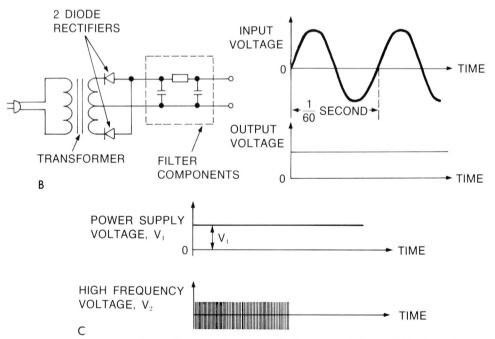

Figure 1–10. A, B, and C, Schematic diagrams of a fully rectified and fully filtered circuit.

Illustration continued on opposite page.

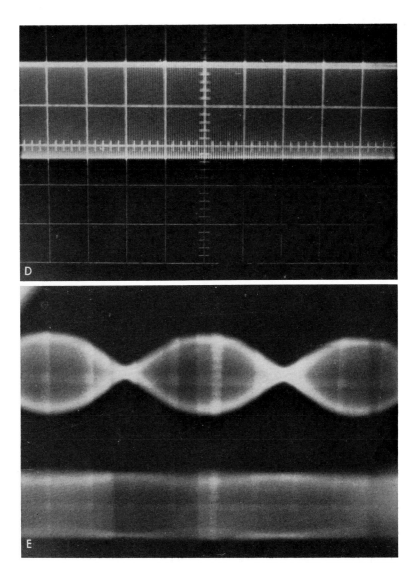

Figure 1–10. Continued. D, Oscilloscopic photograph of this current. *E,* Comparison of currents from fully rectified circuit (top) and continuous wave (fully rectified, fully filtered) circuit (bottom). Note absence of constrictions at half cycles (bottom). *F,* Comparison of two fully rectified units. The oscilloscopic screen showed that the unit with the lower current density (top) produced half as many oscillations as the unit with the higher current density (bottom); power settings were the same on both machines. *F*

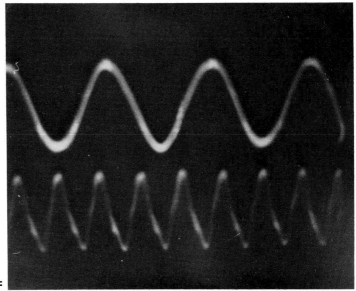

THE THERAPEUTIC ELECTROSURGICAL CURRENTS

There are four therapeutic electrosurgical currents:

1. Electrodesiccation ⎫ Dehydrating Currents
2. Fulguration   ⎭
3. Electrocoagulation ⎫ Coagulating Current
4. Electrosection   ⎭ Cutting Current

The first two—electrodesiccation and fulguration—are dehydrating currents produced by the Oudin current generated by a spark-gap circuit, or by mutated electronic current that has been weakened to simulate the effects of Oudin current when applied to the tissues.

When this highly damped high-frequency Oudin alternating current is applied to the tissues monoterminally, the current flows from the surgical electrode directly into the tissues because the patient's body attracts the current to "ground." The electrode remains cold, but the heat generated by the Oudin current is purported to be approximately 1800 degrees Fahrenheit. If the electrode point is inserted into the tissues (Fig. 1–11A) it produces deeply penetrating tissue dehydration called *electrodesiccation.*

In addition to the actual zone of cellular dehydration produced by this current, there is a variable degree of dehydration of the adjacent underlying tissues which may cause further total or partial destruction of their cellular viability. Because the body resistance to current is believed to vary from 4000 to 40,000 ohms in the 24-hour period, the degree of dehydration and heat penetration that results from electrodesiccation is unpredictable, which makes it difficult for the operator to gauge with accuracy the exact depth and extent of coagulation being achieved with this modality.

From a purely electronic standpoint, electrodesiccation and fulguration are merely variations of the same current, and many medical therapists as well as electrical engineers refer to them interchangeably as the dehydrating currents, since the same electrical energy is used for both; only the manner in which the energy is employed differs. Although it is true that the difference is not due to inherent variations in current characteristics and waveform, as is the case with the other currents, the respective tissue responses are so totally unlike that the therapeutic differences, especially for dentistry, are critically important. In order to create an orderly nomenclature and clear-cut clinical differentiation, the author has felt compelled to establish the fact that for dentistry these are two totally different modalities, as though they were totally dissimilar currents derived from different sources, for the following reasons.

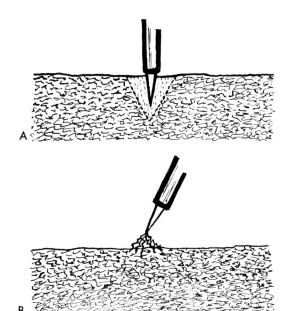

Figure 1–11. Schematic drawings of *A*, electrodesiccation; *B*, fulguration.

Electrodesiccation

When spark-gap Oudin current or simulated spark-gap current is applied monoterminally (without use of a dispersive indifferent plate) and if the surgical electrode tip is inserted into the tissues and permitted to remain unmoved in situ while activated, all the energy being potentiated radiates outward from the tip into the adjacent tissues, producing a potent dehydrating effect on the tissues. Since the electrode remains embedded in situ in the tissues throughout the entire period of electrodesiccation, the heat being generated accumulates and penetrates deeply into the adjacent and subjacent tissues, causing widespread destruction far beyond the site of physical contact of the electrode with the tissues.

This widespread penetrating heat destruction makes electrodesiccation unsuited for all but three clinical uses in dentistry, and it is by far the most dangerous of the therapeutic electrosurgical modalities for dentistry. This is especially so if applied to gingival mucosa, which is attached to periosteum, which in turn is attached to viable bone usually containing vital teeth.

Each instance in which electrodesiccation appears to be indicated, or even justifiable, revolves around its ability to provide very potent hemostasis by dehydration. One instance is when a patient is hemorrhaging so severely that unless a carotid tie-off were performed promptly he would be in dire danger of exsanguination. If there are neither personnel nor facilities to perform surgery, the need to halt the hemorrhage and prevent exsanguination takes priority over the factor of local tissue destruction. Electrodesiccation is also useful for obliterating cavernous hemangiomas in order to avoid danger of profound hemorrhage while attempting their surgical removal, and the tissue destruction may be less hazardous than that produced by injection of chemical sclerosing solutions. Its third area of usefulness, for obliteration of lymphangiomas, also revolves around the fact that electrodesiccation may be safer to use for obliterating these neoplasms than surgery or sclerosing solutions, and its effectiveness for dehydrating the tissues outweighs the local destruction it causes.

Fulguration

The same dehydrating current is employed monoterminally, but this time, instead of implanting the electrode into the tissue and permitting it to remain in situ while activated, the electrode tip is brought toward the tissue surface just close enough for the sparks to emanate from the tip and jump the intervening air-gap to reach the surface of the tissue, producing a superficial dehydration. This is called fulguration (Fig. 1–11B). In fulguration, the operator keeps the electrode moving above the tissue surface, usually in a rotary motion, while the electrode remains activated. In this way destructive penetrating concentration of heat is avoided. The surface dehydration eventually causes charring and carbonization of the surface layers of tissue cells, or the formation of a tough, leathery mass of superficial cells called an eschar. The carbon produced thereby has an inherent insulating quality which helps to make this current self-limiting to a noteworthy degree.

Fulguration, unlike electrodesiccation, can be controlled by the operator to a great extent and has many practical clinical uses in dentistry. Its destructiveness is self-limiting, in part because of the air-space the sparks must jump, in part because of the minimal potency of the current output, and largely because of the insulating effect of the carbon or eschar and the movement to prevent cumulative heat destruction. This modality is especially invaluable in dentistry for destroying undesirable necrotic or cystic tissue fragments that are tightly wedged between teeth and bone in areas totally inaccessible to other methods of instrumentation. It is also useful for destroying fistulous orifices and their tracts, for destroying papillomatous tissue tabs, for destroying the surface layers of cells of the tissue bed from which suspicious neoplasms have been resected, and for controlling bleeding from nutrient foramina on the surface of bone after the mucoperiosteal flap has been elevated. This bleeding can be controlled by application of coagulating energy, but the electrode would have to remain in contact with the bone surface for a perceptible period, which would cause a slight amount of local surface bone sequestration. When the sparking is applied without touching the bone, it causes the blood to clot and seal off the foramina without applying heat to the bone to cause destruction.

Owing to the active sparking, neither electrodesiccation nor fulguration should be used with nitrous oxide analgesia or anesthesia.

Electrocoagulation

This current must be employed biterminally. Electrocoagulating current can be provided by either the spark-gap generator or the electronic equipment, but for dentistry the latter is better suited. When this current is applied properly, the current density becomes sufficiently concentrated at the site of contact to coagulate the organic contents of the tissue surface without penetrating deeply into the adjacent tissues. The resultant zone of coagulation necrosis is limited to the surface of the area to which the current has been applied. The operator can control the extent of tissue destruction by regulating the current density and the period of electrode contact with the tissues, and by use of sound electrosurgical technique. Electrocoagulation destroys tissue by coagulating the organic contents. It is a more potent current than either of the dehydrating currents, and many of its uses are similar to those of fulguration. It is effective in producing hemostasis and is highly effective in sealing off bleeders in soft tissue, eliminating the need to tie them off. This modality is useful for destroying papillomatous and other undesirable tissue masses, for destroying leukoplakia, and for destruction of inoperable oral cancerous masses. It is also excellent for controlling tissue healing by destruction of superficial blood vessels that may be forming in granulation tissue or by controlling their tendency to proliferate. It is especially useful for desensitizing hypersensitive teeth, bleaching discolored teeth, and for drying and sterilizing root canals. Its use for gingival retraction in restorative dentistry, however, is *not* recommended, since it very frequently results in unpredictable and often extensive gingival recession.

Since cellular dehydration and coagulation destroy the diagnostic value of tissue, neither electrodesiccation, fulguration, nor electrocoagulation is a suitable electrosurgical current for performing biopsy.

Electrosection (Acusection)

When undamped fully rectified high-frequency current is applied to the tissues by biterminal application and the surgical electrode is moved along the surface of the tissue as it makes contact, the current density becomes so concentrated along the site of contact that individual cells in the line of cleavage undergo molecular disintegration and volatilize, creating a precise surgical incision. This cutting current, known as *electrosection* or *acusection* is self-limiting in its destructiveness and fully under the control of the operator at all times.

This is by far the most important of the electrosurgical currents for dentistry, and it is used in at least 90 per cent of the dental electrosurgical techniques. When this energy is properly utilized, it is capable of cutting tissue either with a needle electrode to create pure surgical incisions or with a loop electrode to resect tissue masses, without any accompanying coagulation. Electrosection results from the total disintegration and volatilization of tissue cells in the line of cleavage. When partially rectified current is employed, it is accompanied by an inherent degree of surface tissue coagulation, usually only a matter of several layers of cells along the surface of the cut margins. When fully rectified current is properly employed the incision is totally free of any clinical coagulation and looks like tissue that has been incised with an incredibly sharp knife. When the large loop is used there often will be a very thin marginal edge of coagulation at the initial site of contact of the activated electrode with the tissues. Although the output of cutting energy is instantaneous, there is apparently a momentary time-lag at the initial contact when the energy is not potent enough to totally disintegrate and volatilize the cells. The remainder of the tissue segment that has been resected and the bed from which the tissue has been removed are totally free of any coagulation, *if the cutting energy is potent enough to totally disintegrate and volatilize the cells* (see Color Plate I). If the cutting power is inadequate, even though fully rectified current is being used properly, it is incapable of disintegrating and volatilizing the cells, but is powerful enough to cook and coagulate them as would happen with coagulating current (see Color Plate I). If the patient inadvertently loses contact with the indifferent plate the electronic circuit is mutated, owing to loss of power, and the cutting that is performed is inefficient. The healing from such wounds is atypical; it is slow and often there is considerable postoperative pain.

Electrosection is useful for making incisions ranging from simple incisions for drainage to sophisticated incisions for mucoperiosteal flaps. Tissue can also be cut with loop electrodes either to resect a mass of tissue with a single stroke or to shave the tissue in thin layers by planing with the loop in a manner similar to planing a plank of wood with a wood plane to simultaneously reduce and recontour masses of redundant tissue. Electrosection is ideally suited for most of the dental procedures and is uniquely suited for performing what students of cancer term "properly conducted biopsy."

FOOTNOTE REFERENCES

1. Wyeth, G. A.: Surgery of Neoplastic Diseases by Electrothermic Methods. New York, Paul B. Hoeber, 1926.
2. Andrews, G. C.: Clinical and electrical aspects of endothermy in dermatology. J. Radiol., 6:475–480, Dec., 1925.
3. Bierman, W.: Electrosurgery. Amer. J. Surg., 50:768–775, Dec., 1940.
4. Blech, G. M.: Clinical Electrosurgery. New York, Oxford University Press, 1938.
5. Cipollaro, A. C.: Electrosurgery in dermatology. Med. Records, 143:437–440, May 20; 471–472, June 3, 1936.
6. Cumberbatch, E. P., and Hames, W. D.: Fulguration and desiccation. Practitioner, 135:71–82, 1935.
7. Karsner, H. T., in Mock, H. E.: Electrosurgery. J.A.M.A., 104:2341–2350, June 29, 1935.
8. Kime, E. N.: Electrosurgery. New Eng. J. Med., 30:83–87, Feb., 1929.

9. Kovacs, R.: Electrosurgery and Light Therapy. Philadelphia, Lea & Febiger, 1938.
10. Krusen, F. H., and Elkins, E. C.: Electrosurgery. South. Surg., 7:61–67, Feb., 1938.
11. Schmidt, W. H.: High frequency currents in surgery. Surg. Clin. N. Amer., *19*:1545–1556, 1939.
12. Shutt, C. H.: High frequency currents in surgery. J. Missouri M.A., *12*:410–413, July, 1945.
13. Cipollaro, A. C., and Watkins, A. L.: Physical Medicine in General Practice. Philadelphia, J. B. Lippincott Co., 1946.
14. Krusen, F. H.: Physical Medicine. Philadelphia, W. B. Saunders Co., 1941.
15. Mock, H. E.: Electrosurgery. J.A.M.A., *104*:2341–2350, June 29, 1935.
16. McKee, G. M.: Handbook of Physical Therapy. Chicago, American Medical Association, 1936.
17. Kelly, H. A., and Ward, G. E.: Electrosurgery. Philadelphia, W. B. Saunders Co., 1932.

OTHER REFERENCES

Kelly, H. A.: Endothermy, the new surgery. M. J. & Rec., *122*, 1925.
Kowarschik, J.: Electrotherapie. 2nd ed. Vienna, 1923.
Otto, J. F., and Blumberg, T. T.: Techniques in Office Electrosurgery. Cincinnati, Liebel-Flarsheim, 1949.
Ward, G. E.: Electrosurgical Treatment of Neoplastic Diseases, in Pack, G. T., and Ariel, I. M.: Treatment of Cancer and Allied Diseases. 2nd ed. New York, Paul B. Hoeber, 1958.

Chapter Two

DENTAL ELECTROSURGICAL EQUIPMENT AND INSTRUMENTATION TECHNIQUES

Introduction

It has been established that electronic surgery results from conversion of high-frequency RF current into heat energy as a result of resistance the tissues offer to passage of the current. The amount of RF current required for effective electronic surgery is determined by the degree of resistance the tissues offer. The latter is determined by the size and character of the tissues themselves and the physical dimensions of the surgical electrodes used to perform the surgery.

Medical electrosurgery very often involves the cutting of muscles, fascia, ligaments, tendons, fatty tissues, and visceral organs, and urologic wet-field surgery. These tissues offer very high resistance to the passage of the RF currents and require use of large solid blade and heavy-gauge large loop electrodes. To perform such heavy duty medical electrosurgery effectively, very high current densities or power output is required.

Hemostasis is extremely important for effective heavy duty medical electronic surgery. Thus, electrosurgical equipment has been developed especially to fulfill heavy duty medical electronic surgery's dual requirements of very high power output and effective hemostasis. Medical electrosurgical units such as the Liebel-Flarsheim Bovie, Birtcher Blendtome, Cameron-Miller 280, Valleylab, and Electro-Medical Systems units are typical equipment capable of fulfilling the heavy duty medical electronic surgery requirements admirably.

42

For electronic surgery of skin and mucous tissues the situation is quite different, however. These, especially mucous tissues, offer relatively low resistance to the RF currents, and hair-thin wire needle and loop electrodes are used almost exclusively to perform electronic surgery on these tissues. As a result the RF current densities or power output required for optimal electronic surgery of these tissues are so much lower than for the heavy duty medical procedures that use of the heavy duty medical electrosurgical equipment to perform electronic surgery on these tissues is equivalent to using an elephant gun to shoot a rabbit.

Hemostasis is of course desirable and valuable in treating these tissues. However, their lower resistance to the passage of the RF currents and the fact that gingival mucosa is in very close proximity to viable bone and vital teeth make the factor of lateral heat penetration through these tissues of far greater importance.

Inasmuch as the dentist deals largely with the oral mucosa, and especially with gingival mucosa, heavy duty medical electrosurgical equipment is not only unnecessarily large and expensive, but too powerful for optimal use by the dental profession. Special electrosurgical equipment has therefore been developed to meet dentistry's lower current density needs, and to provide versatility and current refinements to minimize lateral heat penetration.

Just as the tissue characteristics and current output involved in heavy duty medical and dental electronic surgery differ, the techniques of instrumentation in using the respective currents most effectively differ greatly. Since potent hemostasis is essential in heavy duty electronic surgery and lateral heat penetration is not of paramount importance, speed of instrumentation is not critically important here. But with the skin and mucous tissues, the importance of lateral heat penetration and damaging effects from cumulative heat retention on these relatively delicate tissues make speed of instrumentation and brief periods of contact of the activated electrodes with the tissues essential for safe, efficient electronic surgery.

Dental electrosurgical equipment that is capable of providing current densities powerful enough to overcome any resistance skin and mucous tissues can offer to the RF currents without coagulating or burning them, without penetrating far beyond the site of application of the currents, and of providing all the useful therapeutic electrosurgical currents is ideally suited to this method of instrumentation.

However, the term "dental" electrosurgical unit is in a sense a misnomer. Medical electronic surgery is not limited to heavy duty cutting. A number of important medical disciplines deal with tissues that require the same current output and special features offered by the dental units, and while their unique electronic *surgical* techniques may differ, the techniques of instrumentation with these currents are for the most part similar or identical. Thus, for the ear, nose, and throat surgeon and the head and neck plastic surgeon, who deal with skin and nasal, oral, and pharyngeal mucosa, and for the gynecologist and proctologist, who treat mucous tissues very similar to oral mucosa, as well as for the neurosurgeon and the ophthalmologic surgeon, who deal with very delicate tissues, the "dental" types of electrosurgical equipment and techniques of instrumentation are better suited than the heavy duty "medical" equipment and techniques of instrumentation. Nevertheless, the designation "dental" electrosurgical equipment, since it helps to differentiate from the very powerful heavy duty type of equipment, serves a useful purpose.

PART 1 — DENTAL ELECTROSURGICAL EQUIPMENT

Electrosurgical circuitry, like electrosurgical technique, has not remained static. The manufacturers of dental electrosurgical equipment make improvements in their products from time to time. These improvements often make evaluation of earlier models obsolete.

If published in this text, such obsolescence would be perpetuated uselessly and unfairly. Evaluation of the various makes of equipment that are currently available will therefore not be published here. In its stead, the author offers a simple, infallible method (to be described) whereby each individual practitioner can quickly and efficiently determine the efficacy of the cutting and coagulating currents provided by any electrosurgical equipment that is marketed. Such personal evaluation should serve a far more useful purpose than an outmoded evaluation or a lack of evaluation of equipment that will be marketed after this text has been published.

ELECTROSURGICAL POWER GENERATORS

Electrosurgical equipment falls into two broad categories: the spark-gap generators and the electronic circuits. All spark-gap generators are basically similar circuits. The electronic circuits vary and differ considerably from one another in design and function. Each type shall therefore be listed separately.

Spark-Gap Generators

The spark-gap generators were the first and most primitive of the high-frequency electrosurgical devices. After D'Arsonval demonstrated that high-frequency current could be safely applied to living tissue without electrocuting the recipient, tumor surgeons, motivated by their desire to destroy malignant tissue more efficiently and effectively than could be achieved with electrocautery, initiated development of the spark-gap equipment. Dermatologists and other medical specialists still use it extensively.

The spark-gap generator produces a "highly damped" or intermittent flow of high-frequency alternating current that is called Oudin current.

Operating on the principle of condenser discharge across a spark-gap, Oudin current produces unrectified current of highly damped waveform similar to that of the single cycle of alternating current shown in Figure 1–5.

With each condenser discharge, a series of oscillations are set up. The voltage peak of the first is highest; then each subsequent oscillation of the series diminishes in voltage right down to zero (Fig. 1–6A). This current produces a concentration of heat energy at the site of contact of the single surgical electrode sufficient to cause marked cellular dehydration. The breaks in the surging, make-and-break pattern of current flow produce peaks of heat that tend to have a thermal shocking effect on the local tissues. When used monoterminally, the spark-gap current produces excellent electrodesiccation and fulguration. Used biterminally, it produces electrocoagulation.

The sparks produced by Oudin current are large—that is, when directed to the surface of tissue, the sparks are seen as lilac-purple in color and are capable of arcing across a wide air-space between the electrode tip and the tissue surface. The sparks often are capable of bridging across as much as a half centimeter or more of space between the electrode tip and the tissue surface.

True Oudin current is the least potent of the high-frequency currents. Thus, although the sparks are capable of spanning across a fairly wide air-gap, they are not sufficiently potent to effectively char and carbonize the tissue surface when employed for fulguration. In most instances they tend to produce enough surface dehydration to create a tough, leathery surface eschar, which then acts as an insulator and prevents destruction of undesirable tissue remaining under the eschar.

The spark-gap generator is incapable of producing true "surgical" cutting current.

Typical Units: The Hyfrecator (Fig. 2–1); Bantam Bovie; Electricator.

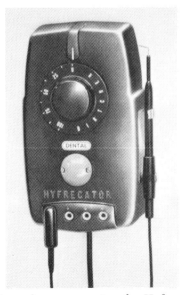

Figure 2–1.   A spark-gap generator, the Hyfrecator (Birtcher).

Electronic Instruments (Radioknives)

With the advent of DeForest's vacuum-tube oscillator, or "radio-tube," a new high-frequency current of different waveform was demonstrated. The vacuum-tube oscillator is capable of producing continuous wave oscillations (i.e., of equal voltage and without interruptions). This type of current produced an entirely new electrosurgical effect on tissue—*it cut like a knife!*[1]

Electronic surgical instruments vary in design and circuit. They range from single power vacuum-tube units to units built with three or more tubes, transistors, or rectifiers. Some units are designed to deliver partially rectified current; others, fully rectified current, and, most recently, continuous wave current. Still others are built with dual or multiple circuits designed to deliver the electronic currents plus unrectified spark-gap current (Fig. 2–2), or a mutant form of damped electronic current. The electronic instruments have one common denominator—they all can perform electrosection.

Electronic electrosurgical equipment converts ordinary commercial 60-cycle alternating current (AC) into high-frequency RF current and delivers this current between the surgical electrode and the indifferent or ground plate (Fig. 1–1). The frequency of electrosurgical alternating current power usually ranges from 1 to 6 million cycles, better known as megacycles, or oscillations per second.

All electronic units have one common denominator: all are powered by an electronic power generator—either the three-element vacuum-power tube generator or solid-state substitutes for the vacuum-tube generator.

The "input" power supply of commercial electricity generates the correct operating voltage and currents that are necessary for the operation of the high-frequency generator. This is essential because the high-frequency generator must receive a positive voltage in order to operate. Since the commercial alternating power from the AC wall outlet is alternately positive and negative 60 times per second, it must first be converted into the necessary positive voltage. Furthermore, the magnitude or "amplitude" of the positive voltage must be correct for the high-frequency generator. The circuitry achieves this in the following manner:

The input power from the AC wall outlet is first routed to the input power transformer of the power supply. This transformer changes the magnitude of the 60-cycle AC power to the proper magnitude to operate the high-frequency oscillator or output power generator. The current at this stage is, however, still 60-cycle AC current. To convert it into the DC or unipolar voltage needed to operate the high-frequency power generator, it is passed through devices known as diodes. Diodes may be either vacuum-tube, mercury-vapor tubes or the more modern semiconductor diodes such as silicon or selenium rectifiers.

The diode possesses the unique property of conducting electric currents in one direction and not permitting them to flow in the other direction. When such diodes are attached to the output of the transformer, they convert the alternating voltages and currents to DC or uniform pulsating voltages or currents. When a single diode is used, it will permit current to flow in the correct

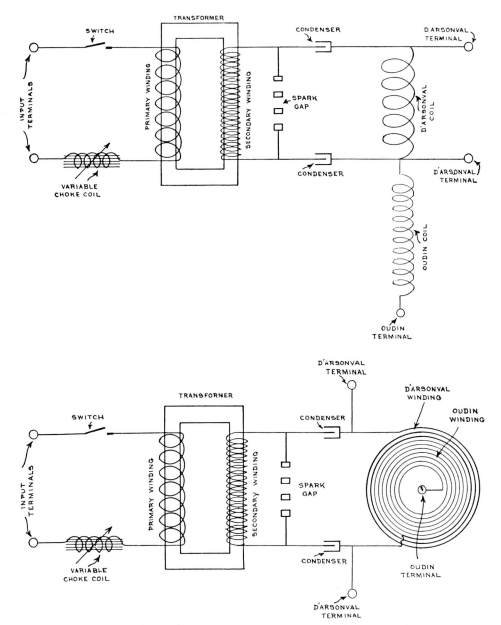

Figure 2-2. Schematic diagram of typical spark-gap circuit.

direction for only one of the half-cycles of the input alternating current. While the input current and voltage of the other half-cycle is in the wrong direction it is shut off completely. This was shown in Figure 1–7A.

Such a power supply is called a half-way rectifier power supply, or a partially rectified power supply. As shown schematically in Figure 1–7B, it delivers a positive pulse of current, or the high-frequency current that is capable of producing a cutting effect on the tissues, for only one half the time, and no current and voltage during the other half. When such voltages are applied to a high-frequency oscillator, it begins to oscillate and deliver its high-frequency signal. When no voltage is supplied to the oscillator, it cannot deliver the signal. Thus the output of the high-frequency oscillator consists of bursts of high-frequency power only while the positive half-cycle is being delivered by the half-way rectifier or partially rectified circuit.

If, instead, two diodes are used, as shown in Figure 1–8A, both halves of each alternating current cycle are correctly switched by means of the diodes, so that each of the half-cycles of the input AC power from the power plug will be of correct positive polarity, as seen in Figure 1–8B. This is known as a full-wave rectifier power supply, or a fully rectified circuit. When these voltages are delivered to the high-frequency oscillator, the latter will deliver successive bursts of RF power uninterruptedly, as seen in Figure 1–8C. The reason why the high-frequency energy comes in bursts is that during each individual cycle of the alternating current of the input AC power from the wall plug, the voltage drops to zero at each half-cycle, creating a constriction (Fig. 1–8D). This describes the fully rectified or full-wave current flow.

There is a third type of power supply which consists of a full-wave rectifier power supply plus an additional set of components to which the full-wave rectifier power is delivered. These components consist of capacitors (condensers) and inductances (coils) which smooth out the pulsations from the positive voltage, so that instead of a positive pulsating voltage the power supply voltage remains constant in level and constant in time, as seen in Figure 1–10C. If such a constant voltage is applied to the high-frequency oscillator, the latter will turn on and deliver its high-frequency power to the surgical electrode. The level or magnitude (amplitude) of the power supply will be constant in time, as seen in Figure 1–10D. This type of power supply is called a fully rectified and fully filtered power supply. The output high-frequency power from the high-frequency oscillator now is constant in time and is called a constant-level high-frequency constant-wave power supply, or CWRF power.

The differences in voltages and currents available from each type of high-frequency oscillator are shown diagrammatically and in oscilloscopic photographs in Chapter 1. Depending upon the power supply, such outputs can be pulsating outputs which are off half the time (partially rectified power supply, Fig. 1–7); pulsating outputs which pulsate all the time (fully rectified power supply, Fig. 1–8); or, finally, output voltages from which the pulsations have been filtered out, and which therefore are constant in time (fully rectified plus fully filtered power supply, Fig. 1–10).

All electrosurgical equipment has an additional component that is part of the high-frequency oscillator. This is the power control for the high-frequency power. This control, usually available on the front panel of the instrument, permits the surgeon to change the magnitude of the power necessary to perform electrosurgery. (The external knob for the power control is referred to elsewhere as the output power control rheostat.)

Although the operator must have control so that he can vary the magnitude or potency of the power, there are certain variations it would be distinctly preferable not to have, particularly unexpected fluctuations in power output.

When the power control knob is set at a given setting, the full amount of that power should be *uniformly* available at all times. Moreover, this precise amount of power should be repeatable without variation or fluctuation from day to day, minute to minute, and even from a brief fraction of a second to fraction of a second, so that the power supply remains *constant* while the activated electrode is in contact with the tissues. Unfortunately, even with the power output at an established setting, a number of internal and external factors can create interferences that produce variations in current magnitude or in the potency of the current being delivered to the tissues at the site of contact of the activated electrode with the tissues.

Variations in magnitude of the commercial voltage entering the circuit through the input AC power plug cause the internal variations that affect the high-frequency power output magnitude. Ideally, the electrosurgical equipment should compensate automatically for any variations in power of the commercial current entering the circuit or should eliminate them as a factor in the magnitude of the current output of the power oscillator.

Fluctuations in input power caused by variations in voltage of the commercial current entering the circuit appear to affect the continuous waveform (CWRF) circuit current output somewhat less than the current output of fully rectified circuits.

The Coles Radiosurg Electronic Scalpel IV units include line voltage meters, called line monitors, to indicate fluctuations in input current power, and a built-in voltage regulator that can be adjusted to compensate for fluctuations in commercial current input. With fully rectified circuits that do not provide comparable devices, fluctuations in current input become known only by sudden changes in the behavior of the activated electrode while it is in contact with the tissues. When the need arises, compensations must be made by manual adjustment in power output of the power oscillator, instead of by adjustment of the power input current entering the circuit. With experience the necessary adjustments can easily be made by the therapist, but it does require more knowledge and skill than does adjustment of power input current.

External factors such as electric household appliances in use can also influence the magnitude or potency of the high-frequency current output and thereby alter the efficiency of the cutting or coagulating currents. Air conditioners, refrigerators or comparable electrical devices create transient or temporary drop or rise in voltage as they are turned on and off and thus affect the high-frequency current potency. Other external factors that can influence the magnitude of the currents include surgical wire leads that become looped or coiled or are excessively long or in close proximity to a large water pipe or conduit. These cause a reduction in the magnitude of the power output being delivered to the surgical electrode.

Ideally, the electrosurgical equipment should have built-in electronic regulation to automatically compensate for such external variations. Such built-in electronic regulation, by use of the principle of coaxial shielding, has been a well-known technique in electronics for 30 years and has been used extensively in television for many years. Coaxial shielding protects the surgical leads from outside influences, so that the only influence on the high-frequency oscillator and the magnitude of current output at the surgical electrode tip will be variations in the thickness and density of the tissues and in the size, shape, or thickness of the surgical electrodes. These create need for variations in the density or potency of cutting energy for different tissues and electrodes.

PARTIALLY RECTIFIED "SINGLE-TUBE" UNITS

The earliest and simplest of the electronic electrosurgical circuits were the partially rectified single-tube units. Many such circuits remain in use, largely by medical therapists.

As was established earlier in the chapter, this type of circuit can convert only the first half of each cycle of current to high frequency; the second half of each cycle, referred to electronically as the second half of the envelope of current, remains inactive. The inability of this circuit to convert the second half of the envelope results in a drop in current density (amplitude) during that period, or a "moderate damping effect," as was seen in Figure 1–7. This damping effect gives the circuit and the current it produces the designation "partially rectified, moderately damped" current.

This loss of continuity of the cutting effect owing to the damping during the second half of each current cycle produces a characteristic coagulation of several layers of cells on the surface of the cut tissue. This coagulating effect is inherent and cannot be avoided or eliminated. When this current is properly utilized the coagulating effect is often so superficial and minimal that it is not likely to interfere appreciably with primary healing. However, it has been established that this current produces an appreciably greater degree of lateral heat dispersion into the contiguous surrounding tissues than fully rectified current, and it appears to result in a slower rate of healing in the deeper structures.[*] Thus, if instrumentation falls short of perfection, any tissue damage superimposed on the inherent coagulation will not only prevent primary repair but will be more likely to result in sloughing and even sequestration.

The inherent coagulating effect of partially rectified current is eminently suited to the needs of many medical specialists. Indeed, in many instances the medical therapist needs much more coagulation than is provided by the inherent amount of coagulation of this current, to reduce danger of surgical metastasis during cancer surgery, and to minimize bleeding. To meet that need,

---

[*]See the Harrison and Kelly reports in the section on Electrosurgical Research.

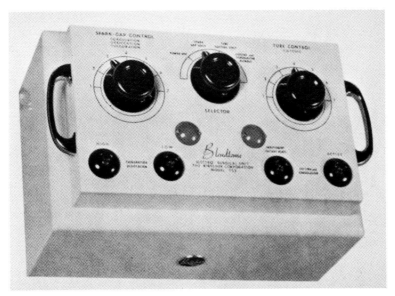

A

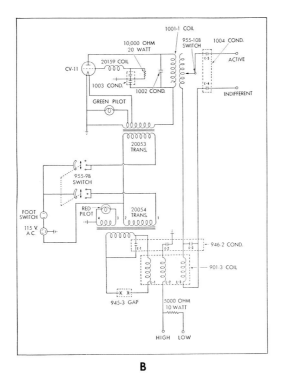

B

Figure 2-3.   A, A dual-circuit (electronic single-tube plus spark-gap) unit, the Blendtome (Birtcher). B, Schematic diagram of the Blendtome dual-circuit unit.

special electrosurgical circuits have been developed that provide cutting and coagulating currents individually, or a simultaneous blend of both currents.

For treatment of mucous and other delicate tissues in various parts of the body, and especially in dental electrosurgery, the situation is vastly different, particularly when gingival mucosa is involved. Gingival tissue normally is about 1 to 1½ mm. in thickness and is attached to periosteum, which is attached to viable bone that usually contains vital teeth. A clinically appreciable degree of lateral heat dispersion could wreak havoc with these structures, and the thin labial gingiva is not apt to tolerate even superficial coagulation. The inherent coagulating effect and greater lateral heat dispersion of partially rectified current and the blending of cutting and coagulating current are therefore not ideally suited for dental use.

Typical Single-Tube Units: Cameron-Miller 255; Siemens Radiotome.

Typical Blended Current Unit: Birtcher Blendtome (Fig. 2–3).

FULLY RECTIFIED UNITS

These electronic devices are RF transmitters built with vacuum-tube power generators or transistors* and either mercury vapor rectifying tubes, dry selenium rectifiers, silicon rectifiers, or other rectifiers, and condensers. Their circuitry is designed to deliver fully rectified (RF) current of undamped waveform. RF current has a slightly modulated or pulsating pattern of current flow that is free of pulsating peaks of heat** and is therefore nonshocking and noncoagulating. Fully rectified current provides clinically desirable hemostasis without accompanying cellular coagulation. When it is used properly its usefulness for surgery is clinically comparable to the best attainable with cold steel cutting instruments.

To differentiate between the various types of fully rectified equipment, it is necessary to subdivide them into the following categories:

Single-circuit fully rectified units. These circuits provide cutting and coagulating currents only. They do not provide either Oudin spark-gap or simulated spark-gap current for fulguration or electrodesiccation. They consist of power components and rectifiers that produce fully rectified (RF) current.

Typical Units: Cameron-Miller 26–230, 26–240, and 255; Parkell Electronic Electrosurgery Dental Model 225 ME.

Cameron-Miller 26–230 (Fig. 2–4) and **26–240** (Fig. 2–5) **units.** These units are powered by vacuum-tube power generators and deliver the currents by linear output.

Parkell Electronic Electrosurgery Dental Model 225 ME (Fig. 2–6). This compact 25-watt unit is manufactured by the same division of Gebrueder Martin of West Germany that manufactures their Elektrotom units but is

---

*Conversion of dental electrosurgical units from tube power generation to solid-state (all-transistorized) power generation and other circuitry refinements are progressing at a rapid pace in the electrosurgical industry. It is quite likely that by the time this text is published the circuitry features of some of the units being reviewed will have undergone varying degrees of revision.

**This phenomenon is due to conversion of the alternating current to pulsating direct current by the electronic power tube or transistors, then reconverted by the rectifying components to high-frequency current that is surge-free.[2]

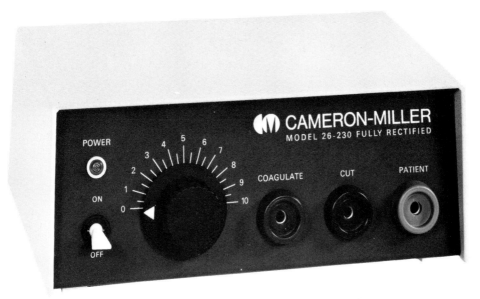

Figure 2-4. Cameron-Miller 26-230 fully rectified unit.

distributed in the United States and Canada by Parkell. The unit is powered by a vacuum-tube power generator with silicon rectifiers.

Single-circuit units produce electronic cutting and coagulating currents. They provide neither Oudin nor simulated spark-gap dehydrating currents. There is a *pervading misconception* that by increasing the cutting current excessively, the sparks and resultant charring of tissues become the equivalent of fulguration. Realistically, charring due to sparking from use of excessively powerful cutting current should not be confused with sparking dehydration produced by fulgurating current, since excessive cutting current output generates substantially greater penetration of lateral heat dispersion into the tissues than is produced by Oudin or simulated spark-gap currents and cannot therefore be safely substituted for either of them.

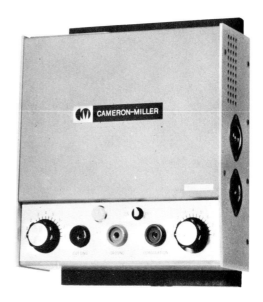

Figure 2-5. Cameron-Miller 26-240 fully rectified unit.

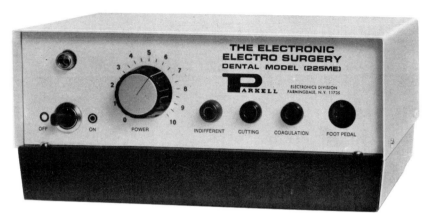

Figure 2–6. Parkell Electronic Electrosurgery Dental Model 225 ME.

Dual-circuit fully rectified units. This type of equipment consists of a fully rectified circuit similar to the ones just reviewed, plus a separate Oudin spark-gap generator, both housed in the one unit. Thus, this type of unit provides all the therapeutic electrosurgical currents.

Typical Units: Martin Elektrotom 70-D (Fig. 2–7); Cameron-Miller R265.

The **Martin Elektrotom 70-D** is their dental electrosurgery unit. It is capable of producing 70 watts of heat energy. It delivers fully rectified cutting, coagulating, and spark-gap fulgurating-desiccating currents. The unit is reputed to feature an alarm buzzer signal that becomes activated when the patient indifferent electrode is not properly connected with the circuit.

Multiple-circuit fully rectified units. In addition to the electronic cutting and coagulating currents, these units provide a simulated spark-gap type of dehydrating current. The latter is created by addition of electronic components that decrease the density of the simulated fulgurating-desiccating current sufficiently to simulate the characteristics of true Oudin current to a workable degree, without generating excessive heat into the tissues. Thus

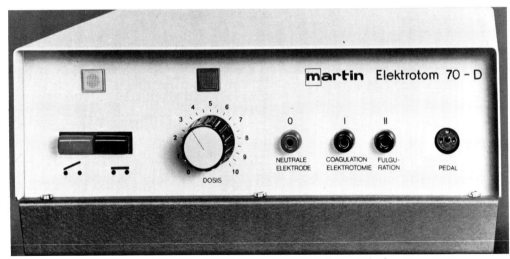

Figure 2-7. Martin Elektrotom 70-D fully rectified unit.

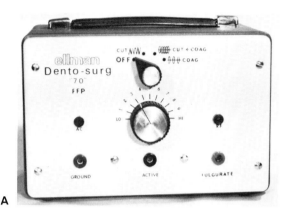

Figure 2–8. A, Ellmann Dento-Surg 70. Fully rectified unit. *B,* Ellman Dento-Surg 90 FFP. Fully rectified and continuous wave unit.

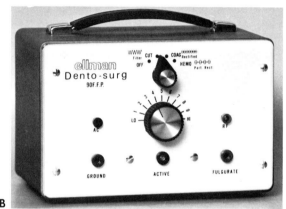

this mutated electronic current provides energy that is clinically suitable for fulguration and electrodesiccation of the oral tissues.

The fully rectified cutting and coagulating circuits of these units are similar to those of the single-circuit and dual-circuit units. Although the density of their mutated dehydrating currents is greatly reduced, it remains somewhat more potent than true Oudin spark-gap current, apparently without clinically significant increase in lateral heat dispersion. Its greater current density results in effective fulguration by controllable charring of the tissue surface. Undesirable oral tissues can therefore be destroyed in situ efficiently.

Typical Units: Ellman Dento-Surg 70 (Fig. 2–8A); Coles Electronic Radiosurg Scalpel IV (Fig. 2–9).

Ellman Dento-Surg 70. This is a compact unit with a vacuum-tube power generator and solid-state components. It delivers fully rectified cutting, coagulating, and simulated spark-gap fulguration-desiccation by linear output.

Coles Radiosurg Electronic Scalpel IV (Fig. 2–9). The manufacturer has discontinued production of this unit. However, many of these excellent units are still in use and giving satisfactory service. Therefore, for the benefit of its users, this unit will be reviewed.

It is a 100-watt unit that delivers all four therapeutic electrosurgical currents: cutting, coagulating, fulgurating and desiccating. It has a built-in line monitor to indicate the amount of current entering the unit and a voltage regulator to adjust the current internally, as required, to compensate for

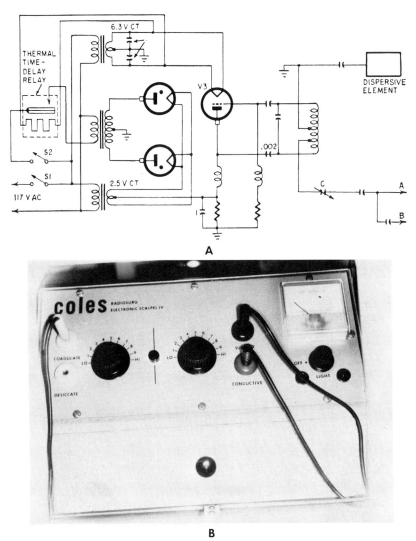

A

B

Figure 2–9. A, Schematic drawing of multiple-circuit electronic unit, Coles Radiosurg Electronic Scalpel IV. *B,* This multiple-tube unit model is portable. The meter in the upper right hand corner of the panel indicates amount of commercial current entering the power generator. Switch on back serves as a voltage regulator and is used to adjust current as required. It has a separate circuit for insertion of a transilluminating lamp which functions independently from the electrosurgical currents.

fluctuations in input line electric current. The unit delivers the high-frequency currents by linear output. It is powered by a vacuum power generator with silicon rectifiers. Its on-off switch serves as the power rheostat output for a transilluminating lamp that can be plugged into the unit's instrument panel.

Fully rectified and filtered (CWRF) circuit units

In these units special electronic components have been introduced into the fully rectified circuit to filter out the slight amount of pulsation (modulation) in current flow as each cycle or "envelope" forms. This results in a uniform, nonpulsing or unmodulated, uninterrupted continuity of current flow that is called a "continuous wave" current.

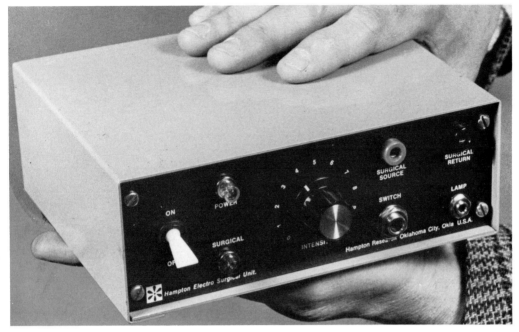

Figure 2–10. Hampton Electro Surgical Unit.

Single-circuit rectified and filtered units. These devices produce continuous wave cutting and coagulating currents. Like the single-circuit fully rectified units, these also provide neither Oudin nor simulated spark-gap current.

Typical Units: Beta Engineering's Dental Electrosurge MK2 D; Hampton Industries Electro Surgical Unit (Fig. 2–10); Whaledent Strobex (Fig. 2–11); Strobex Mark II; and L.A.S.E.R. (Italy).

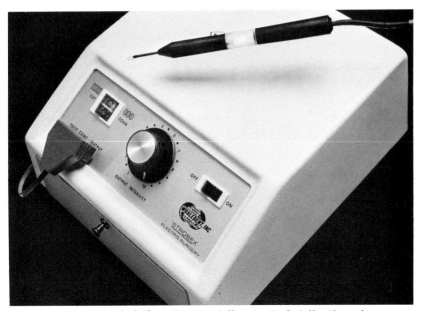

Figure 2–11. Whaledent Strobex fully rectified, fully filtered unit.

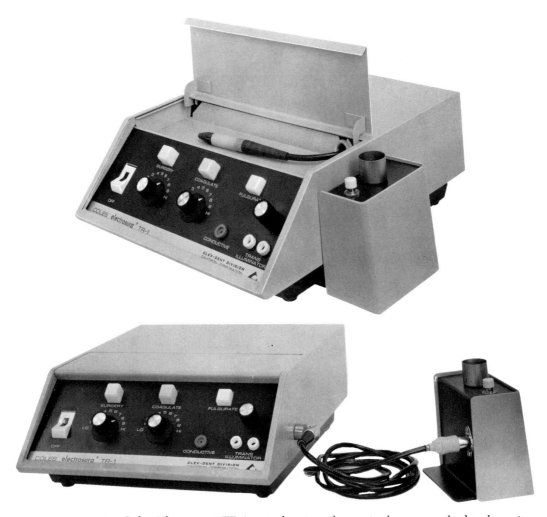

Figure 2–12. Coles Electrosurg TR-1 unit showing ultrasonic cleaner attached to the unit (upper) and separated, attached with an umbilical cable (lower).

Beta Engineering's Dental Electrosurge MK2 D is a compact solid-state unit manufactured in Israel. It features a 110V–220V voltage selector switch on the back panel.

Hampton Electro Surgical Unit is also a compact solid-state unit.

Whaledent (Majeska) Strobex is a compact solid-state unit that features a choice of foot switch power control or an electrode handpiece fingerswitch. The circuit is said to be coaxially shielded. Strobex Mark II is a simpler, less expensive model.

Multiple-circuit rectified and filtered units. These devices produce continuous wave cutting, coagulating, and simulated spark-gap currents.

Typical Units: Coles (Cavitron) Electrosurg TR-1 (Fig. 2–12); Ellman Dento-Surg 90 FFP (Fig. 2–8B); Siemens Sirotom.

Coles Electrosurg TR-1. This is a solid-state unit that provides coaxially shielded continuous wave cutting, coagulating, and simulated spark-gap currents, delivered by linear output. This unit features a retractable electrode handpiece cable and a small ultrasonic electrode cleaner as accessory attachments. The latter is of the split-unit variety. It can be either attached directly to the side of the unit or separated and attached to the unit with an "umbilical" cable. It retains the transilluminating lamp circuit described in the Radiosurg Electronic Scalpel IV. The Electrosurg TR-2 is a simpler, less expensive model.

Ellman Dento-Surg 90 FFP is a compact unit that is powered by a vacuum-tube power generator and a vector board of rectifiers and other components. It has a 90-watt output capability and produces fully rectified cutting, continuous wave cutting, coagulating, and simulated spark-gap currents that are delivered by linear output.

Siemens Sirotom. This is a compact solid-state unit made by Siemens in West Germany that features a finger-switch power control in the electrode handpiece and a cylindrical patient indifferent hand electrode.

Coaxial shielding

A number of circuits have successfully combined coaxial shielding with their constant-wave circuitry. Coaxial shielding eliminates fluctuations in potency of cutting current output due to outside influences such as interference from other electrical devices and the other sources of interference previously mentioned. When coaxial shielding is combined with constant-wave (CWRF) output, the current being delivered to the electrode at the site of tissue contact is virtually impervious to sudden fluctuations or cutbacks in commercial input electricity voltage. This assures uninterrupted flow of current density at the desired level of potency.

Four sophisticated heavy-duty medical electrosurgery units and a new dental unit with unusual safety features also merit mention here. All are solid-state units, coaxially shielded that produce continuous (constant) wave current.

Ritter Bovie. This old hospital favorite has been completely redesigned and revised. It is now a compact, sophisticated unit that signals an alarm if the patient indifferent electrode is not incorporated into the circuit at the start of the surgery.

Electromedical Systems unit also is a compact solid-state heavy-duty medical unit.

Valleylab SSE 1 and SSE 2 electrosurgery units. Both units are solid-state fully rectified and filtered circuits with coaxial shielding. Both are designed specifically for medical electrosurgery and deliver extremely potent current output; the SSE 1 is for office use, the SSE 2 for hospital use.

Ritter Mode[4] electrosurgical unit. This newly developed unit incorporates what promises to be a major breakthrough in dental electrosurgical circuitary. The Ritter Company engineers have developed a circuit that incorporates a number of unique automatic self-regulating built-in safety features that apparently eliminate the hazards that have always been associated with inexpert use of electrosurgery. They expect the unit to be in full production by the time this text is published (Fig. 2–13).

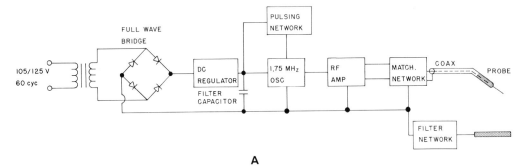

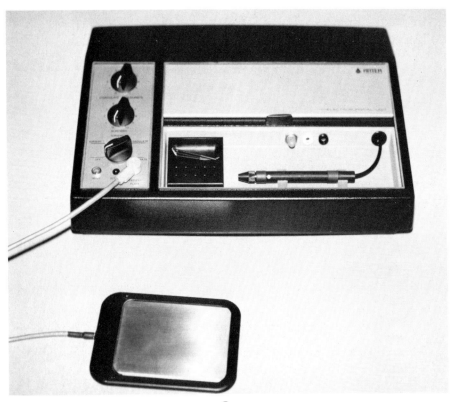

Figure 2-13. A, Circuit diagram, and B, pilot model of Ritter solid-state fully rectified, fully filtered and partially filtered, coaxially shielded automatically monitored unit.

Despite its universally acknowledged invaluable advantages for dentistry, many dentists have continued to abstain from use of electrosurgery in their practices. Their abstinence stems mostly from the fear that through misuse of the currents they might cause serious tissue sloughing, bone sequestration, or pulp necrosis. Such destructive electrosurgical results invariably must be attributed to one or more of the following factors: failure to use the proper amount of current to cut or coagulate tissue efficiently under all clinical conditions; improper electrosurgical instrumentation that causes destructive heat penetration and cumulative heat retention in the tissues; and failure to employ the cutting and coagulating currents biterminally.

The Mode[4] appears to neutralize all these factors effectively. When the existing electrosurgical circuits are used, it is necessary to manually adjust the power output needs created by differences in thickness and density of the tissues being treated, and in the size, shape, and thickness of the surgical electrodes. The fact that the operator must decide how much change is needed for optimal results places a premium on the user's electrosurgical expertise. The Mode[4] eliminates need for this expert judgment by making the current power adjustments automatically self-regulated, so that cutting and coagulation can be performed without need for manual changes in power output settings, regardless of the tissue or electrode variations enumerated above.

The author has verified this experimentally. A perfect incision or loop excision can be performed with this circuit without manual adjustments, regardless of whether cutting is performed with a fine needle or a solid metal blade electrode, or with a narrow U-shaped or J-loop electrode or a 12-mm. round loop electrode. Also, the cutting result seems equally efficient whether the tissue being cut is thin or thick, normal or engorged, friable or dense; thus, the need to depend on expert judgment as to how much to increase or decrease current densities to obtain optimal results is eliminated.

This circuit incorporates a second safety feature — a timing device that limits to one second the period of current flow while the activated electrode is in contact with the tissues; the electrode then becomes automatically deactivated for five seconds. At the end of that interval there is an audible beep which indicates that instrumentation can be resumed for another one second of active electrode contact with the tissues. The enforced five-second rest intervals eliminate the hazard of destructive heat retention in the tissues due to prolonged continuous instrumentation. It also minimizes the damage potential created by slow instrumentation to such a degree that it would virtually require deliberate, willful misuse to cause serious tissue damage. Use of this time device is optional, and it can be switched on or off as desired.

The unit's third safety feature is an automatic cut-off of current flow to the surgical electrode if use of cutting or coagulating current is attempted without use of the conductive circuit. If the operator forgets to plug in the conductive circuit, the surgical electrode remains inactivated until biterminal application is provided; if the biterminal application is interrupted during a procedure through accidental inadvertent loss of patient contact with the indifferent plate, the current flow to the surgical electrode is cut off until contact is restored.

Tissue damage and impaired tissue healing due to reduced cutting efficiency and power resulting from inconsistency of the current densities when the cutting and coagulating currents are used monoterminally are eliminated by this automatic current flow regulation.

In addition to these safety features this unit also provides a unique new cutting current waveform that appears to retain the best characteristics of fully rectified currents *and* continuous wave. Clinicians have found that the continuous wave current fails to provide the hemostasis that is enjoyed with fully rectified current. As a result the tissues tend to ooze or bleed freely following incision or excision with continuous wave cutting current. Such bleeding is apt to be highly undesirable, particularly in preparation of the subgingival tissues for restorative dentistry. The Ritter engineers have developed a modification of the continuous waveform that retains most of the smooth, nonpeaking surgically pure quality of continuous wave current yet provides hemostasis that approximates the hemostasis obtained with fully rectified current.

In addition to these unique major circuitry features, this unit also provides a number of conventional clinically desirable features. It is coaxially shielded, provides a handpiece with a finger control switch as well as the foot control, a single handpiece and cable on a retractable reel, and a built-in surgical electrode holder.

Prior to the advent of the continuous waveform current, the author hypothesized that since fully rectified current provides effective hemostasis without producing clinical or histologic evidence of coagulation, the hemostasis must be resulting from plugging of the lumina of the severed capillaries with the atomic carbon released by volatilization of the tissue cells in the line of cleavage. Since the carbon is washed out by the fixing and processing of the tissue for microscopic examination, this could not be verified histologically, but must remain a justifiable conclusion until other means such as histochemical or radioisotope studies may verify or disprove it. However, the fact that no hemostasis occurs when the capillaries in the cut tissue are enlarged due to inflammation or engorged by stasis would appear to substantiate the author's hypothesis, since under such conditions the lumina of the severed capillaries are too large to become completely and effectively filled with the carbon.

With the advent of the continuous waveform current, however, the author and many of his colleagues have noted that electrosection with this current fails to provide comparable hemostasis, and the cut tissues tend to bleed freely, although this cutting also releases atomic carbon. This suggests that the atomic carbon alone is incapable of completely sealing off the capillaries, but that some additional factor must be involved in producing the hemostasis.

Since the only difference between the fully rectified current (Fig. 2–14A) and the continuous waveform current (Fig. 2–14B) is the elimination in the latter of the indentations at the beginning of each half cycle of current flow, one can only conclude that this produces a slight diminution of current density at the beginning of each half cycle and a subclinical and submicroscopic surface coagulum not tangibly visible but enough to complete the sealing off of the capillary ends that have become plugged, but not sealed, by the atomic carbon.

The modified continuous waveform produced by the Ritter engineers (Fig. 2–14C) therefore would be particularly beneficial clinically if its minimal nonpeaking interruptions in the continuity of the continuous waveform will preserve the purity of the surgical incision produced by continuous wave current yet provide the same hemostatic effect that the half cycle indentations of the fully rectified current flow produces and eliminate blood seepage that creates a clinical disadvantage. The uniform level of

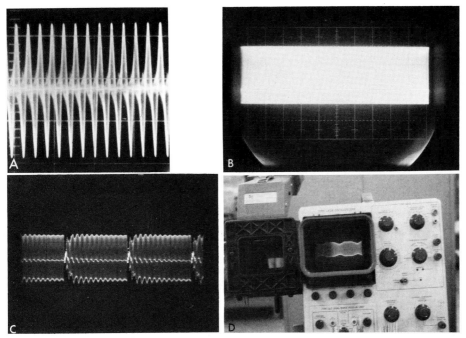

Figure 2-14. Comparative oscilloscopic photographs of *A*, fully rectified current in a half cycle; *B*, continuous wave current; and *C*, modified continuous wave current of Ritter unit (see text for explanation). *D*, Oscilloscope showing pattern of waveform of current on screen.

current amplitude seen in the oscilloscopic illustration of the modified current that has been made available to the author for this text suggests smooth, nonpeaking cutting current that should produce surgically pure cutting when performed properly.

These new features of the Ritter unit constitute a real breakthrough toward making dental electrosurgery universally safe to use. However, they do *not* eliminate the need to develop a high degree of skill in electrosurgical instrumentation nor the need to learn the specific dental electrosurgical techniques to derive *maximum benefit* from its use. But they should make it safe for the novice to achieve both objectives and go a long way toward assuring that, short of deliberate willful misuse, dental electrosurgical cutting and coagulating currents should be safe even in the hands of the untrained novice.

Claims have been made by some manufacturers of dental electrosurgical equipment that with their units efficient electrosurgical cutting can be achieved without the use of the patient indifferent electrode.* A similar claim has been made in a recently published dental electrosurgical text.†

---

*Assertions to that effect for the Martin Elektrotom, Parkell, and Whaledent Strobex instruments.
†Schoen, F.: Electrosurgery in the Dental Practice. Die Quintessence, Berlin, 1971.

Technically, from the electronic standpoint, it is possible to cut or coagulate tissue without having to use the indifferent patient electrode. Extensive clinical experience has demonstrated conclusively, however, that *consistent, efficient* electrosurgical cutting cannot be achieved without the use of the indifferent patient electrode, so that *clinically,* and *therapeutically,* claims to the contrary are erroneous. An experiment that is reported in the section on electrosurgical research of this text substantiates that unless the cutting current is delivered to the tissues and then returned directly to the electrosurgical circuit's power source via the indifferent patient electrode, the cutting current loses reliable consistency, potency, and cutting efficiency. Failure to use the indifferent patient electrode with the cutting current will almost inevitably result in inconsistent electrosurgical performance, tissue damage, and impaired tissue healing. Neither fully rectified constant-wave current nor this current combined with coaxial shielding eliminates need for biterminal application of cutting and coagulating currents and use of the indifferent electrode. Substitutes for the indifferent plate that provide grounding but fail to return the current directly into the circuit will not provide the patient $\leftrightarrows$ power output source direct connection that assures instantaneous maximum current density output needed for maximum clinical efficiency and safety.

LINEAR AND NONLINEAR POWER OUTPUT

One additional related factor must be considered to properly complete this review of the various types of electrosurgical circuitry and their respective power outputs—the manner in which the high-frequency current produced by the circuits is delivered to the surgical electrodes from the power oscillators. In other words, when the need for a change in power output is anticipated clinically, can the operator obtain an immediate, accurately predictable increase or decrease in power output proportionate to the increase or decrease of the power output rheostat dial setting on the instrument panel as the knob is adjusted by the therapist? Although this problem has greatly diminished as the circuitry has been improved, it is still a significant factor with some of the equipment.

Linear Power Output

If, as the dial adjustment is made, the response in power output is instantaneous, proportional, and predictable, the output is linear. Linear output permits the operator to properly and accurately control the density of current output to meet varying clinical requirements to compensate for changes in size, shape, or thickness of the surgical electrodes, thickness and density of the tissues, or similar factors that create need for changes in power output to assure cutting efficiency at all times, under all conditions.

Nonlinear Power Output

If the dial setting of the power oscillator knob on the instrument panel is changed and there is no immediate corresponding change in power output when the knob is turned until a considerable change in dial setting has been made, and if there is then a sudden marked rise or drop in power output, the delivery of the current is nonlinear. It is much more difficult for the operator to be able to maintain a smooth continuity of cutting efficiency essential for favorable electrosurgical results if the instrument cannot deliver power output instantaneously, predictably and consistently in proportion to the dial setting on the panel.

PART 2 – EVALUATION OF ELECTROSURGICAL EQUIPMENT

The author has, in his official capacity as consultant for electrosurgical devices to the Council on Dental Materials and Devices of the American Dental Association, made comprehensive surveys and evaluations of the various dental electrosurgical units that have become available to the profession. The Council published a report of his survey in the Journal of The American Dental Association.[3]

As a teacher of dental electrosurgery he has tried to keep abreast of all new developments in electrosurgical circuitry and of new equipment as it becomes available. The frequency at which new equipment is being introduced, by newcomers and by established electrosurgical manufacturers, is so great that it is becoming impossible to evaluate all the equipment being developed and rushed into the electrosurgical sweepstakes. It is obvious that new units will continue to enter the field long after this text is published. As a result, the omission of emerging equipment in this text is to be anticipated as inevitable. Failure to review such equipment should not be construed as a reflection on their merits.

Since the Coles patent expired, the basic circuitry of the equipment that is currently available has until now been essentially similar, solid state versus power tube claims and counterclaims notwithstanding. Competition has therefore been directed either pricewise or toward incorporating attractive clinical convenience features. With the advent of the new Ritter circuit, the trend of future competition will undoubtedly be in the direction of safety rather than convenience features. Thus, evaluation of the present-day electrosurgical equipment is likely to soon become outdated, and since such evaluations cannot be continually updated in this text, they would soon become obsolete and serve no useful purpose. Therefore, instead of offering such evaluation, a simple method will be described later in this chapter that will enable each reader easily to arrive at an accurate personal evaluation and choice of equipment.

MISCONCEPTIONS

About Current Factors That Influence Electrosurgical Instrumentation

Inasmuch as the electrosurgical currents are the key to electrosurgical instrumentation and its end results, clarification of common misconceptions about them should precede review of specific techniques of instrumentation.

One popular misconception among the electrosurgically uninformed and many neophytes is the assumption that the weaker the high-frequency current, the easier it is to control and the more self-limiting is its destructiveness. This assumption may sound reasonable and logical but it is totally incorrect. Precisely the opposite holds true. The more potent the current, the more self-limiting is its destructiveness and the more fully under the control of the operator, therefore the more efficient and safer to use.

Another popular misconception is that as long as the cutting currents of the various electrosurgical circuits are fully rectified, they are equal in efficiency. Rectification influences the character of the current; it does not influence the power output of the circuit. All fully rectified circuits therefore do not necessarily produce equally powerful current output. The situation is somewhat analogous to the internal combustion engine and the power output of automobiles. All automobiles are powered by internal combustion engines, but surely no one is naïve enough to believe that the combustion engines in all automobiles are equally potent in their power output or in their efficiency.

It is likely that the author was responsible to some degree for the misconception that rectification is the sole criterion for electrosurgical current efficiency. When the first edition was being compiled, and until quite recently, the Coles Radiosurg Scalpel units were the only electrosurgical circuits capable of providing fully rectified current. Having concluded on the basis of many years of clinical experience and observation that fully rectified current is essential for safe, efficient dental electrosurgery, the only comment that appeared necessary was to specify its advantages over partially rectified currents and emphasize its advantages and desirability for dental therapy.*

Since the first edition was published, dental electrosurgery has gained enormously in popularity, with an ever-increasing number of dentists using it in their daily practice. The constantly expanding market for electrosurgical equipment naturally resulted in an increase in the number and variety of fully rectified electrosurgical devices available to the profession in the United States, Canada, and in Europe. There is now a rather wide choice of fully rectified circuits instead of just one type of unit, and the number is increasing almost daily. It therefore becomes necessary to evaluate the significance of power output and its effect on the performance of electrosurgical circuits.

---

*Substantiation by laboratory research is reviewed in the section on research.

About Wattage

Since many of the devices vary considerably in wattage, it seems logical to begin with a brief discussion of this factor.

There appears to be a general consensus that efficient electrosection requires a power output of 70 watts or more. Thus, presumably, any device that is capable of producing 70 or more watts should be capable of delivering adequately potent cutting current.

If all the watts a circuit can produce are delivered in full to the tip of the surgical electrode this would hold true. Unfortunately, this is not necessarily the case. A circuit can produce 70 or more watts, yet *deliver* substantially less to the tissues at the surgical site. Thus the listed designation of an instrument's wattage is not necessarily conclusive. (See Chapter 2, Part 1 for discussion of wattage.)

About Equipment

Invariably, at some point in his teaching sessions, seminars, or lectures, the author is plied with such typical questions as: "Which unit should I buy?" Or, "Unit X costs very little. Will it do?" Or, "I expect to use electrosurgery only to prepare the subgingival tissues for impression-taking. Do I need an expensive, sophisticated unit for that?"

The last question can be best answered with the reminder that the marginal gingiva is one of the most delicate, invaluable, nonexpendable tissues in the oral cavity and deserves to be treated accordingly. In treating marginal gingiva there is very little margin for error. Therefore the most efficient and reliable currents that are available should be used to treat this tissue.

As for the first two questions, obviously a direct unequivocal answer would invite legal harassment. They can therefore be answered best with the reminder that electrosurgical equipment is made of a surprisingly large number of delicate, sophisticated electronic components that can vary greatly in quality and reliability. The components must be assembled with meticulous care to create a reliable circuit. A poorly assembled or improperly insulated circuit may produce current leakage that can result in accidental shock or burns on contact with the outer casing of the unit. A tiny speck of solder or a loose screw can disrupt the safety, efficiency, and reliability of performance of even the best designed electrosurgical circuit. Very high internal impedance in a circuit can reduce cutting efficiency and result in clinical operating failures.

These are not imaginary possibilities; they have been encountered clinically and in laboratory evaluations. At an American Academy of Dental Electrosurgery panel symposium of the 1972 A.D.A. Scientific Program Session, one of the panelists, Dr. Kelly, reported in his presentation a series of experimental evaluations of electrosurgical equipment that Dr. J. D. Harrison and he have conducted at the Southern Illinois University School of Dental

Medicine.[4] He reported that they found a significant number of carelessly assembled units that could prove hazardous to the patient and the operator. They have also found a number of instances in which identical units of a particular model did not perform uniformly and required different current outputs for identical cutting conditions, as well as other similar disquieting factors. They also found that some units appear unable to deliver adequate cutting current power to meet all requirements.

The experiences and observations of Harrison and Kelly parallel and substantiate those of the author, who, in his capacity as consultant to the A.D.A. Council on Dental Materials and Devices for electrosurgical devices, has evaluated most of the available electrosurgical equipment. The reader should therefore be cautioned to beware of permitting price alone or the size of the electrosurgical device to be the major determining factor in choosing an electrosurgical unit.

Electronic components such as coils and transformers vary greatly in size. Transformers in particular may vary greatly, and sturdy, high quality transformers are likely to be bulky and weigh 4 to 8 pounds. Thus, it is conceivable that subminiaturization may be achieved at the expense of durability and reliability of performance of the components. As for price, an inexpensive unit that performs inconsistently, inefficiently, and unreliably could prove very costly in the long run.

The factors of price and size of electrosurgical equipment are in many respects analogous to those relating to the automobile industry. It would be utterly naïve to assume that the only difference between luxury cars such as the Cadillac or Lincoln and subcompact or compact autos is "status symbol." True, luxury cars do enjoy status symbol popularity. The real difference, however, lies in their respective performance, reliability, *safety*, and riding comfort. A further analogy can be drawn between automobiles and electrosurgical equipment:

Greater riding comfort is conducive to more frequent and longer auto trips. Comparably, clinical convenience features in an electrosurgical unit are conducive to more frequent and more universal use of the modality in daily practice. Disentangling loose handpiece cables is a time-wasting nuisance. Equally so is the footswitch that tends to slide around unpredictably. Groping around with the foot blindly to try to locate it, or having to look around for it is very distracting, time consuming, and quite annoying. Replacement of the tangle of cables with a single handpiece and cable on a retractable reel and replacement of the footswitch or supplementing it with a fingerswitch control in the handpiece are worthwhile clinical convenience features, but they add to a unit's price.

Unquestionably, clinical convenience features offered by a unit are desirable, but these too should not become the sole determining criteria. The two considerations that loom above all others, and should take unqualified priority in choosing an electrosurgical unit, are *consistent efficiency* of performance and, above all, *safety* to the patient. In addition to everything else, the reassurance and peace of mind these can bring to the user are priceless assets.

EQUIPMENT PURCHASING GUIDE FOR THE NOVICE

How to Choose Electrosurgical Equipment

The most important function of an electrosurgical unit is its ability to provide cutting and coagulating currents that are consistently efficient and safe under any and all clinical conditions.

It should be a very simple matter for a prospective purchaser of electrosurgical equipment to establish the cutting efficiency of the instrument in a very few minutes by testing its cutting ability on a slab of beef. However, cutting into the beef with a very fine needle electrode, which is the usual method of demonstration, is a very poor and inconclusive way to perform the test. The minute area of contact of a fine needle electrode with the tissues creates so great a concentration of heat energy that even the weaker fully rectified circuits will provide adequate concentration to cut the tissue cleanly. But if a large round loop is substituted, since the cutting energy is distributed over a vastly greater area of tissue, the concentration of heat is decreased proportionally. As a result, if the circuit is capable of delivering adequately potent current output at the surgical site when the power output is increased sufficiently, the activated loop will slice off a segment of tissue even several millimeters thick effortlessly, with no coagulation or searing of the cut surfaces. If despite progressive power output increase the wattage delivered to the surgical site remains inadequate, and the loop fails to cut into the tissue at all or coagulates the tissue at the initial site of contact to the degree that its progress through the tissues is retarded and causes clinically visible coagulation of the cut tissues, the current output is likely to prove inadequate for many dental procedures.

If so inclined, the reader can easily and quite accurately determine the extent of lateral heat penetration into the surrounding and subjacent tissues of any electrosurgical cutting current by excising a thin slice of tissue from a slab of beef with a narrow U-shaped loop electrode measuring approximately 1 cm. in length and 1 to 1.5 mm. in width, or with a J-loop electrode, or with a 17-mm. periodontal loop electrode. Because the latter penetrates so deeply into the tissue, results obtained with it are particularly conclusive.

If the activated loop electrode can excise a translucently thin slice of tissue without altering or destroying its normal color and firm, resilient texture, it will be able to dissect out tissue to create subgingival troughs without damage to the marginal gingivae or teeth. If the tissue becomes blanched and tends to disintegrate readily on gentle manipulation, it has been cooked by the heat; this current would therefore be destructive to marginal gingivae.

The efficiency of coagulating currents can be ascertained with equal facility by applying activated small and large coagulating ball electrodes momentarily to the tissue surface. If a small white dot appears on the tissue surface immediately on contact, this demonstrates that it is effective for performing spot coagulation. To determine the depth of penetration of the coagulating effect, the coagulated white area can be incised with a fine needle electrode. When the incised margins are spread apart, the depth of penetration of the coagulating effect becomes apparent. If the coagulating effect has been limited to the surface layers of cells, the current will be effective clinically for superficial spot coagulation. If the coagulation has not been limited to the surface layers, but has penetrated more deeply, clinically it would be difficult to control the depth of destructive heat penetration of this current.

Some dentists feel that they will make very limited use of electrosurgery and thus may not need the most efficient and sophisticated equipment. Others are being persuaded that "the general practitioner never needs to use a large loop electrode—only an oral surgeon would ever need it."

Both assumptions are equally erroneous and invalid. The practitioner who at the outset expects to make very limited use of electrosurgery nevertheless may encounter clinical factors such as edematous, engorged or hyperplastic proliferative tissue; densely fibrous tissue; profuse persistent hemorrhagic bleeding; or similar conditions that necessitate use of potent current output. Or he may find it necessary to remove obstructive redundant tissue or resect a relatively small lesion for biopsy, for which he will need to use a large round loop electrode in order to be able to include the all-important perimeter of normal tissue with the pathologic specimen. Usually the anticipated use is mostly for crown and bridge, especially for creating subgingival troughs. The marginal gingiva is a very thin, delicate tissue and it can be destroyed easily be excessive heat penetration. Moreover, as the individual uses his electrosurgery more and more and gains confidence in his mastery of the instrument, he invariably finds himself using it for many more procedures than expected.

It is also advisable, for more or less identical reasons, that the electrosurgical circuit provide the user with all the therapeutic electrosurgical currents, so that should the need for fulguration arise, suitable fulgurating current will be available. To be suitable, the current must provide localized tissue destruction by carbonization, without appreciable penetration of heat into the adjacent tissues.

Although fulguration may be necessary only infrequently for a general practitioner, as is claimed by some salesmen, there may be a time when the need does arise and fulguration alone will serve the purpose. It is therefore vitally important to have it available. The automobile again offers an excellent analogy: A spare tire is included as standard equipment in every new automobile. It would be foolhardy to venture on a cross-country trip without one. The likelihood is much greater that the general practitioner will have need for the use of fulguration than the motorist would a spare tire. Thus, electrosurgically speaking, fulguration may well prove to be the clinically indispensable "spare tire."

PART 3—ELECTROSURGICAL INSTRUMENTATION TECHNIQUES

It has been established that there are four therapeutic electrosurgical currents as far as dental electrosurgery is concerned. Each of these currents requires a different method of instrumentation and application to the tissues. The respective methods are presented in inverse order, starting with the least important of the therapeutic currents.

Electrodesiccation (Monoterminal Current)

Electrodesiccation is a dehydrating current that is used without the indifferent electrode. Thus all the energy being potentiated by the current radiates outward from the electrode into the tissues. For electrodesiccation the electrode tip is inserted into the tissues and permitted to remain in situ without movement during the entire period of electrode activation. Electrodesiccation is the only therapeutic electrosurgical current that is delivered to the tissues with a stationary electrode throughout the current application. As the dehydrating current enters the tissues the tissue fluids may sometimes be observed to bubble up to the surface of the tissue. The heat being generated by the current is retained in the area. The cumulative heat retention is very destructive to the adjacent and subjacent tissues, with the destruction extending considerably beyond the actual electrode contact with the tissues. Moreover, it is impossible for the operator to accurately control the amount of destruction. The fact that normal gingival mucosa is approximately 1 to 1½ mm. in thickness and is attached to periosteum which is attached to viable bone usually containing vital teeth makes electrodesiccation the least useful and the most dangerous of the currents for dentistry. There appear to be only three conditions for which electrodesiccation is indicated or even justified. One is for the control of severe hemorrhage that would otherwise require a carotid tie-off to prevent exsanguination of the patient. When there are neither personnel nor facilities to perform this surgical procedure, the mass tissue destruction produced by the dehydrating current occludes the bleeding vessel, thereby producing effective hemostasis that controls the hemorrhage and eliminates need for the carotid tie-off. In such instances the local tissue destruction is secondary in importance to keeping the patient from bleeding to death. Another use of electrodesiccation, basically for hemostasis, as in the previous instance, is to dehydrate and thereby destroy cavernous hemangiomas. When these neoplasia are removed surgically there is always danger of severe hemorrhage which, again, might require a carotid tie-off to prevent exsanguination. Although the local tissue destruction cannot be accurately predicted and controlled by the operator, it is likely that the dehydrating current will destroy the tissues more discreetly and effectively than the sclerosing solutions and the destructive action of the electrodesiccating current is more readily controlled by the operator than is that of the sclerosing solution. For much the same reason electrodesiccation may be used more effectively for destroying lymphangiomas than can be done with the sclerosing solutions. With the exception of these three conditions there does not appear to be any other dental use for which the dehydrating current used in this fashion would be indicated or justifiable.

Fulguration (Monoterminal Current)

The same high-frequency dehydrating current may be safely employed if instead of inserting the electrode into the tissues and permitting it to remain there while the current is activated, the activated electrode tip is gradually brought toward the surface of the tissue to be treated until the sparks become visible as they jump the air-gap between the tip of the electrode and the tissue surface. As the sparks contact the tissue surface they produce a gradual dehydration of the surface layers of cells. As a rule the electrode is kept moving in a rotary direction, sometimes combined with an in and out jabbing motion; but in all instances the electrode is kept moving over the surface of the tissue rapidly during the application of current. After a little while the surface of the tissue becomes dehydrated enough to form either a tough leathery mass called an eschar, or it becomes charred and carbonized. Both the eschar and the layer of carbon act as insulators to prevent heat from penetrating deeply into the tissues. The air-space between the tip of the electrode and the tissue surface also acts as an insulator that helps to prevent deep penetration of the heat. Movement of the electrode while in use prevents cumulative retention of the heat that does penetrate, thereby preventing any appreciable destruction to the adjacent and subjacent tissues from fulguration.

The difference in the range of dental usefulness of fulguration as compared with electrodesiccation could not be greater if these were two totally different modalities produced by two different power sources. Thus, therapeutically, for *dentistry* the author feels that they should be regarded as two totally separate and independent, unrelated high-frequency currents.

Fulguration is useful for destroying the orifices of fistulae and their tracts down to the alveolar bone. It is also useful for destroying papillomatous and other undesirable tissue tabs, more especially fragments of necrotic or cystic tissue tightly wedged between teeth and bone in areas that would be totally inaccessible to other methods of instrumentation, but where the sparks can enter and destroy the tissue by carbonizing it. Another use would be for destroying the surface layers of cells in the bed from which a suspicious lesion has been resected to reduce the danger of possible surgical metastasis of malignant tumor cells. Fulguration also can be employed to control bleeding from nutrient foramina on the surface of exposed bone. When a mucoperiosteal flap incision is made and the flap is elevated, nutrient vessels that emerge from the nutrient foramina often are torn and bleed persistently. Such bleeding can be controlled by applying pressure to crush the bone and seal the foramina, or by applying electrocoagulation to seal off the bleeder. However, to do the latter effectively it would be necessary to keep the activated ball electrode tip in contact with the bone for a few seconds. Either of these would result in formation of a small sequestrum of dead bone. With fulguration the electrode does not come into contact with the bone to damage it. Instead the sparks jumping the air-gap make contact with the blood and soon form a hard crust of carbonized blood that effectively seals off the bleeder without affecting the bone. Fulguration is also useful for treatment of one type of pulp exposure. As has been previously noted, the fulguration produced by the simulated spark-gap current is more potent, and thus more efficient than that produced by the Oudin current of the true spark-gap generator; it is also more self-limiting in its destructiveness and hence more under the operator's control at all times. This, plus the smaller size of the simulated sparks, makes its safe use possible even when applied to apices of interdental papillae in tight embrasures.

Electrocoagulation

This current must be used biterminally. Electrocoagulation may be performed in either of two ways, depending upon the type of coagulation that is sought. If a large mass of tissue must be destroyed and a deep penetration of coagulating energy is needed, the electrode is placed against the tissue and held immobile in situ for several seconds. In dentistry this type of electrocoagulation is rarely indicated. The other type results in superficial penetration.

Most dental tissue electrocoagulation is superficial in nature and is performed most efficiently as superficial spot coagulation. The electrode, usually a small ball-tipped type, is brought into momentary contact with the tissue surface and immediately withdrawn. The contact is repeated as many times as is deemed necessary. With this type of application the operator has complete control over the tissue destruction and can literally limit it to several layers of cells at a time.

For electrocoagulation the tissues should be dried lightly to remove all but the normal surface tension moisture; they should not be excessively moist. The electrode should be kept clean. If a minute layer of tissue adheres to the surface of the ball electrode it acts as an insulator and prevents controlled, effective surface coagulation. The tip of the electrode should be permitted to make very light momentary contact with the tissue surface, without jabbing into the tissue.

When the amount of coagulating current needed to produce instantaneous visible surface coagulation is unknown, the method for determining the proper amount is exactly the opposite of that needed for electrosection. Here it is advisable to start with a minimal amount of current applied momentarily, and gradually increase it until a small white spot appears immediately when the electrode tip makes contact with the tissue surface. Momentary contact with an inadequate amount of current is quite harmless. But if the contact is maintained for several seconds with current too weak to produce any visible coagulating effect, it is much more destructive and the destruction is much more penetrating than when an excessive amount of coagulating energy is properly employed for momentary contact. (See Fig. 5–2 in Chapter 5.)

The coagulating current should never be applied to the tissues with a scrubbing back and forth movement over the tissues. It should be applied with a light tapping or patting motion.

The electrocoagulating current can also be used very advantageously for desensitizing hypersensitive dentin, bleaching discolored teeth, drying and sterilizing root canals, and for conservative pulp capping treatment of one type of pulp exposure.

Electrosection (Acusection): Electrosurgical Cutting Current

This current must be used biterminally. Three essential ingredients are necessary for safe, efficient electrosection. These are *adequate proper cutting energy; speed of instrumentation;* and *a light, deft, pressureless cutting stroke.*

It is highly advisable to review mentally what should be done and to then practice the cutting strokes with the inactivated electrode to achieve a free-flowing wrist rhythm, much as one practices a golf swing before hitting the ball. It doesn't matter how much time is spent planning and practicing the procedure, but when the activated electrode makes contact with the tissues the cutting must be performed as quickly as the electrode can slice through the tissues without pressure and with the hand moving as rapidly as the electrode will permit. *It is impossible to perform efficient electrosection with slow deliberate strokes and prolonged contact with the tissues.* Such contact inevitably leads to tissue destruction, undesirable postoperative sequelae and poor healing through no fault of the cutting energy.

Since the cutting energy disintegrates and volatilizes the tissue cells it encounters, no pressure is required to create the incision. All that the operator must do (except with use of self-regulating current) is adjust the power output to the desired intensity and control and guide the electrode as it is applied to the tissues. The operator must control the depth to which the electrode is permitted to penetrate into the tissues rather than to push the electrode into the tissues to the desired depth. Otherwise, the electrode, by nature, will penetrate its full depth into the tissues, trying to cut through toward the energy at the indifferent plate.

When a single cutting stroke is feasible, a light brushing or wiping stroke with a free-flowing wrist movement is best. When a single stroke would be clinically impractical, short wiping or brushing strokes with a clean electrode are most effective. After each cutting contact of the activated electrode 5 to 10 seconds should be permitted to elapse before repeating the cutting stroke. By doing this the lateral heat will become completely dissipated and danger of tissue damage from cumulative heat will be avoided.

When the proper amount of cutting energy is being used, tissue shreds that may adhere to the electrode can be cleaned off rapidly and effortlessly by simply wiping the electrode with the fingertips or with a moistened 2×2 gauze sponge. If the tissue shreds adhere so tenaciously that they must be scraped off forcefully, an inadequate amount of cutting energy is being used.

When the anatomic contours or the amount of tissue to be removed make a single cutting stroke impractical, and multiple cutting contacts must be made, after each two or three strokes the surface of the cut tissue should be remoistened to restore the normal surface tension, since the moisture normally present on the tissue surface has been vaporized by the cutting heat. Failure to do so would result in slight dehydration of the cut surface tissue, producing a variable thickness of surface coagulum on the cut surface as the tissue heals. The remoistening can be easily accomplished by simply picking up a drop of saliva from the floor of the mouth with the ball of the finger tip and applying it to the cut surface, then wiping off the excess moisture with a light wiping contact of the thumb.

When the operator is in doubt as to how much current to use when it is necessary to cut tissue for which the proper cutting power has not been previously ascertained (and the circuit's power output is not automatically self-regulated), it is safer initially to use more cutting power than not enough. As soon as the electrode makes contact with the tissues, the observant operator will be able to tell whether he is using the proper amount of current by the reaction of the tissues. If the surface of the tissue turns brownish and sparking occurs it indicates that he is using too much current. If an inadequate amount of current is being used, the tissue will adhere tenaciously to the electrode and will blanch and turn white. If the proper amount of energy is being used the electrode will glide through the tissues effortlessly and cut cleanly.

If the tissue turns brownish as the electrode makes contact, immediate removal from the tissue will result in no real damage from the momentary contact. On the other hand, if an inadequate amount of current was used and the tissue adhered to the electrode even momentarily, the disengagement of the activated electrode is slowed and tissue destruction continues until the disengagement is completed.

When the gingival mucosa is normal, the amount of current necessary with the cutting power that is available may be predetermined, and this remains as a norm for all gingival mucosa that is normal in texture and tone. Predetermining the proper amount of current is a relatively simple matter that takes but a few minutes to do. The necessary current density is determined by cutting into a slab of meat that has approximately the same texture and resistance as gingival mucosa. Since the latter has no muscle fibers, its texture appears to be best simulated by the texture of flank steak, shoulder or shin beef, when the meat is incised by cutting *with the grain* of the muscle fibers (*not transversely*). When it is incised with a fine needle electrode, the least amount of cutting energy required to produce a perfect incision without any evidence of coagulation or tissue adherence to the electrode will become the norm, that is, that which is required to cut normal gingivae.

The electrosurgical cutting stroke should be performed with a free-flowing loose wrist movement. The electrode handle should be held in a manner similar to that of an artist holding a camel-hair paintbrush. It should be held lightly, loosely enough to permit it to be easily pulled from the fingers, yet firmly enough to use it precisely without wobbling. Holding the electrode handle with a strangle-hold grip and tightly locked wrist, and performing the cutting stroke with rigid finger movement is NOT conducive to efficient electrosection.

The activated electrode should *always* be kept moving rapidly while in contact with the tissues. It can never be safely employed with slow, deliberate movements. The premise that if the cutting current is reduced to low intensity it can be used safely at slow speed is totally fallacious, and inevitably invites disaster.

It is perfectly safe to contact viable bone, vital teeth, or metal restorations with an activated electrode, *providing the contact is only momentary.** It is not *what* we contact, but *how long* the contact is maintained. If it were in-

---

*Substantiation by laboratory research is reviewed in the section on electrosurgical research.

herently dangerous to contact these structures with an activated electrode, it would obviously be impossible to cut through mucosa and periosteum in order to create an incision for a mucoperiosteal flap.

Tissue Resistance

The number of watts or density of power output needed for efficient cutting is not constant. To assure an uninterrupted continuity of electrosurgical cutting efficiency, in the absence of automatic electronic regulation it is necessary for the clinician to vary the current density manually to meet the demands of different tissue conditions as they are encountered during an electrosurgical procedure.

It would perhaps be easiest to appreciate this if we equate the cutting current with the hand pressure required to cut tissue with a steel scalpel. If one must make an incision in labial gingival mucosa for a mucoperiosteal flap, a certain amount of hand pressure would have to be exerted in order to cut the tissues. If a similar incision had to be made in palatal mucosa with the same scalpel, a much greater amount of pressure would have to be exerted to do so. Or, if in an emergency it became necessary to use a kitchen utility knife to make an abdominal incision, it would require far greater pressure than if the incision were made with a surgical scalpel.

Thus it is obvious that factors such as the thickness and density of the tissues and size and shape or thickness of the cutting instrument create a demand for different amounts of energy to achieve equally effective cutting. When high-frequency current is used instead of the steel scalpel unless the electrosurgical circuit can automatically compensate and regulate the current for us, it is equally necessary, for the identical reasons, to vary the amount of current density of the cutting current in order to compensate for the differences and thus maintain a continuity of cutting efficiency throughout the electrosurgical procedure.

Many factors contribute to alterations in tissue resistance that necessitate compensatory proportional increase or decrease in current density. These include the following:

a. Differences in thickness and density of the tissues.

b. Differences in size, shape, and thickness of the surgical electrodes.

c. Alterations in pH of the tissues due to inflammation or local disease condition.

d. Severe edema or stasis.

e. Alterations in electrolyte balance.

f. Tissue changes due to systemic diseases such as amyloid degeneration.

g. Flooding of the operative field with blood or saliva.

h. Surface dehydration of tissue owing to air exposure, vaporization of the normal surface moisture by instrumentation, or xerostomia.

Obviously, when tissue is full of intra- or extracellular fluids, or when it is engorged with blood, much of the potency of the cutting current needed to disintegrate and volatilize is dissipated by these fluids. When such conditions are encountered it therefore becomes necessary to increase the power output enough to compensate for the dissipation of energy in order to maintain consistent cutting efficiency. By the same token, when the tissue surface is dry as a result of exposure to the air, xerostomia, or vaporization of the normal surface tension of the tissue moisture by instrumentation, unless a normal surface tension is restored or created, the cutting power that would normally be required would have to be reduced to avoid sparking and charring of the dry tissue.

Normally, cutting energy causes sparking only when it is too powerful, when the tissues are too dry, or when the electrode contacts metal restorations. But when a patient has suffered an alteration in electrolyte balance, sparking is likely to occur with a normal amount of current for no clinically apparent reason. The relation of alteration in electrolyte balance to sparking can easily be demonstrated by a simple experiment. A slab of meat or a calf mandible is soaked in a concentrated brine solution for an hour or more. It is then thoroughly rinsed in clean water several times to wash off the brine solution, and partially dried to remove excess moisture. Despite thorough rinsing, when the activated electrode makes contact with the meat, even a relatively minimal amount of current causes a considerable sparking, owing to the retention of an excessive concentration of the sodium chloride in the tissues. Injection of the brine into the meat produces a similar result because of the artificially created electrolyte imbalance.

Power Adjustment Guideline

This discussion of manual power output adjustment to meet varying conditions cannot be terminated without a word of caution to the neophyte using electrosurgery.

It is possible to predetermine precisely the ability of a power oscillator of an electrosurgical unit to instantaneously increase or decrease the current density delivered to the tip of the electrode commensurate with changes in the power control knob dial setting. The performance of the power oscillator can therefore be standardized.

The amount of changes in current density that the variations in electrodes or tissues will require *cannot* be comparably predetermined or standardized, nor can a blueprint be created to show just how much change will be required in any given instance. Unless the circuit can automatically regulate the power output each operator must decide for himself, on the basis of his personal clinical judgment, how much more or less current density will be required for a given change in tissue resistance, and act accordingly.

The specific dental electrosurgical techniques that will be reviewed throughout this text are described in detail in reports of practical clinical cases. In these reports the author mentions the specific amounts of change in dial setting that were required for various conditions. These statistics are mentioned solely as a *reminder* to indicate that these conditions required the changes in power output. They may also be of some help to indicate *approximately* how much change given conditions may require. They definitely were

NOT intended to serve as a tabulated formula or blueprint of specific amounts of change for the reader to follow.

Electrosurgical effects produced by the various high-frequency currents are determined by the type of current and waveform employed. The extent and quality of the tissue responses to these currents is determined by the manner in which the current is applied to the tissues. Improperly applied, the current does *not* achieve the same results as are obtained when it is used properly. Therapeutically, therefore, electrosurgery is based upon *proper use of the proper equipment.* Any deviation from this formula inevitably results in unsatisfactory electrosurgical performance.

PLACEMENT OF ELECTROSURGICAL EQUIPMENT

After an electrosurgical unit has been purchased, the question arises as to where to keep it.

The one factor to be considered above all else in choice of location is *convenience* — its visibility and ready accessibility in the operatory.

Electrosurgical equipment should never be located in an inaccessible area; especially not behind an immovable object such as a floor-fixed dental unit or in a wall cabinet drawer that is distant from the dental chair. Low compartments in wall cabinets close to floor level where the unit can be neither easily seen nor reached are especially unsuitable.

When feasible, an excellent arrangement is to keep the unit on a small mobile stand or cabinet that can be wheeled to and from the dental chair at will as it is needed, then wheeled out of the way when not in use. For this arrangement either the upright mobile type or the flat modular drawer type of equipment is suitable.

If the unit must be kept in a wall cabinet compartment that is close to the dental chair, in a Ritter Sigma or Pelton-Crane Executive Module, or in the cabinet of a four-handed dentistry set-up, a particularly advantageous arrangement is to have the unit seated on a sliding tray in the compartment that can be pulled out into view and become fully visible and accessible. If the sliding tray cannot be installed it is wise to install a fail-safe switch (Fig. 2–15)* that will make contact with the door of the compartment. Thus if the input current to the unit has inadvertently been left on, the house current will be cut off as soon as the door is closed.

ADVANTAGES OF ELECTROSURGERY

Advantages Over Cold-Steel Instrumentation

1. Ability to perform incisions quickly and precisely without need to exert pressure against the tissues.

---

*Device used by Dr. Charles J. Miller.

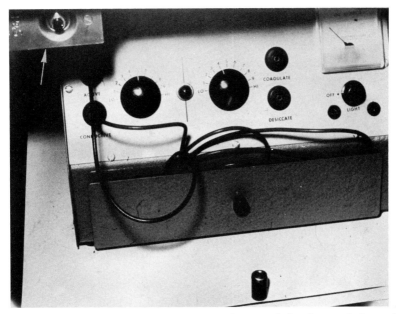

Figure 2-15. Electrosurgical unit on tray showing fail-safe switch (arrow).

2. Ability to reshape needle and loop electrodes quickly and effortlessly to meet unique requirements for gaining easy access to areas difficult to reach with scalpels or other cutting instruments.

3. Painless incisions for drainage under topical anesthesia.

4. Ability to perform biopsy and resection of suspicious neoplasms without danger of surgical or mechanical dissemination of tumor emboli to distant parts of the body.

5. Ability to resect hypertrophic tissue in layers by shaving with loop electrodes.

6. Ability to control hemorrhage or to perform bloodless surgery with a clear operative field.

7. Ability to operate safely in areas of acute infection.

8. Ability to control deep-seated bleeding from bony sockets or bone crypts.*

9. Telangiectases can be destroyed easily and safely without producing profuse hemorrhage.

10. Tissue contours and normal gingival architecture can be restored or corrected easily and accurately by planing the tissues with loop electrodes.

11. Interproximal self-cleansing concave sluiceways can be created easily with appropriate loop electrodes.

12. Surface keratinizations or ulcerations can be eliminated readily by superficial coagulation, resection in layers, or by fulguration.

---

*An attachment made by Cameron, which can be adapted for use with any electrosurgical unit, is especially useful for these cases. It serves as a suction tip when attached to the aspirating unit and, when the occluding blood has been siphoned off, serves as a coagulating electrode to seal off the bleeding point (Fig. 1–2).

13. Coagulation or fulguration of the bases of neoplasms is easily performed to seal off all avenues of metastasis and to destroy any deeply invaginated tumor cells that may be present in the tissue bed.

14. Total destruction of pathological tissue *in situ* can be achieved rapidly and safely with minimal sacrifice of adjacent normal tissue structures.

15. Electronic surgery produces healing by primary and *secondary* intention, with normal tissue repair that is completely free of cicatricial contraction.

16. The reparative scar tissue is identical in color, texture and function with the normal adjacent tissues and is therefore virtually invisible within a short time. This is cosmetically advantageous, while the soft suppleness of the scar tissue insures minimal functional impairment.

Advantages Over Caustics and Escharotics

The electronic "radioknife" also offers incomparable advantages over chemical caustics and escharotics, which destroy tissue by nonselective mass coagulation of the albumin in the tissue cells. Being for the most part liquids, these agents are especially difficult to control in the oral cavity, bathed as it is with saliva. Inability to demarcate the activities of these chemicals frequently causes widespread, indiscriminate destruction, not only of the diseased tissue but also of normal tissue, with massive sloughing of necrotic tissue a common sequela. Such tissue damage, if repeated, can ultimately cause serious tissue deterioration, including malignant degenerations.

When caustics destroy tissue, the surface of the tissue becomes raw and denuded of epithelium and usually bleeds copiously. Raw tissue surfaces are highly susceptible to secondary infection. Electronic coagulation can be accurately pinpointed and completely demarcated. No comparable raw surfaces are produced by use of electrocoagulation. The coagulated surface tissue behaves much the same as mildly sunburned skin, if it is left undisturbed. When tissue regeneration is complete, the surface coagulum peels off exactly like sunburned skin, leaving a clean, healthy, normal-appearing surface of new tissue.

DISADVANTAGES OF ELECTROSURGERY

Although the numerous unique advantages of electrosurgery completely overshadow unfavorable features, the latter must be mentioned and evaluated for the sake of objectivity. They are:

1. The need to learn a new, precise and exacting technique of instrumentation. However, the need for constant alertness during instrumentation is not a requirement unique to electrosurgery. It is equally applicable and essential to all other methods of instrumentation.

2. It cannot be used in the presence of inflammable or explosive anesthetic mixtures. However, with the advent of intravenous anesthesia this no longer is a serious factor.

3. Profound anesthesia is required to protect against pain impulses generated at the moment of circuit closure. Since very few dental procedures are performed without anesthesia, this cannot really be considered a detrimental requirement.

4. The fumes and odor of scorched tissue sometimes created by release of atomic carbon as the tissue cells become volatilized during the instrumentation are disagreeable, and may even be acutely distressing to some patients. However, both the odor and fumes can be greatly minimized by proper instrumentation technique and suitable clinical operating conditions, and use of hygroscopic agents such as Ozium can eliminate them as distress factors.

5. Initial expense of the instrument. However, the increase in patient load due to the elimination of unproductive chair operating time loss that electrosurgery makes possible more than compensates for the investment.

COMMON CAUSES OF FAILURE AND UNDESIRABLE TISSUE REACTIONS

Like the old adage that all coins have two sides, it would be inappropriate not to mention the possibility of failures and undesirable tissue reactions. It would be equally improper to do so, however, without scrutinizing the reasons for failures and undesirable tissue reactions.

The most universal cause of failures and untoward postoperative sequelae unquestionably stems from the failure to recognize that electrosurgery is a *discipline* and not "just another instrument." And that, as with all other disciplines, efficient use of electrosurgery requires special training. The reasons for such failures, listed here, verify this fact:

1. The most frequent is faulty instrumentation. This may be a result of
   a. Lack of understanding of the basic principles of electrosurgery, or,
   b. Lack of understanding of the functions of the electrosurgical currents
2. The therapist may fail to maintain proper regulation of current output and intensity to meet needs created by varying oral conditions or by special operative requirements, such as
   a. Thickness and density of the tissues to be treated.
   b. Size, shape, and thickness of the surgical electrode.
   c. Loss of normal surface tension of the tissues due to prolonged exposure to the air, vaporization of the surface moisture by repeated instrumentation without reconstituting the normal surface tension, or abnormal dryness of the tissues due to systemic diseases such as xerostomia.
   d. Excessively viscous saliva.
   e. Flooding of the operative field by saliva or blood.
   f. Alterations in pH of the blood due to inflammation or disease conditions.
   g. Edema, engorgement, or stasis in the tissues to be treated.
   h. Alterations in intracellular and extracellular tissue fluids.

     i. Alterations in electrolyte balance.

     j. Cellular hyperpermeability.

     k. Systemic diseases such as amyloid degeneration that alter the cellular texture.

3. Lack of speed in instrumentation.

4. Fluctuations in line voltage of input electric power to the equipment.

5. Inadvertent accidental loss of patient contact with the indifferent plate, resulting in monoterminal instead of biterminal current application.

FOOTNOTE REFERENCES

1. Kowarschik, J.: Electrotherapie. 2nd ed. Vienna, 1923.
2. Coles, W. A.: Personal communication.
3. Oringer, M. J.: Evaluation of dental electrosurgical devices. Council on Dental Materials and Devices, J.A.D.A., April, 1969, pp. 799–802.
4. Harrison, J. D., and Kelly, W. J., Jr.: Verbal communication. Report in panel symposium, A.D.A. Scientific Meeting, Oct. 30, 1972.

Chapter Three

INDICATIONS AND CONTRAINDICATIONS

INDICATIONS

Electrosurgery can be used to great advantage in all the dental disciplines. Its principal use is for surgery of the oral soft tissues. However, it also offers extraordinary advantages in treatment of hypersensitive dentin, bleaching discolored teeth, drying and sterilizing root canals, and comparable procedures that involve treatment of the oral hard structures.

Fully rectified electrosurgery can be used to facilitate, accelerate, and improve therapeutic results. The following are among the more important specific dental electrosurgical techniques that have been developed or improved by the author for use in specific areas.

OPERATIVE DENTISTRY. Desensitizing hypersensitive dentin; bleaching discolored teeth; conservative management of traumatic and mechanical pulp exposures; rapid, bloodless exposure of subgingival caries; elimination of polypoid proliferations of marginal gingiva from caries or tooth preparations.

PEDODONTICS. Resection of covering tissue to assist eruption of unerupted or partially erupted deciduous or permanent teeth; locating and sterilizing pinpoint pulp exposures in deep deciduous tooth caries; pulp capping without pulpotomy; frenectomy-frenotomy to prevent facial distortion from abnormal frenal torque.

ENDODONTICS. Tissue resection from retained roots and fractured or carious teeth to facilitate rubber dam isolation and for root canal obturation; drying and sterilizing root canals; root end resection, and definitive one visit treatment of chronically suppurating canals.

CROWN AND BRIDGE PREPARATION. Elongation of clinical crowns by loop planing to restore or retain a 1:2 crown-root ratio; preparation of subgingival troughs around teeth being prepared for full or partial coverage; exposure of key retained abutment roots for functional use; reduction of redundant tissue from edentulous alveolar areas in the dental arch to permit use of normal-size pontics; mucoperiosteal flap incisions for insertion of blade or other implants.

ORTHODONTIA. Resection of tissue to facilitate eruption of permanent teeth in normal alignment; exposure of malposed impacted permanent teeth for orthodontic realignment; elongation of clinical crowns of teeth for banding; frenectomy-frenotomy; pushbacks to eliminate low muscle attachments that interfere with labial arch bar insertion.

PERIODONTIA. Conservative management of advanced periodontal disease by gingivoplasty and infrabony pocket debridement; management of bifurcation and trifurcation involvements; frenectomy; repositioning of marginal gingiva to eliminate gingival clefts, and pushbacks for apically repositioned flaps.

PROSTHODONTIA. Resection of redundant tissue masses from edentulous alveolar ridges and/or vestibules; submucous dissections; mucoperiosteal flap incisions for plastic reconstructions; labial pushbacks (vestibulotomy) to re-create vestibular spaces; reduction of abnormal tuberosities.

ORAL SURGERY. Painless incisions for drainage of acute abscesses; mucoperiosteal flap incisions for surgical procedures ranging from simple surgical removal of retained or fractured roots to sophisticated plastic surgery procedures; frenectomy-frenotomy; loop planing to eliminate papillary hyperplasia; treatment of leukoplakia and ranula; sialolithotomy and similar surgical procedures.

BIOPSY. Properly conducted biopsy by needle or loop excision to eliminate or greatly reduce the hazards of surgical or mechanical metastasis of tumor cells during the biopsy surgery.

CANCER THERAPY. Treatment of "inoperable" oral cancer by electrocoagulation.

This list by no means exhausts the areas of practical usefulness for which the author has developed or modified and improved specific electrosurgical techniques. The latter, as well as those that have been enumerated, will be thoroughly reviewed in the succeeding chapters dealing with these disciplines.

The scope and range of practical clinical usefulness of dental electrosurgery is limited only by limitations of those who use it. With skillful, knowledgeable use, it can be employed safely as well as effectively for most dental procedures. There are a limited number of specific instances, however, in which electrosurgery is distinctly contraindicated and should be carefully avoided. There are also a few isolated instances in which its use is not automatically contraindicated, but in which special precautions must be employed when it is to be used.

CONTRAINDICATIONS

Use With Cardiac Pacemakers

Probably the single most important contraindication is for the patient with a cardiac pacemaker of *unknown* specifications. Moreover, not only would the use of electrosurgery on that patient be contraindicated, but even use of electrosurgery on *other* patients within a 16 foot range of the individual wearing the device would be contraindicated.

Many of the pacemakers are now being made with coaxial shielding that protects against interference. With shielded pacemakers it would be safe to use electrosurgery for the patient. However, in the *absence of specific information* about the frequencies of these instruments, and until such time as all the cardiac pacemakers in use are of the shielded variety, electrosurgery is distinctly contraindicated for wearers of pacemakers of unknown frequencies.

Biopsy of Maxillary Antrum and Parotid Gland

The chapter on biopsy will elaborate on the remarkable advantages electrosurgery offers that make it the ideal means for performing what students of cancer have termed "a properly conducted biopsy." However, when malignant disease of the maxillary antrum or of the parotid gland are suspected, electrosurgery is contraindicated. In each of these instances, a needle punch aspirational biopsy is the method of choice.

Aspirational biopsy eliminates need to cut an opening through the antral bony wall large enough to permit instrumentation to obtain the tissue specimen. Thus, this method of biopsy, which creates a tiny puncture through the bony wall with the hypodermic needle greatly minimizes the danger of metastasis of the malignant lesion by direct extension into the adjacent structures. No other method of biopsy, including electrosection, is an acceptable substitute for the aspirational punch biopsy for this reason.

The electrosurgical biopsy is contraindicated and aspirational punch biopsy indicated when a tissue specimen must be obtained from the parotid gland. The facial nerve plexus ramifies throughout the acini of this gland. Incisional biopsy by any means, including electrosection, would inevitably result in surgical severing of some of the branches of this nerve, with paralysis of the facial muscles of expression as the aftermath. Aspirational punch biopsy of the parotid gland virtually eliminates the hazard of this functionally impairing and aesthetically disfiguring result.

Aphthous Ulcer

Electrosurgery is distinctly contraindicated for treatment of this lesion. The aphthous lesion is not caused by bacterial infection. It is a herpetic lesion that tends to recur and undergoes spontaneous regression if not aggravated. The lesion results from irritation to the nerve ends in the oral mucosa at the site of the lesion by a virus. The irritation causes an ulcerative breakdown of the surface tissue in the affected area. As the affected tissue decomposes, alanine, glutamic acid, histidine, lysine, ornithine, proline, tryptophane, and the other amino acids, the end-products of decomposition of organic tissue, are released.

These acids are powerful irritants, and their irritation to the underlying tissues causes distress to the patient, ranging from discomfort to acute pain. Since the aphthous ulcer, if left undisturbed, undergoes spontaneous regression in approximately one week's time, the best formula for treating them has been aptly described by General Shira as "skillful scientific neglect." This consists of treatment to alleviate the patient's discomfort and to reduce the hazard of secondary infection of the ulcerated site, which, owing to the lowering of the resistance of the tissues in the affected area, becomes highly vulnerable to secondary infection by bacterial invasion.

The application of chemical agents, or use of electrocoagulation or fulguration to the aphthous lesion is not only ineffectual, but only serves to further irritate the tissues and disrupts nature's process of spontaneous repair. The author has followed the formula of skillful scientific neglect clinically for many years with the following regimen of treatment: rinse the mouth several times a day with a mild alkaline preparation such as milk of magnesia or one of the liquid antacids such as Mylanta or Maalox, to neutralize the amino acids and thus allay the pain or discomfort. A 2 per cent *aqueous* solution of acriviolet or gentian violet is applied topically at each office visit and may be prescribed for application by the patient 2 to 3 times daily. Aniline dye in aqueous solution is totally nonirritating to the tissues, and since it penetrates through the walls of the bacterial cell and disrupts its oxygenation, thereby killing the organism without any ill effects to the normal tissue cells of the body, it is an ideal agent for reducing the hazard of secondary infection of the lesion. No other treatment is required.

Electrolyte Imbalance

A number of serious systemic diseases produce electrolyte imbalances. Blood and cellular imbalances in sodium, chlorides as NaCl, and potassium, that are likely to be encountered, particularly in cases of preeclampsia and eclampsia, nephritis, cardiac failure, and Addison's disease, are most likely to influence electrosurgery, even in the early stages of the disease before other diagnostic symptoms have begun to be manifested.

When the sodium content of intracellular and extracellular and/or other body fluids is elevated, contact of an activated electrode with the tissues is likely to produce a profusion of large sparks similar to those produced by fulguration, even though the cutting current density used is optimal for normal tissue cutting.

Should such abnormal sparking occur, it would dehydrate the tissue surface and produce charring. If the electrosurgery must be performed, it is necessary to reduce the cutting current as much as is compatible with the ability to cut the tissues without coagulation and to avoid contact of the activated electrode for more than a maximum of 1 second, during which the electrode is kept moving rapidly, followed by a 10-second time interval before reapplying the electrode. It is also necessary to remoisten the tissue surface after *each* electrode contact, since despite the normal moist state of the oral tissues, the sparking quickly dehydrates the tissue surface and causes charring of the tissue being treated.

While these measures make it possible to use electrosurgery safely despite the scintilla, the most important consideration by far is that when excessive sparking is encountered when the proper amount of current is being used properly and no metallic objects are being contacted, an electrolyte imbalance should immediately be suspected and the patient referred for a thorough medical work-up. Such prompt action may lead to the early diagnosis of previously unsuspected disease that could result in death unless early treatment is instituted.

Creation of the Subgingival Trough by Electrocoagulation

Several years ago laboratory investigation demonstrated histologically that when electrocoagulation was applied to the crevicular marginal gingivae of a dog to create subgingival troughs, the marginal gingivae subsequently regenerated to within one tenth of a millimeter of its original level,* an amount of tissue loss that is clinically insignificant.

However, the experiment involved circumscribing of the teeth *once* with a minimal effective amount of coagulating current density to produce superficial coagulation as it was applied to the tissue. From a practical clinical standpoint it is virtually impossible to prepare an *effective* subgingival trough with a single circumscribing application of a minimal dose of coagulating current. To create a clinically effective subgingival trough it is necessary either to substantially increase the coagulating current density, in which event the operator loses control over the depth of penetration of the coagulating effect, or to circumscribe the tooth several times with minimal current density for optimal superficial spot coagulation, until an effective trough has been created.

If the multiple application method with optimal current density is used to avoid danger of excessive coagulation, each time the electrode circumscribes the tooth after the initial application, it either shreds or tears off the layer of coagulum necrosis that had been created by the previous application, causing bleeding that interferes with impression-taking. If the technique of preparing the trough before completing the shoulder preparation is being used, the bleeding obscures visibility in the subgingival area and makes it more difficult to make an ideal shoulder.

It is impossible to predict accurately the final postoperative level of the marginal gingiva at the time of treatment when electrocoagulation is used, since that level will not be evidenced until the tissue under the coagulum has

---

*Klug, R. G.: Gingival regeneration following electrical retraction. Unpublished thesis for degree of Master of Science in Dentistry, St. Louis University School of Dentistry, 1965.

fully healed and the coagulum has peeled off. Despite the experimental evidence of tissue regeneration that was reported, clinically, the loss of tissue following electrocoagulation appears to be relatively irreversible, and when gingival recession occurs, the tissue does not spontaneously regenerate to or almost to its original level. Innumerable cases of marked gingival recession after preparation of subgingival troughs by electrocoagulation have been called to the author's attention. In all instances the recession was permanent, and when it caused exposure of the shoulders of the preparations, required repreparation of the teeth and fabrication of new restorations.

When tissue is resected by electrosection properly, it tends to regenerate toward its original level. From the clinical standpoint the regeneration usually is complete. When somewhat more tissue is resected than had been planned, the tissue regeneration often minimizes the loss to clinical insignificance. Electrosection is therefore a reversible action, and assures that when it is properly employed the gingival level will remain at the level created by the surgical instrumentation, and most likely will regenerate to its original level, if that has been altered.

The greatest objection that has been directed to electrosection is that *more* regeneration may occur than desired, especially when the clinical crown of the tooth has been elongated. However, should more regeneration than is desired take place, the excess can easily be eliminated, whereas loss of gingival height due to recession following electrocoagulation cannot be corrected except by repreparing and remaking the entire case. It is therefore the author's firm opinion that electrocoagulation is contraindicated for creation of subgingival troughs, and that electrosection should be the method of choice.

ADDITIONAL CONSIDERATIONS

Explosive and Flammable Anesthetic Agents

When the only agents available for general anesthesia were the explosive or flammable inhalants such as cyclopropane, ethylene, and ether, the use of electrosurgery with these agents was distinctly contraindicated. Since the intravenous barbiturates have replaced the inhalants almost universally, electrosurgery is no longer automatically contraindicated for patients under general anesthesia. However, when nitrous oxide-oxygen is used for induction prior to the intravenous administration, the same precautions must be observed as when nitrous oxide-oxygen analgesia is being administered.

Nitrous Oxide-Oxygen Analgesia

Despite the flammable nature of oxygen, if special care and sound clinical judgment are used to avoid burn damage to the oral and pharyngeal tissues, electrosurgery can be used safely and effectively with nitrous oxide-oxygen analgesia.

The author recently learned of two cases in which patients under nitrous oxide-oxygen analgesia suffered burns in the mouth and throat due to ignition of oxygen present in the oral cavity during electrosurgery. In one of the cases the dentist invited disaster by indiscreetly using fulguration, which consists of profuse vigorous sparking that can jump a considerable air-gap and is certain to ignite any oxygen present in or about the mouth. The flash fire ignited the cotton gauze of the throat pack that had been placed across the oropharynx, and the burning gauze did most of the burn damage. The facts about the second case are not as yet fully known except that cutting current was used and a spark from it ignited oxygen present in the mouth.

Inasmuch as electrosurgery is being used thousands of times daily in conjunction with nitrous oxide-oxygen analgesia, without untoward effects, it seems reasonable to assume that the operator in this case must have used excessive current density, or permitted the activated electrode to make contact with a metal restoration, or a metal instrument in the mouth, any of which will produce marked sparking that could ignite oxygen present in the mouth. In the first case, poor clinical judgment was the culprit. In the second case it is likely that poor clinical judgment alone, or combined with poor technique, was responsible for the mishap. In both instances, safeguards that are about to be described could have averted or greatly minimized the damage.

RF current, properly used, does not produce appreciable clinically visible sparking. Under ultraviolet light, sparks that are minuscule in size can be seen. The sparks are so tiny that if the proper amount of current is used, and oxygen is not permitted to accumulate unduly in the oral cavity, electrosurgery can be used safely and effectively in conjunction with nitrous oxide-oxygen analgesia.

In view of the fact that in analgesia the gases are delivered in an open system, that is, with mouth open and the patient breathing air that greatly dilutes the oxygen concentration, a hazardous accumulation of oxygen in the oral cavity normally is not likely to occur, despite the fact that the ratio of nitrous oxide to oxygen needed for optimal analgesia is not a uniform constant for all patients. The ratio varies according to the susceptibility of the individual patient to the nitrous oxide. Thus, although a 50–50 mixture of the gases usually is used initially for analgesia, if the patient is highly susceptible, the amount of nitrous oxide must soon be reduced and the oxygen supply increased proportionally, to prevent the patient from entering the surgical plane of anesthesia. Susceptible patients often are maintained splendidly with mixtures of 20 to 25 per cent nitrous oxide and 75 to 80 per cent oxygen. Needless to say, the need for special precautions is greater for such patients than for those receiving a lesser concentration of oxygen.

Special care must also be used when the electrosurgery is to be performed in the posterior part of the mouth, since the gases pass through the nasopharyngeal orifices on their way to the lungs, and some of the gases can enter the oral cavity at that point, increasing the possibility of oxygen being present in the posterior part of the mouth.

In either event, the most important precaution is to prevent oxygen from entering the oral cavity and accumulating there. This can be accomplished effectively by placing a pharyngeal throat pack across the oropharyngeal open-ing, so that it blocks the entry of oxygen to the mouth while passing through the nasopharyngeal orifices.

A second precaution is to avoid use of excessive current density, so that the sparking will be subclinical and thereby reduce the hazard of igniting any oxygen present in the oral cavity.

A third precaution, that is especially important when instrumentation in the posterior part of the mouth is to be performed, is to insulate any metal res-torations in the mouth with oral bandage material such as Orahesive, or with a lubricant such as petrolatum or topical anesthetic ointment, to prevent spark-ing even when an activated electrode accidentally makes contact with the res-torations. For the same reason, wherever possible, nonmetallic instruments, such as plastic aspirator tips, or insulated instruments should be used, or polyethylene tubing slipped over the metal to insulate it.

Inasmuch as an accidental oxygen flash fire would ignite the cotton gauze of the throat pack, it is extremely important to *moisten* the pack slightly before placing it into the mouth. Moistened gauze will not readily ignite, and thus will prevent serious burn damage to the oropharyngeal and nasopharyngeal tissues.

As far as the oral mucosa is concerned, in view of the extremely brief duration of an oxygen flash fire, plus the natural protection provided by the saliva present in the mouth and the normal moist state of the oral tissue sur-faces, little if any appreciable burn damage will be done to these tissues if the gauze throat pack does not become ignited.

The throat pack should be placed carefully to effectively block the oropharyngeal opening. It is therefore important to avoid moistening the pack to the degree that it becomes a soggy mass unable to retain its shape. Avoiding excess moistening will also eliminate the danger of water dripping from the wet pack down the throat and being accidentally aspirated into the lungs.

Electrosurgery and the Epileptic Patient

Use of electrosurgery on epileptic patients is by no means contrain-dicated. It is, however, advisable that the dentist wear a rubber glove on his nonoperating hand, particularly if the patient is subject to frequent seizures.

The lips, cheek, or tongue should be grasped firmly with the gloved fingers, to maintain control over the mouth, and to retract these structures ef-fectively. In the event that a seizure should suddenly occur, he will be able to maintain control over the area of the mouth, and neither the oral tissues nor his glove-insulated fingers will be accidentally injured by the activated elec-trode.

Section Two

PRECLINICAL INSTRUMENTATION EXERCISES

Chapter Four

PRELABORATORY PRACTICE FOR THE UNDERGRADUATE DENTAL STUDENT

Introduction

Despite continual, often rapid procedural changes in dental therapy, certain methods are controllable, predictable, and almost routinely applicable. Electrosurgery has been shown to fulfill these requisites.[1-8]

Modern dental education is committed to expanding the scope of general dental practice through the teaching of sound efficient procedural methods in depth. Electrosurgery is one of these procedural methods.

In developing a curriculum of undergraduate instruction in dental electrosurgery, a definite sequence of lectures and laboratory exercises should be developed to properly prepare the student for the clinical uses of electrosurgery.[9-10] A proper progression of study involves three preliminary stages of instruction, in the following order:

1. A didactic course of instruction in the basic physics of the electrosurgical currents.

2. Preclinical training exercises to familiarize the student with the special physical requirements that are unique to electrosurgical instrumentation.

3. Laboratory exercises utilizing tissue specimens so that the student can "get the feel" of the electrode as it cuts the tissue.

The ideal final stage in the progression of a course in electrosurgical training would be supervised minor clinical use of the modality by the student.

93

THE RATIONALE FOR "PRECLINICAL" EXERCISES

"Can you offer a formula for electrosurgery that is consistently safe, efficient, and unfailingly successful?" The author has repeatedly been asked this question, and the answer is YES, but the formula is very precise and inflexible. It consists of a combination of skills and knowledge that are inseparably interrelated:

1. Knowledgeable, efficient electrosurgical instrumentation.
2. Sound dental technique.
3. Mature clinical judgment.

Regardless of how good the dental technique used, if the electrosurgical instrumentation is inefficient or the current unsatisfactory, the end result will be failure. By the same token, if the basic dental technique is unsound, no matter how skillful the instrumentation, the result will still be failure. And, despite excellence in both instrumentation and dental technique, if poor clinical judgment was exercised in the management of the case, the outcome will again be failure. The ingredients of this trinity are truly indivisible.

Two of the ingredients can be acquired through instruction. The third, mature clinical judgment, cannot be taught; it must be acquired through experience. Inasmuch as electrosurgical instrumentation efficiency and sound dental technique *can* be taught, this text is dedicated to that endeavor.

It is essential to develop knowledgeable, skillful instrumentation before attempting to perform specific dental electrosurgical techniques. Therefore the undergraduate dental student who will eventually be given the opportunity to use electrosurgery clinically should first be introduced to methods that will facilitate development of efficient techniques of electrosurgical instrumentation. The ideal time for this introduction is, as shall be seen, *before* he begins his clinical training, not after it.

This preclinical section has been included in the hope that it will prove equally beneficial for instruction of the freshman or sophomore dental student, and for the instructor who will subsequently have the responsibility of teaching them clinical uses of electrosurgery in his discipline.

The objectives of the exercises to be described are to help the student develop the light touch, rapid instrumentation, free-flowing wrist movement, and effortless digital dexterity that are essential for efficient electrosurgery. In order to achieve these objectives it is necessary to initiate the exercises before the student has been exposed to instruction in manual cold-steel instrumentation, which requires hand pressure and relatively deliberate movement to be effective. Once he has been exposed to the use of hand pressure, the task of retraining the student to perform electrosurgical instrumentation without pressure becomes infinitely more difficult. Therefore, the best time to initiate these exercises is before the student begins his clinical training program.

In fact, these exercises should even predate his introduction to the electrosurgical equipment, so that by the time he begins his laboratory training for specific dental electrosurgery techniques he will know the basics of good electrosurgical instrumentation. Needless to say, the student's instruction in the basic physics of the electrosurgical modality should precede all other instruction.

FIRST EXERCISE

For the first preclinical exercise each student must provide himself with a very fine camel-hair artist's brush, a supply of India ink, and a sheet of white paper or Bainbridge bristle board. He is instructed to moisten the brush with the India ink and proceed to draw a fine, straight line across the paper with the tip of the brush, without bending the bristles in the process and without blotting the paper. He should be required to repeat this until he is able to do it consistently with ease.

This exercise sounds so simple that it tends to create the illusion that it is too elementary to be important. Factually, however, it has proved an ideal means for developing the essential technique for successful electrosurgery. It teaches the student the importance of a light touch and the need to avoid the use of pressure. It also helps him to develop rapid, controlled movement and, perhaps most important of all, the free-flowing wrist movement that is so essential for efficient electrosurgical instrumentation. Thus this exercise actually is the ideal foundation upon which to base his subsequent training.

After he has satisfactorily demonstrated his proficiency in this exercise he is ready to advance to the second one, in which he is taught to simulate the electrode instrumentation that will be performed when he begins to work with the electrosurgical currents.

SECOND EXERCISE

This simple exercise was originally developed as preliminary instruction in electrosurgical instrumentation used in restorative dentistry. However, it is equally applicable for all the other areas of dental therapy. Its purpose is to simulate grossly, on a model, the basic electrosurgical techniques that are used clinically.

Methods and Materials

This basic exercise is performed on diagnostic casts or on previously used inlay die models (Figs. 4–1 and 4–2). The study cast selected should include edentulous spaces. These study casts (and die models) are covered with modeling clay up to and around the clinical crowns (Fig. 4–3). The modeling clay is adapted between the trimmed die models to simulate interdental papillae (Fig. 4–4). Modeling clay cutting points can be fabricated easily from stainless steel orthodontic wire and buccal tube material. The stainless-

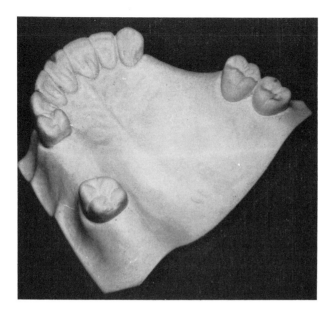

Figure 4-1. Diagnostic cast with edentulous spaces.

steel wire is bent to the shape and configuration of the types of electrosurgical cutting points and spot-welded into hollow stainless-steel buccal tube material (Fig. 4–5). The handle utilized for these modeling clay cutting points can be either a pin vice or an endodontic broach holder.

In this laboratory exercise, the modeling clay, when warmed and in a softened state, will afford ease of cutting with the fabricated cutting points. If the

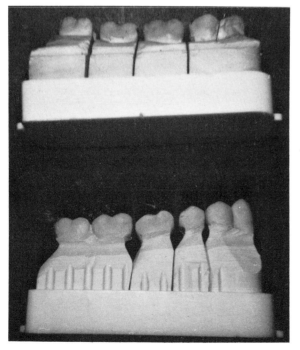

Figure 4–2. Inlay die model trimmed and untrimmed.

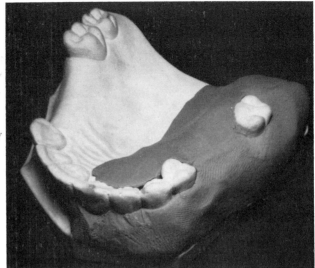

Figure 4-3. Modeling clay adapted to diagnostic cast.

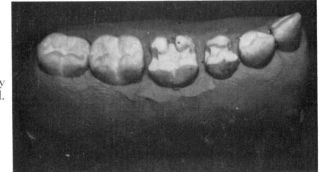

Figure 4-4. Modeling clay adapted to trimmed inlay die model.

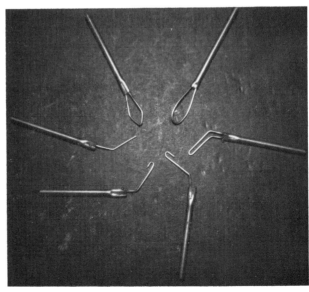

Figure 4-5. Modeling clay cutting points.

clay becomes too rigid, it can be moistened with water to allow for greater ease in cutting. As a training method, if the clay is cut too slowly, the points will drag and if too much pressure is utilized, the points will bend, or the modeling clay will become detached from the model. The modeling clay has the advantage in that it can be cut, remolded and contoured during use, and it is reusable.

Procedure

After preliminary explanation and illustration of some of the uses for electrosurgery in restorative dentistry have been presented, the specific uses of certain cutting points are demonstrated on the modeling clay that had been contoured to the study casts. For example, the instructor demonstrates the use of the loop electrodes and straight cutting points for removal of the free gingival tissue in the elongation of a clinical crown (Fig. 4–6). The student then proceeds to duplicate the cutting procedures with the modeling clay loops and cutting points on his own diagnostic cast. Gingival recontouring of the interdental papillae (Fig. 4–7) and gingival trough formation is then demonstrated by the instructor and repeated by the dental student (Fig. 4–8). As an additional exercise, the modeling clay can be cut with the simulated electrodes for residual ridge reduction in pontic edentulous areas and for the removal of hyperplastic tissue from cariously involved teeth.

Manipulation of Cutting Points

The electrode handle is held in a pen grasp. Only the tip of the cutting point and one lateral surface of the loop electrodes other than the narrow

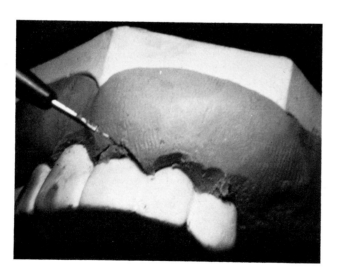

Figure 4-6. Straight modeling clay cutting point utilized for clinical crown elongation.

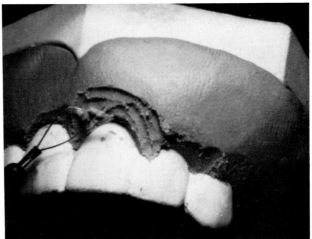

Figure 4-7. Loop modeling clay cutting point utilized for free gingival papilla recontouring.

U-shaped and J-loops should be brought in contact with the modeling clay. The lateral surfaces of the cutting point should not come in contact with the clay.

This basic preclinical laboratory exercise in the teaching of dental electrosurgery is a step in the development of a way of teaching this modality prior to tissue specimen laboratory exercises and final clinical application. It is hoped that through the repeated utilization of this basic exercise the students will become more adept in this type of instrumentation and will be stimulated to progress more rapidly in its clinical use with less apprehension.

Conclusions

1. The instruments, methods, and materials for this exercise are economically and easily procured and understandable.

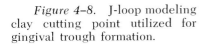

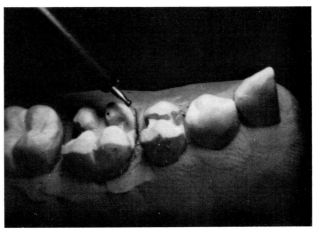

Figure 4-8. J-loop modeling clay cutting point utilized for gingival trough formation.

2. The laboratory time involved is minimal in expenditure and maximal in progress gained.

3. This exercise can be taught in conjunction with any of the specific dental procedures.

4. This approach can stimulate student interest in anticipation of the total concept in restorative dentistry and other areas of dental therapy.

Having successfully completed these preclinical training exercises the student is ready for the next phase of training, the experimental practice techniques.

FOOTNOTE REFERENCES

1. Oringer, M. J.: Electrosurgical aids in operative and restorative dentistry. Dent. Clin. North Amer., March, 57–77, 1966.
2. Klug, R. G.: Original tissue regeneration following electrical retraction. J. Prosth. Dent., 16:955–962, 1966.
3. Kelly, W. J., and Harrison, J. D.: Gingival heat generation and penetration using electrosurgical technics. Scientific Programs, ADA Annual Meeting, Dallas, November 13, 1966.
4. Podshedley, A. G., and Lundeen, H. C.: Electrosurgical procedures in crown and bridge restorations. JADA, Number 6, 77:1321–1326, December, 1968.
5. Stein, S. R.: Pontic-residual ridge relationship, A research report. J. Prosth. Dent., 16:251–285, 1966.
6. Heen, J. H., and Gilmore, N. W.: Management of gingival tissue during impression procedures. JADA, 75:924–926, 1967.
7. Brecker, S. C.: Electrosurgery in restorative dentistry. N.Y. J. Dent., 25:295–299, 1955.
8. Weinfield, E.: Table Clinic Presentation 4th Mid-Annual Meeting, AADE, Southfield, Michigan, 1968.
9. Pipko, D. J., Oringer, M. J., and El-Sadeek, M.: Laboratory exercise for teaching dental electrosurgery in restorative dentistry. J. Dent. Educ., April, 1972, pp. 16–18.

Chapter Five

PRACTICE TECHNIQUES FOR THE PRACTITIONER AND STUDENT

Introduction

The surest way to run into difficulties with electrosurgery is to think of it, and use it, as just another instrument in the dental armamentarium.

The reason for this is quite simple. Electrosurgery is not "just another instrument," but a *discipline*, in the fullest sense. True enough, it is a discipline that is totally dependent upon the availability of a special instrument. But this requirement is not unique to electrosurgery; it applies equally to a number of other important disciplines. For example, where would pathology be without the microscope? roentgenology or radiology without x-ray equipment? or anesthesiology without anesthetic equipment?

Electrosurgery, as is the case with these others, is a discipline that transcends but contributes beneficially to all the other disciplines of dentistry. And again, in common with the others, electrosurgery cannot be mastered by merely purchasing the necessary equipment and attempting to develop the necessary expertise to use it efficiently by self-taught, haphazard trial-and-error methods.

A well-organized and illustrated instructional text may help to minimize the haphazard approach and reduce the potential for error. But it is amazing how often and how much readers of the same text will differ in their respective interpretations of the contents. The frequency and degree of difference between the author's intention and the readers' interpretation thereof are equally surprising.

For these reasons, plus the fact that it is extremely difficult for a reader to be able to invariably visualize accurately or fully appreciate physical dimensional facts solely from verbal descriptions or photographs, no text can completely supplant or fully substitute for the advantages to be derived from the visual demonstrations and supervised practice participation that are integral parts of a worthwhile continuing academic course in dental electrosurgery.

Nevertheless, the author believes that this chapter is not only important but can prove beneficial for the reader who has not had the benefit of prior instruction as well as for the one who has, for quite different reasons. Despite the handicap of the lack of visual instruction, it should prove helpful to the former, because it offers him far more detailed information and technique instruction than can be derived from the usual manual with which the purchaser of electrosurgical equipment is provided. As for the reader who has attended a course in electrosurgery, although this may have taught him the proper techniques, it has not eliminated his need to practice the instrumentation and specific dental techniques diligently so as to develop the digital dexterity and *confidence* needed to translate these newly acquired skills into consistently safe, clinically practical usefulness.

The author, therefore, is confident that this chapter will serve a useful purpose both as a training manual and as a reference source, and should, at least to some degree, benefit all who take the trouble to read it.

THE NEED FOR EXPERIMENTAL PRACTICE

If the rapid rate of increase in the number of dentists who are making use of electrosurgery in their practice is a trustworthy criterion, it appears reasonable to predict that it will not be too long before the profession will be using this modality as universally as it is now using high-speed equipment and central suction.

Still, there are many dentists who want to use electrosurgery but are depriving themselves and their patients of its innumerable advantages because they doubt their ability to learn to use it safely and efficiently. Their lack of confidence stems largely from two interrelated and understandable uncertainties:

1. Uncertainty about how to acquire the training and special skills that are needed for its successful clinical use.

2. Equal uncertainty about whether they, having acquired the rudiments of training, will be able to translate their new skills into efficient clinical application.

Nothing, as has been mentioned before, can fully replace or adequately substitute for a sound basic course in dental electrosurgery. Nevertheless, the uncertainties can be banished if they are counterbalanced by incentive, determination, and diligent application. Even if no other source of training is available, given these three ingredients, a reasonably adequate degree of self-taught electrosurgical skill can often be acquired. To achieve this involves:

1. Diligent study of the fundamentals of electrosurgery: the basic physics of the electrosurgical currents—how they affect the tissues and why the tissues react to the currents as they do.

2. Planned, disciplined, diligent experimental practice in use of the therapeutic electrosurgical currents on meat to develop the proper techniques of electrosurgical instrumentation.

3. The need to develop proficiency in the specific dental electrosurgical clinical techniques that will be described in this and succeeding chapters by practicing them on calf mandibles.

Subsequent to indoctrination in the fundamental physics of the electrosurgical currents and development of adequate digital dexterity, the competent dentist will find that he is able to eventually translate his newly acquired skills clinically into specific practical dental electrosurgical techniques. Many of these are not new but are adaptations and implementations of old proven techniques to new methods of instrumentation. Success with their clinical application imparts self-confidence that opens new horizons which often lead to imaginative boldness to modify and, sometimes, to even expand and develop new original dental applications for electrosurgery.

The time-honored adage "practice makes perfect" is the key to success with electrosurgery. Repeated performance leads to experience; experience is the basic ingredient of success. The safest and surest way to develop dexterity, skill, and confidence is through the medium of preplanned, diligently repeated experimentation with meat and calf mandibles. Such experimentation affords the beginner a splendid opportunity to experience the "feel"—the physical sensation—of the electrode floating through the tissue, and to thoroughly familiarize himself with the behavior of the various electrosurgical currents on tissue and with the operational management of the electrosurgical equipment. The more experienced operator finds such experimentation invaluable for perfecting special techniques and developing original variations of existing techniques.

Maximum operational efficiency demands vigilant control of the electrosurgical equipment at all times. Experimentation affords the beginner an opportunity to develop vigilance in the immediate observation and prompt reaction to the need for regulation of the volume of current output created by the demands of a number of variable factors such as the size, shape and thickness of the electrodes and the texture and density of the tissues. Since such factors also exert a profound influence over the quality of electrosurgical results that are achieved clinically, it is essential for the novice to learn how to cope with them from the outset.

EXPERIMENTAL MATERIALS

Two ingredients are necessary for laboratory experimentation. One is the electrosurgical equipment, including an adequate quantity and variety of electrodes; the other, suitable tissue.

Beef and calf mandibles are the most useful tissues.

The meat should be used at room temperature, and should be fresh and moist. When the surface of the meat becomes dehydrated, excessive sparking and heavy fumes are produced by electrosurgery, with some searing of the tissue surface. Therefore, if the surface of the meat becomes dehydrated from exposure to the air while it is being used, it should be sponged periodically with water or isotonic saline solution to remoisten it. If the dehydration is preexistent and very marked, injecting the saline solution into the meat is more effective than surface sponging. Injection restores the meat's tissue moisture so that the normal cellular moisture of living tissue is more closely approximated. The calf mandibles should have at least 1 to 2 cm. of gingival tissue retained around the teeth, and if possible the calves should be from 4 to 6 months old. If the calf is older the gingival mucosa is likely to be leathery in texture, and if too young the tissue may be too frail, and the teeth may be covered with tissue.

USEFULNESS OF THE CALF MANDIBLE FOR ELECTROSURGICAL TECHNIQUE PRACTICE

The typical rubber typodonts containing plastic teeth or extracted human teeth that are so useful for practicing techniques for operative dentistry and crown and bridge in particular are useless for practicing electrosurgical techniques. Fortunately the calf mandible substitutes admirably as an ideal practice medium for developing skill in crown and bridge electrosurgical technique. The mandibles of calves 4 to 6 months old are most ideally suitable.

The calf mandible is useful for simulating most electrosurgical techniques used in operative, crown and bridge, surgical endodontics, periodontics, and oral surgery, despite the fact that they present a number of important anatomic differences from their human counterpart. The human mandible is a single bone, whereas the calf mandible actually consists of two separate bones that are united by a fibrous union in the midline and by the overlying gingival mucosa. In the calf mandible the area corresponding to the bicuspid area in the human jaw is edentulous. Whereas human molars are individual units with round buccolingual and mesiodistal contours and flat occlusal surfaces with more or less modified cusps, the calf molar crowns taper sharply buccolingually to form a serrated occlusal sharp line with razor-sharp exaggerated cusps. These molars are connected subgingivally and have many sharp spurlike cusps projecting subgingivally. The gingival mucosa of the calf mandible is considerably more fibrous than its human counterpart, and is much thicker and more densely fibrous on the lingual aspect, which resembles the human maxillary palate when the calf mandible is held upside down. Finally, the human alveolar ridge is bony and convex in contour, whereas the alveolar ridge of the calf mandible is a combination of bone and cartilage and is somewhat concave in contour on the labial aspect.

Despite these differences, the calf mandible in many respects simulates to an astounding degree the human dentition and its gingivae, and serves ideally for the laboratory practice needed to perfect the techniques and specific instrumentation they involve, in crown and bridge, surgical endodontics, periodontics, and oral surgery, as the following illustrations demonstrate.

EXPERIMENTAL PROCEDURES

Experimental practice should be carefully planned and should include use of both monoterminal and biterminal currents.

Unless the current output of the unit is self-regulating, the first thing the untrained novice with unfamiliar electrosurgical equipment should do is ascertain the exact amount of cutting and coagulating current output that is needed for optimal performance of his equipment with the available input current voltage.

There is no *average* amount of current that should be used. This is due to the fact that although all the units of a given model of electrosurgical equipment are identical in their circuitry, their individual circuit components often vary somewhat. Thus, just as automobiles from the same assembly line vary in their individual performance, electrosurgical devices from the same source tend to vary somewhat in their individual performance. Since the input commercial current supplies also are variable, the current requirements for each unit must be determined individually unless the unit can provide automatic self-regulation.

The necessary determination is easily accomplished by two simple experiments. To determine the amount of cutting current output for optimal performance, a fine needle electrode, preferably the 45-degree-angle type, is locked into the cutting electrode handpiece, the unit is activated, and the cutting current is activated. The power output dial on the instrument panel is set at a lever higher than what is likely to be needed to determine the amount of cutting current, and the electrode is applied to the tissue with a rapid wiping stroke. This will create a clean incision into the tissue, although the incised tissue edges may be slightly seared. The incising is repeated, and with each repetition the current is reduced progressively until the electrode begins to drag slightly and tissue fragments adhere to it tenaciously. The dial setting that immediately preceded this effect will provide the optimal cutting current output needed to cut cleanly without adhering tissue fragments. This amount of current becomes the norm for the amount of current required to cut normal gingival mucosa with a fine needle electrode and the same input current voltage.

To determine the amount of current output needed for optimal electrocoagulation, the initial current setting is reversed; it is set at a very low setting, the small ball electrode is locked into the coagulating electrode handpiece, the circuit is activated, and the electrode is applied momentarily to the tissue surface. If there is no tangible visible evidence of surface tissue coagulation, the current is increased progressively about one half degree at a time until the output level is reached where contact of the activated electrode produces a distinct, small white spot on the tissue surface. This is the norm for the current output required for efficient superficial spot coagulation.

Unless there is a change in input current voltage, or in the known factors that create need for variations in current output, the optimal values that have been established by these simple experiments remain constant for basic electrosection with the fine needle electrode, and coagulation with the small ball electrode, so that there will be no need to re-evaluate them clinically for each patient.

Monoterminal Currents

In Chapter 2 it was established that electrodesiccation and fulguration are derived from the same spark-gap current and that from a purely *electrical* standpoint they are identical phenomena, which is why many medical experts regard electrodesiccation and fulguration to be merely slight variations in spark-gap electrosurgical therapy.

Owing to the variety in the methods of application of the spark-gap current, for dentistry in particular, the tissue responses to electrodesiccation and fulguration are so vastly different that it is imperative to regard them as two distinctly separate *therapeutic* modalities, just as though they were derived from totally different electrical sources. The physical evidence of the marked difference in tissue response elicited by the respective methods of application of the current can be clearly established and readily demonstrated by employing these methods on a slab of beef.

FULGURATION. To produce fulguration or tissue carbonization, physical contact of the electrode with the tissue surface must be carefully avoided. When fulguration is used, the high-frequency electrical circuit that produces it is completed while tissue and electrode are separated by an air-space. When the electrode is brought close enough to the surface of the tissue for the current to jump across the gap, electric sparks emanate from its tip and arc across the air-space to make contact with the tissue surface, thereby completing the electrical circuit. The sparks produce *superficial* surface dehydration that results in carbonization of the dehydrated cells when the fulguration is continued for 30 to 60 seconds or more (Fig. 5–1A).

If the electrode is kept in constant rotary motion while fulguration is being applied, the underlying tissue remains unaffected for two reasons:

1. Insulation provided by the air-space helps to reduce heat energy produced by the sparks. The sparks therefore are not sufficiently potent to penetrate deeply into the underlying tissues and effect heat changes there.

2. The carbon that forms on the surface of the tissue acts as an effective insulating medium and also helps to protect against heat penetration, thereby providing effective protection against cellular alteration due to heat.

As a result of these factors there is no alteration in the fluid content of the cells in the underlying deeper tissues, which therefore remain normal.

True Oudin spark-gap current is the weakest of the high-frequency currents. Simulated spark-gap electronic current also is much less potent than the nonmutated cutting and coagulating currents. Thus both types of sparking current require a high volume of current output to perform effective electrodesiccation and fulguration.

Oudin and simulated spark-gap currents can readily be distinguished clinically because of their unmistakable physical differences. Oudin current produces large bluish-purple sparks, whereas simulated Oudin current produces small golden yellow sparks. Oudin sparks are very large and can arc across a wide air-gap; as a result, the tip of the electrode can be held well above the tissue surface. Simulated Oudin sparks are considerably smaller and thus cannot arc across as wide an air-gap; the tip of the electrode must be brought closer to the tissue surface to produce the dehydration. This inability to arc across an equally wide air-gap may appear to place the simulated sparks at a disadvantage. Far from being a disadvantage, clinically this is actually distinctly advantageous in dentistry (see Chap. 7). Moreover, owing to their somewhat greater potency, the simulated sparks invariably succeed in carbonizing the tissue surface. Carbonization can be continued to the depth necessary to destroy all undesirable tissue without causing damage to the surrounding tissues. The less potent Oudin sparks often are incapable of carbonizing the tissue; instead, a tough leathery eschar forms as the tissue surface becomes dehydrated and acts as an insulation that prevents further penetration and destruction of undesirable tissue remaining beneath it.

ELECTRODESICCATION. When the same monoterminal spark-gap current is applied to the tissues by inserting the electrode into the tissue and then leaving the electrode in the tissue while activated, the high-frequency current produces tremendous retention of heat energy which literally evaporates the tissue fluids out of the cells (Fig. 5–1B). As the electrode must be in stationary position, the tissue fluids may be seen bubbling up to the surface, leaving behind completely dehydrated tissue cells. Owing to cumulative heat retention the dehydration is not confined to tissue in actual contact with the electrode, but radiates beyond the electrode to variable degrees, as can be observed when the dehydrated areas are incised and inspected (Fig. 5–1C). The extent of penetration of heat into the underlying tissues is determined to a considerable degree by the length of time the activated electrode is kept in the tissues and the amount of current output employed.

Biterminal Currents

ELECTROCOAGULATION.   Electrocoagulation is usually applied to tissue surfaces with ball electrodes of varying sizes with cylindrical or tapered

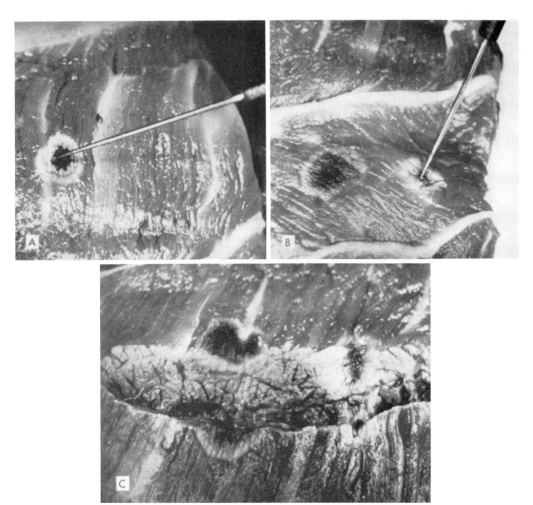

Figure 5-1.   A, Carbonizing sparks of fulgurating current; needle held above tissue. B, Electrodesiccation; needle electrode inserted into the tissue. C, Cross-section of the meat reveals desiccating effect of fulguration is very shallow, while that of electrodesiccation is very penetrating.

solid-rod electrodes such as those employed to create subgingival troughs around teeth in restorative dentistry.

Minimal current output should be used for electrocoagulation. Extent of coagulation achieved should be determined by the *length of time* the electrode is permitted to remain in contact with the tissues rather than by the amount of current intensity. The electrode should be permitted to make contact with the tissue for very brief, frequently repeated periods rather than continuous contact until visible surface coagulation is noted. Typical application of spot electrocoagulation with minimal current output ($\frac{1}{2}$ to 2 with Coles Radiosurg; 25 to 50 with the Birtcher Hyfrecator; 5 with the Cameron Dermatome) can be readily demonstrated on a slab of beef (Fig. 5–2A to D). By incising the coagulated areas the ability to control the extent of coagulation and depth of penetration can be ascertained readily. A very superficial layer of coagulum can be produced, involving only a few layers of tissue cells.

It is rarely advisable to increase the intensity of current output to increase the extent and depth of coagulation. To increase the amount of coagulation it is better to bring the electrode into contact with the tissues more frequently than to have lengthier periods of electrode contact. It is rarely necessary to use coagulating current output in excess of 2 on the Radiosurg, or proportional figures on the other units. Greater current intensities are necessary mostly when the larger ball electrodes are used.

Electrocoagulation can also be applied with bipolar electrodes. When these are used, the tissue between the two electrode tips becomes coagulated (Fig. 5–3). This produces moderately deep coagulation and is unsuited for superficial spot coagulation such as has been described previously. The ill-fated "Webb" technique of bipolar electrocoagulation for periodontal therapy was so disastrously destructive that bone sequestration and tooth exfoliation were common aftermaths. This type of electrocoagulation is totally unsuited for use on gingival mucosa.

One of the most important uses for electrocoagulation is to produce hemostasis and thereby help control bleeding from the soft tissues or from deep within bone crypts and tooth sockets. When an incision is performed with cold-steel scalpel, and a severed capillary, arteriole or venule produces persistent vigorous bleeding, it becomes necessary to clamp and ligate the bleeding vessel. This is time consuming, and when the operative field has been obscured by heavy bleeding, clamping and tying the cut vessel may be very difficult to do. When the incision is performed by electrosection and a blood vessel is severed, or when a blood vessel is accidentally torn when a tissue flap is elevated from the underlying bone and profuse bleeding ensues, electrocoagulation makes it a relatively simple matter to bring the hemorrhage under control promptly. All that has to be done is to clamp off the bleeder with the beaks of a mosquito hemostat and then apply coagulating current to the hemostat. The coagulating current volume usually should not exceed 2 on the Radiosurg, or its equivalents with the other equipment.

The current is applied most effectively with a ball electrode, which should make contact with the beaks of the hemostat for one to two seconds, removed for a few seconds, then reapplied. After about six such applications the hemostat is released to ascertain whether the bleeding has been checked. As a rule this proves to be the case, but if bleeding persists the hemostat

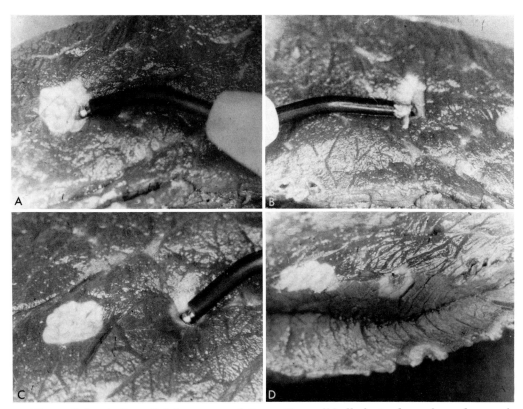

Figure 5-2. A, Superficial spot coagulation with small ball electrode performed properly with minimum amount of current necessary to produce visible coagulation of tissue surface. Current is being applied momentarily, removed, and reapplied to an adjacent spot of tissue. B, The current is excessively powerful but is being applied properly. The electrode tip sinks into the tissue, producing a slight char, and some tissue adheres to the electrode tip. A ring around the coagulated tissue approximately 3 to 4 mm. wide, slightly darker in color, is produced by the lateral heat transmission through the tissues. C, A third spot midway between the previous two is being coagulated. At this site current density is too weak to produce any visible clinical evidence of a coagulating effect when the electrode is brought into contact momentarily as in the previous cases. But the electrode is applied to the site for 4 seconds before it is removed. The electrode tip is penetrating into the tissue, and a small circular area of coagulation has formed. But a dark ring almost 1 cm. in width has developed around the coagulated area, denoting the extent of heat penetration from this minimal amount of current being used improperly — excellent evidence of the importance of speed of active electrode contact, and the destructive hazard of prolonged electrode contact with the tissues even with a very weak current output. D, Cross-section of the three areas of coagulation confirms the results visually. The area treated properly with the proper amount of current shows coagulation to have penetrated about 1 mm., and there is no change in color of surrounding and underlying tissue to suggest lateral heat penetration sufficient to produce destructive tissue changes. The site where an excessive amount of current was properly applied shows approximately 0.6 cm. of coagulation penetration, and a 2-mm. wide circumscribing ring of slightly darker color, indicating the extent of lateral heat transmission and the degree of tissue change. The central spot where minimal amount of current was improperly applied shows coagulation has penetrated almost 1 cm. deeply into the tissue and is surrounded by a dark ring about 0.5 cm. wide, indicating the wide area of lateral heat transmission and the degree of tissue change.

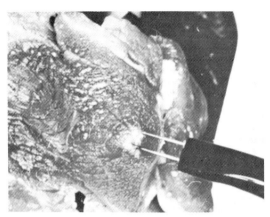

Figure 5-3. Electrocoagulation with bipolar electrode (biterminal application). Note heavy penetrating quality of tissue coagulation.

should be promptly reapplied and the coagulation resumed in the same manner and continued until the bleeding is halted.

This technique can be practiced easily on a slab of beef by clamping the tissue lightly with a mosquito hemostat and applying the ball electrode to the hemostat with coagulating current output set at the required volume (Fig. 5–4). This technique can also be effectively employed to halt bleeding deep in tooth sockets or other bone cavities from nutrient foramina. Here the beaks of the hemostat should be wedged into the bleeding site and the coagulating current applied to the hemostat as described earlier.

In addition to the use of hemostat-ball electrode coagulation just described, hemorrhagic tissue bleeding can also be controlled, even more efficiently, with a special coagulating forceps designed by the author. With the exception of the inner surfaces of its two tips and two small male projections at its other end, the entire forceps is insulated with a coating of Teflon. A twin-wire electric cable connects the forceps to the electrosurgical unit. At one end the cable terminates in a rubber plug containing twin female jack receptacles into which the male projections of the forceps fit, attaching the cable to the forceps. At the other end of the cable its two wires are separated and a male jack is attached to each wire's terminal end (Fig. 5–4E).

One of the jacks fits into the coagulating circuit and the other fits into the conductive circuit of the unit. When the bleeding tissue is pinched between the bare metal tips of the forceps and the coagulating current is activated, one tip serves as the coagulating electrode and the other serves as the indifferent electrode, thereby providing biterminal application of the current to the tissues.

Owing to the very slender shape of the forceps tips and the direct coagulating effect produced on the tissues, the coagulating effect instantly becomes visible. As a result the zone of coagulation necrosis can be minimized much more than with the hemostat-ball electrode coagulation, with much smaller areas of coagulation possible than with the latter (Fig. 5–4 *C* and *D*). The extremely slender taper of the forceps tips makes it possible to apply the coagulating current efficiently even to the apices of interdental papillae in tight embrasures.

As for control of hemorrhage from deep in bone, as from a tooth socket, while it can be performed with the hemostat-ball electrode application as described, it can be performed far more efficiently with the special Cameron-Miller aspirating-coagulating electrode described in Chapter 1 (Fig. 1–2).

Cutting electrodes can also be used with coagulating current to perform so-called bloodless surgery. For such purposes the current output should be approximately equal in volume to that of comparable cutting current for the same electrode and tissue. Some manufacturers have developed multiple circuit units designed to deliver a simultaneous blend of cutting and coagulating

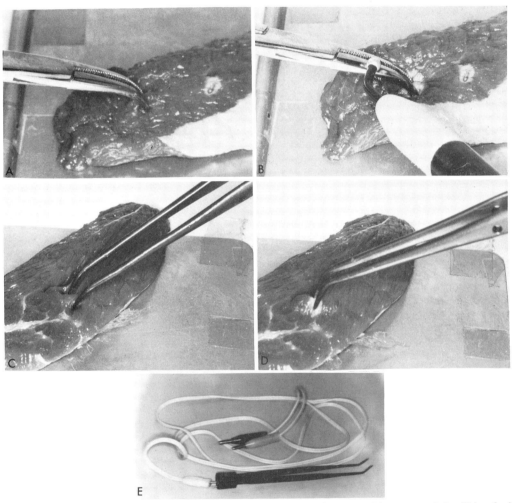

Figure 5-4. Electrocoagulation for control of hemorrhage. *A*, Clamping of the "bleeder" with a curved mosquito hemostat for indirect coagulation of the bleeder off the beaks of the instrument. *B*, Coagulation being performed by applying an activated large ball electrode to the side of a beak of the hemostat. The activated electrode is held against the hemostat until the visual evidence of coagulation becomes evident. *C*, Use of a special coagulating forceps designed by the author. The tips of the Teflon insulated forceps are grasping the "bleeder." *D*, Activated forceps coagulating the tissue by *biterminal* electrocoagulation. The zone of coagulation is much smaller than that created by coagulating off the beaks of the hemostat, and the coagulation can be performed in a precise manner even for the bleeding tip of an interdental papilla. *E*, The author's coagulating forceps with its twin wire cable that provides biterminal application of the current. One terminal jack plugs into the coagulating circuit and the other into the indifferent circuit.

currents for maximum hemostasis during surgery. Such blended current often is admirably suited for medical purposes but is rarely necessary or even desirable for use on the oral tissues.

ELECTROSECTION (ACUSECTION). This is the **only true surgical cutting current.** When it is properly employed, the cut surfaces are entirely free of visible coagulation. The first thing to observe in the use of electrosection is the position of the needle or loop electrode in relation to the surface of the tissue to be incised or resected. It is extremely important to hold the electrode in proper position during electrosection to assure that none of the heat energy being potentiated is dissipated, thereby impairing the efficiency of the cutting current.

When only the tip of the needle electrode is brought into contact with the tissue surface (Fig. 5-5A), all the heat energy potentiated is concentrated at the tip and is sufficient to disintegrate and volatilize the individual cells contacted by the electrode, thereby producing surgical incisions fully comparable to the best that can be produced by cold steel (Fig. 5-6).

When the electrode is not held at right angles to the tissue surface, but at an acute angle so that in addition to the tip some or all of the lateral surface of the needle comes into contact with the tissues (Fig. 5-5B), the heat energy being potentiated is spread along the full length of contact surface instead of being concentrated only at the tip. This results in a marked reduction in heat concentration due to the distribution of heat over a much larger electrode contact area, and thus permits dissipation of a considerable amount of the heat energy so that there is insufficient concentration of energy to volatilize the disintegrated cells. These unvolatilized cells tend to adhere to the electrode tenaciously (Fig. 5-7). This retards the progress of the electrode, impeding its passage through the tissues, and permits the heat energy to penetrate beyond the actual electrode-tissue contact. Undesirable tissue destruction that closely simulates electrocoagulation may result (Fig. 5-5C).

When tissue shreds adhere to the electrode it usually indicates that inadequate current output is being used for the size and shape of electrode or the tissue thickness and density, but it may also indicate that the electrode is not

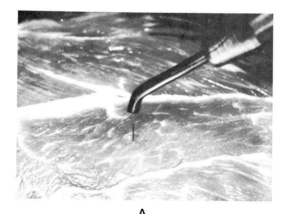

A

Figure 5-5. A, Needle electrode in proper position for electrosection.

Illustration continued on opposite page.

B

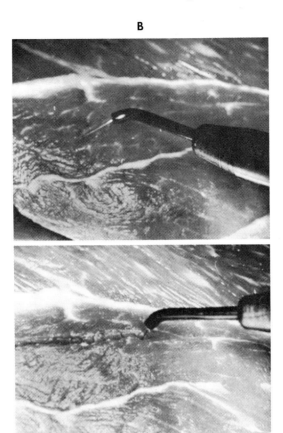

C

Figure 5–5. *Continued.* B, Needle electrode held improperly for electrosection. C, Superficial coagulation of incised tissue surfaces resulting from improper instrumentation.

being held at right angles to the tissue surface. Adherent shreds must be removed from the electrode immediately. The most efficient method of removal is to place the electrode tip firmly on a solid surface and brush it lightly with a small piece of steel wool with short strokes in one direction only.

When loop electrodes are used, the initial sites of contact cannot be pin-pointed, since an arc of the loop is in contact with the tissue surface instead of a fine point. The larger the loop and the more circular its shape, the larger the arc area of contact. Heat energy potentiated in the area of the electrode-tissue contact tends to become dissipated along the line of initial arc contact.

For this reason some otherwise well-informed individuals are convinced that the size of the loop is the factor that determines the quality of tissue excision by electrosection. They are fully convinced that when a large round loop electrode is used it is not possible to excise tissue without some accompanying coagulation of the cut surfaces and perhaps damage to underlying structures.

However, clinical experience has repeatedly and conclusively demonstrated that while the size of the electrode is a factor, it definitely is not the determining factor. The amount of cutting current employed and the

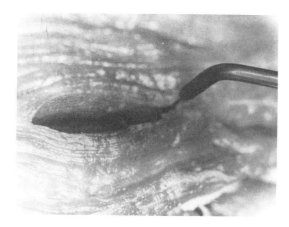

Figure 5-6. Surgical incision by electrosection using fine needle electrode. Note lack of coagulation and smooth tissue surface.

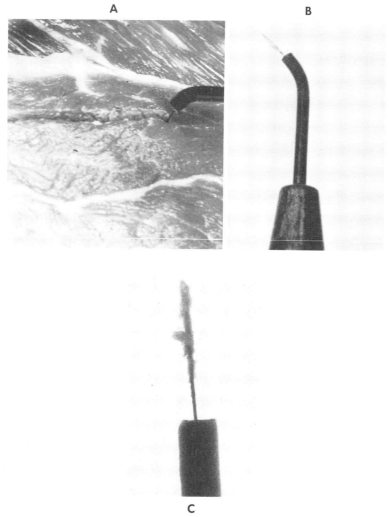

Figure 5-7. A, Improper instrumentation for electrosection; electrode moved too slowly. Note surface coagulation of cut tissue. *B*, Tissue shreds adhere to electrode after it is used too slowly. The same result is obtained when inadequate current output is used. *C*, Adherent coagulation (enlarged).

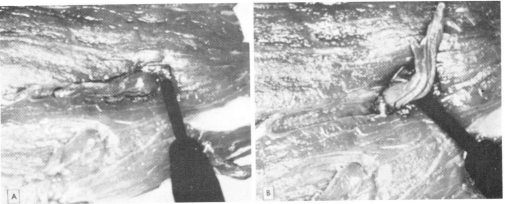

Figure 5–8. *A*, Resection by electrosection with small U-shaped loop electrode. *B*, Tissue segment reflected; underlying tissue and base of the tissue segment are free of coagulation.

speed of instrumentation in performing the excision are the real determining factors.

If enough cutting current power is used to fully disintegrate and volatilize all the cells along the line of electrode contact, and the electrode is moved as rapidly as the tissue resistance permits, the tissue cleavage is just as efficient and free of coagulation as tissue cut with a fine needle electrode.

Another consideration is the gauge of the loop wire. The larger the diameter of the loop electrode, the more important does the gauge of the loop wire become. If the wire gauge is very thin, even a 12-mm. round loop electrode will resect the tissue efficiently without any clinical evidence of coagulation (Fig. 5–8). If the gauge is somewhat thicker, it may become difficult to excise tissue cleanly without coagulation with a 7- to 8-mm. round loop electrode. If, in addition to the increased thickness of wire gauge, the electrode is not moved through as rapidly as the tissues permit, tissue excised with even a 3- to 4-mm. U-shaped loop electrode may produce coagulation of the cut surfaces (Fig. 5–9).

The angulation at which the electrode is brought into contact with the tissue surface is also a factor. A needle electrode cuts most efficiently when brought into contact at, or nearly at, a 90-degree angle to the tissue surface;

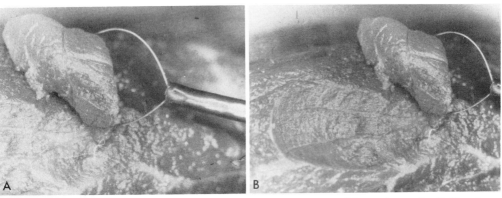

Figure 5–9. *A*, Resection by electrosection with large round loop electrode. *B*, Cut tissue surfaces exposed to view. There is no visible coagulation.

PLATE I

A. Laboratory Technique

Figure 1a. An incision is being made into a slice of beefsteak by electrosection. The 45-degree-angle fine needle electrode is being used with the proper amount of cutting current and proper speed of instrumentation.

Figure 1b. The incision is being extended manually with a disposable Bard-Parker scalpel. Note the smoother surface of the tissue cut by electrosection owing to the disintegration and volatilization of the tissue cells in the line of cleavage, as compared to the surface of the tissue where cleavage results from crushing of the cells as the steel blade is forced through. Note the absence of clinical coagulation throughout the incision.

Figure 1c. Appearance of tissue being cut with the same electrode but with cutting current that is too weak to disintegrate and volatilize all the tissue cells. Note the coagulation of the cut tissue surfaces and the adhesion of the tissue to the electrode.

Figure 2a. Tissue being cut properly with a small loop electrode by electrosection. Note the absence of coagulation on the cut tissue surfaces.

Figure 2b. Tissue being cut properly by electrosection with a 12 mm. round loop electrode. Note that when the proper amount of current is properly employed, cutting can be performed as perfectly with a large loop as with a small one. Note the smooth surface of the cut tissue and absence of clinical evidence of coagulation.

Figure 2c. Tissue being cut improperly with a medium-width loop electrode. Note the cooked appearance and brownish color of the tissue surfaces due to use of excessive amount of cutting current.

B. Experimental Research

Figure 3a. Demonstration of illumination of an electric bulb by cutting current being used monoterminally, without direct current return to the unit through the indifferent plate electrode. The bulb is dimly lit, and onset of the illumination is slow.

Figure 3b. Bulb is illuminated by the same amount of current output, but by biterminal application, with the current returning directly to the unit through the indifferent plate electrode. Note the greater amount of illumination, representing greater cutting efficiency, when the indifferent electrode is employed. The bulb illumination occurs almost instantly as the current is activated.

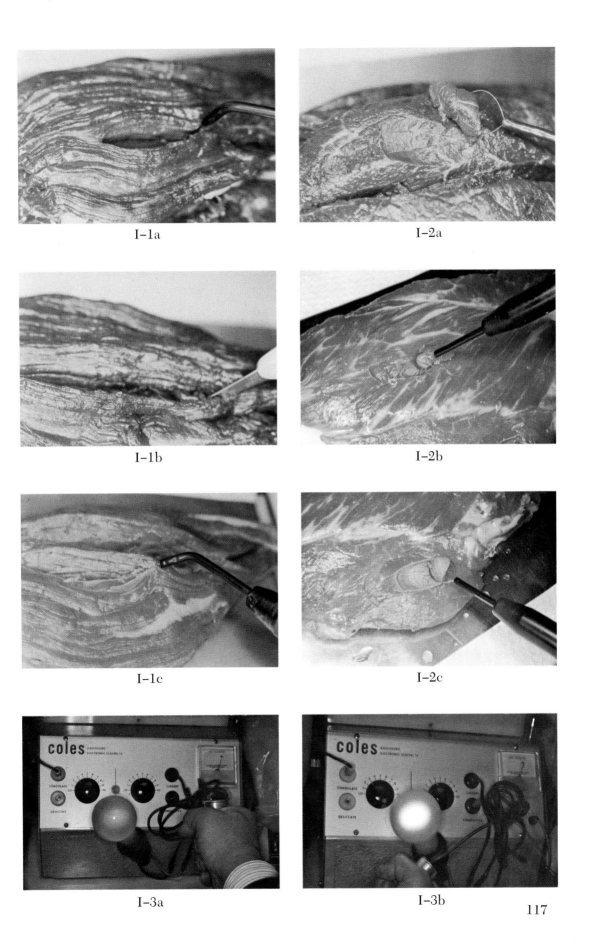

I-1a

I-2a

I-1b

I-2b

I-1c

I-2c

I-3a

I-3b

if a round loop electrode is brought into contact at a comparable angle, before it can begin to excise it must first penetrate into the tissue in order to engage it. While the loop is sinking into the tissue it cannot be moved rapidly. As a result, the *initial site* of electrode penetration is likely to show slight superficial coagulation (Fig. 5–10A). For optimal loop cutting the electrode should be brought into contact at a 45- to 60-degree angle to the tissue surface with a rapid wiping or brushing motion. When the electrode is brought into contact at this angle and the tissue is planed in thin layers, the excision is performed with no clinical evidence of coagulation at the initial site of contact, or along the cut tissue surfaces (Fig. 5–10B).

When an excessive amount of cutting current power is used, the surface of the tissue becomes slightly charred and the cut surfaces have a light brown color, but no tissue adheres to the electrode (Fig. 5–11). Should the cutting current power be too weak, either the electrode will be unable to cut the tissue and will barely penetrate the surface and stick there, or the cut surfaces will become coated with a layer of white coagulum, and some of the coagulum will adhere tenaciously to the electrode.

The electrode should *always* be activated before it makes contact with the tissues. Applying the loop to the tissue surface after it has been activated, instead of activating it while the loop is in contact with the tissue, helps to minimize or prevent coagulation. If the marginal coagulation is very minimal, when it does occur, it does not impair the value of such tissue for histopathologic interpretation or interfere with the normal repair of the basal tissue bed from which it was removed.

Tissue cuts best when it is stretched taut. When a segment is to be removed from a large mobile tissue mass, the removal can be expedited and searing minimized by holding the tissue stretched taut. Tissue hooks are available for this purpose, and the tissue can readily be engaged and pulled taut with a simple half twist of the hook. When the tissue hook is employed, it is first inserted through the eye of the loop electrode, inserted into the tissue with a half turn, then the electrode is activated and used to perform the resection (Fig. 5–12).

After the neophyte has acquired a reasonable degree of skill and dexterity in the techniques of instrumentation with the various electrodes and electrosurgical currents, it is time to advance to practice sessions of experimentation with specific dental electrosurgical techniques.

The calf mandible serves this purpose admirably. The anterior teeth of a calf closely resemble human dentition, and are ideally suited for experimentation with electrosurgical techniques used in restorative dentistry such as elongation of the clinical crown (Fig. 5–13), and for creating a subgingival trough (Figures 5–14, 5–15, and 5–16) with a 45-degree-angle narrow U-shaped loop electrode and with the J-loop electrode (Fig. 5–14). Both types of electrode should be held parallel to the long axis of the tooth as it is being circumscribed by the electrode to excise the subgingival trough. The anterior portion of the calf mandible is also useful for practicing the V-Y frenectomy procedure (Fig. 5–17).

The posterior portion of the calf mandible provides an excellent medium for practice of periodontal electrosurgical techniques such as shall be described in detail in the section on periodontia. It is even possible to simulate

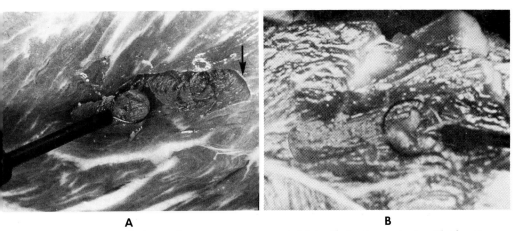

A   **B**

Figure 5–10. *A,* Slight surface coagulation at initial electrode contact with the tissues (arrow). *B,* Planing tissue in thin layers with loop electrode. No coagulation noted even when the resected tissue is so thin it is translucent.

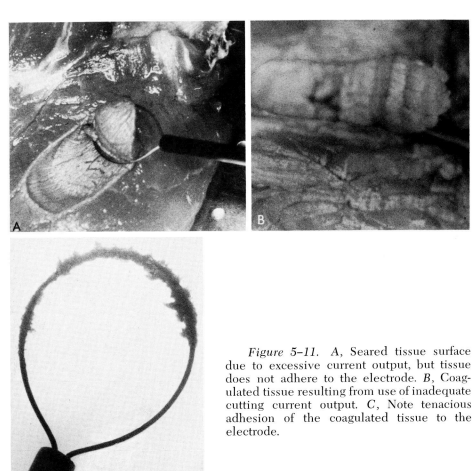

Figure 5–11. *A,* Seared tissue surface due to excessive current output, but tissue does not adhere to the electrode. *B,* Coagulated tissue resulting from use of inadequate cutting current output. *C,* Note tenacious adhesion of the coagulated tissue to the electrode.

119

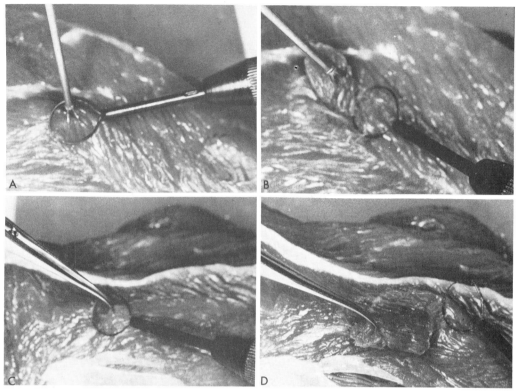

Figure 5-12. Loop excision biopsy techniques. *A*, Shows tissue being pulled taut for excision with a tissue hook through the eye of a 1.2 cm. round loop electrode hooked into the surface tissue. *B*, Shows the completed loop excision. Note the slight "comet-tail" shape of the tissue that often results from the lifting motion of the excision. *C*, Shows a curved ophthalmic tissue forceps being used instead of the tissue hook. The slightly curved slender beaks of the ophthalmic forceps also has been passed through the eye of the loop electrode and is poised for the tissue excision. *D*, Shows the completed excision. Note the smooth character of the tissue specimen and the bed from which it was removed, and the absence of clinical evidence of coagulation.

an infrabony pocket by cutting downward along the side of a tooth with a narrow knife blade or chisel. Techniques for gingivectoplasty and gingivoplasty combined with infrabony pocket debridement may be seen in Figures 5–18 and 5–19. In Figure 5–20 the technique for creating a self-cleansing concave sluiceway in an embrasure can be seen. This portion of the calf mandible also lends itself to a limited degree for practice of numerous surgical incisions for flaps and for removal of pericoronal flaps and exposure of crowns of third molars (Figs. 5–21 and 5–22).

The expert as well as the neophyte can benefit from electrosurgical experimental practice sessions.

The expert in electrosurgery finds many invaluable uses for the calf mandible experimentation. It is especially useful for developing ideas relating to original techniques, or original variations of existing, proven techniques. He will find that with some practice he can soon develop the same degree of skill and confidence with the new procedures that he already enjoys with the techniques he uses daily.

Finally, the experimental practice sessions provide the ideal opportunity to observe the characteristic behavior of the electrosurgical currents when

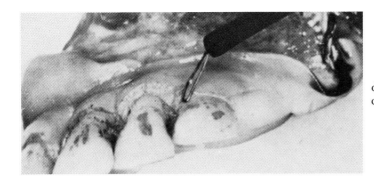

Figure 5-13. Calf mandible: practicing elongation of clinical crowns of teeth.

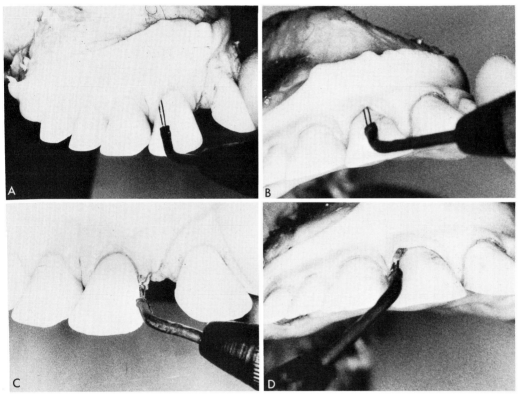

Figure 5–14. U-shaped loop excision. *A,* The U-shaped loop electrode is being held parallel to the long axis of the tooth, and rotated 15 degrees off the horizontal. Note that the loop is almost in a flat horizontal position, with both legs of the loop parallel with the horizontal plane of the labial enamel of the tooth. *B,* The loop is beginning to excise a thin strip of the inner tissue of the marginal gingiva, equivalent in thickness to the width of the acute angle formed by tilting the electrode 15 degrees off the horizontal. The tilting of the electrode to form this angle may be compared to the tilting of a butter knife being used to spread butter on a slice of bread, and the electrode is used with a similar wiping motion to excise the tissue. *C,* The excision of the trough to the mesial embrasure has been completed. Note that by tilting the electrode to a 15- or 20-degree angle the strip of tissue being excised is so thin that there is no shredding of the marginal gingiva, and the level of the gingiva has not been elevated. *D,* Excessive rotation has created an obtuse angle with the tooth surface. Failure to rotate the loop properly resulted in excision of a wide strip of tissue from the marginal gingiva, thereby performing a gingivectomy that is raising the level of the marginal gingiva.

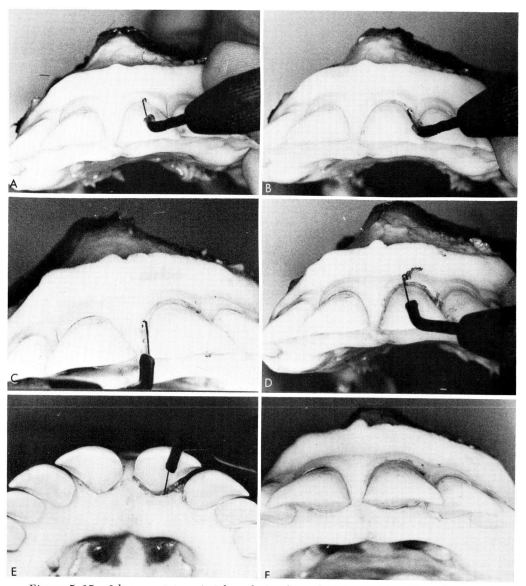

Figure 5–15. J-loop excision. *A*, J-loop being brought into position. Note that the short shaft of the loop is going to be against the tissue, and the long shaft against the tooth. *B*, The subgingival excision has been performed from the midline of the tooth to the distal embrasure, completing the trough preparation of the distolabial quadrant of the tooth. *C*, The mesiolabial quadrant is being excised. *D*, The excised strip of tissue from the mesiolabial quadrant being lifted out of the trough with the J-loop. *E*, The trough being created on the palatal aspect in a similar manner. *F*, A ventral view of the subgingival trough circumscribing the tooth.

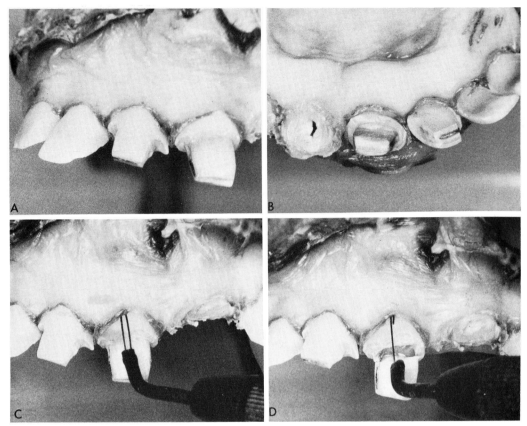

Figure 5–16. Anterior teeth of a calf mandible have been prepared to demonstrate the author's new technique of preparation of subgingival trough before completing shoulder preparation. *A*, Right central has been reduced mesially, distally, and incisally; left central has also had the labial enamel removed. *B*, Ventral view of prepared teeth. *C*, U-shaped loop in position for creating the trough. *D*, J-loop in position for creating the trough.

they are applied to the tissues, and to determine the reasons for any unfavorable results without inflicting damage to living tissue. Adequate experimental practice is the finest insurance against unfavorable results in the patient's mouth.

INSTRUMENTATION AND TECHNIQUE TRAINING

Cutting into tissue with an activated electrode is a totally different sensation from cutting manually with a steel scalpel. Instrumentation methods with the respective modalities also differ greatly.

Efficient cutting with a steel scalpel requires application of firm manual pressure against the tissues with the cutting blade as it is used with a relatively slow deliberate cutting motion. With the activated electrode no pressure need be, indeed, should not be, applied. When the proper amount of cutting cur-

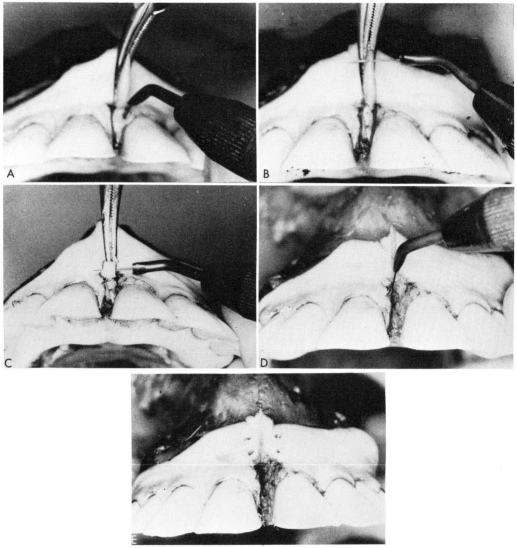

Figure 5–17. Frenectomy-frenotomy. *A*, The simulated frenum, consisting of mucous membrane in the anterior of the calf mandible, has been clamped with the curved mosquito hemostat as it would be in the mouth. The 45-degree angle fine needle electrode is being used to incise along the lateral borders of the "frenum" as the first step in performing the author's ectomy of the attached frenal fibers, and otomy of the areolar fibers at the superior end that control the movements of the lip. *B*, The lateral mucoperiosteal incisions around the fibers have been incised; the tissue projecting from the beaks of the hemostat is being resected from the external surface of the hemostat beaks with the needle electrode. *C*, The resection of the frenal tissue from the surface of the beaks of the curved mosquito hemostat is being completed. *D*, The frenal fibers being "ectomized" having been eliminated, the fibers that invaginate into the median suture line are being destroyed by running the needle electrode down the suture line as rapidly as possible. Immediately after the suture line has been scored with the electrode, the full 10-second time interval between applications of the activated electrode is observed. The electrode is used to score the suture line 5 to 6 times. The superior portion that is being "otomized" can be seen as a crushed line of tissue. *E*, The final appearance of the tissues. The lower half has been ectomized and the upper half otomized. The four black dots seen in the "otomized" upper portion represent the sites where sutures would be inserted, if needed. Clinically the dark portion would be filled with a blood clot.

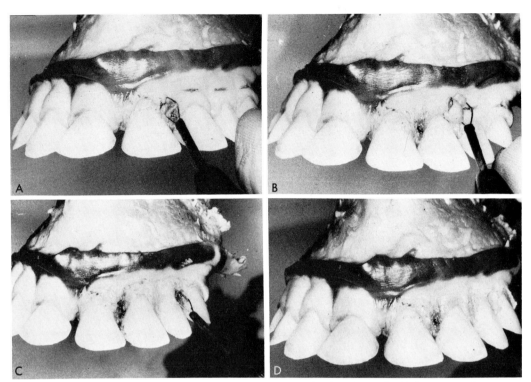

Figure 5-18. Periodontics: Gingivectoplasty. *A*, The level to which the gingival mucosa is to be resected has been marked off with horizontal lines. The gingivectoplasty is seen being performed on the first tooth, by loop planing the tissue with a flame-shaped loop electrode. *B*, The resection of redundant tissue and simultaneous recontouring of the gingival architecture to normal feather-edge marginal gingiva is being continued on the next tooth. *C*, Recontouring of the interproximal papillae to form concave self-cleansing sluiceways in the embrasures is being performed with the flame-shaped loop electrode. The loop is used with a planing motion directed incisally, to assure against accidentally resecting the papilla as might occur if the cutting were directed apically. *D*, The gingivectoplasty has been completed as planned. The gingival tissue has been resected to the desired level, and the normal gingival architecture has been simultaneously restored. The new marginal gingivae are feather-edged and are normal in contour, with no sharp line angles of tissue. This technique is equally suitable for elongation of clinical crowns for fixed prosthodontics and for periodontal surgery.

rent has been used, the electrode literally floats through the tissue effortlessly.

The proper methods of electrosurgical instrumentation to achieve the most desirable effects can be developed only by diligent practice. The knowhow and dexterity to use the currents safely, deftly, and efficiently for specific dental electrosurgical techniques likewise can be developed only through conscientious practice.

For electrosurgery the practice must be performed on organic tissue. Fortunately, two types of organic tissue that are ideally suited for the necessary practice are readily available. The effects of the currents can be appraised and the instrumentation techniques to achieve the desired results efficiently can be practiced most effectively on slabs of meat. The specific dental electrosurgical techniques can be practiced most effectively on calves' mandibles.

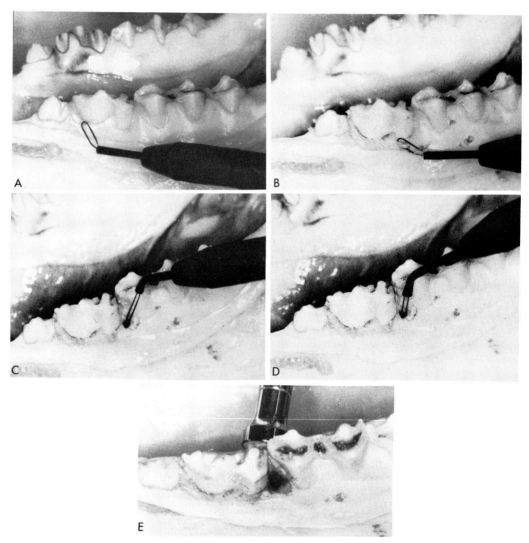

Figure 5–19. Periodontics: Combined gingivoplasty-infrabony pocket debridement. *A*, Gingivoplasty being started in a postero-anterior direction with a 45-degree angle medium width U-shaped loop electrode. *B*, The gingivoplasty being continued to recontour the marginal gingivae. *C*, The 17 mm. periodontal loop electronic curet being introduced into a simulated infrabony pocket. (The pocket is created by punching a hole into the alveolar bone.) *D*, The loop curet is introduced to the base of the pocket with an up and down-rotary motion, so that the loop makes contact with all the internal surfaces of the defect. *E*, After the debridement has been completed the effectiveness is determined by digital examination with the inactivated electrode, then by visual examination with a transilluminating lamp. The lamp is placed on the lingual aspect and the light directed so that it will produce an internal glow in the defect. If any fragments of tissue remain in the defect the transillumination will show them as dark spots that are readily seen and located.

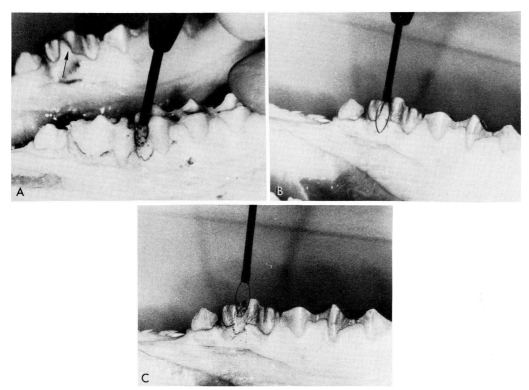

Figure 5-20. *A*, Sluiceway is being created in embrasure on buccal aspect. Arrow points to papilla that requires reduction and recontouring. *B*, Flame-shaped loop electrode in position for the papilla reduction and creating the sluiceway. Note that the dissection is performed toward the apex of the papilla. *C*, The tissue has been simultaneously excised and recontoured into a concave self-cleansing area.

The practice meat should ideally offer approximately the same resistance to the passage of the RF current that is offered by normal gingival mucosa. Gingival mucosa does not contain any muscle fibers, whereas typical practice meat is made up of bundles of striated muscle fibers. The author has found that two cuts of beef are particularly useful. One is shoulder shin beef sliced parallel to the long axis of its muscle fibers. The other is flank steak.

When these cuts of meat are incised or loop excised parallel to the long axis of their muscle fibers the resistance is almost identical to that of the gingivae. When the optimal current output has been determined on practice meat that is at room temperature and not at refrigerated temperature, the same setting will also be proper for use on the human gingivae. When these tissues are cut transversely to the long axis of their muscle fibers, their resistance to passage of the RF current is quite comparable to that offered by the thicker, denser palatal mucosa, and requires a comparable increase in cutting power output for efficient cutting effect.

The effects of electrocoagulation, fulguration, and electrodesiccation also can be studied, and use of these modalities can be practiced on the meat. The steaks should be cut approximately 0.5 to 1.0 inch thick, and 3×5 inches in

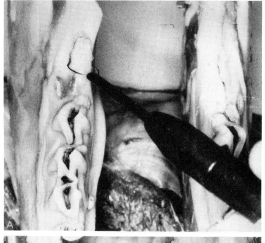
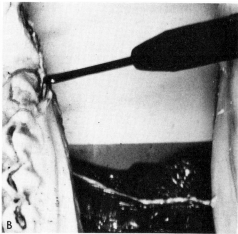
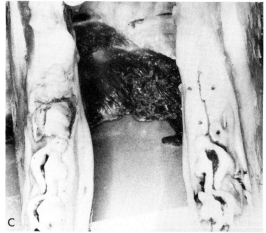

Figure 5-21. Operculotomy of mandibular third molar. *A*, The covering overlying tissue is resected with a round loop electrode to fully expose the crown of the tooth. *B*, The tissue around the exposed crown has been recontoured to restore normal contour to the tissue. The tenaciously adherent Nasmith's membrane is being removed with a narrow U-shaped loop electrode. *C*, Appearance following resection of the embryonal capsule.

dimension. Figures 5–23 to 5–25 demonstrate the usefulness of the meat for practicing the effects of the therapeutic electrosurgical currents.

The practice meat also serves one other useful purpose: to provide the conductivity necessary for efficient use of the currents on calves' mandibles. When the latter are obtained from the abattoir or meat packing plant, all the meat, with the exception of a rim of gingival mucosa about 1 cm. wide, has been trimmed away. The masseter and other muscles having been removed, the bare ramus and angle of the jawbone come into contact with the indifferent electrode. Since bone is a very poor conductor much of the energy is lost and the result is comparable to that obtained when the indifferent electrode is not employed. When the practice meat is placed on the indifferent electrode and the ramus or angle of the mandible is brought into contact with the meat, the necessary conductivity is restored and efficient cutting achieved.

Skillful efficient electrosurgical instrumentation requires total control by the operator of the performance, and the effects, of the RF currents. Such control can only be achieved by practice and observation.

The most important factors relating to efficient electrosection and elec-

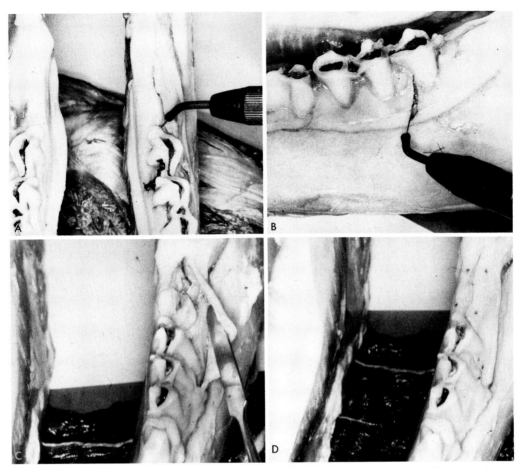

Figure 5-22. Removal of impacted mandibular third molars. *A*, A horizontal incision being made along the edentulous ridge from the anterior border of the retromolar pad anteriorly to the distal of the second molar with a 45-degree angle fine needle electrode. *B*, The activated electrode creating the vertico-oblique incision from the distobuccal angle of the first molar downward and anteriorly to the junction of the alveolar and areolar mucosa, to complete creation of the mucoperiosteal flap to expose the surgical field. *C*, The flap elevated and reflected, exposing the external oblique ridge of bone and the portion of the tooth projecting above the bone. Note the easy access provided, and the facilitation of bone removal, and if necessary, splitting of the impacted tooth for removal in sections. *D*, The tissues restored to normal position. The black dots designate the sites for insertion of the sutures to secure the flap into position.

trocoagulation are the time factor — how long the activated electrode is kept in contact with the tissues — and control of the depth of penetration into the tissues of the effects produced by the currents.

The time factor is governed by the speed of instrumentation. The electrode should be drawn across and through the tissues as rapidly as is possible without application of pressure to try to increase the speed. If the needle electrode or loop bends as it is drawn through the tissues it indicates either that manual pressure has been applied unnecessarily, or that an inadequate current output has been used to permit maximum speed of cell disintegration, or, most commonly, the combination of both.

The operator's control of the instrument is not reduced when pressure is carefully avoided. Indeed, to the contrary, effective control is not possible when pressure is applied. When cutting with an activated electrode it is important to remember that the RF energy is doing the cutting for us, and therefore our function is limited to directing the energy to create the desired tissue cleavage and to controlling the depth to which *we* permit the electrode to penetrate into the tissues. If it is left to its own devices, the current tries to penetrate through the entire thickness of the tissue intervening between the surgical electrode and the indifferent plate. The operator must therefore be able to control the depth of penetration so as to be able to create incisions ranging in depth from small fractions of a millimeter to the total depth of the tissue being treated.

The ability to control the depth of incision is well demonstrated in Figures 5–23 through 5–25. In Figure 5–23A we see a slice of beef with two fairly deep incisions side by side that have been made with a needle electrode. Both incisions had been made through a thin surface terminal portion of fascial sheath of the muscle, and we see a very superficial incision intended to penetrate through the fascial sheath without penetration into the underlying muscle tissue being performed with a fine needle electrode. In Figure 5–23B we see that the incision has penetrated the precise depth of the thickness of the thin surface fascial sheath, without penetrating into the underlying tissue.

Figures 5–23A and B demonstrate the ability to limit the depth of penetration when cutting through relatively fibrous tissue. Figures 5–24A and B demonstrate that comparable control of depth of penetration can be maintained even when the tissue being cut is only microns in thickness, translucent, and extremely delicate. Figure 5–24A shows a piece of meat with an extremely thin delicate membrane covering the muscle. The membrane has been pulled taut so that it can be visualized. Figure 5–24B shows the incision of the membrane with the needle electrode, and we see that the surface membrane has been successfully incised without penetrating a second equally thin and delicate membrane that remains intact over the muscle tissue. Total control of depth of penetration of the cutting effect is invaluable in developing the dexterity and skill of instrumentation that is so important to successful electrosurgery. However, it has definite clinical usefulness as well as technique practice usefulness, since this is the type of depth penetration control that is essential when incising the surface epithelium of the vermilion mucosa of the lip in order to enucleate a mucocele, or similar precise, delicate surgical incisions. Such control can be achieved through repeated painstaking practice.

Electrosurgery is remarkably effective for cutting soft tissue but is completely ineffectual for cutting bone. Thus, when it is necessary to make an incision for a mucoperiosteal flap, the need to control the depth of penetration of the incision is eliminated, since as soon as the electrode penetrates through the soft tissue and makes contact with the underlying bone, it cannot penetrate further. Thus, for mucoperiosteal incisions, all that need be done is to permit the electrode to penetrate as deeply as it can, while drawing it across

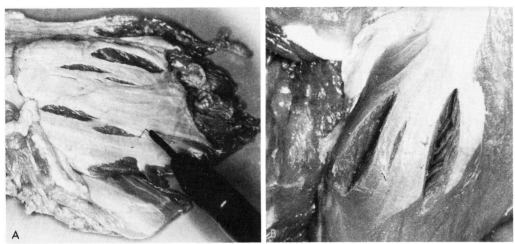

Figure 5-23. A, A very shallow incision being created through a thin but fibrous tendinous muscle sheath with a 90-degree-angle fine needle electrode. The depth of incision is being controlled to permit incision through the tendinous sheath without cutting into the underlying muscle fibers. *B*, The slab of meat with three incisions through the tendinous sheath of different depths. The center incision has cut through the tendinous sheath without cutting into the muscle fibers beneath it. The left hand incision is approximately 0.5 cm. deep, and the one on the right side is approximately 1.5 cm. deep. The depth of each incision was predetermined and precisely controlled. Each incision showed the characteristic remarkably smooth cut margin surfaces and total absence of clinical evidence of coagulation.

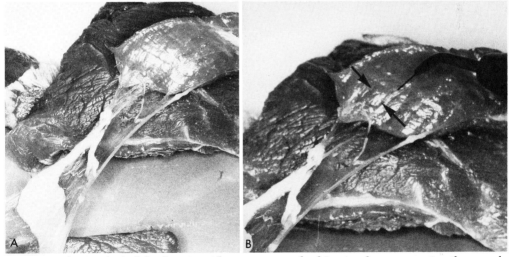

Figure 5-24. A, A slab of meat with a transparently thin membrane covering the muscle fibers. *B*, The surface membrane being incised with a fine 45-degree angle needle electrode. The depth of incision is being controlled to permit incision through the surface membrane without cutting into the muscle fibers, and *without cutting through a second covering membrane.* Arrows to incision.

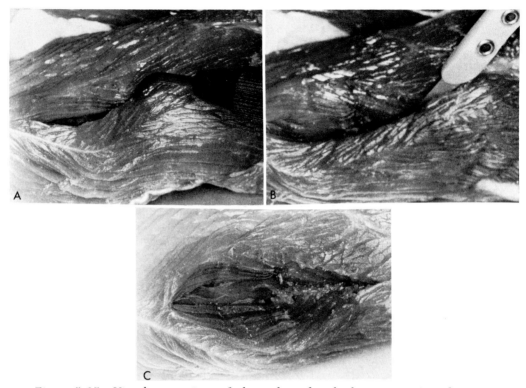

Figure 5-25. Visual comparison of electrode and scalpel incisions. *A*, A deep incision being made by electrosection with fully rectified cutting current with a 45-degree angle fine needle electrode. *B*, The incision being extended by manual cutting with a new Bard-Parker disposable scalpel. *C*, The incision spread wide shows the total absence of coagulation from the part of the incision created by electrosection, and the smooth character of the tissue surface that had been cut with the electrode, in contrast to the slightly rough irregular appearance of the tissue cut with the steel scalpel.

and through the tissue it has penetrated as quickly as possible without bending the electrode by exerting manual pressure to do so.

Reference has been made repeatedly to the traumatic nature of steel scalpel incisions, and the totally atraumatic nature of incisions by electrosection. The contrast in the character of the incision by electrosection and that by steel scalpel is admirably demonstrated in Figure 5–25. Figure 5–25*A* shows an incision being made with a needle electrode by electrosection. Figure 5–25*B* shows the incision being extended with a new Bard-Parker disposable steel scalpel, and Figure 5–25*C* shows the appearance of the respective portions of the incised tissue. The atraumatic character of the electrosurgical incision is demonstrated by the remarkable smoothness of the cut tissue surfaces and the precise sharp line of cleavage, whereas the incision with the scalpel is seen to have created a slightly ragged line of incision and rough surfaces of cut tissue. The total absence of clinical coagulation of the tissue cut by electrosection is noteworthy and clearly demonstrated.

Section Three

ELECTROSURGICAL RESEARCH

PART 1

INDICATIONS AND STANDARDS FOR RESEARCH

Introduction

Research is basic to developing excellence in dentistry. We must continually strive to improve our knowledge in diagnosis and treatment procedures. Many procedures have developed empirically and must be confirmed, improved, or corrected through clinical and basic research.

A well-structured research investigation always provides some meaningful information. A negative result does not necessarily indicate failure of a project, since useful information is usually obtained. Significant results, either positive or negative, can lead to additional investigations of value and often provide improved treatment procedures. For example, several investigations have shown that certain chemicals used in tissue retraction are damaging to the sulcus epithelium and that other chemicals incorporated into retraction cords are not injurious. Thus, the clinician can use certain chemicals in displacing tissue to expose the cavity margin for elastic impression procedures without fear of tissue damage or recession. Clinical and histologic investigation has shown that electrosurgery can be used more effectively and safely for tissue troughing to expose the cavity margin.

The important factor in a research investigation is a "control" with which to compare the results of the study. Since a material, procedure, or instrument under investigation can be improperly applied and provide misleading results, such a "control" is a necessity. In electrosurgical research, as in all other research, the instrument must be used correctly if the study is to be scientifically accurate and meaningful.

A correctly structured research investigation states the problem to be solved, the methods and materials used to complete the project, the control or norm used for interpretation of the results, and the results themselves. Therefore, the reader knows "how" and "why" the investigation was done and provides the clinician with a valid base for evaluation of the results.

JAMES D. HARRISON

135

Chapter Six

RELATIONSHIP OF RESEARCH TO CLINICAL ELECTROSURGERY

The author became aware of the interdependence of clinical electrosurgery and research at the very outset of his involvement with the modality more than a quarter of a century ago.

There were no reliable instruction manuals on dental electrosurgery at that time, and there was very little written about dental electrosurgery in the current literature. A survey of the then existing dental and medical literature revealed that the few electrosurgical techniques being used in dentistry were predicated largely upon techniques developed by physicians for medical electrosurgery.

In view of the vast difference in the characteristics of gingival tissue and other oral mucosa with skin and skeletal musculature, the techniques being used did not appear ideally suited for use on the tissues of the mouth. Equally disturbing was the fact that both the medical and dental literature stressed the admonition to avoid cutting into the tissues more than once with the electrode to make an incision. Despite the universality of this admonition there were no accompanying explanations for why repetition of an incision must be avoided.

A very large part of dental electrosurgery is performed on gingival tissue. The gingival architecture is irregular. It is therefore not conducive to efficient instrumentation with a single stroke of the cutting electrode. Inability to repeat the cutting would restrict the usefulness of electrosurgery for dentistry so much that it would scarcely be worthwhile, since it would limit its use essentially to creation of simple incisions for drainage, and simple short shallow straight line incisions into the tissues.

Inasmuch as no reasons were advanced for the admonition to refrain from duplicating the cutting stroke, the author proceeded to do so experimentally to try to establish the rationale for the admonition. His initial experiments were performed on a slab of beef. He noted that when the cutting was repeated immediately, without an interval of time lapse, the tissue margins showed evidence of coagulation or charring. When the cutting was performed with fully rectified current, and the current was applied for a few seconds and followed by a few seconds of time interval before being repeated, no demonstrable unfavorable effects resulted. However, when the same was done with partially rectified current, the cut margins showed clinical evidence of surface coagulation.

He then proceeded to repeat the experiment on live tissue, first on a dog, then on a rhesus monkey. Both animals responded favorably to the cutting stroke repetition, and both proceeded to heal favorably where the cutting current application was limited to 2 to 3 seconds followed by a time lapse of equal duration. Both animals appeared to be free of distress or ill effects from the repeated experimental cutting and showed no clinical evidence of scar tissue repair.

These observations subsequently led to his development of the technique of planing the tissues with a loop electrode to reduce the bulk and simultaneously recontour the tissues. This eliminated need to resort to block dissection of a wedge of tissue, undermining the adjacent tissues, and attempting to coapt the margins and suture them in the hope of achieving primary repair.

The apparent effectiveness of the formula of current application for 2 to 3 seconds followed by a comparable period of time lapse before resuming the cutting or coagulating action that resulted from these early experiments led over the years to his developing the innumerable other techniques now in use, which until quite recently were based on clinical evidence alone.

For many years lack of experimental facilities and qualified research personnel made it impossible to substantiate histologically the clinical evidence of the remarkable safety and efficacy of competent electronic electrosurgery. Until these became available we could only deduce, theorize, or empirically hypothesize, on the basis of clinical observation and experience, how and why favorable and unfavorable electrosurgical phenomena occurred. Thus for a long time it was impossible to prove indisputably that fully rectified current does not burn tissue when properly utilized. It was equally impossible to prove that fully rectified current is more suitable than partially rectified current for treatment of gingival and other mucous tissues.

Happily, all that is past. Research facilities and personnel are becoming increasingly available. The problem now is to make certain that the research is unbiased, is scientifically accurate, and contributes to better electrosurgery and better dentistry.

GROUND RULES FOR RESEARCH

Mark Twain was, in his inimitably humorous way, a rather profound philosopher. One of his philosophically humorous gems was "T'ain't what we *don't* know that's bad, but what we *know*, that just *ain't so!*"

This aphorism is particularly applicable to the myths and misinformation about dental electrosurgery that still crop up from time to time, in one form or another, even in such unlikely places as laboratory research.

Like General MacArthur's "old soldiers," myths and misinformation never die; but unlike them, they do not fade away. Fear engendered by these twin enemies of progress continues to be the main reason why many dentists continue to deny themselves, and their patients, the innumerable and invaluable advantages that electrosurgery can offer.

These deterrents to progress are diminishing steadily, but traces of them, nurtured by occasional blurbs of misinformation, still linger on. Although it is true that the misinformation is not always mischievously inspired, good intentions often only add to the difficulty of coping with it.

Although research is unique in many respects, it shares one thing with all other spheres of activity. It is subject to and influenced by variables. When these variables exist, they must be recognized and taken into account, and allowances must be made for them.

By the same token, research is also governed by a number of constants—ground rules that never vary. One rule is that no investigator regardless of his or her professional prestige or skill in other disciplines, can improve on the maximum performance or efficacy of the electrosurgical modality or technique being evaluated, regardless of his technical skills. The other side of the coin is, of course, that lack of proper skill can degrade and unfavorably alter the performance.

These factors lead, by logical sequence, to another constant: When an investigation is in the nature of a comparative evaluation and the investigator is not fully qualified to conduct such an investigation, his results become misleading and scientifically invalid.

When multiple comparative investigations of a relatively identical nature are conducted and the respective investigators arrive at completely opposite conclusions, with one reporting unfavorable results and the other reporting unimpeachable, histologically substantiated favorable results, there can be but one conclusion. Obviously, the investigator who reports unfavorable results has failed to utilize the modalities or techniques being investigated skillfully enough to achieve maximum efficacy of performance.

There have been several instances in the recent literature in which the investigators reported results completely opposite from the results being reported here. It is regrettable that the investigators are respected and the publications in which the reports appeared are ethical responsible journals, since that makes it so much more difficult to counteract the effect on the profession of their unfavorable experimental conclusions.

Two typical examples were published in responsible journals in recent years. One, a comparative evaluation of electrosurgical versus steel knife wound healing, purported to be an evaluation of electrosection with fully rectified current. Yet the equipment listed as used in the investigation, a Cameron-Miller #255 unit, is listed by the manufacturer as a partially rectified unit that is incapable of delivering fully rectified current. Moreover, the results described are compatible with results obtained with partially rectified currents.[1] Despite this misleading information, the report is frequently quoted as a reference.

An investigator in another, more recent report defended the results of the investigation and conclusions predicated thereon on the basis of electrosurgical experience and favorable results achieved in a shallow soft tissue cutting phase of the investigation.[2]

To dogmatically equate experience with expertise is specious reasoning. Experience is essentially quantitative, relating to time. One can use electrosurgery with indifferent skill for a long time and qualify as "experienced." Expertise, on the other hand, is a qualitative factor, relating to skill and know-how acquired through *special training* plus experience.

This investigator's assumption that a favorable result with use of electrosection for shallow soft tissue cutting is infallible evidence of skill and know-how is equally specious. Unless the tissues are abused unconscionably, shallow soft tissue cutting by electrosection without coming into contact with bone is highly unlikely to cause irreversible or even appreciable damage such as sloughing of tissue and sequestration of bone. Thus, favorable results are very likely despite lack of expertise. When the cutting by electrosection is performed on tissue and the activated electrode comes into contact with *bone*, comparable lack of expertise is very likely to result in tissue sloughing, bone sequestration, and irreversible gingival recession. It is therefore entirely possible to achieve a favorable result when dealing with soft tissue alone, despite a lack of expertise, but it is highly unlikely to be able to achieve comparable results when bone is involved, in the absence of an expert's skill and know-how.

The fact that comparable comparative investigations, soundly structured and skillfully conducted by qualified investigators, have repeatedly achieved histologically proved favorable results even when the electrodes contacted bone tends to fully substantiate this.

It becomes inescapable that the basic criteria for conducting scientifically meaningful accurate comparative evaluations of electrosurgical instrumentation with any other methods of instrumentation must include, in addition to the other ingredients that make up the efficient investigator, the following:

1. Use of proper item purportedly being investigated.
2. Comparably trained skilled instrumentation with all the methods under investigation.

Electrosurgical instrumentation is entirely different from manual instrumentation with the steel cutting instruments. The results achieved with electronic cutting with fully rectified current reflect the efficiency with which the modality is used rather than the capabilities of the modality. Thus, no matter how skillful one may be in other disciplines or with other methods, unless equally skilled in both, the results must be attributed to the deficiencies of the user and not of the modality. It is unfortunate that high degree of skill with other methods of instrumentation fails to alter this, and cannot substitute for efficient, knowledgeable electrosurgical technique.

Research is relatively infinite in scope. Nevertheless, it falls into the following categories:

1. Abstract Laboratory Experimentation

2. Clinical Laboratory Experimentation
   a. Clinical experimentation
   b. Combined clinical and clinical laboratory experimentation

"Ars Gratia Artis"—art for art's sake—has for many years been the attractive slogan of a major motion picture company. But even the motion picture industry, as a whole, has found this philosophy thoroughly impractical.

A philosophy of pure research, that is, research for its own sake, with no regard to practical application or significance, is equally impractical. Research cannot be divorced from practical considerations. The most esoteric abstract type of research, with surprising frequency, ultimately is reciprocal with realistic practical usefulness. Thus, most of the important technical advances, from the radio to atomic energy and nuclear fission to the laser, have resulted from abstract research. Yet some dental research investigators appear to follow this chimerical philosophy of esoteric research with apparent disregard for practical application.

To the author, as a clinician interested in the practical contributions that research can make toward better dentistry, research for its own sake is a waste of facilities, funding, and trained personnel man-hours of effort.

Regardless of whether research is in the form of clinical investigation and evaluation or of laboratory investigation and evaluation, the ultimate objective of dental research should be its contributions to better dentistry. All the research reported in this chapter, clinical and laboratory, fulfills this objective.

Methodology for conducting experimental investigations is as diverse as is the subject matter. Thus there can be no single formalized blueprint formula that a research study must follow. However, all the investigations being reported here do have one common denominator: all were conducted by investigators who were trained to use the electrosurgical currents competently.

Only the first three of the investigations being reported were conducted by the author. All the others were performed by colleagues who have been kind enough to provide the author with their research data. In several instances the data are original and are being published here for the first time.

Uniformity in presentation of these investigations is difficult owing to the variations in the amount of data provided by each contributor. Thus there will be some degree of difference in the comprehensiveness of the reports. When necessary, the author has interjected obvious conclusions based on the research findings.

Since all things must have a beginning, a logical starting point for this review of electrosurgical research appears to be investigation of the behavioral characteristics of the electrosurgical currents used in dentistry.

FOOTNOTE REFERENCES

1. Pope, J. W., Gargiulo, A. W., Staffileno, H., and Levy, S.: Effects of electrosurgery on wound healing in dogs. Periodontics, 6:30, Nov. 1, 1968.
2. Glickman, I., and Imber, T. R.: Comparison of gingival resection with electrosurgery and periodontal knives—A biometric study. J. Periodont., 41:142, 1970.

EXPERIMENTAL RESEARCH REPORTS

Chapter Seven

BEHAVIORAL RESEARCH

1. INVESTIGATIONS OF BEHAVIORAL CHARACTERISTICS OF THE ELECTROSURGICAL CURRENTS

Comparative Evaluation of Fulguration with Oudin Spark-Gap and Simulated Spark-Gap Current

As a rule genuine things are superior to imitations. But apparently there are exceptions to every rule, one of which the author had observed with regard to one of the therapeutic electrosurgical currents.

Clinical evidence suggested that fulguration performed with simulated spark-gap current appeared to be more efficient, better suited, and easier to manage for dental therapy than fulguration performed with Oudin current sparks produced by spark-gap generators.

141

The clinical evidence was predicated on two factors:

1. Although the true Oudin sparks are larger and can jump across a wider air-space between the electrode tip and the tissue surface, the surface dehydration produced by these sparks usually appeared inadequate to actually carbonize the surface layers of cells, but instead tended to form a tough, leathery eschar. The eschar then appeared to act as an insulator that prevented destruction of undesirable tissue beyond it. The simulated sparks carbonized the tissue and continued to do so as long as the sparks were directed toward the tissue, so that all undesirable tissue could be destroyed in depth, without any clinical evidence of undue lateral heat transmission or undesirable tissue damage.

2. When fulguration is required in confined areas, the Oudin current sparks, owing to their larger size and ability to leap from the electrode tip to the tissue surface, tend to bounce off the tissue and spatter over adjacent teeth or bone. Thus, when the Oudin sparks are directed into an embrasure toward the interdental papilla, they spatter over the adjacent teeth. Needless to say, if metal fillings or other metal restorations are present, the sparking becomes distinctly violent.

Although these clinical impressions were consistent and distinct, the evidence remained somewhat inconclusive because the currents being produced by different equipment were not used concurrently on adjacent teeth or tissues. To overcome this, the author, in addition to his regular stock model of the Coles Radiosurg Electronic Scalpel IV unit (Fig. 7-1-1A), had a special experimental unit built for his use by the Coles Electronic Company. This unit combined the typical Coles Radiosurg Electronic Scalpel IV circuit, which provides the mutated simulated spark-gap circuit, with a true Oudin spark-gap generator housed within the same unit (Fig. 7-1-1B), so that either the true or simulated current provided by this unit could be used interchangeably.

The two currents were then used in adjacent embrasures and also to destroy necrotic or cystic tissue shreds in areas offering only extremely difficult access; for the typical uses of fulgurating current in dentistry, such as destroying fistulous orifices and their tracts down to alveolar bone; and in bifurcation and trifurcation involvements and infrabony pockets, on adjacent teeth or in respective quadrants, so that accurate comparative evaluation of the results achieved with the respective currents could be made.

These tests confirmed the previous clinical findings, and in most instances in which the undesirable tissue penetrated deeply and had to be destroyed in depth, treatment with the Oudin spark fulguration failed and the tissue had to be reoperated, so that it could be completely and effectively eliminated.

CONCLUSIONS

The results observed in this experiment offer conclusive evidence that the simulated sparking is better suited for dental fulguration than is the sparking Oudin current of the spark-gap generator.

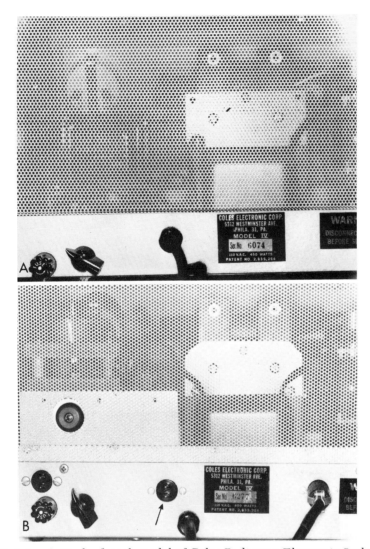

Figure 7–1–1. A, Back of stock model of Coles Radiosurg Electronic Scalpel IV. B, Experimental unit that contains an additional true Oudin spark-gap generator circuit in the same housing (see text). Arrow points to Oudin circuit.

Oscilloscopic Evaluation of Fully Rectified Cutting Currents

Three objectives motivated the author to conduct this investigation:

1. To obtain photographs of the waveform images produced by different fully rectified circuits from the fluorescent screen of an oscilloscope.

2. To ascertain whether fully rectified currents are identical in all respects or whether they differ electronically and in the efficiency of their clinical performance, despite the fact that they all deliver fully rectified RF current.

3. To compare the waveform patterns and efficiency of clinical performance of fully rectified cutting current with that of fully rectified and fully filtered constant wave cutting current.

The equipment and materials used in the investigation included

a. A Tektronix oscilloscope.
b. Fully rectified electrosurgical units A and B.
c. Fully rectified and fully filtered electrosurgical unit C.
d. Two identical 45-degree-angle fine needle electrodes.
e. Two identical round loop electrodes, 10 mm. in diameter.
f. Clinical camera (Exakta VX 1000, with Steinheil Macro-Quinon 55 mm. f. 1.9 lens).
g. Two similar slices of raw beef (shoulder-shin beef, 1 in. x 3 in. x 5 in.).

Identical power settings on the instrument panel power output dials were used with the three units in each of the series of experiments to be described.

Inasmuch as this investigation was not conducted as a comparative evaluation of *all* the fully rectified electrosurgical units that are now available to the profession, and was neither conceived nor initiated for that purpose, the units that were used in these experiments are designated as units A, B and C, instead of by their trade names.

The oscilloscope was connected to a wall socket and activated. Unit A was connected to the oscilloscope and a fine needle electrode was locked into its surgical handpiece. The unit was activated, its cutting current circuit was activated, and several incisions were made into the slice of beef, with cutting current power output set at 3 on the dial. As soon as the cutting current was activated, a pattern of wavy lines appeared on the fluorescent screen of the oscilloscope. These lines produced the characteristic waveform image of fully rectified current as it has been diagrammatically visualized in electronics. This oscilloscopic image was photographed by the author.*

Unit A was deactivated, and unit B was connected to the oscilloscope. The second fine needle electrode was locked into its surgical handpiece and the cutting power output set at 3 on the instrument panel dial. The unit was activated, the cutting current circuit was activated, and several incisions were made into the slice of beef. The wavy lines formed a slightly different waveform image, in that there was more space between the individual oscillations and less oscillations in a half-cycle envelope.

Unit A was then reconnected to the oscilloscope and both cutting current circuits were simultaneously activated, producing simultaneous images of their respective waveforms on the oscilloscope screen (Fig. 7–1–2A).

Unit B was then disconnected from the oscilloscope and replaced with unit C, and the needle electrode was transferred from the surgical handpiece of unit B to that of unit C. Cutting power output was set at 3 on the power output panel dial, the unit was activated, the cutting current circuit was activated, and several incisions were made into the slice of beef. The cutting current from this unit produced a waveform pattern on the oscilloscope screen that differed from the waveform images produced by units A and B, in that the constrictions at the beginning and end of each half-cycle of fully rectified current

---

*Each set of photographs for each experiment was taken at the same lens opening and shutter speed, and the oscilloscope settings were identical for each set of photographs.

flow were missing, so that there was no interruption in the amplitude of the current. Instead, there was a continuous, uniform, uninterrupted current amplitude (Fig. 7–1–2B).

Units A and C were then both activated, power output of both set at 3, and their cutting current circuits activated simultaneously. The cutting currents produced by the two units created their respective waveform images simultaneously on the oscilloscope screen and were photographed (Fig. 7–1–2C).

All the experiments that have been described were then repeated with the power output settings increased uniformly on the respective units one full degree on the dial each time until the maximum output, 10, was reached. The differences in waveform image continued to be manifested proportionally.

The experiments were then repeated, with the round loop electrodes replacing the needle electrodes. Cutting current output with unit A failed to provide enough power to cut into the tissue at all until the dial setting was increased to 5. At that setting the edge of the electrode penetrated slowly into the tissue about 1 mm. and stopped. The tissue in contact with the electrode turned white and adhered tenaciously to the electrode when the latter was lifted from the tissue surface. When the current output was increased to 6 and the electrode was applied to the tissue at an approximate 45-degree angle to the surface, a slice of tissue approximately 3 mm. in thickness was sheared off cleanly, without visible evidence of coagulation and with no tissue shreds adhering to the electrode. When the electrode was applied to the tissues at a 90-degree angle and a thick slice of tissue was engaged, the electrode penetrated about 2 mm. and stopped, unable to cut through the tissue. When the current output was increased to 8, the electrode, applied to the tissue surface at 90-degree angulation, sheared out a slice of tissue about 6 mm. thick, cleanly, effortlessly, and rapidly, without evidence of coagulation and without tissue shreds adhering to the electrode. When the current output was increased to 10 (maximum), some sparking and smokelike fumes were produced when the electrode made contact, and the cut margins appeared brownish and seared instead of the natural fresh color evident when the cutting was done with less current.

The experiment was then repeated with unit B. When the electrode was held at a 45-degree angle to the tissue surface it failed to penetrate into the tissue until the current output was set at 8. Up until then, each time the electrode made contact the cutting current pilot light on the instrument panel became completely dimmed, and the electrode glanced off the tissue surface as it was applied with the required wiping motion. With the current power output set at 8, the pilot light became somewhat less dim and the edge of the loop penetrated into the tissue approximately 2 mm. at which point its progress stopped and the tissue around the electrode became white and adhered tenaciously to the electrode when the latter was lifted from the tissue surface. When the current output was set at 9, the electrode penetrated about 5 mm. before it stopped, and again the tissue around the electrode turned white and adhered tenaciously. When the current power output was set at 10 (maximum) the electrode penetrated into the tissues slowly, with most of the

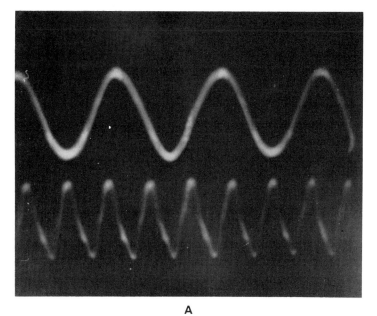

A

B

Figure 7–1–2. A, Characteristic waveform of fully rectified current from unit A *(top)* and waveform produced by unit B, at same power setting, showing alteration in number of waves per envelope *(bottom)*. B, Waveform produced by unit C.

(Illustration continued on opposite page)

advance being the result of exertion of physical pull great enough to distort the electrode into a slightly elliptical shape. The tissue segment that was removed, and the base from which it came were both white in color due to coagulation. When the electrode was applied to the tissues at a 90-degree angle and excision of a thick slice of tissue was attempted, the loop was unable to penetrate more than about 2 mm., even with the maximum current output.

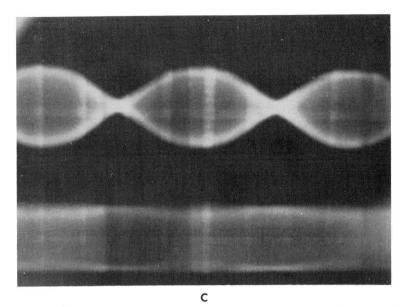

C

Figure 7-1-2. Continued.   C, Simultaneous waveform patterns of units A *(top)* and C *(bottom).*

The entire experiment was then repeated with unit C, with almost identical results. With the electrode applied to the tissues at a 45-degree angle and maximum power setting, the electrode sheared off a slice of tissue about 3 mm. thick a little more rapidly and effortlessly than with unit B, but the tissue turned white and adhered tenaciously to the electrode. When the electrode was held at a 90-degree angle to the tissue and excision of a thick slice of tissue was attempted, the current's power output at the maximum setting (10) failed to cut through, but, as had occurred with unit B, it penetrated only a few millimeters and was unable to progress further, even with considerable physical pull applied. And, as had occurred with unit B, the tissue turned white and adhered tenaciously to the electrode.

SUMMARY AND CONCLUSIONS

Identical experiments were performed with three different electrosurgical units that produce fully rectified currents. One of the three also provides fully filtered current. The same amount of current power output was used with all three in each of the experiments. Identical electrodes and slices of beef were used for each unit in each experiment. The same oscilloscope was used in all the experiments. The same camera, lens opening, and shutter speeds were used for all three units in each experiment.

Despite the identical operative conditions and despite the fact that all three units provide fully rectified currents, differences in their respective waveform patterns as well as in the cutting efficiency of the currents were noted. Units A and B differed electronically in their current density; when visualized on the oscilloscope, the number of oscillations differed within an equal period of time and within each individual half-cycle of current. Unit C differed in waveform from both A and B, with more continuous uniform amplitude, denoting a smoother continuity of cutting current output. Clinically, however, the efficiency of the cutting current of unit C was not appreciably greater than that of unit B, and the current output of neither unit B nor unit C proved as efficient as that of unit A. This was observed not only on the basis of the cutting performance with the loop electrode but even when the needle electrode was used. Although all three cutting currents appeared to be adequately potent to cut the tissue effortlessly and rapidly with the fine needle electrode, on examination it was noted that the electrode used with current from unit A was totally free of adherent tissue shreds whereas with current from both units B and C, a thin film of tissue was found tenaciously adherent to the electrode after use, although the tissue had appeared to be cleanly cut.

The results indicate that the ability to cut into normal tissue with a needle electrode is not an effective means for determining the efficiency of an electrosurgical cutting current, and that cutting with a loop electrode of medium to large diameter is much more revealing.

The different electronic and clinical values produced by these fully rectified currents provided by different fully rectified circuits, despite identical current output settings and identical clinical conditions, appear to prove conclusively that fully rectified currents produced by different electrosurgical circuits *do* vary in potency and efficiency of performance.

Full rectification of the cutting current remains the fundamental prerequisite for dental electrosurgery. But this is obviously not the sole criterion. Nor does it ensure that because the currents are fully rectified they automatically become functionally equal and suitable for dental electrosurgery. It indicates that even full current filtration, although perhaps desirable, does not determine or materially influence the potency and efficiency of the cutting current.

The results of this investigation substantiate the author's premise, based on clinical observation, that when the cutting current is sufficiently powerful to match the resistance offered by the tissues, it will perform most efficiently, be most self-limiting in its destructiveness, and be most completely under the operator's control at all times.

Evaluation of the Role of Biterminal Current Application

The author conducted this experiment to demonstrate three separate but closely related electrosurgical phenomena:

1. To demonstrate visually the function of the indifferent plate and the role of biterminal application of fully rectified cutting current.

2. To demonstrate the need to activate the surgical electrode before making contact with the tissues.

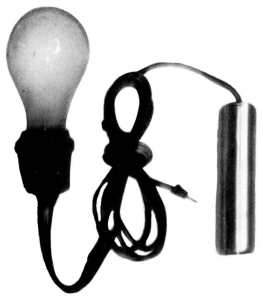

Figure 7-1-3. The hand electrode, rubber socket, and light bulb assembly used in this experiment.

3. To demonstrate the role that impedance (tissue resistance) plays in the electrosurgical cutting phenomenon.

The following equipment was used in the experiment:

a. A Coles Radiosurg Electronic Scalpel fully rectified electrosurgical unit.

b. A hard rubber electric light socket with twin lead wires, and a 75-watt bulb. One lead wire is attached to a male jack to fit the unit's cutting current circuit; the other is attached to a cylindrical metal hand electrode (Fig. 7-1-3).

c. The flat metal indifferent plate supplied with the unit.

The unit was activated and the male jack was plugged into the cutting current circuit on the instrument panel. The cutting current power output was set at 4, with the cylindrical hand electrode in the right hand and the rubber socket and light bulb in the left hand, and the circuit was activated. After approximately 3 seconds the filament in the electric light bulb began to glow dimly (see Color Plate I). The left hand was then placed on the indifferent plate, which had been attached to the conductive circuit of the unit, and immediately the filament glow intensified greatly. The left hand was removed from the indifferent plate, and immediately the filament glow became dim again. The experiment was then repeated, but this time the right hand, holding the hand electrode, was placed on the indifferent plate, to permit the author to photograph the result, with the same results, except that the filament glow appeared somewhat brighter (see Color Plate I, Fig. 8). Again, as soon as the hand was removed from the indifferent plate the filament glow immediately became greatly diminished.

The experiment was then repeated once again, only this time the contact with the indifferent plate was made before the cutting current circuit was activated, and the filament glow was almost immediately at maximum degree.

Since the same amount of power output of cutting current was used each time, this simple experiment proves that the direct current return flow to the power generator via the indifferent electrode greatly increases the current density or potency; in the case of the light bulb, a much brighter and more instantaneous glow resulted. When the same power output was applied monoterminally, with indirect current return flow by way of the earth ground connection instead of via the indifferent plate, much less current density resulted, and the current flow was much slower as seen in the dimmer glow and slower onset.

SUMMARY AND CONCLUSIONS

The results of this experiment, translated into practical clinical terms, indicate that although it is possible to produce a monoterminal flow of cutting current by omitting the indifferent plate from the circuit, the density or potency of the current is significantly diminished. Thus, clinically, if the tissue to be cut is thick, dense, engorged, or edematous, or when the cutting procedure will require use of a large loop type of electrode, the monoterminal current application would be inadequate to perform cutting efficiently, if indeed at all, if the indifferent plate were omitted from the circuit.

The difference in speed with which the power output is delivered also has distinct clinical significance. Nevertheless, although the maximum power output is much more rapid with the biterminal application of current, the slight time-lag before maximum power is attained proves the need to always activate the surgical electrode before applying it to the tissues to make sure that the maximum power output has been attained before contact is made.

When the large hand electrode was introduced into the cutting current circuit, it became a surgical electrode; however, no perceptible heat was generated from it into the hand that was holding it. This is because the area of contact with the large hand electrode is so large that there is no appreciable increase in impedance and therefore no increased concentration of the RF current to convert it into heat energy.

If a small surgical electrode were held in the hand in the same manner, owing to the far smaller area of contact, and if the cutting current were activated and delivered monoterminally, the current density, although it might not be great enough to cut the tissues, would scorch them. If the current were applied biterminally through the indifferent plate, the electrode would, of course, cut into the tissues of the hand holding it.

The cutting effect, therefore, must be attributed to the increase in impedance. Obviously, the smaller the surgical electrode, the greater will be the impedance and concentration of current at the contact site. The fine needle electrode, which presents the smallest possible contact site, therefore requires the least amount of current density to cut efficiently. The larger the electrode used, the greater the area of contact and the less the concentration of current at the site of contact, hence the greater the amount of current density to compensate for the decrease in heat concentration.

This explains why acceptable cutting can be achieved with a fine needle electrode with a cutting current circuit that does not produce very potent cutting power output. But, when this current is used with a moderately large loop electrode that makes contact over a fairly wide area of tissue, and the concentration is much less at the site of contact, the current is not powerful enough to disintegrate and volatilize the tissue cells as it makes contact, and it either fails to cut the tissues or causes tissue coagulation instead of cellular disintegration and volatilization.

The same condition results when the tissues require more than the average amount of cutting power for efficient electrosurgery on normal gingival tissue. It is also the reason why monoterminal application of the current under such conditions would be completely ineffectual.

2. CARDIAC RESPONSES TO ELECTROSURGERY

by James D. Harrison, D.D.S., and William J. Kelly, Jr., D.D.S.

It has been suggested that the electrosurgical currents at higher intensity settings might produce cardiac arrhythmias or complete cardiac arrest. The purpose of this investigation was to see whether electrosurgical techniques could cause any deviations in heart patterns of dogs being continuously monitored on a physiological recorder.

Dogs were anesthetized with phenobarbital and continuously monitored before, during, and after each electrosurgical procedure by a continuous electrocardiogram (EKG) pen recorder. Tissue electrodes for the EKG monitoring were placed over the right and left rib cage and the indifferent or dispersive plate and the active electrode of the surgery unit applied over different areas of the chest, neck, and head. Coagulation and electrosection current was applied, raising the current from minimum to maximum intensity.

DISCUSSION. The following areas of electrode application were used:

Dispersive Plate Area	Electrode Area
Right Rib Cage	Left Rib Cage
Left Rib Cage	Right Rib Cage
Left Front Paw	Right Front Paw
Right Front Paw	Left Front Paw
Left Front Paw	Left Rib Cage
Spine	Left Rib Cage
Spine	Right Rib Cage
Spine	Oral Mucosa
No Plate	Left Rib Cage

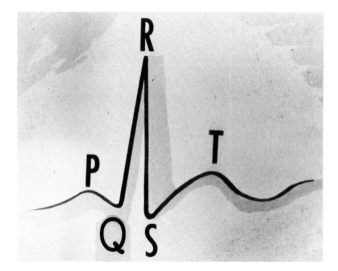

Figure 7-2-1.   A normal electrocardiogram.

The normal EKG is shown in Figure 7-2-1. The P wave results as the atria depolarizes to contract and this is followed by the QRS complex wave, which is recorded by the currents generated when the ventricles depolarize prior to contraction. The T wave or repolarization wave is caused by currents generated as the ventricles recover from the state of depolarization, and the vagus nerve is parasympathetic inhibitor to the heart.* The Q waves in Figures 7-2-2 and 7-2-3 are not prominent because of the electrode position for EKG recording. The results of this investigation were essentially negative.

---

*Guyton, A. C.: Textbook of Medical Physiology. 4th Ed. Philadelphia, W. B. Saunders Co., 1966.

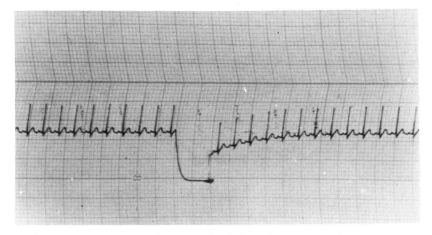

Figure 7-2-2.   An EKG recording: on the left is the monitored pattern; in the center, a short activation of the electrosurgical machine; and on the right, the continued pattern.

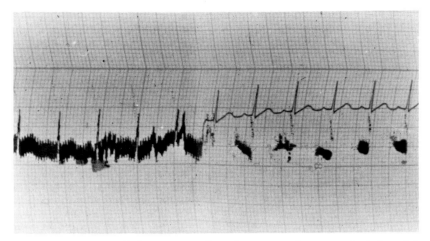

Figure 7–2–3. Prolonged electrosurgical application is shown on the left and the normal EKG pattern on the right.

There was essentially no change in wave magnitude, the time interval change is very slight, and no P or T wave inversion was observed. There was some T wave dimension change; however, this could be attributed to stress. The respiration rate remained essentially unchanged and as the machine's intensity was increased, no heart blockage, fibrillation, or cardiac arrhythmias were noted. The heart rate remained at 120 plus or minus 5 beats per minute.

CONCLUSION. The energy or current is at a high enough frequency so that no physiologic effects on polarization or depolarization of the heart tissue could be observed.

Chapter Eight

LABORATORY EXPERIMENTAL EVALUATION OF EFFICACY OF CLINICAL ELECTROSURGICAL TECHNIQUES

1. HEAT GENERATION AND PENETRATION IN GINGIVAL TISSUES USING ELECTROSURGICAL CURRENTS

by William J. Kelly, Jr., D.D.S., and James D. Harrison, D.D.S.

Introduction

Although various forms of electrocautery had been used prior to the 1920's, the discovery of the three-element vacuum tube by DeForest made possible the development of the electronic scalpel. This electronic scalpel or radioknife uses a high-frequency current which causes a disintegration of the tissue when the activated electrode is drawn across the surgical area.

The principle of electrosurgery is based upon the utilization of an alternating current oscillating at a sufficiently high frequency so that it can be passed through living tissues without shock. When this current radiates through the tissue, it meets resistance to its passage and some heat is produced within the tissues. The type of current and method of application determines the amount of heat generated. Literature reports that properly employed currents will not cause necrosis; only dehydration or volatilization of individual cells occurs from the use of a proper cutting current.[*]

---

[*]Oringer, M. J.: Electrosurgical aids in operative and restorative dentistry. Dent. Clin. N. Amer., March, 1966, pp. 57–77.

Electrosurgical procedures were performed on buccal or facial surfaces of dogs.

A Tele-Thermometer (6 channels) and a Beckman Type R Dynograph Recorder were used to record tissue temperatures resulting from each type of current when an incision was made. The rise in tissue temperature was recorded at the site of incision and at sites 1, 2, 3, and 5 mm. adjacent to it.

To measure heat generation and penetration, the thermistors were connected to a physiological record and inserted into the gingiva; incisions were made at right angles to the thermistor probes and the temperature elevations recorded. Tissues were biopsied at weekly intervals to measure the affected area.

For this experiment, three types of electrical units were used: a spark-gap generator (monoterminal application), a partially rectified or single-tube unit (monterminal and biterminal application), and a fully rectified unit (monoterminal and biterminal application).

The spark-gap generator produced severe destruction of the tissue at the site of application. Coagulation current using the partially rectified unit and the fully rectified unit produces similar results clinically and histologically. Cutting current (electrosection) from the partially rectified unit and the fully rectified unit produced similar immediate clinical results; however, the amount of heat generated, affecting zone and histologic repair, were shown to favor the use of the fully rectified unit.

Method and Materials

As mentioned, three types of electrical units were used: a spark-gap generator, which produces an unrectified current of highly damped waveform which will be referred to as Unit A; a single-tube unit, which delivers a partially rectified high-frequency current with a moderately damped waveform which produces a pulsating pattern of flow, Unit B; and a fully rectified unit, which delivers a filtered, fully rectified high-frequency current of undamped waveform, Unit C.

Four dogs were used for this experiment because of convenience and similarities between their gingiva and that of the human.* After anesthetizing with Nembutal IV, electrosurgical procedures were performed. In the anterior portion of the maxillary and mandibular arches, the spark-gap generator, Unit A, and the electrocoagulating currents of Units B and C were applied biterminally.

Biterminal application refers to the use of two electrodes, the surgical or active electrode and the passive or dispersive electrode. The dispersive electrode in this report was in the form of a plate which was placed under the subject.†

---

*Waerhaug, J., and Zander, H. A.: Reaction of gingival tissues to self curing acrylic restorations. J.A.D.A., 54:760–768, June, 1957.
†Strock, M. S.: The rationale for electrosurgery. Oral Surg., 5:1167–1172, Oct., 1952.

Thermistor probes were connected to a continuous physiological pen recorder and were inserted into the gingiva to measure heat generation and penetration (Figs. 8–1–1 and 8–1–2). Two measurements for distance were made from the site of the original incision to the tip of the thermistor probe. One consisted of laying a wire in the base of the incision, placing a millimeter grid over the roentgenograph, and exposing the dental film using a long cone technique. The other method consisted of a surgical cut down from the site of the original incision to the tip of the thermistor probe. Both methods of measuring the distance from the incision to the probe proved to be correct.

Photographs were taken at the times of surgery and areas biopsied at zero, 7, 14, and 21 days. The tissues were stained with a hematoxylin and eosin preparation. Using a micrometer eyepiece, affected areas were measured and tissue repair noted.

ELECTRODESICCATION

Using electrodesiccation, the following was recorded:

Unit	Dial Setting	Biterminal Application	Time (Sec.)	Distance (mm.)	Temp. Rise (°F.)*
A	1	No	2	3	43.2
A	1	No	3	1	54.9
A	1	No	6	3	64.8

*Above base temperature.

As one increases time of electrode application to the tissue, there is an increase in temperature. This is a potentially destructive modality on tissues and the resulting carbonization causes it to have a self-limiting effect. On zero day, histologic specimens were not obtained because of the necrosis and inability to determine the exact area of electrode contact (Figs. 8–1–3). The tissues at 7 days showed incomplete healing of epithelium and underlying tissue with round cell infiltrate, plasma cells, and lymphocytes. At 14 days, the clinical picture showed a mature gingival tissue; however, repair of the underlying tissue was incomplete. At 21 days, the tissue was essentially normal when viewed histologically and clinically.

Using the coagulating current of Units B and C, the self-limiting effect of coagulation may again be observed.

At zero day, coagulation necrosis was seen at the site of the incision and surrounding tissue showed the radiating effect of heat (Fig. 8–1–4A). Photomicrographs of the seventh-day specimens showed a surface epithelium which was not completely formed, the basement membrane was beginning to become differentiated, and the deeper tissues were undergoing active regeneration with repair (Fig. 8–1–4B).

(Text continued on page 160)

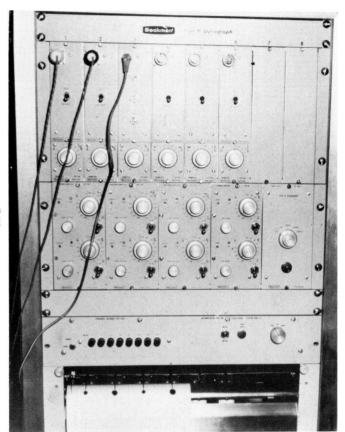

Figure 8–1–1. Photograph of a continuous physiological pen recorder.

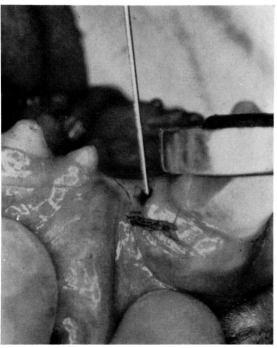

Figure 8–1–2. Photograph showing a thermistor probe being inserted into the gingiva with an incision at right angles to the probe tip.

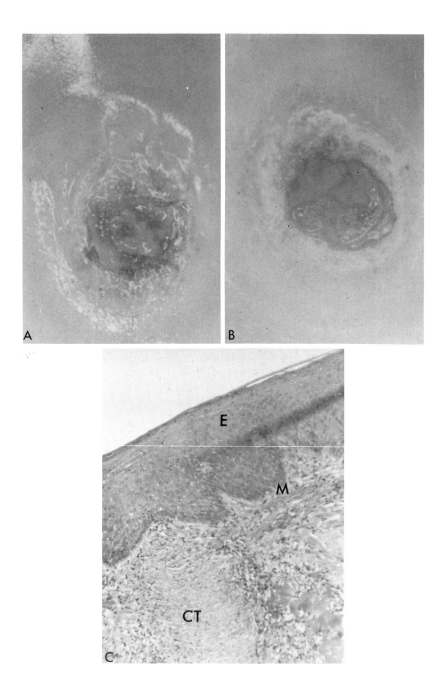

Figure 8–1–3. A, Photograph at zero day after electrodesiccation. Two-second application with machine setting at 1. B, Photograph at zero day after electrodesiccation. Three-second application with the machine setting at 1. Note the wide area of dehydration and necrosis. C, Photomicrograph fourteen days after electrodesiccation: (E) surface epithelium; (M) basement membrane; (CT) immature submucosa.

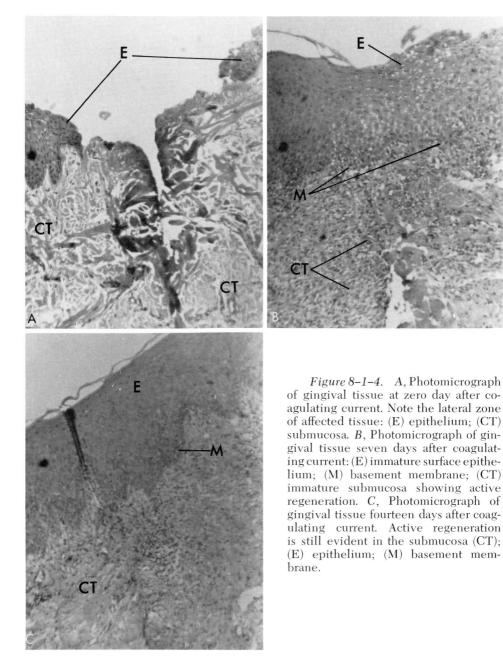

Figure 8–1–4. A, Photomicrograph of gingival tissue at zero day after coagulating current. Note the lateral zone of affected tissue: (E) epithelium; (CT) submucosa. B, Photomicrograph of gingival tissue seven days after coagulating current: (E) immature surface epithelium; (M) basement membrane; (CT) immature submucosa showing active regeneration. C, Photomicrograph of gingival tissue fourteen days after coagulating current. Active regeneration is still evident in the submucosa (CT); (E) epithelium; (M) basement membrane.

ELECTROCOAGULATION

The following chart is a summary using coagulating current for both the partially rectified and fully rectified units:

Unit	Dial Setting	Biterminal Application	Time (Sec.)	Distance (mm.)	Temp. Rise (°F.)*
B	1.5	Yes	2	3	5.4
			3	1	23.4
B	6	Yes	2	3	32.4
			3	1	43.2
C	1.5	Yes	2	3	16.2
			3	1	24.3
C	6	Yes	2	3	28.4
			3	1	37.8

*Above base temperature.

At 14 days, the surface epithelium is intact and mature and the basement membrane is easily defined. The deep tissue organization is not complete and active regeneration is evident (Fig. 8–1–4C).*

After 21 days the sections appeared essentially normal, with mature organization of the collagen fibers, basement membrane, and surface epithelium.

Clinically and histologically, tissue repair was very similar using both Units B and C for coagulating current.

ELECTROSECTION

Using the *partially rectified cutting current*, the following was recorded:

Unit	Dial Setting	Biterminal Application	Time (Sec.)	Distance (mm.)	Temp. Rise (°F.)*	Affected Area (Microns)
B	1–2	Yes	2	3	16.2	
			3	1	37.8	330.0**
B	2–2	Yes	2	3	27.2	
			3	1	59.4	197.8
B	3–2	Yes	2	3	21.6	
			3	1	72.4	301.0
B	4–2	Yes	2	3	28.8	
			3	1	86.4	314.0

*Above base temperature.
**Lateral dispersion.

The zero-day sections showed a clean, well-defined incision, with a wide zone of laterally affected tissue. Some carbon was demonstrated along the margins (Fig. 8–1–5A). At seven days, the epithelium was generally intact;

*Klug, R. G.: Gingival tissue regeneration following electrical retraction. J. Prosth. Dent., 16:955–62, Sept.–Oct., 1966.

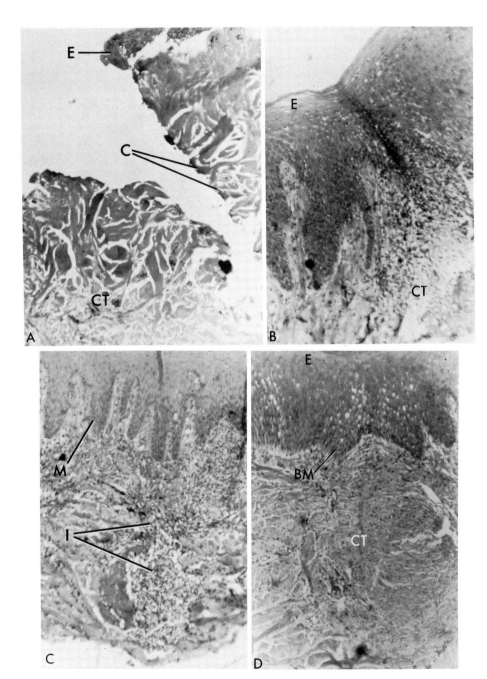

Figure 8–1–5. A, Photomicrograph at zero day after the use of the cutting current of a partially rectified unit. Note the lateral zone of affected tissue: (C) carbon; (E) surface epithelium; (CT) submucosa. B, Photomicrograph at seven days after the use of the cutting current of a partially rectified unit. Note that the surface epithelium (E) has regenerated; however, active repair is evident in the submucosa (CT). C, Photomicrograph fourteen days after the use of the cutting current of a partially rectified unit: (M) basement membrane; (I) inflammatory response in submucosa. D, Photomicrograph twenty-one days after the use of the cutting current of a partially rectified unit: (E) epithelium (BM) basement membrane; (CT) submucosa.

however, the basement membrane was not well defined and active repair was taking place within the deep tissue (Fig. 8–1–5B). The 14-day sections exhibited a mature epithelium, and the basement membrane was becoming well organized; however, in the underlying deeper tissue, there was a lack of organization in the collagen fibers and heavy round cell infiltrate was evident (Fig. 8–1–5C).

At 21 days, the histologic sections showed a complete mature surface epithelium and basement membrane; however, the deeper tissue showed immature cells and active regeneration was present (Fig. 8–1–5D).

The following shows the results using a *fully rectified cutting current:*

Unit	Dial Setting	Biterminal Application	Time (Sec.)	Distance (mm.)	Temp. Rise (°F.)*	Affected Area (Microns)
C	−1	Yes	2	3	13.5	
			3	1	18.0	123
C	1	Yes	2	3	13.5	
			3	1	31.2	102
C	3	Yes	2	3	35.1	
			3	1	47.4	145
C	6	Yes	2	3	36.8	
			3	1	48.6	411**

*Above base temperature.

**Author's Explanatory Note: With Unit C the power setting at 3 represents the ideal cutting energy for this unit. A power output of 6 with this unit is excessively high and far too potent for optimal results. With Unit B, however, a power setting at 5 to 6 is ideal for optimal results.

Within the proper power range, at settings 1 to 3, using biterminal application, it can be seen that the area affected and the amount of heat generated are less using the fully rectified unit as compared to the partially rectified unit.

Histologically, the zero-day sections showed the incision with the laterally affected tissue. Note that the lateral heat dispersion is considerably less with the fully rectified unit (Fig. 8–1–6A). At 7 days, regeneration of the surface epithelium and basement membrane is near completion. Active repair is taking place within the deeper tissue (Fig. 8–1–6B). At 14 days, the sections exhibited a histologic and clinical picture very similar to the 21-day specimens, except for an increase in the number of isolated areas or "nests" of inflammatory cells (Fig. 8–1–6C). The 21-day sections may be regarded as normal in this research animal (Fig. 8–1–6D).

Discussion

In order to have a relative scale to begin from, all electrical units were calibrated, so that the units produced the same dehydrating effect on the sur-

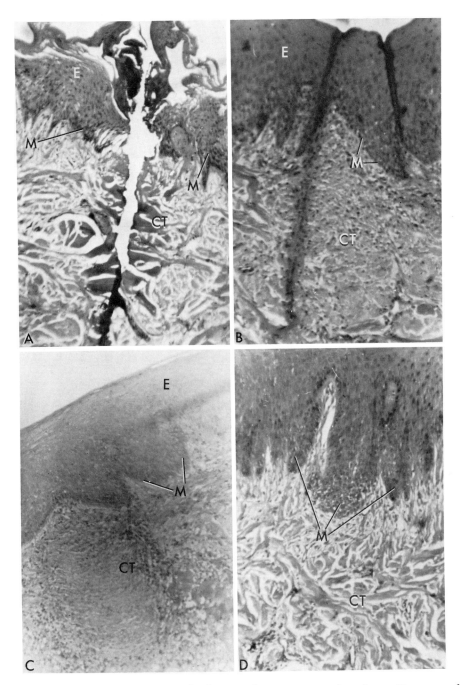

Figure 8-1-6. A, Photomicrograph of gingival tissue at zero day after cutting procedures using a fully rectified unit: (E) surface epithelium; (M) basement membrane; (CT) submucosa. B, Photomicrograph of gingival tissue seven days after cutting procedures using the fully rectified unit: (E) surface epithelium; (M) basement membrane; (CT) immature submucosal tissue. C, Photomicrograph of gingival tissue fourteen days after cutting procedures using the fully rectified unit: (E) surface epithelium; (M) basement membrane; (CT) submucosal tissue. D. Photomicrograph twenty-one days after use of cutting current using the fully rectified unit. This tissue is essentially normal for this research animal: (M) basement membrane; (CT) submucosa.

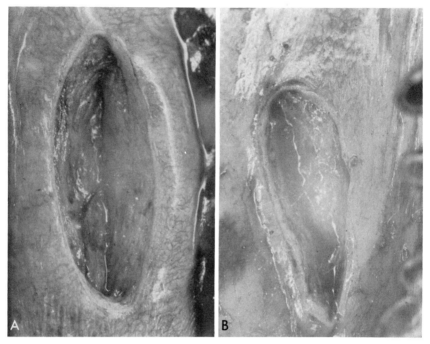

Figure 8-1-7. A, Photograph showing an incision made in the attached gingiva to demonstrate the bloodless field obtained and the lack of searing along the margins of the incision. B, Photograph showing the searing along the incision margins. The investigator allowed the electrode to drag slightly through the tissue instead of using a rapidly flowing movement.

face epithelium for 1-second contact when viewed through a dissecting microscope. Tissue repair was the slowest following the use of electrodesiccation. At 21 days, the underlying tissues were not completely healed.

Comparing Figure 8-1-5C (partially rectified current) and Figure 8-1-6C (fully rectified current) histologically, the healing pattern using the fully rectified current was more rapid in the underlying tissue. This amount of heat generated in the tissue and zone of affected tissue overall was less with the fully rectified unit. Clinically, the *surface epithelium was formed* in most of the 7-day specimens when using coagulating or electrosection current; however, at the time of histologic preparation, tissues that were exposed to the coagulating and the partially rectified current separated rather easily.

If the activated electrode is allowed to remain in the area too long, a marked rise in temperature could be recorded and, histologically, the repair delayed. Clinically, the main difference which could be noted was the amount of searing of the tissue margins which delayed tissue repair (Fig. 8-1-7).

In conclusion, the most consistent results were with the fully rectified unit, which delivers a fully rectified high-frequency current of undamped waveform (Unit C). There was less temperature rise in the tissue and the least amount of lateral heat dispersion to the adjacent tissue, and healing was most rapid and uneventful (Fig. 8-1-8).

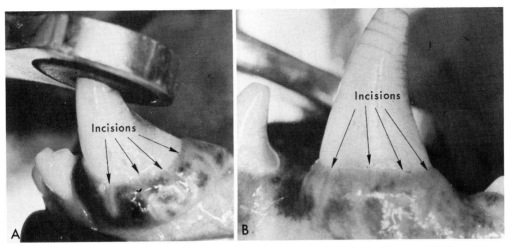

Figure 8–1–8. *A,* A seven day postoperative photograph showing the epithelial regeneration after the use of proper cutting currents using a fully rectified unit. Arrows point to four incisions. *B,* A fourteen day postoperative photograph showing the surface epithelium. As in the previous photograph, four incisions had been made.

2. GINGIVAL TISSUE REGENERATION FOLLOWING ELECTROSECTION

by William J. Kelly, Jr., D.D.S., and James D. Harrison, D.D.S.

Today there is much discussion about the relative merits of electrosection for gingival surgery. This investigation was conducted to evaluate conflicting claims as to the differences in healing between traditional surgery and electrosection, with regard to gingival regeneration.

Procedures

For this investigation, four adult old-world primates, *Macaca nemestrina,* were used, since their tissues are histologically similar to those of *Homo sapiens.*[1, 4, 5, 10, 11, 17, 21, 22, 24] All primates exhibited a full adult dentition and weighed between 18 and 24 pounds (Fig. 8–2–1).

The primates were anesthetized before each procedure. The first procedure consisted of an oral examination, including periodontal charting, scaling, and polishing of all teeth. Following a two-week period after the first procedure, the animals were again anesthetized, and buccal and lingual reference notches similar to a Class V cavity were prepared. The gingival floors of the notches were placed even with the gingival crest using a dissecting microscope. The reference notches were restored to normal contour using zinc oxyphosphate cement. After the cement had hardened, all gingival crevices were marked using Crane-Kaplan pocket markers (Fig. 8–2–2). Gingivec-

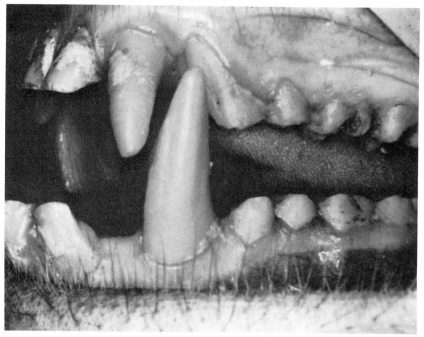

Figure 8–2–1. Animals upon receipt at the animal care center. The tissue presents a healthy clinical view of the marginal gingivae with shallow gingival crevices.

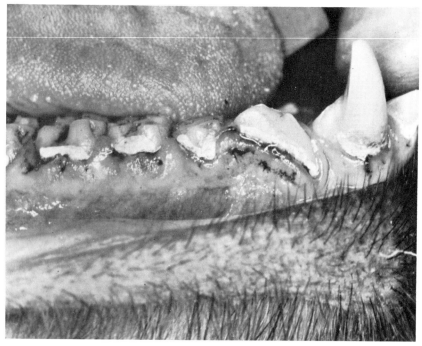

Figure 8–2–2. Bleeding points following pocket marking utilizing Crane-Kaplan pocket markers. This procedure was done for both electrosection and traditional surgery procedures.

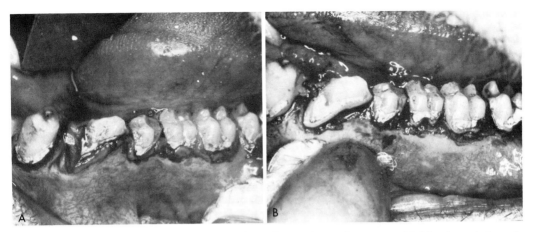

Figure 8–2–3. A, Gingival incision line for traditional surgery. Kirkland periodontal knives were employed in this procedure. B, Elimination of the gingival crevice through traditional surgery techniques. Note the exposed cavity margin.

tomies were performed using either sharpened Kirkland periodontal knives or electrosection (Figs. 8–2–3A and *B*).

A unit which produces a fully rectified high-frequency current of undamped waveform was employed. When the current is applied to the tissues by biterminal application and the surgical electrode is moved along the surface of the tissue as it makes contact, the cells in the line of cleavage undergo molecular disintegration and volatilization.[13, 18]

Biterminal application refers to the use of two electrodes, the passive electrode or dispersive plate, which is placed under the subject, and the smaller active or surgical electrode. Appropriate loops, Coles E–6–A or E–6–B, were used as the active electrodes to perform the quadrant gingivectomies on the facial surfaces (Fig. 8–2–4). The unit dial was set at a reading between 2

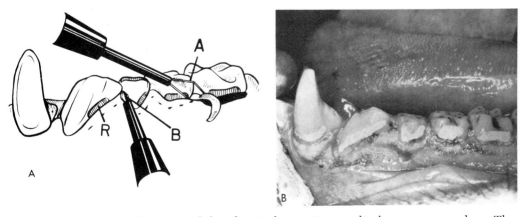

Figure 8–2–4. A, Drawing of the electrical retraction or displacement procedure. The loop electrode E-6-A (A) has been drawn mesially past the reference notch (R). Loop electrode E-6-B (B) is about to be applied to the interproximal gingival area. *B*, Gingivectomy using electrosurgery techniques. Note the relatively bloodless field.

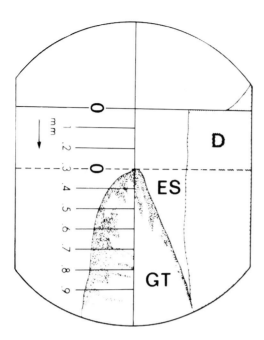

Figure 8-2-5. Drawing of the micrometer measurement. The micrometer scale is superimposed on the tooth and tissues: (D) dentin; (ES) enamel space; (GT) gingival tissue. The horizontal cross hair has been moved down from the floor of the reference notch to approximate the gingival crest, and in this drawing would give a reading of 300 microns or 0.3 mm.

and 4, depending on tissue resistance and fluctuations of line voltage. The opposite side of the arch was then subjected to the traditional surgical methods using the previously mentioned periodontal knives. Care was taken to assure that the most occlusal portion of the remaining gingival tissue in both quadrants was apical to the original gingival crevice.[6, 7, 8] The facial tissues and the lingual control areas were coated with an antiseptic consisting of equal portions of tincture of myrrh and benzoin. The animals were then returned to their quarters for maintenance. The opposing arch was treated in the same manner with the exception of a different time schedule. On one of the four animals, the surgical procedure was varied. Surgery was performed on the buccal and lingual surfaces of the same quadrant and controls were established on the opposite quadrant of the same arch.

Immediately following euthanization, block sections of the maxillary and mandibular arches were removed, fixed in a 10 per cent formalin solution, and then decalcified using a 5 per cent solution of nitric acid. All sections were cut at 6 microns and stained with hematoxylin and eosin[15] or Gomori's trichrome stain.[9]

Crestal height regeneration was measured by using a 10× micrometer eyepiece. This enabled the tissues to be measured in thousandths of a millimeter using the external cross-hair adjustment knob (Fig. 8-2-5).

Results

Histologic examinations of the one-week specimens showed a healing pattern consistent for both methods of surgery. New free gingiva had formed,

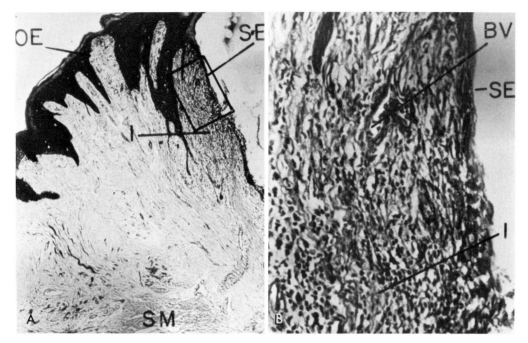

Figure 8-2-6. A, Photomicrograph one week after traditional surgery: (SE) sulcus epithelium; (I) inflammatory response; (OE) oral epithelium; (SM) submucosa (×16). *B*, Area indicated in A: (SE) sulcus epithelium; (I) inflammatory response; (BV) blood vessel (×103).

the outer gingival surface was completely epithelialized, and the sulcus area demonstrated almost complete epithelialization. The connective tissue in the newly formed marginal gingiva was highly vascular and contained many fibroblasts and numerous lymphocytes, especially in the crevicular part of the free gingiva. In a few sections, occasional polymorphonuclear leukocytes and macrophages could be observed. Inflammatory response was most marked in the connective tissue adjacent to the epithelium at the base of the gingival crevice. Inflammation was based on the following criteria: the number and types of inflammatory cells in the submucosa and sulcus epithelium, the degree of vascularity, the presence or absence of epithelial proliferation, and the thickness of the sulcus epithelium (Figs. 8-2-6A and B).

The specimens from the electrosurgically treated quadrant showed a slightly more mature tissue. The rete peg formation (basal cell organization) was more developed and newly formed collagen fiber bundles were more easily demonstrated (Figs. 8-2-7A and B).

The two-week specimens showed a mature surface and crevicular epithelium with well-formed rete pegs. For both series of specimens, thickening of the stratum corneum was seen. The sulcus was lined by epithelium, there was an increase in the collagen bundles in the free gingiva, and the capillaries were somewhat smaller than those viewed in the one-week specimens. However, the capillaries were often surrounded by numerous lymphocytes (Figs. 8-2-8 and 8-2-9).

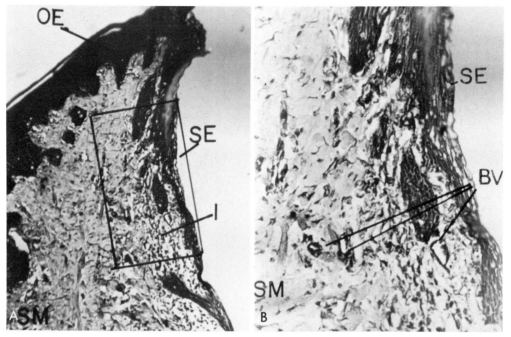

Figure 8-2-7. A, Photomicrograph one week after electrosection: (SE) sulcus epithelium; (OE) oral epithelium; (I) inflammatory response; (SM) submucosa (×43). B, Area indicated in A: (SE) sulcus epithelium; (SM) submucosa; (BV) blood vessel (×103).

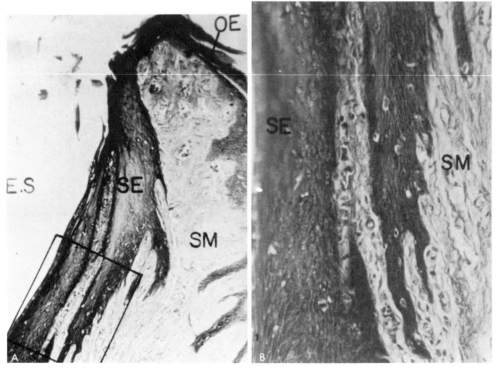

Figure 8-2-8. A, Photomicrograph two weeks after traditional surgery: (SE) sulcus epithelium is extending into the gingival connective tissue; (ES) enamel space; (SM) submucosa; (OE) oral epithelium (×43). B, Area indicated in A, illustrating thickening of the sulcus epithelium (SE) adjacent to the base of the gingival crevice; (SM) submucosa (×103).

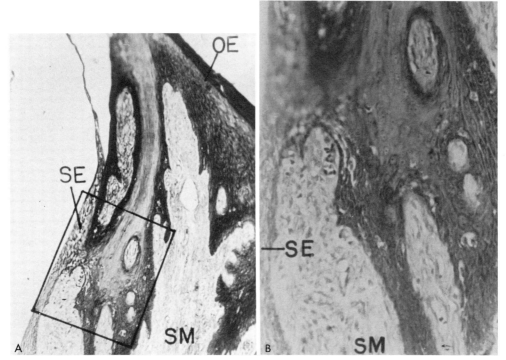

Figure 8–2–9.   A, Photomicrograph two weeks after electrosection: (SE) sulcus epithelium, making extensions into the gingival connective tissue (SM); (OE) oral epithelium (×43). B, Area indicated in A: (SE) sulcus epithelium; (SM) submucosa (×103).

The three-week specimens still showed an inflammatory response, especially in the sulcus area. Vascularity had not appreciably decreased for traditional surgery specimens; however, connective tissue was becoming well organized. The three-week specimens for traditional surgery showed an increase in round cell infiltration when compared to the two-week specimen. This was evident through the entire gingival cuff and not in the tissue adjacent to the sulcus area. This may have been due to individual animal variation.

At four weeks, the epithelium of the marginal and sulcus gingiva was complete and the connective tissue indistinguishable from the connective tissue of the untreated control area. At the base of the gingival sulcus in some of the specimens, inflammatory cells, primarily lymphocytes and plasma cells, were evident. Also, the vascularity had decreased (Figs. 8–2–10 and 8–2–11).

Six- to eight-week specimens were essentially normal when compared histologically and clinically. Inflammation which persisted in the connective tissue was reduced with an increase in time. The eight-week specimens showed the least amount of inflammation. The electrosurgery photomicrograph does show a small area of concentrated round cell infiltration, which can be considered as normal for this experimental animal. Thickness of the epithelium at the gingival crest with electrosurgery and keratin layer depth favored electrosurgery techniques (Figs. 8–2–12, 8–2–13, and 8–2–14).

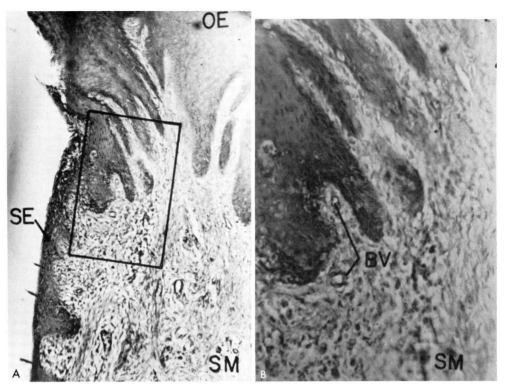

Figure 8-2-10. A, Photomicrograph four weeks after traditional surgery: (OE) oral epithelium; (SE) sulcus epithelium; (SM) submucosa (×43). B, Area indicated in A: (BV) blood vessel; (SM) submucosa (×103).

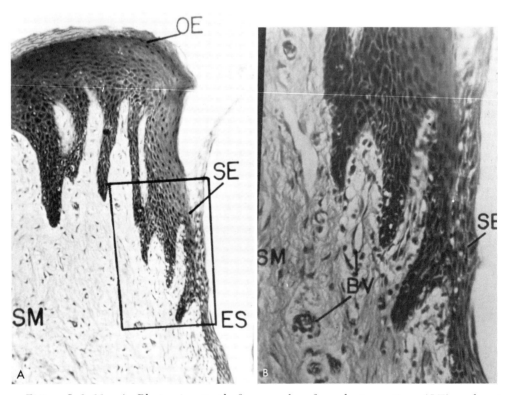

Figure 8-2-11. A, Photomicrograph four weeks after electrosection: (OE) oral epithelium; (SE) sulcus epithelium; (ES) enamel space; (SM) submucosa (×43). B, Area indicated in A: (SE) sulcus epithelium; (SM) submucosa; (BV) blood vessel (×103).

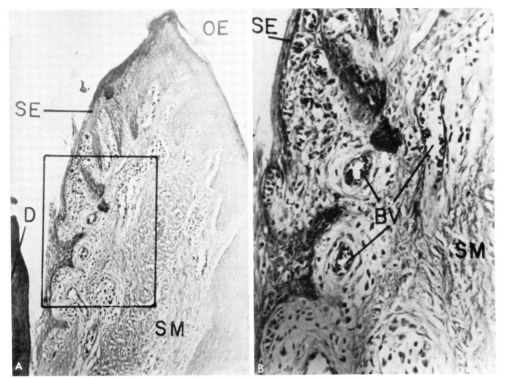

Figure 8-2-12. A, Photomicrograph eight weeks after traditional surgery: (SE) sulcus epithelium; (OE) oral epithelium; (D) dentin; (SM) submucosa (×43). B, Area indicated in A: (SE) sulcus epithelium; (SM) submucosa; (BV) blood vessel (×103).

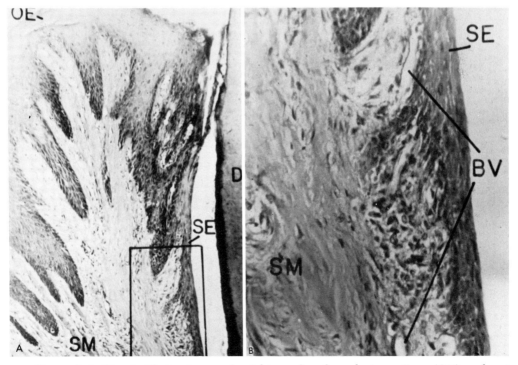

Figure 8-2-13. A, Photomicrograph eight weeks after electrosection: (OE) oral epithelium; (SE) sulcus epithelium; (SM) submucosa; (D) dentin (×43). B, Area indicated in A: (SE) sulcus epithelium; (SM) submucosa; (BV) blood vessel (×103).

173

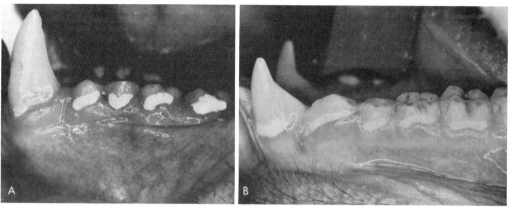

Figure 8–2–14. A, A photograph of the marginal gingiva after eight weeks following traditional surgery techniques, immediately prior to euthanization. B, A photograph at eight weeks following electrosurgery techniques, immediately prior to euthanization.

Table 8–2–1 shows the average inflammation response in the marginal gingiva. Following surgery, the two-week specimens showed a marked decrease in inflammatory response. However, there was marked proliferation of the sulcus epithelium in all histologic specimens. In each animal, all sections were graded with an average of 108 slides read for each quadrant (Figs. 8–2–15 and 8–2–16).

Discussion

This investigation has shown that electrosurgical cutting procedures using a fully rectified current of undamped waveform is fully comparable if not superior to those obtainable when using cold steel instruments. Clinically, little difference could be seen between the methods of surgery except for crestal height regeneration. Also, a comparatively bloodless field was evident when using electrosection as compared to traditional surgical removal. Histologically, the tissue appeared to mature more rapidly when using elec-

Table **8–2–1.** *Average Postoperative Inflammation Response of Marginal Gingiva*

Time	Control	Traditional Surgery	Control	Electrosurgery
1	Mild	Severe	Mild	Moderate
2	Normal	Normal*	Normal	Mild*
3	Moderate	Moderate	Moderate	Moderate
4	Normal	Mild	Normal	Mild
6	Normal	Mild	Normal	Normal
8	Normal	Normal	Normal	Normal

*Sulcus epithelial proliferation.

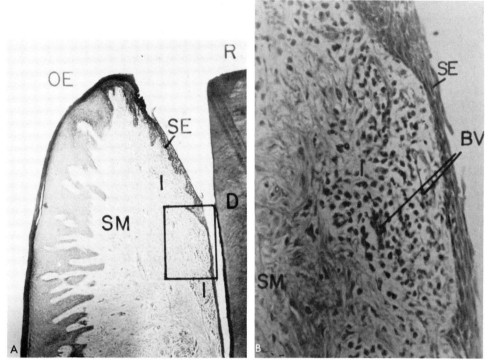

Figure 8-2-15. A, Photomicrograph of the control specimen after two weeks: (R) reference notch; (D) dentin; (OE) oral epithelium; (SE) sulcus epithelium; (SM) submucosa; (I) a few inflammatory cells are adjacent to the sulcus epithelium (×16). B, Area indicated in A: (SE) sulcus epithelium; (I) inflammatory cell; (BV) blood vessel; (SM) submucosa (×103).

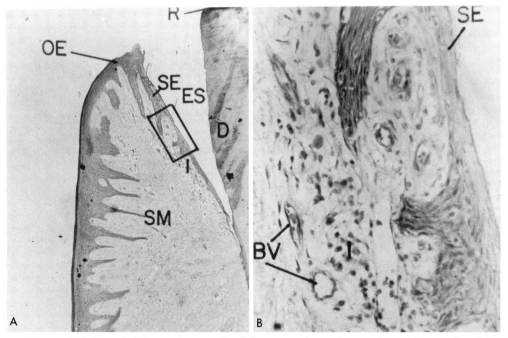

Figure 8-2-16. A, Photomicrograph of the control specimen after eight weeks. A few inflammatory cells are adjacent to the sulcus epithelium: (R) reference notch; (D) dentin; (SM) submucosa; (ES) enamel space; (SE) sulcus epithelium; (OE) oral epithelium; (I) inflammatory cell (×16). B, Area indicated in A: (BV) blood vessel; (SE) sulcus epithelium; (I) inflammatory response (×103).

Table 8–2–2. *Gingival Loss*

| Duration | Methods | |
	Traditional	Electrosection
6 Weeks	0.375 mm.	0.310 mm.
8 Weeks	0.310 mm.	0.115 mm.

trosurgery, this being based on inflammatory cell response, basal cell organization, proliferation and thickness of epithelium and keratinization.

The rapid tissue regeneration of the primate may be due to one or more factors. The animals were in excellent health and were maintained on a carefully controlled diet. Since no periodontal dressing was applied, the tissues were able to epithelialize at their maximum potential and keratinize very quickly, as evidenced in the one-week specimens.

The findings for the traditional methods of surgery closely correspond in time sequence to those reported by others.[2, 3, 12, 14, 16, 19, 20, 23]

At the onset of this experiment, it was felt that electrosurgery procedures could cause retarded healing because of the coagulation potential of this modality. From the histologic and clinical findings, it can be stated that properly employed electrosurgical procedures do not retard tissue regeneration (Table 8–2–2).

Conclusion

Having a modality which gives an almost completely bloodless field following gingival crest removal for fixed prosthodontic impressions is an advantage for the dental practitioner. The results of this investigation show that electrosurgery does not retard gingival tissue regeneration; in fact, the tissues showed a more rapid degree of maturity histologically when compared at one- and two-week intervals. A more nearly similar picture histologically was observed and except for greater crestal height regeneration of the tissues cut by electrosection no differences could be noted in the six- and eight-week specimens.

BIBLIOGRAPHY

1. Bernick, S. and Friedman, N. Microscopic Studies of the Periodontium of the Primary Dentition of the Monkey Anterior Teeth During the Mixed Dentition Period. *Oral Surg., Oral Med., and Oral Path.*, 6:1239–1247, 1953.
2. Bernier, J. L. The Histologic Changes of the Gingival Tissue in Health and Periodontal Disease. *Oral Surg., Oral Med., and Oral Path.*, 3:1194–99, Sept., 1950.
3. Bernier, J. L. and Kaplan, H. The Repair of Gingival Tissue after Surgical Intervention. *J.A.D.A.*, 35:697, 1947.
4. Chacker, F. M. and Cohen, D. W. Regeneration of Gingival Tissue in Non-Human Primates. *J.D. Res.*, 39:743–744, July-Aug., 1960, abstract.

5. Engler, W. O., Ramfjord, S. P., and Hiniker, J. J. Development of Epithelial Attachment and Gingival Sulcus in Rhesus Monkeys. *J. Periodont.*, 36:44–56, Jan.–Feb., 1965.
6. Glickman, I. Clinical Periodontology. *J.A.D.A.*, 66:636–647, May, 1963.
7. Glickman, I. Healing of the Periodontium after Mucogingival Surgery. *Oral Surg., Oral Med., and Oral Path.*, 16:530–538, May, 1963.
8. Glickman, I. Clinical Periodontology, 3rd. Edition, W. B. Saunders Co., Phila., 1964.
9. Gomori, G. A Rapid One-Step Trichrome Stain. *Amer. J. Clin. Path.*, 20:661–664, 1950.
10. Haigh, M. V. et al. Some Radiological and Other Factors for Assessing Age in the Rhesus Monkey Using Animals of Known Age. *Lab. Anim. Care.*, 15:57–73, Feb., 1965.
11. McHugh, W. D. The Development of the Gingival Epithelium in the Monkey. *D. Pract.*, 11:314–324, May, 1961.
12. Orban, B. and Archer, E. Dynamics of Wound Healing Following Elimination of Gingival Pockets. *J. Orthodont. and Oral Surg.*, 31:40, Jan., 1945.
13. Oringer, J. J. Electrosurgery in Dentistry. W. B. Saunders Co., Phila., 1962.
14. Periodontal Workshop, Committee I – Report of Evaluating Behavior of Gingival and Supporting Tissue. *J.A.D.A.*, 45:2, 1952.
15. Permar, Dorothy. Laboratory Outline for Microtechnique. The Ohio State University, Columbus, Ohio. Revised, 1958.
16. Persson, Per-Allen. Healing Process in the Marginal Periodontium after Gingivectomy with Special Regards to the Regeneration of Epithelium. *D. Pract.*, 11:427–437, Aug., 1961.
17. Ramfjord, S. P., Engler, W. O., and Hiniker, J. J. A Radioautographic Study of Healing Following Simple Gingivectomy. *J. Periodont.*, 37:179–189, May–June, 1966.
18. Saghirian, L. M. Electrosurgical Gingivoplasty. *Oral Surg., Oral Med., and Oral Path.*, 2:1549–1557, Dec., 1949.
19. Schultz-Haudt, S. D. and Aas, E. Dynamics of Periodontal Tissues. Part I. Epithelium. *Odont. T.*, 69:431–460, 1961. Part II. The Connective Tissue. *Odont. T.*, 70:397–428, 1962.
20. Schultz-Haudt, S. D. Observations of the Status of Collagen in Human Gingiva. *Arch. Oral Biology*, 2:131–142, July, 1960.
21. Waerhaug, J. New Concepts of the "Epithelial Attachment" and the Gingival Crevice in Health and Disease. *Austral. D.J.*, 4:164–173, June, 1959.
22. Waerhaug, J. Depth of Incision in Gingivectomy. *Oral Surg., Oral Med., and Oral Path.*, 8:707–718, June, 1955.
23. Waerhaug, J. and Zander, H. A. Reaction of Gingival Tissues to Self-Curing Acrylic Restorations. *J.A.D.A.*, 54:760–768, June, 1957.
24. Zander, H. A. Tissue Reaction to Dental Calculus and to Filling Materials. *J.D. Med.*, 13:101–103, 1958.

3. HISTOLOGIC REACTION OF THE VITAL PULP TO ELECTROSURGICAL DESENSITIZATION

by James D. Harrison, D.D.S.

The effective use of electrosurgery for desensitization of hypersensitive dentin has been well established. The use of chemicals such as silver nitrate, thymol crystals, formalin and fluoride paste has not always been completely effective or long-lasting. Oringer has demonstrated the effective use of electrocoagulation current in combination with 10 per cent formalin solution (see page 268. The heat of the current vaporizes the formalin which penetrates the dentinal tubules and fixes the organic material to prevent its breakdown for extended periods of time. This technique combines the advantages of electrocoagulation and fixation.

This study was done, using dogs as the experimental animal, to determine if the heat generated during the desensitization procedure penetrated the dentin sufficiently to cause pulpal damage. The results indicated that the pulp temperature increase varied from 2° F. to 9° F., depending upon the thickness

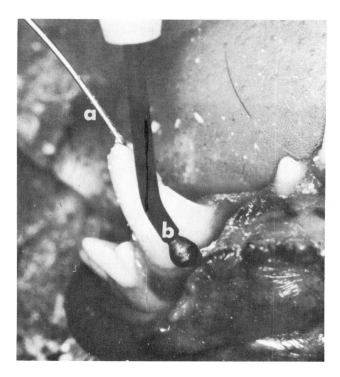

Figure 8–3–1. (a) Temperature probe sealed in canine of experimental animal. (b) Ball electrode in area of application.

of the dentin over the pulp and using the procedure recommended by
Oringer. A small ball electrode, with electrocoagulation current set between
0.5 and 1.0 on the Coles Radiosurg unit, was used to burnish the 10 per cent
formalin solution on the affected area, 1 second on and 1 second off, for 50
applications. Clinical application of this procedure has been modified to 1
second on and 5 seconds off, for 30 applications.

The pulp temperature was recorded by sealing a temperature probe in
the pulp chamber with the tip under the area of application (Fig. 8–3–1)
which was connected to a continuous monitoring Beckman Recorder (Fig. 8–
3–2). The temperature changes were recorded to plus or minus 0.5° F. The
same procedure was repeated on an adjacent tooth and histologic slides were
made from specimens obtained immediately and after 7, 14, and 21 days.

Figure 8–3–3 shows a representative recording of the pulp temperature
increase (range 2° F. to 9° F.) during the desensitization procedure. Pulp temperature increases of less than 12° F. do not cause permanent pulp damage.
The histologic examination of the pulp sections were normal in all specimens
examined. Figure 8–3–4 shows a representative photomicrograph section of
the pulp after electrosurgical desensitization.

The same procedure was repeated using a 5-second application of the
electrocoagulation current and 10 per cent formalin for 20 applications. These
results showed temperature increases ranging from 28° F. to 40° F. (Fig. 8–3–
5) and severe pulp damage did result (Figs. 8–3–6 to 8–3–8); therefore, proper
application of the ball electrode is necessary to prevent pulp damage.

The investigation shows that electrosurgical desensitization of hypersensitive dentin can be safely used under properly controlled applications of 1

(Text continued on page 182)

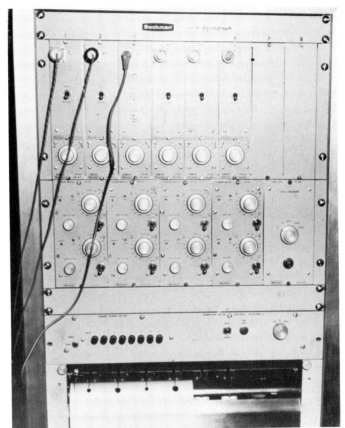

Figure 8–3–2. Beckman Dynograph Physiological Recorder.

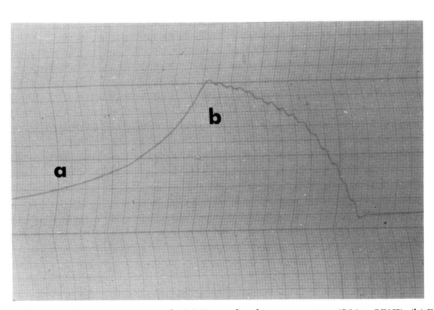

Figure 8–3–3. Temperature graph. (a) Normal pulp temperature (92° to 95°F). (b) Recording of temperature increase (range 2° to 9°F). During periods of desensitization procedure.

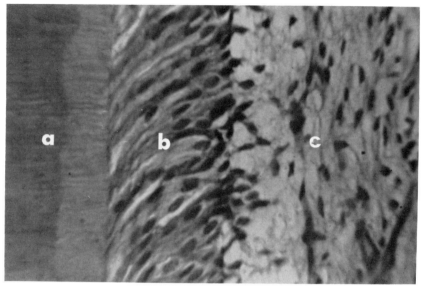

Figure 8–3–4.   Photomicrograph (×430) of representative pulp section, stained with hematoxylin and eosin; (a) dentin, (b) odontoblasts; (c) pulp.

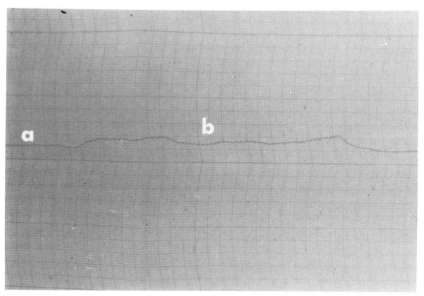

Figure 8–3–5.   Temperature graph showing 40°F increase using incorrect application of ball electrode; (a) normal temperature, (b) 40°F increase.

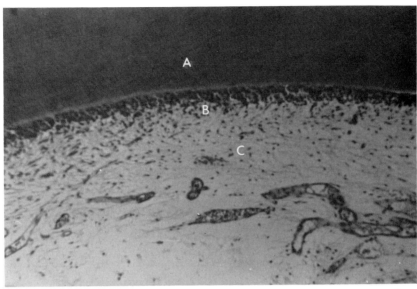

Figure 8–3–6. Photomicrograph (×100) of representative pulp section at 7 days showing hyperemia; (a) dentin, (b) odontoblasts, (c) inflammatory cells in pulp. (Stained with hematoxylin and eosin.)

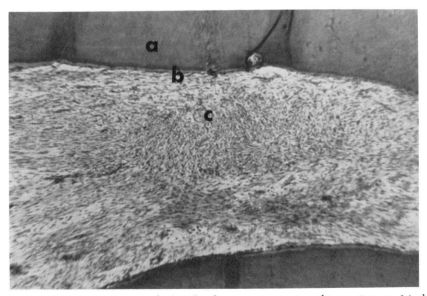

Figure 8–3–7. Photomicrograph (×35) of representative pulp section at 14 days; (a) dentin, (b) note loss of odontoblasts, (c) fibrotic pulp. (Stained with hematoxylin and eosin.)

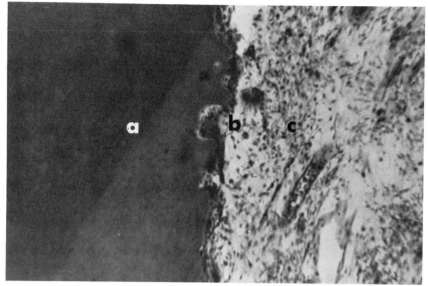

Figure 8–3–8. Photomicrograph (×430) of representative pulp section at 21 days; (a) dentin, (b) loss of odontoblasts and odontoclastic activity, (c) chronic inflammatory cells. (Stained with hematoxylin and eosin.)

second on and 5 seconds off with the ball electrode. This result points up the advantages of the procedure and the necessity to control the time of application for desensitization procedures.

4. ALVEOLAR BONE RESPONSE TO THE ELECTROSURGICAL SCALPEL[*]

by James D. Schieda, D.D.S., Thomas, J. DeMarco, D.M.D., Ph.D., and Lysle E. Johnson, Jr., D.D.S., Ph.D.[†]

It had originally been the author's intention to limit this chapter to reports based on original data made available to him by the investigators for that express purpose. The results obtained in this investigation and the conclusions drawn therefrom have such important clinical significance that if the original data had not been made available the author would have felt justified in deviating from his original intention in this instance, to include at least a review of the report. However, the original data and illustrations have graciously been made available by the investigator for inclusion here in toto or as an abstract.

[*]This study by James D. Schieda was as partial fulfillment of the requirements for the degree of Master of Science in Dentistry.

[†]Dr. Thomas J. DeMarco, Associate Professor and Chairman, Department of Periodontics, and Dr. Lysle E. Johnson, Jr., Associate Professor and Chairman, Department of Orthodontics, Case Western Reserve University School of Dentistry, Cleveland, Ohio.

The report, recently published in the *Journal of Periodontology** describes an excellently structured and executed research investigation of the response of alveolar bone to the application of electrosurgical cutting current. The fact that this investigation paralleled closely the investigation reported in 1970 by Glickman and Imber[1] and produced diametrically opposite results and conclusions adds greatly to its interest and significance.

This investigation helps to disprove the fallacious concept that damage must inevitably and automatically result if an electrode activated by RF cutting current is brought into physical contact with alveolar bone. To the contrary, the results further confirm the author's premise that the type of current used, the period of activated electrode contact, and the technique of instrumentation employed in applying the activated electrode to the bone are the factors that determine the outcome of the contact.

The following pertinent data have been abstracted from the detailed original report.

This research study was submitted by Dr. Schieda in partial fulfillment of the requirements for the degree of Master of Science in Dentistry. It was conducted under supervision of Dr. DeMarco, Chairman of the Department of Periodontology, and Dr. Johnson, Chairman of the Department of Orthodontics, Case Western Reserve University School of Dentistry.

Dr. Schieda's experiment was performed on four healthy male adult dogs to investigate the response of the alveolar bone crest to direct contact with fully rectified current applied with an electrosurgical needle electrode scalpel (Fig. 8–4–1).

Full-thickness gingivo-mucoperiosteal flap procedures were performed on the four quadrants of each dog and reference points were made in four pos-

---

*Schieda, J. D., et al.: Alveolar bone response to the electrosurgical scalpel. J. Periodont., 43:225, April, 1972.

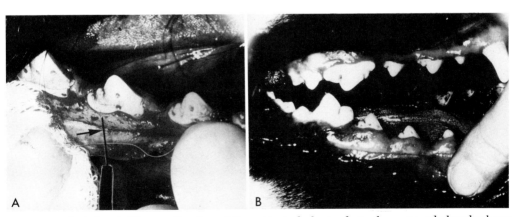

Figure 8–4–1.   A, The application of the activated electrode to the exposed alveolar bone crest (arrow). B, Appearance of the tissues on the 70th postoperative day. Healing is complete and the gingival margin is at its normal level as indicated by its relation to the guidelines in the teeth.

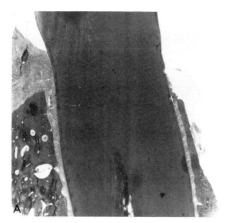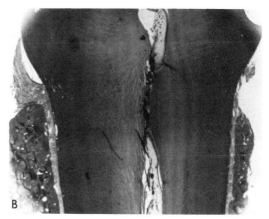

Figure 8–4–2. A, Photomicrograph of a histologic section taken from the mandibular experimental site, where the activated electrode was brought into contact with the exposed alveolar bone crest. The section obtained on the 70th postoperative day shows normal alveolar crestal bone. The tooth guidelines show that there has been no loss of height of the bone crest. *B,* Photomicrograph of a histologic section taken from the control side, where the *inactivated* electrode had been brought into contact with the crestal bone. This 70th day specimen showed normal crestal bone, but the guidelines show that there has been a slight, although clinically insignificant lowering of the height of the bone crest.

(Illustration continued on opposite page)

terior teeth per quadrant from which measurements were made to the alveolar crest (11 maxillary and 14 mandibular measurements per quadrant). After the measurements were obtained, one maxillary and one mandibular quadrant were treated by either the control treatment (bone contacted by an inactivated electrode) or the experimental treatment (bone contacted by an activated electrosurgical scalpel electrode). After seventy days of healing, full-thickness flaps were again reflected and the measurements were repeated. The total measurements taken at the two time periods (0 days and 70 days) were 400. From the two time periods, the first measurement was subtracted from the 70 day measure and a difference of the distance was determined. A mean difference was calculated for each quadrant, and the analysis of variance was used to analyze the information. Histological specimens were prepared for examination of the osseous tissues (Figs. 8–4–2 and 8–4–3).

The pertinent findings were as follows:

1. The maxillary arch showed a greater amount of bone crest loss on both the experimental and the control quadrants compared to either treatment area of the mandible. This was confirmed by the analysis of variance which showed the maxillary response (the combined control and experimental maxillary treatment areas versus the combined results from the mandibular treatment areas) of alveolar bone crest height loss to be statistically significant ($p > 0.01$).

2. All control quadrants (maxillary and mandibular) displayed more crestal bone loss as compared to the experimental quadrants regardless of the respective arch. However, when the difference between the two treatments was analyzed statistically, no significant difference was found ($p > 0.05$).

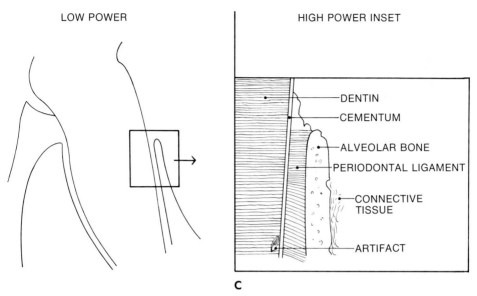

Figure 8-4-2. Continued.   C, Experimental: Mandibular left premolar area, 70th day specimen.

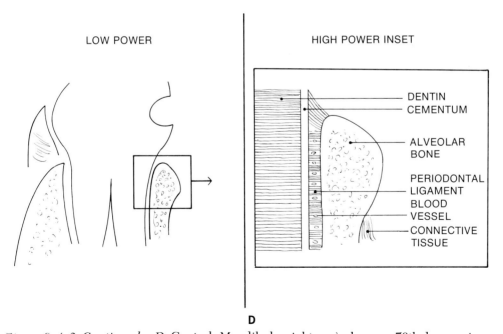

Figure 8-4-2. Continued.   D, Control: Mandibular right premolar area, 70th day specimen.

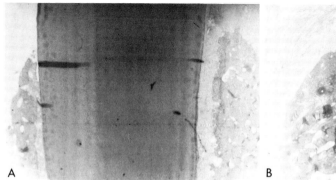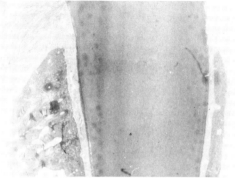

A B

Figure 8–4–3. A, Photomicrograph of a histologic section taken from the maxilla, where the activated electrode had been brought into contact with the alveolar bone crest. This 70th day specimen showed a slight amount of crestal loss not of clinical significance and probably due to the very thin buccal alveolar bone in the maxilla. B, Photomicrograph of a histologic section taken from the control side of the maxilla, where the inactivated electrode had made contact with the exposed alveolar bone crest. This 70th day specimen showed a slightly greater amount of crestal height than the experimental side, but this too was clinically insignificant.

(Illustration continued on opposite page)

3. The alveloar crest bone loss was found to vary among the four dogs in response to the two treatments. This variance was found to be statistically significant among the dogs (p > 0.01).

4. An analysis of the possibility of treatment-arch interaction revealed no significant interaction (p > 0.05).

5. Histological examinations failed to show bone necrosis, sequestration, or any demonstrable destruction of the bone.

"The mean reduction of the alveolar crest bone height of the maxillary controls (0.66 mm. ±0.15) and maxillary experimental areas (0.50 mm. ±0.08) compares closely with other surgical flap studies (Kohler and Ramfjord, 1960;[2] Donnenfeld et al., 1964;[3] Tavtigian, 1970;[4] Donnenfeld et al., 1970).[5] These investigators evaluated alveolar crest height following the employment of a gingivo-mucoperiosteal procedure and found a mean reduction of the crest height of 0.27 mm. (Kohler and Ramfjord, 1960); 0.63 mm. (Donnenfeld et al., 1964); 0.47 mm. (Tavtigian, 1970); and 0.80 mm. (Donnenfeld et al., 1970). However, the mandibular crest height changes on the control (0.13 mm. ±0.09) and the experimental (0.03 mm. ±0.05) areas found in this study are in contrast to the findings reported in other surgical flap studies. A significant difference between the maxillary and mandibular arches was found in this study as well.

"The results from this particular study indicate less alveolar crest bone height reduction following direct contact with the electrosurgical scalpel than other investigators have reported following other surgical procedures: (1) an alveolar bone denudation surgical procedure – Wilderman et al., 1960;[6] Costich and Ramfjord, 1968;[7] Glickman et al., 1963;[8] (2) a muco-gingival split-thickness or partial-thickness surgical flap procedure – Ramfjord and Costich, 1968;[9] and (3) the use of rotary stones and burs on the bone – Lobene and

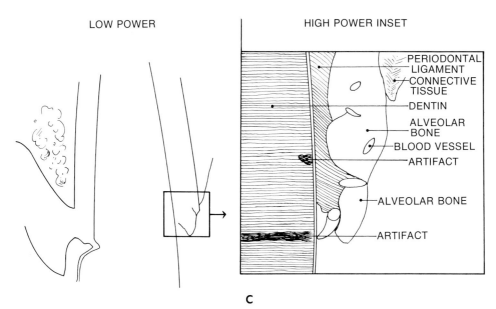

Figure 8–4–3. Continued.   C, Experimental: Maxillary right premolar area, 70th day specimen.

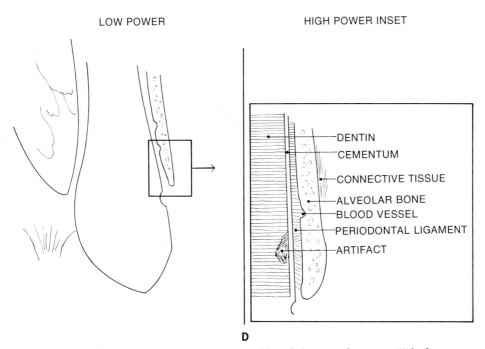

Figure 8–4–3. Continued.   D, Control: Maxillary left premolar area, 70th day specimen.

Glickman, 1963;[10] Calderwood et al., 1964;[11] Pennel et al., 1967;[12] Hiatt et al.,[13] 1968; Donnenfeld et al., 1970.[5]

"An analysis of Glickman and Imber (1970) study showed an analysis of variance was used on the twelve quadrants treated by a shallow gingival resection with the knives and electrosurgery and a t-test was used on the deep resection. Only one of the six areas showed necrosis and sequestration of this small sample size. The deep resection could likely have resulted in bone denudation in the area of bone damage and it is possible that this is what they observed. The statistically significant arch difference revealed in the present study could account for the statistical difference which they found in their study.

"In the present study the 'sham' control procedure (contact of the crest with an inactivated electrosurgical electrode) can be assumed to be essentially similar to just a flap procedure without the 'sham,' since the pressure contact of the inactivated electrode did not seem to be significant.

"Benefits from electrosurgery in periodontics may be as great as the benefits of the high-speed handpiece in operative dentistry. Some skilled surgeons have perfected their techniques during many years of practice and find no benefits from electrosurgery. However, it may be possible for the novice to develop and master sooner his surgical techniques and abilities with the use of electrosurgery. The enhancement of these abilities would enable him to provide his patients with better therapeutic results."

Conclusions

"The observations made in this study indicate that when the electrosurgical scalpel comes into contact with the alveolar crest, no greater detrimental effects to the crestal bone may take place than that which occurs following the reflection of a full-thickness gingivo-mucoperiosteal flap. These observations hold true only:

1. If the electrosurgical scalpel is used judiciously and with the proper brush-like stroke.

2. If soft tissue can adequately cover the area(s) contacted by the electrosurgical scalpel and not leave the bone denuded.

3. If the electrosurgical scalpel contacts the alveolar crest one time and only for the most fleeting moment, since this study did not evaluate the resulting effects which might occur from multiple contacts or the length of time the electrosurgical scalpel could remain in contact with the bone without damaging effects.

4. For the effects noted at the 70-day postoperative period and do not apply for any other time interval.

"One may assume that these results may apply in humans, but no definitive statement can be made, since the osseous tissue response may vary from that observed in dogs."

The report of this investigation was concluded with the following observation:

"It may be concluded that the use of the electrosurgical instrument in periodontal surgery provides a safe and effective instrument, even if contact with the bone occurs. Its use can provide the novice with a means for performing periodontal surgical procedures which may require many years for the skilled surgeon to develop."

The author takes the liberty of adding a few interpretive comments: It appears reasonable to assume that the investigator did not mean by the term "novice" one who is unskilled in electrosurgical instrumentation and know-how, since he stressed the importance of using the proper brush-like stroke, etc. An equally reasonable assumption would appear to be that he did not mean by "novice" one who is uninformed and uninitiated in the methodology of the various periodontal surgical procedures, but rather an individual who, although familiar with electrosurgical instrumentation and also with the specific periodontal surgical procedures, has not acquired the expertise necessary to perform them efficiently.

Throughout this text the author has repeatedly stressed, on the basis of many years of clinical observation, that when tissue is properly cut by electrosection with fully rectified current it subsequently tends to regenerate to or toward its original level. The hypothesis for this phenomenon is that the atraumatic character of the surgery results in absence of the fibrous scar tissue contractile repair produced by traumatic steel scalpel cutting.

The observation of the investigators in this experiment that they had found less alveolar bone crest height loss than had been experienced following incisions with steel scalpels for mucoperiosteal flaps to denude the bone, and for split-thickness or partial-thickness mucoperiosteal flap procedures, and when rotary stones and burs were applied to the bone indicates clearly that the bone reaction to the atraumatic character of electrosurgery is comparable to that of the reaction of the soft tissues.

In view of the fact that the investigators had found *more* alveolar bone crest reduction in the control quadrants where the inactivated electrode had been used than had occurred in the experimental quadrants where the activated electrode had been applied to the bone suggests that although the trauma from the inactivated electrode was extremely minimal, since virtually no pressure had been applied to the fine needle electrode, the greater height of the alveolar crestal bone in the experimental quadrants may well be attributable to stimulation of the tissues to regenerate when the wound heals.

REFERENCES

1. Glickman, I., and Imber, T. R.: Comparison of gingival resection with electrosurgery and periodontal knives—A biometric and histologic study. *J. Periodont.*, 41:142, 1970.
2. Kohler, C. A., and Ramfjord, S. P.: Healing of gingival mucoperiosteal flaps. Oral Surg., 13:89, 1960.
3. Donnenfeld, O., Marks, R. M., and Glickman, I.: The apically repositioned flap—A clinical study. *J. Periodont.*, 35:381, 1964.
4. Tavtigian, R.: The height of the facial radicular alveolar crest following apically repositioned flap operation. *J. Periodont.*, 41:412, 1970.

5. Donnenfeld, O. W., Hoag, P. M., and Weissman, D. P.: A clinical study on the effects of osteoplasty. *J. Periodont.*, 41:131, 1970.
6. Wilderman, M. N., Wentz, F. M., and Orban, B. J.: Histogenesis of repair after mucogingival surgery. *J. Periodont.*, 31:383, 1960.
7. Costich, E. R., and Ramfjord, S. P.: Healing after partial denudation of the alveolar process. *J. Periodont.*, 39:127, 1968.
8. Glickman, I., Smulow, J. B., O'Brien, T., and Tannen, R.: Healing of the periodontium following mucogingival surgery. *Oral Surg.*, 16:530, 1963.
9. Ramfjord, E., and Costich, E. R.: Healing after exposure of periosteum on the alveolar process. *J. Periodont.*, 39:199, 1968.
10. Lobene, R. R., and Glickman, I.: The response of alveolar bone to grinding with rotary diamond stones. *J. Periodont.*, 34:105, 1963.
11. Calderwood, R. G., Hera, S. S., Davis, J. R., and Waite, D. E.: A comparison of the healing rate of bone after the production of defects by various rotary instruments. *J. Dent. Res.*, 43:207, 1964.
12. Pennel, B. M., King, K. O., Wilderman, M. N., and Barron, J. M.: Repair of the alveolar process following osseous surgery. *J. Periodont.*, 38:426, 1967.
13. Hiatt, W. A., Stallard, R. E., Butler, E. D., and Badgett, B.: Repair following mucoperiosteal flap surgery with full gingival retention. *J. Periodont.*, 39:11, 1968.

Chapter Nine

CLINICAL RESEARCH
ON HUMAN SUBJECTS

1. HISTOLOGIC COMPARISON OF
COLD-STEEL AND ELECTROSURGICAL
SUBGINGIVAL CURETTAGE

by Richard Evans, D.D.S.

A number of comparative evaluations of surgery performed with both cold-steel and electrosurgical instruments and the effectiveness of wound healing in laboratory animals have been reported in the recent literature. This investigation of comparative wound healing in gingival tissue was conducted on a human patient, a white adult male with a moderately severe periodontal involvement of the anterior mandibular marginal gingivae.

The objective of this experiment was an accurate comparative evaluation, histologic as well as clinical, of the tissue responses to subgingival curettage: manually, with conventional cold-steel periodontal curets; and electrosurgically by electrosection with fully rectified cutting current and a small, narrow 45-degree-angle, U-shaped loop electrode serving as an electronic curet. Being equally well trained in the use of both modalities, Dr. Evans was well qualified to conduct an accurate, scientifically meaningful investigation.

The experiment was preceded by the customary preoperative preliminary preparation of the field, including a thorough prophylaxis and elimination of all occlusal traumatizing prematurities. The operative field, extending from the mandibular right second bicuspid to the left cuspid, was then prepared and anesthetized using local anesthesia.

The gingivae around the right second bicuspid to and including the right lateral incisor were then subjected to electrosurgical curettage. The unit and cutting current circuits were activated, current output set at 4 on the instrument panel dial and, using the electrode at an acute angle in a manner very similar to that for preparing a subgingival trough around a full crown preparation, the internal diseased epithelial tissue lining the gingival sulci and shallow periodontal pockets was resected electronically. The curettage of this tissue from the right central to left cuspid was performed manually with a steel periodontal curet.

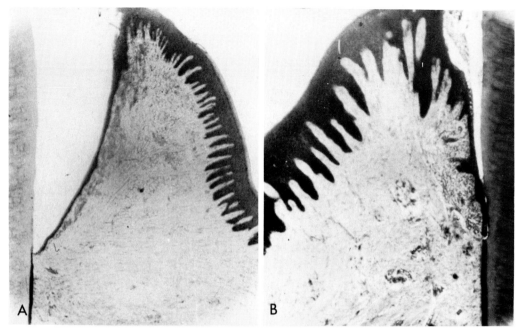

Figure 9–1–1. A, Illustrates typical histologic appearance of normal, healthy crevicular epithelium. B, Illustrates typical histologic appearance of inflamed or diseased crevicular epithelium.

The curettage having been completed, tincture of myrrh and benzoin was applied topically to the curetted areas and the patient was reappointed.

He was seen on the fifth postoperative day, and a small segment of marginal gingiva was excised from the right side where the electrosurgical curettage had been performed. The tissue was processed, stained, mounted, and examined microscopically for histologic evaluation. Two histologic specimens, one, a perfect example of normal marginal gingiva, the other, an equally classic example of diseased, inflamed gingiva (Figs. 9–1–1A and B), were used

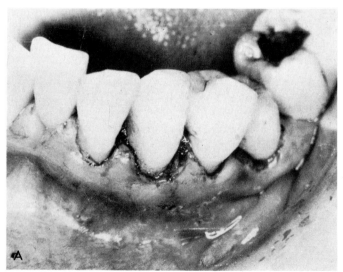

Figure 9–1–2. A, Clinical appearance of some of the tissues that have been treated by the investigator. The gingivae in the right quadrant to the mesial of the right lateral have been treated by manual curettage with steel periodontal curets. The gingivae of the two centrals (seen in this photo) and the left quadrant were treated by electrosection with electronic curets.

Illustration continued on opposite page.

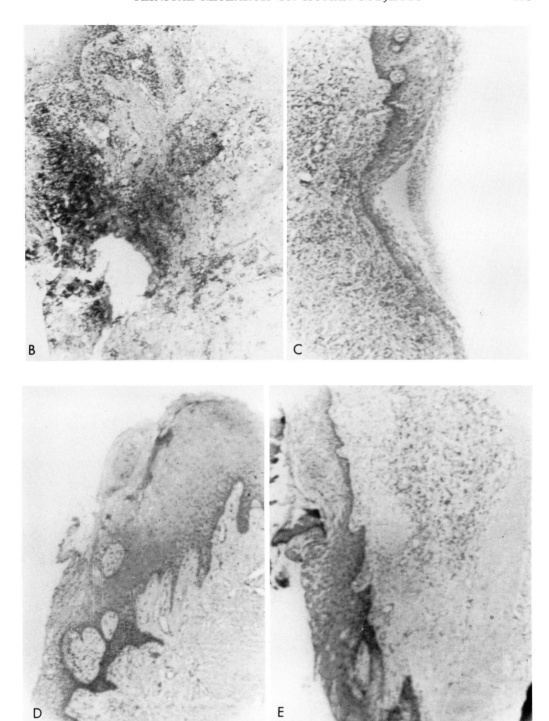

Figure 9–1–2. Continued. B, Histologic appearance of tissue treated by manual curettage on the seventh postoperative day. Note the resemblance to Figure 9–1–1B. C, Histologic appearance of tissue treated by electrosection on the fifth postoperative day. Note the smooth downgrowth of the regenerating epithelium. D, Histologic appearance of the tissues treated by manual curettage on the twelfth postoperative day. There is still vacuolation and immature development of the rete pegs. E, Histologic appearance of the tissue treated by electronic curettage on the twelfth postoperative day. Note the more mature appearance of the rete pegs.

as standards in evaluating the excised tissues. Histologically, the first specimen showed typical inflammation, an infiltration of round cells, and early
evidence of downgrowth of new epithelial lining (Fig. 9–1–2C).

The patient was seen again on the seventh postoperative day, and a small
specimen of tissue was excised from the left side, where the hand curettage
had been performed. This tissue was also processed and compared histologically with the typical histologic specimens. Although this tissue had been
repairing for two days more than the first specimen, the evidence of inflammation was more pronounced, and the epithelium was not as smooth and advanced in downgrowth as the tissue taken two days earlier (Fig. 9–1–2B).

The patient was seen again on the twelfth day, and similar tissue specimens were excised from both sides. The tissue taken from the right side
where the electrosurgical curettage had been performed showed almost completely normal epithelial regeneration. The downgrowth of sulcus epithelium
was complete, with normal rete pegs, no vacuolation, and very few round cells
still present (Fig. 9–1–2E). The specimen taken from the left side (that treated
by manual curettage) showed incomplete and irregular epithelial downgrowth, with much vacuolation and some round cells still present (Fig. 9–1–
2D).

Summary

This investigation was a comparative evaluation of the respective responses of human marginal gingiva to manual subgingival cutting with a steel
periodontal curet and electrosurgical cutting with fully rectified current and a
loop curet serving as an electronic curet.

The investigation was conducted by an investigator who is equally competent in use of both modalities. Since the experiment was performed under
identical clinical conditions, on identical tissues in the same patient's mouth,
any differences in rate and quality of tissue repair that might be evidenced
could be attributed solely to the effects of the respective modalities used.

The tissue specimens presented conclusive histologic evidence that electrosurgical cutting does not burn the tissues when it is performed properly.
On the contrary, the histologic evidence was unmistakable that the rate and
quality of tissue repair was more rapid and more favorable in the tissues
treated electrosurgically than in the tissues treated by conventional cold-steel
manual cutting.

Conclusions

This investigation and others conducted under similar conditions help to
confirm that the tissue response to atraumatic electrosurgical instrumentation
is rapid and eminently favorable. They also help to confirm that the electrosurgical tissue burning and unfavorable tissue repair still being reported by

some investigators have resulted from shortcomings in the ability of the investigators to utilize electrosurgery efficiently, and not from shortcomings of the modality.

2. ELECTRON MICROSCOPE HISTOLOGIC EVALUATION OF COLD-STEEL AND FULLY RECTIFIED ELECTROSURGICAL CUTTING

by William F. Malone, D.D.S., Dale Eisenmann, D.D.S., and Judith Kusek

Introduction

Until the advent of the elctron microscope histologic evidence provided by the 144× high-power oil immersion lens of the light microscope was considered most conclusive and revealing. In the experiments to be described next, the investigators used the electron microscope at powers ranging from 5,700 magnification to 47,400 magnification, which reveal cellular detail in a totally new dimension. The ability to see a single cell so enormously enlarged and showing incredibly minute detail opens new horizons that now make it possible to establish beyond challenge the fantastically self-limiting cellular destruction produced by totally atraumatic fully rectified electrosection properly applied to the tissues. The clinical evidence strongly suggested this, and the light microscope helped to substantiate it; now the electron microscope confirms it completely.

The following experiments involved cutting human marginal gingivae with cold-steel scalpel and by electrosection for comparative evaluation histologically with the light and electron microscopes. By far the most significant of the histologic studies by this team of investigators are the two single tissue cells, each of which had had a portion of the cell sheared off as the tissues were incised. The idea of scanning all the tissue specimens to try to find one or more cells that had been partially cut was inspired by a report published in the Dental Times of a biopsy specimen containing a number of partially sheared cells in the line of cleavage, with the remainder of the cells intact and readily distinguishable histologically.[1, 2]

Their search was rewarded with two perfect specimens: one a mast cell of connective tissue that had been sheared in half; the other a cell from which about one fourth had been sheared away, with the remainder of the cell remarkably intact. Both specimens show dramatically that all the cellular

---

[1]Oringer, M. J.: Lecture, Dec., 1968, at the American Academy of Dental Electrosurgery Annual Scientific Meeting.

[2]Dental Times, Vol. 12, No. 2, Feb. 15, 1969.

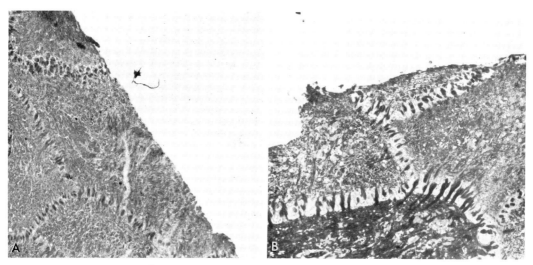

Figure 9–2–1. Histologic appearance of tissue edge cut by knife surgery. *A*, Magnification ×7,200; *B*, Magnification ×12,500. (From J. Prosth. Dent., 22:555, 1969.)

components are completely undamaged and unaltered by the cutting energy that had actually sectioned part of the cell (Figs. 9–2–1 and 9–2–2).

Nothing can possibly be more conclusive than the evidence provided by these two cells to prove two facts: First, that the fully rectified cutting current, properly used and adequately potent, is entirely self-limiting in its destructiveness. And second, that investigators can no longer blame fully rectified cutting current for their own shortcomings that result in tissue damage, cellular destruction or alteration, and slow, unfavorable tissue repair.

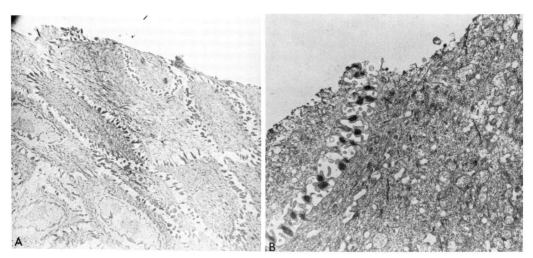

Figure 9–2–2. Histologic appearance of tissue edge cut by electrosurgery. *A*, Magnification ×5,700; *B*, magnification ×16,500 (from J. Prosth. Dent., 22:555, 1969).

Interceptive Periodontics with Electrosurgery[*]

Interproximal tissue was removed from four patients and utilized to record the reaction of a fully rectified electrosurgical instrument (Cameron-Miller). Cutting current with a needle electrode was used to remove the specimen with electrosurgery and a Bard-Parker scalpel was used for the conventional incision. Tissue specimens measuring 1.0×2.5 mm. in breadth were removed from the lower incisor area and placed in fixatives, glutaraldehyde and osmium tetroxide, within 10 to 21 seconds after removal. All specimens were divided into halves. One half was to be used for electron microscopy; the other was stained with hematoxylin and eosin for examination with a light microscope.

The primary purpose of the study was to compare the initial incision of the tissue and the postoperative healing. Seven days postoperatively, all previously cut surfaces were subjected to additional tissue removal with a scalpel to view the progress of the healing. The healing after conventional knife incision was compared with the healing after fully rectified electrosurgical instrument incision.

A third part of the study was to intentionally retard the rapidity of the passage of the electrode through the interproximal tissue. One of the authors was the subject for this portion of the study.

---

[*]A complete, verbatim abstract of the pertinent data in a preliminary report of an electron microscope comparative study of tissue cut with a steel knife and by electrosurgery published in the *Journal of Prosthetic Dentistry*, with original photomicrographs provided by Dr. Malone for this text.

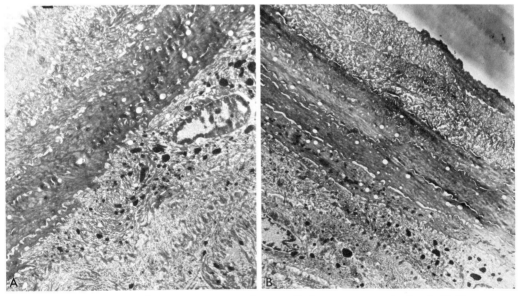

Figure 9–2–3. Histologic appearance of tissue 7 days postoperatively. *A*, Knife surgery result; *B*, electrosurgery result. (From J. Prosth. Dent., 22:555, 1969.)

Discussion

The results of the electron microscope studies illustrate that electrosurgery is a safe, effective method of tissue retraction and removal. These results are in definite contrast to those reported by Pope and colleagues but in agreement with the results of Klug, Harrison, Kelly, and Oringer. Further research is in progress which should shed light on the interim tissue repair and offer further evidence concerning the evaluation of the clinical application of electronic surgery. We hope that this additional research will confirm the insistence of Odland and Ross[11] that the initial trends in healing are most critical.

Results

The tissue edge along the incision showed no appreciable difference between the knife cut and electrosurgery. This similarity was viewed and compared under the electron microscope. The cell membrane, tonofibrils, mitochondria, and glycogen granules showed no signs of disturbance with either means of tissue removal. The results of electrosurgery were indistinguishable from those of the conventional knife cut.

The healing of all specimens illustrated no appreciable cellular alterations which could be interpreted as "delayed healing." However, neither method could be claimed as superior when evaluated by means of electron micrographs. Slow movement of the electrode through the tissues resulted in

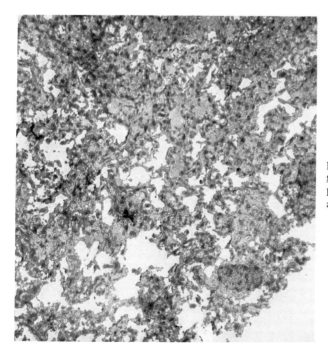

Figure 9-2-4. Histologic appearance of tissue cut by electrosurgery when electrode contact was prolonged (×6,800). Note mass coagulation necrosis.

complete destruction of cellular identification except for the dehydrated appearance of the nuclei (Fig. 9–2–4).

Any extensive tissue contouring should be accomplished with a fully rectified electronic instrument and should be done by a dentist who is familiar with the instrument. The partially rectified instruments are usually accompanied by slight coagulation due to lateral heat dispersion. This factor is considered insignificant when the instrument is merely used to augment restorative procedures in which considerable tissue removal is not anticipated. Employment of a coagulation current should be limited to desensitizing exposed cementum, pulpal extirpation procedures, and possible fulguration to inhibit bleeding.

A partially rectified instrument should not be routinely used as a means of periodontal therapy in which the periosteum is in constant contact with the electrode point.

Summary

Electron microscope pictures of interproximal tissue removed with a fully rectified electrosurgical instrument have shown the initial incision to be noninjurious at the cell level. The healing of tissue after a seven-day period failed to show any difference between the usual knife cut and electrosurgically treated tissue (Fig. 9–2–3). Conservative removal of traumatized interproximal fibrotic tissue is recommended. This can be effectively accomplished by the use of an electrosurgical instrument after the tooth is prepared and before making the impressions.

Included in this discussion is a histologic section of tissue cut by electrosurgery and photographed under 47,400× magnification (Fig. 9–2–6).

Figure 9–2–5. Histologic appearance of connective tissue properly cut by electrosurgery, including mast cell (×5,700). (From Oral Surg., Oral Med., Oral Path., to be published.)

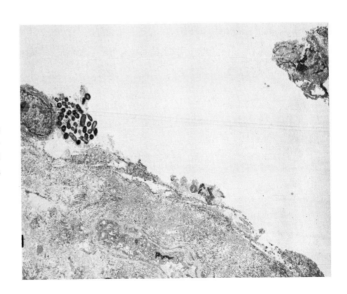

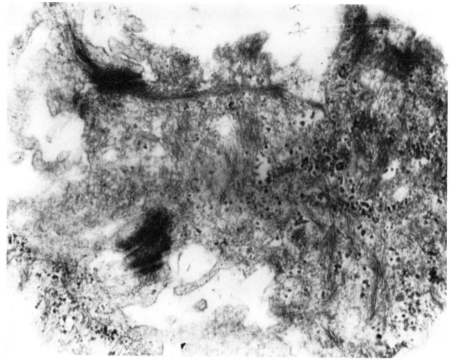

Figure 9–2–6. Electron microscope photomicrograph at 47,400× magnification of remaining portion of a single cell that had been partially cut away by electrosection. The cell
components, tonofibrils, mitochondria, and glycogen granules, are intact.

3. COMPARATIVE EVALUATION OF WOUND HEALING FOLLOWING STEEL SCALPEL AND ELECTROSURGICAL GINGIVECTOMY OF DILANTIN HYPERTROPHY

Overgrowth of the gingival mucosa may be induced by a variety of causes.
The latter may be local or systemic in origin. Localized gingival proliferation
or hyperplasia often is triggered by inflammation. The overgrowth may be in
response to a systemic pathologic condition such as Paget's disease, or it may
be nonspecific in nature, as a localized fibromatosis.

Gingival overgrowth is often manifested as a response to administration
of Dilantin to reduce and minimize the epileptic seizures of victims of grand
mal. As long as the patient continues Dilantin therapy, definitive treatment for
permanent eradication of the hypertrophic tissue cannot be achieved, and
surgery provides only temporary relief. However, when the overgrowth
causes physical distress and/or interference with eating the surgical reduction
is indicated despite the temporary nature of its benefits.

When the gingivectomy is performed to reduce the Dilantin hypertrophy
with a conventional steel scalpel, profuse hemorrhage usually ensues. When

the gingivectomy is performed by electrosection the hemorrhage is greatly minimized or eliminated. Nevertheless, many periodontists proclaim loudly and widely that the gingivectomy should be performed with the steel scalpel rather than by electrosection because they have found that the tissues cut with the scalpel healed more rapidly and favorably than the burn wounds created by electrosurgical methods.

Despite overwhelming evidence that tissue cut *properly* by electrosection is totally free of burn charring, or coagulation, their reports create the impression that electrosection inherently and automatically burns the tissues. The investigation to be reviewed next effectively disproves this myth.

This comparative clinical investigation of the respective efficiency and rate and quality of healing of wounds created by steel scalpel incision and comparable wounds created by electrosection with fully rectified current was performed on a human patient by Dr. Charles W. Conroy of Columbus, Ohio, and is presented here through his considerate cooperation.

This investigator is a highly competent periodontist with an impressive research background who has had excellent training in periodontal use of steel instruments and has also been trained in proper use of fully rectified electrosurgical cutting current. He is therefore uniquely qualified to conduct a comparative evaluation of both modalities.

The patient was a white female in her early twenties. She had experienced grand mal in her early teens and has been on Dilantin medication ever since. The Dilantin therapy produced the classic gingival Dilantin hypertrophy associated with this medication, and eventually it became necessary to reduce the tissue overgrowth surgically to enable the patient to eat more comfortably and to improve the aesthetics and tissue tone.

After a lapse of several years the interdental papillae were again greatly enlarged and the marginal gingivae thickened and engorged (Fig. 9–3–1). Dr. Conroy decided to treat this case as a comparative clinical evaluation between the efficacy and postoperative effects of steel scalpel surgery and those of electrosection, by treating the two mandibular quadrants with the respective modalities: a Bard-Parker steel scalpel was utilized for the cold steel intervention in one quadrant, and loop electrosection with fully rectified cutting current was employed in the other quadrant. Both quadrants were to be treated during the same visit.

A thorough prophylaxis was performed. The tissues were then prepared for an inferior alveolar-lingual nerve block, administered in the mandibular left quadrant.

A gingivectomy was performed by incisional excision with a Bard-Parker scalpel to resect the coronal two thirds of each interdental papilla. When a uniform papillary level was achieved, the cut marginal edges of the individual papillae were beveled with the scalpel blade to recreate a reasonably normal tissue contour. Owing to profuse and persistent bleeding from the cut tissues the speed of instrumentation was hampered and its efficiency was impaired. After the bleeding was controlled and clotting had occurred, tincture of myrrh and benzoin was applied in air-dried layers.

An inferior alveolar-lingual nerve block was then administered to anes-

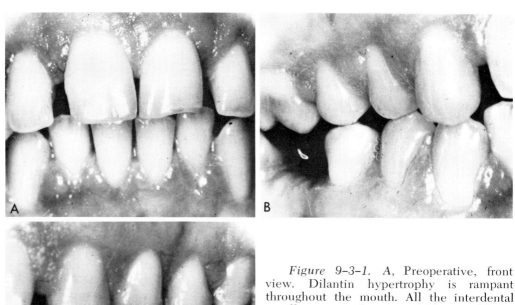

Figure 9-3-1. A, Preoperative, front view. Dilantin hypertrophy is rampant throughout the mouth. All the interdental papillae are grossly enlarged. The mandibular right lateral-cuspid papilla is somewhat larger than the adjacent or contralateral papillae. B, Preoperative, right side lateral view of the tissues. C, Preoperative, left side lateral view of the tissues.

thetize the right quadrant. A flame-shaped loop electrode (Coles E-6-A) was selected, cutting current was set at 6 on the Coles Radiosurg Scalpel IV instrument panel, and the circuit was activated.

The activated electrode was used with short wiping strokes to resect and simultaneously recontour the hypertrophied interdental papillae to reduce the height and restore the gingival architecture in the embrasures. Each application of the activated electrode was very brief, a mere fraction of a second. After two or three such applications, instrumentation was halted for 5 to 10 seconds to permit dissipation of any heat retained in the tissues, and during this period the cut tissue surfaces were remoistened to restore a normal surface tension and prevent dehydration.

The electrosurgical instrumentation was almost totally bloodless. Only a slight amount of oozing from the tissue surface occurred in a few areas. Figure 9-3-2 shows the difference between the two surgical fields very well.

Very soon after the loop planing was completed and surface oozing stopped, the blood clotted. Tincture of myrrh and benzoin was then applied to this quadrant. A periodontal pack was applied to the entire surgical field, home care instructions were given, and the patient was reappointed.

When she returned on the fifth postoperative day the cement pack was removed, the tissues were cleansed by very gentle irrigation with saline solu-

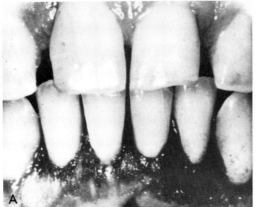
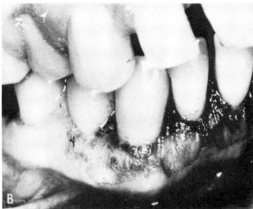
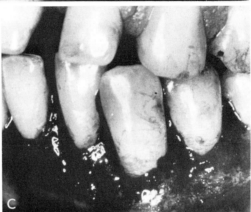

Figure 9-3-2. *A,* Operative appearance of the tissues that have just been treated by gingivoplasty. The tissues of the right central to first bicuspid have been reduced and recontoured by loop planing by electrosection. The tissues of the left central to left first bicuspid have been reduced by steel scalpel gingivoplasty. Note the free bleeding on the left side. *B,* Operative, a right lateral view of the surgical field. *C,* Operative, a left lateral view of the surgical field.

tion, and a second final cement pack was applied. The second pack was removed on the tenth postoperative day, and the tissues were cleansed by irrigation and carefully examined. The tissues in the right quadrant that had been cut by electrosection appeared somewhat more advanced in healing and the tissue tone appeared better than the comparable tissues cut with the steel scalpel. The difference in rate and quality of the tissue repair in the respective areas persisted until the tissues were fully healed (Fig. 9-3-3).

Postoperatively after several months renewed evidence of hypertrophy became clinically visible. The hypertrophy appeared to be slightly more pronounced in the left quadrant that had been treated by steel scalpel excision, despite the fact that the right quadrant hypertrophy had been slightly greater originally, before the surgery had been performed (Fig. 9-3-1). However, it is obvious that in due time, the hypertrophy will have advanced in both quadrants to the degree that another surgical intervention will become necessary to enable the patient to eat more efficiently and comfortably.

The results obtained in this case are interesting but they are also puzzling and contradictory. It has been repeatedly substantiated that when healing, tissues cut properly by fully rectified electrosection tend to regenerate toward their original level, whereas similar tissues cut with a steel scalpel tend to contract, owing to fibrous cicatricial scar repair. But in this case the opposite

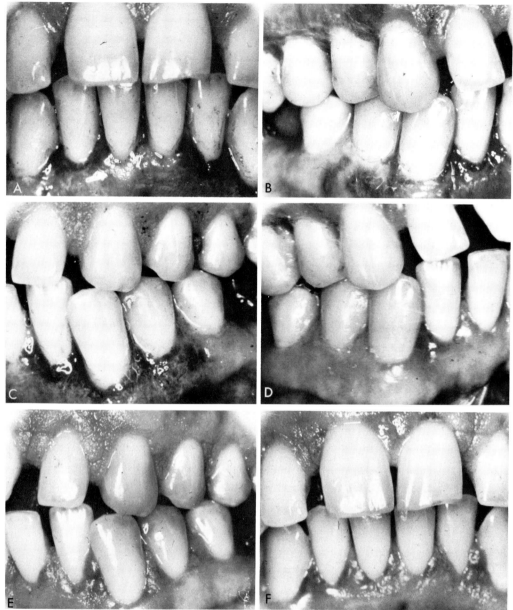

Figure 9–3–3. A, Postoperative appearance of the tissues, front view, one week later. The tissues on the right side, where the electrosurgery had been performed, are beginning to show initial evidence of healing. B, Postoperative appearance of the tissues, right lateral view, one week later. The tissues show unmistakable evidence of healing progress. C, Postoperative appearance of the tissues, left side, lateral view, also one week later. The tissues here show very little clinical evidence of healing progress. D, Postoperative appearance of the tissues fourth postoperative week, right lateral view. The tissues in this area appear well healed and maturely re-epithelialized except in the lateral-cuspid embrasure, where the tissue healing appears slow and the tissue appears immature. E, Postoperative appearance of the tissues, fourth postoperative week, left lateral view; the tissues in this area appear to have healed to a lesser degree and appear not as maturely re-epithelialized as the right side. The tissue in the left central-lateral and lateral-cuspid embrasures appears to be beginning to reproliferate. F, Postoperative appearance one year later; the tissues have reproliferated throughout the mouth. However, the proliferation does not appear quite as marked on the right side where the electrosurgery had been performed.

result was observed. Neither the investigator nor the author can offer any logical explanation for this seeming contradiction. At best one can only surmise that perhaps the bizarre tissue response to the dilantin medication, which is unique to this chemical only, may also produce an equally inexplicable tissue response following periodontal treatment.

What is infinitely more significant and to the point is the fact that this case once again demonstrates dramatically that when the therapist is *equally* competent in use of electrosurgery and cold steel, the tissue repair of the electrosurgical wound healing is less painful and more favorable than that of the tissues cut with the steel scalpel. Results such as were achieved in this comparative evaluation re-emphasize the inescapable conclusion that when similar investigations produce tissue burning and unfavorable tissue repair, or tissue repair that is slower and painful, such results are a reflection of the failure to achieve maximum efficiency and performance from the electrosurgical instrumentation, and not due to inherent deficiency in the electrosurgical modality.

4. EXPERIMENTAL ABORTION OF MANDIBULAR THIRD MOLARS BY ELECTROCOAGULATION

Cephalometric x-ray examination of the skull makes it possible to plot the growth and development of the human jaws from childhood to the adult state. Taking advantage of this possibility, Dr. Ricketts, an eminent orthodontist, has perfected a technique for feeding the cephalometric measurement data to a computer which he has programed to interpret such data and predict the exact adult size of the jaws when the child is still 8 or 9 years old.

On the basis of these computerized predictions, Dr. Ricketts is able to determine when a child's jaw growth and development will be insufficient to permit the normal eruption of the third molars, so that those teeth will be doomed to remain impacted and malposed and a potential source of future problems.

Dr. John E. Flocken, Professor of Restorative Dentistry and Director of Continuing Education, U.C.L.A. School of Dentistry, has made use of such predictability to develop with Dr. Ricketts a technique to abort the development of the third molar while it is only a tooth bud, thereby preventing future trouble from impacted mandibular third molars, by destroying the tooth bud by electrocoagulation.

Dr. Flocken is currently working on expansion of his original experimental objective of aborting third molar germinal tooth buds while in the gelatinous state to aborting impaction of mandibular third molars that would be unable to erupt normally, by retaining and transplanting the partially or fully calcified tooth buds and putting them to good use, instead of destroying them while in the gelatinous state.

He reported on his most recent experiment with tooth buds in a panel symposium at the 1972 A.D.A. Annual Session, using partially or fully calcified third molar tooth buds as transplants for first molars that must be extracted. He pointed out that transplantation of fully developed, or almost fully developed, third molar *teeth* into first molar sockets has been only partially successful. In almost all instances the roots of the transplanted teeth undergo extensive progressive resorption, and in a matter of a few years this usually results in loss of the transplants.

If a partially or fully calcified tooth *bud* instead of a fully developed tooth is implanted deeply into the first molar socket and permitted to develop and erupt in situ, the prospects for normal maturation and a normal life expectancy for the tooth appear far more favorable. Of course, the final judgment of the efficacy of such transplantation will depend on the recorded results of such transplantations over the next decade.

Dr. Flocken's abortion technique consists of two procedures utilizing electrocoagulation. The first procedure is performed in soft tissue only. The second involves the gingival tissue and alveolar bone.

The two procedures differ in that the tooth bud initially is located in the gingival tissue. As the bud develops it burrows into the bone and eventually is completely encased in the bone. There the bud proceeds to develop into a tooth. As the roots develop the tooth begins to push up against the bone until the crown of the tooth erupts through the bone and gingival tissue.

The physical consistency of the tooth bud differs in each stage. In the first stage the bud is a gelatinous germinal tissue that is radiolucent; thus the tooth bud cannot be seen on an x-ray. To locate the mandibular third molar bud at this stage it must be pinpointed anatomically. Dr. Flocken describes the use of a straight rigid wire placed over the buccal cusps of the bicuspids and molars so that the posterior end of the wire comes into contact with the tissue posterior to the second molar. This is the precise site where the bud in the germinal stage is located. A cone-shaped coagulating electrode is inserted into the tissue at this point, and coagulating current is activated, with the same amount of power output to produce immediate superficial spot coagulation. The coagulation is completed in about 2 seconds when used at the correct power setting, without causing appreciable damage to the adjacent or subjacent tissues.

In the second stage the bud can be located roentgenographically. If it is still in the germinal stage it can be seen on careful scrutiny as a small radiolucent spot about three times the size of the head of a pin located distal to the second molar. To verify that the exact site has been located, a metallic marker can be inserted into the tissues where it is believed the bud is located and an x-ray taken with the marker in situ. The roentgenogram will reveal whether the marker has penetrated to the bud. If a metallic marker is being used, the coagulating current can be applied directly to it for about 2 seconds to destroy the bud without causing damage to the surrounding tissues. Or the marker can be removed and the conical electrode reintroduced into the same site where the marker had been and the bud destroyed by direct electrocoagulation.

When the bud has become calcified and, because of premature loss of the permanent first molar it is necessary to remove it and transplant it into the first molar socket, it is essential that it be removed from its bony crypt without damaging it. This is extremely difficult to do when the surgical field is flooded with blood and visibility in the area is severely impaired. When the incision is made by electrosection the hemostasis eliminates the hemorrhagic bleeding or reduces it to a controllable degree, thereby increasing the potential for an atraumatic removal and transplantation.

He emphasized the importance of electrosurgery's contribution to the success of the procedure. Bleeding in the surgical field would impair visibility and make it virtually impossible to remove the delicate tooth buds atraumatically from their cypts without damage. Even aspiration of blood, or sponging to remove the blood is likely to damage the bud and would seriously hamper the delicate instrumentation that is required. Incising the tissue for a mucoperiosteal flap to expose the tooth bud by electrosection with fully rectified cutting current provides the hemostasis without tissue destruction that assures optimal conditions for maximum surgical efficiency.

The author feels that there is another critically important reason why electrosurgery offers the maximum prospect for successful transplantation. Extraction of the mandibular first molar in a child invariably becomes necessary owing to extensive pathologic involvement of the tooth. After extraction and debridement of the socket by manual curettage with surgical steel curets the socket remains contaminated. This seriously jeopardizes the ultimate success of the transplantation. If, after the tooth has been extracted, the socket is thoroughly debrided by electronic curettage with loop electrodes, supplemented, if necessary, by fulguration, the socket becomes sterilized as the diseased area is being eliminated, thereby greatly enhancing the prospects for a successful outcome.

Dr. Flocken offers the prediction that the computerized ability to predict accurately when and where third molar tooth buds should be eliminated to prevent future trouble from impactions, combined with the ability to remove the buds atraumatically by bloodless mucoperiosteal incisions by electrosection and eventual successful neutralization of transplant rejections by the body, will in all probability lead to development of tooth bud banks, similar to eye and other organ banks, for use where needed. This is a very exciting and hopeful prospect for the future that is being made possible by electrosurgery, combined with ingenious, constructive thinking.

Despite the ardent and enthusiastic commitment of our profession to preventive dentistry for the past half century, disappointingly little has been accomplished, and the search for caries prevention, prevention of periodontal disease and of malocclusion, and the numerous other problems of a comparable nature continues unabated.

This technique is a real contribution in the realm of prevention, since it effectively aborts one of the more agonizing problems of young adults, and eliminates not only the pain and need for surgical relief but also a frequent cause of malocclusion, thanks to the unique characteristics of electrosurgery.

5. ELECTROCOAGULATION FOR ENDODONTIC STERILIZATION

On several occasions at scientific meetings of the American Academy of Dental Electrosurgery, Dr. John H. Mullett of Toronto, Canada, has reported his experiments with use of electrocoagulation for sterilization of root canals prior to their obturation.

His original experiments were performed with extracted teeth that had been endodontically prepared, autoclaved, contaminated with measured amounts of *Streptococcus viridans*, then implanted into slabs of meat, treated by electrocoagulation, and cultured to determine the degree of sterility achieved or failure to do so. He found the electrocoagulation to be successful in about 95 per cent of the experiments, with very little evidence of lateral heat penetration into the investing tissue.

He subsequently reported duplicating the experiments in experimental laboratory animals, using dogs as the subjects, and finally investigated the effectiveness of electrocoagulation for treating contaminated teeth in humans. For these experiments he flooded the canals with Jayvex Water, which appears to be similar to Clorox. The electrocoagulation vaporizes the chlorine solution, releasing nascent chlorine. It is difficult to ascertain with certainty to what degree his success should be attributed to the electrocoagulation, and to what degree, if any, to the chlorination. But his results have been reported as extremely favorable and impressive.

Unfortunately Dr. Mullett has not made available to the author x-rays, laboratory reports, or comparable data that are essential for a factual report, but his experiments are interesting enough to deserve mention. It is regrettable that they cannot be reported here in detail.

Section Four

INTERRELATED NONELECTROSURGICAL FACTORS

PART 1

ANESTHESIA

Introduction

This edition devotes much more attention to the matter of anesthesia; specifically to the various techniques for administration of local anesthesia.

There are two very sound basic reasons for the expanded coverage of this subject matter. First, because it is impossible to perform precise, skillful, efficient electrosurgical instrumentation on a patient who is squirming violently because he is in agonizing pain. Performing electrosurgery under such conditions greatly increases the potential for unfavorable electrosurgical postoperative sequelae due to inefficient use.

The second, and in some respects even more compelling reason, is that severe postoperative pain and sometimes retarded poor healing due to tissue trauma created by improper injection technique invariably are unjustly attributed to electrosurgical instrumentation.

Faulty injection technique very often results in severe postoperative pain and unfavorable tissue response that simulates improper use of electrosurgical currents. Those who have used electrosurgery properly are aware that owing to the totally atraumatic nature of electrosection there is a remarkable *lack* of postoperative pain even after extensive oral surgery.

Although absence of the usual unfavorable postoperative sequelae experienced with traditional steel scalpel surgery is one of the many advantages we enjoy with electrosurgery, nevertheless, when a patient reports severe postoperative pain after having experienced electrosurgery, the therapist almost instinctively tends to blame the electrosurgery and often becomes wary of using the modality, even though the pain really was due to poor injection technique. The author therefore feels that it is urgently necessary to review the techniques of local anesthesia as thoroughly as the electrosurgical techniques.

211

Chapter Ten

PHARMACODYNAMICS
OF THE LOCAL
ANESTHETIC DRUGS

PROFUNDITY OF ANESTHESIA

INDICATIONS. It is imperative that the prospective user of electrosurgery recognize the essential need for profound anesthesia if electrosurgery is to be performed safely and satisfactorily. No matter how skillful and dexterous an operator may become, it is impossible to perform electrosurgery delicately, skillfully and accurately upon a fearful patient squirming from acute pain. Furthermore, just as accidental injury can be inflicted with cold-steel scalpels, burs, disks and stones, or as hypodermic needles may break accidentally if the patient squirms or moves with a sudden jerk, accidental injury can be inflicted with an activated electrode under such circumstances.

For consistently painless electrosurgical instrumentation the profundity of the local anesthesia must be fully comparable to the depth of anesthesia required for painless extirpation of vital pulp tissue from a root canal.

CONTRAINDICATIONS. An old adage says that "exceptions prove rules." In electrosurgery there are two noteworthy exceptions to the need for profound anesthesia. One is that surface topical anesthesia usually suffices to permit relatively painless incision of fluctuant acute abscesses. The other is that surface topical anesthesia is usually adequate for performing light superficial spot postoperative coagulation on pinpoint areas of healing granulation tissue.

The reasons for these exceptions are as follows:

1. When an acute alveolar abscess forms, the tissues become distended with pus. The gingival mucosa becomes detached from the underlying bone and becomes severely compressed and thinned out by the pressure and distention. Little if any normal nerve innervation remains in the affected tissue. In such an area, pain stimuli are triggered mostly by pressure exerted against the distended tissue, as is created by incision with a cold-steel scalpel. When an

212

activated surgical electrode is brushed lightly over such an area the tissue parts painlessly as the electrode floats through without pressure.

2. When biterminal coagulating current is used with minimal effective current-intensity output, and a small ball electrode is just barely brought into momentary contact with the surface of incompletely healed, healthy mucosa to which topical anesthesia has been applied, virtually no pain is felt. Little pain is likely to be felt by the average patient when similar spot coagulation is applied to newly granulating tissue in which nerve regeneration has not yet occurred even if the topical anesthetic is omitted. Topical anesthesia therefore is more than adequate to make superficial postoperative spot coagulation quite painless.

LOCAL ANESTHESIA

When anesthesia *is required*, in the absence of specific contraindications local anesthesia is the administrative method of choice. There are three major specific contraindications to use of local anesthesia:

1. Allergy to local anesthetic drugs. This is quite rare, opinions to the contrary notwithstanding.[1]

2. Presence of massive, diffuse, acute intraoral infection.

3. Some systemic diseases, often cardiovascular or renal in nature.

The efficacy of local anesthesia is determined by twin factors: (a) Ability to deposit the anesthetic solution at the proper anatomic site; and (b) the influence of the *pharmacodynamics* of the local anesthetic drugs on the ability of the anesthetic agent to perform its function properly.

CHOICE OF ANESTHETIC ADMINISTRATION. All surgical procedures, irrespective of the nature of the surgery, have one common denominator: all require effective anesthesia. Dental electrosurgery is no exception in this respect. However, it differs from most other surgical procedures in the type of anesthesia that can be most advantageously employed for it.

Visceral and most other forms of medical surgery require total muscle relaxation. Patient mobility or cooperation not only is unnecessary but would be highly undesirable during such procedures. This type of surgery is therefore performed most efficiently on patients who have been rendered unconscious in the surgical plane of general anesthesia.

For dental electrosurgery the situation is reversed. Not only is patient cooperation desirable, it is almost essential for optimal electrosurgical results. The patient who has been rendered unconscious in the surgical plane of general anesthesia, being totally unable to cooperate, must have his jaws propped open during the anesthesia. To avoid injury to the temporomandibular joint the opening usually is limited to approximately 3 to 4 cm. This limited, fixed jaw opening, combined with the patient's inability to turn or tilt the head to improve access and visibility in the operative field, severely hinders the therapist's instrumentation, particularly in the posterior part of the mouth and on the palatal and lingual tissues, and thereby hampers his ability to perform the electrosurgery carefully and competently. Thus, except when clinical conditions dictate specific need for it, surgical plane general anesthesia appears to be contraindicated for dental electrosurgery.

The contraindication is not applicable to the analgesic plane of general anesthesia. Since nitrous oxide-oxygen analgesia merely blunts the patient's pain perception without rendering him unconscious, he remains cooperative and the handicaps encountered with surgical plane anesthesia are eliminated. However, since electrosurgery requires profound anesthesia, analgesia alone is likely to prove inadequate. Analgesia can therefore be employed for electrosurgery most advantageously when used in preplanned balanced combination with local anesthesia. Local anesthesia, properly administered, is by far the most universally advantageous and suitable type of anesthesia for electrosurgery.

The efficiency of administration of the local anesthesia influences dental electrosurgery profoundly in three different but interrelated respects:

1. It is impossible to perform efficient electrosurgical instrumentation on a patient who is physically squirming from pain.

2. Operative pain experienced by the patient due to poor anesthesia is usually mistakenly attributed to the electrosurgery.

3. Postoperative pain resulting from traumatic improper administration of the local anesthesia invariably is improperly attributed to the electrosurgical procedure that had been performed.

Since these three factors can profoundly influence acceptance of electrosurgery by both the patient and the therapist, a brief review of local anesthesia will be included in this text.

IMPORTANCE OF ANATOMIC SITE. If the anesthetic solution is deposited precisely at or very close to the foramen from which the nerve to be anesthetized emerges, the anesthetic solution bathes the nerve sheath and penetrates rapidly to the innermost fibers of the nerve. This results in rapid onset of anesthesia and a very profound, adequately lasting anesthetic effect.

Should the anesthetic solution be deposited in the general vicinity of but not close to the nerve, some of the anesthetic solution will eventually penetrate through the intervening tissues by osmosis and affect the outer sheath of the nerve sufficiently to produce anesthetic symptoms, without penetrating to the innermost fibers. Such an injection produces an anesthetic effect which is of slow onset, poor quality, and usually only transitory.

INFLUENCE OF THE PHARMACODYNAMICS OF LOCAL ANESTHETIC DRUGS. The local anesthetic drugs most commonly used in dentistry belong to either the procaine or lidocaine families of anesthetic salts. The former consists of an anesthetic base combined with an acid radical, the latter of an anesthetic basic amide with an acid radical. The sole function of the acid radical is to maintain the stability of the anesthetic drug. It therefore does not play an active role in producing anesthesia, but prevents the anesthetic salt from functioning until the acid radical has been neutralized.

The alkaline buffers needed to neutralize the acid radical can be provided only by the blood and tissue fluids. If an excessive amount of anesthetic solution is deposited at the injection site the acid radical overwhelms the alkaline buffers present in the area. As a result, the onset of anesthesia is retarded, and the anesthesia is ineffectual. Comparable results occur when anesthetic solution is deposited into an area where the pH of the tissues is on the acid side because of inflammation, stasis, or low-grade chronic infection.

It is noteworthy that when an excessive amount of anesthetic solution has been injected, characteristically the onset of anesthesia is slow and the profundity inadequate during the surgical procedure; however, the patient reports subsequently that although the instrumentation was painful the anesthetic symptoms persisted for many hours postoperatively.

Methods of Administration

Local anesthesia may be administered by infiltration, regional block injection, or by a combination of both.

INFILTRATION ANESTHESIA

Local anesthesia by means of infiltration should be administered only when the tissues are in normal health. Under such conditions subperiosteal infiltration can be safely administered if the injection is made *slowly, a drop at a time,* to guard against traumatic detachment of the periosteum from the bone. When subperiosteal infiltration is administered in this manner the onset of anesthesia is rapid, is acceptably profound in effect, and will not cause postoperative traumatic pain.

Submucous infiltration usually fails to provide adequately profound anesthesia and tends to be transitory in duration. If the anesthetic solution is injected rapidly, the pressure has a traumatic tearing and crushing effect on the tissues, causing considerable postoperative pain. If an excessive amount of solution is injected it tends to cause marked ballooning of the tissues, usually with a traumatic, painful postoperative reaction.

Since infiltration may properly be used only in normal healthy tissue and subperiosteal infiltration provides much more desirable anesthesia, this would appear to be the preferred method of administering infiltration anesthesia.

REGIONAL BLOCK ANESTHESIA

The entire maxilla and mandible can be surgically anesthetized very effectively by regional block anesthesia if the various block injections are properly performed at the proper anatomic sites. The author's personal anesthetic preference for electrosurgery is regional block anesthesia, fortified where and when indicated with subperiosteal infiltration.

PRECAUTIONS TO PREVENT OR MINIMIZE ANESTHETIC SHOCK

Shock, irrespective of its origin, is potentially lethal.

Shock reaction to the administration of local anesthesia is one of the more common and disruptive emergencies encountered in the dental office.

Most anesthetic shock reactions can be prevented by taking the following few simple basic precautions.

Aspiration

Aspiration prior to injecting is one of the most effective means for preventing shock. Since aspirating syringes are now available commercially even in the disposable variety, administration of local anesthesia without first performing aspiration is as inexcusable as it is injudicious and unnecessary.

Aspiration reveals whether the tip of the needle has punctured into a blood vessel. In the latter event, since all local anesthetic salts are protoplasmic poisons to a greater or lesser degree, injection of the local anesthetic solution into the blood vessel is very likely to induce a shock reaction.

If aspiration reveals that a blood vessel has been punctured, the needle should be removed, reinserted at a nearby site, and aspiration repeated until a negative aspiration is obtained. The injection can then be performed without danger of inducing shock from injection into the bloodstream.

In the unlikely event that no aspirating syringe is available, after inserting the needle tip into the tissues 15 to 20 seconds should be permitted to elapse before proceeding with the injection. If the needle has penetrated into a blood vessel, a trace of blood will slowly trickle into the cartridge by capillary attraction and be seen within that period of time, indicating need to withdraw and reinsert the needle.

Blood Contamination of the Anesthetic Cartridge

Injection of local anesthetic solution from a cartridge that has become contaminated by the entry of blood is unequivocally contraindicated, since it is very likely to act as an allergenic agent and induce moderate to severe allergic shock reaction. Thus, even if only a faint trace of blood has seeped into the cartridge it should be discarded and a fresh cartridge of solution used for the injection.

Temperature of the Anesthetic Solution

Injection of cold anesthetic solution into the tissues can induce a shock reaction. The anesthetic solution should therefore be used at or nearly at body temperature. If because of refrigeration or low room temperature the anesthetic solution is cold, it is neither necessary nor advisable to warm the solution by passing it through a Bunsen flame or immersing it in hot water. If the cartridge is cradled in the palm of the hand during the 2 to 3 minute wait for the topical anesthetic to take effect, the warmth of the hand will bring the solution to body temperature without risking breakage of the glass cartridge or chemical decomposition of the anesthetic salt, and without loss of time.

REGIONAL BLOCK ANESTHESIA

MAXILLARY REGIONAL BLOCK INJECTIONS
The posterior superior alveolar block

This is one of the simplest of the regional block injections to administer. However, owing to the close proximity of the pterygoid venous plexus to the injection site, it is essential to exercise great care in administering it (Figure 10–1). The close proximity of this blood plexus creates the hazard of accidentally piercing a vessel in the plexus if contact with the bone is lost, with hemorrhage and hematoma formation ensuing, in addition to shock if the anesthetic is injected into the plexus.

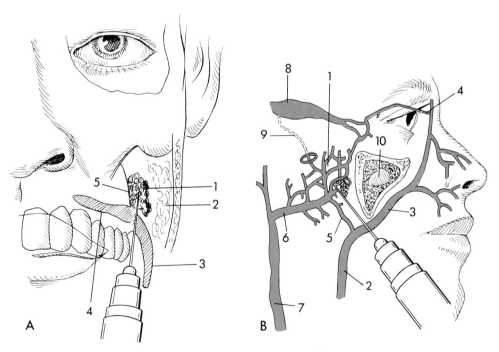

Figure 10–1. A, A transverse section of the pterygoid venous plexus danger area. The needle has penetrated the plexus. (1) Pterygoid venous plexus. (2) Adipose and areolar tissue in the cheek. (3) Buccinator muscle. (4) Origin of the buccinator muscle on the alveolar process of the maxilla. (5) Small superficial head of the medial pterygoid muscle. B, Lateral view of danger areas in pterygoid plexus: (1) Venous pterygoid plexus. (2) Anterior facial vein. (3) Angular vein. (4) Orbital emissary vein. (5) Deep facial vein. (6) Internal maxillary vein. (7) Posterior facial vein. (8) Cavernous sinus. (9) Emissary vein connecting pterygoid plexus and cavernous sinus. (10) Maxillary sinus.

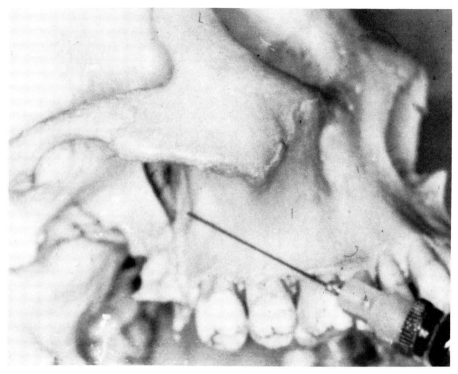

Figure 10-2. Depicts on an anatomic dry skull the proper direction and depth of penetration of the needle for a successful posterior superior alveolar block injection.

This hazard can be neutralized in part by introducing the needle so that it hugs the alveolar bone in the tuberosity area closely (Fig. 10-2) as it is introduced, by avoiding excessive insertion beyond the foramina (Fig. 10-3), and by using an aspirating syringe so that aspiration is performed before the anesthetic solution is deposited. The needle is inserted into the areolar tissue over the apex of the distobuccal root of the maxillary first molar (Fig. 10-4A). Having ascertained by aspiration that the pterygoid plexus has not been invaded, the needle is directed backward, upward, and inward at approximately a 45 degree angle and advanced 3 to 4 cm. (Fig. 10-4B); the anesthetic solution is then deposited slowly, a drop at a time, until about 0.5 cc. of solution has been injected. Tilting the patient's head toward the side opposite the injection site helps to assure the success of this injection by enlisting the force of gravity to direct the flow of the anesthetic solution toward the bone.

The infraorbital block

This block anesthetizes the maxillary anterior teeth. Administered bilaterally it anesthetizes from bicuspid to bicuspid and the labial alveolar bone and mucosa. This is a much more difficult injection to perform than is the previous block. Owing to the anatomic conformation of the buccal aspect of the maxilla in the region of the canine eminence, it is difficult to insert the needle toward the foramen without making premature contact with the bone if the needle is directed posterosuperiorly from the apex of the central incisor

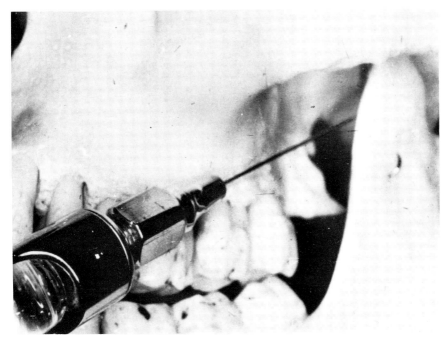

Figure 10–3. Depicts on the dry skull excessive penetration of the needle which in the live patient would most likely result in hemorrhage from the pterygoid venous plexus and might anesthetize the ophthalmic branch of the trifacial nerve and cause drooping of the eyelid.

toward the foramen (Fig. 10–5). Both the infraorbital nerve and artery emerge from the infraorbital canal and foramen and lie under the levator labii superioris muscle of the face. If premature contact with the bone occurs, it not only impairs the ability to reach the foramen but also increases the hazard of piercing the artery, with hemorrhage and hematoma formation similar to the traumatic "black eye" resulting therefrom.

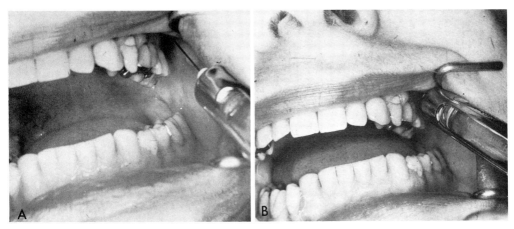

Figure 10–4. *A,* The direction of the needle and syringe for a clinical posterior superior alveolar injection. *B,* The needle penetration to the site of the foramen.

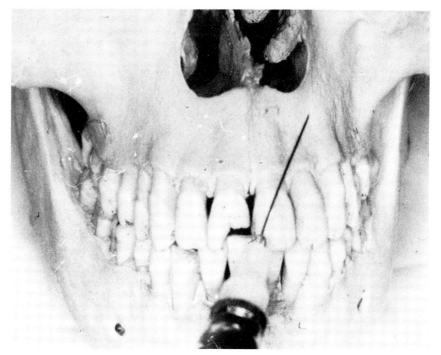

Figure 10–5.   The needle in contact with the canine eminence of the maxilla. This prevents the needle from penetrating to the infraorbital foramen.

The author has found that this hazard can be reduced by inserting the needle over the apex of the cuspid or first bicuspid (Fig. 10–6), at a point approximately 1 cm. labial to the alveolar bone (Fig. 10–7A). When the foramen is reached approximately 0.5 cc. of solution is deposited (Fig. 10–7B).

This injection should always be performed with an aspirating syringe, and aspiration should be performed before completing the injection. If blood is aspirated the needle should be withdrawn, the anesthetic cartridge discarded, and the injection attempt repeated with a fresh cartridge. When the infraorbital block is administered in the manner that has been described, the hazard of causing hemorrhagic hematomas and failure to achieve effective anesthesia is greatly minimized.

It is possible for the infraorbital foramen to be atypically located or to run in an atypical direction (Fig. 10–8A and B). In the event that the foramen cannot be located by intraoral injection in the customary manner it is possible to perform the block via the extraoral route (Fig. 10–8C), but such cases are encountered quite infrequently.

When administered bilaterally, the two blocks that have been described effectively anesthetize the entire labial and buccal aspects of the maxilla. To complete the anesthesia of the maxilla it is necessary to also anesthetize the hard palate.

THE PALATAL REGIONAL BLOCKS

The anterior palatal or nasopalatine block

The nasopalatine block anesthetizes the anterior part of the hard palate.

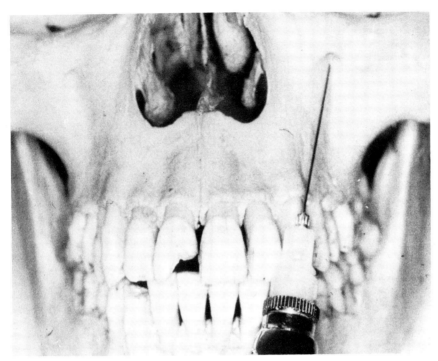

Figure 10–6. The author's preferred point of entry from over the first bicuspid with an unimpeded path to the foramen.

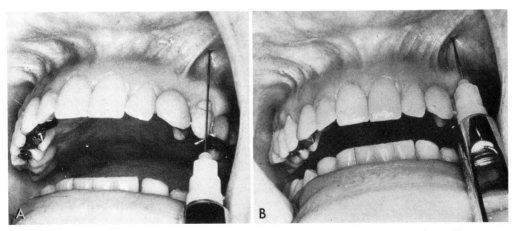

Figure 10–7. A, The needle is beginning to penetrate the mucosa clinically to perform an infraorbital block injection. *B,* The completion of the penetration. The tip of the needle is now at the orifice of the foramen.

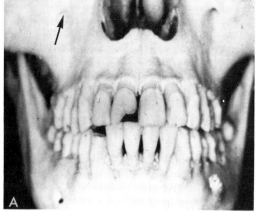
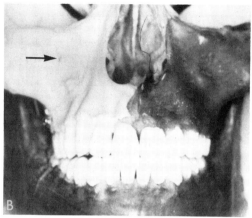
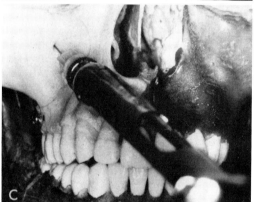

Figure 10–8. A, On a dry skull we can see the lack of uniformity of the infraorbital foramina that may be encountered. The foramen on the right side is open and slanted at approximately 45 degrees. The foramen on the left side is almost entirely closed and slants at about 75 degrees (arrow). It would be impossible to perform an infraorbital block into this foramen. *B*, Another dry skull shows a foramen directed horizontally into the bone and the tiny slitlike opening at the orifice (arrow). *C*, The horizontal direction of the needle as it penetrates into the infraorbital canal. This type of foramen and canal would require an extraoral injection.

According to Gray's *Anatomy*, this area is innervated by the left and right anterior palatine nerves which emerge through the foramina of Scarpa. The left nerve emerges through the more anterior of the two foramina that lie in the midline immediately posterior to the maxillary central incisors, and the right nerve emerges from the foramen located posterior to it. *Clinically*, however, and as can be noted in most dry specimen skulls, there appears to be just one fairly large nasopalatine foramen, located approximately 1 cm. posterior to the palatal aspect of the maxillary central incisor, in the exact midline (Fig. 10–9).

In administering the nasopalatine block it is important to guard against use of excessive pressure to inject the solution into and through the thick, fibrous nasopalatine papilla. Forceful injection usually results in severe postoperative pain, and may even cause sloughing of the papillary tissue.

To avoid these hazards the injection is initiated by carefully introducing the needle tip into the tissue at one side of the papilla and slowly depositing 2 or 3 drops of anesthetic solution into the mucosa (Fig. 10–10A). This produces sufficient anesthesia to permit careful insertion of the needle into the foramen (Fig. 10–10B), so that the anesthetic solution can be injected very slowly without pressure. Injecting 2 to 3 drops of solution through the *labial* interdental papilla between the maxillary central incisors (Fig. 10–10C) often

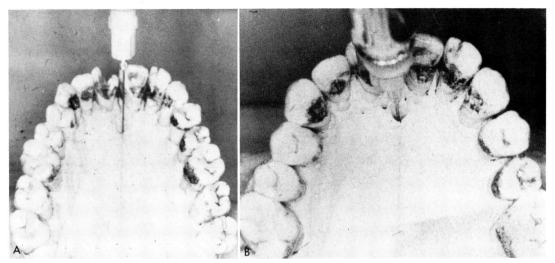

Figure 10–9. *A*, The needle is seen being inserted into the canal. *B*, The location of the nasopalatine foramen on a dry skull and the depth of the canal. The needle has penetrated its full depth.

helps to further assure painless needle insertion through the papilla and thus makes it easier to avoid forceful pressure while injecting.

The posterior palatine block

The injection site to anesthetize the posterior palatine nerve, which innervates the posterior part of the hard palate, is at the anterior palatine foramen. This small foramen is located approximately 1 cm. medially and slightly distal to the maxillary third molar (Fig. 10–11). Injections made anterior to this foramen (Fig. 10–12) provide infiltration anesthesia that usually is adequate, but will not block the entire posterior portion of the hard palate. Should the latter be required, it is usually necessary to probe around with the needle until the foramen is located and then insert the needle approximately 1 cm. into the foramen and inject 6 to 8 drops of anesthetic solution slowly, a drop at a time, without pressure. This block, administered bilaterally, completes the anesthesia of the maxilla.

It is also possible to anesthetize the entire maxilla with just one block administered bilaterally—the second division block, which anesthetizes the maxillary division of the trifacial nerve at the foramen rotundum. This block can be performed intraorally with a long 45-degree-angle needle via the posterior palatine canal through the posterior palatine foramen (Fig. 10–13), or via the extraoral route. This block is, however, a very difficult and hazardous one and is therefore very rarely used, so that the maxillary regional blocks that have been described are the ones that are clinically significant.

THE MANDIBULAR REGIONAL BLOCKS

The inferior alveolar-lingual block

This block, administered bilaterally, effectively anesthetizes the entire mandible. The long buccal branch of the inferior alveolar nerve, which innervates the buccal gingival mucosa in the molar region, sometimes fails to become fully anesthetized. In that event, 2 to 3 drops of anesthetic solution

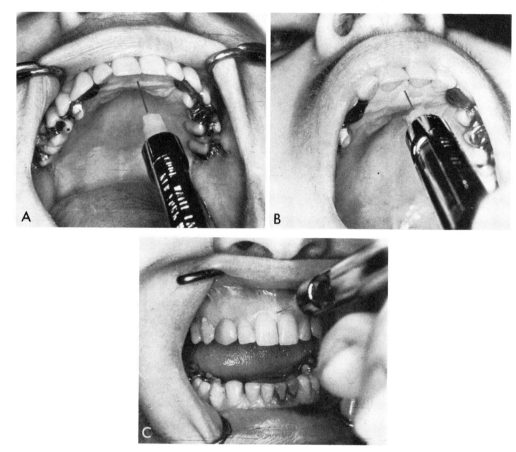

Figure 10–10.   *A*, A clinical injection for a nasopalatine block. The needle has penetrated into the mucosa immediately lateral to the nasopalatine papilla to provide infiltration anesthesia that will make penetration into the papilla painless. A 25-gauge needle 1 inch long is being used. *B*, The nasopalatine injection into the foramen is being performed. As a result of the infiltration anesthesia provided by the previous injection, this final phase of the block injection is totally painless and atraumatic since the anesthetic solution can be deposited very slowly, a drop at a time, to assure that no tissue damage will result. *C*, A few drops of anesthetic are being injected into the interdental papilla between the centrals at the crest of the interseptal bone, to provide supplemental anesthesia to the infiltration performed in *A*. If this supplemental injection is used, it precedes the actual injection into the nasopalatine canal.

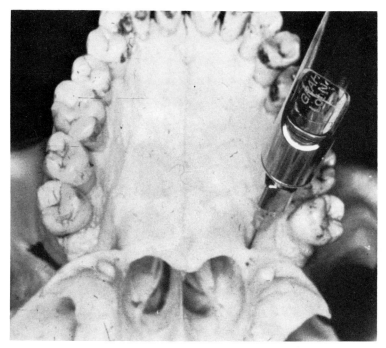

Figure 10–11.   The anterior palatine foramina as seen on an anatomic dry skull. The hypodermic needle is seen deeply inserted into the foraminal canal.

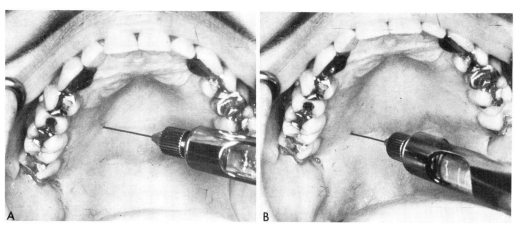

Figure 10–12.   A, A clinical injection *anterior* to the anterior palatine canal is being performed, to provide infiltration anesthesia. B, The clinical injection being performed properly. The needle has been inserted 1 cm. distally and 1.5 cm. superiorly toward the midline to the third molar, and has penetrated to the anterior palatine canal, where a few drops of anesthetic are being deposited.

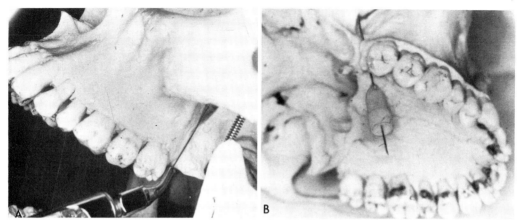

Figure 10–13.   A, A 45-degree angle needle that has been inserted to the foramen rotundum to provide block anesthesia of the entire half of the maxilla. *B*, The site of insertion of the needle to perform this injection via the intraoral route.

deposited into the areolar gingival mucosa in the region of the mesiobuccal root of the second molar effectively completes the anesthesia.

Since the lingual nerve is almost invariably anesthetized as the needle is advanced toward the ascending ramus (Fig. 10–14), the one injection pro-

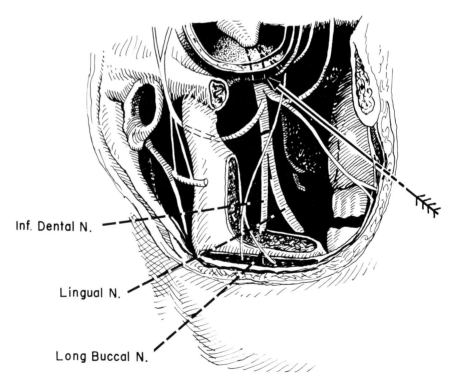

Inf. Dental N.

Lingual N.

Long Buccal N.

Figure 10–14.   Depicts the anatomic structures and the three divisions of the trifacial nerve after its emergence from the skull and the lingual nerve that will be blocked as the needle penetrates toward the foramen.

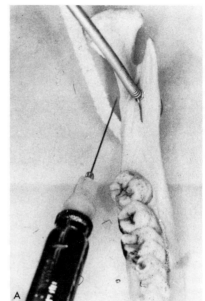
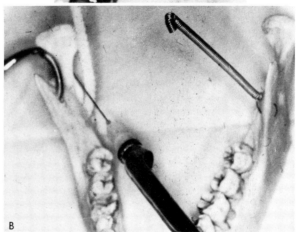

Figure 10–15. A, Depicts on a mandible the proper site for the tip of the needle to penetrate for the inferior alveolar injection. A pipe cleaner has been inserted into the foramen to represent the entry of the inferior alveolar nerve into the mandible. B, Depicts the penetration of the needle far beyond the foramen in the ramus. If introduced this far, the needle will penetrate into the parotid gland and produce a temporary paralysis of the facial muscles of expression.

duces an effective block of both the lingual and the inferior alveolar nerves, so that they are treated as one block. Figure 10–15A shows the needle accurately inserted to the foramen. Figure 10–15B shows the needle inserted beyond the foramen, which results in anesthetic failure or very delayed onset and poor anesthetic result.

This block may be performed either by direct or indirect thrust. The direct thrust technique will be discussed here. To perform this injection the forefinger is placed in the area posterior to the retromolar pad at the internal angle of the jaw and the external oblique line palpated, after an effective topical anesthetic has been applied to the tissues for 2 minutes. The syringe is directed toward the tissues from a point over the crowns of the cuspid and first bicuspid on the opposite side (Fig. 10–16A) and the needle tip is inserted at a point that bisects the fingernail of the palpating forefinger. Two to 3 drops of

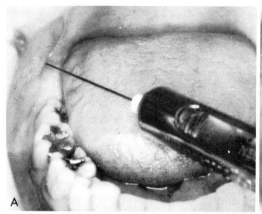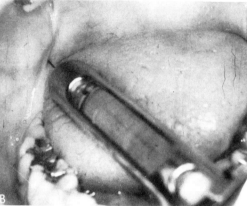

Figure 10–16. A, The tip of the needle has just punctured the tissue and a drop of anesthetic is being deposited ahead of the needle tip to make the penetration toward the foramen painless. B, With the barrel of the syringe parallel to the occlusal surface of the mandibular teeth the needle has been advanced by direct thrust to the foramen and 0.5 to 1.0 cc. of anesthetic solution is being deposited slowly, a drop at a time.

anesthetic are deposited, and the needle is advanced toward the foramen. As the needle penetrates, additional solution is deposited very slowly, and the lingual nerve block occurs before the foramen is reached. When the needle has been introduced about 3 cm. (Fig. 10–16B) the tip should be in the immediate vicinity of the foramen and about 0.5 cc. of anesthetic solution is deposited there.

The proper level at which the needle should be introduced into the tissues is attained by simply resting the barrel of the hypodermic syringe on the occlusal surfaces of the teeth in the dental arch. For the aged edentulous patient, tilt the needle slightly upward, since the foramen usually is at a higher level due to senile resorption of the alveolar ridge. For the very young patient it is best to tilt the needle slightly downward, as the foramen usually is at a slightly lower level in the young.

One of the hazards to guard against in administering this block is to avoid inserting the needle too far posteriorly, since it is then likely to penetrate the parotid gland, which lies on the medial aspect of the posterior part of the ramus near the angle of the jaw. This would traumatize or anesthetize one of the innumerable branches of the facial nerve plexus which ramifies throughout the gland, producing transitory paralysis of some of the facial muscles of expression, usually in the nature of a drooping of the angle of the lips on the affected side, resembling Bell's palsy (Fig. 10–17). Another hazard, seen less frequently, results from injecting at too high a level, so that the ophthalmic branch of the trifacial nerve is anesthetized, and the eye on that side is affected for the duration of the anesthesia. Both hazards are merely minor inconveniences of temporary duration, but both can be avoided by good technique.

Although the entire mandible can be fully anesthetized by bilateral inferior alveolar block injection, the tongue is also anesthetized and it is therefore

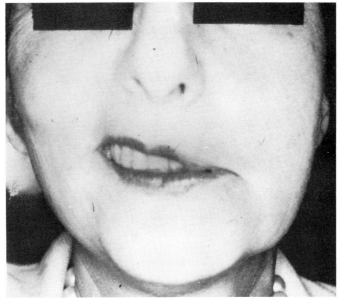

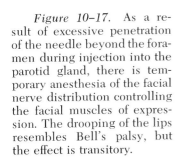

Figure 10–17. As a result of excessive penetration of the needle beyond the foramen during injection into the parotid gland, there is temporary anesthesia of the facial nerve distribution controlling the facial muscles of expression. The drooping of the lips resembles Bell's palsy, but the effect is transitory.

usually preferable to anesthetize one side at a time. If the surgical procedure does not involve the molars, and anesthesia from second bicuspid to second bicuspid is desired, the bilateral mental block provides adequate anesthesia of the labial structures. If the lingual surface is also involved, lingual infiltration usually can provide adequate anesthesia to perform the electrosurgical instrumentation on the lingual *tissues* without pain.

The mental block

The mental nerve emerges from the foramen in a posteroanterior direction and fans out under the periosteum. The foramen is usually located midway between the marginal level of the alveolar bone and the inferior border of the mandible, in the vicinity of the second bicuspid tooth (Fig. 10–18). If the disposable needle is carefully bent to approximately a 45-degree angle and introduced into the areolar mucosa at the base of the buccal vestibule over the apex of the first bicuspid and is directed posteriorly and inwardly to hug the bone, the foramen usually can be reached without too much difficulty. It is advisable to infiltrate the gingival mucosa at the site of needle insertion to permit painless penetration and exploration toward the foramen. When the foramen has been reached, 5 to 6 drops of anesthetic solution deposited slowly, drop by drop, is adequate to provide good anesthesia. Gentle massage of the tissues over a block injection site or the side of the face where the injection has been made helps to stimulate the blood circulation, thereby bringing additional alkaline buffer to the area to help neutralize the acid radical and accelerate the anesthetic effect.

To summarize, effective anesthesia for painless electrosurgical instrumentation can be readily and most effectively achieved by the proper administration of local infiltration or regional block anesthesia or in balanced combination with analgesia.

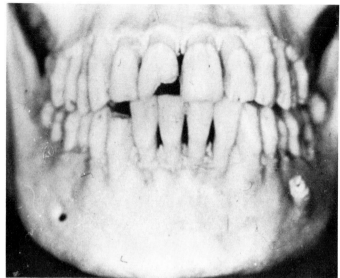

Figure 10–18. The mental foramina seen on a dry skull. A short length of pipe cleaner has been inserted into the left foramen to demonstrate the direction of the canal in the bone and the posteroanterior direction in which the nerve emerges from the canal.

Anesthetic Armamentarium

It may be helpful at this time, before concluding this review of the various regional block injections, to briefly discuss the hypodermic needles used for administering local anesthesia in the mouth.

There appears to be an increasing tendency among dental surgeons to use needles of 27 or 30 gauge, owing to the misconception that the finer-gauge needle will cause less pain as it is inserted into the tissues than would a 25-gauge needle.

In truth, the gauge of the needle plays little part in the pain caused by needle puncture to perform an injection. The causative factor is the *manner* in which the needle is introduced into the tissues. If the needle is *thrust* into yielding tissue such as areolar mucosa, pain will be experienced as the needle punches through the surface of the tissue. If instead of pushing the needle into the tissues, *the tissue is pulled over the tip of the needle,* and if the solution is then deposited *slowly,* a drop at a time, the injection will be painless regardless of the gauge of the needle. When it is not feasible to pull the tissue over the tip of the needle the likelihood of causing pain is minimized by stretching the tissue taut, so that the needle tip will penetrate rapidly without creating drag against the tissues. Use of an effective topical anesthetic applied to the injection site for 2 minutes prior to injection will further ensure against pain.

On the other hand, the finer the gauge of the needle the greater will be the amount of pressure required to expel the fluid through its lumen. Hence the greater will be the force with which the fluid is forced into the tissues. Use of a fine-gauge needle thus actually increases likelihood of traumatizing the tissues by forceful ejection of the fluid, which in turn increases the likelihood of considerable postoperative pain resulting therefrom.

Another consideration is that the fine-gauge needles are so thin that they are excessively flexible. This is of particular importance in administration of regional block anesthesia. Due to the limber flexibility of these needles, especially the 30-gauge needle, even slight resistance encountered in the tissues as the needle penetrates toward the anatomic site is likely to cause the needle to be deflected away from the foramen sufficiently to result in poor anesthesia or injection failure.

TOPICAL ANESTHESIA

Good injection technique minimizes the pain felt from needle penetration into the tissues, as has been described. Use of an effective topical anesthetic applied to the injection site for 2 minutes prior to needle puncture in conjunction with good technique virtually eliminates the pain potential.

Topical anesthetic in ointment form tends to roll away from the site, especially if the tissues are moist. When this happens, the topical anesthetic application is ineffectual. Topical anesthetic in oil suspension tends to remain on the application site long enough to produce effective anesthesia, especially if the site has been gently dried with a sterile sponge before the topical anesthetic has been applied.

The topical anesthetics in oil suspension usually are packaged in spray bottles or cans. The spray effect is activated by Freon gas, which is a potent tissue irritant. Thus, although the topical anesthetic per se may be totally bland and nonirritating, spraying it onto the injection site may result in local tissue sloughing. The author therefore prefers to take a sterile cotton applicator, fluff the cotton so that it will absorb an adequate amount of the fluid, then spray the topical anesthetic on the cotton, wait about one minute to permit the Freon gas to dissipate, and then apply the applicator to the injection site.

In performing regional block anesthesia aspiration should always be performed immediately after initial insertion of the needle, to make sure that the anesthetic solution will not be injected into a blood vessel, since the latter is one of the major reasons for shock occurring during anesthesia. Most aspirating syringes are reusable, metal sterilizable syringes. However, it is now possible to purchase disposable plastic aspirating syringes alone, or complete with needle and anesthetic cartridge, with which aspiration can be performed. It is also possible to use anesthetic cartridges with disposable needles attached for use in the sterilizable metal aspirating syringes (Fig. 10–19).

JET INJECTION ANESTHESIA. No discussion of local anesthetic armamentarium would be complete without comment about the jet-powered anesthetic syringes.

Jet injections are considerably more painful and traumatic to the tissues than a properly administered conventional hypodermic injection owing to the explosive force with which the anesthetic solution is ejected from the jet syringe. It is also likely to cause more postoperative soreness or pain for the same reason. Nevertheless, the jet injection can be used advantageously in conjunction with electrosurgery.

Jet injections can provide effective infiltration anesthesia suitable for minor elective electrosurgery of brief duration, such as resection of tiny, superficial tissue tabs or superficial spot coagulation, and for postoperative

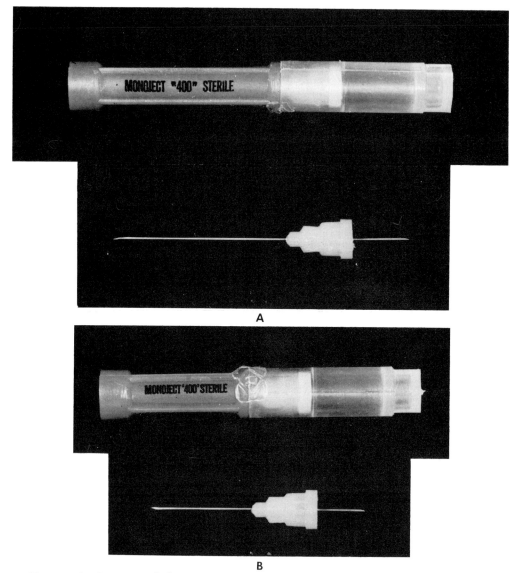

Figure 10–19. Typical disposable needles and Monoject Dental Injector (Sherwood Medical Industries, Inc.). (Astra of Canada has developed a disposable aspirating syringe that is still being evaluated and is not yet commercially available.)

A, Long syringe for block injections. *B*, Short syringe for infiltration.

Illustration continued on opposite page.

treatment of the gingival mucosa. It is therefore often eminently suitable for superficial gingival electrosurgery and for deep scaling and removal of dead cementum from root surfaces in infrabony pockets, prior to periodontal electrosurgery. When used for such purposes, excessive pressure should be avoided, to minimize the tissue trauma. The jet injection can also be used advantageously for more profound intraosseous anesthesia by increasing the amount of jet pressure and directing the spray to the interseptal bone. For proper injection with a jet syringe the tip should always be held gently but

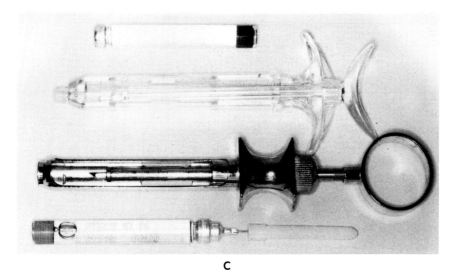

C

Figure 10–19. Continued. C. Typical metal aspirating syringe and plastic disposable syringe, and a unitized disposable needle and anesthetic cartridge.

firmly against the tissues. It is particularly important to do so for effective supplementary intraosseous injections.

Jet injection syringes are made in two styles: one provides for use of anesthetic cartridges like the manual syringes, the other provides a tank into which the anesthetic solution is placed.

It is not the author's intention to attempt to evaluate the merits of the various jet syringes available. However, from the standpoint of ability to maintain an intact chain of sterility, it is his impression that this may be more readily achieved when the solution remains intact in its original cartridge. For this reason the author's personal choice leans toward the cartridge type of jet injection syringes (Fig. 10–20).

Contraindications

This discussion of local anesthesia would be incomplete without brief consideration of the contraindications to its use and the matter of anesthetic emergencies. Local anesthesia is contraindicated in the presence of massive local infection. It is also contraindicated for patients with certain types of renal, allergenic, metabolic, and cardiac diseases. When such systemic condi-

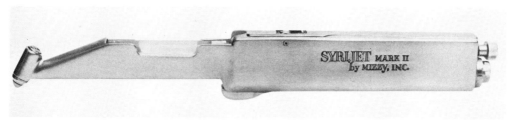

Figure 10–20. An example of jet syringes that utilize individual anesthetic cartridges.

tions contraindicate local anesthesia the victims have invariably been instructed by their physicians to inform their dentist to that effect.

Control of Local Anesthesia Emergencies

Local anesthesia emergencies range from mild allergic reactions and syncope to severe cardiac arrhythmias, angioneurotic edema, or anaphylactic shock. True drug allergy to the anesthetic salts are relatively rare and can easily be verified or ruled out in a matter of minutes by simple patch tests.

By far the most common emergencies encountered with local anesthesia result from failure to premedicate the unduly apprehensive tense patient. Usually these are mild and transitory in nature. Undue apprehension resulting in excessive adrenalin production may induce a mild shock syndrome.[2] The resultant syncope or shock usually is accompanied by temporary ischemia of the brain, with mild hypoxia. For this reason inhalation of pure oxygen is highly effective for treating these conditions. Inhalation of ammonia or inhalation or ingestion of aromatic spirits of ammonia also are helpful. Use of the residual blood supply present in the patient's lower extremities as a source of immediate autogenous blood transfusion is highly effective and usually results in almost immediate recovery.

The autotransfusion is performed by placing the patient in the prone or preferably in the Trendelenburg position in the chair and elevating the legs, one at a time, to a right angle with the trunk of the body. This pours approximately 500 cc. of blood present in each limb directly into the brain case. Normal pink color replaces the waxen pallor almost immediately and recovery is complete, without unfavorable after-effects.

Should the patient show clinical evidence of angioneurotic edema or anaphylactic shock the immediate intravenous or intramuscular injection of methylprednisolone sodium succinate (Upjohn's Solu-Medrol, 40 mg., Emergency Kit) can truly be a lifesaver. This kit, and the less heroic Novol type of emergency kit containing caffeine, adrenalin, sodium benzoate, ammonia, metrazol, and similar types of emergency drugs, should be part and parcel of the armamentarium of everyone who administers local anesthesia. It is hoped that these drugs will never be put to use; but in the infrequent true emergency they are indispensable.

GENERAL ANESTHESIA

Choice of general anesthetic agents suitable for use with electrosurgery is of necessity somewhat limited. Use of combustible gases and explosive anesthetic mixtures is automatically ruled out. The general anesthetic agents of choice are nitrous oxide, an inert gas, and the intravenous agents. These may be used alone or in combination. Brevital sodium, Fluothane mepergam, pentothal sodium, thiopental sodium, surital sodium, and viadril are popular agents used for producing surgical stage anesthesia.

FACTORS THAT INFLUENCE ANESTHETIC RESULTS

It has been estimated that general anesthesia is indicated for approximately five per cent of all cases requiring dental anesthesia. Local anesthesia, therefore, is the administrative method of choice for approximately ninety-five per cent of all dental procedures; this ratio also applies to electrosurgical procedures.

There are numerous instances, however, where despite absence of specific contraindications unfavorable local conditions may prevent local anesthetics alone from providing adequate anesthesia. Such unfavorable results are most likely to be encountered when acute inflammatory conditions such as acute pericementitis or chronic low-grade infections are present in the operative field.

Acute and subacute inflammatory tissue reactions and chronic infection are usually accompanied by engorgement and stasis of the blood circulation in the affected area. Alteration in pH of the alkaline buffers of the tissue fluids in the area toward the acid side usually results. This tends to retard onset of anesthesia. It also appears to create interference with the ability of the anesthetic agent to completely block out all pain impulses, particularly those that are triggered primarily by pressure. Thus it is not uncommon to find that despite excellent anesthesia in the surrounding normal tissues, inadequate anesthesia is encountered in the affected areas where the need is greatest.

BALANCED LOCAL – GENERAL ANESTHESIA

When, due to unfavorable local factors, or the apprehensive hypersensitive patient with a low threshold for pain, local anesthesia alone is likely to prove inadequate to provide completely satisfactory surgical anesthesia, use of a *preplanned* balance of local anesthesia and general anesthesia, or analgesia, provides effective surgical anesthesia.[9, 10]

FOOTNOTE REFERENCES

1. Adriani, J.: Selection of Anesthesia. Springfield, Ill. Charles C Thomas, 1955, p. 107.
2. Selye, H.: Adaptation syndrome. (Synonyms: Selye's syndrome; adaptation syndrome; general adaptation syndrome; stress syndrome; specific alarm syndrome.) J.A.M.A., 139:1119, 1949.
3. Ibid., Science, 122:625, 1955.
4. Selye, H., and Stone, H.: On the experimental morphology of the adrenal cortex. Amer. Lecture Series No. 74, Springfield, Ill., Charles C Thomas, 1950.
5. Selye, H., and Horava, A.: Annual report on stress. A-2, 1952; A-3, 1953.
6. Selye, H., and Heuser, G.: Annual report on stress. A-4, 1954.
7. Selye, H.: Living With Stress. New York, McGraw-Hill Book Co., 1958.
8. Durham, R. H.: Encyclopedia of Medical Syndromes. Baltimore, Paul B. Hoeber, Inc., Medical Division of Harper & Row, 1960, p. 504.
9. Oringer, M. J.: Anoci association: a preplanned balance of local – general anesthesia for the ambulatory patient. D. Items of Interest, March, 1953.
10. Douglas, B. L., and Kresberg, H.: Use of regional anesthesia with general anesthesia in oral surgery practice. J. Oral Surg., Anes. Hosp. D. Soc., 17:83–90, Sept., 1959.

MEDICATION

The drugs, old and new, that are useful in the modern practice of dentistry are myriad in number and bewildering in variety. An attempt at their *exhaustive* review here would be inappropriate and impractical. The rationale for the use of the most useful drugs for preoperative, operative, and postoperative medication will be discussed.

Many of the drugs that will be considered will undoubtedly be old friends. Some will be less familiar and others will be new drugs, or drugs that are still in the stage of clinical evaluation and not now commercially available.

The plenitude and variety of useful drugs makes an orderly and systematic presentation difficult. Subdivision according to method of administration and therapeutic function offers the best prospect for a satisfactory approach.

Chapter Eleven

USE OF SYSTEMIC AND LOCAL DRUGS

A. **Drugs Used Systemically**
   These fall, almost without exception, into one of the following categories:
   1. Preanesthetic-preoperative drugs
      a. Antisialagogues
      b. Tranquilizers
   2. Premedication and postmedication drugs
      a. For pain control
      b. For control of infection: antibiotics and chemotherapeutics
   3. Drugs used for cardiac management

    4. Drugs used for allergy and respiratory management (emergency drugs)
    5. Hemostatic agents (control of hemorrhage)
    6. Vitamins and dietary supplements
B. **Drugs Used Locally**
    1. Topical anesthetics
    2. Local hemostatic agents
    3. Anti-inflammatory drugs
    4. Physiological stimulants
    5. Antiseptics and astringents
    6. Oral bandages
    7. Heterogenous graft materials
    8. Sterilizing agents

A. DRUGS USED SYSTEMICALLY

1. Preanesthetic-Preoperative Drugs

ANTISIALAGOGUES. The autonomic nervous system which innervates the salivary glands reacts to apprehension. Thus apprehension occasionally results in a depressant effect on the salivary glands and temporary cessation or marked reduction in salivary flow. Most often, however, apprehension causes autonomic stimulation of the salivary glands, with excessively copious salivary flow.

When the patient salivates excessively it is difficult if not impossible to keep the operative field from becoming flooded uncontrollably. The urologists have developed a technique for wet-field electrosurgery. Dental electrosurgery, however, cannot be performed efficiently in a flooded surgical field. When electrosurgery is to be performed for a patient who salivates excessively, it is advisable to premedicate him with an effective antisialagogue.

Artane (trihexyphenidil HCL, Lederle) has a direct inhibitory effect on the parasympathetic nervous system and a specific antisialogogue effect. It may produce mild side effects of temporary blurring of vision, dizziness, and nausea. Other useful drugs are as follows: Banthine bromide (methantheline bromide, Searle), a true anticholinergic preparation for control of salivation that can be administered intramuscularly by injection, or by ingestion of tablets ½ to 1 hour preoperatively. For the unusually apprehensive patient the combination of Banthine with 15 mg. phenobarbital is particularly effective.

This drug, as well as Pamine (methscopolamine bromide, Upjohn) and other anticholinergic agents, tends to cause blurring of vision and sometimes drowsiness as side effects. It is therefore necessary to caution the patient against driving an automobile and to recommend that someone accompany him home. These drugs should not be administered to patients with glaucoma, severe cardiac disease, or markedly enlarged prostate glands.

TRANQUILIZERS. These may range from mild neuromuscular relaxants such as mephenesin carbamate (Tolseram, Squibb*) to the extremely potent central nervous system depressants such as the ataraxics (Atarax, Compazine, Equanil, Thorazine, Trancopal, Ultran, Vistaril).

Librium (chlordiazepoxide HCL, Roche)[1] is the first of a new class of tranquilizers that is unrelated chemically and pharmacologically to the other types of tranquilizers. It is a versatile therapeutic agent of proven value for a broad spectrum of anxiety and tension. It is classified as one of the safer of the effective pharmacologic compounds available, and is therefore considered ideally suitable for long-term therapy. Its quick action also makes it a very valuable drug for premedication of the apprehensive dental patient.

Use of this drug is contraindicated for patients who have previously demonstrated sensitivity to the drug. It is also contraindicated for alcoholics and when the patient has been under active therapy with other potent CNS depressant drugs. Its use should also be avoided for patients who are addiction-prone, or who have a known history of drug addiction.

Although it is an excellent tranquilizer, paradoxical reactions to it have been reported. With some types of psychiatric patients and some aggressive, overactive, overstimulated children, instead of tranquilizing, it may produce excitement, stimulation, or acute rage. Its use for premedication of such patients, particularly the overactive, aggressive child, should either be avoided or limited to very minimal dosage, and the patient then observed to detect evidence of untoward reactions.

One of the most highly regarded drugs for premedication of apprehensive patients who suffer from hypertension, cardiovascular diseases or angina pectoris is phenobarbital. Owing to its antispasmodic properties, Phenobarb Theocalcin (Knoll) is useful for treatment of this type of patient.† The drug is administered orally in ¼ to ½ gr. doses approximately one-half hour preoperatively.

Another drug that may prove useful for management of the apprehensive hypertensive individual both pre- and postoperatively is rescinnamine (Moderil, Pfizer). This drug is made of a recently isolated pure crystalline alkaloid of rauwolfia that appears to overcome many of the drawbacks of earlier rauwolfia and reserpine preparations. The drug appears to be relatively free of notable unfavorable side-effects, and is very effective for both tranquilizing and reducing hypertension. It is administered orally in 0.25 to 0.50 mg. doses twice daily after meals.

---

*Manufacture of this excellent drug has recently been discontinued owing to low sales volume, and it is no longer available.

†The patient's physician should be consulted in all cases where systemic therapy with potent drugs is indicated.

An excellent drug for sedating the average apprehensive patient is Seconal Sodium (Lilly). It can be administered either intramuscularly or orally. Intramuscular administration is used primarily for preanesthetic medication, and is given 1 to 1½ hours preoperatively. Oral administration is in capsule form, ¾ gr. for sedation, 1½ gr. for hypnotic effect, taken 15 to 20 minutes preoperatively.

Inordinately apprehensive patients who are emotionally distressed may require the potent tranquilizing effect of ataraxics. A useful drug of this type is Vistaril (Pfizer), a rapid-acting tranquilizer with a wide margin of safety. It induces a calming effect without impairing mental alertness, and provides the secondary benefit of muscle relaxation and has antisecretory qualities. It is quite effective by oral administration in doses of 50 to 100 mg., depending upon the patient's anxiety state.

When very fast sedation of short duration is desired, or when use of barbiturates is undesirable or contraindicated, Valmid ethinamate (Lilly) is very useful. Dosage is 1 or 2 tablets 20 minutes before treatment is begun. There are no contraindications to use of this drug, and the effects disappear within 4 hours. There are no after-effects such as depression, and this drug can be used even in the presence of liver or kidney damage.

Premedication of the very apprehensive patient who is also a gagger always presents a management problem. Compazine (Smith, Kline & French) provides a combination of tranquilizing effect and antiemetic action which markedly reduces the tendency for nausea and vomiting. Oral administration of 15 mg. for adults, and 2.5 to 7.5 mg. for children (determined by age and weight), is a safe, effective dose.

Patients who require premedication for pain relief as well as to reduce the anxiety state can be treated with oral and injectable medicaments. For oral dosage, Darvo-Tran (Lilly), a combination of Darvon (Lilly) (dextro-propoxyphene hydrochloride), reported *by its manufacturer* to be a codeine substitute, with Ultran (Lilly) (phenaglycodol), provides the analgesic effect of Darvon, with the tranquilizing effect of Ultran.

Patients who require more potent pain relief plus tranquilizing effect may do well on premedication with Mepergan (Wyeth) injected intramuscularly.

Patient tolerance for potent CNS depressant drugs varies with the individual. In the event that a patient should unexpectedly manifest drug-induced lethargy from overdosage of tranquilizers, barbiturates, or antihistamines, the abnormally depressant reaction can be effectively combated by administration of Ritalin HCL (methylphenidate HCL, USP, Ciba) orally or by injection. Use of this drug should, however, be avoided for patients with a history of epileptic seizures, since it tends to lower the convulsive threshold.

2. Premedication and Postmedication Drugs

FOR PAIN CONTROL. Although patients usually report remarkably little pain following electrosurgery, postmedication is occasionally necessary for relief of pain that may be inherent to the surgical procedure or may be due to the variability of the individual's pain threshold.

Technically, all drugs that provide relief from pain are analgesics. The potency of the analgesic drugs varies so greatly, however, that subdividing them into three categories may provide a helpful appraisal of their potency.

Most analgesics are equally useful for pre- and postmedication. It would be pointless to re-evaluate those drugs in this category that have already been discussed.

Analgesics. In this subdivision, "analgesics" refers essentially to the multitude of common popular drugs running the alphabetical gamut from Anacin through Zactirin. Many are household words; included are aspirin, Bufferin, Empirin, Excedrin, A.P.C.'s and similar drugs. Analgesics are effective medicaments for relief of reactions ranging from moderate discomfort to mild pain. All those mentioned are far too well known to need further elaboration.

Sedatives. The drugs that fall into this category are somewhat more potent than the analgesics and are therefore better suited to provide relief from, or control of, moderate to severe pain. A large number of the drugs that fit into this subdivision are drugs formulated in combination with acetylsalicylic acid or other salicylates.

Some people are allergic to, or have an intolerance for, aspirin and other salicylic acid derivatives. For such people it is necessary to prescribe drugs that do not contain the salicylates. One such drug is Valadol (Acetaminophen Tablets, N. F., Squibb). Darvon, previously mentioned, provides a reasonable degree of relief from moderate pain, yet does not contain salicylates. Double strength Darvon (65 mg.) is presumed to provide pain relief equivalent to that provided by ¼ gr. of codeine. (Darvon Compound and Darvon Compound 65 are combinations of this drug with aspirin; Darvo-Tran, its combination with Ultran.) Two recent additions are Darvon N and Darvon N with ASA (propoxyphene napsylate, and propoxyphene napsylate with aspirin).[1] Darvon is structurally related to the narcotic methadone. The combination of Darvon with aspirin and/or phenacetin results in greater analgesia than that achieved with either drug administered alone. It is indicated for relief of mild to moderate pain. This agent should not be used in children, since adequate data to establish safe conditions of use are lacking. Darvon N should not be taken when it is necessary to drive a car or operate machinery or other potentially hazardous tasks, as it may impair the mental and/or physical abilities, especially during the first few days of therapy. The patient should be cautioned accordingly.

Although codeine pharmacologically is a narcotic, it is the least potent of those that are medically useful. Its relatively mild potency relegates it primarily to use as a sedative. A.P.C. with codeine is a favorite combination that is effective for relief of moderate pain.

Patients who require sedation of the degree afforded by codeine, but who have an idiosyncrasy for codeine and/or aspirin, may do well on Percodan (Endo Labs), a synthetic codeine with potency equivalent of A.P.C. with codeine. Side-effects are minimal, mostly nausea.

Narcotics. When pain of organic or neurological origin proves intractable despite medication with these various sedatives, use of a more potent type of drug is indicated. This situation calls for administration of effective narcotics.

Morphine and demerol hydrochloride require no elaboration. Both may be administered intramuscularly, subcutaneously or orally. A synthetic morphine derivative, Numorphan (Endo Labs), is reputed to provide greater potency than morphine or demerol hydrochloride, with less side-effects. This drug provides effective narcotic sedation with euphoria, but minimal narcosis (drowsiness and disorientation). It is effective for preanesthetic medication of ambulatory patients and for postmedication for intractable pain in patients trying to continue their normal activities.

Numorphan is rated a class A narcotic with several more desirable characteristics than morphine or demerol. An oral tablet form of this drug was investigated by the author. It proved unsatisfactory and was not marketed. When used in intramuscular or intravenous injection it is effective, but it is unsuited for administration to ambulatory patients.

FOR CONTROL OF INFECTION: ANTIBIOTICS AND CHEMOTHERAPEUTICS. The single most important factor by far to consider in the choice and administration of drugs is the need to think in terms of *the total patient,* rather than of just the dental problem. This factor is particularly important when antibiotics or chemotherapeutics are to be administered parenterally as an integral part of management of severe dental infections, or when such medication is to be prescribed for prophylactic use.

A number of startling and alarming new developments in drug therapy underline the need to think of the total patient. There has been a dramatic increase in bacterial resistance to drugs. There is incontrovertible proof that certain bacteria can transmit to one another the ability to resist the bacteriostatic and bactericidal effects of drugs. This ability, known as "infectious resistance," allows bacteria to quickly acquire immunity to not just one, but many antibiotics. Some bacteria have been reported to be resistant to as many as nine different antibiotic drugs.[9] Among the antibiotics rendered at least partly ineffectual by infectious resistance are tetracycline, streptomycin, leomycin, kanamycin, methicillin, chloramphenicol, and the sulfa drugs.

Infinitely more important than the multiple resistance, however, is the fact that this infectious resistance also enables relatively innocuous bacteria to infect and render drug-resistant far more virulent varieties of antibiotics that had not themselves been exposed to the antibiotic therapy. When this transfer of multiple resistance phenomenon (R-Factor) was first reported by Japanese investigators some years ago it was greeted with skepticism by Western scientists, but infectious resistance is now universally accepted factually.[5-13] Thus, the prognosis for treatment of even mild infections that had formerly responded readily to antibiotic therapy is now relatively unpredictable. Even more significant is the fact that bacteria involved in a dental infection, usually staphylococci or streptococci, that develop resistance to antibiotic therapy, may transfer their resistance to far more virulent organisms and thereby complicate greatly the body's ability to combat and control serious systemic diseases.

Another significant recent development in drug therapy is the Food and Drug Administration's reappraisal of the efficacy of many of the popular drugs and antibiotic combinations that had been used extensively for presumed greater efficacy due to synergistic action, but have failed to live up to the therapeutic claims that had been made for them.[4] This drug reappraisal makes it necessary to take a long hard look at the value of the antibiotic drug combinations that have been used extensively in endodontics and other areas of dental therapy.

In view of the doubtful efficacy of many of the most widely used antibiotics and chemotherapeutics, and the hazards of transferral of drug resistance, the ability of the electrosurgical currents to sterilize as they cut becomes an increasingly important factor. This ability of the electrosurgical current to disintegrate and volatilize bacteria as well as tissue cells reduces the patient's dependence upon antibiotics and greatly improves the prognosis following electrosurgical therapy in contrast to comparable treatment by other modalities that are unable to provide this auto-sterilizing capability.

Needless to say, this does not mean that premedication and postmedication can be neglected, or that antibiotics and chemotherapy are not still important factors in proper management of the dental patient.

When antibiotic or chemotherapeutic prophylactic protection against infection or transitory bacteremia is indicated, in the absence of contraindications to allergy penicillin is still the most universally useful antibiotic drug. From the outset, however, many people showed allergic tendencies toward this drug. As a result of widespread and often indiscreet use, penicillin allergy has become relatively commonplace. There has been an unfortunate corresponding increase in severity of the allergic manifestations accompanying the increase in incidence. A number of fatal anaphylactoid (allergy) reactions to administration of penicillin have been reported.[2] This has discouraged intramuscular (IM) administration, and has increased use of the long-acting oral tablets such as Pen-Vee K (Wyeth), Pentids (Squibb), V-Cillin (Lilly), and others. While the oral penicillin does not obviate the possibility of allergy reactions, when they do occur they are usually somewhat milder and less likely to prove fatal than when penicillin is administered intramuscularly.

When allergy symptoms such as urticaria, edema, and itching are manifested, adrenalin and antihistamines such as Chlor-Trimeton Maleate (Schering) may be injected intravenously or intramuscularly. In the event of anaphylactoid reaction or severe angioneurotic edema of the glottis, immediate intravenous injection of antagonists such as Solu-Cortef (Upjohn) or Cortisone Hemisuccinate (Merck, Sharp & Dohme) can neutralize the allergic reaction and prove life-saving.

Fear of anaphylactoid reaction to penicillin has resulted in enormously increased dependence upon use of the broad-spectrum antibiotics for prophylactic and therapeutic antibiotic medication. The broad-spectrum drugs are not entirely devoid of producing allergic reactions and variable degrees of toxic side-effects. The allergic reactions appear to be limited largely to cutaneous rashes and edema. The most serious side-effects are blood dyscrasias that have been produced by prolonged administration of Chloromycetin (Parke-Davis), and deafness due to damage to the auditory nerve by administration of streptomycin. Chloromycetin is capable of producing aplastic anemia. When this antibiotic is administered, blood chemistry studies should be made regularly and frequently—several times a week if treatment is prolonged. Chloromycetin is extremely potent and is especially effective against many of the highly resistant staphylococcus and streptococcus strains of bacteria that fail to respond to other antibiotics. Administration of this drug should therefore be reserved exclusively for otherwise unmanageable infection for which culture and bacterial selectivity tests indicate it to be the drug of choice. Since deafness may result from streptomycin and dihydrostreptomycin therapy, use of these drugs should also be avoided whenever possible.

Oxytetracycline (Terramycin, Pfizer), tetracycline (Achromycin, Lederle), demethylchlortetracycline (Declomycin, Lederle) and erythromycin (Ilotycin, Ilosone*, Lilly, and Erythrocin, Abbott) appear to be the least toxic of the broad-spectrum antibiotic drugs. However, even these drugs may produce unfavorable side reactions, usually in the form of distressing gastric disturbances and moniliasis.

A number of recent antibiotic drugs, many synthesized, reputed to be effective against resistant strains of bacteria have become available. Notable among these are:

Ilotycin Gluceptate[2] (erythromycin gluceptate sterile, USP and Lilly) for IV injection. Indications, for treatment of *Streptococcus viridans* infection and for prophylactic premedication against bacterial endocarditis for the dental patient; for *Staphylococcus aureus* infections and for *Streptococcus pyogenes* (group A beta-hemolytic) infections. It is effective for premedication for patients with a history of rheumatic fever or congenital heart disease, who are hypersensitive to penicillin.

Bristamycin[2] (erythromycin stearate tablets, Bristol). Indications are similar to those for Ilotycin Gluceptate. Medication with this drug should be maintained for 10 days and taken on an empty stomach. Contraindicated only for patients who are known to be sensitive to erythromycin.

Bristacycline[2] (tetracycline HCL, Bristol, buffered with ascorbic acid). Intravenous administration. Effective against *Streptococcus pyogenes* and anaerobic streptococcus infections, and *Staphylococcus aureus*. It is especially useful when the patient is penicillin sensitive.

Polycillin-N[1] (sterile sodium ampicillin, 109–IV administration, Bristol). Effective against hemolytic and non-hemolytic streptococci. Patient sensitivity to penicillin contraindicates its use.

Lincocin (lincomycin HCL, USP, Upjohn)[1]—An antibiotic that is reputed to be especially effective for treatment of severe bone infections. Lincocin may be administered in capsule form for oral ingestion, or by intramuscular

---

*The January 1974 FDA Drug Bulletin warns that Ilosone (erythromycin estolate) therapy involves a definite risk of hepatotoxicity. The estolate appears to be the only erythromycin derivative which may produce jaundice as a side effect, especially after long-term therapy. It is more effective than the other derivatives, but because of this adverse effect use of this drug for adults should be limited to situations in which it is clearly justified. It should not be used in patients with pre-existing liver disease or in those suspected of having impaired liver function, even though the jaundice is reversible in patients with normal liver function.

injections. It has a number of undesirable side-effects that may be distressing but not dangerous.

Cleocin (clindamycin HCL hydrate, Upjohn)[1] – Derived from the same source as lincocin, but much more potent, since approximately 90 per cent of the drug is reputed to become absorbed by the blood. Many of the unfavorable side-effects of lincocin are absent or minimized.

Unfavorable reactions to antibiotic therapy are attributable to a major degree to the indiscriminate, nonselective bactericidal activity of these drugs in the gastrointestinal tract. In addition to destroying pathogens, the drugs also destroy the normally indigenous B-complex-producing bacteria. Destruction of the beneficial organisms permits monilial fungi present in the gastrointestinal tract to thrive without competition from the bacteria. Mild to severe moniliasis often results; severe generalized moniliasis can prove fatal.

A number of pharmaceutical firms have combined the tetracycline drug with Nystatin (Mycostatin, Squibb), an antifungal substance produced by streptomycin noursei, in order to curb the tendency to monilial overgrowths following prolonged administration of the broad-spectrum antibiotics and thereby avert moniliasis. Squibb's Mysteclin V (Nystatin) and F (Fungizone) are typical examples of the combination of antibiotics that in addition to providing therapeutic protection also provide protection against gastric disturbances and secondary moniliasis. When administration of antibiotic drugs for more than three days is indicated, these combined antibiotics often are preferred.

Mixed infections that are highly resistant to treatment are frequently encountered in the oral cavity. In view of the plethora of pathogens, usually common, but occasionally rare,[14] found in the average human mouth, this is scarcely surprising. Synergistic combinations of antibiotics have been developed by some of the pharmaceutical firms to combat mixed infections. Almost all of the multitude of "synergistic" antibiotic combination drugs have been denounced by the Food and Drug Administration as ineffectual and have been withdrawn from the market.[4]

When mixed infections are suspected it is now more important than ever to prescribe antibiotics on the basis of culture and sensitivity tests and not on the basis of random choice or "synergistic" shotgun remedies.

Chemotherapeutics, especially sulfonamides, may be combined with penicillin or in sulfonamide groupings for synergistic advantages. Notable are penicillin with sulfadiazine and sulfamerazine (Pen-Vee Sulfas, Wyeth), penicillin with sulfadiazine, sulfamerazine or sulfamethazine (Sulfasugracillin, Upjohn), and the triple sulfas [Sulfa-Trio No. 2 (Rexall) and Tri-Sulfanyl (U.S. Vitamin)].

Antibiotics and chemotherapeutics taken orally must be taken around the clock in order to maintain uniformly effective blood levels. The average dose is 250 mg. of broad-spectrum antibiotic *every six hours* four times a day. It is advisable that they be taken with milk or copious amounts of water to reduce the potential for gastric reactions. It is also advisable to prescribe antibiotics for a minimum of three days to reduce the possibility of developing resistant strains of bacteria and to reduce potential future sensitization of the patient due to inadequate drug maintenance.

3. Drugs Used for Cardiac Management

Persons suffering from angina pectoris, coronary hypertension and vascular diseases are poor-risk patients who usually require vasodilator medication. The most beneficial drug for most of these conditions appears to be nitroglycerin; such patients usually carry a supply of this drug with them at all times. They usually premedicate themselves immediately prior to injection or trying operative procedures by dissolving a tablet under the tongue. The beneficial effects of ordinary nitroglycerin tablets unfortunately are very brief, lasting approximately two to three minutes. The patient remains unprotected usually throughout most of the operative procedure.

The PETN drugs or pentaerythritol tetranitrates such as Peritrate (sustained action) (Warner-Chilcott), Peribar L.A. (Whittier Lab.) and Papavatral (Kenwood) are typical long-acting PETN vasodilator drugs. These provide continuous effective protection to the patient for prolonged periods. Administration of these drugs or Nitroglyn (Key), a long-acting controlled nitroglycerin product, to poor-risk patients preoperatively, provides them with full vasodilator protection for the duration of operative procedure and also for the immediate postoperative period. Use of these drugs should be avoided in cases of glaucoma.

4. Drugs Used for Allergy and Respiratory Management (Emergency Armamentarium)

Ready availability of specific drugs and instruments that can effectively counteract sudden cardiac, respiratory, or allergic office emergencies can spell the difference between full recovery from a distressing experience and fatal termination. Thus, although emergency measures were discussed to some degree in the preceding chapter, the author feels justified in repeating emphasis on need for, and itemizing in detail, a suitable armamentarium with which to meet serious office emergencies. This is particularly so since, in addition to emergencies arising from administration of local anesthesia, emergencies can also arise from premedication of the dental patient, and although premedication is not routine, it is by no means rare or unusual.

Untoward drug reactions can range from mild cardiac arrhythmias and mild syncope to auricular and ventricular fibrillations and moderate shock, and from mild allergenic reactions such as urticaria to potentially lethal reactions such as laryngeal angioneurotic edema, anaphylactoid reactions, and anaphylactic shock.

The milder reactions are almost commonplace, and the severe, dangerous reactions happily occur only infrequently. But the fact is, they *do* occur, and when they do, they are potentially lethal. The best insurance against emergency fatalities is the instant availability of an emergency armamentarium consisting of a supply of suitable effective emergency drugs, airways, preferably disposable, and a tracheostomy set including a catheter, that is available for instant, efficient use in the event an emergency arises.

Mild to moderate allergic and respiratory emergencies are likely to respond rapidly and favorably to inhalation of aromatic spirits of ammonia, or to administration of epinephrine, caffeine citrate or sodium benzoate, and similar agents that are included in the Novocol or comparable prepared emergency drug kits, or to administration of pyribenzamine (tripelennamine HCL, USP, Ciba) tablets or ampuls, or Chlor-Trimeton maleate (Schering) tablets or injectable (IM or subcutaneous; not IV).

Solu-Cortef (hydrocortisone sodium succinate, Upjohn) sterile, for IV administration; hydrocortisone hemisuccinate (Merck) sterile for IV administration; or Meticortelone (prednisolone sodium succinate, Schering) sterile, for IV administration, when administered in conjunction with epinephrine,[2-3] is highly effective for combating laryngeal angioneurotic edema or anaphylactoid or anaphylactic reactions. Metrazol is a quick-acting respiratory and circulatory stimulant and is the pharmacological antagonist to the barbiturates and meprobamate. This drug is therefore very useful for treatment of barbiturate poisoning, and dangerously deep anesthesia. While this drug has no known contraindications, it should be used with caution for treatment of patients with a low convulsive threshold.

The emergency armamentarium would be incomplete without inclusion of one other agent—*oxygen*. Oxygen comes closest to being the universally useful emergency agent. Administration of oxygen under positive pressure, alone, or as a supplement to the emergency drug therapy is most desirable. In the absence of inhalation anesthesia equipment or resuscitators that can deliver positive pressure oxygen flow, artificial respiration and mouth-to-mouth breathing can be life-saving. Availability of the airway and tracheostomy instrument for instant use can be equally life-saving.

5. Hemostatic Agents (Control of Hemorrhage)

Patients who give a history of repeated persistent profuse hemorrhage following exodontia and oral surgery or susceptibility to bruises and discoloration, require prophylactic premedication.

It has previously been established that hemostasis is inherent in electrosection performed with fully rectified current.* When the tissue tone is normal, and the capillaries and lymphatics are normal in dimension, this inherent characteristic of hemostasis greatly reduces, and often eliminates completely, the surgical hazard of hemorrhagic free bleeding. But when the capillaries and lymph vessels are dilated by inflammation or distended by engorgement this hemostasis is inadequate to prevent hemorrhage, and free bleeding ensues despite use of electrosection.

Hemorrhage also is likely to occur despite the hemostasis of electrosec-

---

*This characteristic of inherent hemostasis appears to be lost when fully rectified and filtered continuous wave current is used, so that even tissues that are normal in tone tend to bleed freely following electrosection with the filtered continuous wave currents. Therefore hemostatics are likely to play a far more significant role than when the unfiltered fully rectified cutting currents or a *modified* continuous wave current such as the Ritter Mode[4] Surgery two current is used.

tion if the patient has a transitory or pathological blood dyscrasia, is on anticoagulant therapy due to cardiovascular disease, or when the patient has a capillary fragility or hyperpermeability that permits blood cells to seep into the adjacent tissues, and adequate medication has not been instituted to counteract these various conditions.

If the patient has a definite blood dyscrasia or has been on *anticoagulant* therapy he is aware of his condition and is probably under the care of a physician, who should administer and prescribe the premedication. But if the patient reports that he has been "living on aspirin for weeks," or that he bruises easily or spontaneously, or that he tends to bleed for a long time after extraction but not after cutting himself while shaving, there is a definite likelihood that he will require premedication to prevent postoperative bleeding. Such patients are usually not under active care of a physician. When conditions make the time element a cardinal factor the dentist may properly prescribe and administer the necessary premedication for such patients.

Vitamin K is often prescribed for control of bleeding in the mistaken belief that it is a general hemostat. This drug is effective for overcoming hypoprothrombinemia; it has little hemostatic value other than that. Excessive use of aspirin or other analgesics containing significant amounts of acetylsalicylic acid for prolonged periods tends to destroy the prothrombin in the blood and often produces transitory hypoprothrombinemia. Postoperative hemorrhage may be anticipated with such patients, and vitamin K or menadione (synthetic vitamin K) should be prescribed for two or three days preoperatively.

For most postoperative bleeding tendencies systemic hemostats such as Adrenosem Salicylate (Massengill), in tablet or syrup form, or Adrestat (Orgenon), oral tablets, capsules or intramuscular injectable, provide excellent preventive action when taken two days preoperatively and continued for one or two days postoperatively.

Patients who report that they bruise easily or develop spontaneous subcutaneous hematomas are prone to hemorrhagic extravasations and are likely to develop disfiguring postoperative ecchymoses and hematomas. Such patients most likely have either capillary permeability or capillary fragility, which permits blood cells to pass through the blood vessel walls and seep into the adjacent submucous or subcutaneous tissues. They also are likely to be profuse and persistent bleeders, and are subject to secondary postoperative hemorrhages.

Effective premedication with drugs such as rutin, a vegetable alkaloid, 60 mg., plus ascorbic acid, 250 mg.; the citrobioflavinoids and ascorbic acid (CVP, Duo-CVP, U.S. Vitamin) or hesperidin, citrobioflavinoids and ascorbic acid plus minerals and vitamins (Ominol, Kenwood) provides prophylactic protection. When postoperative hemorrhagic extravasations occur unexpectedly, these drugs accelerate resolution of the ecchymotic areas and hematomas. No known contraindications to average doses of these drugs have been reported.

6. Vitamins and Dietary Supplements

It has been mentioned that antibiotic therapy deprives the body of vitamin B complex by destroying the vitamin-producing organisms in the intestinal tract. Therefore it is sound therapy to supplement the antibiotics with oral or intramuscular administration of therapeutic vitamin B complex alone or in combination with crystalline B_{12}.

In 1947 and 1948 the author reported the advantageous use of clear gelatin powder locally in bone defects to aid healing.[15] In 1959 Dubos reported the results of extensive experiments that established that three elements are essential for normal tissue repair. These are collagen, animal protein, and ascorbic acid.[16] Collagen is inherent in the tissues; animal protein and ascorbic acid can be provided by oral ingestion.

The most easily obtained and easily tolerated form of animal protein is clear gelatin, which can be taken easily and pleasantly dissolved in orange or tomato juice. Ascorbic acid, 150 to 250 mg., one to three times daily, provides these essential ingredients to assure optimal opportunity for normal rapid tissue repair.

Excellent dietary supplements for patients who must be kept on a liquid diet are Sustagen, Nutrament and Metrecal (Mead Johnson). These provide the minimal daily requirements of proteins, carbohydrates and vitamins essential for normal nutritional needs. Patients who are kept on semisolid and soft diets find the junior baby foods excellent supplements.

B. DRUGS USED LOCALLY

1. Topical Anesthetics

The average dental patient dreads the injection for anesthesia more than almost any other phase of treatment. Good technique, as was mentioned in the previous chapter, can make the injection almost completely painless. The application of an effective topical anesthetic to the injection site assures that with good technique the injection will truly be completely painless. The author has found that topical anesthetics in an oil base are usually most effective for anesthetizing the moist oral mucosa. The topical anesthetics in ointment base tend to roll on the moist tissue surface and fail to provide the surface anesthesia being sought at the injection site. The oil remains on the tissue surface without rolling and penetrates to provide effective topical anesthesia. The lidocaine type of topical anesthetic seems to provide the depth of topical anesthesia that is desired.

The tissues should be dried gently with a sponge, and the topical anesthetic applied with a cotton applicator. If the latter is wound very tight, it is best to loosen the cotton so that it will convey an adequate amount of the topical anesthetic to the tissues. The anesthetic should be left in contact with the tissues for two minutes, then removed gently with the sponge before proceeding with the injection.

Topical anesthetic spray applications to the tissues should be avoided, because although most topical anesthetics are nonirritating and nontoxic to the tissues and will not cause tissue sloughing, the aerosol spray is activated by freon gas, which can be toxic to the tissues if the freon gas comes into physical contact with the tissues. If the aerosol spray can must be used, it is best to spray the topical anesthetic onto the cotton applicator, wait a minute or two for the freon gas to evaporate, then contact the tissues with the applicator, thus eliminating the hazard of tissue damage from freon gas irritation.

2. Local Hemostatic Agents

Unlike the hemostatic agents administered systemically, which have been reviewed and which are essentially intended for control of hemorrhage due to systemic blood dyscrasias or capillary fragility or permeability, the local hemostatic agents are useful for management of nonsystemic hemorrhage.

These agents are applied locally to the bleeding site, or introduced into the bleeding oral defect. The most useful ones are as follows:

SURGICEL (JOHNSON & JOHNSON).   A regenerated oxidized cellulose in delicate gauzelike woven texture that is applied topically to the bleeding site, this drug does not become absorbed and act as a graft material, but remains a foreign body, although it is tolerated reasonably well by the tissues.

OXYCEL (PARKE-DAVIS).   This is oxidized cellulose that resembles Surgicel closely in appearance, texture, and function. Oxycel is much more brittle than Surgicel and tends to crumble and shred, so that it is more difficult to manipulate. Like Surgicel, Oxycel is not a graft material and its use should be avoided in closed cavities.

MENADIONE (SYNTHETIC VITAMIN K).   This golden yellow powder can be applied topically to the bleeding site. It is useful in cases of prolonged bleeding due to transitory hypoprothrombinemia resulting from ingestion of large doses of aspirin for prolonged periods (i.e., a patient with toothache who has taken a dozen or more aspirins daily for several weeks before coming in for treatment). This drug is very irritating to the tissues, and if applied carelessly can produce a tissue burn and sloughing.

THROMBIN TOPICAL (PARKE-DAVIS).   A sterile hemostatic powder obtained from bovine blood. The prothrombin is activated with bovine thrombokinase in the presence of calcium chloride and sodium chloride. It is packed in sterile vials in powder form and may be applied in dry powder form or in solution with sterile isotonic solution. Thrombin acts directly on fibrinogen, thus helping to form natural clotting, which seals severed capillaries and controls bleeding locally. It is especially useful for control of capillary bleeding which is not controllable by ligation or suturing.

GELFOAM.   Gelfoam, in both the sponge and powder forms, in addition to its usefulness as a graft material and vehicle for introducing sulfonamides or antibiotics into bone cavities is useful as a hemostatic for mild bleeding, owing to its tacky texture and expansion that results when it becomes moistened by the blood.

3. Anti-Inflammatory Drugs (Steroids)

Steroids are extremely potent drugs. When administered systemically these drugs are capable of producing severe, undesirable reactions. Systemic administration of steroids for dental therapy is therefore very rare. When small doses of steroids are applied topically for local therapy, absorption is relatively negligible. Discreet use of local steroid therapy may prove helpful for persistent inflammation of the oral mucosa that is resistant to other therapy, with relatively little danger of incurring unfavorable systemic reactions. Hydrocortisone acetate ophthalmic ointment (Merck, Sharp & Dohme), Magnacort and Neomagnacort (Pfizer), Cortril and Terra-Cortril (Pfizer), Kenalog and Kenalog in Orabase (Squibb) and Cordent (Graham) are some of the steroids suitable for topical application to the oral mucosa.

When oral topical steroid therapy is indicated, triamcinolone acetonide (Kenalog, Squibb) is effective. Kenalog in Orabase (Squibb) is particularly suitable for use as a postoperative protective pack, especially following gingival electrosurgery. Its progenitor was used experimentally in many of the cases reported. This steroid and emollient adhesive protective ointment in many instances can substitute admirably for protective surgical cement packs.

Another useful cortisone preparation is Cordent (Graham), a cortisone powder in an adhesive denture powder base. This preparation is used like any of the denture adhesive powders. It is particularly useful with immediate dentures and acrylic surgical splints to prevent or reduce inflammation and edema postoperatively.

4. Physiological Stimulants

Some aromatic tinctures made of aromatic volatile oils act as physiologic stimulants and as very mild embalming agents that protect tissue surfaces to which they are applied. Tinctures of myrrh and benzoin combined in equal parts is an especially effective topical agent. Surgeons have used tincture of benzoin or myrrh and benzoin as a "dry dressing" when they have wished to avoid use of gauze dressings after sutures or clips have been removed from incisions. When applied to the oral mucosa this tincture helps to stimulate the healing process and hasten maturation of the surface epithelium.

Another useful combination of drugs that provides both antiseptic action and physiologic stimulation of tissue repair is B.I.P. paste, a combination of:

R

Bismuth subnitrate	1 part
Iodoform	2 parts
Petrolatum	3 parts

This mixture provides emollient action with physiologic stimulation and antiseptic action of iodoform, with the extra quality of being radiopaque, and therefore useable diagnostically as a roentgenographic marker, as well as being therapeutically valuable.

Two other drugs, Lipiodol and Iodochloral, radiopaque iodine preparations used for sialolithographic visualization of the submaxillary and parotid ducts and glands when injected into these structures, have mildly antiseptic action due to their iodine content. If the tissues of the structures into which they have been injected have been damaged by inflammation or mild infection, both of these drugs often also serve as mild physiologic stimulants to accelerate tissue repair.

5. Antiseptics and Astringents

Effective antiseptics that are mild enough to be nonirritating to the oral mucosa are uncommon. The aniline dyes, gentian violet and acriviolet, are ideally suited for oral topical application even though they cause marked transitory discoloration of the teeth and tissues. In addition to their germicidal value, the dyes also have a tanning effect on tissue. (They have even been used for coagulation of extensive tissue-surface damage produced by second and third degree burns.)

These dyes have a particular affinity for many of the common oral pathogens, such as the oral spirochetes (b. Vincenti). When these dyes are used as aqueous solutions instead of alcoholic tinctures they are completely nonirritating to the tissues and have no contraindications other than the transitory objectionable discoloration. They are useful in treatment of gingival infections and ulcerations.

The difficulty in pinpointing local application of potent astringents, escharotics, and styptics has been discussed in Chapter 2. There are times, however, when a mild surface tanning effect is desirable even if the medication cannot be pinpointed. When areas of mucosa require superficial astringent coagulation, a 0.01 to 0.05 per cent dilution of the standard 10 per cent chromic acid solution can be sprayed over the area or applied with an applicator. In such dilutions the medication does not penetrate beyond the epithelial surface of the mucosa. It merely coalesces the uppermost layer of cells if it is washed off within one to two minutes.

Another simple, old, and reliable medication is the combination of ordinary table salt with powdered alum, U.S.P., dissolved in water for lavage of the oral cavity. The resultant solution provides the saline stimulation of healing plus the astringent action of the alum to help shrink, toughen, and mature the surface epithelium. These effects tend to reduce tissue edema, hasten maturation and restore normal tissue tone. The solution is simple to prepare: a combination of ⅓ teaspoonful of powdered alum and 1 teaspoonful of salt to an 8- to 10-oz. tumbler of water at mouth temperature. This lavage should be used five times daily for five days at a time; then lavage with normal saline solution should be substituted for one week before use of the astringent lavage is resumed.

6. Oral Bandages

SURGICAL CEMENT PACKS.   Although research has been dealt with in an earlier chapter, it will be necessary to revert to a brief consideration of this matter before we progress to discussion and review of formulas useful for periodontal and other surgical cement packs.

The excellence of a research investigation is determined only in part by the manner in which the investigation was conducted. Of equal importance are the conclusions the investigator has drawn from his experiment. No matter how excellent the laboratory procedures may have been, if they have not been fully and properly evaluated and interpreted the investigation loses much of its value, and may actually lead to confusion and misconceptions that can be more harmful than the benefits it offers.

An excellent case in point is the recent research report that eugenol is an irritant. This is a fact that has always been common knowledge, and no one in his right mind would dream of dropping eugenol onto the eyeball, or using it as an oral lavage, since it would cause severe stinging or burning irritation that could cause tissue damage. Thus the fact that eugenol is an irritant is by no means the most important aspect of this investigation. Rather, an evaluation of the character of the irritation it produces would have been most significant. Irritants vary in their potency; there is a vast difference in the degree or nature of the irritation produced by eugenol and by silver nitrate or phenol, yet all three would have to be classified as irritants. It therefore becomes necessary to subdivide them according to the degree of their activity. A mild irritant, such as eugenol, produces a degree of irritation in small dosage that acts as a physiologic stimulant and thus stimulates tissue repair and regeneration. A severe irritant such as silver nitrate phenol or trichloracetic acid acts as a pathologic irritant that produces tissue necrosis.

If the irritant is used in sufficiently great dilution, even silver nitrate can be used beneficially, as when it is used prophylactically as an eye lavage for newborn infants. Thus we can see that a quantitative as well as a qualitative analysis is essential to arrive at a complete, meaningful scientific conclusion.

Thus, the mere fact that eugenol is an irritant is not the overriding consideration. The important question is the amount of free eugenol that will be coming into contact with the tissues. This is especially true in the matter of choice of periodontal or surgical cement packs. If the formula is one that can be mixed to only a moderately stiff mix, it will contain a substantially larger amount of free eugenol, which might produce enough irritation to impair tissue repair. If the formula can be mixed to a very stiff mix that is almost totally free of free eugenol, without becoming powdery and disintegrating, the amount of irritation will be very mild, just enough to act as a physiologic stimulant that will encourage and accelerate tissue repair. The great advantage enjoyed by the formula presented here over the numerous other formulas is that it can be mixed hard enough to assure against its flowing as a result of pressure exerted against it by the cheeks, lips, tongue, and tissues of the floor of the mouth, yet it remains sufficiently pliant and plastic to permit its close, accurate adaptation around the teeth and against the gingival mucosa, without containing an appreciable amount of free eugenol. This formula therefore has proved particularly suitable for use following gingivoplasty and gingivectoplasty, resection of pericoronal flaps, and for insertion into dentures to serve as surgical stents. It offers several features that are not found in the prepared commercial products.

Inclusion of tannic acid provides hemostasis which is valuable for control of blood seepage from raw gingival surfaces. Sulfathiazole provides chemotherapeutic protection for the operative field against secondary infection while the tissues granulate. Benzocaine provides excellent obtundant qualities which help to ease the initial postoperative period.

Powder

R

Zinc oxide	48 gms.
Powdered rosin	48 gms.
Tannic acid	24 gms.
Sulfathiazole powder (optional)	6 gms.
Zinc acetate	2 per cent
Benzocaine powder, q. s.	3 per cent

Liquid

R

Eugenol	1 oz.
Powdered rosin	1 oz.
Oil of sweet almond	$1/2$ oz.

The tannic acid, sulfathiazole and benzocaine powders are optional. If any of these are contraindicated for allergy or other reasons, they can be eliminated without impairing the cement mix.

The nurse or assistant should be instructed to mix the cement as stiff as possible for maximum strength and retentive qualities.

ORABASE–KENALOG IN ORABASE. Technically the various periodontal and surgical cement packs might be considered to belong in this category. However, they will be reviewed as a separate special category and will therefore not be considered here.

One of the earliest of the oral bandages was a product developed by the Squibb Institute for Medical Research called Orabase, which the author had the privilege of evaluating, together with its medicated form, Kenalog in Orabase. Orabase is the adhesive bandage material made of tragacanth and other adhesive gums in paste form that is useful for protective covering of irritated or inflamed areas. It is very adhesive; in some respects too much so, since after it is placed over the area to be protected, it tends to adhere tenaciously to the tongue, lips, cheeks, and food that come into contact with it, so that it is displaced or pulled away from the area to which it had been applied. Smoothing the surface of the gel with a wet finger gently until it feels slick to the touch helps to minimize this, and if the gel remains in situ long enough to set, it becomes a firm rubbery consistency and effectively protects the site to which it had been applied for days.

FLEXIBLE COLLODION. Flexible collodion is plain collodion to which a specific amount of castor oil is added to increase the flexibility and decrease the tendency to crack and peel. This preparation has a number of disadvantages and also some advantages. It is necessary that the tissues to which it is applied be thoroughly dry, or it will not adhere at all. Since it contains chloroform, it is a powerful tissue irritant and must be used judiciously. Also, it is difficult to get it to adhere to mobile tissue. But it adheres very well to the palatal tissue, when dry, and to the alveolar ridges. It can be used advantageously as a sealant in combination with dryfoil placed over the area to be protected, in which event it seals the dryfoil to the tissues and makes an excellent bandage.

THE SPRAY BANDAGES (JOHNSON & JOHNSON, BHASKAR). These are liquid chemicals that are applied to the tissues as a spray that coats the tissue surface and acts as a protective bandage. In some instances they substitute effectively for sutures by keeping the cut margins in firm coaptation.

Some of these products have received exhaustive field tests, having been used on battle casualties in Vietnam. Nevertheless, they have not as yet been given production clearance by the Pure Food and Drug Administration.

These materials present two advantages: they are easy to apply, being in a liquid form and sprayed over the area, and they appear to adhere well to wet surfaces. They also have distinct disadvantages, however: They appear to disrupt the repair process and are toxic to the tissues if introduced into the wound instead of applied on the external surface of the wound. And, since the spray expellent is freon, which ejects the spray forcefully, there is the danger of accidentally forcing the bandage material into the wound, despite careful use.

SQUIBB'S ORAHESIVE.* This product, which the author also had the privilege of using experimentally before it became clinically available, is a wax base oral adhesive bandage that is very useful in protecting surgical fields for postoperative periods.

The bandage material, made of a wax base, is easy to handle and to cut to size. It is attached by simply holding it firmly under finger pressure for about one minute, until the adhesive surface of the bandage attaches itself to the tis-

---

*The author has learned that this very excellent invaluable product apparently will be discontinued owing to unprofitably low sales volume. If there is sufficient demand a successor company may be obliged to resume its production. A comprehensive review of Orahesive is therefore being included, motivated by the hope that resumption of production will materialize.

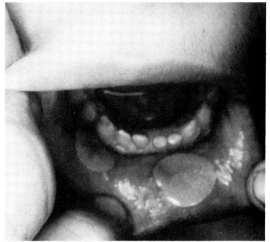

Figure 11-1. Use of thin variety of Squibb Orahesive bandage on mobile mucosa. Since this material is very thin and therefore somewhat flexible, and is very adhesive, it can be used as a dressing when needed.

sue surface; once attached it is tenaciously adherent. It disintegrates spontaneously after a short period, so that the patient does not have to bother about removing it.

This material comes in two thicknesses: a thin type, which is more adaptable to use on mobile tissues (Fig. 11-1) and lasts for about 6 to 8 hours under ordinary circumstances; and a thicker type that lasts for 12 to 18 hours under ordinary circumstances and is useful for application over tooth sockets and other wounds (Fig. 11-2). If longer periods of protection are desired, the author has found that by adding a second layer of bandage superimposed on the first layer, being careful to fuse the edges of the second layer by finger pressure to the first layer, it is possible to increase the protection time to 24 to 36 hours.

This material has a decided advantage over the Orabase and Kenalog in Orabase dressings, which are messy to apply and tend to adhere to the lips,

Figure 11-2. Use of the thicker Orahesive bandage as a dressing over an extraction socket. If the bleeding is not excessive, and the dressing material is kept firmly in contact with the tissues for about one minute, the warmth of the fingers appears to melt the dressing enough to become tenaciously adherent. A double layer has been applied.

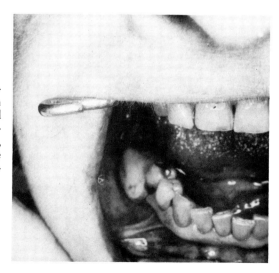

tongue, and cheeks and become easily displaced from the site of application. Orahesive bandage has a slick smooth external surface that is nonadhesive and will not adhere to the various structures of the mouth. Once this bandage becomes attached to the tissues, it is almost impossible to dislodge.

Since this material is made of a wax base, it is important to caution the patient to avoid use of hot lavages or hot foods while the bandage is in situ, since the heat would melt the wax and cause it to disintegrate prematurely. The temperature of lavage liquids or food should not exceed the normal mouth temperature.

The ease with which this material can be cut to size and shape with scissors is a distinct advantage. Low muscle attachments that would displace most other bandage materials or dressings present no difficulty with this material. All that is needed to avoid interference is to cut out a relief for the muscle attachment in the bandage, so that movements of the attachment will not disturb the bandage (Fig. 11–3).

This material is especially useful for brief protective dressings over the tissues that have been treated by electrosection, since very little bleeding results from the electrosurgery. When the Orahesive bandage is to be applied to a bleeding surface it is much more difficult to get it to adhere to the tissues; it is necessary to hold it firmly against the tissues for several minutes in many instances to achieve adhesion, and sometimes the adhesive on the undersurface of the bandage material is dissolved by the blood so that it will not adhere, and another bandage must be cut and applied. But when electrosurgery has been performed and there is little or no bleeding, the bandage material adheres rapidly and effectively. Tinctures of myrrh and benzoin applications to the tissues do not interfere with the adhesion or impair the usefulness of the bandage, so that there is no need to deviate from normal care in order to use the bandage.

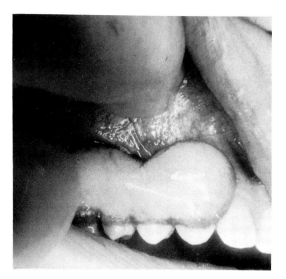

Figure 11–3.   Use of double thickness of the thick Orahesive provides a bandage protection for about 36 hours. The second layer is cut slightly smaller in dimension than the first layer, and then the margins are carefully adapted to the primary layer. If the patient is careful to avoid hot foods or liquids, the dressing often remains for 48 hours.

7. Heterogenous Grafts

A discussion of heterogenous grafts properly should be preceded by the factual observation that the most successful grafts by far are the autogenous grafts — either bone from the crest of the ilium, a rib, or alveolar process, or bone marrow from the ilium or sternum. Experiments with the latter give evidence that bone marrow may be more effective and easier to use in the oral cavity than autogenous bone.[18]

Heterogenous grafts would not be necessary if autogenous grafts could be obtained easily. But this is not the case. Autogenous grafts impose a major handicap — the reluctance of the average dental patient to serve as donor. This reluctance is attributable to the necessity of hospitalization to obtain the graft, except when alveolar bone is involved, and usually moderate to severe postoperative pain and incapacitation. When lack of hospital space for elective surgery and the expense of the hospitalization and surgery are added, the need for heterogenous substitutes for autogenous grafts becomes acute and widespread.

As a result, many substitute graft materials have been conceived and developed. Beube and Silver reported their use of devitalized powdered bone in 1934 and 1936.[19-20] Many heterogenous grafts have been developed and used experimentally in the intervening years, but in all too many instances for one reason or another had to be discarded.

Anorganic bone was discarded as ineffectual after five years of experimental use.[21-24] Freeze-dried bone[25] met a similar fate. Polyvinyl alcohol sponge, initially reported as favorable, likewise was discarded.[26-29] Tantalum gauze also was tried and discarded. Xiphisternal Cartilage (Armour), used by EENT and orthopedic surgeons, has not been used to any extent in oral surgery. Cultured despeciated bovine bone,[30-38] developed by the Squibb Institute for Medical Research and used experimentally by the author very extensively with remarkable success, had to be discarded because of refusal by the U.S. Pure Food and Drug Administration to permit its distribution. This refusal was predicated on the hypothesis that since the graft material contained organic protein it could conceivably induce allergic reactions including anaphylactic shock, although there had been no indications to that effect in the large number of clinical cases in which it had been used experimentally with great success.

There are two other types of heterogenous graft materials that have been reported as used successfully. One is plaster of Paris, which appears to become absorbed when placed into a bone defect and replaced by normal regenerating host bone. However, its use must still be considered in the experimental realm, since the evidence still is not sufficiently conclusive for either unqualified acceptance or rejection.

The second type of heterogenous graft is gelatin. In 1948 the author reported use of powdered gelatin as a heterogenous graft material and vehicle for introducing and holding in suspension relatively insoluble sulfonamides in extraction sockets and alveolar bone cavities.[15] The ordinary household unflavored gelatin originally used by the author has been replaced by a "surgical" gelatin (Upjohn), available either as a sponge or as a fluffy powder.[39] This surgical gelatin is prepared by melting commercial gelatin at high heat until it liquefies, then spinning it in centrifuges, and dehydrating the moisture with dry heat that converts the gelatin into a porous spongy consistency. The sponge is excellent for use in open wounds, but in closed wounds it breaks down and liquefies and is ineffectual. The powdered sponge, on the other hand, is effective when introduced into cystic cavities or comparable bone defects which must be sutured. When the gelatin becomes moistened by the blood present in the defect it swells into an adhesive gelatinous mass that serves as an excellent vehicle for introducing medicaments into the defect. It also helps to retain or restore the normal convex alveolar contours, and it seems to greatly reduce the incidence of surgical dead spaces.

Although they are not available for clinical use, a few of the clinical cases that were reported in the first edition involving the use of cultured despeciated bone have been retained in this edition because they well illustrate specific electrosurgical techniques. In all instances in which these heterogenous grafts were used they served admirably to obliterate bone defects without leaving residual dead spaces and served to maintain or restore normal anatomic contour to the defect areas. All the roentgenographic evidence points to these heterogenous graft materials having become incorporated into and consolidated with the surrounding normal bone.

8. Sterilizing Agents

Drugs for sterilizing the operative field. The number and variety of chemical agents suitable for use in the mouth for preanesthetic or preoperative sterilization of the oral tissues are far too numerous to be exhaustively enumerated and evaluated here. It is therefore advisable to limit the review to a brief résumé of the typical agents and the routine for preanesthetic and preoperative preparation of the operative field that was employed for most of the surgical procedures and their postoperative care that will be described in the following chapters.

Preparation of the patient starts with oral lavage or irrigation with any suitable antiseptic agent to reduce the intraoral bacterial count. Choice of a "suitable antiseptic agent" is a matter of personal preference of the operator. In the author's practice the mouth is irrigated or rinsed with clorpactin WCS-60 (Kasdenol, Guardian). Both this drug and WCS-90 are hypochlorous acid derivatives and potent oxidizing agents. These drugs have been comprehensively investigated, and reported by reliable research investigators and clinicians to be effective bactericides, sporicides, fungicides, and virucides when properly used.[40-50] To provide optimal performance, each mouthful should be held for approximately 15 to 30 seconds, and the final mouthful for two to three minutes.

The injection site or operative field is then gently dried and swabbed with benzalkonium chloride, Zephiran Chloride (Winthrop). The tissues are redried and anointed with a topical anesthetic ointment such as Xylocaine (Astra) or topical anesthetic liquid (oily suspension, Graham) to provide surface anesthesia capable of minimizing sensation from initial insertion of the needle into the tissues for the injection.

If the tissues are irritated, solution of Zephiran Chloride may be substituted for the tincture, or halogens such as aconite and iodine may be substituted for either of these.

STERILIZING AGENTS FOR COLD STERILIZATION OF ELECTRODES. Sterilizing the surgical electrodes presents a more complex problem than that relating to cold sterilization of more conventional types of cutting instruments. In the case of the electrodes, the cutting part—the wire needles, loops or balls—is unimportant, since these are essentially self-sterilizing. Any pathogens that might be present on them share the same fate as the tissue cells through which the ultra-high-frequency current passes; they are either coagulated, disintegrate and become volatilized, or are cremated and carbonized.

The problem is created by the fact that each electrode has a protective guard over the metal shaft, which is usually made of plastic, Bakelite or rubber tubing. The guard serves as an insulator to prevent trauma from accidental contact of the activated electrode shaft with lips, cheeks or tongue. Sterilizing heat and live steam dry out and destroy the usefulness of the guards. These also tend to make the needles and loop wire materials brittle so that they break more readily. The most reliable sterilizing methods, autoclaving and boiling, are therefore contraindicated. Unless Teflon guards are used, sterility must be achieved by soaking the electrodes in a cold sterilizing solution.

Until very recently the quaternary drugs (benzalkonium chloride and similar agents), which have high phenol coefficients, have enjoyed enviable reputations as reliable and effective cold sterilizing agents.

Bacteriologists have recently determined, however, that the quaternary drugs are not as effective cold sterilizing agents as had been believed, since they appear incapable of destroying many of the virulent pathogens often found in the mouth.[50-51] Research investigations have established that the new "tamed iodines," or iodophors, and alcohol-formaldehyde solutions, make efficient cold sterilizing agents which in addition to being bactericidal for gram-positive organisms are highly effective against gram-negative bacteria such as the T.B. bacillus, spores, yeasts, fungi and viruses, which are resistant to sterilizing action of the quaternary drugs.

Wescodyne (West Disinfecting Co.), a detergent iodine complex, is a new "tamed" iodine that is finding favor with many hospitals as a disinfectant and sterilizing agent.[52] It is reputed to provide effective sterilization rapidly, in a matter of five minutes in 75 parts per million concentration. It is handicapped, however, by the fact that it is not suitable for prolonged immersion of metal instruments, since the iodine apparently goes into chemical reaction with the metal and causes discoloration and dulling of sharp cutting edges.

Unlike the iodophors, the alcohol-formaldehyde solutions do not produce chemical reactions with metal instruments. When effective rust inhibitors are added to the solutions it is safe to leave metal instruments immersed in them for extended periods if they are completely free of organic debris.

The sterilizing efficiency of these agents is fully comparable to that of the iodophors, and they produce surgical sterility within 12 to 15 minutes. The following is an excellent formula for an alcohol–formaldehyde solution that is comparatively inexpensive, stable, and not incompatible with the oral tissues if the instruments are either air-dried or dried with sterile sponges before being introduced into the oral cavity.

℞

Ethyl alcohol	960 ml.
Formaldehyde solution ($37\frac{1}{2}$ per cent)	42 ml.
Potassium nitrite (KNO_2)	1.3 gm.

(Sodium nitrite may be substituted as the rust inhibitor)
Sig.: Dissolve the potassium nitrite in the formaldehyde, then add the alcohol. Keep covered.

In addition to being noninjurious to ordinary metallic instruments, this solution also appears to have no deleterious effects on either the fine needle and loop electrode wires or upon the rubber or plastic insulating guards. It is therefore particularly suitable for cold sterilization of electrosurgical instruments.

CIDEX (Johnson & Johnson) is neither a tamed halogen nor of the alcohol-formaldehyde type of cold sterilizing agents. Nevertheless, it is reputed to equal them in sterilizing effectiveness. CIDEX consists of glutaraldehyde, the active ingredient, 2%, and 98% inert matter in powder form and distilled water as the solvent. When the two are combined the solution retains sterilizing effectiveness for 14 days in contrast to the indefinite shelf-life of the alcohol-formaldehyde formula.

FOOTNOTE REFERENCES

1. Physicians Desk Reference to Pharmaceutical Specialties and Biologicals: (PDR) 26 Ed., 1972.
2. 1972 PDR: Supplement A.
3. 1972 PDR: Supplement B.
4. U.S. Food & Drug Administration (FDA) Drug Evaluations: Based on review of drugs by the National Academy of Sciences, National Research Council.
5. Akiba, T.: Mechanisms of Development of Resistance in Shigellae. Proceedings of 15th General Meeting, Japanese Med. Assoc., Vol. 5:299, 1959.
6. Watanabe, T., and Fukasawa, T.: "Resistance Transfer Factor," Anesisome in Enterobacteriaceae. Bio-Chem., Biophys., Res. Commun., 3:660, 1960.
7. Watanabe, T.: Infective heredity of multiple drug resistance in bacteria. Bact. Rev., 27:87, 1963.
8. Anderson, E. S., and Lewis, M. J.: Drug resistance and its transfer in Salmonella Typhimurium. Nature (London), 206:579, 1965.
9. Kabins, S. A., and Cohen, S.: Resistance transfer factor in Enterobacteriaceae. New Eng. J. Med., 275: 248, 1966.
10. Salzman, T. C., and Klemm, L.: Transferable drug resistance (R-Factor) in Enterobacteria. Proceedings of Sixth Interscience Conference on Antimicrobial Agents and Chemotherapy, 46: Oct. 26–28, 1966.
11. Gill, F. A., and Hook, E. W.: Salmonella strains with transferable antimicrobial resistance. J.A.M.A., 198:1267, 1966.
12. Salzman, T. C., Scher, C. D., and Moss, R.: Shigellae with transferable drug resistance: Outbreak in a nursery for premature infants. J. Pediat., 71:21, 1967.

13. Farrar, W. E., and Dekle, L. C.: Transferable antibiotic resistance associated with an outbreak of Shigellosis. Department of Preventive Medical and Community Health, Emory University School of Medicine, 67:6, 1967.
14. Oringer, M. J.: Gaffky's tetrads. Oral Surg., Oral Med., Oral Path., 1:10, 936, Oct., 1948.
15. Oringer, M. J.: Use of drugs and their effects on tissue repair. J. Dent. Med., 3:60, 1948.
16. Oringer, M. J.: Treatment of acute and subacute localized osteomyelitis with chemotherapy. Oral Surg., Oral Med., Oral Path., 1:9, 842, July, 1948.
17. Dubos, R. J.: Nutrition and tuberculosis. Sixteenth Bela Schick Lecture, Mt. Sinai Hosp., N.Y., April 30, 1959.
18. U.S. Naval Dental School, Bethesda, Md.: Personal communication to the author.
19. Beube, F. E., and Silvers, H. F.: Influence of devitalized heterogenous bone-powder on regeneration of alveolar and maxillary bone of dogs. J. Dent. Res., 14:15, 1934.
20. Beube, F. E., and Silvers, H. F.: Further studies on bone regeneration with the use of boiled heterogenous bone. J. Periodont., 7:17, 1936.
21. Boyne, P. J., and Losee, F. L.: Use of anorganic bone implants in oral surgery. J. Oral Surg., 16:53, Jan., 1958.
22. Boyne, P. J., and Lyon, H. W.: Long-term histologic response to implants of anorganic heterogenous bone in man. (Abstr.) J. Dent. Res., 38:699, July-Aug., 1959.
23. Costich, E. R., and Hayward, J. R.: Resorption studies of anorganic bone. (Abstr.) J. Dent. Res., 38:689, July, 1959.
24. Bell, W. H.: Resorption characteristics of autogenous and anorganic bone implants. (Abstr.) J. Dent. Res., 38:698, July-Aug., 1959.
25. Cooksey, D. E.: Application of freeze-dried bone grafts in cysts of the jaws. (Abstr.) J. Dent. Res., 33:655, Oct., 1954.
26. Amler, M. H., Johnson, P. L., and Bevelander, G.: Bone regeneration following grafts with polyvinyl plastic sponge. Oral Surg., Oral Med., Oral Path., 11:654, June, 1958.
27. Grindlay, J. H., and Waugh, J. M.: Plastic sponge which acts as a framework for living tissue. A.M.A. Arch. Surg., 63:288, Sept., 1951.
28. Gale, J. W., Curreri, A. R., Young, W. P., and Dickie, H. A.: Plastic sponge prosthesis following resection in pulmonary tuberculosis. J. Thorac. Surg., 24:587, Dec., 1952.
29. Lewin-Epstein, J.: Use of polyvinyl alcohol sponge in alveoloplasty: a preliminary report. J. Oral Surg., Anes., Hosp. Svc., 18:453, Nov., 1960.
30. Hinds, E. C., and Arnim, S. S.: Use of cultured calf bone paste in oral surgery. (Abstr.) I.A.D.R., 35:90, 1957.
31. Shankwalker, G. B., and Mitchell, D. F.: Response of despeciated calf bone and calcium hydroxide implants. (Abstr.) J. Dent. Res., 37:981, Sept., 1958.
32. Seiffert, D. M., and Swanson, L. T.: Histological evaluation of bone grafts made with cultured calf bone paste. Harvard D. Alumni Bull., 19:121, Oct., 1959.
33. Tucker, E. J.: Studies on the use of cultured calf bone in human bone grafts. Clin. Orthoped., No. 7, 171, 1956.
34. Fisher, W. B.: Clinical use of cultured calf bone grafts. Transplantation Bull., 4:10, Jan., 1957.
35. Clayton, I.: Cultured calf bone; a new bone grafting material. Illinois Med. J., 110:49, Aug., 1956.
36. Fisher, W. B., and Clayton, I.: Surgical bone grafting with cultured calf bone. Quart. Bull. Northwestern Med. Sch., 29(4):341, 1955.
37. Georgiade, N., et al.: Use of calf bones in transplantations. D. Abstr., 4:34, April, 1959.
38. Stallard, R., and Randall, W.: Effects of calf bone on rate of bone regeneration in the tibia of guinea pigs. J. Periodont., 30:348, Oct., 1959.
39. Guralnick, W. C.: Absorbable gelatin sponge and thrombin in oral surgery. J. Oral Surg., 32:792, 1946.
40. DeAlmeida, P. F., et al.: Action of Chlorpactin WCS 90 in microbiology. Rev. Paulista de Med., 43:104, 1953.
41. De Stefano, T. M.: Summary of cases using Chlorpactin WCS 60 for various oral lesions. J. N. Jer. D. Soc., 25:49, April, 1954.
42. Lattimer, J. K., and Spirito, A. L.: Chlorpactin for tuberculous cystitis. J. Urol., 73:1015, 1955.
43. Swanker, W. A.: Use of Chlorpactin WCS 90 as an antiseptic in surgery. Amer. J. Surg., 90:44, 1955.
44. Wolinsky, E., Smith, M. M., and Steenken, W., Jr.: Tuberculocidal activity of Chlorpactin, a new chlorine compound. Antibiotic Med., 1:382, July, 1955.
45. Zwerling, M.: Chlorpactin WCS 90: a new antiseptic. A.M.A. Arch. Otolaryngol., 62:157, Aug., 1955.
46. Conn, H. F.: Editorial in Current Therapy, 1973. Philadelphia, W. B. Saunders Co., 1955, p. 359.
47. Sanders, M., and Soret, M.: Virucidal activity of WCS 90. J. Antibiotics Chemother., Nov., 1955.
48. Oringer, M. J.: Oral medicine and therapeutics. J. N. Jer. D. Soc., 27:36, July, 1956.
49. Kruger, G. O.: Management of impactions. Symposium on Office Oral Surgery, Dent. Clin. N. Amer., 709, 1959.
50. Zubrow, H. J., Spatz, S. S., and Kline, S. N.: Antibiotics in Oral Surgery. Symposium on Office Oral Surgery. Dent. Clin. N. Amer., p. 686, Nov., 1959.
51. Littman, M. L.: Personal communication to the author.
52. Blechman, H.: Personal communication to the author.
53. Mt. Sinai Hosp., N.Y.: Formulatory Facts. Issue 3, Apr. 16, 1962.

CLINICAL ELECTROSURGICAL TECHNIQUES

Before proceeding with a review of the electrosurgical techniques useful in the various dental disciplines, it might prove beneficial to briefly examine some of the reasons why and how electrosurgery can offer so many unique advantages to dentistry.

The most important reason by far is that the practice of dentistry is complicated by a fundamental contradiction that creates unique special problems. *Diagnostically*, the oral cavity is one of the most accessible and visible parts of the body. *Therapeutically*, however, we as dentists know only too well that there are many areas in the mouth where access is limited and visibility obscured even by the normal anatomic structures that belong there, such as the cheeks, tongue, and tissues forming the floor of the mouth. Needless to say, the presence of anatomic abnormalities, neoplasia, or blood in the operative field substantially increases these handicaps.

Inaccessibility and poor visibility inevitably become translated clinically into impaired operative efficiency, loss of chair operating time, and an increase in operator and patient fatigue. Obviously, any modality that can neutralize or minimize these natural handicaps offers dentistry immeasurable advantages. Electrosurgery is precisely such a modality. A brief comparative analysis of electrosurgery versus "conventional" cold-steel instrumentation readily reveals the reasons why this is so.

Cold-steel instruments are rigid; they cannot be reshaped to meet special needs of the individual case. This sharply limits their maneuverability, hence their usefulness, in areas that offer poor access. Cold-steel cutting requires

263

pressure against the tissues with the cutting instrument. The operator must therefore grasp the instrument close to its cutting end to use it effectively. The bunched fingers tend to block the mouth orifice and interfere with access and visibility. Bleeding, often profuse and persistent, that accompanies the cutting further impairs visibility. When the inherent limitations of this method of instrumentation are superimposed on the natural handicaps, they greatly compound our operative difficulties.

By contrast, surgical electrodes are hair-thin wire needles or loops that can easily be bent to any required shape, greatly increasing their maneuverability even in areas that offer poor access. No pressure is required to cut with the activated electrode, since neither the operator nor the electrode does the cutting. As was established in an earlier chapter, the cutting results from conversion of the high-frequency energy radiating through the patient's body into heat energy when the circuit is completed by contact of the activated electrode with the tissues to be treated. Thereupon, the individual cells in the line of cleavage volatilize and undergo molecular dissolution. All the operator need do is guide the electrode and control its activity. With need for pressure eliminated, there is no need to grasp the instrument close to its cutting end; thus neither access nor visibility is impaired. Hemostasis is inherent in electrosurgery. Normal capillaries and lymph vessels are sealed off as they are severed, and capillary bleeding is therefore greatly reduced.

The increased maneuverability and improved visibility that electrosurgery affords the operator greatly simplifies and accelerates treatment. This means *reduced* chair operating time, *superior* operative results, and *reduced* operator and patient fatigue. When we add the further advantage of greatly minimized postoperative reactions, owing to the atraumatic, relatively bloodless instrumentation, and the functional and aesthetic advantages of normal-looking, soft, supple repair tissue devoid of cicatricial contraction, plus the sterilizing quality of the high-frequency current as it cuts, the superiority of electrosurgery over cold-steel instrumentation for surgery of oral mucosa should become self-evident even to an avowed skeptic.

This does not imply, however, that electrosurgery is a panacea. The requirements for good electrosurgery are exacting and precise. The essential ingredients to achieve maximum efficacy and safety with this modality are a balanced combination of sound dental technique, skillful electrosurgical instrumentation, and mature clinical judgment. No one ingredient can substitute for the others, and omission of any one of the trinity more than likely will destroy its usefulness.

PART 1

RESTORATIVE DENTISTRY

Introduction

That phase of dentistry which deals with the restoration of the natural dentition had, until recently, been traditionally subdivided into two separate and independent disciplines: operative dentistry, which often included endodontics until the latter emerged as a full-fledged dental specialty, and crown and bridge prosthodontics.

In the dental school hierarchy operative dentistry and crown and bridge prosthodontics constituted separate departments, each with its own departmental chairman and faculty and its own teaching curriculum. Endodontics often constituted a third department, independent of the other two.

In keeping with this separatism, the electrosurgical techniques developed for use in operative dentistry (including endodontics) and in crown and bridge prosthodontics were included in the first edition as unrelated entities.

Because operative dentistry, endodontics, and crown and bridge prosthodontics are often collectively involved in clinical treatment of the patient, a new trend has recently evolved in dental education. Recognition of the frequent intimate involvement and interdependence of all three, both in the treatment plan and in the clinical treatment, has led to the growing trend in dental education toward combining the three into one all-encompassing department of restorative dentistry, in which each is a contributory subdivision, in order to increase treatment plan coordination and improve clinical efficiency.

In keeping with this trend, and in view of the clinical interdependence of the three categories, they will be reviewed in this edition as related subdivisions under the general heading "Restorative Dentistry." Inasmuch as this interdependence is to a great extent also applicable to pedodontics, the latter is included as a fourth subdivision.

Chapter Twelve

OPERATIVE DENTISTRY

Many techniques uniquely useful in operative dentistry have been developed by the author in the interim since the first edition was prepared. There are now six principal areas in operative dentistry in which electrosurgery can be uniquely useful to simplify and improve operative technique and reduce chair operating time. These are:

1. For desensitizing hypersensitive dentin.
2. To expose deep subgingival caries efficiently.
3. To eliminate redundant proliferative tissues from caries.
4. Subgingival electrosection for inlay preparation.
5. To elongate clinical crowns of teeth for aesthetics or function.
6. To bleach discolored teeth.
7. For pulp capping without pulpotomy.

DESENSITIZING HYPERSENSITIVE DENTIN

Hypersensitivity of eroded enamel surfaces and of extensive tooth preparations is a common irritant to both patient and dentist. Electrosurgical desensitization of hypersensitive dentin is a very simple, rapid, yet highly effective operative procedure.

When the dentin becomes exposed as a result of caries, erosion, tooth fracture or tooth preparation for operative restoration it becomes highly sensitive to thermal, chemical and mechanical stimuli.

Dentin contains innumerable canals, or tubules. Branching processes from the odontoblasts lining the dentinal aspect of the pulp chamber extend into these canals. Many of these projections extend the full length of the canals and on into the enamel at the dentino-enamel junction.[1-7] These projecting processes, known as Tomes' fibers or the dentinal fibers, are

266

reputed to be responsible for sensitivity of the dentino-enamel junction and of exposed dentin.

Dentinal hypersensitivity can be controlled best by coagulating the organic contents of the canals at their exposed terminal ends. Coagulation may be achieved by chemical or thermal action, either alone or combined. Silver nitrate has for many years been the most widely used chemical agent for this purpose. Application of silver nitrate to hypersensitive dentin produces variable degrees of decreased sensitivity for variable periods of time.

Although silver nitrate has been the principal chemical coagulating agent it has several objectionable features which limit its usefulness. One is the unsightly black permanent discoloration that results, which makes it impractical for use in the anterior part of the mouth. A more important objection has been created by recent research reports indicating that silver nitrate applied to dentin often passes through the dentinal tubules and reaches the pulp tissues by capillary attraction[8-16] (or through the "dentinal lymphatic circulation," a hypothesis first propounded by Bodecker[2, 3]). This produces pulpal irritation and deterioration[17, 18] which may lead to ultimate devitalization and necrosis of the pulp tissue in extreme cases.

Thymol crystals melted onto the tooth surface, warm oil applied to the surface with heated instruments, fluoride preparations, and formalin solution applied to sensitive dentin and then evaporated by blasts of warm air, all are among the chemical and thermal methods that also enjoy some popularity and produce varying degrees of improvement for relatively brief periods of time.

Electrocoagulation applied to the exposed dentin provides desensitization for much more extended periods. Electrocoagulation permits complete control of the depth of coagulation achieved, and produces uniform coagulation. It is therefore a highly accurate modality for effectively desensitizing teeth.

The electrocoagulation usually is performed with a small round coagulating electrode. When the desensitization must be carried to the marginal gingiva, or if it is necessary to extend it slightly into the crevicular space, the pointed conical electrode is best suited to perform the electrocoagulation without contacting and coagulating the marginal gingiva. When a hypersensitive groove erosion has been caused by friction of a denture clasp, the conical silver coagulating electrode often fits into the groove best, and thus provides the most effective contact.

Although electrocoagulation overcomes dentin hypersensitivity, this does not completely solve the problem unless it is combined with supplementary collateral preventive treatment. The coagulated exposed ends of the Tomes fibers will, unless prevented, undergo decomposition.

The amino acids, the end-products of decomposition of organic matter, are highly irritating. Since these end-products can flow back through the dentinal tubules to the pulp chamber by capillary attraction, they are likely to stimulate an inflammatory painful pulp response, and conceivably even pulp degeneration. Application of a tissue preservative to the tooth surface immediately prior to the application of the coagulating current can prevent this. Both are therefore necessary for ideal desensitization.

Formalin, a solution of the gas, formaldehyde, in water, is very rapid acting and probably has better penetrating qualities than any of the other fixative agents. Heat vaporizes formalin, releasing the gas, which rapidly permeates and fixes organic matter, thereby preventing its decomposition. The technique to be described utilizes the combined advantages of electrocoagulation and fixation.

(When more than one case is reported herein to describe a specific technique, an unavoidable basic similarity may be noticed. Pointless duplication, however, has been meticulously avoided. Each case has been selected because it presented a different treatment problem, a variation in technique, or a difference in local or systemic factors that influenced the treatment or the tissue responses to the electrosurgical treatment.)

CASE 1

This is a typical case of hypersensitivity of exposed dentin resulting from preparation of teeth for restorative dentistry.

PATIENT. A 49-year-old white female.

HISTORY. She was referred primarily for repair of a palatal defect, which will be described in a subsequent chapter (Chap. 22). Two of her maxillary teeth had been reduced for full-crown coverage to serve as abutments for a fixed bridge. Both prepared teeth had subsequently become extremely sensitive to thermal and mechanical stimuli. The referring dentist therefore requested that in addition to the reparative surgery, electrosurgical desensitization of the two teeth be performed.

CLINICAL EXAMINATION. The maxillary left central incisor and first bicuspid were reduced slightly beyond their dentino-enamel junctions for full-crown coverage.

TREATMENT. An explorer run lightly over the buccal surface of the bicuspid elicited a painful response. The gingival mucosa around the tooth was dried; then topical anesthetic ointment was applied to the gingival mucosa to serve as a protective lubricant to prevent any tissue damage from capillary attraction of the formalin to the tissues and also to desensitize the mucosa.

A small pellet of cotton was moistened with formalin solution, excessive moisture was removed, and the pellet was carefully applied to the tooth surface. Electrocoagulating current was then applied to the tooth with a small ball coagulating electrode (Case Fig. 1–1). A minimal amount of current output was assured by setting the dial midway between 0 and 1 and on the Radiosurg Scalpel unit. (With later models of the Radiosurg Scalpel, current output for visible superficial spot coagulation ranges from 1.5 to 2.5 on the instrument panel; with the Cameron or other single-tube units the equivalent current output can be obtained by setting the dial at about 4, and with the Hyfrecator the current output is set at about 25.)

The coagulating current was applied biterminally for one second, during which time the electrode was kept in constant rapid motion over the tooth surface. The electrode was then removed for five seconds during which time the formalin was reapplied to the hypersensitive area. The electrocoagulation was reapplied for one second as described, and the alternate coagulation–rest interval was repeated for a total of 15 applications. The tooth was then tested for hypersensitivity by scraping the surface with an explorer point, which elicited a slight degree of sensitivity. The elec-

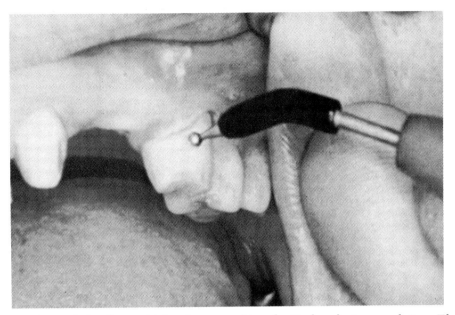

Case Figure 1–1. Desensitizing hypersensitive dentin by electrocoagulation. Electrocoagulation with the small ball electrode. Note: The "bare metal" shaft of the electrode actually is insulated with a clear plastic sleeve; the black portion is bakelite. Exposure of bare metal should be carefully avoided.

trocoagulation and remoistening with formalin during the ensuing rest interval was reinstituted for an additional five times, and the tooth was again tested for hypersensitivity, and this time it failed to react.

The reduced central incisor was then prepared and desensitized in exactly the same manner, but this time the gingival portion of the tooth was treated adequately also. After 15 applications of the coagulating current, this tooth was retested and was unresponsive to the contact of the explorer. Both teeth were then thoroughly cleansed with wet sponges to remove all traces of the formalin solution, and the patient was reappointed for the surgery.

The patient was recalled semiannually for postoperative checkup for two years after the reparative palatal surgery was performed. During that period the patient reported that at no time after desensitization had the two teeth given further trouble, either before or after the fixed restoration was inserted.

CASE 2

This case differs from Case 1 in that the hypersensitivity was localized along the marginal edge of the labial aspect of the crown and extended subgingivally to the cemento-enamel junction. The treatment therefore had to be extended into the gingival sulcus. Obvously subgingival electrocoagulation could not be performed subgingivally with a ball electrode without destroying the marginal gingiva.

If a Coles solid tapered conical type of electrode is substituted and the marginal gingiva is gently elevated from the tooth surface with the *inactivated* electrode in a manner similar to that of a manicurist freeing the cuticle around fingernails, the tapered tip of the electrode can be applied to the tooth surface subgingivally without coagulating the marginal gingiva.

It is also not possible to apply the formalin to the subgingival portion of the tooth in the usual manner, since the chemical would very likely fix the free gingival margin tissue and perhaps the edge of the investing alveolar bone and periosteum, which is distinctly to be avoided. The author has found that by dipping the tip of the conical electrode into the formalin and permitting the excess to drip off before introducing it, it is possible to bring enough formalin to the tooth surface being treated to be effective, without danger of fixing the investing tissues in doing so.

Increased elevation of the marginal gingiva from its close adaptation to the tooth surface can be achieved atraumatically by use of a piece of unimpregnated cord, or rolling a wisp of cotton into a cordlike strand; either material can be tamped under the free margin into the sulcus space gently but firmly and left there a few minutes. When the cord is removed the small end of a double end ball burnisher can be introduced and used to further lift the tissues gently away from the tooth surface, creating the space for the cone-shaped electrode to be applied to the cemento-enamel junction safely.

The following case demonstrates this modification.

PATIENT.   A 49-year-old white female.

HISTORY.   She had been troubled by thermal and chemical sensitivity. The sensitivity was particularly troublesome during mastication or toothbrushing. Although there was no evidence of decay or tooth erosion she consulted her dentist in the hope of obtaining relief. He referred her to the author for help when he found the sensitivity was subgingival rather than coronal.

CLINICAL EXAMINATION.   The patient's oral hygiene was excellent. The sensitive tooth, the maxillary right central incisor, showed no evidence of erosion or caries, but when a fine explorer tip was inserted subgingivally and scraped over the cemento-enamel junction she immediately complained of severe discomfort.

TREATMENT.   Since the patient appeared to have a normal pain threshold, and her reaction was not grossly exaggerated, the desensitization was performed without anesthesia, so that the tooth could act as its own control to determine when the sensitivity was overcome.

The external surface of the marginal gingiva was lubricated with oil-based topical anesthetic. The cuff of marginal gingiva was then lifted slightly with the inactivated conical electrode, and the topical anesthetic was sparingly introduced subgingivally. After two minutes the tissue was sponged gently and a hand-rolled cotton wick was gently but firmly tamped into the gingival sulcus and was kept there for 5 minutes. The wick was then removed, and the small end of a ball burnisher was inserted and used as a lever to gently elevate the tissue further from the tooth surface.

A solid conical tapered coagulating electrode was selected and coagulating current output was set at 2 on the Coles unit power rheostat dial. The electrode tip was then dipped into 10 per cent formalin solution, and the excess was permitted to drip off. Then the tip was inserted and the activated tip was used with a rubbing motion over the sensitive cemento-enamel junction for one second (Case Fig. 2–1), followed by 10 seconds of rest interval, during which time the electrode tip was reimmersed in the formalin solution. The active electrocoagulation was repeated 30 times, and the explorer was applied to the tooth exactly as it had been used initially, but this time it failed to cause any sensitive reaction. The crown of the tooth and especially the sulcus area were irrigated to wash away any trace of the formalin solution, and the patient was dismissed from further treatment.

This technique is applicable in all cases that require subgingival desensitization.

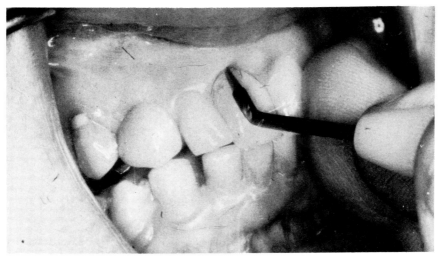

Case Figure 2–1. A solid conical sharp tapered coagulating electrode is being used to extend the desensitization subgingivally. The desensitization on the labial aspect of the tooth having been performed with a small ball electrode to within a fraction of a millimeter short of the marginal gingiva, the latter was elevated by inserting a small ball burnisher under the free gingival margin and gently rotating it with a lifting motion similar to that used to free the cuticle from a fingernail, so that the pointed tip of the tapered electrode could be inserted and used without making contact with the cuff of free gingival tissue. Formalin is *not* applied subgingivally, as it is on the external surface of the tooth.

CASE 3

This is a typical case of hypersensitivity caused by enamel erosion and its treatment.

PATIENT. A 62-year-old white female.

HISTORY. She was referred for reduction of gingival hypertrophy around the mandibular cuspids and desensitization of extremely sensitive deep erosions on the labial surfaces of the two teeth, the result of wear from cast clasps of a partial denture.

CLINICAL EXAMINATION. The mandible was edentulous except for the two cuspids. Each tooth had a deep, highly polished labial groove. Both eroded areas were extremely sensitive to both thermal and mechanical stimuli; running an explorer lightly over the eroded surfaces was unbearably painful to the patient.

TREATMENT. The teeth were isolated with gauze sponges and dried, their gingivae were anointed with lubricant, and desensitization was performed in a manner similar to that described in Case 1, with one noteworthy exception. Whereas in Case 1 drying and the effects of the formalin solution had reduced the sensitivity sufficiently to permit electrocoagulation without need for anesthesia, in this case there was no comparable reduction in sensitivity. Local anesthesia, therefore, was administered by subperiosteal infiltration before the biterminal electrocoagulating current could be applied to the sensitive areas of these teeth.

After a few minutes the explorer could be applied to the eroded surfaces without eliciting painful responses. Formalin solution was applied, and the coagulating current was applied for five-second periods with the cylindrical electrode kept in constant motion (Case Fig. 3–1). After a five-second pause during which the formalin was reapplied, the electrocoagulation was resumed and repeated as described for a total of 20 such applications.

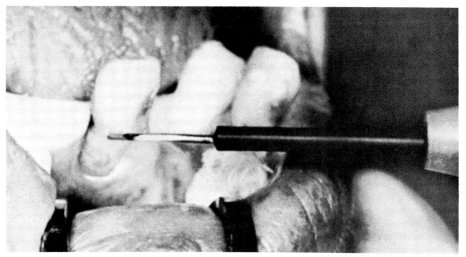

Case Figure 3–1.   Desensitizing painful cervical clasp erosion by electrocoagulation with cylindrical electrode.

Because of the anesthesia it was impossible to ascertain the efficacy of the treatment immediately; therefore it had to be terminated empirically after each tooth had received 20 five-second applications. The teeth were cleansed of formalin and the patient was reappointed for the gingival surgery. When she returned she reported that both teeth were behaving normally. She was seen postoperatively three months later and again six months later. On both occasions the patient reported that both teeth felt comfortable under the denture clasps.

EXPOSURE OF SUBGINGIVAL CARIES, SHOULDER PREPARATIONS, AND FRACTURE SITES FOR DEFINITIVE TREATMENT

Electrosurgery can be used to great advantage to eliminate one of the major sources of unproductive chair operating time loss — the exposure of obstructed caries for definitive treatment. The worst offenders are caries that extend subgingivally and either become filled with friable proliferated marginal gingiva or are located subgingivally and are covered by normal gingival mucosa, and pulp polyps in extensively carious deciduous teeth.

Chemical coagulation has been the most common method of dealing with such tissue. The coagulation is performed with a caustic or escharotic; usually silver nitrate, phenol, or trichloracetic acid is applied. The proliferative tissue is typically so very vascular and friable that as soon as it is contacted by the chemical agent it usually begins to hemorrhage as profusely as when it is scooped out surgically with a surgical curet.

When the coagulation finally is completed and the bleeding stops, the coagulated debris must be removed from the cavity. Bleeding resumes almost invariably as soon as the cavity is washed out, even though care is exercised to irrigate very gently. The bleeding is mostly a persistent oozing that prevents definitive treatment and necessitates a subsequent visit for that purpose, hopefully without recurrence of the proliferation.

Comparable tissue proliferation frequently occurs in the embrasures between proximal inlay preparations. Since good inlay preparations feature parallel or flaring walls and beveled margins, with an absence of undercuts, temporary fillings inserted into proximal inlay preparations tend to become displaced quickly and fall out. When this occurs, proliferation of the subgingival tissues is very likely.

When proliferation does occur, usually manifested by tissue flowing over the axial floor of the cavity, it prevents the seating and cementation of the inlay restorations until the redundant tissue is eliminated. Here again, if this tissue is coagulated chemically, the subsequent oozing of blood will prevent successful cementation of the restoration at that sitting or, at best, involve expenditure of unproductive chair operating time to accomplish it.

The facility with which the proliferative tissue can be removed by loop resection or destroyed by electrocoagulation, without hemorrhagic bleeding and oozing that prevents definitive treatment, must be witnessed or experienced to be fully appreciated. The benefits are time saved and the ability to conclude definitive treatment in one sitting, and hence, improved clinical treatment and improved office economics.

The tooth with caries that extends far beyond the gingival level along the root of the tooth is another source of operative difficulty and unproductive chair operating time loss. In such a case, if the obstructing overlying gingiva is resected with a steel scalpel or destroyed by grinding with a diamond stone or surgical bur, it hemorrhages profusely and cannot be treated definitively until the tissue has healed. If the obstructing tissue is displaced by packing gutta percha into the cavity and overfilling to force the tissue away, it usually produces an acute inflammatory reaction, with swelling and engorgement of the gingiva and considerable pain. Again, definitive treatment must be deferred until the tissue has been displaced and returned to its normal dimension and tone.

Electrosurgery provides a means of removing the offending tissue in all these conditions rapidly and without hemorrhage or postoperative complications. It also permits the recontouring of the margin of the cut gingiva to normal feather-edge architecture, when indicated, and makes it possible to isolate the tooth with a rubber dam, as needed. Thus, immediately after the electrosection has been performed the tooth is ready for cavity preparation and definitive treatment without delay, including gold foil fillings, if desired.

Since the electrosection can be performed in a matter of seconds, and definitive treatment can be concluded during one office visit, this method of treatment eliminates the disruption of the appointment schedule as well as the unproductive loss of much chair operating time. Cumulative time saved from this and the other advantages that electrosurgery offers makes possible an appreciable increase in the patient load and the concomitant increase in income on an annual basis.

Electrosurgery is notably helpful in operative dentistry in one other area—the preservation and restoration of fractured teeth that would become candidates for extraction.

This applies particularly to teeth accidentally fractured longitudinally and although a considerable portion of the tooth crown is fractured in the vertical plane, the fracture does not involve the pulp chamber or the root canal. In such cases it is possible to restore the fractured portion with Markley pins and an amalgam filling, or with a pin inlay, and thereby preserve the tooth for functional use, *if the tissue can be cleared away to provide access to the fractured area* and the restoration can be inserted in a dry field.

Electrosurgery is ideally suited to treat these cases for a variety of reasons. The electrode best suited for use is the 17-mm. U-shaped periodontal curet loop electrode. The lack of physical bulk of the loop, its flexibility, and the ability to bend and reshape it at will all help to assure ready access to the deepest and narrowest parts of the subgingival end of the fracture. The fact that the energy does the cutting, eliminating the need for manual pressure, assures efficient excision of tissue in the most confined areas and makes it possible to dissect away enough of the adjacent tissue after the fractured fragment has been removed to provide adequate access and visibility to the fracture site to simplify and facilitate the restoration of the tooth.

The following cases demonstrate the practical clinical application of these uses of electrosurgery for operative dentistry.

REMOVAL OF PROLIFERATIVE TISSUE FROM GINGIVAL AND INTERPROXIMAL CARIES OR CAVITY PREPARATIONS

The technique for coagulating undesirable proliferative tissue having been well documented in the past,[19-21] it will not be reviewed in this text, particularly since the resection technique appears to provide more efficient results.

CASE 4

This case is one in which a large Class V caries extends into and beyond the gingival sulcus, and irritates and stimulates the gingiva to proliferate into the cavity to fully or partially obscure it and prevent examination or treatment. It is noteworthy that in this particular case the marginal gingiva showed exceptionally severe inflammation with marked edema and engorgement, and the entire large cavity was filled with a mass of friable proliferated tissue.

PATIENT. A 56-year-old black female.

HISTORY. The tooth had been decayed for a long time, but since it did not cause discomfort, the patient did not have it treated. Recently it began to bleed suddenly, the tissues became painful, and the patient went to a dentist to have the tooth extracted. Her dentist thought that the tooth could be filled if the tissue filling the cavity could be removed. He referred her for removal of the tissue polyp, and, if necessary, extraction of the tooth.

CLINICAL EXAMINATION. The mandibular right second molar was an isolated tooth. The buccal marginal gingiva was very swollen and engorged, and the huge cavity on the buccal aspect of the crown was filled with engorged friable tissue (Case Fig. 4–1).

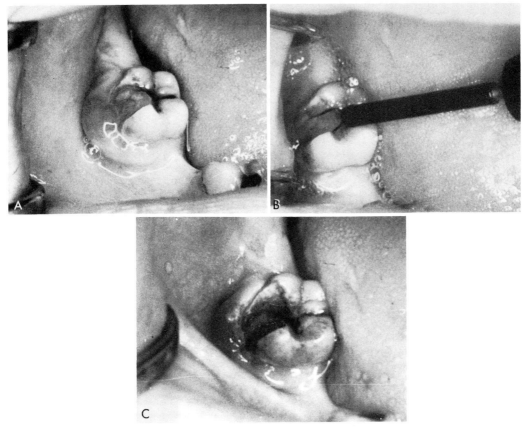

Case Figure 4–1. A, Massive proliferation of inflamed marginal gingiva into a huge cavity in a molar that extends subgingivally. The marginal gingiva is massively swollen and engorged, and its proliferative extension into the cavity is friable and bleeds profusely at the slightest touch. B, A large round loop electrode has been squeezed into an elongated, somewhat oval shape, so that it fits exactly into the cavity to excise the tissue mass without being impeded. Cutting current is set at 8 on the instrument panel, and the entire mass is excised with a single lifting, scooping motion. The electrode is seen in the process of cutting the tissue. C, Immediate postoperative appearance of the tooth and gingiva. The cavity is cleared of tissue. There is no hemorrhagic free bleeding to obscure vision or impair treatment. The cavity can now be inspected and definitive treatment instituted.

TREATMENT. The tissues were prepared and inferior alveolar-long buccal regional block anesthetic was administered. A large round loop electrode slightly narrower than the diameter of the cavity was selected and current output was set at 8.5 on the power output dial. The activated electrode was used with a scooping motion and the entire polypoid mass was resected at the first attempt at resection. There was no free bleeding, despite the severe gingival engorgement, and no tissue burn.

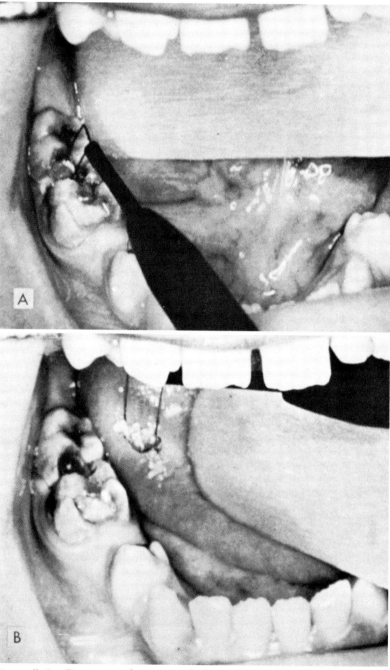

Case Figure 5-1. Resection of tissue occluding proximal cavities (or inlay preparations). A, Tissue resected with U-shaped loop electrode. B, Resected tissue being lifted out with the electrode, leaving cavities accessible to treatment. Note lack of bleeding.

Since the tooth was valuable as an abutment, she was sent back to the dentist for further treatment.

CASE 5

This case is typical of electrosurgical elimination of proliferative hypertrophic gingival tissue from between adjacent interproximal cavities or cavity preparations.

PATIENT. A 39-year-old white female.

HISTORY. The patient was referred for either extraction of two mandibular right molars or removal of hypertrophic tissue that occluded the cavities in order to permit cavity preparation if extraction were unnecessary.

CLINICAL EXAMINATION. The proximo-occlusal cavities in the mandibular first and second molars were completely occluded by a globular mass of hypertrophic tissue which was severely engorged.

TREATMENT. Topical anesthetic ointment was applied to this tissue. A medium-sized U-shaped loop electrode was selected and inserted into the coagulating electrode handle. Coagulating current output was set at 5, and the electrode was brought into position for use (Case Fig. 5–1A). The mass was resected in one stroke by applying the electrode to the base of the embrasure and scooping the mass out with a lifting motion. The mass adhered to the electrode (Case Fig. 5–1B) as it was lifted out. There was no bleeding, and an immediate examination of the cavities was easily performed.

This technique is equally suitable for clearing out proliferating gingival hypertrophic tissue that bulges up into the interproximal space between proximal inlay preparations, obliterates the cavity margins, and prevents seating and cementing of the restorations.

The coagulating techniques referred to above consisted of either inserting the electrode into the tissue to be destroyed and applying electrodesiccation, or applying biterminal electrocoagulation until the mass shriveled beyond the cavity area without causing free bleeding or seepage that would interfere with cementation of the restorations. This coagulating method (the Webb technique) caused a great deal of extensive tissue damage, including bone sequestration and exfoliation of teeth; hazards that are nonexistent in the technique of electrosection that has been described.

CASE 6

PATIENT. A 28-year-old white male.

HISTORY. The patient suddenly began to feel pain in a tooth in the right upper jaw. He consulted a dentist who found caries extending subgingivally beyond an old amalgam filling in the right maxillary first molar. The gingival tissue had proliferated downward somewhat, so that the entire carious area was covered by tissue, making it impossible to prepare or even thoroughly examine the cavity. He was referred for resection of the tissue to expose the cavity.

CLINICAL EXAMINATION. An old amalgam filling was present on the mesio-occlusal aspect of the tooth. A slight amount of decay was barely visible at the superior border of the filling. The gingival tissue dipped downward in the edentulous area where the second bicuspid had been removed, so that the gingival level at the carious site was lower than in other areas of the mouth (Case Fig. 6–1A).

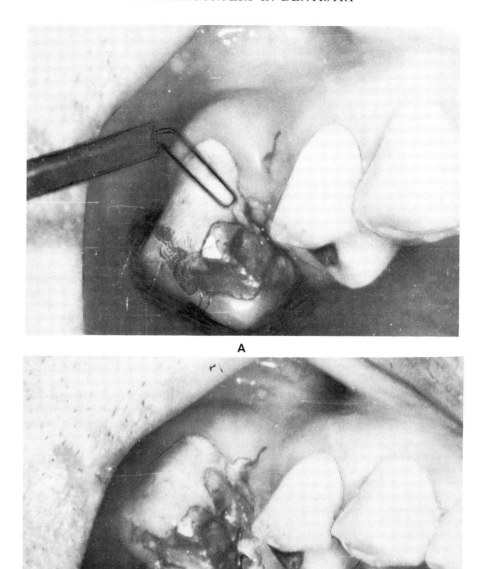

A

B

Case Figure 6–1. A, Exposure of subgingival caries. The maxillary right first molar has a large old MO amalgam filling that has leaky margins. There is evidence of caries extending beyond the axial floor of the filling. The alveolar mucosa in the edentulous second bicuspid area has proliferated downward and dips down to meet the old filling. This tissue will have to be excised to expose the cavity. A 45-degree angle U-shaped loop electrode is poised in position for the excision of the redundant tissue. *B,* The tissue has been excised with a wiping and scooping motion of the activated electrode, with cutting current set at 3.5 on the instrument panel. Some of the excised tissue is brought away with the loop, and some is curled and resting on the gingival tissue. The caries is fully exposed, and ready for definitive treatment. It is now possible to apply a rubber dam if desired.

TREATMENT. The tissue was anesthetized with infiltration anesthesia. A small narrow U-shaped loop electrode was selected and cutting current set at 3.5 on the power output dial. The electrode was activated and used with a few short wiping strokes to resect the tissue and fully expose the cavity to view and provide access (Case Fig. 6–1B). Tincture of myrrh and benzoin was applied, and the patient was referred back to his dentist, who proceeded to prepare and fill the cavity.

CASE 7

PATIENT. A 39-year-old white female.

HISTORY. During a regular periodic dental checkup her dentist found a slight edge of decay immediately beyond the finish line of a porcelain veneer crown, at the neck of a mandibular first bicuspid. He inserted an explorer tip and found that the decay extended downward a considerable distance. The caries obviously extended apically along the facial aspect of the root of the tooth but was completely covered by the gingival mucosa. The patient was referred for loop resection of the overlying tissue rather than dissection with a scalpel or packing with gutta percha to displace the tissue.

CLINICAL EXAMINATION. The gingival mucosa appeared normal and the teeth also appeared normal except for a slight margin of decay barely visible immediately beyond the gingival margin of the right cuspid (Case Fig. 7–1A).

TREATMENT. The tissue was anesthetized with infiltration anesthesia. A flame-shaped loop electrode was selected and cutting current set at 4.5 on the power output dial. The electrode was activated and used with a single wiping stroke to dissect the overlying tissue. This exposed the caries to view (Case Fig. 7–1B). The electrode was then used with short wiping strokes to recontour the marginal gingiva around the caries, to restore a normal feather-edge gingival architecture (Case Fig. 7–1C). Tincture of myrrh and benzoin was applied in air-dried layers, and the patient was instructed to return to her dentist for preparation and filling of the now accessible cavity.

CASE 8

This case offers an excellent example of the usefulness of electrosurgery in treating a vertically fractured tooth that is capable of being restored.

PATIENT. A 62-year-old white male.

HISTORY. The patient felt a sudden sharp pain and heard a crunching sound as his teeth came into forceful contact with a grain of sand while eating a salad. He tugged gently at the tooth to see whether it had loosened and he felt some movement. He immediately consulted his dentist who found a vertical fracture involving the mesial third of the crown of the tooth. The fracture extended well beyond the gingival level, and a periapical x-ray film confirmed that the fracture extended several millimeters beyond the cemento-enamel junction of the tooth. He was referred for electrosurgery to provide access to the fractured area, so that restoration of the tooth could be attempted.

CLINICAL EXAMINATION. The mesial third of the crown of the maxillary left second bicuspid was somewhat mobile, and a dark line, obviously the fracture line, was visible clinically (Case Fig. 8–1A). The fracture appeared to have split off the mesial bulge of the crown plus a small amount of the root on that side. Roentgenographic examination confirmed the dentist's verbal report that a partial vertical fracture of the tooth was visible on the x-ray.

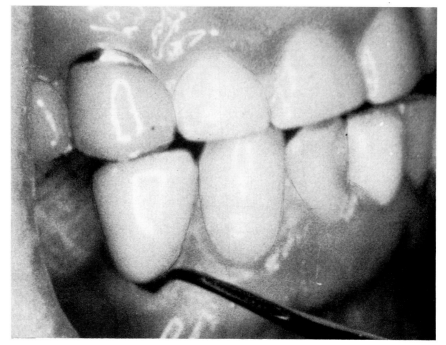

A

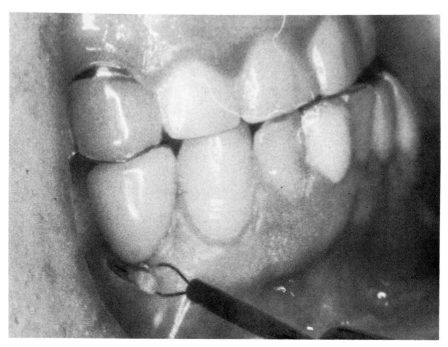

B

Case Figure 7–1.   *A,* Exposure of caries extending deeply along the root of a mandibular cuspid. There is a small narrow space between the edge of the marginal gingiva and the end of an acrylic veneer crown on the mandibular right cuspid. A periodontal pocket probe has been inserted and penetrates almost its full length before it reaches the bottom of the cavity on the facial aspect of the root. *B,* The tissue covering the cavity is resected with a flame-shaped loop electrode, with cutting current set at 4.5 on the instrument panel.

(*Illustration continued on opposite page.*)

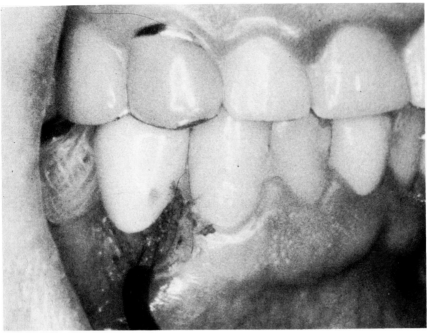

C

Case Figure 7–1 (Continued). C, The cavity has been fully exposed, and the marginal gingiva around the cavity has been beveled to restore a feather edge to the new marginal edge. A 45-degree angle U-shaped loop electrode is being used to scoop out friable tissue that has invaginated into the defect. A rubber dam clamp can now be attached to the root of the tooth immediately below the inferior edge of the cavity, if rubber dam isolation of the tooth should be necessary. There is no bleeding.

TREATMENT. The area was anesthetized with a posterior superior alveolar regional block and palatal infiltration anesthesia. The loose fractured part of the crown was removed by hand instrumentation, after freeing it from its epithelial attachment. A small amount of free bleeding ensued (Case Fig. 8–1B). A 17-mm. periodontal loop electrode was selected and cutting current set at 6 on the power output dial, the higher than normal setting being used in anticipation of loss of energy due to dissipation by contact with the engorged tissue. The tissue was sponged lightly to remove excessive moisture, and the activated electrode was used to resect the soft tissue that had been in contact with the mesial aspect of the tooth (Case Fig. 8–1C). The electrode was used effectively to remove the lacerated tissue at the end. A flame-shaped loop was substituted and used to recontour the gingiva of the fracture deep in the defect. A dressing of surgical cement was then packed into the defect to maintain the space created to provide access to the fracture site, and the patient was reappointed for the following week.

When he returned one week later the cement pack was removed, revealing healthy tissue rapidly repairing by granulation repair (Case Fig. 8–1D). He was deemed ready for restorative treatment and was referred back to his dentist, who successfully restored the tooth.

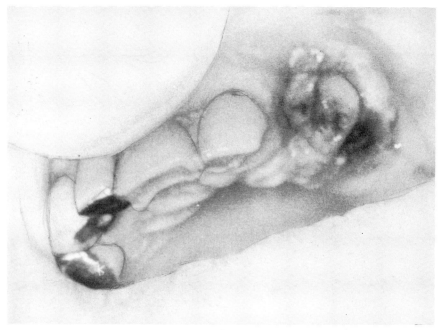

A

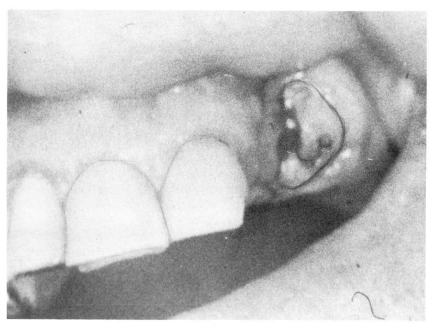

B

Case Figure 8–1. *A,* Restoration of a fractured maxillary first bicuspid crown, preoperative appearance. The mesial third of the crown has been traumatically fractured. The tooth, key terminal abutment for a long edentulous span, is vitally important if a partial restoration is to be used instead of a full denture that would become necessary if the tooth were to be lost. The tissue around the tooth has been traumatized. The tissue trauma is most notable at the distal of the tooth. *B,* The loose fractured portion of the tooth has been removed. The mesial gingiva now sags inward toward the fractured wall of the tooth.

(Illustration continued on opposite page.)

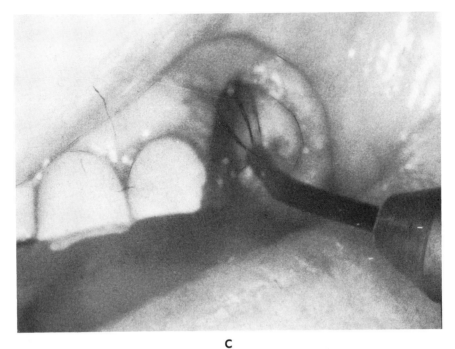

C

D

Case Figure 8–1 (Continued).   C, The portion of the mesial tissue that is now excess is being resected with a medium-width U-shaped loop electrode down to the bottom of the defect, to fully expose the fractured mesial wall of the tooth. Because of the oozing of blood from the traumatized tissue, cutting current had to be set at 6 on the power output rheostat on the instrument panel. *D,* Appearance of the tissues on the fifth postoperative day, after removal of the surgical cement pack that had been inserted to keep the tissue displaced and permit the cut tissue surfaces to granulate. There is no bleeding, and the tissue surface is covered with a translucent film of coagulum that cannot be seen in a black and white photograph. The fractured wall of the tooth is fully exposed and ready for insertion of Markley pins for an amalgam restoration, or for pins for a pin-inlay restoration, and functional use of the tooth as an abutment.

SUBGINGIVAL ELECTROSECTION FOR INLAY PREPARATION

Subgingival loop electrosection has become identified with the preparation of subgingival troughs around teeth being prepared for full crown restoration, since it is used very extensively for just that purpose.

However, this is not its sole area of usefulness. Subgingival electrosection of a tissue channel in the interproximal embrasures is equally useful in inlay preparation. The excision of a smooth trench between two teeth to expose the axial floors of proximal inlay preparations facilitates preparation and beveling of the axial floor of each preparation atraumatically without lacerating the papillary tissue, and therefore without the usual free bleeding that interferes with impression-taking.

Removal of the trench of tissue, in addition to facilitating cavity preparation and impression-taking, avoids impingement of the subgingival portion of the inlay into the embrasure tissue and assures that the excised tissue will regenerate without disruptive irritation.

One important precaution must be taken to ensure the best results. It is necessary to avoid creating abrupt sharp line angles of tissue at the buccal and lingual or palatal terminal ends of the excision. Should that happen, although the papillary tissue would ultimately regenerate, the tissue repair would be much slower than is desirable or attainable.

All that need be done to avoid abrupt sharp terminal ends of the trench is to round off and recontour the tissue in these areas after excising the channel. This can be accomplished very easily by using a flame-shaped or medium-width 45-degree angle U-shaped loop electrode to bevel the tissue inward toward the center of the embrasure. Planing the tissue by electrosection in this manner recontours the tissue so that the tissue regeneration that will occur after the inlay is inserted to restore the tooth will adapt itself very tightly against the highly polished gold, without cratering such as would occur if the sharp line angles at the terminal ends of the embrasure were not recontoured as described. Figure 12–1 demonstrates use of the U- and J-loops.

CASE 9

The next case is the first of a series of cases from the files of Dr. Peter K. Thomas of Beverly Hills, California. Dr. Thomas is world renowned for the excellence of his occlusal carvings. He is equally noted for his preference for use of partial coverage wherever it is practicable.

The first of his cases demonstrates his use of electrosurgery to resect the subgingival tissues, particularly from the embrasure areas between proximal inlay preparations, to facilitate perfect beveling of the axial floor and walls and to permit accurate impressions of the axial floors of the inlay preparations.

PATIENT. A middle-aged white male.

HISTORY. The patient had had many teeth filled with amalgam fillings. Some of the fillings had begun to deteriorate and he was referred to Dr. Thomas for replacement restorative dentistry.

CLINICAL EXAMINATION. All the posterior teeth in the maxilla had been restored with amalgam fillings. Some of the teeth showed evidence of secondary decay.

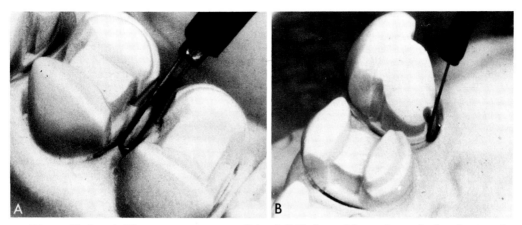

Figure 12–1. A, The proper position of the full U-shaped loop electrode for clearing the tissue in the embrasure that covers and obscures the access to the axial floor of the preparation and would interfere with margin beveling and flow of impression material for accurate impression of the axial floor of the preparations. B, Proper position of J-loop electrode for excising subgingival tissue. Note that the electrode is being held parallel to the long axis of the tooth. (Study models courtesy of Dr. P. K. Thomas.)

The marginal gingivae on the palatal aspect around some of the teeth appeared slightly irritated and engorged, and the apices of the interdental papillae of many of the posterior teeth appeared partially detached and engorged (Case Fig. 9–1).

TREATMENT. The old amalgam fillings were removed and the teeth were reprepared for inlay restorations. The tissues in the embrasures were resected with the narrow 45-degree angle U-shaped loop electrode and with J-loop to expose the axial floor of the preparations and their bevels. A hydrocolloid impression was taken and a working model was poured. The inlays were fabricated after they were waxed up and their occlusal carving performed on the articulated models. The restorations were cemented into their respective teeth (Case Fig. 9–1D). The tissues in the embrasures regenerated rapidly and adapted themselves tightly to the respective restorations.

When the tissues are excised partially to fully expose the axial finish lines, planing the buccal and palatal terminal ends of the tissue toward the center of the embrasures helps to accelerate the flow of the repair tissue into the embrasures. If the planing is not done, the tissue will regenerate anyway, but it will take a little longer to do so.

CASE 10

This is another case made available to the author by Dr. Peter K. Thomas of Beverly Hills, California. Unknown data have been reconstructed by the author from the Kodachrome slides supplied for this case.

This case demonstrates the ability to prepare the interproximal tissues between teeth being prepared for partial coverage with gold inlays and to assure perfect impressions of the axial floors of the cavity preparations in a manner similar to that for preparation of subgingival troughs around teeth being prepared for full crown coverage. It also demonstrates admirably the excellent speedy regeneration and readaptation of the interproximal tissues into the embrasures when the buccal and lingual (palatal) terminal ends of the excised embrasure tissue are bevelled toward the centers of the embrasures. This eliminates the elevated sharp line angles of tissue

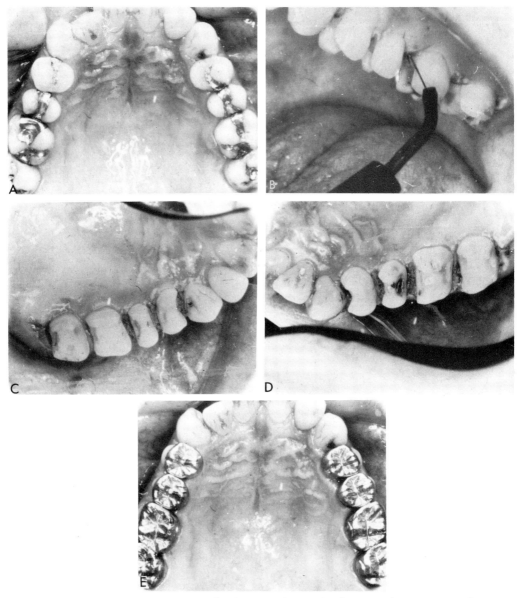

Case Figure 9–1. Preparation of subgingival troughs for partial coverage (J-loop). *A,* Preoperative appearance of the maxilla ventral view. All the bicuspids and molars have been restored with old amalgam fillings. There is also a lingual pit filling in the right lateral and a small distal filling in the left cuspid. *B,* All the old fillings have been removed and the cavities reprepared for inlay restoration. A J-loop electrode is being used to clear the tissue in the embrasures and fully expose the axial floor areas of the proximal inlay preparations. The tissue is being cleared away to form a partial subgingival trough, exposing the axial floor areas of the left first and second bicuspids. *C* and *D,* Appearance of the left and right quadrants as seen from the ventral view, after preparation of the partial subgingival troughs have been completed. *E,* Postoperative appearance of the tissues after insertion of the restorations into the two quadrants.

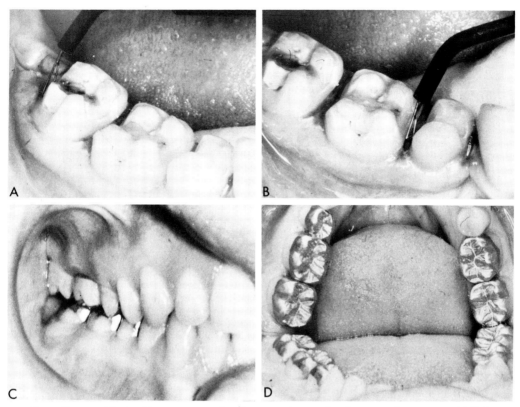

Case Figure 10–1. Preparation of subgingival troughs for partial coverage (full loop).
A, A narrow 45 degree angle U-shaped loop electrode is being used to clear the tissue at the
distal aspect of the mandibular right second molar to expose the axial floor of the preparation
for beveling. The height of the gingival tissue in the edentulous area at the distal of the tooth
has been reduced to eliminate the upward growth of the tissue that obscured the distal portion of the tooth and interfered with preparation of the tooth in that area. *B,* The same electrode
is being used to create the partial subgingival trough between the second bicuspid and first
molar. Note the concave contour of the marginal tissues directed inward toward the center
of the embrasure. This prevents formation of sharp line angles of tissue at the respective terminal ends of the excision. The concave contoured terminal ends such as we see here permit
rapid repair with the tissues flowing into the embrasures and adapting tightly around the inlays. When the terminal ends terminate in sharp line angles the regeneration of the interproximal papillae is much slower and the tissue adaptation may not be equally perfect.
C, Appearance of the tissues after the restorations have been inserted. Note the perfect adaptation of the papillae into the embrasures (lateral view). *D,* Appearance of the tissues as seen
from the ventral (mirror image) view. The tissues have regenerated and fill the embrasure
spaces, and are almost fully matured.

that would otherwise be created, which tend to retard the rate of healing into the
embrasures.

PATIENT.   A white female of unknown age.

HISTORY.   Several of her posterior teeth had defective old fillings that had to be
replaced with inlays.

CLINICAL EXAMINATION.   The mandibular right first and second molars and the
second bicuspid had been prepared for MOD inlay-onlay restoration. The interproximal tissue in the embrasures between the preparations extended upward above the
axial floors of the preparations, making it doubtful whether accurate impressions of

these areas could be obtained. The tissue immediately distal to the distal aspect of the second molar was hypertrophied and extended almost to the occlusal surface of the tooth.

TREATMENT.   The quadrant was anesthetized with an inferior alveolar-lingual regional block injection. A medium-size round loop electrode was selected and bent to a slight curve for better tissue contact. Cutting current was activated and the bulge of tissue distal to the second molar was reduced by loop planing. A narrow 45-degree angle U-shaped loop electrode was substituted, current output was reduced, and the tissue covering the distal axial floor of the second molar preparation was excised with the activated loop (Case Fig. 10–1A). The same electrode was then used to clear out the tissue in the mesial embrasure and the molar-bicuspid embrasure, care being taken to plane the terminal ends of the embrasure tissue toward the centers of the respective embrasures (Case Fig. 10–1B).

The excisions having been completed without tissue shredding or bleeding, accurate impressions were obtained. The subgingival interproximal areas were so sharply reproduced in the working cast that the margins and axial floors of the restorations were easily finished perfectly. The inlays were cemented in and the interproximal tissues regenerated rapidly and adapted themselves tightly into the embrasures and against the restorations (Case Fig. 10–1C and D), with no evidence of any impingements.

Excision of the interproximal tissue greatly facilitates taking accurate impressions of the subgingival portions of inlay preparations. If these tissues extend beyond the level of the axial floors of the preparations, excision of the tissue before preparing the axial floor and the margin bevel will enable the operator to complete the preparation atraumatically and bloodlessly, with a clear view and unimpeded access to the area. As a result, more perfect preparations as well as more accurate impressions are attained.

CASE 11

This case was made available to the author by Dr. Charles J. Miller of Pittsburgh, Pennsylvania.

Dr. Miller has used electrosection to resect enough of the papillary tissue in the interproximal embrasures to fully expose the beveled axial floors of proximal inlay preparations, without sacrificing all the papillary tissue and without the irritation resulting from the chemically impregnated cords he had formerly used to achieve this.

PATIENT.   An adult white female.

HISTORY.   Several of the teeth showed primary caries and secondary caries under old fillings. The affected teeth were to be restored with gold inlays.

CLINICAL EXAMINATION.   The posterior teeth in the mandibular right quadrant required treatment. The second molar had been prepared for an MO inlay restoration, the first molar and second bicuspid for MOD restorations, and the first bicuspid for a DO restoration.

TREATMENT.   A J-loop electrode was selected and cutting current output set at 3.5 on the power output dial on the instrument panel. The activated electrode was then used to resect just enough of the papillary tissues in the respective interproximal embrasures to expose the beveled margins extending beyond the axial floors of the preparations (Case Fig. 11–1A). Care was exercised to avoid removal of excessive amounts of the papillary tissues and to avoid creation of abrupt sharp line angles of

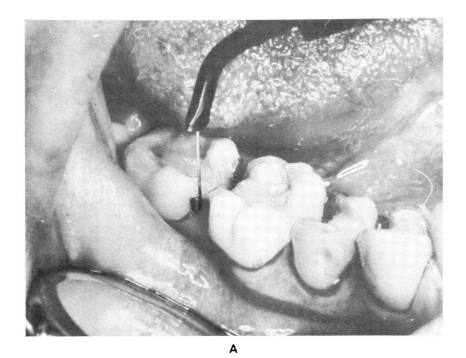

A

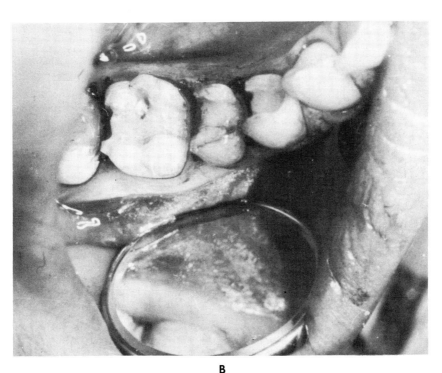

B

Case Figure 11–1. A, The J-loop electrode being used to excise the tissue in the embrasure between proximal inlay preparations to fully expose the axial floors of the preparations, so that proper bevels can be made, and so that impression material will be able to flow into the area and reproduce the preparations faithfully in the working model. *B*, The embrasure tissues have been scooped out sufficiently to adequately expose the axial floor areas of the preparations.

tissue at the buccal and lingual at the terminal ends of the resected tissue. This is easily accomplished by planing the tissues at the terminal ends slightly toward the centers of their embrasures.

The loop resection eliminated the resected tissues cleanly, without bleeding or fragmentation. Perfect impressions can therefore be obtained to provide accurate working models from which precise finish lines of the axial floors of the inlays can be achieved (Case Fig. 11–1B).

GINGIVECTOMY OF INTERDENTAL PAPILLAE TO FACILITATE CAVITY PREPARATION

When a patient presents rampant interproximal caries involving most of his dentition, and the caries extend to and often under the interdental papillae, it is not possible to prepare the cavities or fill and polish them without traumatizing the tissues and causing free bleeding that interferes with the operative procedures.

If the interdental papillae are resected with a steel scalpel, it is not possible to proceed with the operative dentistry until the tissues have healed. When healing occurs, the papillae do not regenerate fully into their embrasures, creating an unaesthetic appearance.

When this resection is performed by electrosection and the tissue tone is reasonably normal, the hemostasis obtained with fully rectified current makes it possible to proceed with definitive operative procedures immediately after the slight gingivectomy. Moreover, since the tissue tends to then regenerate toward its original level, the embrasures fill with normal papillae, and the mouth presents a pleasingly aesthetic appearance.

The following case demonstrates this admirably.

CASE 12

This is a case made available to the author by Dr. William J. Kelly, Jr., St. Louis, Missouri.

PATIENT. An adult white male.

HISTORY. This patient had neglected his dental health and rampant caries developed. A combination of pain and unfavorable aesthetics forced him to seek dental treatment.

CLINICAL EXAMINATION. Virtually every tooth in his mouth was decayed. Most of the teeth had interproximal caries, especially the anterior teeth, several of which had multiple caries, that extended to and beyond the level of the papillae (Case Fig. 12–1). The tissue tone appeared to be normal.

TREATMENT. In order to gain access to the cavities to prepare them, apply a rubber dam, fill them, and then polish the fillings, it would be necessary to cut away a sufficient amount of the interdental papillae. The tissues were anesthetized by infiltration. A fine 45-degree angle needle electrode was selected and current was set at 3 on

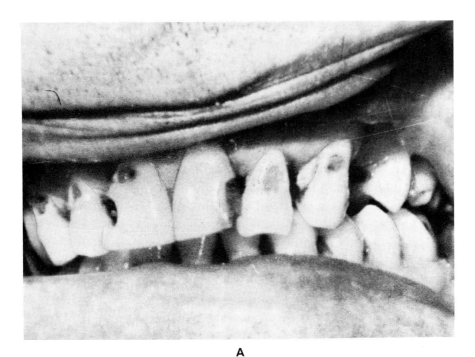

A

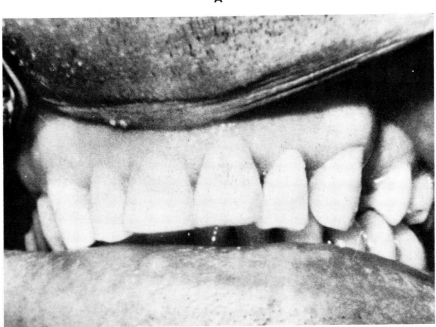

B

Case Figure 12-1. A, Preoperative appearance of rampant caries throughout the maxillary dentition. There are facial cavities on the labial aspect of the right and left laterals and cuspids and the right central incisor, and proximal cavities in each tooth, many extending subgingivally. B, Postoperative appearance of the dentition after amputation of the apical portions of the interdental papillae sufficient to fully expose the proximal caries. All the cavities have been filled with synthetic porcelain fillings. The aesthetics of the mouth as well as the function has been greatly improved. The amputation of the apices of the papillae having been performed with a needle electrode by electrosection, the tissue has completely regenerated to its original level in the respective embrasures.

the instrument panel. The activated electrode was used to resect the necessary amount of papillary tissue by electrosection. A flame-shaped loop electrode was substituted, current output was increased to 4.5 on the instrument panel, and the activated electrode was used with a brushing motion to plane the sharp cut edges to bevel them. Tincture of myrrh and benzoin was applied in air-dried layers.

Rubber dam was then applied to the teeth and the cavities were prepared, filled, and polished, without contact with the gingivae. When the operative procedure was completed the patient was instructed to return for further polishing. Healing and regeneration of virtually the entire missing portions of the papillae proceeded uneventfully, and approximately 2 months postoperatively the tissues appeared fully healed and normal in tone and aesthetics.

CASE 13

This is one of the cases made available to the author by Dr. John E. Flocken of Los Angeles, California. Case details that were not provided to the author have been reconstructed in part from the Kodachrome slides of the case.

Despite the apparent similarity, treatment in this case was not for the purpose of facilitating impression taking as described in the preceding cases. Instead it demonstrates the marked clinical advantage to be derived from being able to eliminate without hemorrhage the proliferative tissue that flows over the axial floors and bevelled margins of inlay preparations and prevents insertion and cementation of the restorations.

PATIENT.   Details unknown.

HISTORY.   The mandibular left second bicuspid and first molar had been prepared for MOD inlay restorations at the previous visit. Impressions had been taken, temporary fillings had been inserted into the preparations, and the patient had been reappointed for insertion of the restorations. Shortly after insertion, the temporary fillings had fallen out.

CLINICAL EXAMINATION.   Proliferations of gingival tissue had flowed over the axial floors of the cavity preparations, preventing the seating and cementation of the inlays. The proliferation was particularly extensive in the second bicuspid-first molar embrasure, and this tissue was engorged and friable (Case Fig. 13–1A).

TREATMENT.   Infiltration anesthesia was administered. A 45-degree angle narrow U-shaped loop electrode was selected and activated with the cutting current. The activated electrode was applied to the redundant tissue with a scooping motion to resect and fully expose the axial floors and bevelled margins of the preparations. The hemostasis provided by the fully rectified current was sufficient to accomplish the resection without bleeding, tissue charring, or coagulation, even in the second bicuspid-first molar embrasure (Case Fig. 13–1B). The toilet of the cavity preparations and cementation of the inlays were therefore able to be performed immediately after removal of the redundant tissue.

ELONGATING THE CLINICAL CROWN

Some procedural similarity and a degree of technique and instrumentation overlapping from one discipline to another is inevitable. Such overlap-

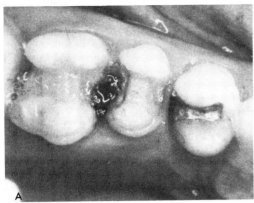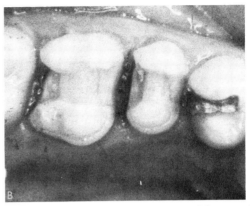

Case Figure 13–1. A, Preoperation appearance. The mandibular right second bicuspid and first molar have been prepared for MOD inlay restorations. The gingival tissues in the first and second bicuspid and first and second molar embrasures have proliferated upward and cover the axial floors and their bevelled margins. The redundant tissues in these embrasures appear relatively normal in color and texture. In the second bicuspid-first molar embrasure, however, the gingival proliferation is so extensive that a polypoid mass of severely engorged friable tissue bulges upward, covering the axial floors of the preparations and almost one third of the mesial wall of the molar. This tissue bleeds freely when it is touched. B, Postoperative appearance. The redundant tissue has been cleared out of the respective embrasures, and the axial floors of the preparations and their bevelled margins are fully exposed. Although there is no evidence of coagulation or tissue charring, there is no bleeding from the cut gingival surfaces, and the teeth are ready for cavity sterilization and cementation of the inlays.

ping is especially likely to be anticipated in operative dentistry and crown and bridge. The basic overlapping between the subgingival resections that have just been reviewed and the preparation of subgingival troughs for full crown restorations are paralleled by overlapping in the elongation of the clinical crowns of teeth in the respective disciplines.

The end result of the elongations is basically the same for both. The rationales for the treatment are multiple, however, and vary from discipline to discipline. For example, in operative dentistry the clinical crowns of teeth usually are elongated to improve aesthetics, to eliminate painful tissue trauma due to incomplete eruption of permanent teeth, or to facilitate application of the rubber dam. While any or all of these may also apply to elongation in crown and bridge, by far the most important reason for the elongation in that discipline is dictated by need either to restore or to create the all-important 1:2 crown-root ratio that will enable the restoration to withstand the torque of function.

The instrumentation methodology usually varies less than the rationales of treatment, but here too important differences are often encountered. Elongation of the clinical crowns of teeth can be accomplished either by gingivectomy, substituting the fine needle electrode and cutting by electrosection for the manual steel scalpel incision, or by the technique of gingivectoplasty that has been developed by the author for simultaneous resection of the tissue for the elongation by loop planing, and simultaneously recontouring the newly cut marginal gingivae to normal feather-edged gingival architecture.

Both methods will be utilized in the next series of cases. However, the specifics of the techniques of instrumentation will be reviewed in detail in Chapter 14.

CASE 14

This case typifies the cosmetic importance of elongating clinical crowns even when only a single tooth is involved.

PATIENT. A 34-year-old white female.

HISTORY. The patient had accidentally fractured all incisal angle from her maxillary right central incisor, causing noticeable shortening of the crown of this tooth. Although the degree of cosmetic disharmony was relatively slight, the patient became extremely self-conscious and was highly distressed by it. She consulted her dentist about restoring the tooth with a porcelain crown.

The dentist found that the fracture was not the sole cause of the poor cosmetics. The tooth was tilted and the gingival margins over the left central and lateral incisors dipped downward beyond the gingival margins of their respective adjacent teeth. He pointed out to the patient that unless the gingival harmony was improved, even a porcelain crown would not completely solve the cosmetic disharmony. The patient was referred for electrosurgical elongation of the left central and lateral incisor crowns.

CLINICAL EXAMINATION. *Extraoral.* Negative.

Intraoral. The maxillary right central incisor was tilted about 10 degrees from the normal vertical plane in a postero-anterior direction. A triangular segment of the mesioincisal angle of the tooth, approximately 2 mm. in height and extending to the center of its incisal edge, was missing. The gingival margins of the left central and lateral incisors dipped down approximately 2 mm. lower than those of their adjoining teeth. The malposition and gingival disharmony exaggerated the cosmetic defect created by the fracture. The combined effect made the tooth with the fractured crown appear conspicuously shorter than the other teeth.

The disharmony was further heightened by poor gingival tissue tone in the area. The gingival tone was normal on the left side and over the right central incisor. Here the tissue was pink, the surface stippled in appearance, and the interproximal papillae firmly attached and normal in contour. The gingivae on the right side, from the lateral incisor posteriorly, appeared hyperemic and the interproximal papillae were hypertrophied, engorged, and detached slightly at the tips (Case Fig. 14–1A). The papilla in the lateral-cuspid embrasure was more engorged and hypertrophied than the others; the mucosa around the lateral incisor appeared more edematous and was shiny and smooth. The localized gingivitis appeared to be the result of a localized malocclusion created by a deviation in the alignment of the mandibular teeth, with the left lateral incisor elevated above the mandibular occlusal plane and the tooth tilted lingually.

TREATMENT. The mouth was prepared for surgery in the usual manner and local infiltration anesthesia administered. The coronal elongations were performed by electrosection. A 45-degree-angle narrow U-shaped loop electrode was selected and current output set at 4.5 for cutting. The electrode was held with the loop pointing downward so that it could be applied to the gingival mucosa of the central incisor at an approximate right angle to the tooth. The electrode was used with short brushing strokes until 2 mm. of the excess marginal gingiva was removed (Case Fig. 14–1B). The lateral incisor was treated in the same manner. After the gingival mucosa of the teeth was reduced the necessary 2 mm., the electrode was replaced with a flame-shaped loop electrode. This was used with a scooping motion directed from above

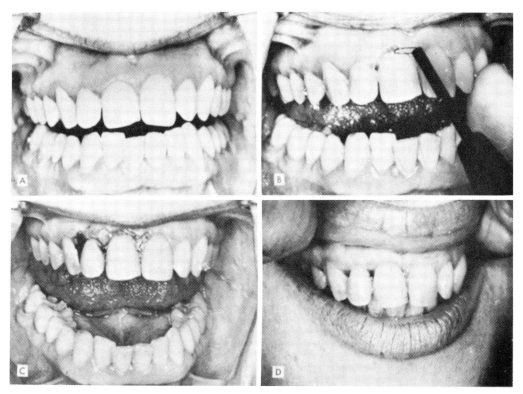

Case Figure 14-1. Cosmetic improvement resulting from elongation of the crowns of two adjacent teeth. *A*, Preoperative view. The gingival margin of the right central incisor is approximately 2 to 3 mm. lower than the left central, and the right lateral is also correspondingly lower than the left lateral. Loss of almost 3 mm. of the mesio-incisal angle of the right central, and a slight angulation increased the disparity in size between the two centrals. *B*, Marginal gingiva resected with short brushing strokes until the gingival margins of the two centrals were at uniform levels.

C, Appearance of the teeth after both the central and the lateral incisors on the right side were elongated to the exact level of the left central and lateral. *D*, Appearance of tissues approximately three weeks postoperatively. Crowns appear uniform and gingivae appear normal except the apices of the central-lateral and lateral-cuspid papillae, which had also been engorged and hypertrophied prior to the surgery.

downward in order to reduce the convexity of the hypertrophic papillae sufficiently to create slightly concave sluiceways.

The entire procedure was performed bloodlessly except at the distoproximal embrasure of the lateral incisor (Case Fig. 14–1C) where a slight amount of superficial oozing of blood was readily halted by pressure with a sterile gauze sponge. Chromic acid, .001 per cent dilution, was applied topically to the oozing surface. The mildly styptic action of the greatly diluted chemical produced very superficial coagulation, but it was sufficient to seal the tissue surface effectively. After 30 seconds the area was cleansed with water and the tissue gently dried. Tincture of myrrh and benzoin was applied to the operative field and the tissues were dried with an air syringe. The tincture of myrrh and benzoin was reapplied several times in this fashion to provide a thick layer of medication over the area. The surgery having been completed, the incisal edges of the two teeth were ground and beveled until incisal harmony was achieved.

The patient was instructed to stay on a soft diet and use a saline lavage. She returned on the fifth postoperative day. The gingival mucosa was healing very satisfactorily, although the distoproximal papilla of the lateral incisor appeared to be healing somewhat slower than the rest of the tissues. The operative field was irrigated with warm Kasdenol solution. Light spot coagulation was then applied to the retarded papilla with a small ball electrode. The electrode was used with current set at 0.5, and was brought into repeated momentary contacts with the tissue surface until the desired amount of coagulation was achieved. No anesthesia was required for this procedure. Tincture of myrrh and benzoin was then applied to the area. She was instructed to remain on a soft diet for two weeks and to return for observation at the end of that period.

Upon her return, examination revealed excellent gingival healing of the cut surfaces and normal labial feather-edged margins. The interproximal papillae had healed but still presented a slight amount of hypertrophy at their extreme tips, particularly the troublesome one in the lateral-cuspid embrasure (Case Fig. 14–1D). The patient was very pleased with the cosmetic results. She was warned, however, of the likelihood that unless the traumatic occlusion were balanced, gingivosis would probably recur in these tissues and again cause hypertrophic deterioration of the marginal and cemental gingivae. Spot coagulation was again applied superficially to the apices of the papillae and tincture of myrrh and benzoin was applied.

Use of a rubber stimulator tip was recommended and she was asked to return again in two weeks. She did not return as requested. Instead, she phoned to say that she did not think it necessary to return, since the tissues had healed fully and the long trip to the office was an inconvenience. Inasmuch as nothing further has been heard from this patient, it is reasonable to assume that the condition of her mouth has remained satisfactory.

CASE 15

This case is an example of the severe aesthetic and social handicaps imposed by abnormally short clinical crowns created by hyperostosis and fibromatosis. It demonstrates the service that can be rendered by elongation of the clinical crowns of teeth in order to create a normal oral appearance.

PATIENT. A 23-year-old white female.

HISTORY. With her mouth closed the patient was a very pretty young woman. When she smiled, however, she exposed a vast expanse of gingival mucosa and prominent alveolar ridge with a disproportionately small amount of visible tooth structure, which gave her a grotesque appearance (Case Fig. 15–4A). This handicap was grave enough to mar her social life and lower her earning capacity because of difficulty in obtaining desirable employment and because of a sense of inferiority stemming from the unflattering appearance of her mouth. She was referred for electrosurgical elongation of her maxillary teeth from second bicuspid to second bicuspid.

CLINICAL EXAMINATION. *Extraoral.* Negative.

Intraoral. The maxillary right lateral incisor was congenitally missing. The crowns of all her teeth appeared abnormally short. The anterior portion of the maxilla sloped downward and outward at about a 30 degree angle from the vertical. The buccal aspect of the maxillary bone was hyperostosed, producing a bulging of the bone which created a rounded overhang from the distal aspects of the cuspids in a posterior direction bilaterally. The left second bicuspid had been restored with an artificial crown.

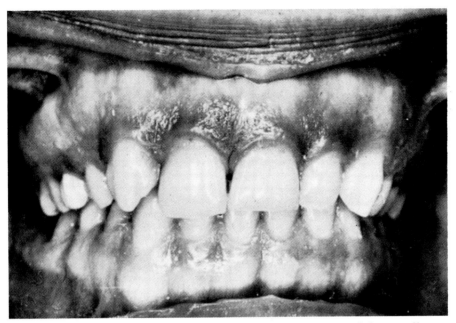

Case Figure 15–1. Marked cuticle-like deep free margins around the maxillary anterior teeth. Note maxillary anodontia; the right lateral incisor is missing and the cuspid occupies its place in the dental arch.

A moderate degree of fibromatosis was superimposed over the hyperostosis. The marginal gingivae around the labial aspects of the teeth were elongated, creating a cuticle-like appearance extending 3 to 4 mm. beyond their gingival crevices (Case Fig. 15–1). The abnormal length of the marginal gingivae and abnormal depth of the gingival crevices were verified by the insertion of a flexible silver probe under the free gingival margin. The probe penetrated upward from 3 to 4 mm. before it encountered resistance from the bases of the crevices.

The tissue tone of the entire gingival mucosa appeared subnormal, and the tissues appeared hyperemic. The patient reported that she frequently found blood on her pillow on arising, and that she could induce bleeding at will by creating a sucking motion with her lips and tongue.

Roentgenographic examination revealed that the teeth were normal in size and in crown-root proportion.

TREATMENT. Consultation with the patient's physician confirmed that she was in normal health. In view of the mild gingivosis, ascorbic acid, 250 mg., twice a day for four days, was prescribed. Knox clear gelatin, twice a day, was prescribed as premedication, and use of a salt-alum astringent mouthwash was recommended.

When she returned for her next visit the mouth was prepared for surgery and bilateral infraorbital block and nasopalatine block anesthesia was administered. This was supplemented with bilateral infiltration in the first molar areas.

A medium-sized 45-degree-angle U-shaped loop electrode was selected, cutting current set at 5, and the labial excess marginal gingivae reduced by looping with short brushing strokes of the electrode, starting with the shorter left central incisor (Case Fig. 15–2A). The labial excess was removed in a similar manner from bicuspid to bicuspid. Then the convexity of the interproximal papillae was reduced by using the same

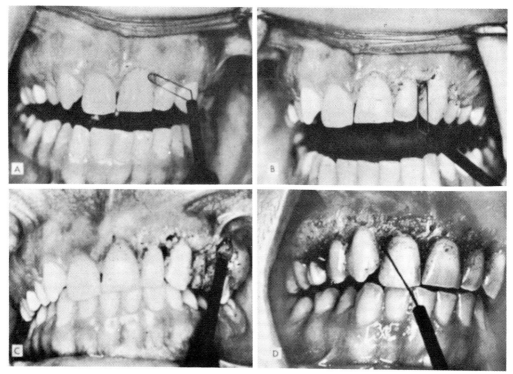

Case Figure 15-2. Electrosurgical procedure. *A*, Gingival margin of the shorter left central raised by looping the cuticle-like tissue away with wiping strokes of a 45-degree angle medium-sized U-shaped loop electrode. Gingival margin raised approximately 5 mm. *B*, Convexity of interproximal papilla between lateral and cuspid reduced by downward stroke of the electrode. *C*, Buccal bulge of tissue reduced with flame-shaped loop electrode. *D*, A spurting bleeder fulgurated. (Fulgurating effect is more superficial than coagulation if the electrode is kept moving. When bleeding is persistent and requires a considerable amount of electrocoagulation, and especially if the bleeder is close to the alveolar bone, fulguration may be safer to use.)

electrode with lightly scooping motions from above downward (Case Fig. 15-2*B*). The papillae were reduced in this manner without encountering bleeding until a spurter was encountered in the right central cuspid embrasure. The bleeder was quickly brought under control by fulguration (Case Fig. 15-2*D*).

The gingival margins having been heightened approximately 4 to 6 mm. from cuspid to cuspid, and approximately 3 mm. in the bicuspid regions, some of the marginal alveolar bone around the bicuspids was exposed and denuded of tissue. The denuded bone was removed from the necks of the teeth by curettage with McCall periodontal curets and flat periodontal files. The greatest convexity of the exposed buccal bone was reduced with a bone file; then the new gingival margins were beveled to a feather edge with the loop electrode.

A flame-shaped electrode was substituted, current output increased to 6, and the buccal alveolar mucosa reduced down to the bulging underlying bone by shaving in layers with wiping strokes of the electrode (Case Fig. 15-2*C*). After the labial-buccal coronal elongation was completed, the excess marginal gingivae were removed from the palatal aspect in the same manner. Since aesthetics was not involved here, only approximately 2 to 3 mm. of excess extending beyond the gingival crevices was removed, without exposing any of the palatal bone.

When the electrosurgical procedure was completed, the tissues were dried with sponges and tincture of myrrh and benzoin was applied in air-dried layers. A surgical cement pack medicated with sulfathiazole crystals and benzocaine powder was applied to the operative field. (Under ordinary circumstances cement packs are unnecessary after simple coronal elongation of normal mucosa, but in this instance, due to the extensiveness of the surgery, the gingivosis and bone reduction, it appeared advisable to provide protection and obtundant medication to the denuded buccal alveolar surfaces and to encourage granulation over the denuded areas. The patient was instructed in proper postoperative care, and reappointed.

She returned on the fifth postoperative day and reported considerable discomfort despite use of the cement pack. The cement was removed and the mouth thoroughly irrigated with Kasdenol used at mouth temperature. The marginal gingivae appeared to be healing very well, but the denuded bone areas were not completely covered with granulation tissue. The mucosa was covered with a thin layer of coagulum, and several patches of blood clot were still present (Case Fig. 15–3A). These tissues were sponged dry and tincture of myrrh and benzoin applied to them in air-dried layers. The cement packs were replaced with a coating of adhesive Kenalog (experimental) ointment; Cosa-Tetrastatin, four times a day, was prescribed for prophylactic antibiotic therapy and Darvo-Tran for relief of pain and for tranquility. She was seen three times a week for the next two weeks, during which time the marginal gingivae ap-

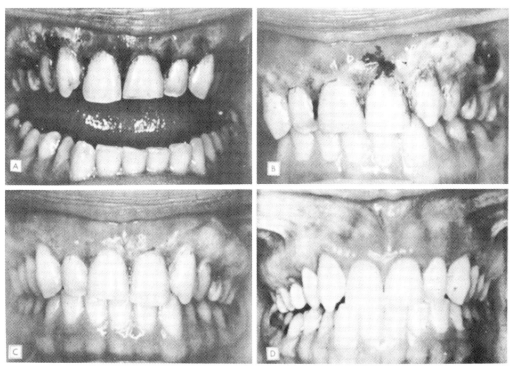

Case Figure 15–3. Postoperative results. *A*, Appearance of tissues on fifth postoperative day. Anterior healing is progressing well. Posterior denuded bone surfaces not yet covered with granulation tissue. *B*, Small sequestra of disk-like flat flakes of cortical bone removed from thinned posterior alveolar cortex and granulating tissue. *C*, Healing progressing well; tissues almost completely normal. *D*, Tissues fully healed as seen three months postoperatively. Gingival margin from left lateral to right cuspid had regenerated 1 mm.

peared to be healing very well; however, the denuded buccal alveolar bone was granulating with hypertrophic, hyperemic, friable tissue which bled freely at the slightest provocation. One week later several small sequestra of flat, disk-like cortical bone appeared and were easily removed from their granulating bed (Case Fig. 15–3B). Within one week the sequestration stopped. Healing proceeded rapidly thereafter without further incident, and the tissues began to appear quite normal again (Case Fig. 15–3C).

The patient continued to return twice a week for one month for postoperative observation and care, then she was reappointed to return in six weeks. When she returned, the gingival mucosa was completely normal, but from left lateral to right cuspid the gingival free margins had regenerated sufficiently to extend downward 1 mm. (Case Fig. 15–3D). The tissue tone was greatly improved, and the patient had a normal smile and appearance (Case Fig. 15–4B).

Perhaps the most important result of improvement was a new sense of self-confidence which helped her to improve her social and economic status immeasurably, and may have been largely responsible for her marriage less than six months after her mouth was fully healed.

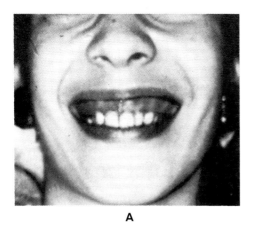

A

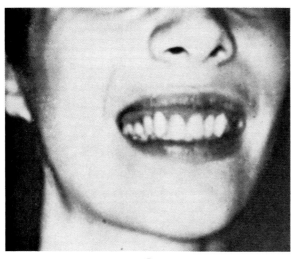

B

Case Figure 15–4. A, Photograph of young woman with an abnormally long, prominent maxillary alveolar ridge and abnormally short teeth creating a grotesque smile. Cosmetic rehabilitation of the mouth by elongating the clinical crowns of abnormally short teeth resulted in the excellent aesthetic appearance shown in B. B, Final healing shows the patient with a charming smile; the teeth are harmonious and gingival tone is excellent.

The fact that sequestration was encountered in this case may give rise to speculation and snap judgments as to the cause. Perhaps it is a natural reaction to blame the electrosurgery. A review of the facts in the case tends to belie this conclusion, however.

The bilateral sequestra were small, isolated, extremely thin bone fragments. They constituted very small portions of the total areas of denuded bone. Had the sequestration been caused by osteitis resulting from electrode contact with the buccal alveolar bone during the electrosurgical procedure, the entire denuded areas would have been equally affected and have become exfoliated.

It appears far more likely that sequestration occurred as a result of excessive thinning of the high spots in the convex portions of the buccal alveolar bone with the bone file. If such excessively thinned out spots did not receive an adequate blood supply to maintain normal metabolic function, the individual islands of thin bone would, as a result, necrose and exfoliate precisely as occurred in this case.

TOOTH BLEACHING BY ELECTROCOAGULATION

When for one reason or another a tooth suffers pulp hemorrhage, blood flows into the dentinal tubules by capillary attraction. As the blood trapped in the tubules decomposes, its hemoglobin deteriorates into methemoglobin. Methemoglobin contains ferric iron, a chocolate brown-colored compound. This dark brown compound present in the dentinal tubules produces bluish to greenish brown coronal discoloration (see Color Plate II, Fig. 2A).

When methemoglobin is exposed to oxidation by nascent oxygen it is reduced to oxyhemoglobin, a colorless compound, thereby bleaching out the discoloration. When aesthetic considerations dictate a need to restore a discolored tooth to normal or near-normal color, a pellet of cotton is moistened with superoxol or a comparably potent oxidizing agent and is introduced into the pulp chamber. Heat is then applied to the oxidizing agent to release the nascent oxygen to combine with the methemoglobin and reduce it.

The traditional technique for applying heat to the oxidizing agent has been to heat a ball burnisher in a Bunsen flame to cherry-red glowing heat and apply the heated instrument to the moistened cotton pellet in the pulp chamber (see Color Plate II, Fig. 2B). Immediately upon contact of the hot instrument with the wet cotton there is a sizzling sound, indicating a sudden sharp rise in tooth temperature, and a release of nascent oxygen. The moisture quickly quenches the heat, however, and the release of nascent oxygen is therefore brief in duration and intermittent. As a result, this method frequently results in postoperative reactions ranging from a mild pericementitis to acute periostitis. Even acute osteitis may result from the sharp increases in heat radiating outward from the pulp chamber into the root canal

PLATE II

A. Operative Dentistry

Figure 1a. A very large bucco-occlusal cavity that extends subgingivally is completely occluded by a proliferative mass of engorged, friable tissue. The marginal gingiva is massively swollen and severely engorged along the edge of the cavity. This is the tissue that has proliferated into the caries.

Figure 1b. The entire friable mass is being engaged with a round loop electrode so that it can be resected with a single scooping, lifting motion of the activated electrode. Note that the loop has been squeezed into a slightly elliptical shape to permit it to engage the entire mass without binding against the walls of the cavity, to assure freedom of movement of the activated electrode.

Figure 1c. Appearance of the gingiva and the tooth immediately after the polypoid mass has been resected. Note the absence of hemorrhagic free bleeding despite the severe engorgement of the tissue. Subgingival caries can be exposed for immediate definitive treatment with equal facility.

Figure 2a. Bleaching discolored teeth by electrocoagulation. Appearance of the discolored tooth immediately before bleaching is instituted.

Figure 2b. A large round ball electrode activated by electrocoagulating current is being applied to a pellet of cotton saturated with Superoxol in the pulp chamber of the tooth to release nascent oxygen needed to bleach the discoloration.

Figure 2c. Appearance of the tooth after bleaching by electrocoagulation has been completed.

B. Endodontics

Figure 3a. A vertico-oblique incision is being made down to bone for reflection of a mucoperiosteal flap to gain access for performing a root-end resection. The incision is being made by electrosection with a fine 45-degree-angle needle electrode. Note that the incision is being made lateral to the interdental papilla, to avoid splitting the apex of the papilla through which a suture will be inserted labio-palatally to secure the flap into position postoperatively. Note the absence of free bleeding or tissue coagulation.

Figure 3b. Appearance of the tissues on the fifth postoperative day, before the sutures have been removed. Note the evidence of beginning of primary healing, and the excellent tissue tone.

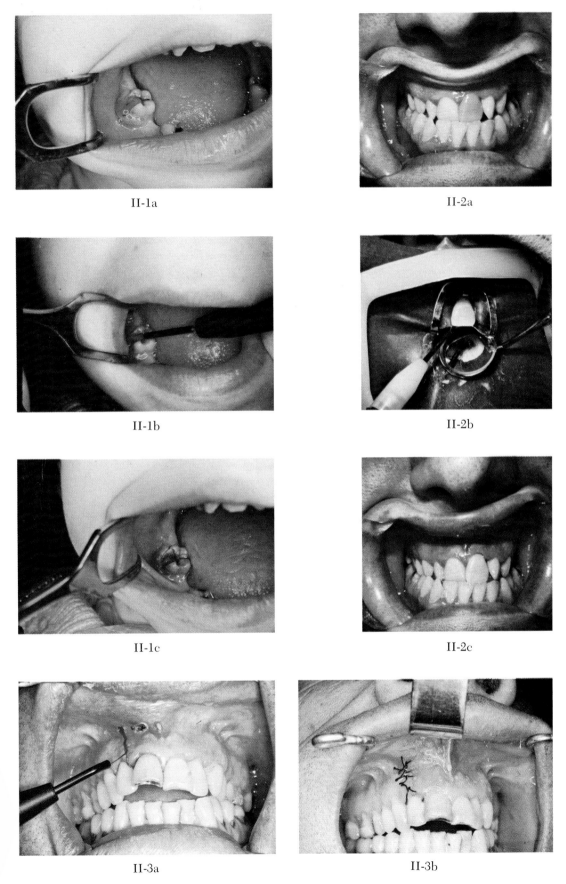

II-1a

II-2a

II-1b

II-2b

II-1c

II-2c

II-3a

II-3b

303

and affecting the investing alveolar structures. Moreover, owing to the brief intervals of intermittent nascent oxygen release, this is inherently a slow and often ineffectual method of oxidizing methemoglobin and often fails to adequately bleach all the discoloration from the teeth.

When a ball electrode activated by electrocoagulation is applied to the moist cotton pellet, the output of heat energy is constant and can be regulated by the operator to assure that the intensity of heat will not be greater than is needed to produce immediate superficial spot coagulation of mucosa. Potential unfavorable postoperative sequelae due to sudden sharp increases of heat in the tooth are thereby eliminated.

Electrocoagulating heat energy continues uniformly and uninterruptedly as long as the activated electrode is kept in contact with the cotton pellet. A steady release of nascent oxygen and more efficient bleaching results therefrom. In order to compensate for the loss of heat energy due to the moisture to which the coagulating energy is being applied, it is necessary to increase the amount of energy utilized; the setting of the power rheostat should therefore be increased to approximately twice the power output normally needed to produce superficial spot coagulation on the surface of mucosa.

When electrocoagulation is applied to the surface of mucosa the tissue does not provide any insulation against penetration of the heat energy, and the application must therefore be only momentary in duration. The thickness and density of the dentin and cementum of the tooth root serve to insulate to a noteworthy degree against penetration of the heat to the investing structures, if cumulative heat effect is to be avoided. The activated electrode may be kept in contact for a full second instead of merely momentarily, such as when contacting tissue. The total number of applications is unimportant; the applications may be repeated safely until complete bleaching has been achieved, *providing that the 10-second interval between applications is scrupulously observed to prevent a cumulative heat effect.*

When the electrocoagulating technique of tooth bleaching is employed as described, it is much quicker and more efficient than the red-hot ball burnisher, and the bleaching effect is more uniform and effective (see Color Plate II, Fig. 2C).

CASE 16

This case, made available by Dr. William F. Trice of Erie, Pennsylvania, provides an excellent demonstration of the author's tooth bleaching technique. Unknown details have been reconstructed by the author from the Kodachrome slides of the case.

PATIENT. Details unknown.

HISTORY. Root canal therapy had been performed on an anterior maxillary tooth several months previously. The tooth began to turn dark soon thereafter and appeared to become progressively more discolored.

CLINICAL EXAMINATION. The crown of the maxillary left central incisor was greenish brown in color, in contrast to the other teeth in the mouth (Color Plate II, Fig. 2). The opening into the pulp chamber on the palatal aspect of the tooth through which the endodontic procedure had been performed was sealed with a synthetic porcelain filling.

TREATMENT. The filling and all the gutta percha down to the root canal opening was removed from the pulp chamber with a large round bur. The tooth was isolated by applying a rubber dam, and a pellet of cotton moistened with Superoxol was inserted into the pulp chamber.

A large round ball coagulating electrode was selected and activated with coagulating current, and the activated electrode was applied to the cotton pellet for 2 seconds. The electrode was removed for 5 seconds, then reapplied for 2 seconds. This was repeated three times. A freshly moistened new cotton pellet was inserted and treatment resumed three more times, after which a fresh Superoxol moistened cotton pellet was applied. The 2-second active coagulation applications provided a steady release of nascent oxygen, and the 5-second pause intervals between applications of the activated electrode prevented a cumulative heat build-up. Changing the cotton frequently assured an adequate source of nascent oxygen needed to bleach the discoloration. After 30 applications of the coagulating current the tooth appeared almost completely normal in color. The cotton pellet was discarded, the pulp chamber was thoroughly dried, and the cavity was filled with a zinc oxide cement.

PULP CAPPING

When caries invades the pulp chamber of a tooth and the pulp tissue becomes contaminated, the prognosis for successful pulp capping is very poor, and endodontic therapy usually is required to preserve the tooth.

When the pulp becomes traumatically exposed and treatment is instituted without undue delay, the prognosis for successful pulp capping is reasonably good. When electrosurgery is utilized in the pulp capping procedure, the prognosis for a successful outcome is greatly enhanced.

If there has been an appreciable time lapse between the exposure and treatment, the prognosis for successful pulp capping is greatly diminished, owing to the sterilizing effect of the cutting current. If adequate parenteral antibiotic therapy has been instituted immediately after the exposure, use of electrosurgery for the pulp capping increases the potential for a successful outcome, despite the adverse time factor.

There are three categories of traumatic pulp exposure. Each category requires use of a different electrosurgical current and a different technique for employing the respective current that is required. (See Figure 12–2.)

1. ACCIDENTAL FRACTURE OF PART OF THE CROWN OF THE TOOTH, WITH A HORN OF THE PULP EXPOSED AND PROTRUDING FROM THE PULP CHAMBER

This type of exposure responds most favorably to electrosection of the exposed protruding portion of the pulp with a loop electrode. Owing to the extreme vascularity of the pulp tissue, it is necessary to use a high output of cutting current to assure efficient disintegration and volatilization of the pulp tissue cells, despite the dissipation of heat energy caused by the excessive

LOOP CUTTING   FULGURATION   ELECTROCOAGULATION

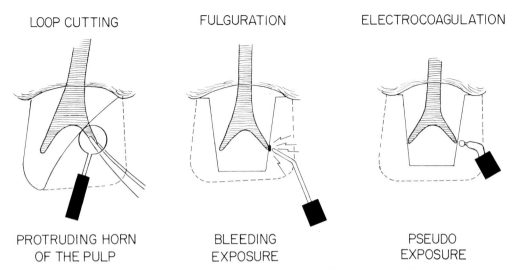

PROTRUDING HORN   BLEEDING   PSEUDO
OF THE PULP   EXPOSURE   EXPOSURE

Figure 12-2.   Treatment by electrosurgical means of traumatic pulp exposure.

moisture present in this tissue. Should an inadequate amount of cutting current be employed, it will be too weak to disintegrate and volatilize the cells but strong enough to cook and coagulate them, and thereby will seriously jeopardize the success of treatment.

The small to medium size round or wide U-shaped loops, depending on the size of the exposed pulp tissue, are the electrodes of choice. The electrode is activated and applied to the exposed pulp tissue with a wiping stroke to shear the protruding pulp tissue away from the tooth structure. The protruding tissue is resected cleanly, rapidly, atraumatically, and bloodlessly. If the proper amount of cutting current has been employed, the pulp tissue still in the pulp chamber remains completely unaffected by the cutting energy and is totally free of coagulation or charring.

The exposed pulp tissue having been resected, a calcium hydroxide dressing is applied over the exposure site and the crown of the tooth is covered with a celluloid or plastic crown form. As the pulp tissue repairs, it recedes, laying down a layer of secondary dentin which effectively seals and protects the exposure site.

2. MECHANICAL EXPOSURE OF THE PULP DURING PREPARATION OF A TOOTH FOR FULL OR PARTIAL RESTORATION, WITH BLOOD OOZING FROM THE EXPOSURE SITE

If electrocoagulation were employed, the presence of blood would cause much of the coagulating energy to be dissipated by the moisture. It would therefore be necessary to use a substantially higher amount of coagulating energy to compensate for the loss, and it would be necessary to keep the electrode in contact with the tooth at the bleeding point for an appreciable amount of time to coagulate and seal off the bleeding. This would result in an unpredictable and uncontrollable amount of heat concentration at the exposure site that would most likely be highly destructive to the pulp tissue. Thus, clinical judgment dictates that fulguration, because of its physical characteristics and method of application, would be the most advantageous current to use for treatment of this type of exposure. Since fulguration consists of using the sparks from the true Oudin spark-gap current or the simulated spark-gap current of the Coles Cavitron equipment to produce superficial dehydration by jumping the air-space between the tip of the electrode and the tissue surface until charring occurs, the need for physical contact between the electrode and the surface to be treated is eliminated. Inasmuch as the electrode is kept moving constantly in a rotary manner while the sparking is performed, there is no need to apply the electrode and there is far less danger of producing heat concentration, particularly in view of the fact that the air-space and the carbon that forms on the surface both act as effective insulators against heat penetration.

As the sparks are sprayed over the bleeding area, the blood is congealed and the surface becomes carbonized, thereby effectively sealing the bleeding point. After the carbonized blood crust has stopped the bleeding, a dressing of calcium hydroxide and protective crown form are applied in the manner described for the previous category; as the pulp repairs, it recedes and lays down secondary dentin that protects the exposure site.

3. Mechanical exposure, or pseudo-exposure, of the pulp during preparation of the tooth for restoration, with a pink spot visible but no bleeding from the exposure site

In this type of exposure, since there is no blood present to dissipate the potency of the coagulating energy, it is possible to employ superficial spot coagulation to the site with a small ball electrode just as effectively as when it is applied to the surface layers of soft tissue for superficial spot coagulation. Each application of the coagulating energy is merely a momentary contact. It is essential that each application be followed by a 10-second interval to permit the heat to dissipate and prevent damage from cumulative heat concentration. As a rule, only two or three applications will be required, but the applications may be repeated as often as is deemed clinically necessary. The amount of coagulating current output is the same as for soft tissue spot coagulation.

If the 10-second rest intervals are observed when more than one application is necessary, there is no danger of destructive heat penetration to jeopardize the viability of the pulp tissue. After the coagulating current application, a calcium hydroxide dressing is applied and the tooth crown protected with a celluloid or plastic crown form as in the previous cases.

All three methods of treatment have one common denominator: there has been no crushing of pulp tissue cells or comparable tissue insult, and because of the sterilizing effect of the three types of electrosurgical current on bacteria that may be present at the exposure site, the prognosis for successful treatment is enhanced. The absence of heat penetration eliminates the hazard of pulpal inflammation and premature aging due to fibrosis or necrosis of the pulp.

The outstandingly advantageous feature of the electrosurgical methods of pulp capping that have been described is that it eliminates need to sacrifice all the pulp tissue from the pulp chamber as is necessary when other methods of treatment are utilized.

FOOTNOTE REFERENCES

1. Noyes, F. B., and Thomas, N. G.: A Textbook of Dental Histology and Embryology. Philadelphia, Lea & Febiger, 1921, p. 144.
2. Bodecker, C. F.: Distribution of living matter in human dentine, cement and enamel. Read before American Dental Association, Niagara Falls, N.Y., Aug., 1898.
3. Bodecker, C. F.: The soft fiber of Tomes, a tubular structure: its relation to dental caries and the desensitization of dentin. J. Nat. D. Assn., 9:281, 1922.
4. Orban, B. J.: The development of the dentin. J.A.D.A., 16:1547, 1929.
5. Orban, B. J.: Oral Histology and Embryology. 4th ed. St. Louis, C. V. Mosby Co., 1957, pp. 108–134.
6. Bevelander, G.: The development and structure of the fiber system of dentin. Anat. Rec., 81:79, 1941.
7. Sicher, H.: The biology of dentin. Bur, 46:121, 1946.
8. Bodecker, C. F.: Diffusional channels in the teeth and their relation to the Hartman desensitizing fluid. New York D. Soc. Tr., 109–122, 1936.
9. Bevelander, G., and Amler, M. H.: Radioactive phosphate absorption by dentin and enamel. J. D. Res., 24:45, 1944.
10. Bodecker, C. F., and Lefkowitz, W.: Concerning the "vitality" of calcified dental tissues. J. D. Res., 16:463, 1937.
11. Fish, E. W.: The circulation of lymph in dentin and enamel. J.A.D.A., 14:1, 1927.
12. Scott, D. B., and Wycoff, R. W. G.: Elctron microscopy of human dentin. J. D. Res., 29:556, 1950.
13. Scott, D. B.: Recent contributions in dental histology by use of the electron microscope. Internat. D. J., 4:64, 1953.
14. Scott, D. B.: The electron microscopy of enamel and dentin. J. New York Acad. Sc., 60:575, 1955.
15. Shroff, F. R., Williamson, K. I., and Berteaud, W. F.: Electron microscope studies of dentin. Oral Surg., Oral Med., and Oral Path., 7:662, 1954.
16. Shroff, F. R.: Further electron microscope studies on dentin: The nature of the odontoblastic process. Oral Surg., Oral Med., & Oral Path., 9:432, 1956.
17. Zander, H. A., and Burrill, D.: Penetration of silver nitrate solution into dentin. J. D. Res., 22:85, 1943.
18. Englander, H. R., James, V. E., and Massler, M.: Histologic effects of silver nitrate on human dentin and pulp. J.A.D.A., 57:5, 621–630, Nov., 1958.
19. Ogus, W. I.: The use of the desiccating current in treating buccal gingival caries. D. Digest, 52:268, 1946.
20. Saghirian, L. M.: Surgical diathermy in office practice. J.A.D.A., 51:573, 1955.
21. Strock, M. S.: The rationale for electrosurgery. Oral Surg., Oral Med. & Oral Path., 11:1166–1172, Nov., 1952.

Chapter Thirteen

USES IN PEDODONTICS – TREATMENT OF DECIDUOUS TEETH AND AIDS TO ERUPTION OF PERMANENT DENTITION

The treatment techniques employed in pedodontics are, for the most part, patterned after and sometimes even overlap those that are used for adult dentistry. The pedodontist is, however, often compelled to vary his techniques from those used in treatment of fully developed teeth because of the special problems created by the prominent horns of the pulps and wide open blunderbuss apical foramina usually present in deciduous teeth and incompletely developed permanent teeth.

Although by far the greatest usefulness of electrosurgery is in the treatment of the oral soft tissues, it also offers the pedodontist many significant advantages that can improve and facilitate his treatment of the teeth typically encountered in the mixed dentition. For that reason, although the treatment procedures may in some instances differ only slightly from those used in adult dentistry that have been or will be reviewed in other parts of this text, some of the procedures that are most uniquely useful are being presented here as a separate special chapter devoted to pedodontics.

FULGURATION TO VISUALIZE AND TREAT PINPOINT EXPOSURES

One of the areas where electrosurgery can be uniquely useful is in the discovery and treatment of pinpoint exposures in deciduous teeth. Although technically this does not differ from treatment of pinpoint exposures in adults that were described in the preceding chapter, it does present a unique problem that requires a major variation in treatment.

When a deciduous tooth has a large deep cavity, the advantage of retaining the tooth as a space maintainer until eruption of the permanent tooth is likely to result in an attempt to treat and fill the tooth rather than extract it. After thorough excavation of the carious material, if there is no clinical evidence of a pulp exposure, the cavity is sterilized and filled with copper cement or with a cement base and copper or silver amalgam.

Despite the absence of clinical evidence of a pulp exposure, in many instances the pulp subsequently dies and putrefies, and an abscess forms, necessitating extraction of the tooth after all. Obviously when this happens, there must have been a minute pinpoint exposure that could not be seen with the naked eye.

Dr. Robert Morrow, a pedodontist of Spokane, Washington, has devised a simple method to make such pinpoint exposures clinically visible and at the same time to sterilize them to reduce the likelihood of subsequent death of the pulp.[1] His technique consists of drying the cavity after completing the excavation and then spraying the cavity surface with sparks from the fulgurating current. When a pinpoint exposure not visible to the naked eye is present, a tiny black spot forms at the exposure site, thereby visualizing and locating it (Fig. 13–1). At the same time, the fulguration also sterilizes the pulp tissue at the exposure site as well as the rest of the cavity.

The cavity is then carefully dried, calcium hydroxide is placed over the exposure site, and the cavity is filled with copper cement or an antibiotic cement. Dr. Morrow reports that a gratifyingly high percentage of cases treated in this manner have remained asymptomatic and the teeth have been successfully retained until replaced by the permanent teeth.

This procedure can also be used advantageously to treat exposures in permanent teeth with incompletely calcified roots and "blunderbuss" open apical foramina that are so very difficult to treat successfully with root canal therapy.

This technique and the three electrosurgical techniques for conservative management of pulp exposures without need for extirpation of all the tissue in the pulp chamber that were described on page 306 are ideally suited for use by the pedodontist for preservation of doubtful deciduous dentition as effective space maintainers.

SURGICAL ASSISTANCE IN DELAYED ERUPTION OF PERMANENT DENTITION

Electrosurgery is especially valuable for surgical assistance in cases of painful delayed eruption of permanent teeth that are in relatively normal alignment but are unable to cut through their overlying gingivae unassisted.

---

[1]Personal communication to the author.

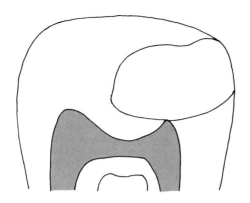

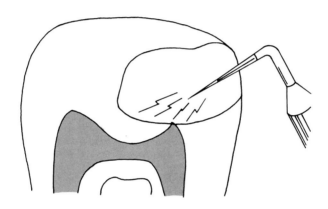

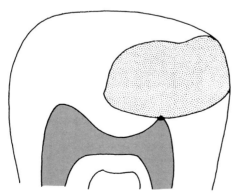

Figure 13–1. Fulguration to disclose and sterilize pinpoint exposure in deciduous tooth. (See text for explanation.)

This condition is apt to occur when the deciduous tooth has been lost some time before the permanent tooth is ready to erupt. It is a very simple matter to render the surgical assistance by resecting a little of the covering tissue to create an unimpeded avenue for the eruption. The assistance can be rendered by manual excision with a steel scalpel of the tissue covering the incisal third of the crown of the tooth, or by electrosection with a needle or loop electrode (see Case 2, Chapter 16).

The tooth will erupt postoperatively in either event without difficulty. The electrosurgical excision offers two distinct advantages to the pedodontist. The child patient can readily identify the steel scalpel and become very apprehensive about what is about to be done to him. The tiny needle or loop electrode is much less likely to register its purpose and as a result the child is more apt to remain calm and amenable to treatment with the electrode. In many instances the very intelligent and inquisitive child will ask about the electrode and, if it is explained to him properly, it is likely to arouse his curiosity to the degree that he becomes intrigued about it rather than alarmed. The second advantage inheres in the hemostasis provided by the electrosection, which results in elimination of the shock reaction of the child when he expectorates blood, such as occurs after resection of the tissue with the steel scalpel. The following cases demonstrate the simplicity of the procedure and its advantages admirably.

When an erupting permanent first molar is still partially covered with tissue on the occlusal surface that is traumatized by the opposing tooth, surgical intervention to eliminate the redundant tissue and fully expose the crown of the tooth is the quickest and most effective means of eliminating the pain caused by the trauma. The following case demonstrates a typical condition and its effective correction.

SURGICAL EXPOSURE IN DELAYED ERUPTIONS

CASE 1

This case typifies the simplest surgical aid to orthodontics: exposing the crowns of teeth in cases of delayed eruption of the normal permanent dentition.

HISTORY.   The patient was a 9-year-old white boy. He was referred for exposure of the crown of his permanent right central incisor which had failed to erupt.

CLINICAL EXAMINATION. *Extraoral.*   Negative.

Intraoral.   The left central and the two lateral incisors were fully erupted and in normal alignment in the dental arch. The right central incisor was not visible. The space where this tooth should have been seen was filled with an expanse of gingival mucosa which bulged outward somewhat.

Roentgenographic examination revealed that the unerupted tooth was in relatively normal alignment, tilted approximately 15 degrees from the vertical.

TREATMENT.   The mouth was prepared for surgery and infiltration anesthesia was administered. A flame-shaped loop electrode was selected and current intensity was set at 6 for electrosection. The electrode was applied to the overlying gingival

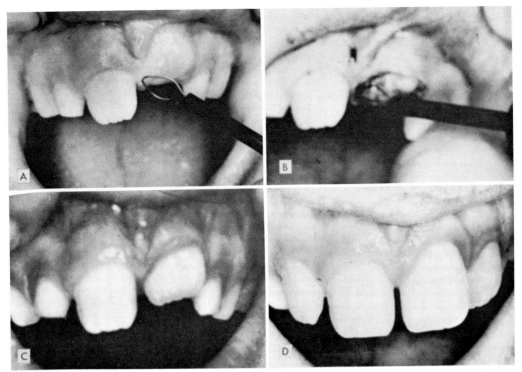

Case Figure 1–1. Exposing unerupted permanent central incisor. *A,* Loop in position at 45 degree angle to the tissues. *B,* Incisal third of the unerupted tooth crown exposed with loop. *C,* Postoperative appearance in two weeks. Tooth half erupted. *D,* Postoperative appearance three months later. Tooth fully erupted and in good alignment.

mucosa at a 45 degree angle starting at the mesio-incisal angle of the unerupted crown (Case Fig. 1–1A). The overlying mucosa was resected to the level of the gingival margin of the fully erupted left central incisor, thereby exposing the incisal third of the unerupted tooth (Case Fig. 1–1B).

The entire procedure was bloodless. Postoperative dressing, therefore, was limited to topical application of air-dried layers of tincture of myrrh and benzoin. Postoperative instructions for home care were given and the patient was reappointed.

He returned two weeks later. The gingival mucosa appeared fully healed and the tooth had erupted about halfway down to the incisal level of the adjacent central incisor (Case Fig. 1–1C). The vertical alignment of the tooth was fairly good but it was rotated mesially. The patient was advised to press his tongue against his "new" tooth to help straighten it, and was told to return in three months for further postoperative observation.

He returned as requested. The tooth was now in normal alignment and fully erupted (Case Fig. 1–1D). The gingival margin around the crown of the tooth was completely normal in all respects and gave no indication that it had recently undergone surgery.

Orthodontic correction is usually a complex and difficult process even under optimal conditions. Unfavorable local factors that will hinder treatment must therefore be eradicated wherever possible before treatment is instituted.

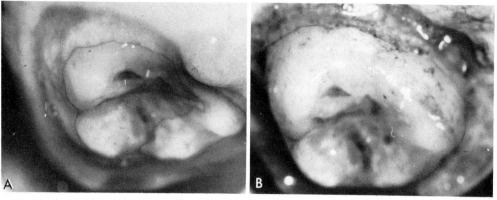

Case Figure 2–1. A, Exposure of a partially erupted molar. The maxillary right molar is partially erupted, with only the distal portion of the cusps of the tooth exposed clinically. The rest of the tooth is covered with gingival tissue; the redundant tissue along the mesial aspect and on the palatal aspect two thirds posteriorly extends over the occlusal surface of the tooth. The palato-occlusal tissue shows traumatized indentations where the cusps of the mandibular opposing tooth made contact with it. B, The tissue all around the crown of the tooth has been resected by loop electrosection. The tissue planing has created a reasonably normal marginal edge around the exposed crown.

CASE 2

This case is from the personal patient files of Dr. Charles Miller.

PATIENT. A 6-year-old child.

HISTORY. The maxillary left first molar began to erupt and shortly thereafter the child began to suffer pain when eating and even with the mouth closed. Dr. Miller, the family's dentist, was consulted and instituted the necessary treatment.

CLINICAL EXAMINATION. The maxillary left first molar was partially erupted; the distal two thirds of the crown of the tooth was clinically exposed, but the mesial third of the crown including the occlusal surface was still covered with gingival tissue. The tissue extended on the palatal aspect of the occlusal surface to the center of the tooth, and this tissue was pitted by indentations created by the traumatic contact of the mandibular tooth during function (Case Fig. 2–1).

TREATMENT. The tissue was anesthetized by infiltration anesthesia, and the redundant tissue was resected by loop planing the tissue with a flame-shaped loop electrode by electrosection. The tissue planing created an approximate 45-degree angle which produced a normal feather-edged gingival margin and fully exposed the crown of the tooth rapidly and efficiently.

EXPOSURE OF PARTIALLY ERUPTED TEETH BY GINGIVECTOPLASTY

The pedodontic patient is likely to have a mixed dentition or a number of permanent teeth that are incompletely erupted. When the partially erupted tooth is malposed and covered with hyperplastic proliferative gingival mucosa, in addition to exposing the tooth, it is also necessary to recontour the gingival tissue to restore or create a normal gingival architecture around the tooth. Loop electrosection makes possible the gingivectoplasty or simultaneous resection of the covering tissue and recontouring to create a desirable architecture. The following case offers an excellent example of the usefulness of electrosurgery in this type of case.

CASE 3

PATIENT. A 10-year-old white male.

HISTORY. The patient had an incomplete cleft of the hard palate, and although there was no clinical opening in the palate, the tissue of the hard palate was subnormal in tone. Many of the teeth were missing from the maxilla and others were only partially erupted or malposed. His maxillary left lateral was malposed and incompletely erupted and was causing him some distress. His pedodontist was consulted and he was referred for surgical exposure of the tooth.

CLINICAL EXAMINATION. The two maxillary central incisors were rotated palatally in the midline, with the distal ends of the teeth rotated labially at an approximate 45-degree angle. The left lateral was covered on the labial aspect with a thick layer of hyperplastic proliferative tissue. The tissue was detached from the tooth at one point, creating a pocket-like opening. The palatal mucosa of the hard palate was dark red in color and had a granular surface texture. This tissue was atonal and extended anteriorly almost to the marginal gingivae of the central incisors. The cuspid teeth were missing from the dental arch.

TREATMENT. The tissues were prepared and anesthetized by infiltration anesthesia. A flame-shaped loop electrode was selected and cutting current output was set at 5.5 on the power output rheostat. The activated loop was used to resect the tissue covering the facial aspect of the tooth crown and simultaneously bevel the tissue to create a feather-edged gingival margin (Case Fig. 3–1). The loop planing was carried

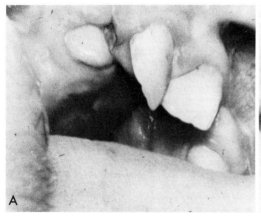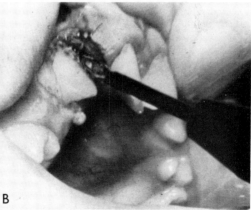

Case Figure 3–1. *A,* Exposure of malposed cuspid. Preoperative appearance. The patient has a bilateral cleft in the anterior part of the palate extending through the edentulous areas where the lateral incisors should be, creating a floating premaxilla. The two centrals are rotated with the distal aspect of the teeth pointing labially, creating a V formation. The cuspid is tilted slightly medially, and only the incisal third of the crown is exposed. The gingival tissue around this tooth is thick, edematous, engorged, and at the mesial aspect, where the cleft extends, a friable mass of proliferative tissue is present. *B,* The tissue is being resected by electrosection with a flame-shaped loop electrode, and as the tissue is being reduced, it is also being beveled and recontoured to create a normal feather-edged margin. Even the friable tissue in the line of cleft is being reduced and recontoured. There is no bleeding even from the friable engorged tissue, nor is there coagulation of the tissues that have been cut.

around to the palatal aspect to expose the crown fully without creating any undercuts that could act as food traps around the tooth. The J-loop electrode was then used with current output reduced to 3.5 to create a sulcus space around the tooth from which the epithelial lining had been removed. Tincture of myrrh and benzoin was applied to the tissues in air-dried layers, and the patient was instructed in postoperative home care. Healing progressed without incidence, and the recontoured tissue remained normal, with no recurrence of proliferation.

FRENECTOMY–FRENOTOMY TO AID ERUPTION OF MAXILLARY PERMANENT CENTRALS

By far the most frequent reason for performing a maxillary frenectomy is to eliminate the diastema created by physical separation of the two central incisors by the ligamental fibers.

The pedodontist occasionally encounters other reasons, unique to his discipline, for performing the frenectomy. One of the reasons is to facilitate normal eruption of permanent maxillary central incisors whose eruption is being impeded by the presence of an abnormally large broad frenum that partially covers the unerupted teeth.

The details of the surgical procedure for the author's technique for combined frenectomy of the attached alveolar fibers and frenotomy of the areolar fibers and the rationale for the technique will be discussed in detail in the part of the text covering routine oral surgery. The following case is being presented to best visualize this type of impediment unique to pedodontics. The surgical procedure will be described very briefly, since it will be reviewed in detail elsewhere.

CASE 4

PATIENT. A 6½-year-old white male.

HISTORY. His mandibular permanent centrals had erupted several months previously, but the maxillary centrals gave no evidence of doing so. The pedodontist was consulted. X-rays revealed that this was not a case of anodontia of the permanent teeth. Both permanent teeth were present and in normal alignment immediately above the deciduous centrals whose roots were almost fully resorbed. The pedodontist decided the eruption of the two centrals was being impeded by a broad large frenum. The patient was referred to the author for frenectomy.

CLINICAL EXAMINATION. The four first molars and the mandibular central incisors were the only permanent teeth in the dental arches. A diastema of approximately 7 mm. separated the two maxillary deciduous centrals, and there was a very large broad labial frenum that extended through the center of the diastema to the palatal aspect, terminating at the anterior border of the nasopalatine papilla. The deciduous centrals were surprisingly firm despite the extensive resorption of their roots (Case Fig. 4–1).

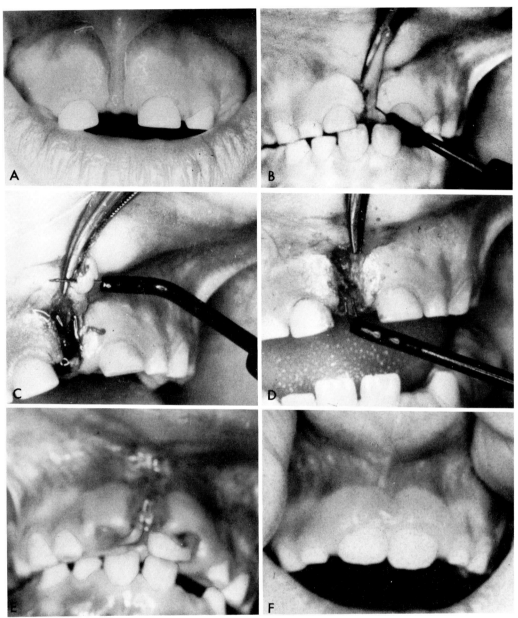

Case Figure 4-1. *A*, Preoperative appearance. Maxillary dentition (except first molars) is still deciduous. There is a 1.5 cm. space between the two central incisors, and an abnormally large, long labial frenum extends between them and terminates at the anterior border of the nasopalatine papilla. The frenal fibers spread laterally about 3 mm. on each side along the crest of the edentulous space. *B*, The frenum has been clamped with a curved mosquito hemostat and the initial incision for the V–Y excision of the attached alveolar part of the frenum is being performed with a fine 45-degree-angle needle electrode by electrosection. *C*, The areolar part of the frenum is being resected from the beak of the hemostat for the frenotomy. *D*, Invaginating frenal fibers are being destroyed by running the activated electrode very rapidly along the median suture line of the maxilla. *E*, Postoperative appearance on the fifth day. The deciduous teeth had been extracted after the completion of the frenectomy-frenotomy, and the permanent centrals can be seen beginning to emerge into their normal position in the dental arch. *F*, Postoperative appearance one month later. The two permanent centrals are fully erupted in the dental arch, but approximately one half of their clinical crowns are still covered with gingival mucosa. The frenal fibers that control the lip movements are present and functioning in the areolar mucosa, down to the mucogingival junction. The alveolar frenectomy site is fully healed with no fibrous scar tissue.

TREATMENT. The tissues were prepared and subperiosteal infiltration anesthesia was administered on the labial aspect, and a nasopalatine block on the palate. The upper lip was extended upward and outward and the frenum was clamped with a curved mosquito hemostat. The alveolar portion of the frenum was incised with a V–Y incision following the outline of the fibers and the freed incised fibers were resected from the beaks of the hemostat. The areolar portion was then also resected, the invaginating fibers were destroyed, and the deciduous teeth were extracted. When the blood in the tooth sockets was clotted, tincture of myrrh and benzoin was applied. When it was dry, flexible collodion was applied to the area.

When the patient returned on the fifth postoperative day the incisal third of the left permanent central was clearly visible, and some of the incisal of the right central could also be seen, although both teeth were almost completely covered with labial gingival mucosa. Three weeks later the teeth had erupted to their normal level, and only the upper half of the tooth crowns was covered with gingival mucosa. The frenal fibers of the areolar mucosa were fully healed and functioning to control lip movements, and the tissue in the alveolar area from which the frenal fibers had been resected was completely healed.

FRENECTOMY–FRENOTOMY FOR FUNCTION AND AESTHETICS

There is one other area in which electrosurgery can be invaluable to the pedodontist. He bears the responsibility of eliminating any developmental factors that could cause distortion of the facial bones and create facial disharmony. Torque from an abnormal maxillary labial frenum can produce distortion of the anterior maxilla and create permanent facial disharmony. The ability to eliminate such frena without massive contractile scar tissue interfering with eruption of the permanent maxillary central incisors and without sacrificing control of lip movement can be achieved by an electrosurgical technique of combined frenectomy-frenotomy developed by the author. This technique will be reviewed in detail in the chapter on minor oral surgery. The effectiveness of this procedure to prevent permanent facial disfigurement is well demonstrated in the following case.

CASE 5

PATIENT. A 1½-year-old white male.

HISTORY. The child's pediatrician had become convinced that the traction of the child's maxillary labial frenum was creating torque great enough to distort his anterior maxilla, causing a bulging effect in the anterior part of his face that was disfiguring and would cause permanent disfigurement if permitted to continue. The child was referred to the author for surgical elimination of the frenum.

CLINICAL EXAMINATION

Extraoral. The upper lip bulged outward in the midline owing to a convex contour of the anterior maxilla, creating the appearance of a swollen upper lip and nose.

Intraoral. The maxilla appeared somewhat elongated in the anterior central segment. An abnormally large, broad labial frenum was present; it extended between the deciduous central incisors, creating a wide diastema between the two teeth, and extended to the anterior border of the nasopalatine papilla into which it merged (Case Fig. 5–1). His other oral structures appeared normal.

TREATMENT. A ¾ gr. capsule of Seconal was perforated at both ends and administered rectally one-half hour before surgery. The labial and palatal mucosa around the frenum was anesthetized by local infiltration. The upper lip was extended upward and outward to pull the frenal fibers taut and was then clamped with a curved mosquito hemostat as closely as possible to the ventral surface of the lip. A fine 45-degree-angle needle electrode was selected, cutting current was set at 3, and the activated needle was used to incise the V portion of the excision of the attached alveolar portion of the frenum by following the outline of the frenal fibers down to and through the diastema, and dissecting them from the nasopalatine papilla at their juncture with the latter.

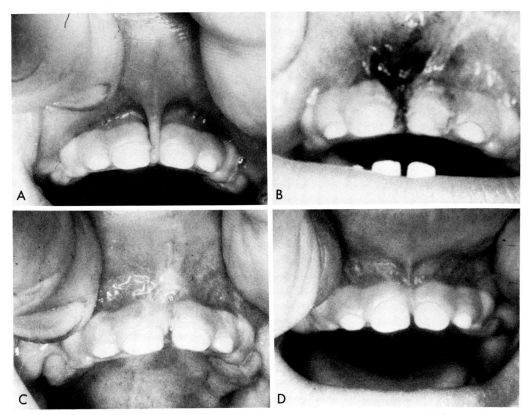

Case Figure 5–1. Combined frenectomy–frenotomy procedure in pedodontics. *A,* An enormously enlarged maxillary labial frenum extends between the maxillary central incisors and terminates at the anterior border of the nasopalatine papilla. *B* The frenectomy has been performed, and the fibers invaginating into the median suture line have been destroyed. Blood has been permitted to fill the surgical field, but there is no free bleeding. *C,* The healing on the tenth postoperative day. The site of the alveolar "ectomy" is covered with a thin layer of coagulum. The site of the "otomy" portion of the procedure, preserving the frenal fibers that control the movement of the lip, is clearly demarcated. *D,* Postoperative appearance three months later. The "ectomized" alveolar portion has healed without any trace of scar tissue. The "otomized" frenal fibers are controlling the movement of the lip but are no longer exerting the abnormal traction that was causing facial disfigurement.

The incised tissue was elevated with a periosteal elevator, and the excised frenal tissue was resected from the mosquito hemostat from the surface of the instrument external to the ventral surface of the lip. The surgical field was sponged to remove a slight amount of blood produced by the tissue manipulation, and the needle electrode was used with a very rapid stroke down the median suture line to destroy frenal fibers that invaginated the suture line. The momentary contact of the activated electrode with the bone was followed by a 10-second rest interval before the scoring effect of the suture line was repeated, five times in all. Bleeding was encouraged in the area and clotting was permitted. The tissue that had been clamped with the hemostat was crushed and sealed tightly by the resection from the hemostat with the cutting current, so that the tissue had not flared wide open, and therefore no sutures were required. When the clotting was completed, tincture of myrrh and benzoin was applied in air-dried layers and the patient was dismissed and reappointed.

Healing proceeded without incidence and without scar tissue adhesions. The tissue in the midline where the frenum had been excised, seen three months postoperatively, was smooth and normal in texture and tone, without any trace of the scar tissue that characterizes repair of frenectomies performed with steel scalpel excisions. The frenal fibers in the areolar tissue had not been sacrificed and remained intact to control the movements of the lip.

The child's reaction to the premedication deserves comment. The child, apparently instinctively aware that something unusual was about to happen, determinedly fought off the effects of the hypnotic and remained hypermobile during the surgery. But as soon as his mother got out of the dental chair and began to walk toward the exit door, his head slumped and he fell soundly asleep for 6 hours.

One other unusual fact is worthy of comment. Due to the very young age of the patient, his mother sat in the chair and held him on her lap during the procedure. The author has had an indifferent seat electrode of his own design built into the upholstering foam rubber of the dental chair. The seat electrode is covered with Naughehyde, the external chair upholstering material, which is a rubber product. Both the child and his mother were fully clothed. Nevertheless, enough energy was conducted into the child through his mother's body that the surgery was performed with the same output of current as is required when the patient alone is in contact with the seat electrode. This suggests that there should be no need for the patient to wear a metal bracelet type of electrode for direct skin contact or for the operator to do so and bring his hand into contact with the patient's face in order to perform effective biterminal electrosection.

Chapter Fourteen

ENDODONTIC USES OF ELECTROSURGERY

Electrosurgery renders invaluable aid in endodontia in three principal areas:

1. To facilitate effective rubber dam isolation of teeth requiring treatment.

2. To dry and sterilize contaminated root canals, including chronically suppurating canals to permit one-visit definitive treatment.

3. For root-end resection.

RUBBER DAM ISOLATION

When decay, coronal fracture, or tapered shape of the tooth crown makes it virtually impossible to apply a rubber dam clamp effectively to the tooth, rubber dam isolation cannot be utilized. There are some instances in which use of rubber dam isolation for endodontia is not essential, as when the patient does not salivate freely and therefore cotton rolls or gauze sponges can satisfactorily isolate the tooth and keep the canal free of saliva. In most instances, however, rubber dam isolation is to be greatly preferred. Electrosurgery by loop resection greatly simplifies and facilitates clearing away of sufficient gingival tissue from the root surface to permit unimpeded application of the rubber dam clamp that must hold the dam in position securely, even when caries extends far beyond the gingival level, when there has been a partial or total fracture of the crown extending subgingivally, or when the marginal gingiva around the tooth is markedly hyperplastic or hypertrophic.

The following case reports demonstrate admirably the facility with which the gingival tissues can be resected by electrosection and a normal gingival architecture simultaneously restored to the affected tissues as an adequate amount of tissue is removed to permit a clamp to be securely applied.

CASE 1

PATIENT. A middle-aged white male in normal health.

HISTORY. The lingual half of the crown of the maxillary right first bicuspid fractured when the patient accidentally bit down on a grain of sand while eating a salad. The fracture extended approximately 3 millimeters beyond the marginal gingival level (Case Fig. 1–1).

TREATMENT. The palatal tissue was prepared for injection of lidocaine in 1:100,000 dilution administered by local infiltration. A 45-degree-angle U-shaped loop electrode was selected, cutting current set on the power output dial at 6, and the tissue was resected in thin layers until the coronal end of the root was exposed (Case Fig. 1–2). The gingival contour was planed as the tissue was reduced to restore a normal feather-edge as the marginal level was lowered. The rubber dam was applied to the tooth and locked securely in place with a rubber dam clamp applied to the exposed root portion (Case Fig. 1–3).

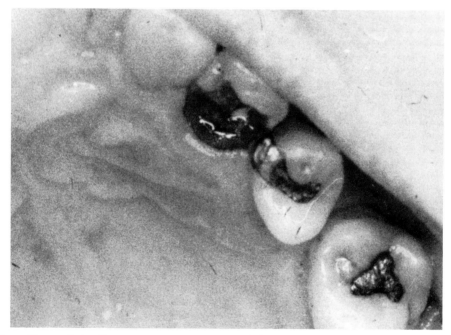

Case Figure 1–1. Preoperative appearance of fractured maxillary first bicuspid crown. The palatal half of the crown has been fractured down to the base of the pulp chamber of the tooth, well below the palatal mucosa.

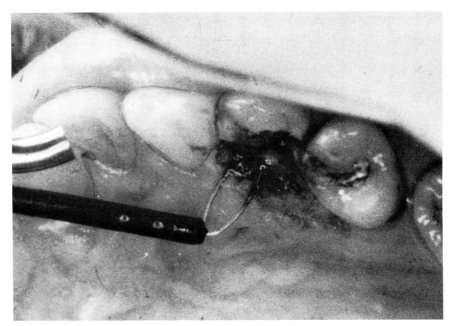

Case Figure 1–2. The palatal mucosa is being reduced in height to expose the fracture fully. The tissue is being reduced by loop planing with a 45-degree-angle elliptical loop electrode and cutting current is set at 5.5 on the instrument panel.

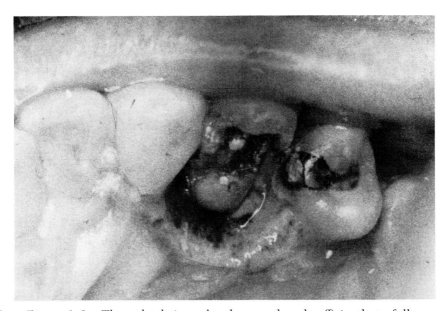

Case Figure 1–3. The palatal tissue has been reduced sufficiently to fully expose the defect and about 4 mm. of the root of the tooth, so that a rubber dam clamp can easily be applied to the tooth. The tissue has been planed to create a very gradual slope that forms a feather-edged new marginal gingiva, and there is no undercut to act as a food trap. A dressing of tincture of myrrh and benzoin applied in air-dried layers is all that is needed to cover the surgical site.

CASE 2

This case is presented courtesy of Dr. Manuel Weisman, Augusta, Georgia.

PATIENT.   A 14-year-old white male.

HISTORY.   The entire crown and a few millimeters of the coronal end of the root were lost by traumatic fracture (Case Fig. 2–1).

TREATMENT.   The tissues were prepared for anesthesia, and labial and palatal injections of lidocaine in dilution of 1:100,000 were administered by infiltration. A flame-shaped loop electrode was selected, cutting current set at 4½ on the power output dial, and the labial marginal gingiva was resected with a wiping stroke, which simultaneously beveled the marginal gingiva to a normal feather-edge contour.

The flame-shaped loop was then replaced with a 45-degree-angle U-shaped loop and cutting current was set at 6 on the power output dial. The palatal marginal gingiva was resected with this loop to the required depth by shaving the tissue in layers, allowing a 10-second time lapse between the cutting strokes. When approximately 3 millimeters of the coronal end of the root was exposed, cutting was discontinued and tincture of myrrh and benzoin was applied in several air-dried layers. The rubber dam was then applied to the exposed root end and secured into position with a rubber dam clamp (Case Fig. 2–2).

After the tooth has been isolated in this manner, treatment becomes routine: The pulp tissue in the canal of the retained root is extirpated with a barbed broach, and the canal is thoroughly irrigated to remove blood that may be present. The canal is then prepared biomechanically by thorough reaming and filing and obturated with gutta

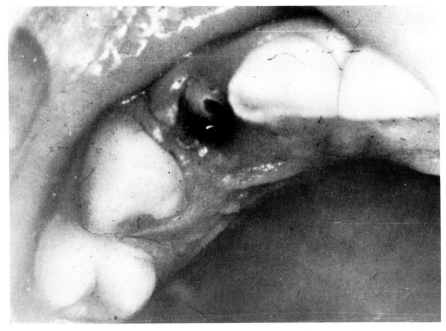

Case Figure 2–1.   A maxillary lateral incisor has been fractured traumatically. All that remains of the crown of the tooth is a thin labial shell. The fracture extends approximately 0.5 cm. below the level of the palatal mucosa, and the base of the pulp chamber is clearly visible.

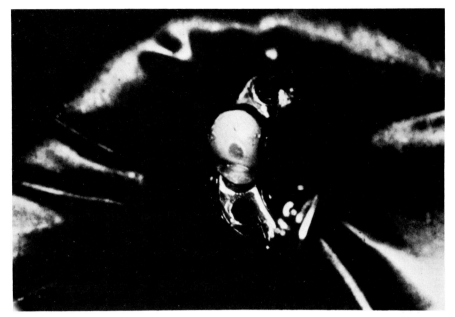

Case Figure 2–2. The tissue of the palate has been planed in a manner similar to that in Case Figure 1–2, until enough of the palatal aspect of the root of the tooth has been exposed, and a rubber dam has been applied to the tooth and is held in place with a rubber dam clamp attached to the fractured tooth.

percha points, condensing the apical half tightly and leaving the coronal half unfilled so that a post can be inserted into the canal. A wax pattern for a metal core for the porcelain crown restoration is prepared and cast, after which the tooth is restored with a porcelain jacket crown.

ROOT CANAL STERILIZATION BY ELECTROCOAGULATION

USE OF ANTIBIOTICS. Antibiotic sterilization of root canals has been utilized for almost three decades.[1-4] After Grossman introduced his poly-antibiotic formula,[5] antibiotic sterilization of the root canal prior to obturation continued until recently to be the traditional method of endodontic therapy.[6] Operative and 72- to 96-hour postoperative cultures to establish the sterility of the canals before obturation became a standardized part of the procedure.

Despite reports of bacterial survival and warnings of development of resistant strains, controversy about the efficacy of antibiotic treatment did not assume major proportions until recently. Now, however, the significance of negative cultures, the importance of canal sterility, and indeed the *ability to achieve sterility in a canal* are being seriously challenged. The matter has become so highly controversial that the American Board of Endodontics is said to have recently conducted a survey among all Board members to determine their use of cultures in their practices and their opinions as to the clinical usefulness of these cultures.

The controversy stems from the fact that many eminently qualified endodontists have found it impossible to consistently achieve sterility of root canals despite treatment with antibiotics after completion of thorough biomechanical preparation of the canals.

The author has neither the desire nor the intent to become involved in any controversy regarding need or desirability of attaining sterilization of contaminated canals prior to their obturation. This text will therefore be confined to consideration of why antibiotic therapy fails to achieve consistent sterility and to presenting a method of treatment whereby total sterilization of root canals can be achieved safely and consistently, regardless of the degree of contamination present in the canals.

The antibiotics used to achieve root canal sterility are known as "broad spectrum" drugs, owing to their remarkable effectiveness against a wide variety of organisms. Nevertheless, they are neither cure-alls nor shotgun remedies. They have specific bactericidal or bacteriostatic effects on susceptible organisms, but are likely to be ineffectual against bizarre organisms such as spores and anaerobes that may be present in contaminated root canals.[7] Even relatively commonplace gram-negative bacteria occasionally found in root canals may prove to be immune to many of the antibiotic drugs. Moreover, even when antibiotics are used against susceptible organisms, *unless the dosage used is adequate to assure total bactericidal or bacteriostatic effect,* surviving organisms become resistant strains and the patient usually becomes sensitized to future administration of that antibiotic.[8-12] Infinitely more serious than the failure to attain root canal sterility is the hazard created by the R factor; those innocuous bacteria which survive the antibiotics and develop resistance to the drugs may transfer their acquired resistance to virulent organisms that have not been subjected to the therapy.[13-15]

The small quantity of antibiotic drugs introduced into the canals and, in most instances, failure to supplement the local therapy with parenteral administration of the antibiotics are also accountable for many of the failures to achieve consistently sustained negative cultures following antibiotic endodontic therapy.[*] Since the culture's function is to indicate the efficacy of the chemotherapeutic attempt to achieve canal sterility, failure to do so consistently has created skepticism as to whether sterilization of the canal is necessary or attainable.

When canal sterility is dependent upon the efficacy of antibiotic therapy this skepticism appears eminently justified. However, this does not alter the fact that consistent sterilization of contaminated canals is clinically attainable. Research investigations reported in an earlier chapter and clinical experience have amply demonstrated this. Bacteria that may be immune to chemotherapy or can survive antibiotic therapy and develop immunity to subsequent treatment with the drug enjoy neither comparable immunity nor the ability to survive when subjected to efficient electrocoagulation within the lumen of the biomechanically prepared root canal. That consistently effective sterilization of contaminated canals can be achieved by electrocoagulation is verified by the demonstrated ability to obtain successive negative cultures if

---

[*]Presence of contaminated hair-fine lateral accessory canals that are not revealed by routine x-ray examination also can be a factor. A method for establishing their presence and coping with them is described later in the chapter.

during the interval between cultures the oral opening into the canal is hermetically sealed with an effective sealing agent.[16]

The problem, therefore, is obviously not a matter of possibility but rather one of specific methodology whereby endodontic sterilization can be safely and effectively achieved by electrocoagulation.

USE OF ELECTROCOAGULATION. The most efficient and rapid method of sterilization is by total coagulation of all living organic matter present. In the autoclave the use of live steam under pressure coagulates and totally destroys all living organisms present, even resistant or otherwise immune strains of bacteria. When this principle is applied to the root canal it is equally effective.

When high-frequency electrocoagulating current is applied uniformly to the walls of a root canal all its organic contents become completely coagulated,[17-20] regardless of the amount or severity of contamination. The coagulation results primarily from direct physical contact of the activated electrode with the internal surface of the canal. Supplementary coagulation may occur as the moisture present in the canal becomes vaporized by the density of heat energy generated by the current, producing live steam. Steam tends to rise as it is being generated. Furthermore, owing to the anatomic conformation of root canals, which taper greatly toward their apices, the lumina of the canals become constricted and the steam cannot readily escape through the apical foramina. In addition, the electrode in the canal acts as a plug, partially sealing the canal. All these factors tend to combine to create live steam under partial pressure within the canal, thereby simulating to some degree an autoclave effect.

Pulp tissue occasionally undergoes dry gangrene. In the absence of natural moisture, pulp chambers and root canals can be moistened with tap water or normal saline solution, so that when the electrode is introduced into such a canal and electrocoagulating current is applied live steam will be generated. Additional methods for creating moisture in the root canal will be discussed further on.

To be clinically practical, endodontic sterilization by electrocoagulation must fulfill two requirements:

1. It must be capable of producing enough heat within the canal to coagulate all the organisms that may be present.
2. It must accomplish this without permitting the heat to penetrate through the canal walls and irritate or destroy the viability of the periodontal membrane and/or the investing bone.

Clinical evidence has been confirmed histologically that damage from cumulative heat penetration can be avoided by the combined precautions of limiting the coagulation to very brief periods of activated electrode contact with the internal walls of the canal, rapid instrumentation in the canal during the periods of contact, and adequate intervals of time lapse between applications of the coagulating current.

Each episode of active electrode contact with the tissues must be rigidly limited. Moreover, the electrode must be kept moving rapidly in the canal during each brief period of active contact to prevent concentration of heat energy from developing at any given point in the canal during the contact period. Permitting an adequate lapse of time between applications is essential to prevent danger of destructively penetrating cumulative heat effect.

Electrocoagulation can be applied to the internal walls of a root canal most effectively and safely with an electrode that can be moved rapidly in the canal while it is activated, so that it will make contact with all the internal surfaces and will not permit the heat generated to penetrate through the walls of the canal to cause damage to the investing periodontal membrane or bone. In order to prevent concentration of heat through the walls of the canal, which could be injurious to the periodontal fibers or alveolar bone and cause pericementitis, periostitis or acute osteitis, the current should *under no circumstances* be applied continuously for more than a maximum of 1 to 2 seconds at any one time. This should be followed by a 5- to 10-second pause before the current is reapplied.

The most effective electrode for this purpose is the regular endodontic barbed broach when it is locked into a special handpiece with a chuck small enough to clamp onto and hold it securely. A barbed broach slightly thinner in diameter than the diameter of the canal is ideally suited for this purpose, since it will permit the up and down and rotary movements that are essential for its safe and effective use. If the canal is tortuous, or the lumen too fine to permit use of a barbed broach, a smooth broach may be substituted, but only if the barbed broach cannot be moved freely in the canal while it is activated (Fig. 14–1).

There is a logical reason for the preference for use of the barbed broach, although admittedly the smooth broach can be manipulated much more easily. When a barbed broach is employed and used with the proper up-down and rotary movements in the canal while it is activated, each of the barbs serves as the equivalent of a separate coagulating electrode tip, and the probability of failure to contact all the internal surface of the canal is extremely remote. Unless the smooth broach fits the lumen of the canal snugly, there is a distinct possibility that some of the internal surface of the canal may not be contacted by the activated electrode, and thus the result is incomplete sterilization.

Many roots are curved or have a dog-leg bend instead of being straight. It is often possible to use a barbed broach in such a dilacerated root freely down

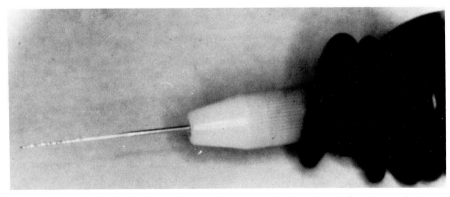

Figure 14–1. Endodontic barbed broach electrode handle. This electrode handle is a shorter version of the Coles Radiosurg Scalpel IV coagulating handpiece. It differs in that the chuck in the tip of the handpiece is small enough to lock tightly onto the barbed broach shaft and convert it into an electrode.

to the bend, but not beyond it. In such cases the barbed broach can be used to sterilize the portion of the canal down to the bend, and then a smooth broach can be substituted and used to complete the sterilization of the remainder of the canal, being careful to avoid forcing the smooth broach through the apical foramen.

Regular needle and loop electrodes are made either of tungsten wire, which can withstand very high heat, or of solid steel in round ball, tapered cone, or cylindrical forms that have considerable physical bulk, which helps them to withstand the heat. Thin steel wires such as the barbed and smooth broaches tend to crystallize when subjected to high heat for long periods. It is therefore imperative to avoid reusing them, since they could become crystallized and fracture, and the result would be a broken broach remaining wedged in the canal.

Sterilization of root canals by electrocoagulation applied indirectly through root canal files or reamers wedged snugly in the canals and contacted by an activated coagulating electrode has been reported in the literature and its use was described in the first edition of this text. Not only is this method of electrocoagulation of root canals *not* recommended, but such use is deplored as being fraught with danger of causing acute periostitis and osteitis, owing to the high lateral heat penetration from the stationary instruments through the walls of the canal and into the investing structures.

The author has been informed of a number of instances in which this indirect method was used and resulted in persistent, agonizing postoperative pain that necessitated extraction of the teeth, and several instances in which the teeth were exfoliated. Such postoperative hazards bar the indirect method as an acceptable electrosurgical endodontic procedure.

The barbed broach enjoys the further advantage that when it becomes necessary to introduce moisture into the canal for proper electrosurgical instrumentation, or if there is any doubt as to whether all the internal surface of the canal has been uniformly contacted, it is possible to wrap a wisp of cotton lightly around the barbs, which will prevent dislogdment of the cotton in the canal, and after moistening the cotton, using the cotton-tipped barbed broach in the canal like a ramrod in a gun barrel, thereby assuring uniform contact with all the internal surfaces of the canal and adequate moisture for good electrical conductivity of the RF current.

The major factor in endodontic sterilization is direct physical contact of the activated coagulating electrode with the internal surfaces of the canal. When the tooth has accessory canals these obviously cannot be sterilized by direct physical contact. However, they may become sterilized by a by-product of the coagulation.

The by-product is the live steam created by vaporization of the moisture in the canal by the coagulating heat being generated in the canal. Even though the amount of steam pressure that can be produced within the canal by electrocoagulation can simulate to only a limited degree the effects of an autoclave, if accessory canals are present and the canal has been cleansed with acetone before coagulation, the degree of steam pressure at the constricted end of the canal is likely to be sufficient to enable the steam to penetrate through the accessory canals and sterilize them.

The increased potential for effective steam penetration through accessory canals after the acetone cleansing is due to the fact that acetone is a lipoid solvent. When the acetone is introduced into the canal it flows into the accessory canals by capillary attraction, dissolving out the lipoids in the pulp tissue that is present in their lumina. This increases their permeability to the penetration of the steam, thereby increasing the potential for their effective sterilization.

To facilitate introduction of the acetone into the canal a tiny wisp of cotton is loosely wrapped around the barbs of the broach, so that it will not detach readily in the canal. The cotton is moistened with acetone and used with a pumping motion in the canal.[21] As the acetone evaporates, the lipoids evaporate with it. Elimination of the lipoid can also be of diagnostic value, since it will permit chloroform-diluted Chloropercha to flow into accessory canals by capillary attraction. Injection of the radiopaque Chloropercha into the canal will reveal the presence of even hair-thin accessory canals and thereby influence treatment, since presence of multiple lateral or interlacing accessory canals in the apical third of the root would make it advisable to perform a root-end resection.

Normally there is enough natural moisture in the canal so that there is no need to introduce moisture into the canal at the outset; however, as the coagulation is repeated a drop of moisture is added from time to time to replace moisture that has evaporated. Mullett has reported a technique of flooding the canal with chlorinated lime solution and applying the coagulating current into the flooded canal.* The nascent chlorine that is released in this technique may be particularly effective when treating canals with one or more lateral canals.

Instrumentation technique. After the biomechanical debridement of the canal has been completed, a smooth broach is measured against the x-ray film of the tooth, and bent at the apparent proper length of the canal to reach the internal aspect of the apical foramen or within 1 millimeter of it. The smooth broach is left in the canal while an x-ray film is taken. This film reveals whether the broach measurement is accurate, so that if it is not, the necessary adjustment can be made in the length of the barbed broach, which is now bent at the incisal or occlusal level of the tooth, thereby creating a measurement control that will prevent forcing the broach through the apical foramen. The tooth is isolated, and the barbed broach is used with a rapid simultaneous up and down and rotary motion for 1 to 2 seconds. This is followed by a 5- to 10-second rest interval to permit the heat to be thoroughly dissipated. The coagulation is repeated as needed. If this formula of instrumentation is followed, it does not matter how many times the treatment is repeated, since it eliminates the hazard of overheating from cumulative effect. Inasmuch as the number of coagulating episodes is in itself immaterial, the author feels that the instrumentation should be repeated about 30 times for the average tooth. Increased dosage is a discretionary matter and can only be determined by the clinical judgment of the therapist.

---

*The tooth to be treated is isolated. Dr. Mullett then introduces into the canal a solution of Javex water diluted 50 per cent with water. Similar results can be obtained by substituting Clorox, Chlorpactin WCS 60 (Kasdenol), or Zonite for the Javex water.

When the number of coagulating episodes deemed necessary by the therapist has been concluded, the canal is thoroughly dried with sterile paper points. A wisp of sterile cotton is wrapped around a sterile barbed broach, moistened with sterile isotonic saline solution, and used to wipe around the internal aspect of the canal. It is then wiped over the surface of the blood agar plate or broth used for culturing.

The sharp tip of another sterile paper point is cut off with a pair of sterile scissors, and the point is inserted into the canal. A small pellet of sterile cotton is then inserted into the pulp base of the chamber. The coronal opening into the tooth is sealed with Cavit or Quickseal, which effectively seals it until it is opened at the next visit. If the culture proves negative, and a second culture obtained 72 to 96 hours later likewise proves negative, the canal can be obturated. If the culture proves positive the sterilizing procedure is repeated until sterile cultures are obtained.

Technique for One-Sitting Treatment of Chronically Suppurating Root Canal

It is by no means rare to encounter a contaminated canal that continues to suppurate profusely despite all attempts to halt it. When such a canal is to be treated it is necessary to consider the alternatives realistically. In most instances the involved apical portion of the tooth has undergone a degree of resorption externally, so that the cementum is badly eroded and pitted. Massive amounts of bacteria are trapped in the pits. Moreover, there is only one way to determine whether the periapical lesion is a degenerated granuloma or a cyst sac and that is by histologic examination. From a realistic practical clinical standpoint, the conclusion is not only that a root end in that condition is expendable but that its resection is imperative if the tooth is to be successfully preserved.

The treatment consists of the total evacuation and arrest of the exudation, sterilization and obturation of the canal, followed by resection of the involved apex to surgically debride the periapical diseased area. Success of the technique is predicated on the fact that the body cannot immediately replace the exudate if the latter has been forcefully evacuated in its entirety. This makes it possible to thoroughly cleanse the canal and complete its biomechanical preparation, sterilization, obturation, and root end resection in one clinical session. Repair is identical with that of root end resections performed for eradication of other types of periapical disease.

OPERATIVE TECHNIQUE.   The bulbous suction tip end of a plastic disposable saliva ejector device is cut off, leaving a length of plastic tubing. Plastic connectors such as are provided with the Monoject saliva ejectors are connected to the two ends. One of the connectors is attached to the central suction line. A Luer-type needle, preferably the blunt 20-gauge Monoject periodontal irrigating syringe needle, is attached to the other connector (Fig. 14–2). The needle is inserted toward the apex of the tooth, and suction is instituted to forcefully evacuate all the pus that is present in the lesion. The needle is then washed clean, detached from the suction device, and attached to the disposa-

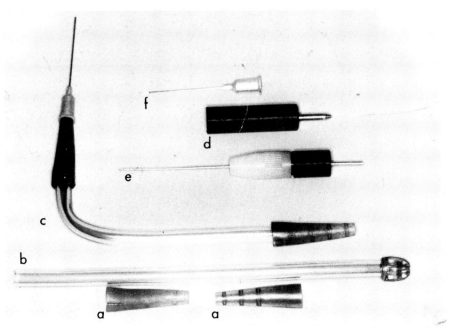

Figure 14–2. The instrument the author has devised for the one-visit definitive treatment of chronically suppurating root canals is shown. Its components, starting at the bottom, are (*a*) two typical plastic connectors for use with the Sherwood Monoject type of disposable plastic saliva ejector tips, (*b*) a saliva ejector tip with its protective bulb at one end, and (*c*) a saliva ejector tip with its protective bulb cut off and a plastic connector attached to each end. A blunt Luer-type suction needle has been attached to one of the connectors. The connector at the other end will be attached to the central suction or aspirator. (*d*) An electrical connector; a nail-like solid wire male plug projects at one end and the other end has an internal channel for insertion of the barb broach electrode handpiece used with electrosurgical units that have externally attached electrode handpiece cables. (*e*) A special barb broach electrode handpiece for use with the retractable universal type of electrode handpieces. (*f*) The special Monoject irrigating needle that is blunt and has a slot opening on one side of the tip for better irrigation and aspiration. (When the purulent exudate is very copious and viscous, an ordinary 18- or 20-gauge needle with the cutting tip removed and rounded is likely to be even better suited.)

able irrigating syringe (see Fig. 10–1). The syringe is filled with liquid, preferably a chlorine solution such as Chlorpactin WCS 60 solution, diluted Clorox solution, diluted Zonite solution, diluted Javex water solution, or saline solution, or, if preferred, hydrogen peroxide solution. The canal is irrigated vigorously with the fluid to wash out the slimy exudate material that adheres tenaciously to the internal walls of the canal. The irrigation-aspiration is repeated until there is clinical evidence that all the adherent purulent sludge has been removed. The canal is then dried and the biomechanical preparation of the canal is completed with canal files and reamers. The canal is then cleansed with acetone, dried, and moistened with a drop or two of the irrigating fluid, and electrocoagulation is instituted as previously described. The coagulating procedure is repeated as many times as clinical judgment dictates. The author recommends application of electrocoagulation for 1- to 2-second intervals, repeated 60 to 90 times.

    The Luer-type of syringe has traditionally been used for irrigations. This type of syringe has no built-in control of pressure and regulation of flow of the

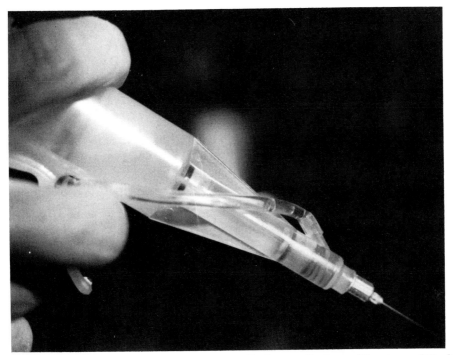

Figure 14–3. Controlled pressure irrigating Endovage Syringe. (Courtesy of Endovage Company.)

fluid, thus the pressure and flow vary with the manner in which the individual uses it. A new type of syringe to provide controlled positive pressure has been designed specifically for endodontic irrigation. The author has been informed that with this syringe the irrigation can be performed much more thoroughly and efficiently than with the Luer syringe. If it lives up to the claims made for it, this device, the Endovage Syringe (Fig. 14–3), would also likely prove advantageous for irrigating narrow, often tortuous infrabony periodontal pockets after debridement by electronic curettage.

When the sterilization by electrocoagulation is deemed satisfactory, the canal is filled, and, if the filling material is gutta percha points, *overfilled.* The overfill will not do any harm, since the root end will be resected and it helps to assure perfect condensation of the obturating material. This is followed by a typical root end resection such as will be described in detail later in this chapter.

The great advantage of this procedure is that it permits definitive treatment in a single session and eliminates the otherwise indefinite period of suppuration.

CASE 3

This is a typical case of persistent suppurative drainage from a canal despite repeated irrigation and medication, which had prevented completion of the endodontic therapy.

PATIENT. A 58-year-old white male.

HISTORY. The pulp chamber of a carious mandibular bicuspid was exposed when the tooth was reduced to a shoulderless stump for full-crown coverage to serve as an abutment for a fixed-bridge restoration. After the canal had been debrided of partially decomposed necrotic nerve tissue, suppuration had been encountered. It persisted despite all efforts to dry and sterilize the canal in the usual manner. The patient was referred for electrosurgical drying and sterilization of the canal.

CLINICAL EXAMINATION. There was no evidence of soft tissue pathology. The mandibular left second bicuspid was missing, and the first bicuspid had been reduced to a conical shoulderless stump for full-crown preparation. A diagnostic wire projected from the canal (Case Fig. 3–1A).

Roentgenographic examination revealed a slight thickening of the periodontal membrane at the apex of the first bicuspid. No other pathology was visible.

TREATMENT. Owing to its conical shape, a rubber dam clamp could not be attached to the tooth, and the dam could not be used to isolate it. The area was thus isolated with sterile sponges. The projecting diagnostic wire was then removed and in a few moments a thick purulent exudate began to ooze from the open canal. A 20-

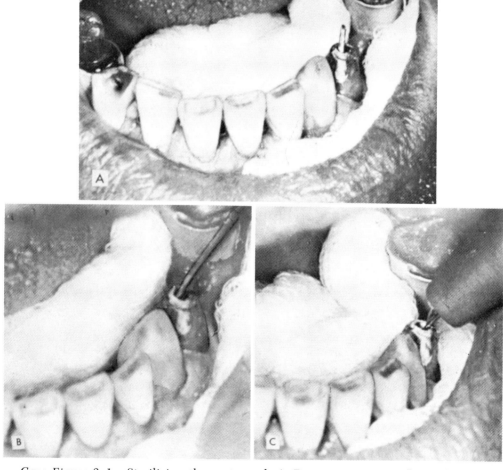

Case Figure 3–1. Sterilizing the root canal. *A,* Preoperative view; diagnostic wire in canal. *B,* Smooth broach inserted, bent to serve as marker and x-rayed for precise measurement of the canal. *C,* Barbed broach electrode in position sterilizing the canal.

gauge Luer-Lok hypodermic needle was attached to an aspirator tip and inserted into the canal; suction was applied for two minutes to siphon off the exudate. The aspirating needle was then removed and the canal was irrigated with Kasdenol solution. Aspiration was performed simultaneously with irrigation. After irrigation was completed, aspiration was halted and a sterile cotton point was inserted into the canal to dry it. Three points showed progressively lesser degrees of moisture; the fourth was dry except at the extreme tip, which still showed a trace of moisture.

The exact measurement of the length of the tooth was established by holding a smooth broach against the roentgenographic image of the tooth and bending it to size at a point corresponding to the occlusal edge of the stump. The broach was then inserted into the canal as a diagnostic wire (Case Fig. 3–1B). A roentgenogram was taken with this diagnostic wire in position; the new film confirmed the accuracy of the original measurement, showing that the wire reached exactly to the apex of the tooth.

A barbed broach slightly narrower than the lumen of the canal was selected and bent to exact length. This broach was inserted into an endodontic broach-holding electrode handle specially designed for use with the Radiosurg Scalpel unit, and the electrocoagulating current output was set at 1.* The barbed broach electrode was inserted into the canal, and the current was applied for three seconds while the electrode was kept in constant motion in circular and up and down directions (Case Fig. 3–1C). Care was taken to keep the electrode in constant contact with the inner walls of the canal. After a two-second pause the current was reapplied for another three-second period† and followed by the pause. This was repeated 30 times for a total of one and a half minutes of actual electrocoagulating time.

At this point the electrode was removed from the canal and a sterile cotton point inserted. Inspection after its removal showed that even the extreme apical tip of the point remained dry. After waiting five minutes another point was inserted to ascertain whether suppuration had resumed. This point also came out completely dry. The dentist, who had accompanied the patient, thereupon proceeded to fill the canal with silver points.

The tooth remained asymptomatic and two weeks later the fixed bridge was inserted. More than three years have elapsed since the canal was sterilized and filled, and the tooth has remained normal in all respects. At no time has the patient experienced pain or discomfort.

Although electrocoagulation can be performed with spark-gap generator current applied biterminally, owing to greater lateral heat dispersion of this type of current, its use is not recommended by the author for endodontic electrocoagulation.

ROOT-END RESECTION

Root-end resection, commonly referred to as root amputation or apicoectomy, is a surgical procedure that is so intimately related to the endodontic

---

*The potency of current output at a power output setting varies from unit to unit. With the electrosurgical unit used to treat this case optimal spot coagulation was obtained with the current output set at 1 on the panel rheostat.

†The period of active coagulation is now being limited to 1 to 2 seconds followed by a 5- to 10-second rest interval.

procedure that it is justifiably regarded by most as being more conservative than extraction of the diseased tooth.[23-26]

Root-end resection is considered successful when the tooth remains asymptomatic and the periapical defect is obliterated by bone regeneration that undergoes maturation and calcification. It must be considered a failure when the regenerating bone fails to mature and remains uncalcified as immature bone, or if it fails to fill in at all and remains as a surgical dead space.

Many factors influence the success or failure of the root-end resection. Some, such as the patient's capacity to heal, are intangible. The majority of factors are tangible; those governed by the efficiency of the operator are

1. Size and location of the incision
2. Thoroughness of debridement of necrotic periapical tissue
3. Smooth rounding off of the cut apical end of the root
4. Smoothing and rounding of the periphery of the buccal bony window
5. Hermetic sealing of the filling material at the cut apex
6. Scoring and roughening of dense sclerotic walls of bony crypts resulting from pressure by expanding cystic sacs
7. Accurate coaptation and readaptation of flap margins
8. Elimination of healing disruptive traumatizing occlusal prematurities

Electrosurgery fulfills an important role in three of these areas (i.e., 1, 2 and 5). Since the other five factors may also bear important influence on the outcome of the procedure, a brief review of these factors will also be included.

SIZE OF INCISION. There is a popular misconception that small incisions are less traumatic and heal more rapidly than larger ones and are therefore safer to use. This is a dangerous fallacy; if anything, the opposite is usually true. The size of an incision does *not* govern the speed or quality of healing at all. Far from being advantageous, small "buttonhole" incisions often allow inadequate access to, and visibility of, the operative field. This necessitates excessive traction and frequently results in laceration of the terminal ends of the incision. Ragged, torn margins repair much more slowly and produce undesirable scar tissue. It is therefore important that the incision be made large enough to provide satisfactory access and visibility without excessive tension on the incised tissues.

Location of the incision also plays an important role in the efficiency of the operative procedure, and may at least in part govern the speed and quality of tissue repair. A semilunar incision of the alveolar mucosa over the root of the affected tooth is deemed by many to be the favored site. A brief review of the histology of the gingival mucosa indicates that the supposed efficacy of this type of incision bears closer inspection.

HISTOLOGY OF GINGIVAL MUCOSA. The gingival mucosa is composed of a layer of stratified squamous epithelium supported upon a tunica propria. These in turn are supported upon a submucous layer composed of a coarse network of white elastic fibers containing the larger blood vessels. The blood supply of the mucosa is very rich, and the blood vessels form two plexuses, both more or less parallel with the surface. The outer plexus is composed of small capillaries forming a small-meshed network; the deeper plexus is composed of large vessels more widely separated.[27-29] The connective tissue bundles of elastic fibers also are arranged parallel to the epithelium.

SEMILUNAR INCISION. If a semilunar incision is to be large enough to provide good access and visibility it must be extended across an area of three teeth or more, with the involved tooth in the exact center of the area. The incision must be carried down through the submucosa and periosteum to bone, and in doing so traverse innumerable capillaries and many larger vessels. The profuse bleeding that ensues usually persists for quite a while and tends to retard the progress of the surgery. Many connective tissue and elastic fibers also are severed by the semilunar incision, as well as numerous muscle attachments extending from the areolar gingiva of the mucobuccal fold into the alveolar or cemental gingiva. When the flap of incised tissue is reflected from the underlying bone it undergoes marked contraction. Upon completion of the surgery, when the flap is restored to position, accurate coaptation of the margins creates considerable tension against the sutures in order to overcome the tissue contraction. Not infrequently (especially if the tissue tone is subnormal), this tension is sufficient to cause the sutures to cut through the atonal tissues and pull the incised margins apart. When the incision is performed with *cold steel*, repair tissue forms as contractile cicatricial scar connective tissue (Fig. 14–4). When incised margins are pulled apart by tension as described, a considerable amount of scar tissue may form which partly obliterates the buccal vestibule, or the defect may fail to heal satisfactorily. The likelihood of failure to heal is greatly increased if the line of incision is not created well below the lowermost border of the bony defect.

VERTICO-OBLIQUE INCISION. On the other hand, when a verticooblique incision is made (Fig. 14–5), relatively few blood vessels are traversed, and minimal contraction of the tissue flap occurs. No muscle-attaching

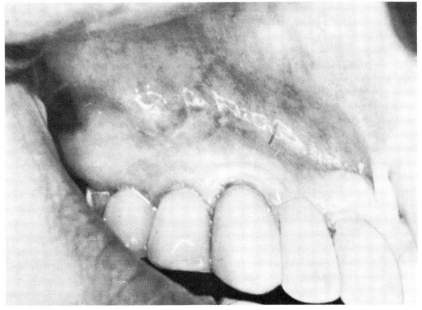

Figure 14–4. Typical cicatricial scar repair following semilunar incision with cold-steel scalpel for root-end resection.

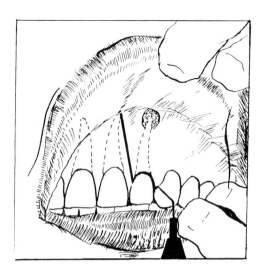

Figure 14–5. Vertico-oblique incision for root-end resection and severance of interproximal attachment.

fibers are severed horizontally. When the incision is extended from the mucobuccal fold to the marginal crest and on under the interproximal papillae, it affords excellent access and visibility with minimal retraction. The flap usually can be reflected and tied out of the way easily by inserting a suture at its edge and tying the latter to a posterior tooth distal to the flap (Fig. 14–6). This procedure eliminates instruments and hands from the operative field. Lack of bleeding, good access, and clear visibility accelerate the operative procedure. Lack of contractile tension and subgingival hemorrhage reduces the tendency for postoperative edema that so often accompanies the use of the semilunar incision.

REMOVAL OF NECROTIC DEBRIS.   The periapical necrotic debris is often readily accessible and easily removed by curettage. Not infrequently, however, some necrotic tissue may extend beyond the limits of the periapical bone defect and invaginate downward along the root surface toward the gingival

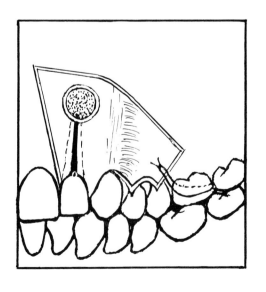

Figure 14–6. Flap of vertico-oblique incision tied posteriorly out of the operative field with a suture. A circular window to provide adequate access to the periapical pathology has been created in the labial bone.

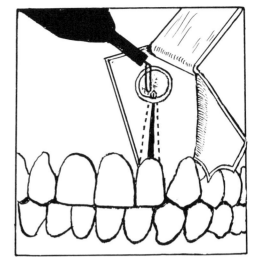

Figure 14–7. Necrotic debris inaccessible or difficult to reach by cold-steel instrumentation without considerable additional removal of alveolar bone, which is being removed in this case with a narrow U-shaped loop electrode.

margin. It is impossible to resect such tissue by ordinary instrumentation without sacrificing so much of the buccal alveolar bone or root length that the prognosis is endangered.

If this necrotic tissue is not fully resected or destroyed it deteriorates and prevents normal repair of the bone defect. In such instances, if electrosurgery is available, the tissue can be resected with small, narrow U-shaped loop electrodes bent to shape (Fig. 14–7), or destroyed *in situ* with fulgurating current applied with moderately fine needle electrodes (Fig. 14–8). The sparking usually makes it possible to destroy such tissue *in situ* without need for excessive sacrifice of either bone or root. Debridement can be completed with a narrow loop electrode.

Fulgurating current should be applied to the invaginating fibers with high current intensity for short periods with the electrode kept in constant

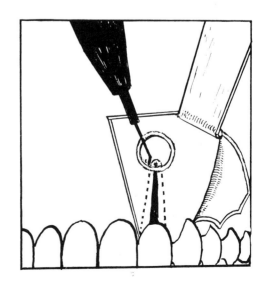

Figure 14–8. Diseased tissue inaccessible even to the loop electrode destroyed *in situ* by fulguration.

motion (as much as the confining area will permit). When it is used in this manner, fulguration, being superficial and largely self-limiting, does no harm to the investing alveolar bone, while the undesirable tissue is carbonized.

If no fulgurating current is available with the electronic unit, the tissue can be electrocoagulated with the fine needle electrode. The current output is set at 2 for biterminal electrocoagulation, the electrode is inserted into the space occupied by the necrotic tissue and moved around as much as possible. The electrode is kept *in situ* until coagulation is completed, but is kept activated for only two or three seconds at a time.

SEALING THE CANAL APEX. Rounding the apex after it has been cut is important in eliminating the irritating effect of the sharp edges on new granulation tissue which initially fills the surgical defect. Sharp jagged bone margins must also be trimmed smooth to prevent irritation of regenerating granulating tissue and the overlying gingival mucosa.

Hermetic sealing of the canal filling at the cut end helps to protect against recontamination from leakage due to loss of adhesion of the filling material to the inner surface of the canal. When root-end resection is performed it is advisable to fill and overfill the canal so that the filling material projects beyond the apex into the bone cavity. After the apex is cut off and the cut margins rounded, the filling should be hermetically sealed at the apex. The latter is necessary because the act of cutting across the root end tends to tear the filling material loose from its adherence to the inner aspect of the canal wall. Apical seal can be performed satisfactorily in a number of ways. It can be sealed with a heated ball burnisher, or some of the apical filling material can be removed with an inverted cone bur and the resulting apical cavity filled with amalgam. If the canal filling material is gutta-percha the apex can be sealed by applying a pellet of cotton moistened slightly with chloroform, eucalyptol, oil of eucalyptus or other gutta-percha solvent and by rubbing this over the cut end. Electrocoagulation applied to the new apex and exposed filling material with a ball coagulating electrode ably serves to seal the apex thoroughly and at the same time sterilizes as it coagulates (Fig. 14–9).

OTHER CONSIDERATIONS. Cystic defects grow by expanding pressure exerted against their bony confines. The process is usually very slow. When the periapical lesion is a radicular cyst the walls of the bony crypt that is formed tend to be sclerotic. In such cases, after the root-end resection has been performed it is usually noted that there is neither bleeding nor evidence of the usual nutrient foramina present in the defect. If the tissue flap is restored without further delay it is more than likely that the periapical space will fail to fill in with regenerative tissue and that a surgical dead space will result. In such cases it is advantageous to roughen and scarify the dense bony walls of the defect by curettage or by scoring with burs or chisels in order to reopen some of the nutrient foramina. It may even be necessary to drill perforations through the dense sclerotic bone with a small round bur to induce free bleeding into the cavity. Scarification and/or perforation of the dense bone assures not only the formation of a blood clot but also a blood supply to bring nutrition to the clot.

The presence of large metallic, ceramic, or acrylic restorations on teeth

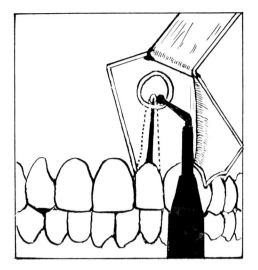

Figure 14-9. Sealing and sterilizing cut apex by electrocoagulation with a small ball electrode.

involved in the flap area often constitutes a handicap to rapid normal tissue healing and interproximal reattachment. Nevertheless, with firm bony support and perfectly coapted margins provided by the vertico-oblique incision, even the presence of such restorations will not as a rule prevent normal reattachment of the flap and interproximal papillae when the tissue tone is normal (Fig. 14-10). But when this handicap is superimposed over the further handicap of poor tissue tone and/or periodontal disease of these tissues, it may be necessary to resort to use of the semilunar incision. When the latter is performed by electrosection instead of by cold-steel instrumentation, a minimal amount of scar tissue or contraction ensues. The semilunar incision also becomes necessary when the alveolar ridge is abnormally short and the root lengths of the teeth are normal or extra long.

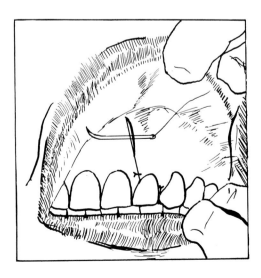

Figure 14-10. Flap restored and coapted margins sutured. Suture also inserted through interproximal papilla for accurate readaptation.

The basic principles of surgical root-end resection vary little. However, the presence of alveologingival fistulas, excessive labial alveolar bone loss, porcelain crowns, gold inlays or other restorations that extend subgingivally, broken instrument fragments in the root canals, perforated roots, and defective old root canal fillings creates special problems and requires operative variations that will be demonstrated in the following case reports.

CASE 4

This is a typical case of root-end resection complicated by the presence of an alveolo-gingival fistula.

PATIENT.   A 37-year-old white male.

HISTORY.   He had received a blow to his upper lip and maxillary anterior teeth. A nonvital central incisor projecting labially took the brunt of the blow. Although his lip swelled badly he did not seek dental treatment until he noticed that the tooth was slightly loose and that a small lump had formed over it.

He consulted his dentist almost two weeks after the injury and was informed that the tooth was abscessed and would require endodontic therapy and periapical surgery, or extraction. He chose the former. The canal was opened and the old canal filling removed to establish drainage. The dentist found no exudate. A formocresol dressing was inserted and sealed into the canal. The patient was referred for root-end resection to be performed immediately after the dentist filled the canal.

CLINICAL EXAMINATION.   *Extraoral.*   Negative.

Intraoral.   A fistulous orifice was present on the labial mucosa in the apical region of the malposed maxillary left central incisor. Rotentgenographic examination showed that the canal had been slightly overfilled as requested and that the filling was well condensed. A large radiolucent area was present periapically (Case Fig. 4–2B).

TREATMENT.   The mouth was prepared for surgery. Kasdenol spray irrigation, 0.5 per cent solution, was followed by application of Tr. Zephiran Chloride to the tissues. The mucosa was dried and a topical anesthetic was applied for two minutes. The area was anesthetized by local infiltration anesthesia.

Monoterminal current output was set for 8 and the fistula was thoroughly fulgurated with a heavy wire needle electrode (Case Fig. 4–1A). Cutting-current output was then set at 3.5 on the Radiosurg, and a vertico-oblique incision was made by electrosection with a fine 45-degree-angle needle electrode. The incision was started at a point slightly distal to the apical aspect of the lateral incisor in the mucolabial fold and carried downward and slightly forward to its termination at the mesioproximal angle of the gingival margin of the lateral incisor (Case Fig. 4–1B).

The tissue medial to the line of incision was undermined with a periosteal elevator and reflected from the bone, exposing the labial alveolar bone plate and the apical defect (Case Fig. 4–1C). The incision caused very little bleeding; just a trace of blood oozed from it. When the flap was undermined and reflected there was considerable bleeding, but this was easily staunched by pressure with a sterile sponge. The operative field remained free of active bleeding thereafter, and visibility was clear throughout the procedure without need for constant sponging. The flap was retracted in a distal direction and retained in that position with a suture inserted at the mesioproximal angle of the tissue, then tied to the right cuspid. This served several useful purposes:

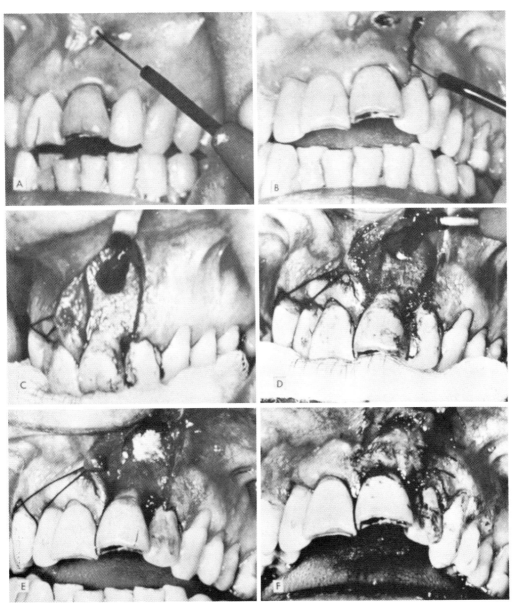

Case Figure 4–1. Root-end resection: surgical procedure. *A,* The fistulous orifice is destroyed by fulguration. *B,* A vertico-oblique incision is made at the mesial aspect of the lateral incisor with 45-degree-angle fine needle electrode. Incision started over apex of the lateral high in the vestibule. *C,* Flap retracted and tied posteriorly with a suture. Labial bone window has been rounded, the apex cut, and debridement completed. Note lack of bleeding from incision. *D,* The new apical end of the root canal filling and the apex sterilized with large ball electrode by electrocoagulation, sealing the gutta-percha filling at the root end. *E,* Medicated mixture of bone paste and surgical gelatin powder inserted into the defect and mixed with blood present. *F,* Flap restored, margins coapted and sutured with interrupted silk sutures. The interproximal papilla also is sutured palatally.

It avoided trauma against the lip and tissues from constant pressure of a retractor to hold the flap out of the way. It eliminated the natural tendency for the flap to slip out from the grasp of the retractor, as well as the tendency for the tissue to contract. The last but by no means least important advantage this offered was the elimination of the need for a hand and instrument (the presence of which would clutter up the operative field), thus assuring better visibility and access with minimal assistance.

The periapical bone defect was approximately 0.5 cm. wide and 1.2 cm. long. The apical portion of the root projected upward into the defect about 4 mm. The supra-apical degenerative granulomatous tissue was removed with curets. The apical projection was reduced about 3 mm. in height by grinding with a round diamond stone. The bone margin was trimmed smooth with a bone file and the surgical field was thoroughly debrided. Then the apical end of the canal filling was sealed by applying coagulating current to it with a large ball electrode (Case Fig. 4–1D) for a total of 15 seconds with the current output set at 3.

A mixture of cultured, despeciated bone paste and medicated powdered gelatin was deposited into the bone defect and mixed with blood in the area (Case Fig. 4–1E). The flap was then restored to position, the tissue margins coapted, and the wound closed with 0000 braided silk interrupted sutures (Case Fig. 4–1F).

Postmedication was prescribed—Panalba,* double strength, four times a day around the clock for three days; Kadenol lavage three times a day; Darvon Compound as required, and ascorbic acid, 250 mg., plus Knox clear gelatin as a dietary supplement. Instructions were given for postoperative care and the patient was instructed to return on the fifth postoperative day for removal of the sutures.

The postoperative instructions and medication prescribed in this case, as well as the preparation of the operative field for surgery, were typical and are therefore being described in some detail. Variations from this regimen will be elaborated in subsequent reports.

Postoperative instructions were: In the event of mild discomfort take two aspirin or Anacins. If this proves inadequate take the Darvon Compound. Use the Kasdenol in the usual way but hold the last mouthful for three minutes. Use saline lavage every two hours at mouth temperature. Bland diet, semisolid for the first 24 hours, soft diet thereafter. In the event of marked swelling apply an ice pack, partially filled with crushed ice and wrapped in a towel, for 10 to 15 minutes, off for 45 or 50 minutes, repeated 5 or 6 times.

The patient returned on the fifth day. He reported that there had been no bleeding and very little swelling. He had had no pain and relatively slight discomfort. He had taken two Anacin tablets when the anesthesia wore off and did not require further sedation.

On examination the tonal quality and healing progress of the tissues appeared excellent; the fulgurated fistula was healthily granulated, with a thin layer of normal coagulum covering it (Case Fig. 4–2A). The sutures were removed and Tr. Myrrh and Benzoin was applied to the area. He was instructed to continue the soft diet and lavage for another two weeks, at which time he was to return for observation.

He returned approximately three weeks postoperatively. Primary healing appeared to be complete, with little clinical evidence remaining of the incision or the fistula. The patient was asked to return again in ten weeks for further postoperative observation. Roentgenographic examination at that time revealed excellent bone regeneration (Case Fig. 4–2B)

---

*Many of the medicaments, such as Panalba, used in treatment of the cases reported in this text have since been superseded by newer drugs or withdrawn from the market because of FDA re-evaluation.

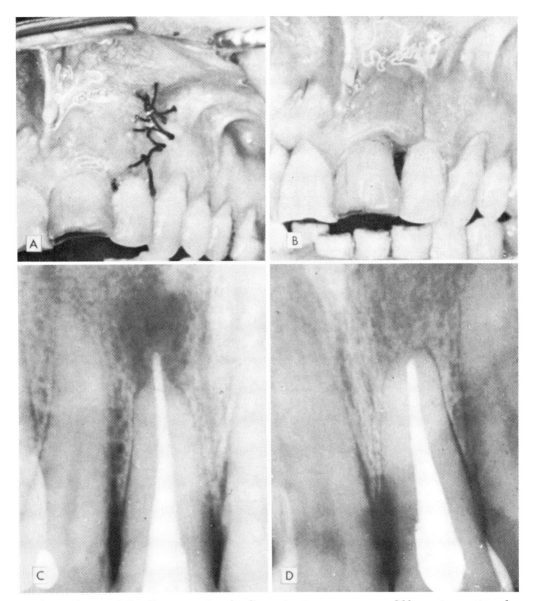

Case Figure 4–2. Postoperative healing. *A,* Appearance on fifth postoperative day, sutures still in position. Fulgurated fistulous lesion has filled nicely, and is covered with a very light layer of healthy coagulum. The line of incision has healed by primary intention. Interproximal and cervical gingival reattachment, and tissue tone are excellent. *B,* Appearance three weeks postoperatively. Primary healing is complete. Tissue tone and reattachment are good. The only clinical evidence that still remains of fulgurated fistula or incision is partial retraction of the interproximal papilla* and a small, very shallow groove on the surface of the labial mucosa. *C,* Roentgenogram showing periapical lesion and canal overfilled and well condensed. *D,* Roentgenogram taken four months postoperatively shows evidence of satisfactory bone repair. The cut apex is seen to be well rounded. Apparent shortness of canal filling from apex is an optical illusion due to angulation.

---

*Malposition of the central undoubtedly contributed to the retraction and helped retard full regeneration and reattachment of this interproximal papilla.

CASE 5

All root-end resections present a number of basic similarities. In all cases there is periapical disease that necessitates the surgical amputation of the affected roots. In all cases either the canal has been obturated prior to the resection or it will have a retrograde filling inserted into the cut apical end of the canal after the apex has been cut off. Frequently, there is a fistulous lesion that communicates from the periapical lesion to the external surface of the gingiva.

The next case was atypical in the latter respect. There was a periapical lesion and a fistulous lesion on the gingival surface. But unlike the usual fistulous tract located over or above the root apex that penetrates directly to the periapical disease (Case 4), the lesion here is located midway between the cemento-enamel junction and the root apex, and the lesion was extremely fibrotic and bluish black in color instead of having the liquefaction necrosis or semi-granulomatous, semi-fibrotic tissue that is usually found in these lesions.

The fibrotic tissue was so tenaciously adherent to the alveolar bone that it was impossible to elevate the mucoperiosteal flap until the adhesion was eliminated by resection of the adherent tissue which was found to extend from the level of the external gingival lesion superiorly to the periapical lesion.

PATIENT.   A 45-year-old white female.

HISTORY.   She had had endodontic therapy and a root-end resection performed on a maxillary central several years ago. She had no trouble with the tooth thereafter, but she noticed that the gingival tissue over the tooth formed a depressed hole from which a very hard knotlike tissue mass emerged. She was fearful that this might be a cancerous lesion and consulted her dentist, who found considerable periapical radiolucence on x-ray examination. He referred her for diagnosis and treatment.

CLINICAL EXAMINATION.   The affected tooth was the maxillary left central incisor. The tooth had been restored with a well-fitted porcelain jacket crown. A blister-like hard nodule was present on the labial gingiva midway between the crown and apex of the tooth along its distal aspect. Contiguous and immediately superior to this mass there was a fistulous tract orifice. The labial gingiva appeared to be slightly swollen and engorged (Case Fig. 5–1A). The dentist had provided his roentgenogram which showed what appeared to be a surgical dead space over the cut apex of the tooth.

TREATMENT.   The tissues were prepared and an infraorbital block plus labial infiltration over the right central and palatal infiltration was administered. A fine 45-degree-angle needle electrode was selected, cutting current was set at 3, and the activated electrode was used to create a vertico-oblique incision. The incision was made about 3 mm. distal to the tissue nodule and extended from the mucogingival level to the mesiogingival angle of the lateral, care being taken to avoid splitting the interdental papilla (Case Fig. 5–1B). The apical attachments of the papilla in the central-lateral embrasure and the papilla in the embrasure between the two centrals were severed with the electrode to create the mucoperiosteal flap. The flap was lifted to free it but proved to be tenaciously adherent to the bone. Several cordlike fibrous structures were tying the gingival tissue to the bone (Case Fig. 5–1C). Scraping with a periosteal elevator was unable to tear the adhesions completely free from the alveolar bone. The adherent tissue had to be resected with a 7 mm. round loop electrode, used with current output set at 5 to remove it completely from the labial surface of the alveolar bone.

When the fibrous degenerative tissue was completely removed it exposed to view the periapical defect, which was filled with more of the degenerative fibrous tissue. A

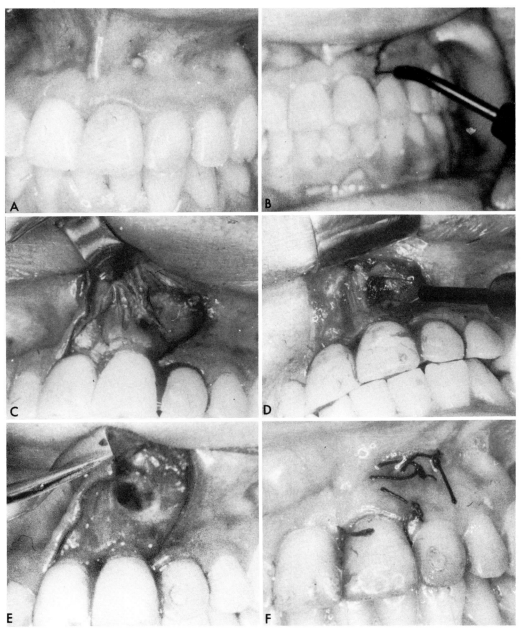

Case Figure 5–1. A, Preoperative appearance. There is a blister-like hard nodule on the labial gingiva midway between crown and apex along the distal aspect of the maxillary left central incisor. Immediately superior to the nodule there is a fistulous orifice, and the tissue over it appears swollen and somewhat reddened. B, A vertico-oblique incision from the muco-gingival junction downward and anteriorly from the region of the apex of the cuspid to the distogingival angle of the central is being created by electrosection with a fine 45-degree-angle needle electrode with current set at 3 on the instrument panel. C, The apical attach-ment of the papilla in the central embrasure having been severed, the flap is elevated and re-tracted, exposing a mass of tough fibrous strands of degenerative tissue firmly adherent to the bone. The tissue appears to be emerging from the site of the ventral surface of the fistulous orifice rather than from the periapical lesion. D, The tightly adherent fibrous tissue is resected from the intact surface of the alveolar bone with a medium-width U-shaped loop electrode, and cutting current is set at 6. E, The large periapical lesion has been debrided and the apex of the affected tooth has been cut and rounded. F, Appearance on the fifth postoperative day, before the sutures were removed. The tissue tone is excellent, and the line of incision shows a sur-prising degree of primary healing.

347

medium-width U-shaped loop electrode was selected and bent to a slight curvature to provide more effective entry into the defect, and the debris was resected almost completely with this electrode (Case Fig. 5–1D). The debridement was completed with a narrow 45-degree-angle U-shaped electrode that was able to be used to debride behind the root portion that projected upward beyond the floor of the bone defect. The mucogingival flap was then everted to expose the ventral surface of the tissue. Some of the degenerative fibrous tissue was also adhering to the tissue and had to be resected from it with the round loop electrode, care being taken to avoid perforating through the tissue in doing this. The tissue surrounding the fistulous orifice and the hard nodule were resected with a fine 45-degree-angle needle electrode and sent for biopsy. At this point the bone defect appeared totally debrided (Case Fig. 5–1E).

The debridement of the organic tissue having been completed, the projecting apex which, with the aid of a transilluminating light directed into the defect, was seen to be badly pitted and jagged at the tip was reduced approximately 2 mm. to where the root surface appeared normal. This remaining projecting root portion was curetted to remove the dead cementum, then sterilized by activating the narrow U-shaped loop electrode and scraping it against the exposed root surfaces rapidly. The freshly cut root end was rounded with a diamond stone, and the gutta percha at the apical end was resealed and sterilized by coagulation with a large round ball electrode. A small pellet of cotton was then moistened with chloroform and the damp-moist pellet was rubbed over the apex to further assure a hermetic seal of the apical gutta percha.

Bleeding was then induced in the bone defect and surgical gelatin was introduced and mixed with the blood. When the blood clotted it filled the defect and created a uniform level with the surrounding bone, thus providing a firm base for the mucogingival flap which was restored to position and immobilized by suturing along the line of incision and also through the papillae in the central and lateral embrasures. On the fifth postoperative day the patient returned for removal of the sutures. Postoperative inspection showed all the sutures intact, with distinct evidence that the coapted tissue along the line of incision was undergoing healing by primary repair. The apices of the interdental papillae also appeared to be reattaching. The tissue tone appeared quite good, despite the fact that the tissues in the surgical field still were slightly darker in color than the surrounding tissue (Case Fig. 5–1F), but greatly improved over their preoperative appearance. The sutures were removed and tincture of myrrh and benzoin was applied. The patient was seen again one week later. Healing appeared to be progressing without incidence. The biopsy report having ruled out cancer, the patient returned to her home and was not seen again by the author. However, he was kept informed of her progress by her dentist, who reported that healing had continued uneventfully and that a roentgenogram taken by him about 6 months postoperatively showed a complete bone regeneration and normal labial gingiva.

CASE 6

Poor oral hygiene, hyperemia, and hyperplasia are distinct handicaps to tissue repair that apply to electrosurgical as well as steel scalpel wounds. The healing response following electrosurgery seen in this case suggests that perhaps the sterilization of the surgical field during electrosurgery helps to minimize the handicaps.

PATIENT.   A 38-year-old white male.

HISTORY.   The maxillary left lateral incisor had required endodontic treatment one and one half years previously. The canal had been treated by a well-qualified en-

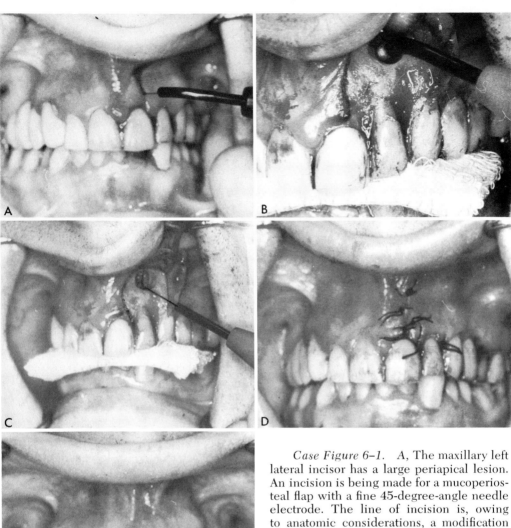

Case Figure 6–1. A, The maxillary left lateral incisor has a large periapical lesion. An incision is being made for a mucoperiosteal flap with a fine 45-degree-angle needle electrode. The line of incision is, owing to anatomic considerations, a modification of the vertico-oblique incision usually created. The incision is being made in a slightly arced direction instead of in a straight line, to avoid cutting into the maxillary labial frenum. The incision extends from the mucogingival junction over the apex of the tooth anteriorly and downward in a gentle arc and ends at the mesiogingival angle of the tooth. Oral hygiene is deplorably poor. There are many heavy deposits of plaque. Gingival tone is very poor and the tissues are severely engorged. Anterior interdental papillae are enlarged and partially detached. Despite poor tone and engorgement there is surprisingly little evidence of bleeding. B, Debridement having been completed, the gutta percha at the cut end of the root is being resealed by coagulation with a large ball electrode. C, The apical attachment of the lateral-cuspid papilla has been severed and the mucoperiosteal flap elevated and reflected, exposing a large round perforation in the labial alveolar cortex. The granulomatous debris having been removed and the apex of the tooth cut and rounded, a few fragments of tissue not removed by loop excision are being destroyed in situ by fulguration. Absence of bleeding allows the area to be thoroughly inspected. D, Bleeding is induced in the defect and powdered Gelfoam mixed with the blood; the mucoperiosteal flap has been restored and sutured into position with interrupted silk sutures through the interdental papillae and the embrasures to the palatal papillae, as well as along the line of incision. E, Three week postoperative appearance. The line of incision is fully healed and only a slightly more pink appearance denotes its location. The tissue tone in the surgical field is somewhat better than the surrounding tissue tone. The central, lateral, and cuspid are badly discolored from frequent applications of air-dried layers of tincture of myrrh and benzoin, which will disappear when the patient receives prophylaxis and maintains reasonable home care as instructed.

349

dodontist, and the x-ray appearance of the obturated canal appeared excellent. Several weeks ago he suddenly began to feel pain in the tooth while eating, and soon the pain was constant. He consulted his dentist who found on x-ray that a large periapical lesion was present around the apex of the lateral. He was referred to the author for a root-end resection.

CLINICAL EXAMINATION.   This patient was obviously negligent about maintaining good oral hygiene. There was a heavy film of plaque present on the labial and buccal tooth surfaces, and around the marginal gingivae. The latter showed symptoms of early gingivitis — reddened marginal edges and slight to moderate hyperplasia and hyperemia of the marginal gingivae. The alveolar gingiva over the root of the lateral was intact but was tender to light digital palpation.

TREATMENT.   The proposed surgical field was cleansed of plaque and prepared for surgery; infraorbital and nasopalatine block anesthesia was then administered.

A 45-degree-angle fine needle electrode was selected and cutting current output was set at 3 on the power output rheostat dial. The activated electrode was then used to incise the tissues in a vertico-oblique direction starting at the mucogingival junction and extending downward and anteriorly to the distal aspect of the papilla in the lateral-cuspid embrasure (Case Fig. 6–1A). The apical attachments of this papilla and of the papilla in the central-lateral embrasure were severed with the electrode, and the mucoperiosteal flap was elevated and reflected, revealing the periapical lesion which had destroyed a circular area of the overlying bone 0.5 cm. in diameter. The granulomatous necrotic debris was partially resected with surgical curets by manual instrumentation. Approximately 0.5 cm. of the root projecting into the defect was then resected with a fissure bur. The new root end was rounded with a small round diamond stone, and the gutta percha canal filling at the cut end was resealed by electrocoagulation with a large ball electrode (Case Fig. 6–1B). Debridement was resumed with the curets, and all but a bit of debris that was firmly wedged between the root and bone was removed manually. The remaining fragments were destroyed in situ by fulguration (Case Fig. 6–1C), without need to remove any more bone or tooth structure. The sparks were directed toward the tissue for one-second intervals followed by 10-second pause intervals to prevent cumulative heat damage.

Debridement having been completed, bleeding was encouraged in the area and powdered Gelfoam sponge was introduced and mixed with the blood. As soon as the mixture was partially clotted, the tissue flap was restored to position and sutured with interrupted silk sutures (Case Fig. 6–1D). The patient was instructed in home care and told to return on the fifth postoperative day. When the sutures were removed on the fifth day, the incised tissues gave evidence of favorable healing. The patient was seen at weekly intervals postoperatively. At the end of the third week the incised tissues appeared fully healed (Case Fig. 6–1E). From the amount of plaque present and the degree of tooth stain (exaggerated by the applications of tincture of myrrh and benzoin) it was obvious that the patient was not cooperating with regard to maintaining a reasonable degree of oral hygiene, and he was instructed to either make an effort to be more cooperative or further treatment would be pointless.

He did not return for further treatment, but his dentist informed me that a periapical film of the tooth taken about 6 months later showed complete bone regeneration in the periapical area. The patient has apparently had no further trouble with this tooth.

This case demonstrates the ability to discourage tissue proliferation and reduce proliferative tissue bulk by use of superficial spot electrocoagulation.

When proliferative tissue is coagulated superficially the coagulum serves as a protective surface cover that shields the healing tissue from mechanical, chemical, and thermal irritation while tissue repair takes place. When healing is complete the coagulum peels off spontaneously, exposing the normal repaired tissue surface.

CASE 7

PATIENT. A 34-year-old white male.

HISTORY. Approximately one year previously the maxillary cuspid was treated endodontically. Several weeks ago the patient suddenly began to feel tenderness in the apical region of the cuspid. The tenderness persisted despite lavage and massage, so he consulted his dentist. A periapical x-ray film revealed a large periapical radiolucence around the cuspid apex. He was referred for a root-end resection.

CLINICAL EXAMINATION. There was no swelling, but the areolar mucosa over the apex of the cuspid appeared darker red in color. The reddened tissue was markedly tender to even gentle palpation. The tooth was also very sensitive to percussion.

TREATMENT. The tissue was prepared and infraorbital block and palatal infiltration anesthesia was administered. A 45-degree-angle fine needle electrode was selected, cutting current was set at 3 and used to create a vertico-oblique incision for a mucoperiosteal tissue flap (Case Fig. 7–1A). The incision extended downward from the apex of the lateral incisor to the mesiogingival angle of the cuspid. The apex of the interdental papilla in the cuspid-first bicuspid embrasure was then incised to permit the tissue flap to be adequately elevated. The mucoperiosteal flap was then reflected to fully expose the apical area of the cuspid (Case Fig. 7–1B).

The labial cortex of the alveolar bone over the cuspid root apex had been almost completely destroyed, with a translucent membranous thin remnant remaining, through which a dark greenish brown mass could be seen filling the apical defect. The granulomatous debris was removed with a surgical curet. Resistantly adherent fragments of tissue were removed by resection with a fine U-shaped loop electrode with cutting current set at 4. A few fragments that resisted even loop resection were destroyed in situ by fulguration, after the pitted protruding apical end of the root had been resected with a cross-cut fissure bur and the cut end rounded with a round diamond stone. The gutta percha at the cut root end was then resealed by electrocoagulation with a ball electrode and current set at 2 on the instrument panel coagulating dial.

Debridement having been completed (Case Fig. 7–1C), bleeding was encouraged in the apical defect. Powdered Gelfoam was introduced and mixed with the blood. The mucoperiosteal flap was replaced, and the coapted margins were sutured with interrupted silk sutures and the papilla was sutured through the embrasure. Tincture of myrrh and benzoin was applied to the tissues in air-dried layers, and the patient was instructed in home care and reappointed.

He returned on the fifth postoperative day, and the sutures were removed. A slight amount of tissue proliferation had occurred at the suture sites (Case Fig. 7–1D). Small bulges of proliferative tissue were reduced to normal dimension by momentary superficial spot electrocoagulation with a small ball electrode and coagulating current output was set at 2 on the instrument panel dial (Case Fig. 7–1E). Tincture of myrrh and benzoin was then applied to the gingival tissue in air-dried layers. The patient was cautioned to continue with the regimen of postoperative care that had been prescribed and to return five days later.

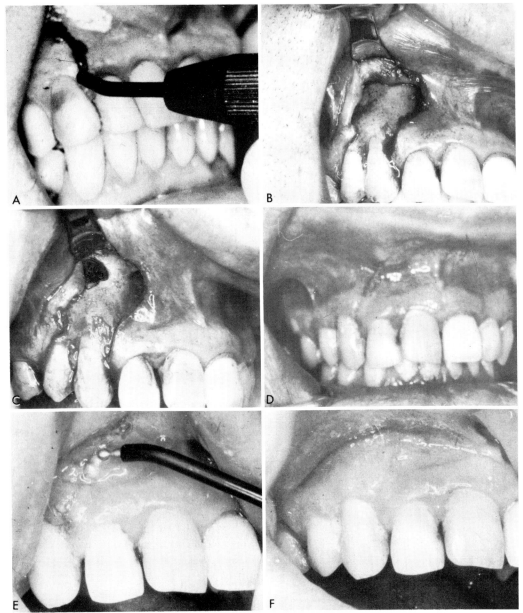

Case Figure 7–1. A, A vertico-oblique incision is being made with a 45-degree-angle fine needle electrode from the mucogingival junction over the apex of the maxillary right lateral incisor antero-posteriorly downward to the mesiogingival angle of the cuspid. B, The cuspid-bicuspid papilla has been severed from its apical attachment and the mucoperiosteal flap has been elevated and is being retracted with a tissue retractor, exposing the alveolar bone, which has been thinned out over a large apical area. The thinned bone is considerably darker in color than the normal bone. C, The parchment-thin bone has been removed and the periapical lesion thoroughly debrided. The involved apical portion of the root has been removed and the cut end has been rounded slightly, as have the edges of the bone around the defect. D, The tissues immediately after the sutures were removed. The line of incision is healing, but there is a proliferation of tissue along the upper half of the line. E, The proliferating tissue is being destroyed by careful spot coagulation with a small ball electrode and current output set at 2. F, Appearance of the tissues two weeks after coagulation of the proliferative tissue. The proliferation has disappeared and the entire line of incision is undergoing uniformly excellent repair.

When he returned, the tissue repair was found to have progressed considerably. There was no evidence of tissue proliferation and the tissue tone appeared normal. The line of incision was slightly depressed, owing to the absence of surface keratin, but primary repair appeared to be progressing satisfactorily. He was seen postoperatively at weekly intervals for three more weeks, at which time he was dismissed from further observation, since the healing which had been progressing uneventfully appeared complete (Case Fig. 7–1F). The patient was seen again four months postoperatively, at which time the bone repair was found to be complete, with no apical radiolucence.

The author has observed for many years the clinical response to superficial spot coagulation to control the tendency of repairing tissue to proliferate. Results such as in this case occur invariably unless there is a systemic underlying reason for failure of normal tissue repair. Since the proliferative tissue destruction can be pinpointed and limited exclusively to the tissue that requires treatment, the benefits derived from the electrocoagulation are not diluted by damage to adjacent normal tissue.

CASE 8

If the periapical pathology is so extensive that the root-end resection would destroy the 1:2 crown-root ratio necessary for the tooth to withstand the torque of function, the tooth must be extracted. If the pathologic condition does not involve the entire root surface circumferentially, but affects the mesial or distal surface only, it may be possible to cut the root "on the bias" at a slant that will retain enough root length of the unaffected half to retain the crown-root ratio. This case demonstrates the effectiveness of retaining the unaffected portion of the root.

PATIENT.   A 62-year-old white male.

HISTORY.   The patient, a very eminent and very busy physician, had had time for only emergency dental treatment consisting largely of very large class V cavities in the anterior maxillary teeth that had been restored with large silicate fillings. A lateral incisor broke off a few days previously. He felt tenderness in the region of the broken tooth, so he consulted his dentist. A clinical examination by the dentist revealed a fistulous orifice slightly distal to the broken lateral, and roentgenographic examination revealed two large radiolucent areas involving the lateral and cuspid. He was referred for root-end resection of the two teeth which had both been treated endodontically some years earlier.

CLINICAL EXAMINATION.   Large silicate restorations, several with leaky margins, were present in the six maxillary anterior teeth. The left lateral incisor crown was missing, but a fragment of the marginal edge of the crown and about 2 mm. of the retained root projected beyond the gingival tissue. A fistulous orifice was present almost midway between the lateral and cuspid on the labial aspect about 1.5 cm. beyond the marginal gingiva and slightly closer to the cuspid tooth.

TREATMENT.   The tissues were prepared and infraorbital block and palatal infiltration anesthesia was administered. A heavy long wire needle electrode was selected and the fistulous orifice was fulgurated (Case Fig. 8–1A) with the current output set at 8 on the power output dial. A fine 45-degree-angle needle electrode was then selected, cutting current set at 3, and the activated electrode used to make a

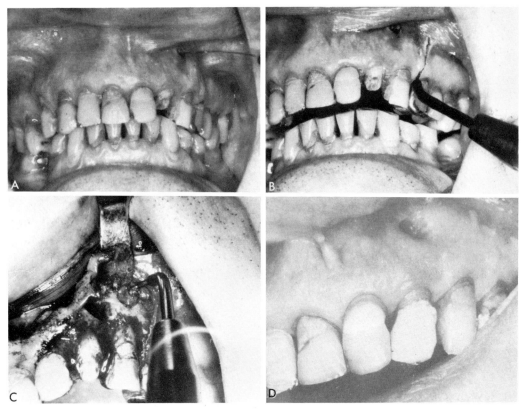

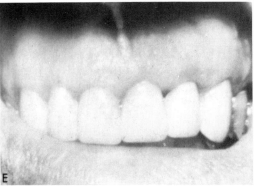

Case Figure 8–1. *A,* Preoperative appearance of maxillary left retained lateral incisor root and left cuspid. A fistula with its external orifice midway between the apices of the two teeth is being destroyed by fulguration. *B,* The fulguration having been completed, a vertico-oblique incision for a mucoperiosteal flap is being incised from the mucogingival junction downward and slightly anteriorly to the mesiogingival angle of the first bicuspid with a fine 45-degree-angle needle electrode, cutting current set at 3. *C,* The apical attachments of the papillae having been severed, the mucoperiosteal flap has been elevated and is being retracted with a tissue retractor, exposing two huge bone defects in the alveolar labial cortex over the two teeth. The apical half of the incisor retained root has been resected at a 45-degree angle "on the bias," so that as much of the root length as possible would be retained, and the granulomatous debris has been thoroughly resected. The fistulous tract has been found to communicate with this defect. There is only about 2 mm. of alveolar bone left covering the retained root. Granulomatous debris is being resected from the cuspid defect with a 45-degree-angle U-shaped loop electrode. Although there is a band of alveolar intact labial bone about 3 mm. wide remaining over the root of the cuspid, this bone is thick enough to help hold the tooth firmly. *D,* Three month postoperative result. The retained root has been restored with a temporary crown that will serve until all the anterior teeth have been restored with permanent porcelain jacket crowns. The line of incision is fully healed, but the site of the fistulous orifice is depressed, and the tissue, which had broken down soon after the surgery, is filling in by secondary granulation repair. *E,* Two year postoperative appearance of the restored mouth. The six anterior teeth have been restored with porcelain jacket crowns. The retained lateral root had been built up with a gold core and the porcelain crown was cemented to the gold core restoration, without fixation to the adjacent teeth. The lateral is now aesthetically as well as functionally useful. The defect from the fistulous lesion that had undergone secondary repair is now completely healed and there is only a barely discernible depression on the surface of the alveolar gingiva less than 1 mm. deep to mark the site. The bone repair is equally good.

354

vertico-oblique incision extending posteroanteriorly from the mucogingival fold anteriorly to the mesiogingival angle of the first bicuspid, being careful to avoid splitting the cuspid-bicuspid papilla (Case Fig. 8–1B). The apical attachments of the papillae in the embrasures on either side of the lateral and cuspid were then severed to complete the incision for a mucoperiosteal flap. The flap was elevated and retracted. This revealed two huge areas where the alveolar bone had been destroyed over the apices of the two teeth, and that the periapical defects were filled with granulomatous debris. The alveolar destruction over the lateral was so extensive that at the distal edge less than 1 mm. of bone covered the otherwise denuded root, owing in part to the alveolar recession that had occurred. The recession had denuded the cuspid of almost 1 cm. of bone and the periapical defect extended downward so far that all the bone that remained over the cuspid was a ridge that was only about 2 mm. wide in the center of the root. The bone that remained was, however, thick and apparently healthy.

The granulomatous debris in the two defects was removed mostly by curettage with surgical curets. Fragments that remained wedged between the roots and the bone were resected with narrow U-shaped loop electrodes (Case Fig. 8–1C) and such tissue fragments as this electrode was unable to remove were destroyed in situ by fulguration. Since the disease appeared to involve only the distal half of the lateral root the root resection was performed longitudinally "on the bias" rather than as a root-end resection, leaving a slender shaft of mesial half of the root intact. The cuspid apex was cut off and the remainder of the root that extended into the defect, but was not badly pitted, was curetted to remove the dead cementum and detritus. The sharp edge of the lateral was rounded slightly and the gutta percha of both teeth was coagulated at the cut areas with a ball coagulating electrode. Bleeding was induced in the two defects, and surgical gelatin was introduced and mixed with the blood, creating spongy masses that filled each defect. The tissue flap was replaced, and the margins were coapted and sutured. The respective papillae were then sutured through the embrasures to complete the immobilization of the flap. Tincture of myrrh and benzoin was applied to the surgical field and the patient was reappointed for removal of the sutures.

He returned on the fifth postoperative day. Healing appeared to be progressing favorably. The line of incision was healing by primary intention, and the fistulous site was covered with normal-looking coagulum. The sutures were removed and tincture of myrrh and benzoin was applied; the patient was cautioned to continue the postoperative regimen as directed, and he was asked to return at weekly intervals for postoperative observation. Two weeks after the sutures were removed the gingival mucosa at the fistulous site began to break down again. The deterioration appeared to be tubelike and did not extend to the rest of the tissue repair in the periapical defect. The area was anesthetized by infiltration, the new defect was irrigated with a solution of Kasdenol, then it was debrided by electrosection with a narrow U-shaped loop electrode. Bleeding was induced, and a little surgical gelatin was mixed with the blood, which formed a firm clot. A small piece of adhesive dry foil was placed over the clot and attached to the tissue with flexible collodion to provide a protective cover which remained undisturbed until he was seen again five days later. At his next visit the dry foil-collodion bandage was removed, and the site inspected. Some breakdown had again occurred, but there had apparently also been some improvement. The defect was treated by scarification at 2-week intervals and the defect gradually filled with healthy granulation tissue from underneath by secondary intention. By the end of the third month the defect was almost fully repaired; only a shallow crater remained (Case Fig. 8–1D). The root, which had been restored with a gold core and post, had been restored with a temporary crown. The restored tooth was successfully withstanding the torque of function and showed no evidence of pathological mobility. The patient was asked to return in three months for further postoperative observation. When he returned, six months after the surgery had been performed, there was a total absence of roentgenographic or clinical evidence of the original pathologic condition except for a shallow crater of less than 2 mm. depth where the secondary granulation repair had occurred, and the gingival tissue appeared completely normal in all respects. At this time the dentist proceeded to prepare the teeth for porcelain jacket crowns, which were fabricated and inserted.

The patient was seen again at 6-month intervals. At the 2-year visit the gingival tissues were in excellent condition and completely normal except for an almost imperceptible surface depression of less than 1 mm. where the fistulous site had been. The marginal gingivae were tightly adapted around the jacket crowns and the line of incision was totally indistinguishable from the adjacent tissues (Case Fig. 8–1E).

More than 10 years have elapsed since the surgery was performed, and the patient has had no trouble in all that time. Most of the credit for the successful outcome in this case really belongs to the patient, since the author had advised extraction of the retained lateral root and replacement with a fixed bridge. Fortunately the patient insisted that the attempt be made to preserve the tooth. This is another of the many clinically "hopeless" cases that have responded favorably to treatment. The author is firmly convinced that the sterilization of the surgical field as the tissue cutting is being performed is an important contributing factor.

CASE 9

Cases that appear clinically to have a hopeless prognosis frequently respond favorably to electrosurgical treatment. Two phenomena appear to be responsible for the successful treatment. One phenomenon is that, as electrosection is performed, the cutting current simultaneously sterilizes the surgical field. This increases the likelihood that the blood clot and subsequent repair tissue will not undergo deterioration due to bacterial contamination. The second phenomenon is that osteoblastic regeneration of alveolar bone appears to emanate from the periosteum. As a result even when the entire labial alveolar bone over a tooth has been destroyed by disease, complete regeneration of the lost bone and repair of periapical defects can occur.

Both phenomena are well demonstrated in this case.

PATIENT.   A 42-year-old white female.

HISTORY.   She had had a root-end resection performed on a maxillary cuspid approximately two years previously. Several weeks before she was seen by the author she began to feel pain in the tooth while eating and tenderness in the gingival tissue over the tooth. She consulted her dentist, and his roentgenographic examination revealed a large area of periapical radiolucence, apparently a surgical dead space. He referred her to the author for another root-end resection or extraction of the tooth.

CLINICAL EXAMINATION.   The marginal gingivae had receded approximately 0.5 cm. around the labial and buccal aspects of most of the teeth in the two arches. The gingival tissue over the apex of the right maxillary cuspid was swollen, and the tissue was dark red in color. A second area of swelling was present about 1 cm. above the gingival margin. A fistulous opening was present in the center of this swelling. The tooth was tender to light percussion. A sterile silver endodontic point was introduced into the fistulous orifice and directed upward until it met resistance (Case Fig. 9–1A). A roentgenogram taken with the silver probe in situ showed it to be in contact with the superior surface of a large periapical area of radiolucence.

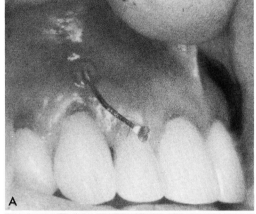
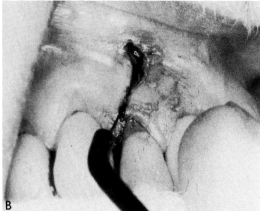
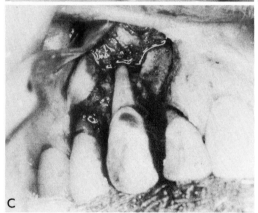

Case Figure 9–1. A, Preoperative appearance. There is a large periapical swelling over the maxillary right cuspid, and a second smaller swelling about 1 cm. above the gingival margin. This second smaller lesion has in its center the orifice of a fistulous tract. A sterile endodontic silver point has been introduced into the fistulous tract to serve as a radiopaque x-ray marker. B, Reveals the considerable gingival recession ranging from .5–1 cm. present throughout the maxilla. An activated 45 degree angle fine needle electrode is being used to create the vertico-oblique incision for a mucoperiosteal flap. The incision is being made to curve along the external mesial edge of the fistulous defect, and terminates at the distogingival angle of the lateral, carefully avoiding splitting the papilla. C, The apical attachment of the cuspid-bicuspid interdental papilla having been severed to release the tissue, the mucoperiosteal flap has been elevated, revealing a huge periapical defect filled with granulomatous debris.

TREATMENT. The ease with which the probe had penetrated suggested that the labial alveolar bone had been destroyed. However, even if the tooth would have to be extracted it would be necessary to debride the diseased tissue thoroughly, so the treatment plan was to proceed on the basis that a root-end resection would be performed and extraction reserved as a last resort.

The tissues were prepared and infraorbital regional block and palatal infiltration anesthesia was administered. A fine 45-degree-angle needle electrode was selected and cutting current output was set at 3 on the power output control. The electrode was activated and used to create a somewhat curved vertico-oblique incision for a mucoperiosteal flap, care being taken to avoid splitting the papilla (Case Fig. 9–1B). The incision was curved around the anterior edge of the fistulous tract and a second incision was performed to excise the fistulous tissue. The apical attachment of the cuspid-first bicuspid papilla was then severed with the electrode and the mucoperiosteal flap was elevated and retracted (Case Fig. 9–1C). This revealed that the entire labial alveolar bone had been destroyed and a large periapical defect filled with a fibrotic mass of tissue that appeared also to be partially granulomatous in texture.

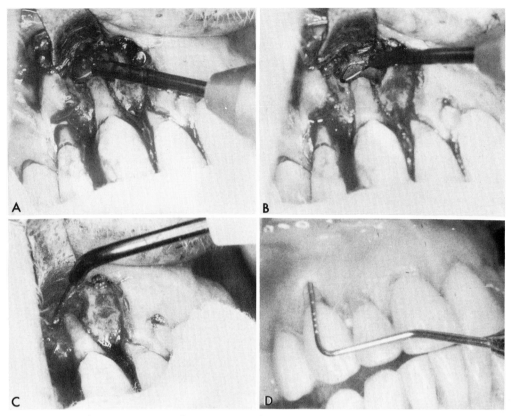

Case Figure 9–2. A, A medium (7 mm. diameter) round loop electrode has been bent slightly to provide most effective means for debridement. The activated electrode is being used to perform gross debridement. B, The major part of the granulomatous debris having been resected, the round loop is replaced with a flame shaped loop that has also been bent to a slight curvature and is being used to complete the debridement. C, Shows use of fulguration to destroy in situ a few tenaciously adherent tissue shreds the loop resection has not been able to eliminate. Note the sparks as the tissue is being carbonized in situ (arrow). D, The final postoperative result. The labial bone has undergone repair by bone regeneration. Reattachment of the gingival mucosa is verified by insertion of the tip of a periodontal probe subgingivally. The probe has penetrated to the base of the gingival sulcus, and can not penetrate further, despite enough pressure to produce marked gingival blanching.

A 7-mm. round loop electrode was selected and curved slightly to permit its use with a scooping motion in the periapical defect. Current output was increased to 5 and the activated electrode was used to debride the fibro-granulomatous tissue from the periapical lesion (Case Fig. 9–2A). Fragments of fibrous tissue remained wedged between the distal aspect of the root and the investing bone. A flame-shaped loop was curved and used to try to remove this tissue (Case Fig. 9–2B). A few remaining fragments that still remained wedged were then destroyed in situ by fulguration (Case Fig. 9–2C).

Debridement having been completed, the root apex was freshened and the sharp edge rounded with a round diamond stone to restore as much as possible a normal apical contour. The gutta percha at the apex was resealed and sterilized by coagulation with a large ball electrode. Bleeding was then induced in the periapical defect, and surgical gelatin was introduced into the area and mixed with the blood, creating a spongy mass that would provide support for the mucogingival flap and prevent it from sagging into the defect and also help to avert a surgical dead space. The flap was replaced, and the margins were coapted and sutured with interrupted silk sutures. Finally, sutures were inserted labiopalatally through the apices of the interdental papilla, tincture of myrrh and benzoin was applied to the surgical field and the patient was reappointed for removal of the sutures. The sutures were removed on the fifth postoperative day and the patient reported she had been remarkably free of postoperative reactions. She was seen at weekly intervals for one month, then reappointed for a final six month postoperative examination. When she returned the clinical condition defied detection as to where the surgery had been performed. The tissue was normal in all respects and there was no scar evidence of where the incisions had been made. The tooth was comfortable when percussed and the roentgenogram taken at that visit showed that the periapical lesion had filled with normal bone, with no evidence of the preoperative radiolucence. A periodontal probe was inserted under the free gingival margin and directed upward toward the base of the sulcus with forceful pressure. The probe penetrated to the base of the sulcus and was unable to penetrate further despite marked blanching of the tissues due to the pressure being exerted (Case Fig. 9–2D).*

CASE 10

One of the presumed drawbacks of the vertico-oblique incision is marginal and interproximal reattachment in the presence of cervical restorations or gold or ceramic crowns in the operative area. This case demonstrates that when the tissue tone is normal preoperatively, tooth alignment is good, and the flap is accurately readapted and sutured, the presence of gold cervical restorations need not be a contraindication for this technique.

This case also affords a typical example of the excellent use that can be made of electrosurgery to destroy *in situ*, or to resect diseased tissue in close proximity to the maxillary antrum, where curettage could result in an oroantral perforation.

PATIENT. A 49-year-old white male.

HISTORY. His maxillary right first bicuspid had been devitalized and root canal therapy performed approximately four months previously. The tooth suddenly became painful and sore to touch, and his face swelled slightly. His dentist x-rayed the area and found a periapical radiolucent area around the apex or apices of the devitalized tooth. The patient was referred for root amputation of one or both roots.

CLINICAL EXAMINATION. *Extraoral.* There was a slight amount of swelling in the right cheek immediately adjacent to the ala of the nose. The swollen area appeared slightly reddened.

Intraoral. The mucosa at the junction of the alveolar and areolar gingivae in the vicinity of the apex of the tooth was engorged and tender. The tooth reacted with moderate severity to light percussion. The maxillary right cuspid and first bicuspids had been restored with large cervical inlays which extended under the free gingival

---

*Occasionally the question is raised whether obliteration of the defect is caused by bone regeneration or reattachment of the epithelial attachment. Labial bone regeneration has been demonstrated experimentally; comparable proof in human patients usually is impossible. Histologically this is regrettable, but to the patient and the clinician the question is a matter of relatively inconsequential academic semantics, in view of the effectiveness and permanence of the clinical functional results.

margins of the teeth. The second bicuspid was restored with a porcelain crown with gold coping that also extended under the free margin.

Roentgenographic examination revealed a large periapical radiolucent area involving the apices of the first bicuspid.

The treatment plan was to perform the root-end surgery, then have the dentist, who planned to be present, prepare and insert a retrograde amalgam filling to seal the canals after they had been sterilized by electrocoagulation.

TREATMENT. The mouth was prepared for surgery and infraorbital block anesthesia was administered. A 45-degree-angle fine needle electrode was selected and current output set at 3.5 for electrosection. A vertico-oblique incision was made with the electrode starting high in the mucobuccal fold, over the apex of the lateral incisor, and then downward and slightly posteriorly to terminate at the mesial aspect of the cuspid (Case Fig. 10–1A).

The apical attachments of the interproximal papillae were severed with the electrode tip and the flap was elevated and retracted. This procedure revealed a bone defect in the apical region of the first bicuspid (Case Fig. 10–1B). The defect margins were trimmed smooth to enlarge the opening slightly. This revealed the apices of the first bicuspid and considerable necrotic debris. There was very little bleeding from the incision or the elevation of the flap. The necrotic debris was removed with curets and a narrow U-shaped loop electrode, then the apices were cut with a cross-cut carbide bur. There were some tenacious necrotic fragments between the two roots and also behind the palatal root, where they were inaccessible even to the loop electrode. These were destroyed *in situ* with fulgurating current (Case Fig. 10–1C). The apices had been cut on the bias for better access and visibility. The dentist proceeded to prepare cavities in the canal portions of the cut root ends, which were sharply undercut. A strip of selvage gauze was packed into the bone defect and around the roots to prevent any amalgam from dropping into the open bone defect. The retrograde cavity preparations were sterilized by electrocoagulation with a flexible cylindrical electrode. The amalgam fillings were then inserted and well condensed (Case Fig. 10–1D).

Debridement having been completed, bleeding was induced in the defect; then medicated surgical gelatin powder was deposited into the defect and mixed with the blood present. The flap was restored and the coapted margins sutured with interrupted 0000 braided silk sutures. Sutures were then inserted through the interproximal apices anteroposteriorly through to the palate and tied securely through the interproximal spaces.

The usual postoperative instructions were given and, in view of the clinical evidence of infection originally noted, Panalba antibiotic therapy was prescribed for three days.

The patient returned on the fifth postoperative day and reported very little discomfort. The healing was well advanced. The incision was healing by primary intention and was almost fully healed. Interproximal reattachment appeared to have occurred (Case Fig. 10–1E). The remarkable rate and quality of healing was verified when the sutures were removed. Healing was almost complete. Tincture of myrrh and benzoin was applied to the area and the patient was reappointed for the following week. He was seen at weekly intervals for the next three weeks, during which time the healing progressed rapidly and uneventfully. By the end of the third weekly visit, healing was virtually complete. The line of incision was fully healed and almost completely obliterated. The gingival marginal and interproximal reattachment was excellent despite the presence of the cervical restorations (Case Fig. 10–1F).

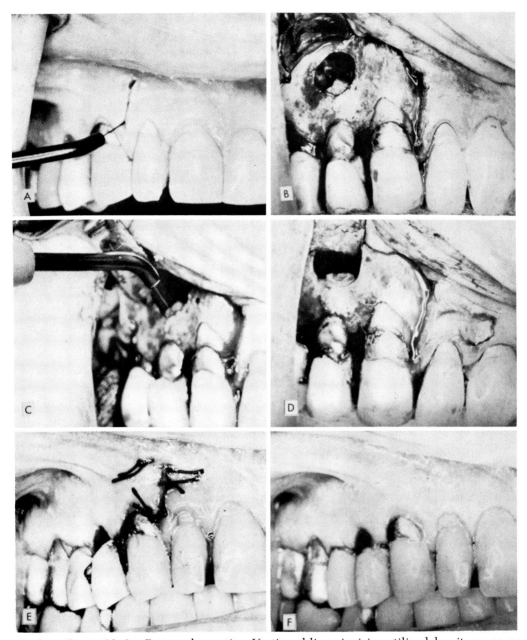

Case Figure 10–1. Root-end resection. Vertico-oblique incision utilized despite presence of large cervical inlays in cuspid and first bicuspid, and coping veneer crown on second bicuspid that extends beyond the gingival margin.

A, Incision by electrosection with fine 45-degree-angle needle electrode. Vertico-oblique incision started over apex of lateral and carried downward and posteriorly to the mesial aspect of the cuspid. The attachments of the interproximal papillae in the cuspid and bicuspid embrasures are severed. B, Flap reflected revealing perforation of buccal alveolar plate through which bicuspid apices and granulomatous detritus can be seen. Note remarkable freedom from bleeding from incision or flap retraction. C, Tenacious necrotic fragments between the apices are fulgurated with moderately fine needle electrode. D, Retrograde filling has been inserted into the apex, which has been cut on the bias. E, Appearance on the fifth postoperative day. Tissue tone excellent; healing by primary union is well advanced; interproximal reattachment appears favorable. F, Appearance three weeks postoperatively. Healing is virtually complete. The line of incision is fully healed and almost completely obliterated. Gingival marginal reattachment is excellent despite presence of the cervical restorations.

CASE 11

This case is an example of local factors that may make it necessary to use a semilunar incision instead of the vertico-oblique type.

PATIENT.   A 53-year-old white female.

HISTORY.   She had suddenly developed extra- and intraoral swelling, and a maxillary cuspid abutment tooth for a fixed bridge restoration had become mobile and sore to the touch.

Her dentist established drainage on the labial aspect with a stab incision and inserted a selvage gauze drain. Because of the presence of a cast gold crown on the tooth he made no attempt to establish drainage through the old root canal, filled many years previously. The patient was placed on massive antibiotic therapy and was referred for the root-end resection. The treatment plan provided for insertion by the dentist of a retrograde amalgam apical filling at the time of surgery to seal the apex.[30]

CLINICAL EXAMINATION.   *Extraoral.*   Negative.

Intraoral.   An oval granulomatous mass of scar repair tissue was seen bulging from the site of recent drainage (Case Fig. 11–1A). The mass was located on the labial aspect of the left maxillary cuspid near the mucolabial fold of an abnormally short alveolar ridge. The cuspid was quite mobile.

Roentgenographic examination revealed extensive periapical radiolucence around the cuspid root. The root lengths of the teeth appeared normal despite the short alveolar ridge height.

TREATMENT.   The operative field was prepared for surgery and anesthetized with an infraorbital block and palatal infiltration. A medium-sized round loop electrode was selected and current output set at 6 for electrosection. The bulging mass of scar tissue was reduced to the level of the adjacent normal tissue with a wiping stroke of the electrode, revealing a narrow slit base from which it had emerged. The loop was replaced with a fine 45-degree needle electrode and the cutting current was reduced to 3.5 to perform the incision. A semilunar incision was made immediately superior to the slit defect. This incision, made with a single wiping stroke of the electrode, extended from the left central incisor to the left second bicuspid. A second, paralleling incision was made immediately beneath the slit defect, thereby dissecting it out.

The flap was retracted upward, exposing the alveolar bone plate. A perforation was visible over the apex of the cuspid. Two millimeters of the root end were cut off with a cross-cut carbide fissure bur, then the cut apical end was beveled and rounded.

Case Figure 11–1.   Root-end resection utilizing semilunar incision, necessitated by presence of an extruding mass of proliferating hypertrophic tissue.

A, Preoperative view. A bulging mass of proliferating scar tissue projects from site of a recent stab incision for drainage of an acute periapical abscess. B, Incision has been made by dissecting out the remainder of the hypertrophic mass. After debridement of necrotic debris from bone defect, fragments lying distal to the root are fulgurated to avoid need to reduce the length of the root, which would be required to permit other methods of instrumentation at that site. C, Debridement complete, root end trimmed smooth and cut on bias for insertion of retrograde amalgam filling. D, Immediate suturing of wound with interrupted silk sutures. E, Appearance of tissues on fifth postoperative day, with sutures *in situ*. Healing is progressing favorably by primary union. A very light superficial coagulum is present along the line of incision. F, Appearance three months postoperatively. Healing is complete. There is no evidence of cicatricial contraction, and there has been no loss of vestibular height. The tissue tone is normal, and there is virtually no evidence of scar tissue.

teeth is much more difficult and hazardous and is far from routine. The reason for the difference between them is anatomic.

There is a degree of risk of accidental perforation into the nasal fossa or the maxillary antrum inherent in the procedure, but they can be readily visualized on the roentgenogram and the relation of the root of the affected tooth to these structures can easily be established, so that unless the periapical lesion has perforated into and communicates with these anatomic sites, the risk of accidental perforation is inconsequential if the operator is careful and skillful.

The fact that the labial-buccal maxillary cortical plate is very thin is the main reason why the risk is minimal. The periapical disease often perforates the cortical bone, making it a very simple matter to pinpoint the site of the lesion. Enlarging the opening to create a surgical window in the bone for the root-end resection can easily be done with a rongeur forceps. If the cortex has not been perforated by the lesion, it usually has been thinned out sufficiently to be translucent and darker in appearance than the surrounding bone, simplifying the location of the exact site for the surgical window, and the bone can be cut easily with a round bur to do so. In either event the ability to establish the precise site for the bone window greatly minimizes the risk of accidental perforation into the fossa or antrum.

The situation is definitely not as favorable in the mandible. The labial-buccal cortical bone is thick and very dense, and rarely does the lesion perforate through this cortex. Locating the precise site for the surgical window through the bone is far more difficult and is easily missed. When this is in the cuspid-bicuspid area the mental nerve plexus that emerges from the canal and extends anteriorly in that area creates a decided risk of severing the nerve and causing a prolonged paresthesia of the lip. If the affected tooth is a molar, there is a distinct danger of accidentally perforating into the mandibular canal, which can cause postoperative complications ranging from paresthesia of the inferior alveolar nerve distribution to development of an amputation neuroma (see chapter on major oral surgery).

The most effective way to avoid such complications is to establish the precise site of the lesion before attempting surgery, then to exercise great care in making the incision for a mucoperiosteal flap in the cuspid-bicuspid region to avoid injury to the mental nerve plexus, and equal care in elevating and reflecting the flap after it has been cut to avoid accidentally tearing the nerve or blood vessel that emerges from the mental canal.

The author recommends use of a radiopaque marker to help establish the precise location of the lesion. In the cuspid-bicuspid area the flap can first be incised and reflected, then a round bur used to cut a shallow indentation into the surface of the bone into which a speck of BIP paste (formula in the chapter on medication) is placed immediately prior to taking the x-ray film. Localization of the molar lesion can be performed in an identical manner, unless for some reason it may appear desirable to establish the exact site before incising the mucoperiosteal flap, in which event the surface of the tissue must be thoroughly dried before placement of the BIP paste, and then the cheek must be kept away from the tissue while the x-ray is being taken.

The radiopaque marker makes it possible to pinpoint the precise location of the periapical lesion and, even more important, to orient the affected tooth apex with the mental canal and mandibular canal to assure against accidental perforation.

It has been the author's experience that the best way to avoid injury to the mental nerve is to begin the incision at the mesial aspect of the cuspid and direct the incision anteriorly in an arclike direction instead of vertico-obliquely. The incision may be started at the mesiogingival angle of the cuspid and carried downward toward the base of the buccal vestibule, or begun at the lower level and directed upward in an arclike direction toward the mesiogingival angle of the cuspid, as clinical conditions and the surgeon's judgment dictate.

Creating the incision in an arc instead of vertico-obliquely assures that the incision will be anterior to the anteriormost portion of the mental nerve plexus that emerges from the mental foramen in an anterior direction, thus avoiding surgical trauma to the nerve. If the mucoperiosteal flap that is thus created is elevated from the bone and rotated posteriorly carefully, the flap displacement can be performed without mechanical injury to the nerve. The alveolar bone having been exposed, the slight depression can be created with a round bur, the BIP paste inserted as the radiopaque marker, and the roentgenographic localization achieved without difficulty. The following case demonstrates this technique for minimizing the risk of accidental surgical injury to the mental nerve.

CASE 12

PATIENT. A 43-year-old white female.

HISTORY. She had had her mandibular right first bicuspid devitalized about one year ago. About one month ago she began to feel discomfort in the tooth. The discomfort became progressively more distressing so she consulted her dentist. He x-rayed the tooth, found a periapical radiolucent area, and referred her to the author for a root-end resection.

CLINICAL EXAMINATION. The gingival tissue appeared normal and there was no swelling or other clinical evidence of disease except the tenderness of the tooth to even light percussion. Another x-ray of the tooth confirmed the presence of the periapical radiolucent area.

TREATMENT. The tissues were prepared and anesthetized by inferior alveolar block injection. A 45-degree-angle fine needle electrode was activated with cutting current set at 3 and used to create an anterior arcing incision in the gingival mucosa extending from the base of the buccal vestibule upward to the mesiogingival angle of the cuspid (Case Fig. 12–1A). The apex of the cuspid-first bicuspid interdental papilla was severed with the electrode to permit elevation of the mucoperiosteal flap. The shape and location of the incision assured that the mental nerve plexus would not be injured, and careful elevation and reflection of the incised tissue flap was performed without traumatizing the nerve. This exposed the cortical bone which was intact and offered no visual evidence of the exact location of the periapical lesion.

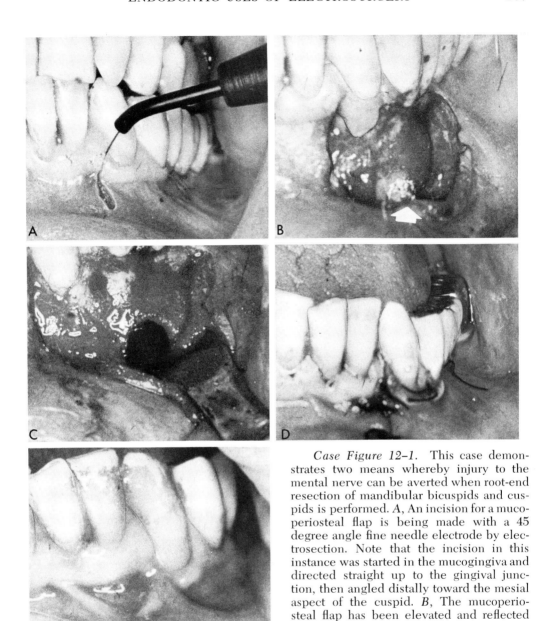

Case Figure 12–1. This case demonstrates two means whereby injury to the mental nerve can be averted when root-end resection of mandibular bicuspids and cuspids is performed. *A*, An incision for a mucoperiosteal flap is being made with a 45 degree angle fine needle electrode by electrosection. Note that the incision in this instance was started in the mucogingiva and directed straight up to the gingival junction, then angled distally toward the mesial aspect of the cuspid. *B*, The mucoperiosteal flap has been elevated and reflected from the bone and a shallow depression has been cut into the cortical surface of the mandible with a large round bur at a point that had been determined roentgenologically to be the site of the periapical lesion, which appeared to be midway between the cuspid and bicuspid. Some BIP paste has been inserted into the depression to serve as a radiopaque marker to verify that the exact site for the surgery has been established. *C*, The x-ray film having confirmed the site, the window through the bone has been cut and the affected apex has been cut off and rounded, leaving a surgically clean opening into the jawbone. *D*, Appearance of the tissues immediately after completion of the suturing. *E*, Appearance of the tissues one month postoperatively. The tissues are fully healed and firm, with excellent tone. Except for the plaque accumulation on the teeth, due to lack of toothbrushing, it is difficult to find the incision site. Note: the discoloration of the teeth is due to the tincture of myrrh and benzoin that had been applied frequently during the postoperative period, which has stained adherent plaque.

A shallow indentation was made in the surface of the bone with a large round bur at the site suggested by the roentgenogram, and a small quantity of BIP paste was inserted into the depression (Case Fig. 12–1B). The roentgenogram taken with the radiopaque marker confirmed that this was in fact the exact site of the periapical lesion and not the mental foramen.

The bur was then used to perforate through the cortex and open a window through which the root-end resection could be performed. The granulomatous debris was removed partly with a small surgical curette and mostly with a 45-degree-angle medium-width U-shaped loop electrode, especially after the pitted, eroded apex of the tooth was cut off with a cross cut fissure bur. The cut end was rounded with a round diamond stone and the gutta percha at the cut end was resealed by electrocoagulation with a ball coagulating electrode. When the debridement was completed (Case Fig. 12–1C), powdered surgical gelatin was introduced into the defect and mixed with the blood, forming a spongy mass that filled the cavity without compression. The tissue flap was restored and sutured with interrupted silk sutures (Case Fig. 12–1D). The clot of blood and gelating powder provided a firm support for the tissue so that it did not sag into the defect. The sutures were removed on the fifth postoperative day, and healing progressed rapidly and uneventfully, except that traction from a high muscle attachment slightly anterior to the cuspid lowered the mesiogingival level of the marginal gingiva at angle of the cuspid about 1 or 2 mm. The gingival tissue was fully healed without a scar, and the only clinical evidence that the patient had undergone treatment was discoloration of plaque on some of the teeth from the applications of tincture of myrrh and benzoin (Case Fig. 12–1E).

Broken Instruments; Accidental Perforations

The technique described for performing root-end resection and retrograde amalgam filling of the cut apex can also be advantageously employed for treatment of cases involving broken instrument fragments that are impacted at the apical end of root canals and that cannot be displaced downward. In such a position they prevent proper debridement, sterilization and filling of the canals. In these cases the canal may be throroughly prepared as far up as the impacted fragment will permit, and the filling inserted after the apex has been resected.

If the broken instrument fragment involves *less* than one third the total root length, the entire involved portion can be cut off without unduly jeopardizing the stability of the tooth. The new apex can then be rounded off with diamond stones or round burs. If the canal has been filled with gutta-percha the apex can be sealed by electrocoagulation with a ball electrode. Regardless of the nature of the filling material, the apex can also be sealed effectively by preparing an undercut recess for insertion of a retrograde amalgam filling.

If the broken instrument fragment involves *more* than one third the total root length, resection of the entire involved portion becomes impractical, since this would create an inadequate crown-root ratio with resultant abnormal functional torque stresses. In such cases it is advisable to remove a safe amount of the apex, cutting the segment on the bias at an approximate

45 degree angle, with the inferior border on the anterior surface of the tooth. Vibration created as the carbide bur or knife-edged diamond stone hits the impacted metal sometimes jars the metal loose and permits the displacement of the fragment downward through the canal. If the fragment remains firmly impacted, a trench can be cut around it with a small, round or inverted cone bur so that some of the fragment projects upward out of the trench. The projecting portion may then be able to be grasped with a curved mosquito hemostat and removed by pulling it upward out of the canal. If it still cannot be displaced, the projecting portion can be ground down to the base of the trench with a small diamond stone, and an undercut cavity prepared in the apex for insertion of a retrograde amalgam filling to seal the apex.

When the lateral wall of a canal is accidentally perforated and the canal is then filled, some of the filling material usually escapes through the perforation into the surrounding tissues. This material is likely to produce a foreign-body reaction. Necrotic debris which usually results from foreign-body reaction to projecting filling material can be removed easily from relatively inaccessible areas by use of slender loop electrodes bent and shaped to meet the particular needs of the specific case.

CASE 13

This case demonstrates a method of treatment by electrosurgery of root perforations in normally inaccessible areas.

PATIENT. A 34-year-old white woman.

HISTORY. Her mandibular right first molar had been devitalized as a preliminary to coronal reconstruction of the tooth with a cast gold crown. The dentist had accidentally perforated through the medial wall of the distal root, but he proceeded to fill the canals with gutta-percha points and chlora-percha. Shortly thereafter a moderately acute foreign-body reaction occurred; the tooth became somewhat sensitive to pressure and slightly mobile. She was referred for surgical correction of the defect.

CLINICAL EXAMINATION. *Extraoral.* Negative.

Intraoral. The gingival mucosa around the mandibular right first molar appeared normal. The tooth, however, was slightly mobile and somewhat sensitive to digital pressure and percussion with an instrument. The cast crown restoration was very well adapted to the tooth margins.

Roentgenographic examination revealed that practically the entire coronal portion of the tooth including the pulp chamber had been built up with a cast gold core. The casting projected downward approximately 1 mm. into the mesial root canal and approximately 3 mm. into the distal root canal. The latter projection was positioned more vertically than the root itself, which slanted at about a 30 degree angle from the vertical posteriorly. At the junction in the distal root between the distal projection and the medial aspect of the canal, approximately 3 mm. below the bifurcation, a considerable amount of radiolucence was noticed. A perforation of the medial aspect of the root was clearly visible. The radiolucence of interseptal bone extended about 2 mm. below the site of perforation.

TREATMENT. The operative field was prepared and anesthesia administered by inferior alveolar regional block. A 45-degree-angle fine needle electrode was selected and cutting current output was set at 3.5 on the selector dial. A specially designed wire frame was inserted to retract the cheeks and lips, and a vertico-oblique incision was performed by electrosection. The incision was started at the distogingival angle of the first bicuspid and extended downward and slightly posteriorly to the mucobuccal fold in the approximate center of the second bicuspid region (Case Fig. 13–1A).

The flap was undermined with a periosteal elevator, reflected from the underlying bone and retracted downward and posteriorly in order to expose the buccal alveolar plate. The overlying bone was so thin that a small round area over the mesial root of the tooth had lifted away with the flap. The bone in the interradicular area appeared somewhat discolored. This bone was removed with a round bur, creating a window through the cortical bone (Case Fig. 13–1B).

A long, slender U-shaped loop electrode was selected and contoured to form a slight curve. The electrode was bent to provide easier entry into the bone defect. The necrotic debris was removed from the bone defect by electrosection applied with a scooping motion of the loop (Case Fig. 13–1C). A perforation on the medial surface of the distal root became visible. Gutta-percha could be seen projecting through the perforation. The excess gutta-percha was removed; the perforation was sealed over by electrocoagulating the area with a small ball electrode which was applied to the gutta-percha (Case Fig. 13–1D).

Thorough debridement was performed and the crest of the interseptal bone was curetted smooth. The defect was filled with a mixture of despeciated cultured bone paste and medicated gelatin powder which was then mixed with blood present in the area. The incised margins were coapted and sutured with 0000 interrupted braided silk sutures (Case Fig. 13–1E). Cosa-Tetrastatin antibiotic therapy was prescribed, to be taken every six hours for three days, and the customary postoperative directions were given, including recommendation of dietary supplements.

The patient returned on the fifth postoperative day for removal of the sutures. The gingival incision appeared almost fully healed by primary union, and the tissue tone was excellent (Case Fig. 13–1E). The sutures were removed, tincture of myrrh and benzoin applied, and the patient was instructed to continue the postoperative regimen until her next visit. She returned one week later. By that time healing was almost complete. Tincture of myrrh and benzoin was applied topically. She returned at weekly intervals; by the end of the fifth week the line of incision was fully healed and clinically invisible. The tissue tone was excellent, although a slight hyperemia of the interproximal papilla between the two bicuspids was noted. The patient was instructed to use the rubber stimulator tip of her toothbrush to massage the interproximal papillae, and to return again the following week.

When she returned as requested, the hyperemia was no longer visible and the papillae all looked normal. She was instructed to return in three months for further postoperative observation. When she was seen at this final visit, there was no longer any visible evidence of where the incision had been and the marginal gingivae of the teeth were firmly reattached. The tissue tone was excellent (Case Fig. 13–1F). Roentgenographic examination revealed reasonably favorable evidence of bone regeneration in the formerly radiolucent area.

It is not always necessary to perform root-end resection to eliminate periapical granulomatous debris. In cases where there are no undercuts into which the necrotic tissue can invaginate and the apex is easily accessible,

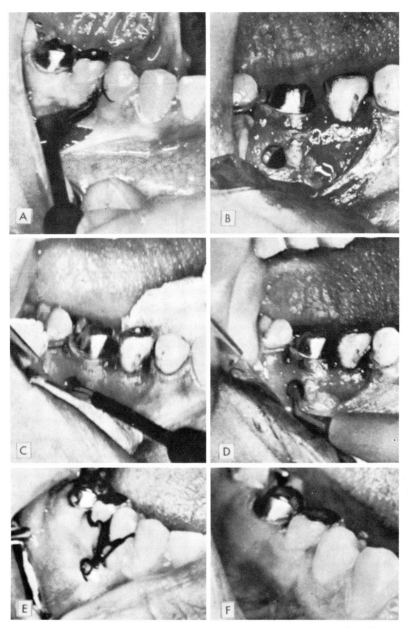

Case Figure 13–1.   Repair of root perforation, with intraradicular alveolar deterioration. *A*, Profuse bleeding as incision is performed. *B*, Bleeding had been brought under control by coagulation. Flap reflected and small bone defect enlarged. The perforation of the medial surface of the distal root of the first molar can be seen as a white area along distal margin of the bone window. *C*, Necrotic debris removed by curets, and inaccessible fragments are scooped out with a slender, curved U-shaped loop electrode. *D*, Debridement completed, the gutta-percha at the perforation site is sterilized and sealed with a long-neck small ball electrode.

E, Appearance of the tissues on the fifth postoperative day. The tissues appear almost fully healed by primary union. Interproximal reattachment appears excellent. The tissue tone is excellent. *F*, Appearance of tissues four months postoperatively. Healing is complete and there is no visible clinical evidence of where the incision had been made.

periapical debridement by curettage may suffice. In such cases the surgical technique is basically the same as has been described for the resections. Use of electrocoagulation is often particularly advantageous in such cases in order to assure thorough destruction of occasional adherent granulomatous tissue shreds that resist displacement by curettage. The latter often can be performed more efficiently with loop electrodes than with cold-steel curets.

It seems likely that at least some of the cases that have been described might not have been performed with such efficiency, facility, quality, or rate of repair if instrumentation other than electrosurgery had been employed.

Intangible Factors Involved in Root-End Resection Failures

The root-end resection is a simple surgical procedure. Under normal conditions if the tangible factors relating to the efficiency of the resection that were enumerated earlier in this chapter are meticulously observed a successful outcome of treatment is assured, barring postoperative secondary infection.

If these tangible factors have not been observed treatment failure is predictable but preventable. But when there are intangible factors present that defy preoperative detection the failure of treatment is unpredictable and cannot be averted.

Undiagnosed, unsuspected systemic disease that precludes normal healing is such an intangible factor. The difficulty of accurate roentgenographic diagnosis of three-dimensional pathologic tissue from a one-dimensional x-ray film is another of the disruptive intangible factors, especially when eye-arresting disease is present and is in the maxilla, which, owing to the confusing welter of anatomic configurations, is at best difficult to interpret roentgenographically.

CASE 14

This case is an example of the diagnostic limitations of the roentgenogram and the unexpected complications that may remain unrevealed even after the tissue flap is reflected. Roentgenographs reveal periapical and lateral bone loss, but if the loss occurs along the labial or palatal (lingual) aspect of the tooth it may remain unrevealed. Similarly, incomplete vertical or oblique fractures of roots often cannot be seen on the roentgenogram due to superimposition of sound radiopaque structure. Indistinct oro-antral fistulous tracts that are unsuspected are also likely to escape detection.

PATIENT. A 38-year-old white male.

HISTORY. A root-end resection had been performed on his maxillary left central incisor two years previously. The result had seemed to be satisfactory until a few days prior to referral when he suddenly noticed a small "pimple" on the gum over this tooth and that the tooth seemed to be becoming loose. His dentist x-rayed the area and found that periapical breakdown had recurred and apparently was responsible for a fistulous orifice on the labial gingiva. The old root canal appeared to be inadequately condensed. The patient was referred for endodontic surgery, with a retrograde amalgam filling to be performed by the dentist at the time of surgery.

CLINICAL EXAMINATION. *Extraoral.* Negative.

Intraoral. There was a fistulous orifice present on the labial aspect of the left central incisor about 0.5 cm. above the gingival margin (Case Fig. 14–1A). Roentgenographic examination revealed periapical radiolucence (Case Fig. 14–1B).

TREATMENT. The mouth was prepared for surgery, and infraorbital regional block anesthesia supplemented by infiltration in the midline was administered. A long heavy needle electrode was inserted into the coagulating electrode handpiece and current output was set at 8 for fulguration. The fistula was thoroughly fulgurated with the electrode kept in constant motion until the surface was carbonized. A fine 45-degree-angle needle electrode was selected and current output set at 3.5 for electrosection. The electrode was applied to the tissues, and with a light wiping motion an incision almost vertical in direction was made. The incision was started in the mucolabial fold over the center of the lateral incisor and extended downward and slightly forward to the mesioproximal angle of the gingival margin of the lateral. There was virtually no bleeding as a result of the incision (Case Fig. 14–2A). When the tissue flap was undermined and reflected from the bone some bleeding occurred, but this was readily halted by pressure applied with a sterile gauze sponge. The flap was retracted posteriorly and kept out of the operative field by tying it firmly in a posterior direction to the cuspid with a silk suture.

When the operative field was fully exposed to view it revealed that all the labial alveolar bone had been lost except a small spur shaped like half of a cast clasp arm. This bone fragment embraced the tooth on its distal surface at a point midway between the gingival margin and the apex. The remainder of the root was completely denuded of bone and fully visible. The patient was informed of the almost complete loss of bone, advised that the prognosis appeared hopeless, and that extraction was indicated. He insisted, however, that since the root-end resection had been started he preferred to attempt to save the tooth rather than to extract it forthwith, and was willing to take the chance that it might succeed, knowing that it was a calculated risk.

All the necrotic granulomatous tissue was resected with curets and narrow U-shaped loop electrodes (Case Fig. 14–2B). The apex was cut on the bias, creating an approximate 25-degree angle, posteroanteriorly, with the highest point at the palatal aspect of the root. The freshly cut root end was beveled and rounded; then the root was isolated by packing selvage gauze into the bone defect. The patient's dentist then proceeded to prepare the apical end for insertion of a retrograde amalgam filling.[21] After the cavity was sufficiently undercut it was sterilized by electrocoagulation (Case Fig. 14–2C). The dentist then inserted and thoroughly condensed the amalgam filling (Case Fig. 14–2D).

The selvage gauze, which had served to prevent amalgam particles from being deposited into the bone defect, was then removed and the cavity was filled with a mixture of cultured despeciated bone paste and medicated gelatin powder. These were thoroughly incorporated with blood that had been induced to flow in the cavity. The flap was restored to position and the coapted margins sutured with interrupted 0000 braided silk sutures. Cosa-Tetrastatin was prescribed, four times a day for four days, and the patient was given full postoperative instructions.

He returned on the fifth postoperative day for removal of the sutures. The tissue repair under the circumstances appeared nothing short of remarkable. The fulgurated

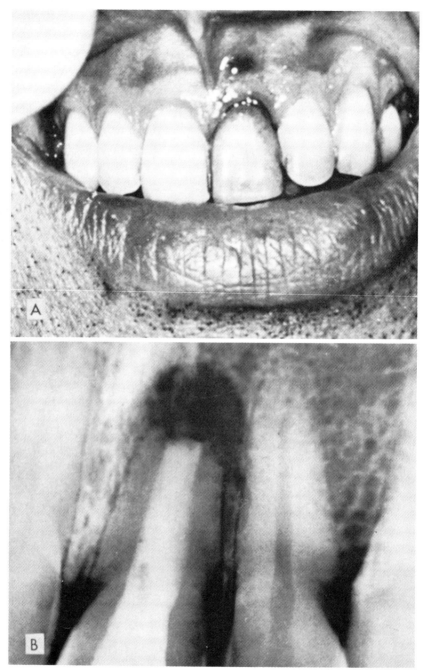

Case Figure 14-1. Root-end resection of tooth with fistulous orifice and large periapical lesion or surgical dead space following unsuccessful prior endodontic surgery. *A*, Clinical view of mouth showing fistulous orifice about 1 cm. above the gingival margin. The marginal gingiva is hyperemic and slightly detached. *B*, Roentgenogram reveals large periapical radiolucent area. There appears to be evidence of apical resorption, and root canal filling is poorly condensed.

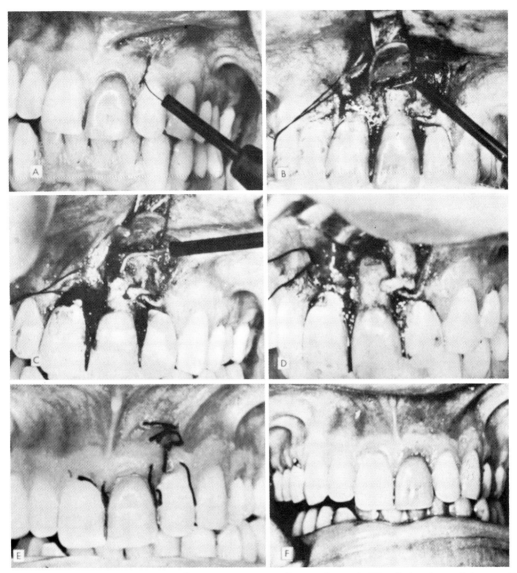

Case Figure 14–2. Root-end resection: surgical procedure. *A*, Fistula has been fulgurated. Vertico-oblique incision with a fine 45-degree-angle needle electrode is started high in labial vestibule over apex of the lateral and terminated at the mesiogingival angle of the lateral. *B*, Flap has been reflected and tied posteriorly, revealing almost total loss of labial alveolar bone. Two bony projections hug the mesial and distal aspects of the root like short clasp arms. Extensive necrotic debris is resected with a narrow U-shaped loop electrode. *C*, Debridement has been completed. Preparation in apical end of the root for retrograde amalgam filling is sterilized by electrocoagulation with a cylindrical electrode. *D*, A retrograde amalgam filling has been inserted at the apex and well condensed. *E*, Appearance of tissues on fifth postoperative day. Fulgurated area of fistula granulating satisfactorily and covered with a light layer of healthy coagulum. Line of incision is healing by primary intention. Interproximal papillae appear to be reattaching satisfactorily. Tissue tone normal. *F*, Appearance in sixth postoperative week. Incision completely healed and almost imperceptible. Interproximal reattachment complete. Tissue tone excellent except for slight marginal hyperemia. Unfortunately this evidence of repair is not a true index of the repair status. The labial gingiva has again become detached from the tooth, proliferative submucous tissue has reappeared, and although the original fistula site is now fully healed a new fistulous orifice appears to be forming about 3 mm. superiorly and slightly distal to the former site. Obviously the healing that had begun so favorably has broken down, and the tooth will have to be extracted.

area was filled with granulation that was covered with a thin layer of healthy coagulum. The tissue tone appeared excellent and the line of incision appeared almost fully healed by primary intention (Case Fig. 14–2E).

The sutures were removed and the patient was instructed to return at weekly intervals for postoperative follow-up observation. For six weeks the outcome appeared completely successful (Case Fig. 14–2F). Then suddenly the tissue immediately over the root end deteriorated and a fistulous orifice reappeared. It was destroyed by fulguration, and a French sliding-flap closure of the defect was attempted. The plastic repair also failed and the tooth had to be extracted.

Inasmuch as the initial healing response of the gingival tissue had been excellent, but the repair process broke down a few days later, it appeared that some factor unrelated to the extensive alveolar destruction and large periapical lesion might perhaps be responsible for the unfavorable delayed reaction. With this in mind, before extracting the tooth the roentgenogram was carefully re-examined under magnification, with special attention paid to the bone beyond the periapical lesion and the tooth.

The anatomic configurations of the maxillary bone are irregular and confusing, but close scrutiny revealed a thin black line extending upward from the superior edge of the defect to and apparently through the floor of the maxillary sinus. This suggested an oro-antral fistulous communication that would account for the delayed breakdown after initial favorable tissue repair. After the tooth was extracted and the granulomatous debris removed by curettage, a flexible silver lachrymal probe was inserted into the defect and directed upward. After some probing exploration the silver probe suddenly penetrated upward into the antral cavity. To assure normal healing of the tooth socket coagulating current was applied to the silver probe with a ball electrode to destroy the fistulous tract.

Postoperative healing of the extraction site progressed without incident. Perhaps if the oro-antral fistula had been observed initially and the coagulation of the fistulous tract performed during the endodontic surgery, the outcome of treatment might have been successful despite the extensive alveolar bone loss. But this case was a good example of not being able to see the trees for the forest, owing largely to the limitations that lack of three-dimensional visualization places on x-ray interpretation.

The endodontic surgical procedure failed to save this tooth. But the initial tissue response to the electrosurgery was an excellent example of the quality of healing that may result even when local conditions are scarcely conducive to ideal repair.

The case previously reviewed demonstrated the use of fulguration to destroy a fistulous orifice and tract prior to surgical incision of a mucoperiosteal flap to expose the periapical area. The case that is about to be reviewed demonstrates the advantageous use of fulguration to eliminate undesirable periapical disease that would be inaccessible to instrumentation without additional resection of bone and/or tooth structure that would jeopardize the successful outcome of the case.

FOOTNOTE REFERENCES

1. Stewart, G. G.: Preliminary report on penicillin in root canal therapy. J.A.D.A., 33:1281, Oct., 1946.
2. Bender, I. B.: Penicillin in root canal therapy, a report of 53 cases. J.A.D.A., 34:99, Jan., 1947.
3. Grossman, L. I.: Treatment of infected pulpless teeth with penicillin. J.A.D.A., 37:141, Aug., 1948.

4. Grossman, L. I., and Stewart, G. G.: An effective penicillin-streptomycin suspension for endodontic treatment. Oral Surg., Oral Med., & Oral Path., 2:374, March, 1949.
5. Grossman, L. I.: Polyantibiotic treatment of pulpless teeth. J.A.D.A., 43:265, Sept., 1951.
6. Grossman, L. I.: Root Canal Therapy. 4th ed., Philadelphia, Lea & Febiger, 1955, pp. 249–281.
7. Thoma, K. H., Holland, D. J., and Rounds, C. E.: The use of antibiotics in mixed infections. Am. J. Orth. & Oral Surg., 33:5, 337, May, 1947.
8. Oringer, M. J.: Use of drugs and their effects on tissue repair. J. Dent. Med., 3:60–69, 1948.
9. Behrman, S. J.: The development of antibiotic-resistant organisms: its significance to the dentist. N.Y.D.J., 21:297, 1955.
10. Jawetz, S. J.: The rational use of antimicrobial agents: reason versus emotion in chemotherapy. Oral Surg., Oral Med., & Oral Path., 8:982, 1955.
11. Lane, S. L.: A review of current opinion on the hazards of indiscriminate antibiotic therapy in dental practice. Oral Surg., Oral Med., & Oral Path., 9:952–961, Sept., 1956.
12. Seltzer, S.: Verbal communication; lecture, Midtown Dental Society, N.Y., 1960.
13. Watanabe, T., and Fukasawa, T.: Episome-mediated transfer of drug resistance in Enterobacteriaceae. II. Elimination of resistance factors with acridine dyes. J. Bacteriol., 81:679–683, 1961.
14. Kabins, S. A., and Cohen, S.: Resistance-transfer factor in Enterobacteriaceae. New Eng. J. Med., 275:248–252, 1968.
15. Kabins, S. A., and Cohen, S.: Unusual patterns of tetracycline resistance in Shigellae mediated by resistance-transfer factors. Antimicrob. Agents & Chemother., 1968, pp. 25–29.
16. Parris, L., Kapsimalis, P., Cobe, H. H., and Evans, R.: Effects of temperature changes on sealing quality of temporary filling materials. Oral Surg., Oral Med., & Oral Path., 17:771–778, June, 1964.
17. Ogus, W. I.: Sterilizing root canals by desiccation: electrosurgery (presenting the work of M. K. Baklor). Am. J. Orth. & Oral Surg., 27:185, 1941.
18. Tomura, J.: High frequency currents — dental pulp and root canal. Dent. Abstr., 1:645, 1956.
19. Kjaer, E. W.: The use of high frequency currents in root canal treatment. Dent. Practit., 6:274, 1956.
20. Oringer, M. J.: Electrosurgery in Dentistry. 1st ed., Philadelphia, W. B. Saunders Co., 1962, pp. 68–94.
21. Albert, H.: Personal communication to the author.
22. Synott, E. C., Scher, E. A., and Keith, J. E.: Some clinical applications of a high frequency current in dental practice. Irish Dent. Rev., July, 1959.
23. Kennedy, D. J.: Root amputation — conservative surgical therapy. N.Y.D.J., 17:251, June–July, 1951.
24. Luks, S.: Root canal therapy. J.A.D.A., 41:184, Aug., 1950.
25. Salman, I.: Roentgenographic changes following root amputation: report of 100 cases. Dent. Digest, 38:356, Oct., 1932.
26. Wakefield, B. G.: Root canal therapy and resection technique. Oral Surg., Oral Med., & Oral Path., 3:743, June, 1950.
27. Noyes, F. B., and Thomas, N. G.: A Textbook of Dental Histology and Embryology. 3rd ed., Philadelphia, Lea & Febiger, pp. 289–290, 1921.
28. Miller, S. C.: Textbook of Periodontia. Philadelphia, Blakiston Book Co., 1938, pp. 32–34.
29. Orban, B. J.: Oral Histology and Embryology. 4th ed., St. Louis, The C. V. Mosby Co., 1957, pp. 221–223.
30. Luks, S.: Root end amalgam technic in the practice of endodontics. J.A.D.A., 53:424–428, Oct., 1956.

Chapter Fifteen

CLINICAL TECHNIQUES FOR CROWN AND BRIDGE PROSTHESIS

The fantastic usefulness of electrosurgery in dentistry has been recognized, appreciated, and utilized clinically to a greater degree in the disciplines of restorative dentistry than in any of the other dental disciplines. Within the realm of restorative dentistry electrosurgery's usefulness has been utilized most universally and its acceptance has been most noteworthy in the discipline of crown and bridge prosthodontics. The reason for its appeal in this discipline is obvious; it offers unique advantages in every aspect of fixed prosthodontics; from the simple undramatic repair of broken down crowns and bridges, to such highly sophisticated uses as creation of mucoperiosteal flap incisions for implantology.

Given such a wide range of clinical usefulness there is bound to be a degree of overlapping of uses. All the uses are reviewed in this chapter, rather than in a series of separate chapters, to assure efficient comprehensive demonstrations and evaluation of each area of crown and bridge respectively and in conjunction with its related areas. The chapter is subdivided into the following component parts for maximum coordination:

I. Crown and Bridge Repairs
II. Elongation of the Clinical Crown
III. Preparation of the Subgingival Trough
IV. Exposure of Retained Key Abutment Roots
V. Reduction of Redundant Tissue from Edentulous Areas in the Dental Arch
VI. Implant Mucoperiosteal Flap Incisions
VII. Crown and Bridge Failures: Reasons and Corrections

The component parts have been further subdivided in some areas, as you will see later.

378

CONTRIBUTIONS OF ELECTROSURGERY

The first edition listed four areas in which electrosurgery makes outstanding contributions that greatly improve the art and science of crown and bridge restorative dentistry. These are

1. Elongating the clinical crowns of abutment teeth to maintain or restore the 1:2 crown-root ratio that is critically essential if abutment teeth are successfully to withstand functional torque.
2. Preparation of effective subgingival troughs around full-crown preparations so that unimpeded impressions of the subgingival areas can be obtained and reproduced so accurately that perfect subgingival finish lines can be fabricated.
3. Exposure of key retained abutment roots for functional use.
4. Reduction of redundant tissue in edentulous areas in the dental arch to permit use of normal-size pontics with minimal grinding. In addition to saving chair time, this also reduces the hazards of weakening the pontics or spoiling their aesthetics.

These contributions are particularly valuable in full-crown coverage for occlusal reconstructions and extensive periodontal splinting and for exposing axial floors of inlay preparations to facilitate perfect finishing of inlay margins when partial coverage is employed.

Many new electrosurgical uses and techniques have been developed in the intervening years since the first edition was published. Two of them have expanded the usefulness of electrosurgery in crown and bridge prosthodontics into two new areas:

5. Crown and bridge repairs.
6. Creation of mucoperiosteal flap incisions for implantology. Electrosurgical hemostasis facilitates obtaining accurate subperiosteal impressions for fabrication of subperiosteal implants and accurate channeling of the bone for snug insertion of blade implants.

Still another new area has been introduced in this edition. This area does not relate to new techniques. Instead, it deals with what *not* to do, and why:

7. Crown and bridge failures and how to avoid them.

Four major reasons for fixed bridge restoration and splinting failures have been recognized and universally acknowledged.[1] These are

1. Failure to restore proper functional occlusion and provide occlusal harmony of the entire dentition.
2. Poor clinical preparation of crown abutments.
3. Improper fitting and finishing of castings at the gingival margins.[2]
4. Improper mesiodistal and/or buccolingual crown contours.

With the increased use of full-crown coverage in the techniques of complete mouth rehabilitation and multiple splinting of teeth, a fifth reason that has been largely overlooked has assumed major significance. This fifth reason is the failure to provide adequate subgingival space to accommodate the crowns without severe impingement against the subgingival periodontal structures.

Bartlett[3] and others have emphasized that durability is *not* the only criterion of success in fixed-bridge construction. The most serious type of failure, despite durability, is one that results in further loss of teeth. Iatrogenic (man-made) periodontal disturbances all too often lead to such losses.

Deepening and widening the gingival free-margin crevice has been widely accepted as the most effective method for facilitating impression-taking of prepared teeth and for preventing subgingival impingement, with its concomitant periodontal hazards. Many methods have been devised or improvised to create the necessary subgingival space. In alphabetical sequence W. W. Dolan,[4] J. E. Flocken,[5] J. D. Harrison,[6,7] W. F. Malone,[8,9] C. J. Miller,[10] I. F. Miller,[11] L. D. Pankey,[12] R. S. Stein,[13] and P. K. Thomas[14] are among the leading prosthodontic exponents for creating subgingival troughs around crown preparations electrosurgically. L. Fox,[15] as a prosthodontist and a periodontist, also favors this method. The late S. Charles Brecker[16,17] also was an ardent early exponent of this method. Even the late Irving Glickman,[18] although not an exponent for electrosurgical periodontal therapy, when given the choice between gingival retraction with chemically impregnated cords and subgingival electrosurgery publicly expressed preference for the latter method. The pros and cons for the other methods, and techniques for creating subgingival troughs electrosurgically, will be fully elaborated later in this chapter.

REDUCTION IN CHAIR OPERATING TIME. Electrosurgery can make a very positive contribution in this area by eliminating many of the causes of unproductive chair time. The hemostasis inherent in the electrosurgical procedures offers an excellent example of this. Control of bleeding is at best a frustrating, time-consuming chore. Electrosurgery performed with fully rectified cutting current results in hemostasis that eliminates or greatly reduces free bleeding by sealing off normal size capillaries and lymph vessels as the tissues are cut. Bleeding that ensues when somewhat larger vessels are severed can usually be brought under control rapidly and efficiently by coagulating the bleeders with the beaks of a mosquito hemostat or with coagulating forceps. This method of treatment eliminates need to spend time tying off bleeders and sponging and aspirating the blood, or to use hemostatic chemicals that may prove destructive and cause tissue sloughing. It also provides a clear operative field that is conducive to more rapid and efficient instrumentation.

Electrocoagulation can also be used effectively to control bleeding in the subgingival trough that prevents obtaining accurate impressions of the subgingival area. Such bleeding can occur even though the trough was created atraumatically by loop electrosection, since such bleeding usually results from severing nutrient capillaries in the base of the gingival sulcus. This type of bleeding can sometimes be halted by simply tamping a wick of cotton or of unimpregnated cord into the sulcus and applying light finger pressure against the wick in the direction of the base of the sulcus for 2 to 3 minutes. If this fails to stop the bleeding completely, it invariably arrests it long enough to locate the exact bleeding sites in the sulcus. Each bleeder can then be "spot welded" effectively by electrocoagulation. The latter is performed by contacting the tip of an activated solid cylindrical 90-degree-angle coagulating electrode momentarily to the bleeding site and repeating the spot coagulation as required until the bleeding stops completely. Rarely are more than three or four such momentary applications required. The slender shape and lack of bulk of the electrode make it possible to insert it into the trough without touching the marginal gingiva, and the flat circular disclike tip end makes perfect contact with the bleeding site. Thus the coagulation can be performed without damage to either the gingival or subgingival tissues, and accurate impressions can be taken without further treatment or loss of time.

Operating time is also appreciably reduced because electrosurgery using loop electrodes greatly simplifies and facilitates recontouring of the gingival architecture and re-creation of normal, feather-edged gingival margins. Furthermore, when the gingival tissues are normal preoperatively, topical applications of tincture of myrrh and benzoin usually provide all the obtundent and protective action needed. Time consumed in preparation and application of protective surgical cement packs is therefore saved.

BETTER COSMETIC RESULTS. It is usually possible to restore normal coronal and gingival harmony by elongating the clinical crowns of abnormally short teeth. Notable cosmetic disfigurement may ensue when gingival and coronal harmony is disrupted by downward dip of the gingival margin, even when only a single tooth is involved. Better cosmetic appearance is also assured by creating adequate subgingival space to accommodate seating of full-crown restorations without tissue impingement and without exposure of metal.

SIMPLIFIED IMPRESSION TECHNIQUES. Space created around a tooth by formation of a subgingival trough prior to preparing the crown, or around the shoulder after it has been prepared, permits subgingival flow of impression materials. This allows accurate impressions of multiple-tooth preparations and their subgingival areas in single, reversible or irreversible impressions of entire dental arches.

CREATE STRONGER ABUTMENTS. The crown of a tooth normally is one third the length of the entire tooth. In cases of abnormally short clinical crowns or where abrasive action of bruxism reduces the clinical crowns, the normal 1:2 crown-root ratio is upset. Teeth-bearing restorations built on such abnormally short crowns are subjected to severe abnormal torque stresses that are injurious to their investing alveolar and periodontal structures. Restoring the normal ratio by elongating the clinical crowns eliminates such torque, making them stronger and more durable abutments.

ABILITY TO MAINTAIN NORMAL GINGIVAL HEALTH AROUND FULL-CROWN RESTORATIONS. It is not uncommon to find that insertion of well-constructed full-crown restorations is followed by severe periodontal deterioration (Fig. 15–1B). It is ironic that restorations prescribed and constructed specifically for stabilization of periodontally involved teeth frequently serve as the triggering mechanism for greater and more extensive periodontal deterioration than the original condition.

The triggering factor is constant, but the nature and degree of the prosthetic impropriety is variable. It can range from the deceptively innocuous appearance of the restoration itself, which is nevertheless damaging owing to

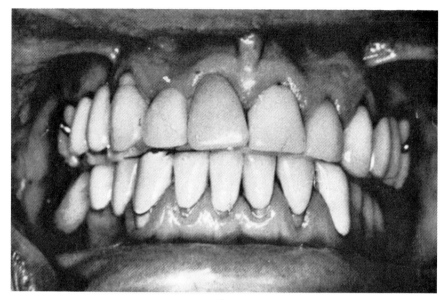

A

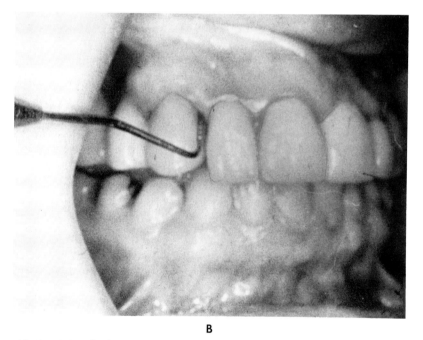

B

Figure 15–1.   *A*, Marked iatrogenic periodontal deterioration that is obviously attributable to poor restorative dentistry. Occlusal disharmonies, poor buccolingual diameter of the crowns, and subgingival impingement are the triggering mechanisms for the breakdown of the gingivae and supportive structures. *B*, Iatrogenic periodontal deterioration despite excellence of the supragingival portion of the restoration. The aesthetics are excellent, and the mesiodistal and buccolingual diameters of the crowns are also excellent. Nevertheless, there are deep periodontal pockets and poor gingival tissue tone owing to failure to provide and *maintain* subgingival accommodation for the subgingival portion of the restoration.

lack of subgingival accommodation, to the deplorably bad dentistry seen in Figure 15–1A that is unquestionably responsible.

Inasmuch as secondary factors can influence the *degree* of tissue response to the irritant, the extent and severity of the periodontal deterioration is not always in direct ratio to the degree of irritation produced by the restoration. In the absence of secondary influencing factors, it is axiomatic that the more poorly conceived and executed the restoration the greater the severity of the tissue reaction it will produce. This is well demonstrated in Figure 15–1B.

Most full-crown restorations are constructed with full or partial shoulders. Some are also made with narrow gold copings that extend slightly below the shoulders. Unless adequate subgingival space is created to accommodate their subgingival bulk, the crowns tend to impinge against, and compress, the marginal gingivae. The resultant irritation sets off a chain reaction: Irritation produces inflammation; inflammation produces swelling, engorgement, and stasis of the blood circulation in the affected areas. The tissue response to these pathological reactions usually is rapidly demonstrated: Clinical evidence of acute periodontal breakdown accompanied by gingival hypertrophy or gingival recession is soon manifested.

Needless to say, electrosurgery makes many other contributions to the field of fixed prosthodontics, but these listed are the areas in which it makes a unique and consistently invaluable contribution.

Before entering into discussion of the uses of electrosurgery in these areas, one important ground rule should be established—no attempt should be made to restore the dentition with fixed prostheses when the investing gingival tissues are inflamed and subnormal in tone or diseased. Although tissues cut by fully rectified electrosection heal rapidly and ideally and tend to regenerate toward their original level, the tissues must be healthy at the start of treatment. If the tissue tone is sub-par at the outset of treatment, the repair tissue is very likely to also be sub-par, proliferative, and friable (see Case 3, Chapter 17). Thus, to obtain optimal results with electrosurgery, it is essential that (1) thorough prophylaxis be performed first to ensure against irritation from subgingival calculus that can disrupt tissue healing, and (2) the tissue tone be improved as much as possible by vigorous gingival massage and good oral hygiene by the patient.

The time invested in preliminary treatment of the tissues to improve their tone is well repaid by the speed and quality of tissue repair, with no need for prolonged postoperative curettage or other palliative treatment.

FACTORS THAT INFLUENCE TISSUE TOLERANCE OF THE RESTORATION

These include the occlusion, anatomic contours of the artificial restoration, anatomic contour and tone of the gingival tissues, and the systemic health of the patient.

If the patient is a victim of anemia or other blood dyscrasia or of diabetes or other metabolic disease that impairs the ability of the tissues to maintain and repair themselves, the systemic condition should be corrected or at least brought under control before extensive restorative dentistry is instituted if the outcome is to be successful (see Case 8 in this chapter).

Unfavorable local conditions such as poor tissue tone or gingivitis should be eliminated before treatment is instituted if a favorable response to the restoration is to occur.

The occlusion is not a matter for consideration in this text other than to stress the importance of maintaining or creating a balanced occlusion with the fixed prosthesis in order for the investing structures to remain healthy. This brings us to the matter of local anatomic factors that deserve comment.

LOCAL ANATOMIC FACTORS. By far the most important of these is the matter of *tooth contour of the artificial crown*. The crown that provides a bullet-shaped tooth contour provides adequate "Lebensraum" for the inter-dental papillae in their embrasures. Thus these tissues are likely to remain healthy. On the other hand, failure to provide adequate space in the embra-sures impairs the blood supply and almost inevitably triggers inflammatory responses, with hyperemia, hyperplasia, and detachment of the interdental papillae as likely end results.

Buccolingual tooth curvature also influences the response of the gingival tissues to the artificial crown. Gingival tissues react more favorably to artificial crowns that reproduce the normal labial curvature of the natural tooth than to the artificial crown that presents a flat surface or bulging exaggerated labial convexity.

The *gingival contour* also influences the response to the artificial restora-tion. When the crest of the marginal gingiva is thick and rounded it will usually react unfavorably to the artificial crown. When the marginal gingiva is very thin, as in the maxillary cuspid region, restoration of a normal labial cur-vature to the artificial crown, if it deviates even slightly from that of the origi-nal crown form, is likely to cause unfavorable tissue responses because its cuff of marginal gingiva is too avascular to tolerate any deviation from its original tooth-tissue relationship. This is one of the reasons why the labial marginal gingiva of the maxillary cuspid almost invariably recedes after restoration with an artificial crown.

MARGINAL PLACEMENT. The dilemma of where to end the artificial crown—in the gingival crevice (subgingivally) or completely short of the gingival tissues (supragingivally)—is one of the main reasons for the notable and often dogmatic differences in conceptual preference between the perio-dontist and the prosthodontist.

To be sure, both are equally desirous of a favorable response of the in-vesting tissues to the fixed prosthesis and of the maintenance of healthy in-vesting structures. The periodontist, because of the frequency of unfavorable reaction of the investing structures to insertion of fixed prostheses, usually prefers to have the artificial crowns terminated supragingivally, so that they will not come into direct contact with the marginal gingivae. But the prostho-dontist must concern himself with the matters of aesthetics, patient accep-tance, and functional usefulness of the restoration, in addition to the matter of the health of the investing structures.

Most patients are intolerant of the visible band of gold that is inescapable when the crown is terminated supragingivally and reject this method of restoration. This is especially true when the anterior teeth are to be restored. When the crown finish line is placed supragingivally, the cement at the finish line loses the protective cover provided by the marginal gingiva. This makes the tooth highly vulnerable to decay as the exposed cement begins to disintegrate and washes out. These are among the reasons why the prosthodontist favors the subgingival termination of the crown whenever and wherever possible.

Electrosurgery can eliminate most of the troublesome problems encountered with subgingival termination of the crown, including tearing and mutilation of the subgingival tissues either from forceful seating of tissue retracting cords or from the forcing of copper bands too deeply in the hope of obtaining a good impression of the subgingival part of the tooth. Perhaps this accounts for the enthusiastic acceptance and widespread use of electrosurgery by most prosthodontists, which is so aptly described by Coelho: "The use of electrosection for prosthetic needs is increasing rapidly. This modality permits for better technic in impression procedures, regardless of the type, and improves the tissue tone in the marginal area of the restoration."

It is factual that no matter how meritorious it may be, unless a method or technique can be used by all who make the effort to learn it, it becomes academic and clinically useless, and suggestion that it is useful in the hands of only the developer is a certain kiss of death for its universal acceptance.

The author has been teaching techniques of electrosurgery for restorative dentistry for many years in this country and abroad, and the techniques are being used effectively by all who made the effort to learn how to perform them. The thousands of dentists who are using electrosurgery daily to good advantage are incensed by the suggestion of some diehard skeptics that only an elite few exceptional electrosurgical experts can perform the electrosurgical techniques for restorative dentistry safely and competently. To help dispel this myth some of the men the author has been privileged to teach have very generously made available for this text reports of typical practical clinical uses of these techniques in their daily practices. Their reports will be featured in the discussions of the various procedures involved in crown and bridge prosthodontics.

CLINICAL ELECTROSURGICAL TECHNIQUES

I. CROWN AND BRIDGE REPAIRS

It is virtually axiomatic that the more complex and difficult the dental procedure, the more significant and invaluable is electrosurgery's contribution to achievement of successful treatment.

Electrosurgery's usefulness is, however, by no means limited to major and heroic procedures. There are many instances where its contributions are comparably invaluable for relatively simple and unsophisticated procedures such as the repair of a pontic or replacement of a full crown.

The following cases are typical examples of electrosurgery's usefulness in these areas.

Single Crown

CASE 1

This case has been made available by Dr. Brian F. Pollack of New York City.

This case involves replacement of a unit-built porcelain crown that was complicated by extensive secondary decay extending subgingivally.

PATIENT.   A 62-year-old white female.

HISTORY.   Her dentition had been restored ten years previously with extensive fixed bridges of the unit-built variety, with removable porcelain crowns. The solder joints between the units made interproximal cleansing difficult. This, combined with the patient's overindulgence in consumption of caramels and other sweets, resulted in decay that caused the loosening of one of the crowns. She consulted Dr. Pollack for recementation or replacement of the loose crown.

CLINICAL EXAMINATION.   The maxillary left second bicuspid crown was loose and could be removed effortlessly. The gingival tissues around the restorations appeared atonal and edematous. Upon removal of the loose crown, a gold collar and post were exposed, as well as extensive decay on the buccal aspect of the root that undermined the post and extended subgingivally. On further examination it became evident that the decay extended into the root canal (Case Fig. 1–1A).

TREATMENT.   Normally the procedure would be to remove the post and collar, thoroughly excavate the decay, then replace and recement the post into the root canal. This was attempted, and proved unsuccessful since force was avoided. Rather than applying force and risking a fracture of the coronal end of the root, an attempt was made to remove the decay without removing the post from the canal.

The soft decay on the buccal aspect was excavated to the crest of the gingiva. In order to complete the excavation it became necessary to resect some of the marginal gingiva. The marginal edge of the gingiva was resected with a narrow U-shaped loop electrode by electrosection, with power output set at 2.5 on a Coles Radiosurg Electronic Scalpel IV unit.

Alternate gingival resection and excavation was performed 4 times before the base of the caries was reached. Each time, the activated electrode was brought into momentary contact with the periosteum and bone with a light wiping motion in order to remove the tissue. When the base of the caries was reached the coronal end of the root and a band of investing bone were denuded of tissue and exposed clinically (Case Fig. 1–1B).

Thorough examination of the tooth and post was now possible. The remaining proximal tooth structure was sound, but it was impossible to determine whether the tooth structure behind the post was also sound. Rather than take it for granted that no further decay was present, and risk leaving any decay untreated, the tooth was carefully dried and 30% stannous fluoride was flooded into the canal for 1 minute. The tooth was then carefully dried and the buccal cavity was filled with silicophosphate cement to provide sustained fluoride release.

The crown preparation was then recontoured and a hydrocolloid impression taken. The tooth was restored with a veneer crown. (See Case Figures 1–1C to F.)

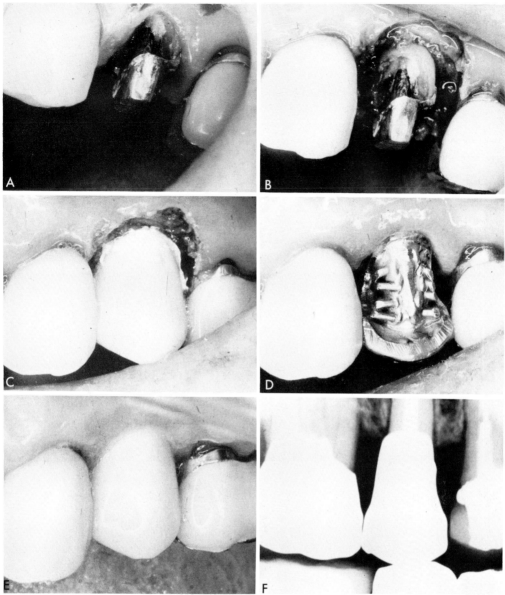

Case Figure 1–1. *A,* Gingivectomy for repair of a broken down veneer crown and root. Preoperative condition. Extensive decay has occurred around the post and gold core restoring the maxillary left second bicuspid retained root and loosened the veneer crown restoration that had been placed over it. Two punctures have been made in the gingival mucosa on the buccal aspect of the tooth to denote the height of a gingivectomy that will be performed to fully expose the area that would have to be debrided and built up with a new post and core. *B,* The gingivectomy has been performed by needle electrosection and the tooth and soft tissue debris has been thoroughly removed. The absence of free bleeding has facilitated debridement and assured its thoroughness. To assure adequate access, the gingivectomy was extended beyond the bone margin, and the activated electrode was in contact with the bone during the brief moment that the tissue was being incised. *C,* A temporary veneer crown has been inserted over the new gold core and post that has been cemented into the root. Note the fact that the gingival level is approximately 2 mm. beyond the finish line of the veneer crown. *D,* The new veneer crown casting has been inserted. Note the adaptation of the gingival tissue around the casting, and the fact that the marginal gingiva has regenerated to its original level almost entirely. *E,* The acrylic facing of the veneer crown has been inserted, completing the restoration of the tooth. Note that except for a slight lack of keratinization of the regenerated surface epithelium, the marginal gingiva is normal in all respects. *F,* Bite wing x-ray shows that the crown casting extends apically about 4 mm. beyond the level of the molar restoration, and that the contour is excellent, with no overhanging margins. This result, which assures that there will be no subgingival irritation from the casting, was made possible by the excellent access and visibility of the field during debridement.

387

Bridge Repair: Anterior

CASE 2

This case has been made available by Dr. William J. Kelly, Jr., of St. Louis, Missouri.

This case presents an atypical but very useful version of the electrosurgical elongation of the clinical crown. It is atypical since it involves the resection of redundant tissue from the backing of a Steele's facing pontic of a fixed restoration to permit the reinsertion of a suitable porcelain facing for which there is inadequate space.

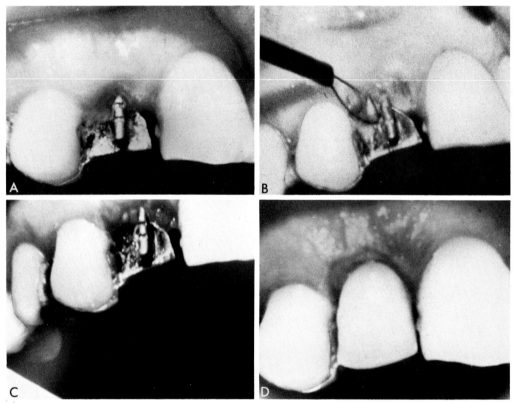

Case Figure 2-1. A, Preoperative: A Steele's facing is cantilevered as an extension of a fixed bridge attached to the maxillary right cuspid and bicuspid porcelain veneer crowns. The porcelain facing of the Steele's facing is missing, and the gingival mucosa has proliferated downward over the top third of the metal backing. Either the redundant tissue is removed to make room for a replacement facing, or the porcelain pontic facing will have to be ground so much that it will weaken it and ruin its aesthetics, and consume much time. *B,* The redundant tissue is being resected from the edentulous alveolar ridge area and the metal backing with a flame shaped loop electrode. Contact with the activated electrode is only momentary and each is followed by an adequate rest period to avoid accumulation of heat that could be damaging. *C,* Most of the redundant tissue has been removed, and the entire metal backing is being cleared of the obstructive tissue. *D,* An aesthetically acceptable and functionally effective new porcelain facing has been prepared quickly and easily. The porcelain fits snugly against the tissues without traumatic pressure, and is ready for permanent cementation.

PATIENT.   A white male of undetermined age.

HISTORY.   The porcelain Steele's facing of an old bridge fractured and fell off. The gingival tissue immediately superior to the pontic proliferated downward. By the time the patient came to Dr. Kelly for replacement of the facing there wasn't enough space left to fit in an aesthetically acceptable and functionally useful facing. To do so it was necessary to remove the redundant tissue.

CLINICAL EXAMINATION.   The maxillary left central facing was missing. The marginal gingiva had proliferated downward and around the metal backing (Case Fig. 2–1A).

TREATMENT.   The tissue was anesthetized by infiltration. A medium width U-shaped loop electrode was used to resect the redundant tissue (Case Fig. 2–1B and C). The gingiva was recontoured to conform around a new normal size facing; tincture of myrrh and benzoin was then applied to the area.

At the next visit the tissue was sufficiently healed to permit insertion and cementation of the new facing (Case Fig. 2–1D).

By being able to remove the undesirable tissue without free bleeding and to recontour the tissues to conform to the contour of the new facing it eliminated need to do a great deal of grinding of the porcelain in order to be able to use a pontic facing of normal dimension.

Bridge Repair: Posterior

CASE 3

This case has been made available to the author by Dr. John E. Flocken of Los Angeles, California.

This case is in some respects similar to the preceding case. In both cases porcelain pontics had broken and been lost, leaving edentulous spaces in the dental arches. In both cases the pontics were cantilevered from single abutments and the gingival tissues had proliferated and partially filled the edentulous spaces so that it would be impossible to insert new pontics without first eliminating the redundant tissue.

The two cases did differ in one important respect. In the preceding case as soon as the redundant tissue had been cleared away from the metal backing and the new Steele's facing had been ground to fit against the gingiva, it was a simple matter to fit and attach the new facing without further ado. In this case, however, in addition to eliminating the redundant tissue, the edentulous saddle area had to be recontoured in order to fit the new pontic against the ridge, and at the same time have the pontic fit properly against the gold occlusal casting so that it could be properly inserted and attached. The preparation of the soft tissue and of the porcelain pontic therefore had to be much more precise in this case.

PATIENT.   Details unknown.

HISTORY.   A porcelain pontic had broken and fragments had fractured off from time to time creating an empty space into which food particles wedged.

CLINICAL EXAMINATION.   The mandibular right first and second bicuspids were missing from the dental arch, but the edentulous space had been restored with a single bicuspid pontic. The pontic was cantilevered off a cast gold crown on the first molar by means of a cast gold occlusal extension. The porcelain portion of the pontic

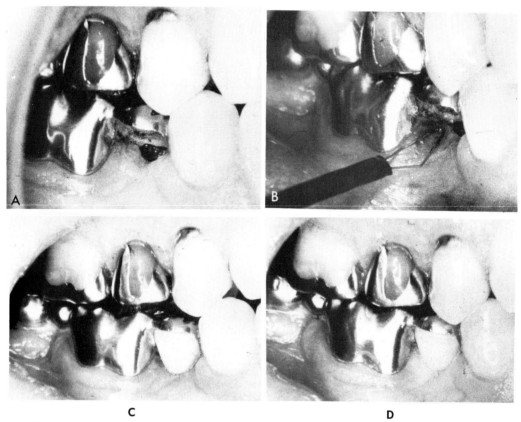

C   D

Case Figure 3–1.   Bridge repair: Replacement of a broken posterior porcelain pontic.
A, Preoperative appearance of broken pontic, which is the cantilevered anterior terminal end
of the restoration. The occlusal gold casting is intact but the gingival mucosa in the now edentulous saddle area has proliferated superiorly at either terminal end of the edentulous space
to almost totally fill the original space for the porcelain pontic with redundant tissue. *B*,
Redundant tissue is being excised and the saddle area restored to normal contour by loop
electrosection with a triangular-shaped loop electrode. *C*, Restoration and gingival tissues
one week postoperatively. The gingival mucosa of the saddle area is almost fully healed. The
porcelain pontic has been ground in slightly and fits into the area perfectly, with the glazed
saddle portion of the porcelain butted snugly against the tissue and the top in perfect contact
with the occlusal gold casting. *D*, Two week postoperative appearance of the tissues. The
gingival mucosa is fully healed and indistinguishable from the surrounding mucosa.

was missing, and the gingival mucosa had proliferated superiorly at either terminal end of the edentulous space so that most of the original space for the porcelain pontic was filled with redundant tissue (Case Fig. 3–1A).

TREATMENT. The tissue was anesthetized by infiltration anesthesia. A triangular-shaped loop electrode was selected, activated with cutting current, and used to resect the redundant tissue from the edentulous saddle area (Case Fig. 3–1B). When the redundant tissue had been adequately resected and the ridge saddle area suitably recontoured, tincture of myrrh and benzoin was applied in air-dried layers and the patient was reappointed. At the next visit one week later the gingival tissue on the saddle area was almost fully healed. The porcelain pontic was then ground so as to fit accurately against the tissue and also against the gold occlusal casting (Case Fig. 3–1C). The pontic was cemented in and the patient was again reappointed to return in one week. At the next visit the gingival tissue appeared fully healed and the healed tissue appeared totally indistinguishable from the surrounding tissues (Case Fig. 3–1D).

(Case details that were not provided have been reconstructed by the author from the Kodachrome slides of the case.)

II. ELONGATION OF THE CLINICAL CROWN

Coronal elongation may be indicated for cosmetic or functional reasons. Need for it may be limited to a single tooth or may be indicated for a substantial portion of the dentition. Regardless of the reason or the number of teeth involved, the basic concept for the technique of elongation remains the same.

The author's personal observations and experience (corroborated by those of many of his students) indicate that the best electrosurgical results of coronal elongation are usually achieved by electrosection performed with loop electrodes. However, when the gingival tissues are severely engorged and friable, or if there is a history of hemorrhagic tendencies (particularly of the secondary type), biterminal electrocoagulation performed with wire loop or solid coagulating electrodes may be advantageously substituted, because of the advantages of the greatly increased hemostasis this modality affords.

Coronal elongation by a number of methods other than electrosection or electrocoagulation have been advocated by some men. Some experts in restorative dentistry advocate coagulation of the unwanted gingival tissue with monoterminal desiccating current instead of cutting it away, and claim excellent results. Advocates of this method usually give two reasons for their preference: first, that for a beginner coagulation is easier to learn than the cutting technique; second, that monoterminal coagulation insults the tissues, thereby promoting repair by tough, fibrous, contractile cicatricial scar tissue, which is less likely to regenerate and will undo the results achieved by the elongation.

This type of reasoning appears rather specious. Thorough scrutiny and careful assay of these reasons is indicated and justified. Motivation for this evaluation does not stem from any desire by the author to dissuade the reader from using techniques that have proved successful and have produced consistently excellent results. It is motivated by the fact that this text has been designed to guide those readers who either have had no previous experience with coronal elongation by electrosurgical techniques, or who have used coagulating or monoterminal desiccating techniques and feel that these techniques leave room for improvement.

Let us scrutinize the first premise. Does accurate destruction of tissue by desiccation or coagulation really require less skill than the cutting technique? The fact is that it is extremely difficult to accurately predetermine the precise end result of tissue loss due to coagulation necrosis. On the other hand, it is a simple matter to predetermine exactly how much tissue will be lost by cutting. The cutting technique permits the operator to visualize the end result at the time of surgery. It is, therefore, much easier for the average operator to use cutting techniques accurately than coagulating or desiccating techniques, the end results of which are difficult to gauge or to control.

Now let us examine the second premise: the desirability of obtaining repair by contractile cicatricial scar tissue to assure that there will be no undesirable regeneration of the marginal gingivae that had been removed. It is debatable whether repair with abnormal tissue can be preferable under any circumstance to normal repair. When potentially undesirable consequences of the respective techniques are compared it is even more debatable.

If the cutting technique is used and undesirable regeneration of marginal tissue does occur, it is usually gradual, minimal, and easily controlled or corrected by superficial spot coagulation with very low current intensity, for which topical anesthesia in most instances is quite adequate. The worst consequence conceivable would be that a modicum of supplemental corrective surgery might have to be instituted. On the other hand, when coagulating or monoterminal desiccating current is utilized and excessive contraction and recession of the marginal gingivae results, the damage is irreversible. The contracted tissue cannot be restored to its proper height. The aesthetic loss which ensues when the subgingival portions of the restorations and their juncture with the roots of the teeth become exposed to view cannot be corrected except by entirely remaking the restorations.

Based upon these considerations it seems valid to conclude that the successful use of coagulating or desiccating current for elongating clinical crowns of teeth is by no means an accurate index of the simplicity or efficacy of the method. Rather, it is a great tribute to the individual skill of the operators who employ it successfully.

We shall, therefore, devote our attention primarily to the technique of elongating clinical crowns of teeth by electrosection with loop electrodes and, to a lesser degree, the use of biterminal electrocoagulation to accomplish this.

Loop electrodes are available in a large variety of shapes and sizes. Selection of electrodes is a matter of individual preference based upon the operator's conception of what will best suit the needs of a particular case. The flame-shaped loop electrode comes closest to being universally useful for gross preliminary resection of the marginal gingivae. This electrode is ideally suited for resecting the marginal gingivae from the labial aspect of anterior teeth to elongate their crowns by gingivectoplasty (Fig. 15–2A). It can also be used advantageously for the same purpose on the palatal aspect if the loop is bent around a firm round object to create a curve that will facilitate optimal tissue contact for increasing the coronal exposure by planing to shave the tissue in layers and thus avoid scooping out a trench of tissue that will become a food trap and cause irritation. This electrode also is ideally suited for re-contouring the interproximal papillary tissues after the coronal exposure has been increased, to restore these tissues to normal architecture. When it is used for this purpose, the loop should be bent slightly to create a very gentle curve in it. This facilitates its use (Fig. 15–2B).

The medium-width 45-degree-angle U-shaped loop electrode closely rivals the flame-shaped loop in usefulness for elongating the clinical crowns of teeth, and in some areas is somewhat more efficient. It can be used with al-most equal facility to elongate the clinical crowns on the labial aspect and is especially well suited for use in the posterior part of the mouth, where it pro-vides excellent access and maneuverability without need to bend it to any special shape (Fig. 15–2C). It can also be used efficiently for elongating the crowns on the palatal aspect by planing to shave the tissue in layers (Fig. 15–2D).

After gross tissue resection has been performed, further contouring re-finements can be attained by supplementary use of the narrow U-shaped loop electrodes, since these provide more favorable access and maneuverability in the interproximal areas and other areas of limited access and maneuverability. Combined use of the flame and wide U-shaped loops with the narrow U-shaped loops usually produces optimal results.

The manner in which the loops make contact with the tissues plays an important role in the efficiency of the gingivectoplasty. If the gingival tissue is to be resected by loop planing to shave it away in thin layers, the electrode should be brought into contact with the tissue at an acute angle to the tissue surface. Only one side of the loop should be in contact with the tissue; the other side of the loop should be elevated slightly above the tissue surface. The more obtuse the angle the electrode makes as it comes into contact with the tissue, the thicker the slice of tissue it will resect. If the tissue is to be re-moved with one or perhaps two tissue contacts, the electrode should create a 45- to 60-degree angle with the tissue surface and be used with a wiping stroke. If the tissue is to be resected by shaving it in thin layers, the electrode should be used with short brushing strokes as the electrode side that comes in contact with the tissues creates an acute (15 to 30 degree) angle to the tissue surface.

It has been stressed that only one side of the loop should make contact with the tissues. There is one important use where this does not hold true. When it is necessary to recontour the interproximal tissue in the embrasures, the flame-shaped loop, which is ideally suited for this purpose, should be

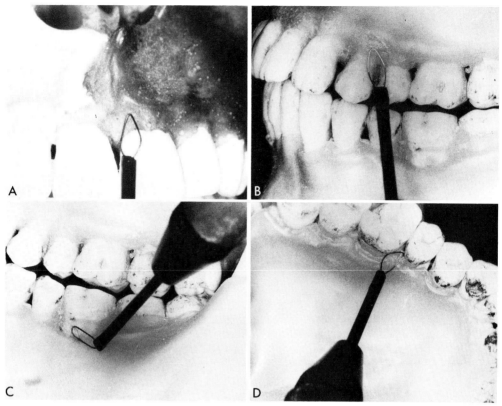

Figure 15–2. Elongation of clinical crowns of anterior and posterior teeth by loop electrode gingivectoplasty. (Demonstrated on specially prepared anatomic dry specimen, with pink base plate wax simulation of the gingival tissues.) *A,* Proper position of the flame-shaped loop electrode for resecting labial gingiva from anterior teeth by gingivectoplasty (simultaneous resection of marginal gingiva and recontouring of the cut tissue to normal gingival architecture). Note that only the left side of the loop is in contact with the tissues. The electrode is held at a slight anteroposterior angle with the right side of the loop elevated slightly above the tissue surface as the electrode is applied with a lateral wiping motion. *B,* Proper position of the flame-shaped loop electrode for recontouring the interdental papillae to form self-cleansing sluiceways. Note how well the flame-shaped loop conforms to the contour of the embrasure space. The loop has been bent slightly to create a gentle convexity, and the anterior half of the *convex* surface is brought into flat contact with the tissue as the loop is pulled coronally toward the apex of the papilla. *C,* Use of the flame-shaped loop electrode for elongating the crowns on the palatal aspect, especially in the posterior part of the mouth. For this purpose the loop is bent to form a marked curvature for optimal tissue contact. Note that the lower half of the loop is in contact with the tissue, to shave the tissue in thin layers so that the crown will be exposed without gouging out a trench of tissue that would create a food collecting undercut. Used properly, the tissue planing results in restoration of normal gingival architecture with feather-edge marginal gingivae, even on the palatal aspect. *D,* Correct position of the 45-degree-angle medium-wide U-shaped loop electrode for elongation of the clinical crown of a posterior tooth. Note that the tip and anterior one-third of the lower half of the loop is in contact with the tissue and the remainder of the loop is elevated slightly above the tissue surface as the electrode is being used.

brought into flat contact with the tissue. The loop should be bent to a slight curvature and the convex surface should be brought into contact with the tissue and used with a light pulling motion directed *toward the apex* of the interdental papilla and NOT toward the root of the tooth. Only the tip half of the loop should make contact with the tissues (Fig. 15–2B). Use of the electrode as has been described here assures that an excessive amount of tissue will not be sheared off accidentally.

The amount of gingival tissue to be removed should be either marked off with punctures or accurately visualized before instrumentation is started. The loop electrode, held at an acute angle to the mucosa, may be used with either free wiping motions or short brushing strokes. The former is preferable when removal of a major portion of the tissue with a single stroke is desired. The latter is preferred if it is deemed safer to remove the tissue gradually or in layers with short strokes, each followed by a rest interval to prevent cumulative heat retention in the tissues.

After the gross coronal elongation has been established, further delicate instrumentation for necessary refinements and finishing touches, such as creating interproximal concave sluiceways and feather-edged margins, should be instituted to assure good aesthetics and function.

Elongation of the clinical crown may range from cosmetic improvement of one or two teeth to functional correction of the entire dentition.

Aesthetic Advantage

CASE 4

This case has been made available by Dr. Charles Jay Miller of Pittsburgh, Pennsylvania.

This case presents the elongation of the clinical crown to derive the aesthetic and functional advantages of gingival harmony. It demonstrates the ability to fully expose an incompletely erupted permanent tooth to the same gingival level as the contralateral tooth which has had the gingival level elevated in the process of preparing it for a porcelain jacket crown restoration. Unless the gingival level harmony is restored in such cases, especially when the maxillary anterior teeth are involved, the disparity is likely to be conspicuous.

The elongation itself is quite similar to the procedures reviewed in Chapter 12 except that the gingival level must match the adjacent tissue level and the elongation must therefore be more precise than is necessary for coronal elongation for operative dentistry.

PATIENT.   A pre-teen age white male.

HISTORY.   He had fallen and fractured off the disto-incisal portion of his maxillary right central incisor. The nature and extent of the fracture made it necessary to prepare the tooth for full crown coverage.

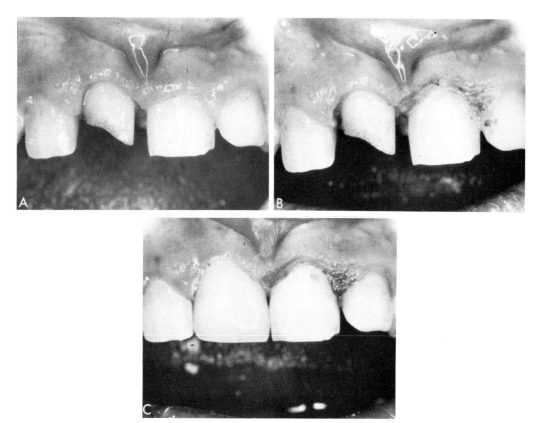

Case Figure 4–1. A, Preoperative appearance. The fractured right central has been prepared for coverage with a porcelain jacket crown. The gingival level over the prepared tooth is
several mm. higher than that of the contralateral central, creating marked gingival disharmony.
B, Enough of the marginal gingiva over the left central has been resected by gingivectoplasty
by electrosection to restore gingival harmony. *C,* Porcelain jacket crown has been inserted,
emphasizing the harmonious level of the marginal gingivae over the two teeth.

CLINICAL EXAMINATION. The maxillary teeth were incompletely erupted. The
gingival tissue that covered approximately one third of the clinical crowns of the teeth
was thick and somewhat engorged and atonal. The fractured tooth was firm and the
horn of the pulp was not exposed despite the loss of tooth structure. The tooth had
been prepared for restoration with a full crown and the labial gingival level of the
prepared tooth was about 3 mm. higher than the gingival levels of the two adjacent
teeth.

TREATMENT. The tissues were prepared and infiltration anesthesia was administered. The fractured right central was prepared for full crown coverage. The finish
line of the crown preparation was extended to the cemento-enamel junction, and a
temporary crown was inserted over the prepared stump and retained with temporary
cement. The gingival tissue had been traumatized in the process of preparing the
subgingival finish line, but when the patient returned one week later the tissue was
almost fully healed. The disparity in the level of the marginal gingivae over the two
centrals was conspicuous. When the crown was removed, the difference in the gingival level appeared even more pronounced (Case Fig. 4–1A), with the prepared
tooth's gingival level about 3 mm. higher than that of the left central.

A flame-shaped loop electrode was selected and activated for electrosection, and enough marginal gingiva was removed by loop planing to elevate the gingival level to that of the prepared right central (Case Fig. 4–1B). The porcelain jacket crown was inserted and cemented for temporary retention (Case Fig. 4–1C). The elongation of the gingival level of the left central had greatly improved the aesthetics of the case. The healing proceeded without incidence and when complete, since the occlusion was satisfactory, the crown was cemented permanently.

(Details not provided were reconstructed from the Kodachrome transparencies by the author.)

Functional Advantages

If a tooth is to have the ability to withstand the stress of functional torque as an effective abutment it is essential that the necessary 1:2 crown-root ratio be maintained or restored. It is very often necessary to elongate the clinically exposed portion of the tooth by resecting enough of the covering gingival tissue and, if necessary, alevolar marginal bone in order to re-create or maintain the proper crown-root ratio.

Alveolar marginal bone removal is only infrequently necessary, in which event it can easily be performed by hand instrumentation with chisels, bone gouges, or cleoid curets. When indicated, it is best to remove the bone about 1 millimeter beyond the new gingival level.

The gingival mucosa can be resected with steel scalpels, periodontal knives, or needle or loop electrodes. By far the most effective and efficient method is loop excision, which creates a perfect feather-edge gingival bevel for the new marginal edge and facilitates perfect recontouring of the gingival architecture in the embrasures. In addition, the hazard of surgical shock is eliminated, since electrosection is achieved without blood loss. Most important by far is the character of the respective tissue repair.

Repair following steel cutting results in typical tough fibrous contractile scar tissue. Repair following electrosection results in supple tissue that is identical in all respects to the original normal marginal gingiva. It was been intimated that marginal gingiva of firm fibrous texture is preferable for subgingival placement of full-crown restorations. The most charitable interpretation for such intimations is that they represent wishful thinking. A more realistic interpretation is that necessity is the motivating factor, since this is the only kind of tissue repair that can be achieved with cold-steel surgery. Needless to say, if a tough fibrous contractile marginal gingiva were ideal, nature would have created normal marginal gingiva of that texture. Despite all the scientific achievements to date, man has been unable to effectively duplicate, let alone improve on, nature's scheme of things.

The following case report is an excellent example of the efficacy of loop electrosection of the gingival mucosa for elongation of the clinical crowns. It also demonstrates the ability of the marginal gingiva to regenerate to or almost to its original level.

CASE 5

This case also was made available by Dr. Charles J. Miller.

PATIENT.   Details unknown.

HISTORY.   The patient had been referred to Dr. Miller for restorative dentistry. This included a fixed bridge extending from the maxillary left first bicuspid to the second molar.

CLINICAL EXAMINATION (MAXILLARY LEFT QUADRANT).   The first molar was missing. The second bicuspid and second molar crowns were restored with large MO temporary cement fillings. The first bicuspid was prepared for full-crown coverage. The marginal level of the buccal gingiva of this tooth was almost 5 mm. higher than that of the second bicuspid. The latter tooth had a large periodontal pocket on the buccal aspect. A periodontal probe, on insertion, penetrated almost 5 mm., revealing that the buccal gingival detachment extended to the same level as the marginal gingiva of the prepared tooth (Case Fig. 5–1A).

TREATMENT.   The anesthesia that had been administered for preparation of the first bicuspid sufficed for the electrosurgery. A triangular-shaped loop electrode was selected and activated with cutting current. The activated electrode was used with a wiping motion to resect the detached buccal gingiva (Case Fig. 5–1B). This simultaneously eliminated the periodontal pocket, recontoured the gingival architecture of the second bicuspid to provide a normal feather-edge gingival margin, and restored a harmonious level to the buccal gingivae of the first and second bicuspids (Case Fig. 5–1C).

(The author reconstructed the above data from the Kodachrome slides of the case.)

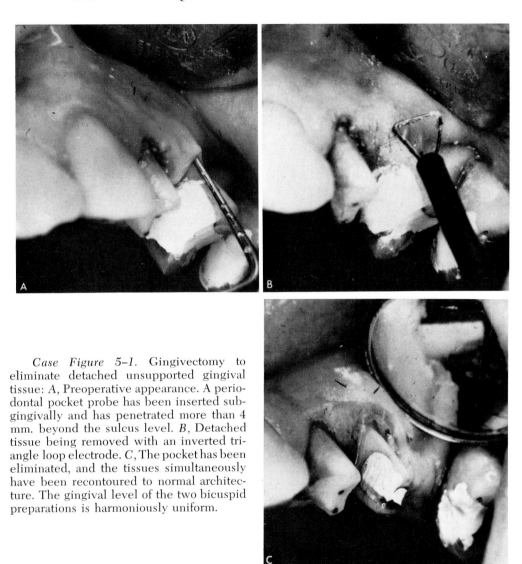

Case Figure 5–1. Gingivectomy to eliminate detached unsupported gingival tissue: *A,* Preoperative appearance. A periodontal pocket probe has been inserted subgingivally and has penetrated more than 4 mm. beyond the sulcus level. *B,* Detached tissue being removed with an inverted triangle loop electrode. *C,* The pocket has been eliminated, and the tissues simultaneously have been recontoured to normal architecture. The gingival level of the two bicuspid preparations is harmoniously uniform.

CASE 6

This case has been made available to the author by Dr. James D. Harrison of Edwardsville, Illinois.

PATIENT.   Data unknown.

HISTORY.   The patient required extensive restoration of the dentition. The overall treatment plan included replacement of a long missing maxillary first molar with a fixed prosthesis extending from second bicuspid to second molar.

CLINICAL EXAMINATION.   Caries was rampant. The maxillary right second molar which would be the posterior anchor abutment for the prosthesis was partially unerupted on the palatal aspect, with the marginal gingiva covering about one half the clinical crown, creating an abnormally short clinical crown.

TREATMENT.   To assure that the second molar would be able to withstand the functional torque to which it would be subjected as the posterior anchor abutment it would be necessary to perform a gingivectomy on the palatal aspect and expose enough of the clinical crown of the tooth to provide the necessary 1:2 crown-root ratio.

The extent of the gingivectomy was outlined with a series of stab incisions around the palatal aspect of the tooth (Case Fig. 6–1), after infiltration anesthesia had been administered. A 45-degree-angle wide U-shaped loop electrode was selected, activated with cutting current, and the gingivectoplasty was performed by loop planing the tissue to expose the tooth crown adequately. As the gingival level was being altered and the exposure achieved the loop planing simultaneously recontoured the new gingival margin to normal architecture (Case Fig. 6–2). Tincture of myrrh and benzoin was applied in air-dried layers. No other dressing was required, and healing progressed without incident.

(Details partially reconstructed from the Kodachrome slides by the author.)

The author's technique for elongating the clinical crowns of teeth by gingivectoplasty, simultaneous resection of the tissue by loop planing and recontouring to a normal feather-edge gingival architecture of the new gingival margins has been demonstrated repeatedly.

This next case demonstrates admirably that it is also possible to elongate clinical crowns of teeth by gingivectomy, but substituting the needle electrode and cutting current for manual steel scalpel incision of the gingival tissue.

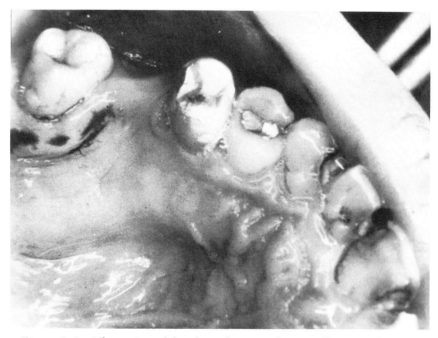

Case Figure 6–1.   Elongation of the clinical crown of a partially erupted maxillary molar. The amount of tissue to be resected has been marked off by stab incisions on the palatal aspect and partly on the alveolar ridge in an edentulous area between the molar and second bicuspid. There is slight bleeding at the wound sites.

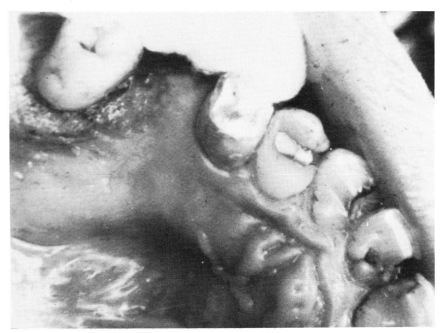

Case Figure 6–2. The tissue resection has been performed by loop planing that recontours the tissue architecture at the same time that the height of the tissue is reduced. There is no bleeding in the surgical field.

CASE 7

This case has been made available to the author by Dr. John E. Flocken of Los Angeles, California.

PATIENT.   A white adult male.

HISTORY.   The maxillary right first and second molars were badly broken down. Coronal destruction was so extensive that restoration of the teeth with full gold cast crowns was chosen as the most desirable treatment plan.

CLINICAL EXAMINATION.   The maxillary right first bicuspid area was edentulous. The first and second molar crowns were extensively decayed. The decay in the first molar involved the mesial, occlusal and distal surfaces of the tooth. The distal and distobuccal half of the second molar crown was missing. The clinically exposed portions of both teeth appeared so short that it was doubtful whether the teeth would be able to withstand the torque of function after restoration with the cast crowns unless more of the coronal structure could be exposed clinically.

TREATMENT.   The additional exposure of the crowns of the two teeth was to be achieved by performing a gingivectomy around both teeth. The level and extent of the gingivectomy incisions were outlined on the buccal and palatal surfaces of the gingivae around the two teeth (Case Fig. 7–1A and *B*) with an indelible pencil.

A straight fine needle electrode was selected, activated with cutting current, and used to incise the gingival tissue on the buccal aspect, directing the incision downward toward the bone at an approximate 45-degree angle, to bevel the tissue as it was being cut (Case Fig. 7–2A). A 45-degree-angle fine long needle electrode was substituted, current power output increased, and the gingivectomy incision on the palatal

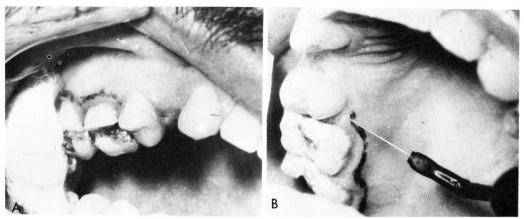

Case Figure 7–1. Gingivectomy to elongate the clinical crowns of teeth that are to be restored with full cast gold crowns. *A,* Preoperative appearance. The maxillary right first and second molars are extensively decayed. The line of incision for a gingivectomy to increase the clinical height of the crowns of the two teeth has been outlined on the buccal gingiva with indelible ink. *B,* The gingivectomy incision has been outlined on the palatal mucosa with indelible ink. The 45-degree-angle needle electrode that will be used to perform the electrosection on the palatal aspect is poised for action.

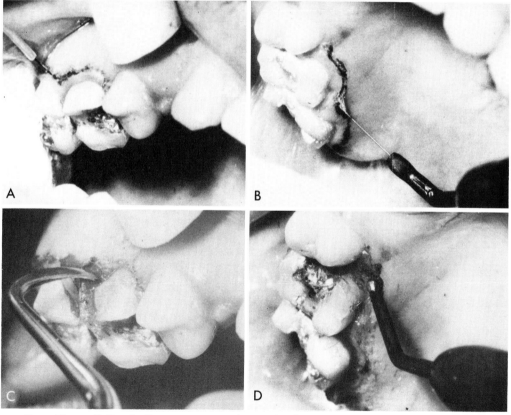

Case Figure 7–2. *A,* Operative procedure. The buccal gingival tissue is being incised along the inked outline. The electrode is tilted to incise the tissue at a 45-degree angle toward the occlusal of the teeth, to bevel the new marginal edge of the tissue. A straight fine needle electrode is being used with the cutting current. *B,* The palatal gingivectomy incision is being performed with the 45-degree-angle fine needle electrode. *C,* The buccal strip of incised gingival tissue is being detached from the alveolar bone with a sickle scaler hand instrument, causing a little free bleeding. *D,* Bleeding at the anterior terminal end of the palatal gingivectomy is being brought under control by spot coagulation with a small ball coagulating electrode.

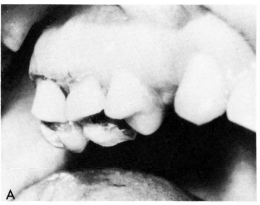
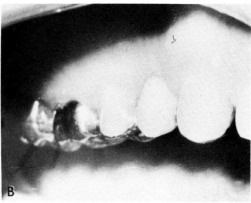

Case Figure 7–3.   A, Postoperative appearance: One week after surgery. The crowns of the two teeth appear to be adequately exposed to make the restorations torque-resistant. The gingival tissues appear to be healing satisfactorily, and the gingival architecture appears acceptable. B, Postoperative appearance: Three weeks after surgery. The cast gold crowns have been inserted. The tissues appear to be perfectly adapted around the crowns, and the healing appears to be complete. The gingival architecture is excellent and the tissue tone is normal.

aspect was performed (Case Fig. 7–2B). The circumferential incisions around the teeth for the gingivectomy having been completed, the incised strips of gingival tissue were detached from the alveolar bone (Case Fig. 7–2C) with a sickle scaler. A slight amount of free bleeding occurred as the tissue was being displaced manually. Bleeding at the anterior end of the palatal gingivectomy was quickly brought under control by spot coagulation with a ball coagulating electrode (Case Fig. 7–2D). After the bleeding was brought under control tincture of myrrh and benzoin was applied to the cut tissue surfaces in air-dried layers and the patient was reappointed for preparation of the teeth. He returned one week later; the cut gingival tissues were healing well and the clinical crowns of the two teeth now appeared adequately exposed (Case Fig. 7–3A). The teeth were prepared for full crown coverage, impressions and bite were obtained, and the patient was reappointed for insertion of the restorations. The crowns were fabricated and inserted one week later. He was seen again the following week, at which time the tissues were fully healed and well adapted around the gold castings (Case Fig. 7–3B) and appeared normal in tone and architecture.

(Unknown details have been reconstructed by the author from the Kodachrome slides of the case.)

CASE 8

This is another of the cases made available by Dr. Charles J. Miller.

   PATIENT.   An adult male.
   HISTORY.   The patient had been wearing an old fixed bridge that had been made many years ago. The alveolar bone under the restoration had undergone considerable resorption and been replaced by redundant gingival mucosa. Dr. Miller had removed the old prosthesis in order to reprepare the teeth for a new, modern fixed bridge (Case Fig. 8–1).
   CLINICAL EXAMINATION.   Removal of the old restoration revealed a large amount of redundant mucosa on the edentulous portion of the dental arch in the maxilla. The maxillary left cuspid, second bicuspid, and second molar teeth which had

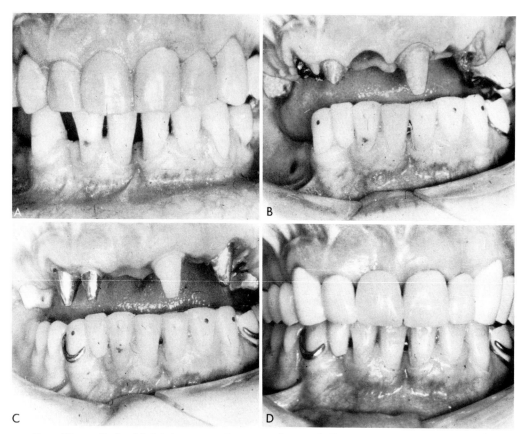

Case Figure 8–1. Multiple restorative procedures. *A,* Preoperative appearance is decep-tively innocuous. There is an acrylic restoration present in the maxilla from cuspid to cuspid, and bilateral fixed bridges extend from first bicuspid to second molar. The mandibular arch is edentulous posterior to the right cuspid and to the left second bicuspid. There is a 3-mm. diastema between the mandibular centrals, 1.5-mm. diastemas between the centrals and lat-erals, and a 7-mm. diastema between the right lateral and cuspid. *B,* The old bridgework has been removed from the anterior and right posterior of the maxilla. The major portion of the crown of the left cuspid has decayed, leaving a retained root of the tooth. The left lateral and right central areas are edentulous, with deep concave grooves where the pontics had dug into the tissues. Downgrowth of gingiva has covered two thirds of the right cuspid crown, and the interdental papilla between the cuspid and retained root of the right first bicuspid is hyper-trophied and detached. There is much redundant tissue present on the edentulous ridge be-tween the bicuspid root and the second molar. The mandibular diastemas have been eliminated by simple tooth movement, and the teeth have been fixed into their new position with Whale-dent horizontal pin splinting, to which a right lateral pontic has been added to fill the large diastema space. *C,* The redundant tissue has been loop resected by electrosection resected from the maxilla, and the teeth and roots have been reprepared for full crown coverage. Note the excellent tissue repair. *D,* The mouth has been fully restored with new restorations (veneer crown restorations in the maxilla and a lingual bar partial in the mandible). The external por-tions of the Whaledent pins have been ground out enough to permit insertion of porcelain fill-ings for better aesthetics. The tissues around the crowns in the maxilla are normal in tone and snugly adapted around the restorations.

been serving as abutments all had considerable redundant tissue covering portions of the clinical crowns of the respective teeth. The molar had some secondary decay.

TREATMENT.   The area was anesthetized. A medium-size 20-degree-angle U-shaped loop electrode was selected and current was set at 4 on the power output dial. The activated electrode was then used to reduce the redundant tissue in the edentulous area to normal dimension and contour.

The same electrode was then used to elongate the clinical crowns of the teeth, particularly the bicuspid, of which almost one half the coronal portion was covered with redundant tissue. The subgingival trough was then prepared around the three prepared crowns and an impression was taken for a master model on which the new restoration was fabricated. When the new restoration was completed, it was inserted into the dental arch. The restoration was perfectly contoured to the alveolar ridge, the crowns fitted accurately subgingivally, and the pontic, normal in size, was aesthetically and functionally suitable.

The use of electrosurgery had eliminated need for time-consuming laborious grinding of the pontic as well as the hazard of weakening the pontic and making it vulnerable to breakage under functional stress, and assured that the abutment crowns would be able to withstand the torque of function without impingement against the subgingival tissues.

Combined Aesthetic and Functional Advantages

CASE 9

This is another of the cases made available to the author by Dr. Charles J. Miller of Pittsburgh, Pennsylvania.

This case demonstrates the advantages to be derived from elongating the clinical crowns of teeth that are to serve as functional abutments. It also demonstrates graphically the enormous amount of tissue proliferation that can be stimulated by poorly designed and ill-fitting prosthetic restorations.

PATIENT.   Details unknown.

HISTORY.   The patient had been wearing an old fixed bridge for a long time. The gingival tissues around the gold crowns gradually grew down and partially covered the abutment crowns and bulged out from under the pontics. This tissue became uncomfortably tender so he consulted Dr. Miller for its treatment.

CLINICAL EXAMINATION.   The maxillary left quadrant from first bicuspid to second molar was restored with a fixed bridge consisting of gold shell crowns and gold and solder-backed porcelain facings. The gingival tissues covered more than half of the first bicuspid and second molar abutment crowns, and dark red friable tissue bulged from under the pontics.

TREATMENT.   The gold crowns were cut and the bridge was removed. This revealed extensive decay of the second molar crown and massive hyperplasia of the tissues around the abutment teeth and on the edentulous saddle area (Case Fig. 9–1A). The quadrant had been anesthetized with a posterior superior alveolar block injection before the bridge had been removed. A medium-size round loop was selected, acti-

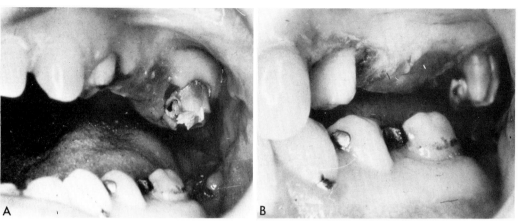

Case Figure 9–1. *A,* Old fixed bridge removed, revealing massive hyperplasia that almost covers the maxillary left first bicuspid and half the second molar and much redundant tissue on the edentulous ridge area. *B,* The redundant tissue has been resected with a loop electrode and the excess tissue planed from the edentulous area. The teeth are now adequately exposed to permit preparation of functionally useful abutments.

vated with cutting current and used to resect the hyperplastic tissue covering the clinical crowns of the two abutment teeth and the redundant tissue on the saddle area, so that normal-size pontics could be inserted (Case Fig. 9–1B). Tincture of myrrh and benzoin was applied in air-dried layers and the patient was instructed in home care and reappointed. When he returned one week later the tissues were healing satisfactorily and repreparation of the teeth and tissues for a new restoration proceeded without incidence.

CASE 10

Although Cases 14 and 15 in Chapter 12 involved the identical technique of elongation, neither one was necessitated by requirements related to crown and bridge restoration. This case, however, demonstrates a typical example of the invaluable role played by this technique in assuring the cosmetic and functional success of extensive restorative dentistry by restoring teeth with abnormally short clinical crowns in order to re-create the normal 1:2 crown-root ratio essential for successful occlusal reconstruction.

PATIENT. A 37-year-old white man.

HISTORY. The patient was a victim of severe bruxism. He was referred for elongation of all the maxillary teeth from second bicuspid to second bicuspid as an essential preliminary to occlusal rehabilitation and bite opening to restore a normal vertical dimension.

CLINICAL EXAMINATION. *Extraoral.* The patient presented classic evidence of marked loss of vertical dimension due to bruxism. His facial appearance presented unmistakable evidence of a closed bite. The mandible was tilted forward and upward into a protrusive excursion. The chin jutted forward, bringing his lips into compressed premature contact, with the lower lip noticeably protruded (Case Fig. 10–1B).

Intraoral. The intraoral appearance confirmed the drastic loss of vertical dimension. The maxillary left central incisor and the right first and second bicuspids

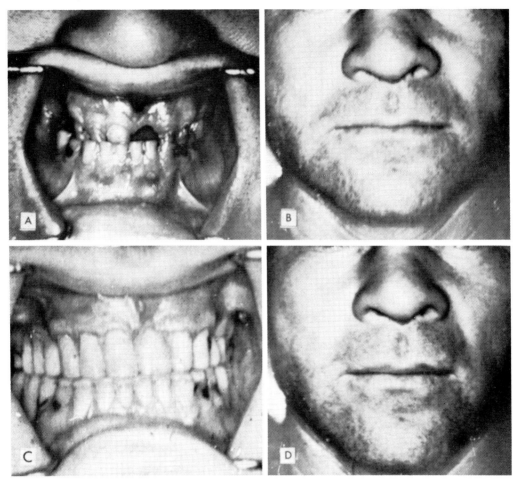

Case Figure 10–1. Elongation of clinical crowns of teeth badly abraded by bruxism, preliminary to full mouth rehabilitation and bite raising. *A*, Intraoral view. Mandibular teeth appear normal in size. Maxillary teeth worn down to approximately one half their original length. There is a wide edentulous space in the left central region, and the labial alveolar bone is markedly concave over the edentulous space. Some scar-like fibrous tissue is present near the crest of the edentulous ridge, and there is some fibromatous piling up of tissue. *B*, Extraoral appearance. Mandible juts forward simulating a Class III malocclusion. Lower lip juts forward, and upper lip is compressed into a straight thin line. *C*, Normal-sized crowns have been created, and a bite plane splint is in position. Fibromatous piling up of tissue is somewhat more marked in the relatively brief time since the restorations were inserted. *D*, Fascial appearance after rehabilitation and bite raising were performed. Mandible no longer is protrusive, and both the upper and lower lips are relaxed and normal looking.

and first molar were missing from the dental arch. The remaining teeth were worn down to somewhat less than half their normal height; the incisal edges were worn flat and the dentin could be seen. The entire labial-buccal mucosa appeared atonal. Instead of the normal, pink, stippled and firm appearance of normal, healthy gingival mucosa, the entire gingivae appeared edematous and engorged, with smooth, shiny tissue surface (Case Fig. 10–1A).

TREATMENT. The mouth was prepared in the usual manner and bilateral infraorbital and nasopalatine block anesthesia was administered. The amount of increase in height required to restore a normal 1:2 crown-root ratio was predetermined and marked off by puncturing the mucosa with the hypodermic needle.

It was evident that when corrected, the new gingival margins would extend rootward considerably beyond the base of their gingival crevices, exposing marginal alveolar bone which would have to be removed. A medium-sized 45-degree-angle U-shaped loop electrode was selected and current output set at 5 for electrosection.

The marginal gingivae were resected by looping off the tissue with short wiping strokes. After the desired labial gingival height was achieved, a flame-shaped loop electrode was substituted, current output increased to 6, and the convex plane of the interproximal papillae reduced. The electrode was used with a downward scooping motion, shaving the tissue in thin layers to create concave sluiceways. The same electrode was then applied to the new gingival margins at a 45-degree angle to bevel them to normal feather edges.

The flame-shaped electrode was then replaced with a straight U-shaped loop electrode which had been bent to contour it into a convexoconcave curve. The current output was increased to 7 and the electrode was applied to the palatal tissues with short brushing strokes, being held at an approximate 90-degree angle to the tissues. The thick, dense palatal mucosa was also shaved off in layers until the crowns of the teeth were properly exposed. This also exposed a narrow rim of palatal marginal bone around the elongated crowns approximately 2 to 3 mm. wide.

The exposed labial and palatal bone was then removed with curets, a bone file and a tapered bone bur, until all the exposed bone plus an additional millimeter of bone from under the newly established gingival margins was removed.

The operative field was thoroughly debrided, the tissues dried with sponges, and tincture of myrrh and benzoin applied in air-dried layers. A protective pack of stiffly mixed surgical cement was inserted over the entire operative field; the patient was instructed in postoperative care and reappointed.

He returned on the fifth postoperative day. The cement pack was removed and the mouth irrigated with Kasdenol and saline solutions. The operative surfaces of the gingival tissues were covered with a thin layer of coagulum, and they appeared to be healing satisfactorily. The tissues were dried, tincture of myrrh and benzoin was applied, and a fresh cement pack inserted. On the tenth postoperative day he returned for further postoperative treatment. The cement pack was removed and the mouth irrigated. The entire operative field appeared to be granulating normally except in two small labial patches, each about 4 mm. in diameter, which were still covered with coagulum. Tincture of myrrh and benzoin was reapplied, and the patient was told to return again in two weeks.

The next time the patient was seen the gingivae were completely healed and their tissue tone considerably improved. A temporary restoration with a clear acrylic occlusal splint for opening the bite had been inserted (Case Fig. 10-1C).

Although the tissue tone was now somewhat improved over its original condition it was still somewhat subnormal and slightly puffy, with a shiny, translucent appearance. He was advised to use an astringent salt-alum mouthwash for five-day periods, alternated with similar periods of saline lavage, to toughen and tan the hypokeratinized surface epithelium of the mucosa.

The patient was seen again three months later. From the appearance of the gingivae it seemed that the astringent lavage had been beneficial. This time the mucosa was firm, normally pink and stippled looking. His extraoral facial appearance

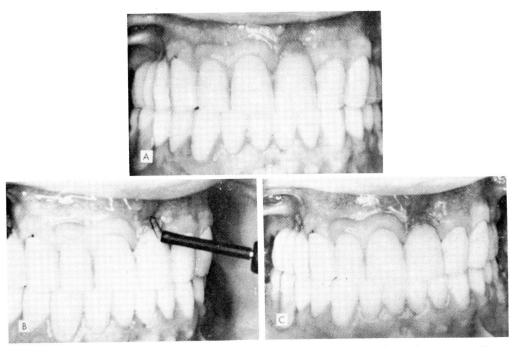

Case Figure 10-2.   Eighteen months after original elongation of clinical crowns had been performed patient returned for further treatment.

A, Preoperative view. There is a bulging mass of angry looking scar tissue present over the left central pontic which is butted against the concave alveolar ridge. *B*, Bulging tissue resected by planing with narrow 45-degree-angle U-shaped loop electrode to the level of the adjacent normal tissue. *C*, Mass completely reduced to normal level. Note lack of bleeding.

had been greatly improved by the restoration of normal vertical dimension. His mandible no longer jutted forward and upward, and the lips were relaxed, giving the face a much more youthful appearance (Case Fig. 10–1*D*).

He was seen again 18 months later. The gingival tone was excellent, although there had been a piling up of hypertrophic fibrotic mucosa. In addition to hypertrophic fibrosis of the marginal gingivae around the crown-bearing teeth, a considerable amount of hypertrophic tissue bulged out from under the left central incisor pontic (Case Fig. 10–2*A*). It was apparent that the fibrosis was a response to the impact of the abnormally heavy bite.

The mouth was prepared, and 4 minims of anesthetic solution were deposited by infiltration into the area of the left central. The excess tissue was then reduced to the level of the adjacent mucosa with a narrow U-shaped loop electrode and the cutting current was set at 5. The tissue was removed bloodlessly with short brushing strokes (Case Figs. 10–2*A* and *B*). The area was painted with tincture of myrrh and benzoin and postoperative lavage prescribed. He was seen again one week later. The tissue was found to have healed sufficiently so as not to require further treatment.

The next case demonstrates particularly well the importance of adequate elongation of the clinical crowns to assure that a fixed-bridge restoration will be able to withstand the torque of function.

This is the type of case in which ability to perform incisions or tissue resections without applying pressure to the structures being cut is uniquely invaluable. The patient was a victim of cleft palate with floating premaxilla that required immobilization with a surgical splint. The usefulness of electro-surgery in such cases is greatly magnified by the fact that the premaxilla usually is attached very precariously to the body of the maxilla. By eliminat-ing need to apply pressure to elongate the clinical crowns of the abutment teeth, electrosurgery eliminates the very real and likely danger of pathologic fracture of the mobile part. Moreover, the ease and uniformity with which electrosurgery permits reconstruction of the grossly irregular gingival architecture to normal contour cannot be duplicated by other methods of instrumentation.

In this particular case the initial attempt to immobilize failed and the splint had to be remade. The need to remake the case did not detract from the usefulness of electrosurgery, since it was in no way responsible for it. Failure resulted from the prosthodontist's failure to utilize fully the addi-tional clinical crown length the electrosurgical gingivectoplasty had exposed. As a result the first crown preparations were much too short to provide the 1:2 crown-root ratio necessary to successfully withstand functional torque. The splint repeatedly became loose and finally had to be discarded and replaced with a new splint after re-elongation of the clinical crowns in a second stage of electrosurgical gingivectoplasty.

CASE 11 – STAGE 1

PATIENT. A 13-year-old Puerto Rican female.

HISTORY. She was a patient at the Mt. Sinai Hospital Cleft Palate Center, New York City, for treatment of a bilateral cleft palate with floating premaxilla which was attached to the body of the maxilla by a very long slender stem and was quite mobile.

The treatment plan for this case was to attach and immobilize the premaxilla to the main body of the maxilla with a fixed-bridge splint constructed with full-crown coverage of all the involved teeth. She was referred for electrosurgical elongation of the clinical crowns of the maxillary teeth in order to create stronger abutments for maximum immobilization and to provide cosmetic improvement by creating har-monious gingival margins for all the anterior teeth.

CLINICAL EXAMINATION. *Extraoral.* The scar of a cleft lip repair was plainly visible.

Intraoral. The maxillary labial vestibule in the midline was partially obliterated by scar tissue adhesions from the lip repair. There was a 4 mm. space between the left lateral incisor and cuspid; the right lateral incisor was congenitally missing. There was a 4 mm. space between the right central and cuspid. Bilateral clefts in the gingival mucosa and underlying bone were plainly visible on the labial aspect. These clefts were long and narrow and ran through the 4 mm. spaces between the teeth in vertical planes (Case Fig. 11–1). There was a palatal cleft located immediately posterior to the nasopalatine papilla. The palatal cleft was larger, irregular and roughly pear shaped.

The premaxilla, containing the three incisors, was quite mobile and responded to very light pressure. The five anterior teeth appeared to have been partially prepared for full-crown coverage. They were covered with celluloid crown forms which were short of the gingival margins of the teeth. The crowns of the left central and lateral were shorter than the other anterior crowns, and the gingival margins of the two

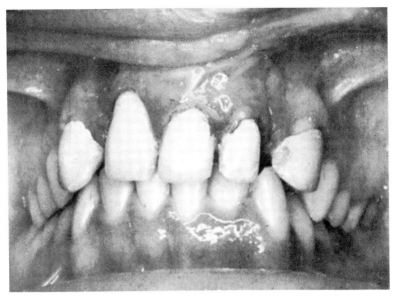

Case Figure 11–1.   Bilateral anterior cleft palate. Floating premaxilla, labial view.

smaller teeth were almost 4 mm. lower than the level of their adjacent marginal gingivae.

Roentgenographic examination with an intraoral occlusal-view film of the maxilla showed that the premaxilla with the three anterior teeth was almost completely detached from the body of the maxilla. It was attached by a very slender stem (Case Fig. 11–2).

ELECTROSURGICAL PROCEDURE.   The mouth was prepared for surgery and bi-

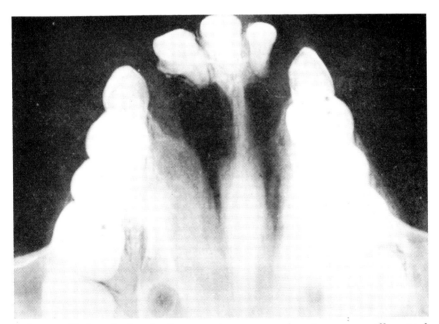

Case Figure 11–2.   Occlusal view roentgenogram showing premaxilla attached by a very slender stem.

lateral infraorbital regional block anesthesia plus palatal infiltration was administered. A narrow 45-degree-angle U-shaped loop electrode was selected and current output set at 4.5 for electrosection. The labial gingival margin of the left central incisor was treated first. The activated electrode, held at right angles to the long axis of the tooth, was applied to the gingival margin with a wiping stroke, removing a 2 mm. strip of marginal gingiva (Case Fig. 11–3A). When 5 mm. was removed in this fashion, the lateral was treated in a similar manner. The new gingival margins of both teeth were now at the same level as the corresponding teeth on the right side. This revealed that the exposed portion of the central was discolored a dark bluish gray and was a rough-surfaced structure notably softer than normal root cementum.

The gingival margins of the right central and the cuspids were raised 2 mm. When the gingival height of the labial aspect of all the anterior teeth was harmoniously equalized, a flame-shaped loop electrode was substituted, current output set at 6, and the newly created gingival margins beveled to a feather edge. The interproximal papillae were reduced to create slightly concave sluiceways by applying the electrode lightly with a downward pulling motion (Case Fig. 11–3B). The original narrow loop electrode was replaced at this point, current output reduced to 4.5, and slight irregularities in the outlines of the new gingival margins eliminated in order to create even marginal outlines.

The labial and buccal surfaces of these teeth having been completed, elongation of the palatal aspects was begun. Current output was increased to 7. The flame-shaped loop electrode was restored and used to raise the height of the palatal gingival margins of the five anteriors from 2 to 4 mm. by shaving the tissue with short brushing strokes. A straight U-shaped loop electrode was selected and bent into a convexoconcave curve. This electrode was substituted for the flame-shaped one, current output decreased to 5.5, and the contour of the palatal mucosa restored (Case Fig. 11–3C). It was then used to reduce the palatal convexity of the interproximal papillae to slightly concave contours. Finally, the narrow loop electrode was used, with current output of 5, to eliminate irregularities of the new gingival margins and create feather edges. The end result was a harmony of the gingival margins of all anterior teeth and increase in the length of the clinical crowns up to 0.5 cm.

The tissues were thoroughly debrided of loose fragments. The marginal alveolar bone around the right cuspid had been exposed slightly by the coronal elongation. Almost 2 mm. of denuded bone plus 1 mm. from under the new margin were removed with curets. This restored a marginal crevice around the tooth. The entire electrosurgical procedure had been bloodless. Tincture of myrrh and benzoin was applied to the operative field in air-dried layers. A medicated protective dressing of adhesive ointment was applied to the tissues and the usual postoperative instructions were given.

The patient was seen again on the fourth postoperative day. The new gingival margins were granulating normally, but the tissue tone was slightly subnormal and the tissues appeared slightly edematous. The patient was instructed to continue the saline lavage, to start using an astringent salt-alum lavage for five days, and to return in one week. The following week the alveolar gingivae appeared relatively normal. Tincture of myrrh and benzoin was applied and the patient was reappointed. When she returned again the following week the tissues appeared fully healed, firm, fully epithelialized and in excellent tone. All the teeth had normal feather-edged margins (Case Fig. 11–3D and E).

The patient was referred back to the crown and bridge department for completion of her fixed-bridge prosthesis. Six weeks later the cast framework was completed, and two weeks after that her completed restoration was cemented into position (Case

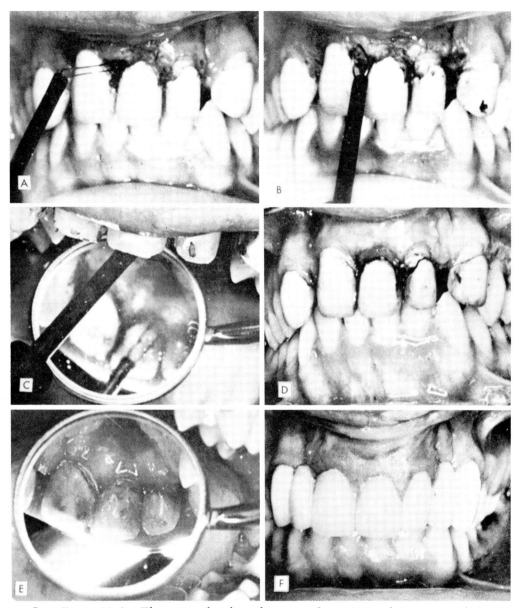

Case Figure 11-3. Elongating the clinical crowns of anterior teeth to serve as abutments for fixed prosthesis to immobilize floating premaxilla.

A, Left central incisor elongated 5 mm. with narrow U-shaped loop electrode. *B*, Interproximal papilla reduced to concave sluiceway with flame-shaped loop electrode. *C*, Palatal tissues recontoured with curved U-shaped loop electrode.

Postoperative healing. *D*, Third postoperative week. Tissues fully healed on labial aspect. Note discolored root of left central. *E*, Same visit, palatal view. *F*, Three months' postoperative appearance. Fixed prosthesis in position, locking floating premaxilla to body of maxilla. Teeth and gingival margins all at harmonious level for good cosmetic effect. Tissue tone excellent.

Fig. 11–3F). The cosmetic and functional improvement was impressive, and the formerly high mobile premaxilla appeared to be solidly immobilized. The ceramic restorations seemed normal in size and appearance, and the gingival tissues were fully healed.

CASE 11 – STAGE 2

The apparently successful outcome was only illusory, however. It soon became apparent that all was not well with the apparent functional improvement. The splint became loose and had to be repeatedly recemented. Finally the patient was referred back to the author for additional elongation of the crown preparations.

CLINICAL EXAMINATIONS. Although the aesthetics left much to be desired, the restoration appeared satisfactory as a splint (Case Fig. 11–4), but when it was removed it became obvious that the crown preparations were much too short to be able to withstand functional torque (Case Fig. 11–4B).

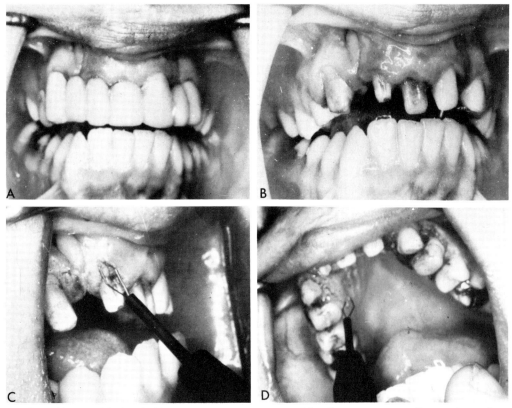

Case Figure 11–4. A, Preoperative appearance. The floating premaxilla resulting from bilateral clefts has been restored with a temporary splint as the first step in immobilizing the premaxilla and fixing it to the maxilla with a fixed splint. The temporary splint keeps becoming loose and becomes displaced despite temporary cementation. Note the irregularity of the crown levels, and of the marginal gingivae. B, The removal of the temporary splint reveals gross hyperplasia of the marginal gingivae, with downward growth that materially reduces the size of the clinical crowns of the teeth, so that they cannot provide the 1 to 2 crown:root ratio necessary for functional stability. C, Gingivoplasty to reduce the bulk and recontour the gingivae being performed with a flame-shaped loop electrode. Note the amount of tooth that is now exposed on the cuspid. D, The gingivoplasty being performed with the same loop on the palatal aspect, with equal facility.

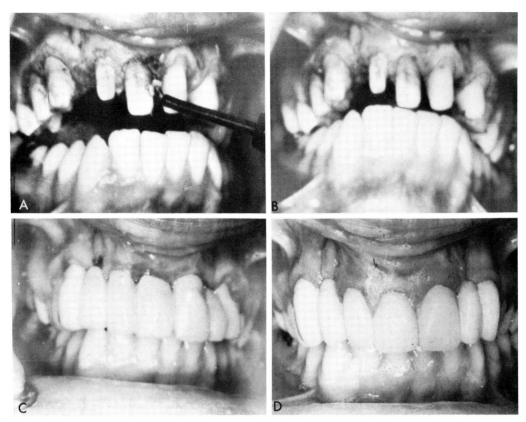

Case Figure 11–5.   A, Subgingival troughs being created around the teeth with a narrow 45-degree-angle U-shaped loop electrode. *B*, The elongations completed. Note the amount of elongation that was necessary, as seen by the darker color of the newly exposed portions. Also note that reasonable gingival harmony has been restored. *C*, One week postoperative appearance with built-up temporary splint in position. Quickcure acrylic was added to the splint immediately after the elongation had been completed the previous visit. *D*, Final appearance of the mouth after the permanent splint was inserted. The splint has locked the premaxilla to the body of the maxilla firmly. The gingivae are healed and normal, and the crowns of the splint are aesthetically acceptable and functionally useful. The gingival level is acceptably harmonious.

TREATMENT.   A flame-shaped loop electrode was selected and after infiltration anesthesia was administered, the electrode, activated with cutting current set at a power output of 5, was used to elongate the preparations on the labial and palatal aspects (Case Fig. 11–4*C* and *D*) by shaving the tissue in thin layers, with 5 to 10 second rest intervals between tissue contacts of the activated electrode.

When the external elongation was completed, the elongation was continued in the embrasure with a 45-degree-angle narrow U-shaped electrode (Case Fig. 11–5*A*). Tincture of myrrh and benzoin was applied to the cut tissues when the elongation was completed, the restoration was inserted and a cement pack applied around it, and the patient was referred back to the Crown and Bridge Department, but instructed to return in one week for postoperative observation. At the next visit the gingival tissues appeared to be fully healed (Case Fig. 11–5*B*). The addition of acrylic to the old crowns of the bridge revealed the amount of elongation that had been provided (Case Fig. 11–5*C*). The additional crown length proved adequate to withstand the functional torque to which the restoration was being subjected, and after approximately 2 months a new permanent fixed restoration was fabricated and inserted. The new restoration (Case Fig. 11–5D) not only provided excellent aesthetics and functional usefulness, but it also served to immobilize the floating premaxilla and eliminated fear of pathological fracture.

Restoration in Adolescent Patient with Amelogenesis Imperfecta

CASE 12

This case has been made available by Dr. William F. Malone, Loyola University School of Dentistry.

This patient presented a number of other serious dental defects in addition to the amelogenesis imperfecta; marked gingival hypertrophy, periodontoclasia, malposition of the teeth in the dental arch, and an open bite.

PATIENT.   A white adolescent female.

HISTORY.   Unknown except the history of amelogenesis imperfecta.

CLINICAL EXAMINATION.   Diastemas separated all the maxillary teeth. The lateral maxillary incisors were in slight palatal version and the cuspids in moderately marked labial version. The interdental papillae were grossly enlarged and partially detached. In the mandibular anterior region they were also severely engorged. The mandibular posterior teeth tilted lingually at an approximate 45-degree angle from the normal vertical position. With the teeth in the closed position there was an anterior open bite approximately 1 cm.

TREATMENT.   The course of treatment was subdivided into three phases: Phase 1, minor orthodontics to improve the alignment of the teeth in the maxillary arch (Case Fig. 12–1); Phase 2, gingival surgery to reduce the hypertrophied tissues to normal dimension; and Phase 3, preparation of the teeth and restoration of the dentition to normal. After Phase 1, the minor orthodontics, was completed, Phase 2 was insti-

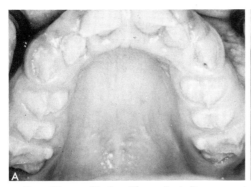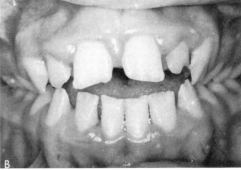

Case Figure 12–1.   Phase 1: *A*, Preoperative appearance of adolescent patient with amelogenesis imperfecta. *B*, Anterior teeth after minor orthodontic treatment to reposition upper lateral incisors.

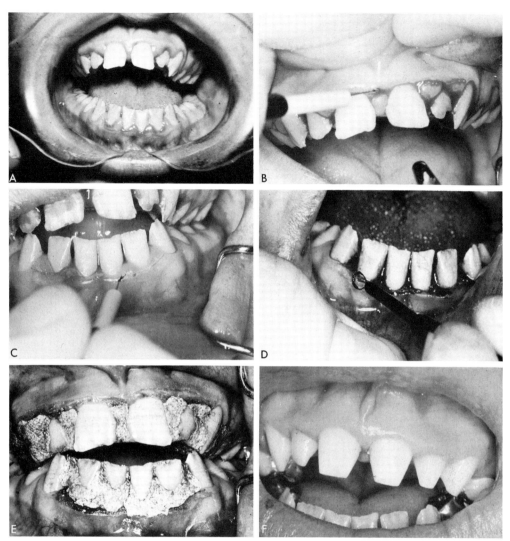

Case Figure 12–2. Phase 2: *A,* Full face view showing morphologic deficiencies of the coronal portions of teeth. The soft tissue is hypertrophied, edematous, and friable. *B,* Needle (thin-diameter) electrode incision is the preferable approach to tissue removal, owing to rapid electrode passage through the tissue. *C,* Tissue treatment of mandibular arch. Note clean incision without tissue accumulation on needle electrode. *D,* Tissue planing with loop electrode, with 10-second intervals between applications of current. *E,* Placement of periodontal pack dressing is encouraged after necessarily deep tissue eradication. *F,* Upper anterior teeth one week after preparation and electrosurgical sculpturing.

tuted (Case Fig. 12–2). A fine needle electrode was selected and activated with fully rectified cutting current. The activated electrode was used to incise and excise the interdental papillae in the maxilla at the level of the necks of the respective teeth. In the mandible, the incisions were made at the level of the cuspids. The sharp, right-angled edges of the cut tissues were then beveled and recontoured by loop planing with a round loop electrode, with care to allow a full 10 seconds to elapse between

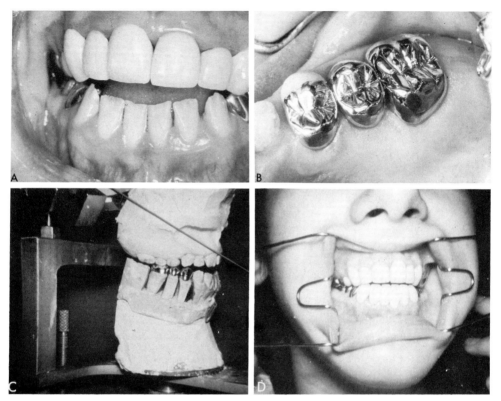

Case Figure 12–3. Phase 3: *A*, Restoration of upper anterior teeth with gold cast core and heat-treated acrylic veneer crowns. The gingival termination is "knife-edged." *B*, Restoration of upper posterior teeth using a modified P. K. Thomas cusp-fossae technique. *C*, Working cast mounted on semi-adjustable Arcon articulator. Note anterior "open bite" due to a tongue-thrust habit. *D*, Six months postoperatively, treatment completed.

reapplications of the activated loop. Periodontal pack dressings were applied to the surgical fields. The following week the cement packs were removed and the maxillary anterior teeth were prepared for full crown coverage. The following week the tissues were fully healed.

A restoration consisting of a gold cast core with heat-treated acrylic veneer transitional crowns was fabricated and used to restore the maxillary anterior teeth (Case Fig. 12–3). The posterior teeth were then prepared and restored with cast gold crowns using a modified P.K. Thomas cusp-fossae technique. The mandibular posterior teeth were then prepared and restored with cast crowns. The cast gold crowns were fabricated on a working cast mounted on a semi-adjustable Arcon articulator. Subsequently, the mandibular anterior teeth were prepared and restored with a gold core and heat-treated acrylic veneer crowns that were built up to close the opening between the teeth in the two arches.

The patient was seen again postoperatively six months later. The mouth was now normal in all respects. The gingival tissues and interdental papillae were normal in tone and contour, and the open bite was eliminated, creating normal aesthetics and function.

III. PREPARATION OF THE SUBGINGIVAL TROUGH

The rationale for the technique was briefly reviewed at the beginning of this chapter. The technique offers restorative dentistry three potential advantages:

1. The subgingival trough assures against tissue compression, impingement, and irritation by providing adequate space for the seating of the subgingival portions of the restorations.

2. Shoulder preparation with full bevel or chamfer can be accomplished without the usual traumatic laceration or maceration of the subgingival tissues by instrumentation, if the subgingival space is created before the tooth is fully prepared.

3. More accurate impressions of all prepared teeth in one jaw can be obtained, since the trenches around the prepared teeth allow impression materials to flow freely into the marginal crevices (Fig. 15–3).

Full Crown Preparation

There are four types of full-crown preparations (Fig. 15–4):
1. Shoulderless crowns.

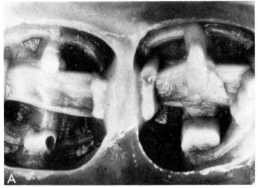
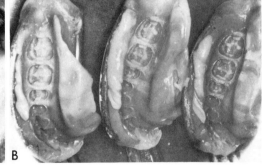
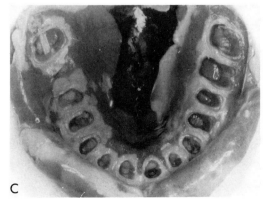

Figure 15–3. A and B, Typical hydrocolloid impressions of the inlay preparations. Note the detail of the impressions in the embrasures. C, A typical injection hydrocolloid impression of an entire arch prepared for full coverage. The subgingival troughs have permitted the impression material to flow unimpeded into the subgingival area, thus providing perfect detailed accuracy that makes it possible to use the model as a working model for fabrication of the restoration.

PLATE III

Crown and Bridge Prosthodontics

Figure 1a. Preparation of subgingival troughs around crown preparations. The first bicuspid and first molar have been prepared for full crown coverage, and the tissue in the edentulous space between the two teeth has been planed to reduce the tissue bulk. Subgingival troughs are being prepared around the two crown preparations with a 45-degree-angle narrow U-shaped loop electrode by electrosection.

Figure 1b. Appearance of the tissues one week later (mirror image view). Tissue healing is practically complete.

Figure 1c. Appearance of the tissues after insertion of the restoration (mirror image view). Note the perfect tissue adaptation around the crowns and absence of tissue impingement.

Figure 3a. Remake of an unsatisfactory fixed prosthesis. The tissues have been planed by loop electrosection to restore a normal tissue architecture. The gingivoplasty having been completed, subgingival troughs are being created around the full crown preparations by J-loop resection.

Figure 2a. Exposure of a key retained abutment root for functional use. The coronal end of the root is being exposed by loop electrosection of the overlying tissue, care being taken to plane the tissues to avoid creating undercuts around the exposed root.

Figure 2b. The exposed root has been built up with a gold core to create a full crown preparation. Note the excellent tissue tone of the now fully healed tissue around the newly exposed root.

Figure 2c. Appearance of the mouth after the retained root has been restored with a porcelain veneer crown that is serving as an effective functional abutment for a partial denture.

Figure 3b. Appearance of the tissues one week after the new fixed prosthesis has been inserted. Note the rapid tissue healing and excellent tissue tone, and absence of evidence of impingements.

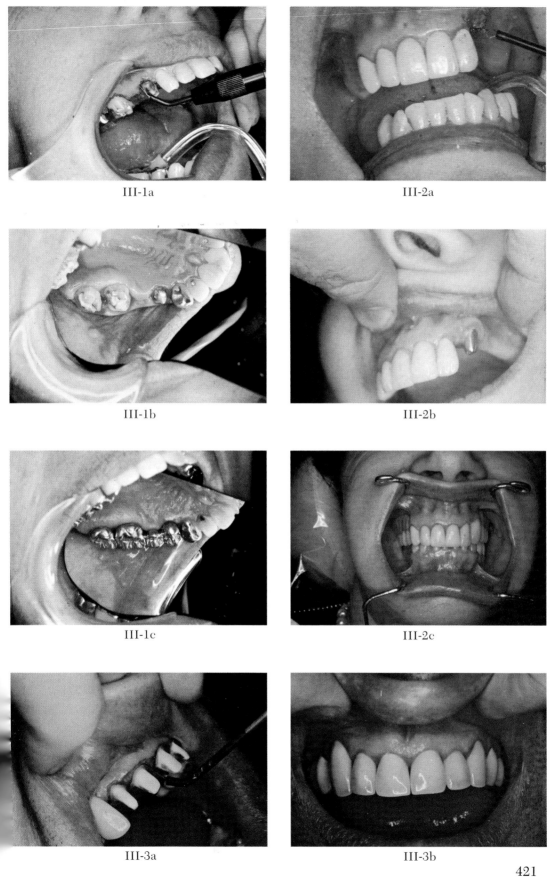

III-1a

III-2a

III-1b

III-2b

III-1c

III-2c

III-3a

III-3b

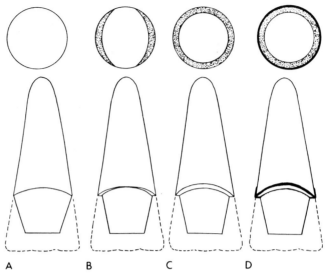

Figure 15–4. Full crown preparations: *A,* Shoulderless crowns. *B,* Crowns with partial shoulders on their mesial and distal proximal surfaces. *C,* Crowns with full shoulders. *D,* Crowns with full shoulders and coping bevels or chamfered shoulders.

2. Crowns with partial shoulders on the mesial and distal proximal surfaces.

3. Crowns with full shoulders (plain or chamfered).

4. Crowns with full shoulders and coping bevels.

All four types have one common feature. No matter what type of preparation is used, unless the crown is to be terminated above the free margin of the gingiva, a subgingival trough is advantageous for some or all of the reasons outlined above.

It is advisable to review the histologic and anatomic characteristics of the gingival and subgingival mucosa before entering into description of the instruments and methods of instrumentation involved in this technique.

The oral mucosa is subdivided into the following anatomic divisions:[3]

Marginal gingiva, or free gingiva (Fig. 15–5A), is made of wedge-shaped extensions that encircle the enamel or cementum at the cervix of the clinical crown. It extends from the rest of the gingiva to the epithelial attachment at the base of the gingival crevice.

Cemental gingiva rests upon the crest of the alveolar process and is supported thereby. It is attached to the cementum and crest of the alveolus and extends from the base of the gingival crevice or epithelial attachment, above, to the crest of the alveolar bone below. In this region is found Kollicker's ligament (circular ligament) which is made up of connective tissue fibers from the upper part of the pericementum which hold the marginal gingiva to the tooth and, proximally, help to keep contacts closed.

Alveolar gingiva covers the alveolar process from the cemental gingiva with which it is continuous rootwise. It blends with the areolar mucosa.

Areolar mucosa overlies the alveolar process below the alveolar gingiva and is attached to the cortical bone by a loose areolar connective tissue.

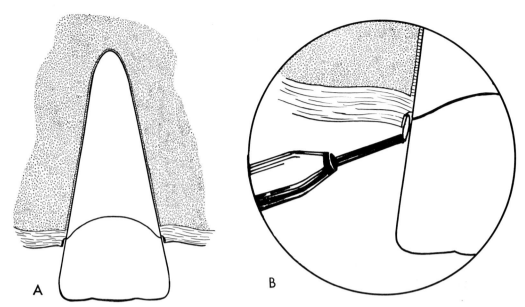

Figure 15–5. The marginal gingiva: *A,* Maxillary central incisor showing marginal gingiva and free margin. *B,* Cutting electrode in position in free margin to create a subgingival trough.

Both the marginal and cemental gingivae are involved in creating the subgingival trough (Fig. 15–5*A* and *B*).

It is virtually impossible to create a subgingival trough efficiently by any method other than electrosurgery. Results obtained by substitution of powerful chemical astringents and pressure packs to increase the gingival crevice space only serve to confirm this fact. Comparison of the results obtained with the astringents with those obtained by skillful use of electrosurgery shows the former to be decidedly unfavorable.

The common nonelectrosurgical method consists of packing a cotton wick impregnated with racemic epinephrine or zinc chloride into the crevice space. Both of these drugs are powerful astringents and markedly shrink the gingival tissues. This produces some increase in the width of the space but cannot increase the depth of the crevice. Furthermore, this method produces severe chemical and pressure irritations of the marginal and cemental gingivae, often with engorgement and hypertrophic reaction as the end result. Since the effects of the astringent action of these chemicals are not under the control of the operator, hypertrophy or excessive contraction of the gingival tissues frequently ensues.

When electrosurgery is skillfully employed there is little or no bleeding; there is no pressure irritation, chemical reaction, hypertrophic or contractile tissue response, or uncontrolled tissue necrosis.

Instruments and Methods of Instrumentation

Two electrodes are especially useful for this technique. One is the straight or angled, very narrow U-shaped loop electrode used for cutting; the shaft may be either straight or at a 45-degree angle. The other is the J-loop electrode, created by cutting a narrow loop so as to leave a 1- to 2-mm. curved, open loop end; the shorter or open portion of the loop is used against the tissues (See Fig. 15–6).

A feature common to both types of electrodes is that they are used in similar positions and directions. They should be held parallel to the long axis of the teeth, with their tips directed rootward.

The J-loop electrode can be used for movement to either left or right for labial and lingual access in full crown preparations. (Fig. 15–6).

The electrode of choice having been selected and suitable anesthesia administered, the electrode is inserted under the gingival free margin to the base of the crevice. The cutting current is set at about 3.5, the instrument is used with a rotating movement to circumscribe the entire circumference of the tooth. The electrode must be kept in constant motion from the moment it is inserted under the free margin and the current is applied. If the electrode is moved very rapidly and not permitted to linger in contact with the tooth, and a full 10 seconds is permitted to elapse before reapplying the activated electrode, the momentary contact of the activated electrode will not cause any clinically meaningful damage to either the pulp of the tooth or the periosteum and investing alveolar bone.

When the U-shaped loop electrode is to be used to create the trough, the width of the trough is determined by the angle at which the electrode is held in the gingival crevice. If the loop is held at right angles to the tooth surface the full width of the loop projects against the inner surface of the marginal gingiva. This will remove so much of the tissue that the height of the marginal gingiva will be reduced even if the narrowest loop is used. But if the loop is held at an approximate 15-degree angle to the surface of the tooth (forming an acute angle), very little of the inner surface of the marginal gingiva is removed. To widen the trough, the electrode is held at a less acute angle, thereby removing more of the inner surface tissue. When the cut J-loop electrode is used, if the electrode is held flat against the tooth surface with the tiny curved loop-end arc facing toward the marginal gingiva, only the 1 mm. end will do the cutting. The width can be determined either by the diameter of the arc end or by holding the latter at an angle to the tooth surface.

The depth of the trough is determined largely by the depth to which we permit the electrode to penetrate. With the loop electrodes the depth is determined by the operator. For a shallow depth, the operator prevents the electrode from penetrating beyond the desired depth. For greater depth, the electrode is permitted to penetrate to the desired depth and then rotated at that depth.

After the subgingival trough has been created to the desired width and depth, the crown preparation can be completed; the colloid, hydrocolloid, rubber base or alginate impression can be taken, and the temporary splint or permanent restoration can be properly seated.

When the embrasure tissue is to be excised to provide access to the axial floor areas of proximal inlay preparations, it is important to avoid scooping out

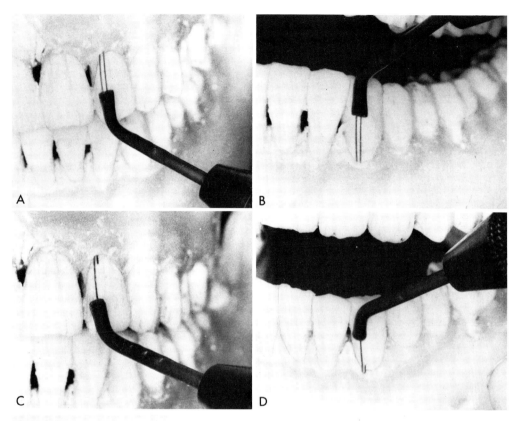

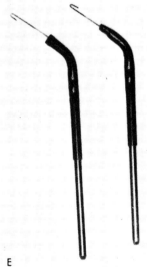

Figure 15–6. Preparation of subgingival troughs with a small narrow 45-degree-angle U-shaped loop electrode demonstrated on the specially prepared dry specimen. *A,* Proper position of the electrode for preparing a trough in the maxilla. The electrode points upward with the loop portion parallel to the long axis of the tooth and directed apically. The electrode has been rotated so that the wire forming the left side of the loop is in contact with the tooth and the right half is elevated from the tooth to create a 15- to 20-degree angle between it and the tooth in a manner similar to the angulation and position of the knife blade when butter is spread on a slice of bread. The angulation is maintained as the loop circumscribes the tooth. *B,* Proper position of the electrode for creating a trough in the mandible. The position of the electrode is reversed and the loop is now pointing downward apically. The angulation and use of the electrode is the same as in the maxilla.

Preparation of subgingival troughs with a J-loop electrode demonstrated on the same dry specimen. *C,* Proper position of the electrode for preparing a trough in the maxilla. The position and use are similar to that of the U-shaped loop, except that the angulation with this loop usually is 30 to 40 degrees, owing to the narrower diameter of the tip of the J. *D,* Proper position of the electrode for preparing a trough in the mandible. The position and use of the loop is similar to that of the U-shaped loop, and if the marginal gingiva is thin, even the angulation may have to be similar. *E,* The J-loop electrode can be used for either labial or lingual access in preparation of subgingival troughs.

the tissue abruptly. Sharp line angles formed at the terminal ends of the excision retard the regeneration of the tissues into the embrasures and may result in failure to obtain close adaptation of the regenerated papillae to the restorations. It is necessary to begin the excision from the external aspect of the buccal gingiva and continue the slightly scooping motion toward the center of the embrasure and then to reverse the direction and, starting from the external of the lingual or palatal surface, carry it toward the center. This creates slightly concave, gently contoured terminal ends that permit the regenerating tissue to flow into the embrasures rapidly and uniformly and adapt against the restorations very tightly.

Value of Subgingival Trough in Fixed Prosthodontics

In order to properly evaluate the role of the subgingival trough in fixed prosthodontics, it is necessary to chronologically review the salient factors that led to development of this technique.

The original full crown restoration, the gold shell crown, required very little tooth preparation. No attempt was made to attain a continuous smooth finish line with the root of the tooth; the subgingival end of the shell was simply crimped with contouring pliers to hug the neck of the tooth as snugly as possible.

When the shell crowns were replaced with the cast crowns, veneer crowns, and porcelain jacket crowns, it soon became apparent that these restorations could not be finished in a similar manner by mere adaptation to the outer surface of the root. Shoulder preparations came into vogue and these progressed from a simple butt joint to shoulders with bevels, chamfers, and beveled chamfers. These sophisticated refinements made it imperative that accurate impressions of the prepared subgingival areas be obtained. The techniques for chemical gingival retraction and subgingival troughing were developed as a means of meeting this need.

By and large, fixed prosthodontists have considered the subgingival trough invaluable for one purpose — to facilitate an unimpeded flow of impression material into the gingival sulcus to obtain a faithful reproduction of the shoulder area or finish line of the restoration on the working model. An accurate finish line was presumed to assure against unfavorable tissue response to the restoration.

This desire to obtain an accurate impression of the subgingival areas prompted the use of chemically impregnated cords to produce gingival retraction to facilitate flow of impression materials subgingivally. When, despite perfect finish lines, the restorations still produced irritation and inflammatory reactions in all too many instances, it was assumed that the unfavorable tissue responses were due in part to the damaging irritation of the chemicals and in part to the mechanical damage caused by packing the cords subgingivally and strangulating the blood supply.

Some prosthodontists began to use electrocoagulation to produce gingival retraction electrosurgically to avoid the damaging effects of the chemical retraction. Unfortunately, the electrocoagulation proved unsatisfactory for a number of reasons. In order to create adequate subgingival space, either the coagulating current had to be powerful enough to coagulate enough layers of cells to provide the space, which created the hazard of lack of control over the depth of penetration of the coagulation, or the normal amount of current had to be used, but the electrode had to circumscribe the tooth several times until enough coagulation was produced to create adequate space, which created the hazard of loss of control of the depth of penetration of the coagulating effect.

Since the end result of electrocoagulation cannot be determined until the tissues have healed fully and the coagulum has peeled away spontaneously, and since the tissues destroyed by electrocoagulation do not tend to regenerate toward their original level to a degree comparable to that of tissues cut by electrosection, prosthodontists all too frequently found that the marginal gingivae had receded several millimeters beyond the finish line of the restorations. Since this is an irreversible result, the only remedy was to reprepare the teeth and redo the restoration. Thus this method also fell into disfavor.

Since tissue properly cut by fully rectified electrosection tends to regenerate toward its original level, the author reasoned that if the trough were created by excising a thin sliver of the marginal gingiva from the inner surface of the sulcus gingiva, the hazard of gingival recession beyond the finish line could be avoided. The technique that he developed of resecting the tissue from the sulcus with a narrow U-shaped loop electrode or with the J-loop (broken loop) electrode, which was described in the first edition, was predicated on this reasoning.

This technique eliminated all the hazards that had been the downfall of the techniques involving chemical retraction and electrosurgical coagulation, and should therefore have provided foolproof results. But subsequent events failed to substantiate this and forced him to reappraise the entire problem.

When the occlusion and biomechanical factors such as buccolingual and mesiodistal contours of the restoration are acceptable, and the only other factor needed to prevent subgingival irritation is a perfect impression of the shoulder area to make possible a perfect finish line, the technique of excisional resection of tissue to form the subgingival troughs should be satisfactory. Factually, however, it is no exaggeration to assert that the majority of dentists nevertheless refrain from permanently cementing permanent restorations, especially multiple units, for prolonged periods, often for many months and even years. The widespread practice of inserting and maintaining a permanent fixed prosthesis under temporary cementation for many months offers unmistakable proof that neither the accurate impression nor the perfect finish line of the subgingival portion of the restoration alone offers the solution.

It would of course be highly injudicious and unwarranted to cement in a restoration permanently without first determining that the occlusion is acceptable. But this can be accomplished in a matter of one or two weeks. What, then, motivates dentists to maintain permanent restorations for prolonged periods with temporary cementation? It is obvious that the motivation is uncertainty as to how the tissues will react to the restoration and fear that it may produce subgingival irritation. In the event that a remake of the restoration is necessary, temporary cementation eliminates the risk of fracturing the coronal portions of the tooth preparations in the process of forcefully removing the permanently cemented restorations. Moreover, very frequently the prosthodontist who risks permanent cementation, immediately after determining that the occlusion is acceptable, often finds it necessary to cope interminably with inflammatory gingival reactions manifested either by proliferation of the marginal gingivae or by gingival recession, or, not infrequently, by a combination of both, coexisting simultaneously around the same restoration.

If the occlusion is satisfactory, the proliferative or recessive tendencies of the marginal gingivae must be attributed to subgingival irritation. If subgingival irritation continues to plague the prosthodontist even though the biomechanical factors are favorable and a perfect finish line of the subgingival portion of the restoration has been achieved, we are forced to conclude that, as important as these are, they do not entirely solve the problem and that despite them, periodontal irritation can still occur. How and why it can occur becomes the crux of the matter.

Subgingival irritation under such circumstances can result from impingement of the subgingival portion of the restoration against the subgingival tissues. Let us examine how and why this can happen.

The space having been created to obtain a perfect impression and the perfect subgingival finish line, the tissue promptly regenerates and fills in the space if it is not maintained, and often the shoulder area is obliterated. By the time the restoration is fabricated and ready to insert into the mouth, the subgingival space has been completely obliterated. Thus, when the restoration is inserted, it impinges against the periodontal ligament and other subgingival tissues and produces gingival irritation and inflammation. In effect, it is impinging against these tissues and acting like a splinter under a fingernail, just as though the space had never been created.

It therefore became apparent to the author that in addition to creating the space that permits the impression material to flow subgingivally, it is imperative to then maintain that space so that the tissue will repair properly against the transitional splint that is inserted while the permanent restoration is being fabricated.

Functional Roles of Intermediate (Temporary) and Permanent Fixed Restorations

Many if not most of the failures experienced in fixed prosthodontics would undoubtedly be avoided if the true functions of the initial, or so-called "temporary," and the final, or permanent restorations were more clearly defined and better understood. Specifically, the initial or temporary restoration fulfills an active functional role, and the permanent restoration a passive role, in the responses of the gingival tissues to insertion of the respective restorations.

The reasons for their respective roles are clear-cut and unmistakable. After the subgingival troughs have been created around the prepared teeth, the cut tissues begin to regenerate and heal. As this occurs, the regenerating tissues adapt themselves around and against the subgingival portion of the initial or temporary restoration. If the subgingival portion of this restoration has been fabricated carefully to provide a perfect subgingival finish line, and has been polished to a smooth external surface, healing progresses uneventfully, the regenerating tissues adapt themselves tightly around the subgingival portion of the restoration, and the repair tissue becomes fully matured.

If, however, the initial restoration is regarded as merely a stop-gap to protect the prepared teeth, and the accuracy of its fabrication is therefore deemed unimportant, the tissue responses invariably reflect this failure and a totally different chain of events takes place. If there is a discrepancy between the finish lines of the prepared teeth and the finish lines of the restoration, the regenerating tissue flows into and fills the intervening spaces. When the permanent restoration is inserted its accurately finished subgingival portion impinges against the redundant tissue that has filled the spaces and produces subgingival irritation. Even if the subgingival finish of the initial restoration is satisfactory, but its mesiodistal and buccolingual contours are poor, the regenerating tissues adapt themselves around and against these contours. When the permanent restoration with excellent mesiodistal and buccolingual contours is subsequently inserted, the fully healed marginal gingivae cannot adapt themselves accurately around the new restoration. If everything else is satisfactory but the subgingival portion of the initial restoration is not polished to a smooth exterior, the regenerating tissues will tend to proliferate or to recede away from the rough surfaces.

Thus it is obvious that the initial restoration is in effect the active device that will determine the rate and quality of the tissue repair, and will influence greatly the subsequent health of the marginal gingivae. By the time the permanent restoration has been fabricated and is ready for insertion as the replacement for the initial appliance, the subgingival repair has been completed and all that is required of the permanent restoration is that it should not alter or disrupt the favorable tissue-restoration relation that has been established by its predecessor. The permanent restoration therefore obviously fulfills the passive role, that of merely maintaining the status quo that has been achieved.

In view of these respective roles, obviously a meticulously accurate subgingival finish and proper contours are of equal importance in both restorations, and both should be fabricated as perfectly as possible in all respects. Factually, therefore, and not merely as a matter of semantics, the initial restoration is infinitely more important than just a stop-gap cover for the prepared teeth, but is the critically important transitional intermediate restoration.

If the permanent restoration is fabricated and finished to duplicate the intermediate splint identically, it fits into the subgingival space precisely, without any possibility of impingement. Under such conditions, as soon as the occlusion has been found acceptable, the permanent restoration can be cemented in permanently, and there will be no subsequent periodontal irritation or deterioration.

ATRAUMATIC CREATION OF SUBGINGIVAL TROUGH

The technique the author has devised that makes this possible also resolves the problem of how to create a bevel or chamfer on a subgingival shoulder atraumatically.

Figure 15–7A shows on a Typodont model the preoperative appearance of a maxillary left central incisor. First the mesial, distal, and incisal surfaces of the tooth are reduced with discs and stones to the approximate shape of the crown preparation (Fig. 15–7B). Then the labial and lingual or palatal surfaces are denuded of their enamel, and the crown preparation is completed to within 2 to 3 mm. of the gingival level (Fig. 15–7C and D). At this point an impression is taken and a model poured, reproducing the supragingival preparation. An acrylic splint restoring the missing supragingival preparation is fabricated.

Now the subgingival trough is created with the full narrow U-shaped or J-loop electrode, by electrosection, using the 2- to 3-mm. ledge of enamel as a guide to assure the proper position and angulation of the electrode and to serve as a fulcrum on which the electrode can be rested and rotated as the trough is cut, thereby eliminating need for freehand circumscribing of the shoulder area, which invariably results in a degree of irregularity and often a slight shredding of the edge of the marginal gingiva (Fig. 15–7E and F).

After the trough has been prepared, the space created by removal of the enamel plus the space created by resection of the sliver of tissue from the internal surface of the gingival sulcus provide adequate space for atraumatic subgingival instrumentation. Free bleeding such as occurs when the tissues are macerated and lacerated by the diamond stones and burs is absent, and therefore clear vision and access that make possible preparation of an ideal shoulder with the aid of loup magnification are provided.

When the shoulder has been completed, a master impression is taken. After a second identical impression is taken, models are poured. This assures that the intermediate and the permanent restorations will be processed on identical models. If copper band impressions are used, the second impression may be omitted and, instead, the model may be duplicated.

If the validity of the premise that a subgingival trough has three functions is accepted, it becomes apparent that to properly fulfill these functions it must be a clean, well-defined space of uniform dimension and free of tissue fragmentation. The most effective way to create such a trough is by electrosurgical

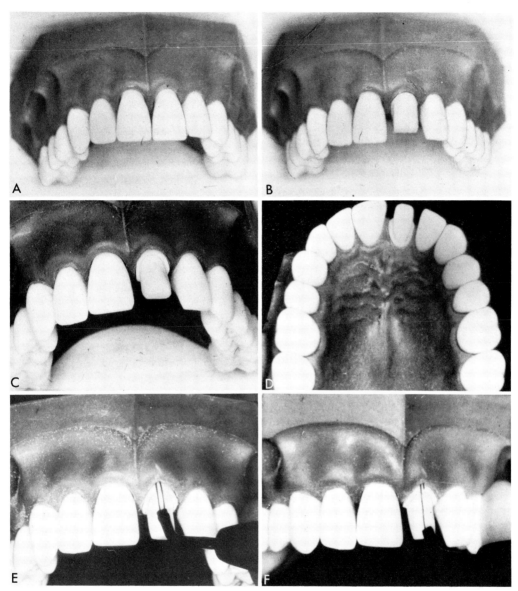

Figure 15–7. A, Typodont showing preoperative appearance of maxillary left central incisor. B, Appearance of the tooth after reduction of the mesial, distal, and incisal surfaces. C, Labial appearance of the tooth after the enamel has been removed to within 3 mm. of the gingival margin. D, Palatal appearance of the prepared tooth. E, Position of the narrow 45-degree-angle full U-shaped loop for preparation of the subgingival trough. The loop is held parallel to the long axis of the tooth and tilted 15 degrees off the horizontal plane, lifting the inner leg of the loop slightly off the tooth surface, with the other (external) leg resting on the remaining 3 mm. ledge of enamel. F, Position of the J-loop electrode for creating the subgingival trough. Note that the open short part of the loop is contacting the tissue.

atraumatic excision of a uniform amount of tissue from the internal surface of the marginal gingiva.

This creates the problem of choice of electrode to excise the trough. The needle electrode is ideally suitable for use as a scalpel to incise tissue for drainage, to incise mucoperiosteal flaps, or for block dissection of wedges of tissue. It is *not* suitable for excising slices of tissue of uniform thickness. The loop electrode is ideally suitable for this purpose. The angle at which the electrode is held as it makes contact with the tissue determines the thickness of the slice it will excise. If the angle is maintained during the brief cutting stroke, the entire slice will be uniform in thickness.

The small narrow U-shaped loop or the J-loop electrodes are most suitable for dissecting out the thin slices of tissue to create the subgingival trough. However, if they are used free-hand to circumscribe the tooth, it is extremely unlikely that even the loop electrodes can excise tissue slices of uniform thickness and create troughs of uniform dimension. If the 2- to 3-millimeter ledge of enamel is used as a rest on which the electrode is rotated around the tooth, as shown in Fig. 15–8, need for free-hand dissection is eliminated, thereby assuring excision of tissue of uniform thickness and creation of a trough of uniform precise dimension. Whether creation of the trough requires two strokes or four to excise the tissue, the contact of the activated electrode with the enamel ledge for each stroke is extremely brief. If, in addition, the 10-second pause interval between cutting strokes is strictly observed to avoid damage from cumulative heat, atraumatic preparation of a trough of uniform dimension without tissue fragmentation or destruction of the marginal edge of the marginal gingiva is assured.

Techniques Using Needle Electrodes

Some prosthodontists wish to avoid use of electrocoagulation because of the likelihood of subsequent recession of the marginal gingivae, yet for one reason or another they are also reluctant to use loop electrodes to cut the subgingival troughs. As a result, several techniques have been devised to create the troughs by electrosection with needle electrodes. Not only are these techniques incapable of creating *precise troughs of uniform dimension* but some are fraught with the danger of unfavorable postoperative sequelae, ranging in severity from gingival recession to acute periostitis and/or osteitis.

The least dangerous of these techniques consists of incising subgingivally with a fine needle electrode to sever the epithelial attachment, so that the tissues can be displaced to facilitate impression-taking. By the time the permanent prosthesis is ready to be inserted, the epithelial attachment usually must be re-incised, so that the subgingival portion of the restoration can be inserted without impingement. This technique does serve well to facilitate impression-taking, but it sacrifices the other two critically important functions of the subgingival trough.

Another technique involves use of a fine needle electrode with cutting

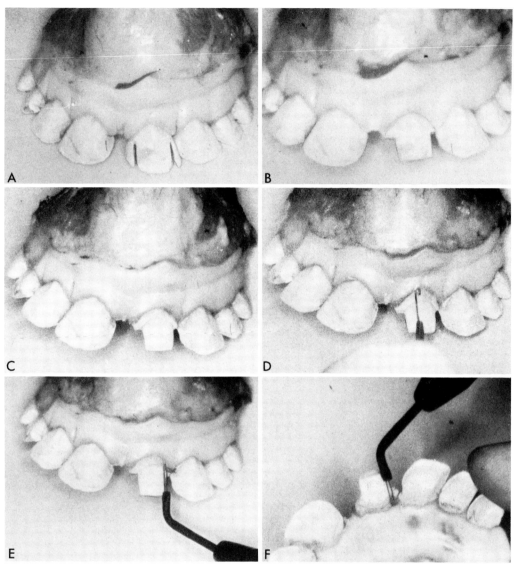

Figure 15–8. A, Beginning of tooth preparation on calf mandible. Parallel vertical cuts have been made with a diamond stone disc to within 3 mm. of the gingival tissue around the tooth. B, The mesial, distal, and incisal portions of the crown have been cut away, providing the basic outline of the crown preparation. C, The enamel has been removed from the labial and palatal surfaces to within 3 mm. of the gingival margin, leaving a 3-mm. ledge of enamel at the gingival end of the crown. D, The J-loop electrode in position is resting on the 3-mm. ledge of enamel that will serve as a fulcrum for a smooth, even circumscribing excision of the tissue to form the subgingival trough. E, The full narrow 45-degree-angle U-shaped loop electrode is being used to excise the tissue to form the subgingival trough on the labial aspect. F, The same loop is being used to excise the tissue to form the subgingival trough on the palatal aspect to complete the procedure. The mesial and distal reduction permits clearance for the electrode to pass through the embrasures and complete the troughing.

current to repeatedly circumscribe the shoulder area until a trench of charred tissue forms around the tooth. The charred debris is then washed out by irrigating with hydrogen peroxide until debridement is completed. In addition to the fact that this method is imprecise and causes tissue fragmentation unless each circumscribing stroke around the tooth is followed by a 10-second pause interval to permit dissipation of the heat being generated, continuous application of the cutting energy until the tissue chars creates a grave danger of acute periostitis and/or osteitis due to cumulative heat damage.

Still another needle electrode technique with a high potential for postoperative problems involves use of a short wire needle electrode that protrudes only 1 to 2 millimeters beyond an insulated shaft that extends from the normal electrode shaft, that fits into the chuck of the electrode handle. The technique consists of resting the end of the insulated shaft tip on the shoulder of the crown preparation, so that the 1- to 2-millimeter exposed needle tip extends beyond the shoulder and makes contact with the subgingival structure to create a groove around the preparation. The rationale for this technique appears to be predicated upon the theory that inasmuch as only the insulated shaft portion of the electrode tip comes into contact with tooth structure while the activated exposed tip portion is circumscribing the tooth to create the trough, this will prevent the irritation of the pulp by the heat being generated during the troughing. The fallacy of this theory is that if the electrode is being moved slowly enough for the heat being generated to cause pulp irritation and necrosis, the marginal gingivae and alveolar investing bone with which the activated needle is in contact are equally susceptible to damage from the heat during preparation of the trough.

If adequate cutting current power to disintegrate and volatilize the cells efficiently is being used, the heat generated by it is likely to char the trough tissue and cause destruction of the thin marginal edge of the gingiva. If a weak cutting current output is used, the heat generated will be inadequate to totally disintegrate and volatilize the tissue cells and, instead, will either partially or completely coagulate them, creating the hazard of irreversible gingival recession that electrosection is supposed to avoid.

It is not beyond the realm of probability that methods of preparing subgingival troughs more efficiently than by electrosection with loop electrodes may some day be developed. Until such time, however, loop electrosection is the most effective and efficient method for preparing the subgingival trough.

Preparation of Subgingival Trough in Thin Marginal Gingiva

The technique to be described is to prevent labial gingival recession around maxillary cuspid crowns. When the typical maxillary cuspid tooth is restored with a full crown, unless the restoration is terminated supragingivally, the marginal gingiva on the labial aspect of the tooth almost invariably recedes. The recession appears to occur regardless of the kind of preparation used, the condition of the occlusion, how well the subgingival portion of the restoration is finished, or whether the restoration is ceramic, acrylic, or ceramic or acrylic on gold.

Recession sufficient to expose the shoulder area is by no means a rarity. Nevertheless, because of the unaesthetic exposure of gold if the crown is terminated supragingivally, this type of restoration is not popular, and most maxillary cuspid crowns are extended subgingivally despite the almost inevitable likelihood that gingival recession will occur.

The typical maxillary cuspid tooth is characterized by its convex contour on the labial aspect, which creates the canine eminence. As a result of the convexity, the labial alveolar bone is so thin that dehiscences are often present, and the marginal bone usually terminates 3 or more millimeters above the cemento-enamel junction. The marginal edge of the marginal gingiva on the labial aspect of the tooth is so very thin that it is translucent and avascular and resembles cuticle rather than normal marginal gingiva. This thin cuticle-like marginal gingiva is unsuited for electrosurgical preparation of a subgingival trough. It is equally unsuited for the instrumentation involved in shoulder preparation or for functional use as the host tissue to accommodate the subgingival portion of the restoration.

Recession of the marginal gingiva is an irreversible process, and the extent of the recession is unpredictable and uncontrollable. If the recession is anticipated and the technique is modified accordingly, it is possible to avoid being victimized by the vagaries of nature. Moreover, by taking advantage of the inherent tendency of tissue properly cut by electrosection to regenerate toward its original level, we can reverse the tendency for recession and expect regeneration of tissue instead. Thus, since all or most of the excessively thin marginal gingiva that is resected by electrosection will regenerate, this tissue becomes expendable.

TECHNIQUE. Gingivectomy of 2 millimeters of the cuticle-like marginal gingival crest is performed by electrosection with either the needle or loop electrode, preferably the latter. (See Figures 15–9 and 15–10.)

The electrode, either a small round loop, an elliptical loop, or a small U-shaped loop, is held parallel to the tooth and gingiva, so that the tissue can be resected at right angles to create a *square* cut edge rather than the beveled cut usually employed to elongate the clinical crown and simultaneously restore a feather-edge to the cut tissue margin. The blunt-edge right-angle cut creates a new crest of marginal gingiva that is thick enough to permit proper instrumentation and a suitable subgingival trough.

The author has found that when marginal gingiva must be resected he is able to control the accuracy of the resection better with loop electrode excision than by needle incision gingivectomy. In addition loop excision makes possible simultaneous beveling of the new gingival margin to restore the normal gingival architecture. But for gingivectomy of the thin cuticle-like marginal gingiva it is necessary to avoid beveling the cut tissue margin, and a

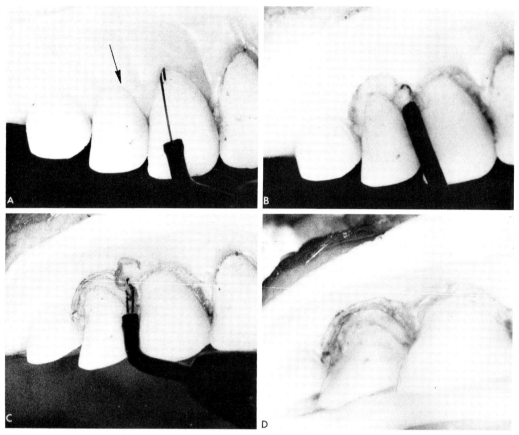

Figure 15–9. Subgingival trough preparation in thin gingiva. Technique using full U-shaped loop electrode and gingivectomy with round loop. *A,* Gingiva over tooth (arrow) is too thin to permit preparation of subgingival trough without removal of some gingival height, as will be seen in *B. B,* A gingivectomy is being performed with a small round loop electrode to remove the cuticle-like thin edge of the marginal gingiva. Note that the J-loop has resected some of the marginal gingiva, owing to the excessive thinness of the tissue. The operator has no control over the inadvertent gingivectomy. *C,* A subgingival trough is being created with the full U-shaped loop electrode. The blunt edge of marginal gingiva is now thick enough to permit the troughing without uncontrolled loss of gingival level. *D,* A perfect trough has been created that will permit accommodation of the restoration in the subgingival sulcus area without impingement. Instead of gingival recession, the tissue removed by the gingivectomy will regenerate to, or very close to, its original level.

blunt square-edged cut margin is needed, as was described in Figures 15–9 and 15–10.

Even when beveled margins are desired many clinicians try to avoid loop resection and prefer to simulate the traditional gingivectomy by substituting the needle electrode and cutting current for the manual steel scalpel incisional gingivectomy. Inasmuch as this particular type of gingivectomy calls for a blunt, square-edged gingival margin, the needle incision gingivectomy can be used very advantageously for this technique.

The new gingival level that is to be created by the gingivectomy is outlined on the tissue with an indelible pencil, or by a series of pinpricks or tiny stab incisions with the tip of the activated needle electrode, after the tissues

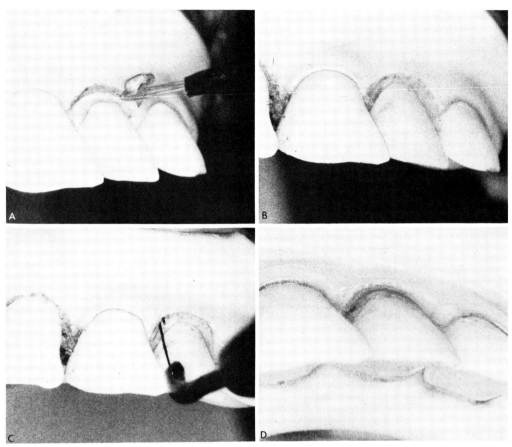

Figure 15–10. Subgingival trough preparation in thin gingiva. Technique using J-loop electrode and gingivectomy with U-shaped loop. *A,* Excessively thin cuticle-like marginal gingiva being excised with a narrow U-shaped loop electrode. A strip of tissue is excised. The strip of tissue beneath it, in contact with the tooth, can then easily be removed with a periosteal elevator. *B,* The appearance of the tooth and tissue after removal of the marginal edge tissue. The new marginal edge is blunt and thick enough to permit the necessary instrumentation for creating the trough. *C,* The subgingival trough is being created with a J-loop electrode. *D,* The appearance of the completed trough as seen from a ventral view. The trough is well defined and the tooth is ready for impression.

have been anesthetized (Fig. 15–11A). The needle electrode is then applied to the tissues at right angles to the alveolar bone surface along the outlined tissue, to create a blunt, square-edged cut margin (Fig. 15–11B). The incised strip of gingival tissue is undermined with a periosteal elevator (or a sickle scaler) (Fig. 15–11C) and removed.

The new gingival margin is now thick enough to permit preparation of the subgingival trough. The needle electrode is replaced with a J-loop (or narrow U-shaped loop, if preferred), and the activated electrode is used to dissect out a thin strip of the inner surface of the new gingival marginal tissue to form a subgingival trough around the tooth (Fig. 15–11D).

The subgingival trough is created in the new marginal edge by dissecting out the sliver of internal aspect of the tissue with a full U-shaped loop or J-loop electrode. Resecting the tissue for the trough also creates a feather-edged

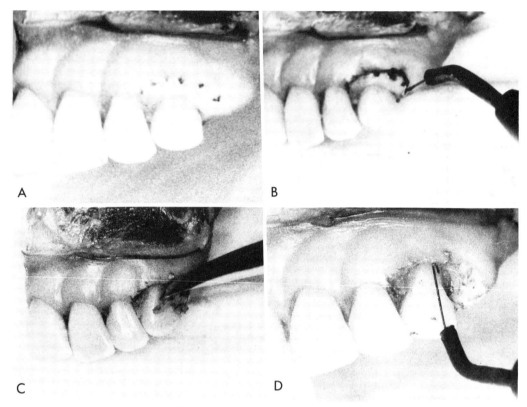

Figure 15–11.   Subgingival trough preparation in thin gingiva. Technique for performing the gingivectomy by needle electrode incision and creating the subgingival trough by J-loop excision. *A*, Gingivectomy outlined on tissue by pinprick stabs with the activated needle electrode. *B*, The incision for the gingivectomy is performed with the needle electrode held at right angles to the surface of the alveolar bone as the incision follows the outline on the tissue. *C*, The incised strip of mucosa is undermined with a periosteal elevator to detach it from the alveolar bone. *D*, A subgingival trough is created in the blunt square-edged new gingival margin with a J-loop electrode.

margin; however, this occurs on the internal surface instead of the external surface, as happens when the usual elongation of the crown is performed. Removal of the tissue to form the trough helps to provide space for atraumatic subgingival instrumentation to prepare the shoulder.

This technique can be used with equal success in areas other than the maxillary cuspid, where the marginal gingiva is also excessively thin.

PROCESSING THE INTERMEDIATE, TRANSITIONAL, OR PROVISIONAL SPLINT

There is no need for the author to spell out the technical laboratory procedures for fabricating the supragingival intermediate splint, since they vary with the physical facilities of the office and personal preferences of the therapist. Those who use the Omnivac type of equipment will prefer to utilize that method of fabrication. Those who use pre-formed acrylic crown forms will no doubt prefer to use that method.

After the subgingival troughs have been prepared, shoulder preparations completed, impressions taken, and work models poured, the previously processed supragingivally terminated intermediate splint is placed on one of the work models. The gap between the gingival end of the splint and the shoulder area on the model is filled with a quick-setting hard acrylic such as Bosworth's Trim or Coe's Raypaque to bridge the gap.

Since grinding and polishing do not cause these materials to warp or buckle, the newly added acrylic can be finished to fit accurately in the shoulder area and polished to a smooth high luster. The intermediate splint is now ready to be inserted into position in the mouth. The accurate fit of the subgingival portion of the splint prevents proliferation of marginal gingiva over the shoulder area. As the part of the crevicular gingiva resected to create the subgingival trough proceeds to regenerate to its original dimension, it becomes intimately adapted around the polished subgingival portion of the splint, thereby eliminating danger of tissue compression or impingement against the subgingival tissues as the regenerated crevicular epithelium matures.

Amsterdam and Fox[*] have described a different method for fabricating an accurately fitted intermediate splint that also appears to have much merit. Their technique consists of fabricating the intermediate crowns on Ney's Zephyr Temporary Splint Bands (Fig. 15–12). The Zephyr Bands are thin, highly malleable gold bands that can easily be contoured to accurate adaptation to the subgingival portions of the crown preparations and thus provide perfect subgingival finish lines for the intermediate restorations.

---

[*]Amsterdam, M., and Fox, L.: Provisional Splinting—Principles and Technics. The Dental Clinics of North America. March, 1959, W. B. Saunders Co.

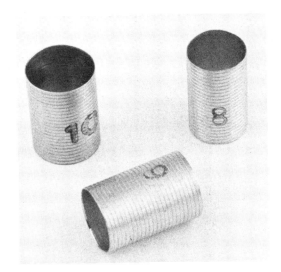

Figure 15–12. Ney's gold Zephyr Temporary Splint Bands. Soft, highly malleable, easily contoured for accurate subgingival finish line. Externally serrated for better bond with acrylic.

If the permanent restoration is fabricated to identical subgingival dimensions as the intermediate splint, whenever it is completed it becomes interchangeable with the latter. When the intermediate splint is removed and replaced by the permanent restoration there is no alteration in gingiva-crown relation. As soon as the occlusion has been determined to be satisfactory, usually a matter of one or two weeks, the final restoration can be permanently cemented without risk of causing subgingival compression or impingement that would trigger inflammatory responses that could ultimately result in iatrogenically induced periodontoclasia.

The following series of cases is being presented through the considerate cooperation of a number of eminent prosthodontists whom it has been the author's privilege to have instructed in the proper use of electrosurgery. Each of these contributors has been utilizing electrosurgery very effectively in his clinical practice for many years. As is to be expected, each utilizes electrosurgery in his own inimitable fashion, but the end results are uniformly effective.

CASE 13

The first of the series is a case that has been made available by Dr. James D. Harrison, Southern Illinois University School of Dental Medicine. It is being presented as the lead-off case because it is an excellent demonstration of the ease with which a subgingival trough can be prepared around a full shoulder crown preparation with a J-loop electrode.

PATIENT.   Details unknown.

HISTORY.   The maxillary left central and lateral incisors had been restored with porcelain jacket crowns. The left maxillary cuspid was to be restored next.

CLINICAL EXAMINATION.   The cuspid had been prepared for a full shoulder jacket crown. The marginal gingiva around the distal half of the tooth appeared to be slightly engorged and proliferated (Case Fig. 13–1A).

TREATMENT.   The fully rectified cutting current was activated. The tissue around the tooth was anesthetized by infiltration anesthesia. The activated J-loop electrode was then used with a wiping motion to dissect out the thin sliver of tissue to create the subgingival trough, circumscribing the entire preparation (Case Fig. 13–1B). It is noteworthy that the subgingival trough that was created is uniform and that there is no tissue fragmentation or free bleeding to interfere with the impression-taking (Case Fig. 13–1C).

CASE 14

This case has been made available by Dr. William W. Dolan of Coral Gables, Florida.

This case serves to demonstrate two things. First, and most important, the superb adaptation of regenerating marginal gingiva around a highly glazed ceramic restoration after electrosurgical excision of a subgingival trough. It also demonstrates, with the aid of the magnification provided by a Deesen extreme close-up lens, the typical

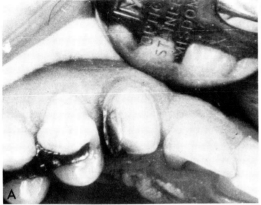

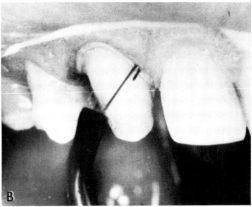

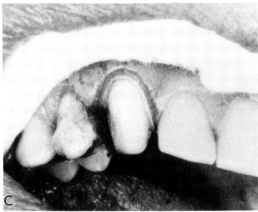

Case Figure 13–1. Preparation of a subgingival trough around a full shoulder crown preparation with a J-loop electrode. *A*, Preoperative appearance. The maxillary right cuspid has been reduced for full crown coverage; a full shoulder has been prepared. The distal of the tooth had been filled previously to eliminate undercuts. A slight amount of engorgement and thickening of the marginal gingiva is present at the distal aspect of the tooth. *B*, An activated J-loop electrode is being used with cutting current to dissect out the subgingival trough on the labial aspect of the tooth. *C*, Immediate postoperative result. A well-defined trough has been created around the tooth, thereby exposing enough of the root surface beyond the shoulder to assure an accurate impression of the subgingival finish line. Note the absence of tissue shredding or bleeding.

irregular, slightly scalloped appearance of the marginal gingiva when the excision of the tissue to create the trough is performed by free-hand circumscribing instrumentation. Although the marginal tissue appears slightly jagged, it heals evenly when in contact with a highly polished restoration.

PATIENT. Details unknown.

HISTORY. The maxillary right central incisor crown had been missing and had been restored with amalgam to create the coronal stump for a porcelain crown restoration. A subgingival trough was to be prepared around the restored tooth.

CLINICAL EXAMINATION. The entire coronal portion of the tooth was made of amalgam, which had been carved to form the coronal stump for a porcelain jacket crown.

TREATMENT. The tissues had been anesthetized by infiltration anesthesia, and a thin sliver of the internal surface of the free marginal gingiva was excised with a narrow U-shaped loop electrode by electrosection (Case Fig. 14–1). A copper-band impression was taken and a porcelain jacket crown fabricated. The crown was inserted with temporary cement, and the patient was reappointed. The following week the crown was removed and the temporary cement was removed from the crown and the tooth preparation prior to permanent cementation. The marginal gingiva had adapted itself very tightly around the highly glazed surface of the porcelain crown and appeared fully healed. When the crown was reinserted, the tissue around the crown was identical in appearance to the free marginal gingiva around a natural tooth.

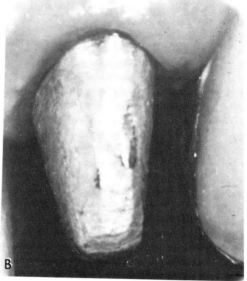

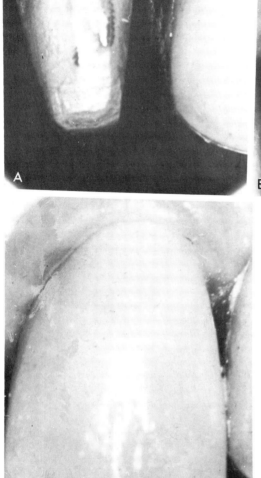

Case Figure 14–1. A, A retained root has been built up with an amalgam stump that has been prepared as a full crown preparation, and a subgingival trough has been created around the preparation. Irregularity of the marginal gingiva is due to free-hand instrumentation in troughing.

B, Appearance of the tissues around the preparation one week later. Note the regeneration of marginal gingiva and adaptation to the porcelain crown that was inserted.

C, Appearance of the tissues a week later, with the porcelain crown in the mouth. Note the tight adaptation of the healing tissues to the smooth glazed surface of the porcelain.

This case demonstrates that when the regenerating tissue is in contact with a highly polished or glazed surface it heals rapidly and uneventfully and is very tightly adherent to the smooth-surfaced restoration.

CASE 15

This is another of the series of cases Dr. Peter K. Thomas has made available for use by the author.

This case demonstrates Dr. Thomas' use of electrosurgery for preparation of the subgingival troughs around teeth prepared for full crown coverage. He obviously had

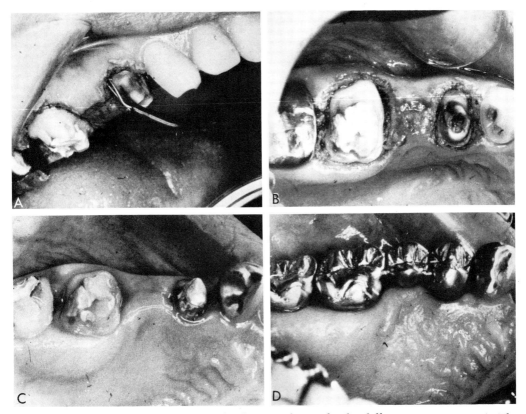

Case Figure 15–1. Preparation of subgingival troughs for full crown coverage. *A,* The maxillary right quadrant is being prepared for full coverage. A subgingival trough has been created around the molar, and a trough is being prepared around the first bicuspid with a full U-shaped 45-degree-angle loop electrode. Enough redundant tissue has been resected from the crest of the edentulous alveolar ridge between the two teeth by loop planing to permit use of normal size pontics that will not require excessive grinding. Note: the ragged appearance of the marginal tissues is inevitable when the trough is prepared free-hand, without resting the electrode against the tooth. *B,* Appearance of the tissues around the teeth as seen from the ventral view. Note the absence of bleeding and of coagulation or charring. *C,* Appearance of the tissues one week postoperatively. The tissue on the crest of the edentulous ridge as well as around the teeth is almost fully healed and has adapted itself as it regenerated snugly against the splint. *D,* Appearance of the tissues with the splint in position. Note the absence of impingement and the perfect adaptation of the tissues around the crowns.

also reduced the bulk of tissue in the edentulous area by planing with a loop, shaving the tissue in layers until the desired ridge contour was achieved.

PATIENT.   A white male of undetermined age.

HISTORY.   A number of his teeth were extensively decayed and were to be restored with full crown restorations. These teeth were to serve as abutments for a fixed prosthesis to replace teeth that had been extracted.

CLINICAL EXAMINATION.   The maxillary right quadrant was to be restored. The second bicuspid was missing from the dental arch. The first bicuspid and both molars were badly broken down and to be restored with full cast veneer crowns (Case Fig. 15–1).

TREATMENT.   The three teeth were prepared for full crown restoration. A bulge of redundant tissue on the crest of the edentulous second bicuspid area in the dental arch was reduced by planing with a flame-shaped loop electrode. Subgingival troughs were then prepared around each crown preparation with a narrow 45-degree angle U-shaped loop electrode.

The troughing was completed without bleeding or burning the tissues. A hydrocolloid impression was taken and a stone model was made. The restoration was fabricated and inserted. The tissues were closely adapted to the crowns, but without impingement against the subgingival tissues. One week after the initial insertion, the occlusion having proved acceptable, the restoration was cemented in permanently.

(The case details have had to be reconstructed by the author from the Kodachrome slides supplied.)

CASE 16

This case also has been made available by Dr. Thomas.

PATIENT.   A white adult male.

HISTORY.   Unknown.

CLINICAL EXAMINATION.   (Reconstructed from evidence provided by Kodachrome slides made available to the author by Dr. Thomas.) The anterior maxillary segment from cuspid to cuspid had been restored with porcelain veneer crowns. The mandibular anterior segment from cuspid to cuspid had not been restored. The maxillary and mandibular four posterior quadrants, from first bicuspid to second molar, required restoration with porcelain veneer crowns to be splinted together as fixed splint restorations.

TREATMENT.   A typical quadrant is demonstrated (Case Fig. 16–1). The teeth in the maxillary right quadrant are being prepared for full crown coverage. After the preparations were completed, a narrow 45-degree-angle U-shaped loop electrode was selected, and the activated electrode was tilted to a slight angle as it circumscribed the tooth to cut out a subgingival trough. Each crown preparation was treated in the same manner. When all the troughs had been created, an injection hydrocolloid impression was taken. The subgingival troughs permitted the impression material to penetrate subgingivally to provide accurate impressions of the area for the finish lines of the crowns.

The splints were fabricated and inserted into the mouth. A mirror image offers an excellent lateral view of the splendid manner in which the tissues adapted around the crowns without any evidence of impingement. Case Figure 16–1C gives a full face view of the appearance of the entire mouth after a few weeks. The tissues are tightly adapted around the crowns and into the embrasures.

The next case is another in the series being presented through the cooperation of Dr. Dolan. This case demonstrates the unfavorable tissue reaction that results when provision has not been made for adequate subgingival accommodation of fixed restorations. It also demonstrates the facility with which optimal tissue contour can be restored and subgingival accommodation provided by electrosection with appropriate loop electrodes.

CASE 17

This case was made available by Dr. William W. Dolan of Coral Gables, Florida.

PATIENT.   A white female of unknown age.

HISTORY.   A maxillary first bicuspid had been restored with a porcelain veneer

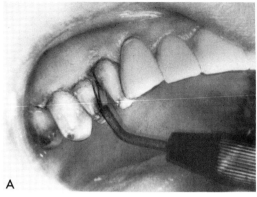

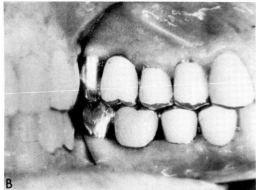

Case Figure 16–1. Preparation of subgingival troughs for full coverage (maxilla). *A*, The maxillary right quadrant is being prepared for full coverage. A subgingival trough is being prepared around the first bicuspid with a 45-degree-angle narrow U-shaped loop electrode. *B*, Mirror image lateral view of the tissues immediately after insertion of the restorations in the maxillary and mandibular quadrants. *C*, Full face view of the restorations and the tissues. All four quadrants have been restored. Subgingival troughs were prepared around all the crown preparations as described in *A*. Note the condition of the gingival tissues around the restoration and how closely they are adapted to the crowns.

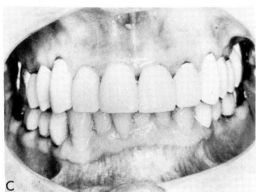

crown. Although a subgingival trough had been created to facilitate taking of the impression for the crown, no provision had been made for retention of the subgingival space, most of which had been obliterated by the time the veneer crown was inserted into the mouth. Shortly thereafter, the papilla in the embrasure between the first and second bicuspid teeth began to swell and became engorged and proliferative. The tissue bled freely on brushing the teeth and often during eating. She was seen by Dr. Dolan and his decision was to remove the crown, resect the proliferative tissue and reinsert the crown.

TREATMENT. Infiltration anesthesia was administered. A narrow 45-degree-angle U-shaped loop electrode was selected, activated with the cutting current, and used to resect the redundant tissue and recontour the external part of the papilla (Case Fig. 17–1*A*). The veneer crown which had been sterilized in cold sterilizing solution was dried and recemented with temporary cement and the patient was reappointed. She returned one week later. The external surface of the papilla was healing rapidly and the following week the crown was removed for permanent cementation. The tissues were fully and normally healed. The papillary tissue had regenerated and had adapted itself tightly against the smooth polished surface of the crown (Case Fig. 17–1*B*). The temporary cement was removed and the crown was recemented with permanent cement. There has been no repetition of the inflammatory proliferation.

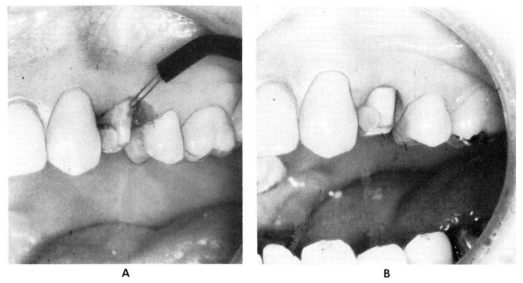

A   **B**

Case Figure 17–1.   *A*, Proliferative tissue in the left maxillary bicuspid embrasure is being removed with a narrow U-shaped loop electrode. The tissue had proliferated in response to irritation from a cast veneer crown. *B*, Appearance of the tissue in the embrasure one week later. The tissue has regenerated and adapted firmly against the polished surface of the crown.

CASE 18

This case has been made available by Dr. Dolan.

This case is very similar to the previous case, with one important exception. Unlike the previous case, the four maxillary anterior teeth in this instance had been restored with porcelain jacket crowns instead of acrylic crowns. This case is therefore being included to emphasize that the unfavorable tissue reaction is not a result of the materials used to fabricate the restorations but of the biomechanical factors created by subgingival impingement, owing to lack of space to accommodate the subgingival portions of the restorations.

PATIENT.   A white female of undetermined age.

HISTORY.   The maxillary four anterior teeth had been restored with porcelain jacket crowns. Subsequently the marginal gingivae began to darken in color and proliferate and failed to respond to localized curettage. She was referred to Dr. Dolan for further treatment.

CLINICAL EXAMINATION.   The marginal gingivae around the four teeth on the labial aspect were inflamed, friable, and proliferative (Case Fig. 18–1) They were equally inflamed and proliferative on the palatal aspect. The remainder of the marginal gingivae throughout the mouth appeared normal.

TREATMENT.   The tissues were anesthetized by local anesthesia, and the marginal gingivae were recontoured to normal anatomic architecture with a narrow U-shaped loop electrode. The external tissues having been recontoured to normal dimension, the crowns were removed, revealing that the shoulders of the preparations had become covered with proliferative tissue. The redundant tissue was resected with the loop electrode, and subgingival troughs were prepared, fully exposing the shoulders.

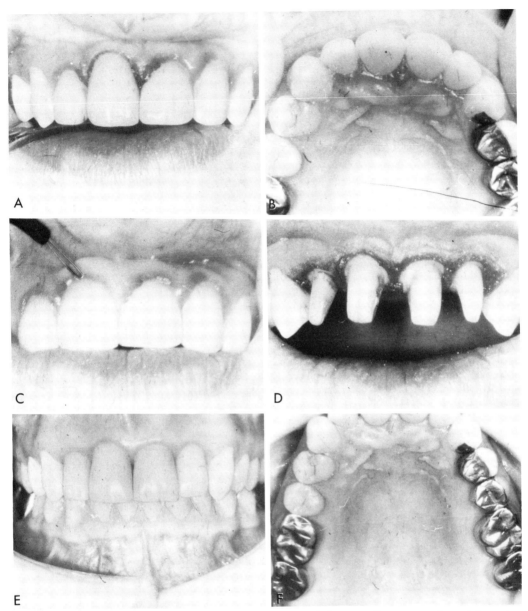

Case Figure 18–1. A, Preoperative appearance of the maxillary centrals and laterals: labial aspect. The four teeth have been restored with porcelain jacket crowns. The marginal gingivae around all four teeth are severely engorged and proliferated, creating thick, partially detached margins and interdental papillae. B, Preoperative appearance: palatal aspect. The gingival engorgement and proliferative tendency is also present here but appears slightly less acute than on the labial aspect. C, Corrective treatment. The redundant proliferative tissue is resected around the crowns to restore a normal gingival architecture. The resection is being performed with a narrow 45-degree-angle U-shaped loop electrode used with a wiping motion. D, Immediate postsurgical appearance. The gingivae have been recontoured to normal architecture, the redundant tissue that had proliferated over the shoulders of the preparations has been removed, fully exposing the shoulders, and subgingival troughs have been created around the preparations. E, Final postoperative appearance of the teeth and new restorations: labial aspect. The tissues are normal in color, tone and contour. The marginal gingivae are tightly adapted around the crowns and there is no clinical evidence of subgingival impingement that might stimulate repetition of the gingival deterioration. F, Final postoperative appearance of the tissues: palatal aspect. The tissues are normal in all respects and snugly adapted around the new restorations. The tissues show no evidence of subgingival impingement or of irritation.

A previously prepared acrylic splint was inserted and used as a stent. Two weeks later, the tissues having healed fully, the new ceramic restorations that had been fabricated were inserted, and there has been no recurrence of inflammation or proliferation since. The gingival architecture, tissue color and tone are normal and the marginal gingivae and interdental papillae are tightly adapted around the new crowns (Case Fig. 18–1E and F).

The next two cases, also from the personal patient files of Dr. Dolan, are almost identical in all but one respect. The only significant difference is the fact that in the first case the restorations were acrylic crowns and in the second case the restorations were porcelain jacket crowns.

These cases are *not* being presented for the purpose of expressing an opinion as to the relative merits of these materials. They are being presented to demonstrate that when adequate space is not provided to accommodate restorations subgingivally, both react identically, and when adequate space is provided, they react identically to the more favorable conditions. This suggests that freedom from subgingival impingement is the deciding factor in the ability of the tissues to tolerate the restoration.

CASE 19

This case also was made available by Dr. Dolan.

PATIENT. A white male of undetermined age.

HISTORY. The central and lateral maxillary incisors had been restored with acrylic crowns and the posterior teeth with veneer crowns. The restorations were maintained in the mouth with temporary cement. Soon the gingivae around the four anterior teeth became red, edematous, and painful. Palliative treatment having failed to provide relief, the patient was referred to Dr. Dolan for further treatment. Dr. Dolan concluded that the condition had resulted from subgingival irritation and that it could be relieved by creating subgingival troughs around the crown preparations (Case Fig. 19–1).

CLINICAL EXAMINATION. The marginal and alveolar gingivae around the four anterior teeth, on the palatal as well as the labial surfaces, were red, inflamed, edematous, and ulcerated in several labial areas.

TREATMENT. The restorations were removed, and the patient was instructed to massage the gums and use a saline mouthwash frequently to reduce the inflammation.

At his next visit the tissues were anesthetized, the restorations were reinserted and the marginal gingivae were recontoured to feather-edge normal architecture. The restorations were then removed, and the tissue that had proliferated over and covered the shoulders of the preparations was resected with a narrow U-shaped loop electrode. Subgingival troughs were then prepared around the preparations with a J-loop electrode (Case Fig. 19–1D), and the restorations were reinserted with temporary cement while the tissue repair and response were kept under observation. A few weeks later, the tissues having returned to normal tone and color, the restorations were cemented in permanently (Case Fig. 19–2). There has been no recurrence of the inflammation or proliferation since then.

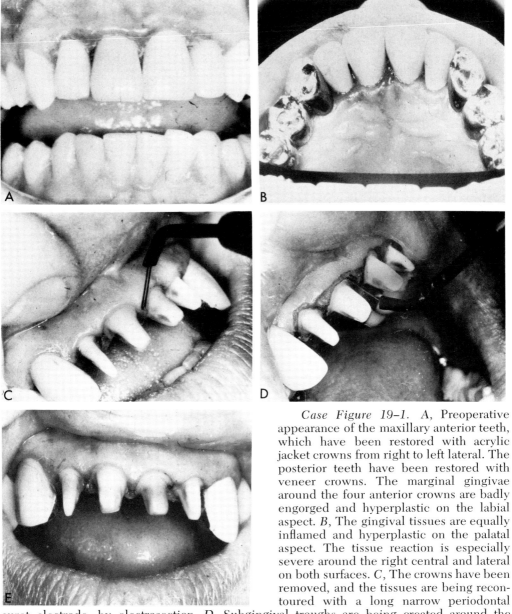

Case Figure 19–1. A, Preoperative appearance of the maxillary anterior teeth, which have been restored with acrylic jacket crowns from right to left lateral. The posterior teeth have been restored with veneer crowns. The marginal gingivae around the four anterior crowns are badly engorged and hyperplastic on the labial aspect. B, The gingival tissues are equally inflamed and hyperplastic on the palatal aspect. The tissue reaction is especially severe around the right central and lateral on both surfaces. C, The crowns have been removed, and the tissues are being recontoured with a long narrow periodontal curet electrode, by electrosection. D, Subgingival troughs are being created around the preparations with a J-loop electrode. The shoulders of the preparations are now well defined. E, Appearance of the tissues the following week. The tissue around the right lateral still shows a little engorgement, but all the tissues are immeasurably improved.

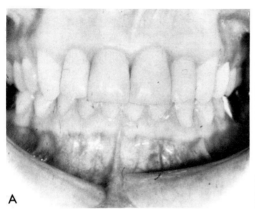
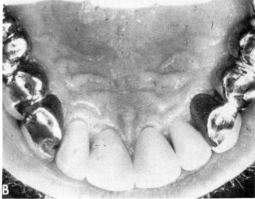

Case Figure 19–2. *A*, Postoperative appearance of the tissues around the crowns several weeks later, labial view. The tissues are normal in tone and contour, and are adapted tightly against the acrylic crowns which now have adequate subgingival space without impingement. *B*, Appearance of the palatal tissues shows an equally favorable result.

CASE 20

PATIENT. An adult white male.

HISTORY. An occlusal reconstruction of the maxillary arch had been performed for him by means of three splints; two restoring the posterior segments, and a third restoring the anterior segment. Apparently no provision had been made for accommodation of the subgingival portions of the restorations. The marginal gingivae around the anterior veneer crowns had begun to undergo periodontal deterioration that had not responded to conservative palliative treatment. The patient was referred to Dr. Dolan who decided to remove the anterior splint, recontour the gingival tissues in that segment, provide subgingival accommodation by creating subgingival troughs around the crown preparations, and fabricate a new splint to fit the recontoured tissues accurately.

CLINICAL EXAMINATION. The maxillary right posterior splint extended from the cuspid posteriorly to the second molar. The anterior splint extended from the right lateral incisor to the left cuspid, and the left posterior splint extended from the first bicuspid to the second molar. The right central incisor crown had a defect on the labial aspect near the center at the gingival margin (Case Fig. 20–1). The marginal gingiva had receded approximately 0.5 cm. beyond the superior edge of the left cuspid. The labial alveolar gingivae appeared slightly engorged. The apical attachments of the interdental papillae on the palatal aspect were slightly proliferative and partially detached (Case Fig. 20–1*B*).

TREATMENT. The anterior splint was removed under local anesthesia. A narrow 45-degree-angle U-shaped loop electrode was selected and cutting power output set at 3.5 on the power output dial. The activated electrode was used with brushing strokes to shave the tissue in thin layers and recontour the gingivae to feather-edged margins (Case Fig. 20–1*C*). A J-loop electrode was substituted and used to prepare subgingival troughs around the crown preparations (Case Fig. 20–1*D*), without any accompanying free bleeding (Case Figs. 20–1*E* and *F*).

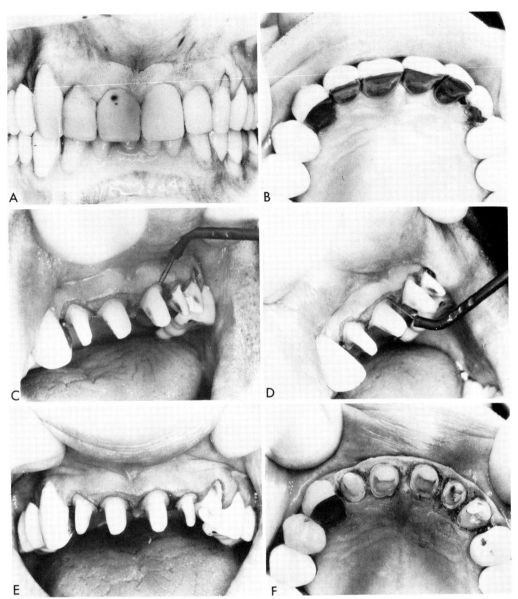

Case Figure 20–1. A, Preoperative appearance of the maxilla from cuspid to cuspid. There is hyperplasia and evidence of deterioration of the marginal edge of the marginal gingivae. B, Palatal view; there is evidence of irritation around the gold castings of the veneer crowns. C, The four crowns have been removed from the right and left centrals and laterals, and the left cuspid has been prepared for crown coverage. The marginal gingivae are being re-contoured with a 45-degree-angle medium-length narrow U-shaped loop electrode. The gingivoplasty is being performed by electrosection. D, The tissue is being excised around the crowns to create subgingival troughs around the teeth. The J-loop electrode is being used to create the troughs. E, Labial view of appearance of the tissues after instrumentation has been completed. F, Appearance of the subgingival troughs as seen from a ventral view. The shoulders of the crown preparations are well defined, and the troughs also are well defined.

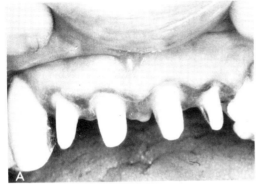
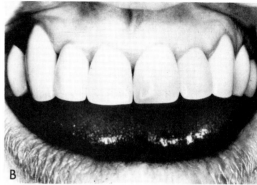
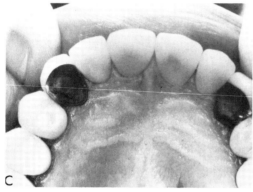

Case Figure 20–2. A, Appearance of the tissues one week later, before insertion of the new porcelain jacket crowns. B, Appearance of the tissues one week after the new restorations have been inserted. The tissues are very tightly adapted around the porcelain jacket crowns and are normal in tone and contour. C, The tissues are equally well adapted on the palatal aspect, and the tissue tone is equally favorable.

An impression was taken and a working model processed. Tincture of myrrh and benzoin was applied to the gingival tissues. The splint, which had been sterilized in cold sterilizing solution, was replaced and sealed into position with periodontal pack cement.

Healing progressed rapidly and uneventfully and one week later was almost fully healed (Case Fig. 20–2A). The new splint was fabricated and inserted. The tissues were tightly adapted around the crowns and there was no evidence of subgingival impingement (Case Fig. 20–2B). Several weeks later, the occlusion having proved satisfactory and the interdental papillae on the palatal aspect having become firmly reattached (Case Fig. 20–2C), the splint was permanently cemented.

CASE 21

This case also has been made available by Dr. Dolan.

This case offers an excellent example of the gingival recession that so often co-exists simultaneously with hyperplasia due to subgingival impingement by a temporary splint that was not properly finished to provide unimpeded subgingival seating for the restoration.

PATIENT. Details unknown.

HISTORY. The patient had had both arches restored with fixed bridges. The restorations after many months were still retained with temporary cement. Irritation from the restorations triggered an inflammatory response, the tissues becoming puffy and tending to bleed readily in some areas, and caused recession in other areas, especially in the lower jaw. Repeated palliative treatments failed to materially improve the condition. The patient finally decided to try another dentist and was referred to Dr. Dolan.

CLINICAL EXAMINATION. *Mandible.* The six anterior teeth were most involved. The splint restoring these teeth appeared aesthetically as well as functionally unsuitable. The acrylic veneer/cuspid abutment crowns were worn through on the incisal surfaces so that the gold of the castings was exposed, indicating occlusal traumatizing prematurities. The acrylic had a spongy appearance that resembled a porcelain biscuit bake rather than a polished finished acrylic. The marginal gingivae on the labial aspect were hyperplastic and the apices of the interdental papillae were partially detached, but the marginal gingivae around the right central and the left central, lateral, cuspid and first bicuspid were receded more than 2 mm., exposing the gold finish lines of the restorations and denuded root surfaces (Case Fig. 21–1A). The tissues on the lingual aspect were in much the same condition (Case Fig. 21–1B).

TREATMENT. The tissues were anesthetized and the bridge was removed. The teeth were cleansed of temporary cement, a narrow 45-degree-angle U-shaped loop electrode was selected, activated with cutting current, and used to reduce the hyperplastic tissue to normal contour by loop gingivoplasty (Case Fig. 21–2A). A right-angle narrow U-shaped loop was substituted and used to reduce the interstitial tissue bulges and expose the finish lines of the preparations (Case Fig. 21–2B). This revealed that the shoulder preparations were not well defined and only partially prepared (Case Fig. 21–2C). The gingival architecture having been restored to normal contour, tincture of myrrh and benzoin was applied, the previously sterilized old splint was re-

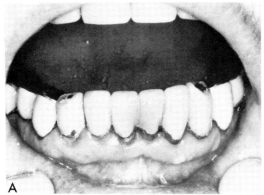

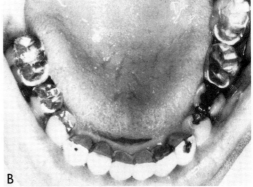

A

B

Case Figure 21–1. A, Appearance of the mandibular teeth and tissues, labial view. This is truly a "temporary" bridge, in its worst connotation. The temporary crowns are short of the gingival tissues in many areas and appear to be impingeing against the subgingival tissues in the embrasures. As a result, the interdental papillae are grossly enlarged and partially detached. B, The tissues on the lingual surface appear engorged and atonal. C, Appearance of teeth and tissues with restoration removed.

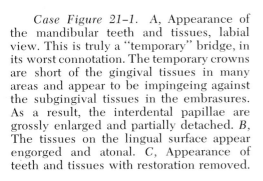

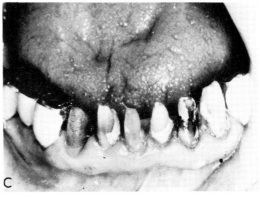

C

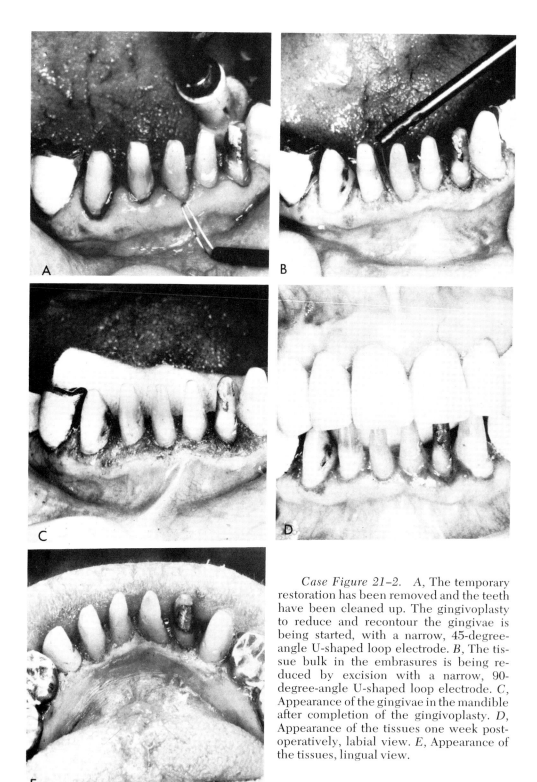

Case Figure 21–2. *A*, The temporary restoration has been removed and the teeth have been cleaned up. The gingivoplasty to reduce and recontour the gingivae is being started, with a narrow, 45-degree-angle U-shaped loop electrode. *B*, The tissue bulk in the embrasures is being reduced by excision with a narrow, 90-degree-angle U-shaped loop electrode. *C*, Appearance of the gingivae in the mandible after completion of the gingivoplasty. *D*, Appearance of the tissues one week post-operatively, labial view. *E*, Appearance of the tissues, lingual view.

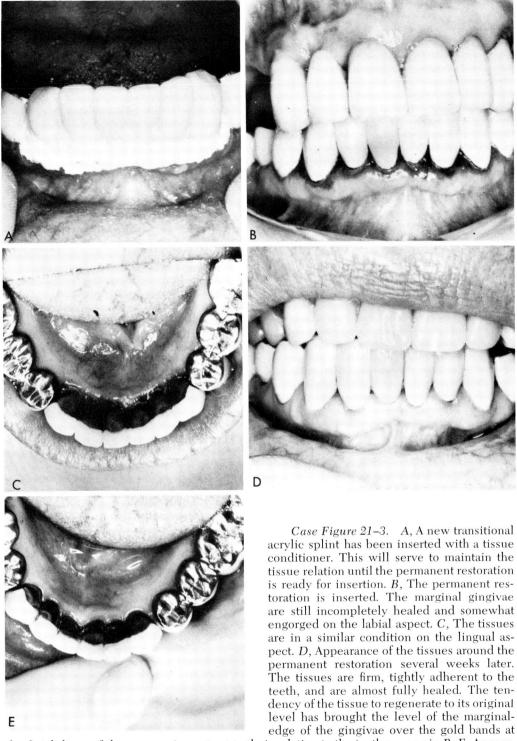

Case Figure 21–3. A, A new transitional acrylic splint has been inserted with a tissue conditioner. This will serve to maintain the tissue relation until the permanent restoration is ready for insertion. B, The permanent restoration is inserted. The marginal gingivae are still incompletely healed and somewhat engorged on the labial aspect. C, The tissues are in a similar condition on the lingual aspect. D, Appearance of the tissues around the permanent restoration several weeks later. The tissues are firm, tightly adherent to the teeth, and are almost fully healed. The tendency of the tissue to regenerate to its original level has brought the level of the marginal-edge of the gingivae over the gold bands at the finish lines of the crowns, in contrast to their relation to the teeth as seen in B. E, Appearance of the tissues on the lingual aspect. The tissue tone appears normal, and the maturation of the tissues appears to be progressing favorably.

inserted, and a periodontal cement pack was applied to cover the cut tissue and retain the restoration. The patient returned one week later and the tissue healing appeared to have progressed very favorably except around the left lateral which had been the worst spot preoperatively. The engorgement was greatly improved throughout the surgical field except in this area which was laggard in healing as compared to the rest of the tissues on the labial and lingual aspects (Case Fig. 21–2D and E).

The crown preparations were reprepared at this visit to create definite subgingival finish lines, an impression obtained, and a new transitional splint was processed in acrylic. The new splint was inserted with a tissue conditioner liner (Case Fig. 21–3A). This splint served to maintain a proper tissue relation until the permanent restoration was fabricated and inserted (Case Fig. 21–3B and C). The new restoration obviously was properly finished and free of subgingival impingement, since the tissues healed rapidly and uneventfully after it was inserted. A few weeks later the restoration was cemented in permanently. The tissues were fully healed on the labial and lingual aspects and completely normal (Case Fig. 21–3 D and E).

This case once again offers dramatic evidence that a temporary splint that is finished poorly and does not fit precisely in the subgingival region because it is "only a temporary splint" and therefore unimportant is an open invitation to dental disaster.

IV. EXPOSURE OF RETAINED KEY ABUTMENT ROOTS FOR FUNCTIONAL USE

There are many instances when the ability to expose and utilize a key retained abutment root spells the difference between being able to restore missing teeth with a partial prosthesis and the need for full-denture restoration. The latter is especially likely if remaining abutment teeth are periodontally involved, or if there is a large edentulous span that would result in an extended free-end saddle.

The following case reports demonstrate various conditions in which the ability to expose retained abutment roots for functional use as abutments was the decisive factor in enabling the restoration of the mouth with a partial prosthesis.

CASE 22

This case typifies the usefulness of the elongating technique for exposing retained roots and reclaiming them for use as key abutments for large restorations.

PATIENT. A 54-year-old white male.

HISTORY. The patient was referred for exposure of a retained maxillary left cuspid root by electrosurgery for use as a key abutment. Availability of this root meant the difference between a partial restoration with bilateral attachment and a full denture.

CLINICAL EXAMINATION. The patient had four maxillary teeth clinically visible. These had been prepared for full veneer-crown restorations. The left cuspid root was also present but buried well below the surface of the gingival mucosa (Case Fig. 22–1A). A temporary splint restoring the six anterior teeth had been processed as well as a

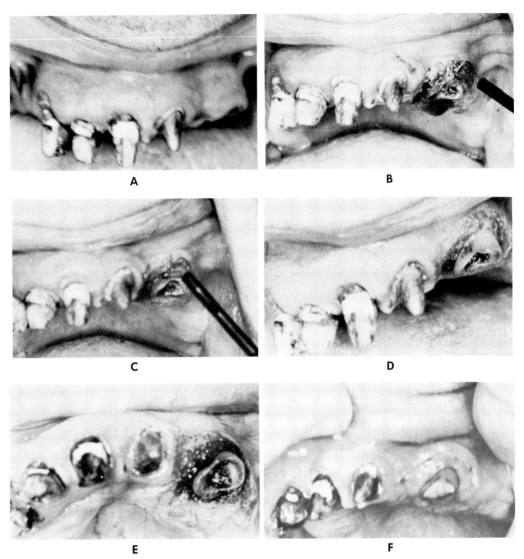

Case Figure 22–1.   Exposure of retained cuspid root for use as a key abutment. *A,* Pre-operative appearance of maxilla. Four maxillary teeth reduced for full-crown coverage are visible clinically. The left cuspid is a retained root lying beneath the mucosa. *B,* Exposure continued with triangular loop electrode used to plane the tissue around the root at right angles to the long axis of the root. *C,* Gingival margin and subgingival trough prepared with narrow U-shaped loop electrode. *D,* Root fully exposed to view, labial aspect. *E,* Root fully exposed to view, palatal aspect. Note wide area of tissue planing on palatal aspect to tissue undercut. *F,* Postoperative healing, fifth day. Tissue is granulating nicely and is covered with a healthy looking thin layer of coagulum.

partial denture to restore the posterior teeth. The cuspids were to serve as the abutments for the partial.

TREATMENT.   The mouth was prepared for surgery and infiltration anesthesia administered. Owing to the amount and density of the tissue to be removed the flame-shaped electrode was selected to start the gross tissue removal. Current output was set at 6 for electrosection.

The electrode was applied to the tissues at a 45-degree angle and used with short brushing strokes to grossly expose the root. The electrode was replaced with a triangular-shaped loop electrode, which was used at a 45-degree angle to the tissues (with current increased to 6.5) in order to plane the mucosa at right angles to the root and eliminate all undercuts, until about 4 mm. of the root was exposed to view (Case Fig. 22–1B). A narrow 45-degree-angle U-shaped loop electrode was selected for completion of the root exposure. Cutting current was reduced to 4.5, and this loop was used to trim the marginal gingiva to a feather edge and to prepare a subgingival trough (Case Fig. 22–1C).

A thin narrow strip of labial marginal alveolar bone was exposed by the tissue removal. This bone was removed with curets and a small bone file to a point 1 mm. beyond the newly created gingival margin. The labial aspect of the root was now fully exposed with harmonious gingival margin (Case Fig. 22–1D). The occlusal portion of the root was somewhat shorter on the palatal aspect due to decay, but the gingival margin of the palatal aspect was harmonious with that of the adjacent tooth (Case Fig. 22–1E). To avoid creating an undercut on the palatal surface, the mucosa there was removed by shaving in layers over a broad expanse from the root medially in order to provide a gradual gingival margin. Although more than 1 cm. of the palatal mucosa was partially denuded, there was little bleeding. The entire area was sponged dry and tincture of myrrh and benzoin applied in air-dried layers. The temporary splint was then inserted into position, and a protective surgical cement pack adapted around the exposed root area. The patient was given postoperative instructions and reappointed.

He returned on the fifth postoperative day. The cement pack was removed, then the splint; the mouth was irrigated with Kasdenol and isotonic saline solutions. The tissue healing was found to be progressing splendidly (Case Fig. 22–1F). The area was painted with air-dried layers of tincture of myrrh and benzoin and the splint reinserted. He was reappointed at weekly intervals and was seen postoperatively for the next four weeks. Periodic superficial spot coagulation accelerated the healing. Each week the tissues showed evidence of progressing maturation. By the end of that period the bridge splint was permanently cemented and the gingival mucosa all around the exposed root was completely healed and firm, with excellent tissue tone.

CASE 23

This case involved exposure of two retained abutment roots. One of the roots required removal of some dense sclerotic bone to expose it adequately. The other did not require removal of bone. The subsequent postoperative healing of the two sites, treated identically except for the bone removal, was interesting but inexplicable. It also unexpectedly made it necessary to treat the patient in two separate surgical stages.

PATIENT.   A 47-year-old white male.

HISTORY.   He had had most of his maxillary teeth extracted and replaced with a partial upper denture. The right second molar and left second bicuspid served as the abutments for an unsophisticated partial denture and the left second bicuspid in particular began to undergo periodontal deterioration. His dentist persuaded him to have two retained roots exposed to serve as additional supportive abutments, and he was referred to the author.

CLINICAL EXAMINATION.   With the teeth in occlusion, the two retained cuspid roots are just barely visible clinically. The right cuspid root is seen as a dark depression on the crest of the ridge. About 3 mm. of the root end of the tooth crown of the left cuspid protrudes beyond the gingival tissue. Both remaining teeth are involved periodontally to a moderate degree, and are somewhat mobile. A full denture is present in the mandible (Case Fig. 23–1A).

TREATMENT.   Infiltration anesthesia was administered. A 45-degree-angle medium-width U-shaped loop electrode was selected, cutting current was set at 3.5, and the activated electrode was used to resect about 4 mm. of the gingival tissue covering the root (Case Fig. 23–1B). The left lateral was then exposed in the same manner (Case Fig. 23–1C).

The loop gingivectoplasty resulted in exposure of thick dense bone that covered the right cuspid root almost to the crest of the ridge. This bone proved too sclerotic to be removed efficiently by hand instrumentation with chisels, and had to be removed by grinding with a surgical bur. Care was taken to avoid overheating the bone by use of a water spray and frequent stops to allow any heat to dissipate. When the bone was removed to a depth of 1 mm. beyond the new gingival margin of the root a J-loop electrode was used with current set at 3 to create a sulcus space around the two roots (Case Fig. 23–1D).

Tincture of myrrh and benzoin was applied to the two areas, and the patient was reappointed at weekly intervals for postoperative observation. It soon became apparent that there would be no problem about the healing around the left cuspid, but the tissue around the right cuspid showed unmistakable signs of poor delayed healing with a tendency for proliferation and very poor tissue tone on the distal aspect of the root. One month later the left side was fully healed, as was the mesial half of the right side, but the distal half of the right cuspid root was covered with tissue down to the crest of the ridge (Case Fig. 23–2A). This tissue would have to be removed in a second surgical intervention.

Second Stage: An infraorbital block was administered. A flame-shaped loop electrode was selected and inserted into the handpiece for the coagulating current. Current output was set at 5, the same as the output that would be required with the cutting current. The activated electrode was then used to dissect away the redundant tissue by shaving it in layers (Case Fig. 23–2B). When the exposure was deemed adequate, bearing in mind that there would be no regeneration of tissue from the coagulating current, tincture of myrrh and benzoin was applied and the patient was instructed to return again at weekly intervals for observation. Healing progressed uneventfully, except that the surgical field was covered with a heavier layer of coagulum. By the end of the third week the tissue was fully healed on the labial and palatal surfaces (Case Fig. 23–2C and D). The patient was referred back to his dentist for the restorative dentistry.

Inasmuch as the treatment of the two teeth had been identical in all respects except the bone removal from the one that failed to heal favorably, it appears reasonable to assume that the bone removal must have been the differentiating influence. Although maximal care was exercised to avoid overheating the bone it was impossible to avoid traumatizing the tissue with the bone bur. Such trauma is very apt to have an unfavorable influence on the tissue repair.

Use of the coagulating current to shear off tissue, sometimes referred to as bloodless surgery, can be justified only when the possibility of gingival recession is not too important, and is superseded by need to try to prevent renewed proliferation.

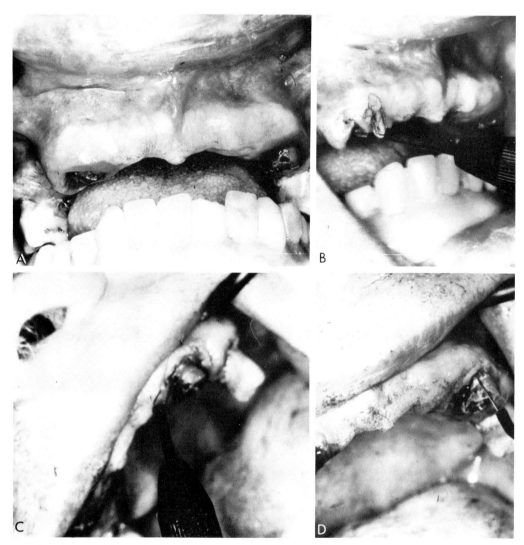

Case Figure 23–1. *A,* Preoperative appearance: the maxilla is edentulous except for the right second molar and left second bicuspid teeth and right and left cuspid retained roots. The discolored, slightly decayed tip of the coronal end of the left cuspid root protrudes slightly beyond the surface of the gingival mucosa, but the right cuspid root is slightly submerged under the gingival level. The gingival mucosa on the crest of the alveolar ridge in the edentulous areas dips down along the mesial and distal of each root, creating an uneven tissue level, which is exaggerated by a downward dip of the alveolar bone and tissue in the midline. *B,* The coronal end of the right cuspid root is being exposed by a gingivectomy performed by loop planing by electrosection. The coronal end of the distal portion of the root is below the level of the labial alveolar bone, which is thick and sclerotically dense. The bone has had to be removed to properly expose the root end. *C,* The coronal end of the left cuspid root is being exposed by loop planing the mucosa with the 45-degree-angle medium-width U-shaped loop electrode. The redundant mucosa on the crest of the alveolar ridge around the two roots has been planed level. *D,* The root end having been adequately exposed, a crevicular space is being prepared by electrosection with a J-loop electrode. No bone removal was required for the exposure of this root.

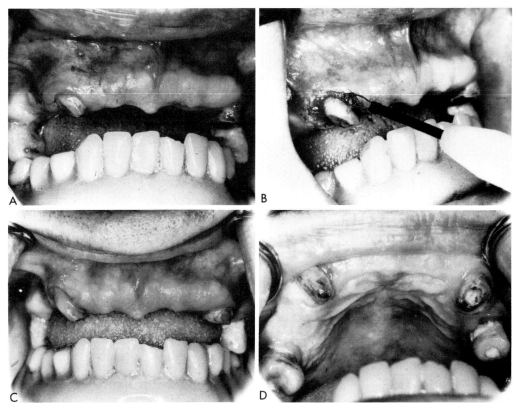

Case Figure 23–2. A, Postoperative appearance of the tissues and exposed roots one month later. The left cuspid root is properly exposed and the gingival tissues around the root are normal in tone and contour. The tissue around the mesial half of the right cuspid root appears normal in tone and contour, but the tissue around the distal half of the root appears edematous and engorged, and it has proliferated downward toward its original level. B, The redundant proliferative tissue is being resected by loop planing, but the coagulating current is being used instead of electrosection, to take advantage of the irreversible character of the tissue repair and reduce likelihood of further proliferation. C, Appearance of the tissues three weeks later, facial view. The tissue at the distal aspect of the cuspid root now appears normal in tone and contour. The tissues are normal in all respects around both roots. D, Appearance as seen from the ventral (palatal) view. This view confirms that there are no undercuts around the exposed roots that could act as troublesome food traps, and the level of the mucosa along the crest of the alveolar ridge is harmonious.

CASE 24

This case demonstrates a number of interesting facts: first, that even when the retained root is substantially beneath the gingival level, it can be exposed and utilized as an effective terminal abutment if the root is long enough; second, that despite the discrepancy between the coronal end of the root and the level of the gingivae of the adjacent teeth, the aesthetic effect is acceptable if the tooth is restored with a porcelain jacket or a veneer crown; and, perhaps most important of all, that when such a root can be exposed for functional use and thereby avert need for a full denture in occlusal contact with the natural dentition, it avoids the excessive resorption that so often accompanies such occlusal impact.

PATIENT.   A 39-year-old white female in normal health.

HISTORY.   The maxillary right molars had been extracted several years pre-

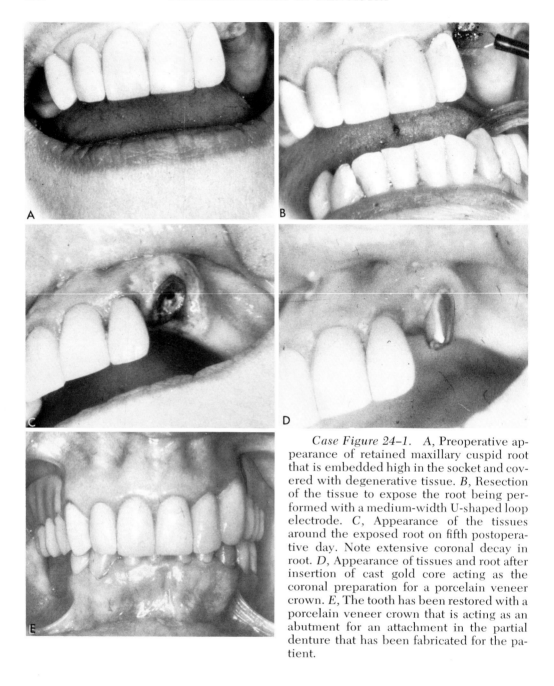

Case Figure 24-1. A, Preoperative appearance of retained maxillary cuspid root
that is embedded high in the socket and covered with degenerative tissue. B, Resection
of the tissue to expose the root being performed with a medium-width U-shaped loop
electrode. C, Appearance of the tissues
around the exposed root on fifth postoperative day. Note extensive coronal decay in
root. D, Appearance of tissues and root after
insertion of cast gold core acting as the
coronal preparation for a porcelain veneer
crown. E, The tooth has been restored with a
porcelain veneer crown that is acting as an
abutment for an attachment in the partial
denture that has been fabricated for the patient.

viously, as well as the left maxillary molars and bicuspids. The central and lateral incisors had been restored with porcelain jacket crowns. The left cuspid had decayed
through at the cemento-enamel junction, and the crown of the tooth had fractured off
some time previously, leaving the retained cuspid root in situ. She sought dental
treatment and was referred by her dentist to have the retained root exposed for use as
an abutment for a partial upper denture.

CLINICAL EXAMINATION. The gingival mucosa had overgrown the coronal end
of the retained root, so that it was completely submerged (Case Fig. 24-1A). The mandibular teeth were present, and with the jaws closed she presented a marked overbite

that would have increased the likelihood of accelerated resorption of the maxillary al-veolar ridge if it were edentulous and bearing a full upper denture that would be traumatized by the impact of her mandibular natural dentition.

TREATMENT. A flame-shaped loop electrode was selected, and cutting current was set at 5 on the power output dial. The tissues were prepared and infiltration anes-thesia administered. The electrode was activated and used with short wiping strokes applied momentarily, with a 10-second pause interval after each contact, until the coronal end of the root was exposed (Case Fig. 24–1B). The gingiva around the root was then recontoured to eliminate undercuts that would act as food traps and impair the healing. When about 3 mm. of the coronal root end was exposed all around, the J-loop was substituted, current was reduced to 3, and the root was circumscribed with the activated electrode in the same way as it is used to create a subgingival trough, but in this instance to create a crevicular space around the root. Tincture of myrrh and benzoin was applied, and a Peripak dressing was applied around the root.

The patient was next seen on the fifth postoperative day. The tissue around the exposed root was healing very well, with a light layer of coagulum covering the sur-face and protecting the granulation repair underneath it (Case Fig. 24–1C). The coronal end of the root was badly decayed.

The patient was referred back to her dentist, who proceeded to clean out the decay and restore the coronal end with a post and gold core shaped to serve as the crown preparation, whereupon she returned to the author for postoperative observa-tion. The tissue around the gold core was fully healed and normal in tone (Case Fig. 24–1D). The next time she was seen, one week later, the tooth had been restored with a porcelain crown. Two weeks later the restored tooth was used to serve as the termi-nal abutment for a partial denture (Case Fig. 24–1E). Despite the height of the re-tained root above the level of the gingivae of the other teeth, the aesthetic appearance was acceptable, and the tooth has been serving as an effective abutment for more than eight years. Since the retained root was located so much beyond the level of the marginal gingivae of the remaining teeth, the author had had serious qualms about the aesthetic factor even if the tooth could be successfully restored for functional use. However, the tendency of the gingivae to regenerate toward their original level after properly performed electrosection with suitable current would render the aesthetics, although not ideal, acceptable.

By far the most important factor in this case, however, is that exposure of the abut-ment root made it possible to construct a stable functionally useful partial denture and thereby to avoid need to resort to a full maxillary denture that would be opposed by natural mandibular dentition and a decidedly unfavorable occlusal relationship that would almost inevitably have resulted in destructive trauma to the maxillary anterior alveolar bone. Such a situation could only lead to disastrous results, especially in so young a patient.

V. REDUCTION OF REDUNDANT TISSUE FROM EDENTULOUS AREAS IN THE DENTAL ARCH

The simplest and most effective method of removing undesirable hyper-trophic tissue from edentulous saddle areas so as to create sufficient space for restoration with normal-sized pontics is to remove the excess tissue with round or flame-shaped loop electrodes by electrosection.

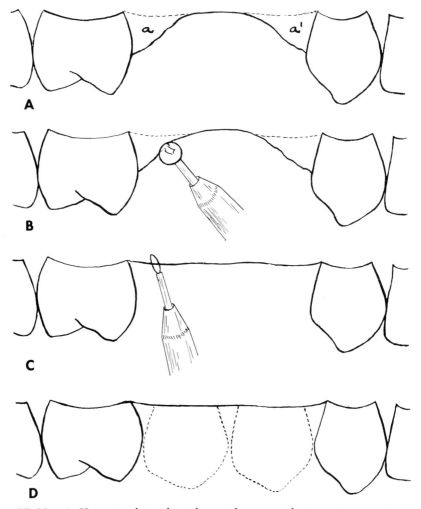

Figure 15–13. A, Hypertrophic edentulous ridge areas that require recontouring. Schematic line drawings of typical case where ridge dips down at each terminal end (*a* and *a'*) along the medial side of abutment teeth. Unless the excess tissue is resected there is not enough room for insertion of normal-sized pontics. B, Resecting the hypertrophic tissue with a loop electrode. C, Alveolar ridge, now reduced to normal height, is beveled with a loop electrode to normal contour. D, There is now adequate space for insertion of normal-sized pontics in the edentulous area.

The excess tissue can easily be reduced to its proper level by shaving in layers with wiping or brushing strokes. The loop electrode can then be used to round off the tissues in order to restore normal convex ridge contour. When this procedure is performed on healthy tissue it is relatively bloodless. In such cases obtundent dressings are usually not required. After the ridge height has been adequately reduced, topical applications of tincture of myrrh and benzoin to the operative field usually provide all the obtundent and protective action necessary (Fig. 15–13).

If the patient has been wearing a partial denture or if a temporary splint has been prepared, a soft mix of surgical cement may be added to the saddle areas. If an obtundent dressing appears to be indicated and no denture or splint is available, adhesive ointments such as Kenalog in Orabase can be applied to the areas as protective dressings. Cement packs and adhesive ointments are also useful as vehicles for local antibiotic or chemotherapeutic medication.

CASE 25

Although this case related to construction of an immediate full upper denture instead of a fixed-bridge restoration, the technique for elimination of gingival mucosa that proliferated downward at the distal aspect of the left cuspid crown was identical to that involved in ridge preparations for fixed-bridge restorations. The purpose of the surgical procedure likewise was identical. For that reason it is being reported in this chapter instead of in the chapter on prosthetic electrosurgery.

PATIENT.   A 52-year-old white female.

HISTORY.   An unfortunate combination of advanced periodontoclasia and maxillary alveolar ridge deformity resulting in malocclusion and very poor cosmetics determined the necessity for multiple extractions and extensive alveoloplasty in preparation for immediate denture insertion.

CLINICAL EXAMINATION.   The maxillary alveolar ridge was markedly elongated in the anterior region and shelved outward labially almost 1 cm. as well as downward 1 cm. This created a marked malocclusion and a rather grotesque facial appearance, particularly when the patient smiled.

The patient was wearing a partial denture restoring the bicuspid-first molar areas bilaterally. The gingival mucosa on the left edentulous alveolar ridge dipped down almost 3 mm. along the distal aspect of the left cuspid crown (Case Fig. 25–1).

TREATMENT.   Elimination of this hypertrophic tissue at the time the posterior teeth were to be extracted would avert an irregular tissue bulge at that site when the anterior teeth are extracted, thereby helping to simplify the anterior alveoloplasty. In a case with marked deformity of the anterior alveolar ridge such as this, simplification of the anterior alveoloplasty becomes an important consideration.

Four minims of anesthetic solution were injected into the labial surface and 2 minims into the palatal mucosa, thus circumscribing the operative field by infiltration. A flame-shaped electrode was selected, cutting current set at 6, and the excess tissue resected by shaving in layers. The electrode was used with short wiping strokes directed postero-anteriorly. The alveolar mucosa was then accurately contoured all around the distal aspect of the cuspid. This operative procedure was very brief and completely bloodless. Tincture of myrrh and benzoin was applied to the operative field in air-dried layers. No other obtundent or protective coating was needed. This procedure preceded extraction of her posterior teeth, which was then performed.

The patient returned on the fifth postoperative day and reported that there had been neither pain nor noteworthy discomfort in the cuspid region. The gingival mucosa on the crest of the left alveolar ridge and around the distal aspect of the cuspid appeared almost fully healed. The tissue tone was excellent. Tincture of myrrh and benzoin was applied to this area as well as to the posterior regions. She was seen again one week later. The tissue in the left cuspid region appeared fully healed and normally keratinized. The alveolar ridge was now uniform in height and normal in contour. Although the posterior extraction sites were not fully healed, this area was healed and no longer required any postoperative care.

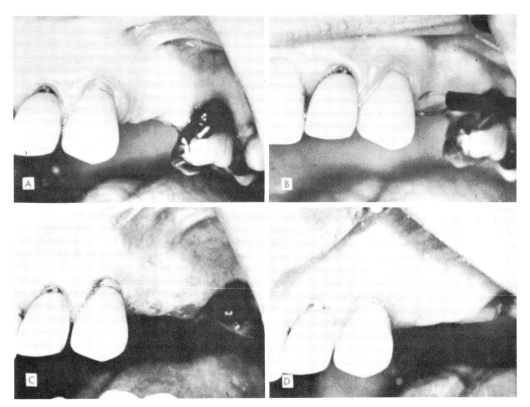

Case Figure 25–1. A, Preoperative view. Edentulous space dips markedly at each terminal end. *B,* Tissue excess planed off with flame-shaped loop electrode. *C,* Appearance immediately following surgery, a bloodless procedure. *D,* Appearance on the twelfth postoperative day. Healing quite complete. Note that socket of tooth that was extracted at the same time is not quite as fully healed.

CASE 26

This is another of the cases made available by Dr. Miller.

PATIENT. Details unknown.

HISTORY. The patient had been wearing a wrought wire clasp partial denture replacing several missing teeth in the maxilla. The tissue in the edentulous areas had proliferated downward, reducing the height of the alveolar ridge. Since this denture was to be replaced with a veneer crown fixed prosthesis, the redundant tissue would have to be removed to eliminate necessity for excessive grinding of pontics.

CLINICAL EXAMINATION. The tissues in the respective edentulous areas in the maxillary right quadrant had proliferated downward along the distal aspects of the anterior teeth and mesial aspects of the posterior teeth in each edentulous area (Case Fig. 26–1).

TREATMENT. The redundant tissue was resected from each edentulous area by electrosection with a medium-width U-shaped loop electrode. The same loop was also used to elongate the clinical crowns of the teeth that were to be prepared to serve as abutments. The tissue was resected uniformly all around the teeth with the loop,

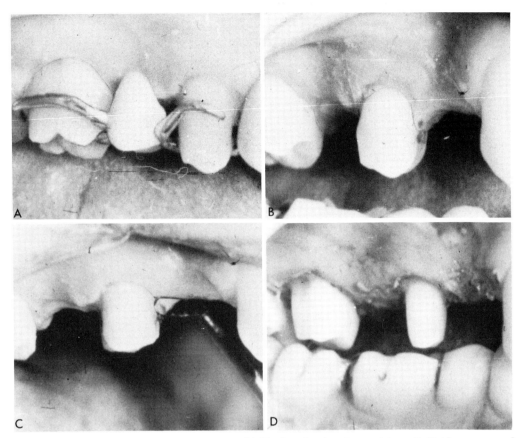

Case Figure 26-1. A, Preoperative; old Nesbitt bridge in position. B, Bridge removed; redundant tissue along mesial aspect of the second bicuspid and first molar and along crests of the edentulous spaces between the teeth that must be reduced. C, Tissue resected with medium-width 45-degree-angle U-shaped loop electrode. D, Appearance of the tissues along the crest of the ridges, and the full crown preparations the removal has facilitated.

planing the tissues so that they presented a feather-edge of marginal gingiva on the palatal as well as on the labial and buccal aspects.

The abutment teeth were then prepared for restoration with veneer crowns, and a dressing of tincture of myrrh and benzoin was applied to the tissues. The patient was seen again on the fifth postoperative day, on the tenth postoperative day, and again 7 weeks postoperatively. Even on the fifth day the rate and quality of the healing were noteworthy.

This case is another example of the innumerable uses Dr. Miller finds for improving his fixed prosthodontics by judicious use of electrosurgery.

In this case he employed electrosurgery to perform three of the five procedures for which electrosurgery has justifiably become invaluable: elongation of the clinical crowns of the abutment teeth, preparation of subgingival troughs around abutment preparations, and reduction of redundant tissue from the endentulous area in the dental arch to permit insertion of normal sized, aesthetically acceptable pontics.

CASE 27

This case also has been made available by Dr. Miller.

PATIENT.   An adult white male.

HISTORY.   He had an old fixed bridge in the mandibular right quadrant. Hyperplasia of the marginal gingivae and periodontal deterioration had occurred around the terminal abutment teeth. The old restoration was therefore to be removed and replaced with a new porcelain against gold fixed bridge after surgical correction of the gingival tissues.

CLINICAL EXAMINATION.   An acrylic veneer bridge was present in the mandibular right quadrant. It extended from the second molar to the first bicuspid. The second molar had a periodontal pocket at the distobuccal aspect and the marginal gingiva around the first bicuspid was somewhat hyperplastic. The mesial half of the anterior abutment crown had been cut away, as the first step in removal of the restoration (Case Fig. 27–1).

TREATMENT.   The area had been anesthetized with an inferior alveolar block injection. The old restoration was removed, exposing the edentulous area of the second bicuspid and the marginal gingivae around the two molars and the first bicuspid. A

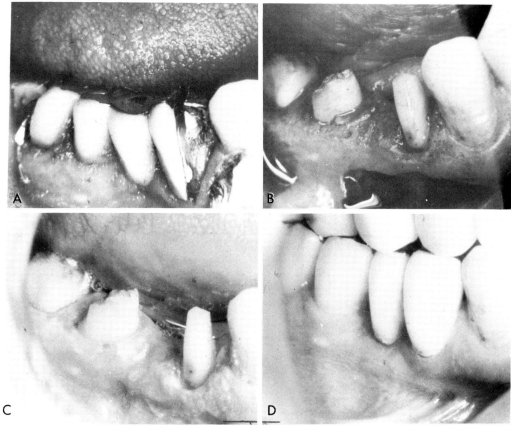

Case Figure 27–1. Gingivoplasty to recontour the tissues. *A,* The old restoration still in position. The crown of the cuspid is being cut to enable the bridge to be removed. *B,* The bridge has been removed and the redundant tissue removed by gingivoplasty performed with a loop electrode. *C,* Appearance of the tissues two weeks later. *D,* Tissues nicely adapted around the new restoration. Note the tissue tone and contour.

20-degree-angle medium-width U-shaped loop electrode was selected and cutting current output was set at 5 on the power dial. The activated electrode was used to recontour the marginal gingivae and the slightly redundant tissue in the edentulous area. A smaller 45-degree-angle, narrow U-shaped loop was substituted, current output was reduced to 3.5, and this activated electrode was used to create subgingival troughs around the abutment teeth and debride the shallow pocket of the second molar. An impression was then taken and a model processed for the fabrication of the new bridge. The remainder of the old bridge, which had been sterilized in cold sterilizing solution, was used as a temporary splint with a periodontal pack to cover the surgical field.

The patient returned the following week and the bridge splint and cement pack were removed, exposing the healing tissues. Healing progressed rapidly and uneventfully, and when the new restoration was inserted the tissues were fully healed and accurately adapted to the restoration. There was a total absence of subgingival impingement and no recurrence of the gingival hyperplasia or periodontal deterioration.

VI. IMPLANT MUCOPERIOSTEAL FLAP INCISIONS

In addition to the advantages electrosurgery offers the clinician in the other areas of restorative dentistry that have been reviewed, this modality also offers noteworthy advantages to accelerate and improve the efficiency of the various implant restorative procedures.

In the use of implants to convert edentulous areas to an artificial dentulous state the initial step is the surgical exposure of the edentulous alveolar bone, irrespective of whether an implant is being utilized to replace a single valuable abutment tooth or multiple implants are to be utilized to restore an edentulous arch with a fixed and partial prosthesis.

When the incision of the mucoperiosteal flap is created with a steel scalpel to achieve the exposure, free bleeding, often profuse and persistent, ensues. Control of this bleeding is not always readily achieved.

Free bleeding obscures the operative field and thereby impairs the efficiency of the operator. It also impairs the accuracy of the critically important impressions of the surgical field. These twin handicaps retard and prolong the operative procedure and jeopardize the ultimate outcome.

Another factor relating to bleeding merits special consideration. Implantology is performed most frequently for patients who fall within the geriatric age range. Postoperative shock due to blood loss is especially hazardous to the geriatric patient.

The hemostasis inherent in electrosection eliminates these handicaps. It makes possible precise and rapid preparation of the exposed alveolar area for implantation of metal blades and/or for impression of the exposed area for fabrication of a metallic framework, without blood loss and its concomitant effects and without damage to the incised tissues.

The clear, unobscured operative field resulting from the electrosurgical mucoperiosteal incisions offers a particularly valuable advantage to the clinician who wishes to demonstrate or to teach implantation techniques.

The case to be reported below involved replacement of a single tooth needed as an abutment. Nevertheless, the advantages electrosurgery offered of working in a relatively bloodless field and being able to see even under loop magnification to prepare the implant site were noteworthy. Needless to say, the value of the advantages increases proportionally when the implants are utilized to restore the entire edentulous arch with a fixed and partial prosthesis.

Although subperiosteal and blade implantology differ somewhat in concept and markedly in technique, they share a common denominator: in either technique it is necessary to incise and reflect the mucoperiosteum and expose the underlying bone onto or into which the implant will be secured.

When the mucoperiosteal flap incision is made with a steel scalpel, free hemorrhagic bleeding ensues that is a decided handicap to the precise performance of either technique. The reasons are self-evident. With subperiosteal implants, success depends largely on fabrication of a very accurately fitted casting that will hug the alveolar bone tightly. When there is hemorrhagic bleeding, it is virtually impossible to obtain a perfect, clean impression of the exposed bone. The potential for fabrication of a casting that is properly adherent to the bone is greatly diminished and optimal results are highly unlikely. With blade implantology, hemorrhagic bleeding obscures the operative field and greatly increases the difficulty of cutting a precise narrow groove into the bone for snug insertion of the blade portion, so that the implant will be firmly embedded and not wobble around loosely. The latter is likely to prove disastrous, since it would result in a fibrous repair around the blade instead of the bone regeneration that is necessary to provide firm abutments that can withstand the torque of function.

When the incision for the mucoperiosteal flap is made with a needle electrode with fully rectified current, the hemostasis inherent in electrosection almost invariably eliminates hemorrhagic bleeding as a factor. If the incised tissues are elevated and reflected *gently,* bleeding is minimal and readily controlled and the surgical field remains clearly visible. This enhances and facilitates maximum efficiency with either implant procedure.

When the flap incision is being made for a blade implant, the alveolar bone being contacted by the activated electrode will subsequently be eliminated as the groove is cut into the bone for the blade insertion. This, however, does not eliminate need for good electrosurgical technique. It is true that cutting out the bone to create the groove eliminates the area of bone most vulnerable to damage, and if the instrumentation should be slightly slower than is normally necessary, there is more margin for error. But if the activated electrode is permitted to linger slowly against the bone by making a very deliberate incision, the lateral heat dispersion produced by the instrumentation will penetrate beyond the portion of bone that will be removed by cutting the groove and postoperative sequestration may result.

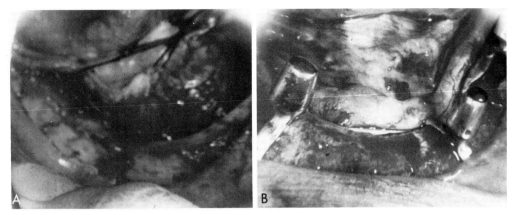

Figure 15–14. Comparative appearance of incisions with steel scalpel for a mucoperio-steal flap for implant insertion. *A,* Tissue has been incised with a steel scalpel and the muco-periosteum has been elevated and retracted to expose the alveolar ridge. Note the profuse hemorrhagic bleeding that obscures the surgical field and impairs visibility and instrumenta-tion. *B,* Free bleeding continues after implants have been inserted. Note that despite the fact that these are subperiosteal implants and that grooves have not had to be cut into the bone, the free bleeding persists.

Should clinical considerations make it necessary to re-incise the tissue several times in order to penetrate through thick fibrous tissue, it is necessary to allow adequate time intervals to elapse between applications of the ac-tivated electrode to prevent damage due to cumulative heat buildup. If, in the desire to avoid any possibility of free bleeding from the incision, the cutting current output is increased enough to char the tissue margins, it is especially important to allow a full 10 seconds to elapse between applications of the ac-tivated electrode to assure against excessive heat damage to the bone.

Figure 15–14 illustrates the typical hemorrhagic bleeding encountered when the incisions are made with the steel scalpel. They provide a dramatic and illuminating contrast to the conditions encountered when the tissues have been incised electrosurgically.

The aforementioned invaluable advantages that electrosurgery makes available for performing implantology are demonstrated admirably in the fol-lowing group of clinical case reports that have been made available to the au-thor by Dr. Peter M. Beck of Toronto, Ontario, Canada.

CASE 28

This case differs from the other cases in this series principally in the fact that the implant procedure was performed soon after extraction of a tooth in the edentulous area being restored.

PATIENT. Details unknown.

HISTORY. Several posterior teeth were missing from the left side of the lower jaw. One of the teeth had been extracted two weeks previously. The implant was be-ing made at the patient's insistence, instead of the usual fixed prosthesis that would normally be indicated.

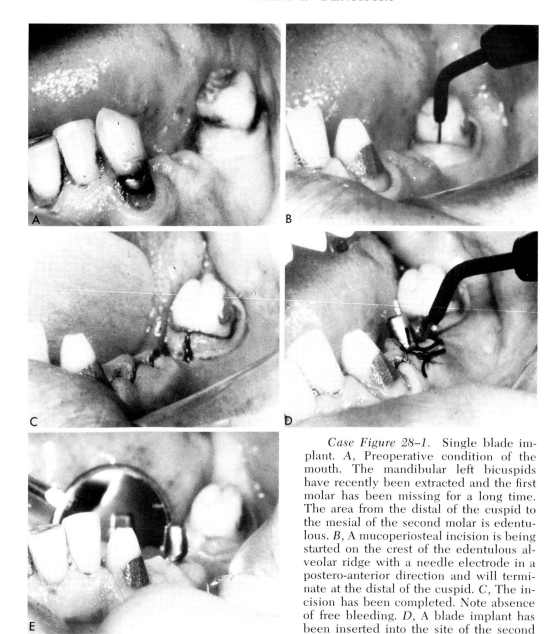

Case Figure 28-1. Single blade implant. *A,* Preoperative condition of the mouth. The mandibular left bicuspids have recently been extracted and the first molar has been missing for a long time. The area from the distal of the cuspid to the mesial of the second molar is edentulous. *B,* A mucoperiosteal incision is being started on the crest of the edentulous alveolar ridge with a needle electrode in a postero-anterior direction and will terminate at the distal of the cuspid. *C,* The incision has been completed. Note absence of free bleeding. *D,* A blade implant has been inserted into the site of the second bicuspid, and a bulge of tissue excess around the implant is being incised for excision to prevent tissue puckering around the implant. *E,* Appearance two weeks after removal of the sutures. The tissues are well healed and very tightly adapted around the implant and are now ready for insertion of the prosthetic superstructure.

CLINICAL EXAMINATION. The mandibular left quadrant was edentulous from first bicuspid to second molar. The socket of the second bicuspid was incompletely healed. A large class V amalgam filling on the labial aspect of the cuspid had decay along the inferior margin (Case Fig. 28-1A).

TREATMENT. The quadrant was anesthetized with an inferior alveolar block injection. A 45-degree-angle fine needle electrode was selected and used to make an incision along the crest of the alveolar ridge with cutting current set at 3.5 to assure hemostasis. The incision was started at the mesial of the second molar (Case Fig. 28–1*B*) and carried to the distal of the cuspid (Case Fig. 28–1*C*). The hemostasis was effective and there was no free bleeding.

The margins of the incised tissue were spread apart, exposing the alveolar bone. A small round bur was used to cut a groove along the crest of the ridge downward into the bone to permit insertion of a blade implant. The blade was seated firmly into the bone and the tissue margins were coapted around the supragingival part of the blade and sutured securely. A small pucker of excess tissue around the buccal aspect of the implant was excised with the electrode (Case Fig. 28–1*D*) to create a harmonious gingival contour around the implant. Healing progressed rapidly and uneventfully, and in less than two weeks the incised tissue appeared fully healed (Case Fig. 28–1*E*).

CASE 29

This case demonstrates the use of blade implants to create artificial abutments that make possible use of a fixed prosthetic restoration with terminal abutments instead of a free-end cantilevered prosthesis. The advantages of a restoration attached to terminal abutments over free-end cantilevered restorations is self-evident.

PATIENT.   Details unknown.

HISTORY.   Details unknown.

CLINICAL EXAMINATION.   The maxilla had a full complement of teeth in normal alignment. The mandibular right quadrant distal to the first bicuspid was edentulous.

TREATMENT.   The patient had an aversion for removable appliances. A blade implant in the second molar area to serve as the posterior abutment for a fixed prosthesis was therefore decided upon.

The quadrant was prepared for surgery and an inferior alveolar-lingual nerve block was administered. The planned line of incision through the tissues to expose the alveolar bone was outlined in indelible pencil. A 45-degree-angle needle electrode was then activated and used to incise the tissues as outlined (Case Fig. 29–1). The incision did not produce free bleeding.

The broad end of a periosteal elevator was then used to displace the buccal and lingual mucoperiosteal flaps, care being taken to detach the periosteum gently and expose the alveolar bone without inducing hemorrhagic bleeding to obscure the operative field.

The respective buccal and lingual mucoperiosteal flaps having been displaced adequately, and a bur was used to cut a narrow groove cleanly and precisely through the cortex and into the cancellous portion of the mandible. A blade implant was inserted into the groove in the bone so that it was snugly wedged without lateral mobility, and the tissue margins were coapted and adapted around the projecting implant and were sutured into place.

Healing was rapid and uneventful. There was evidence of primary repair on the fifth postoperative day, and the sutures were removed. Healing was complete by the time the restoration was fabricated, and it was inserted. After two weeks it was apparent that the occlusion was satisfactory, and the restoration was permanently cemented.

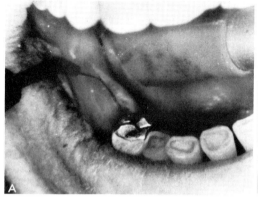
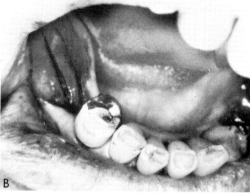
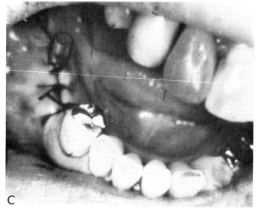

Case Figure 29–1. Mucoperiosteal incision and bone groove for blade implant. *A*, Incision being made with a needle electrode by electrosection in the right mandibular quadrant for insertion of a blade implant. *B*, The incised mucoperiosteum has been reflected and a groove has been cut into the alveolar bone for insertion of the blade of the implant. *C*, The mucoperiosteal flaps have been restored, coapted and adapted around the implant, and sutured into position with interrupted silk sutures.

CASE 30

This case serves to demonstrate the advantages inherent in use of blade implants placed strategically into long edentulous areas to serve as additional abutments that will reduce functional stresses upon the natural abutments created by unsupported long pontic spans. It also demonstrates the facility with which the tissue irregularities often encountered around the implants can be reduced or resected to create harmonious gingival continuity around the implant projections.

PATIENT.   Details unknown.

HISTORY.   Details unknown.

CLINICAL EXAMINATION.   The maxillary teeth from cuspid to cuspid were missing and had been replaced with a partial clasp-bearing denture. The remaining teeth in both jaws appeared healthy and in normal alignment. When the denture was removed it revealed presence of a thick fibrous layer of mucosa on the crest of the alveolar ridge (Case Figs. 30–1 and 30–2).

TREATMENT.   The treatment plan provided for insertion of two blade implants in the anterior region to provide simulations of the central incisors. The thickness and density of the overlying mucosa made it evident that it would in all probability require multiple reincisions to create the mucoperiosteal flaps to expose the bone.

A 45-degree-angle needle electrode was selected and activated with the cutting current. The activated electrode was used to incise the tissues across the edentulous span. As anticipated, it was necessary to repeat the incision several times; however,

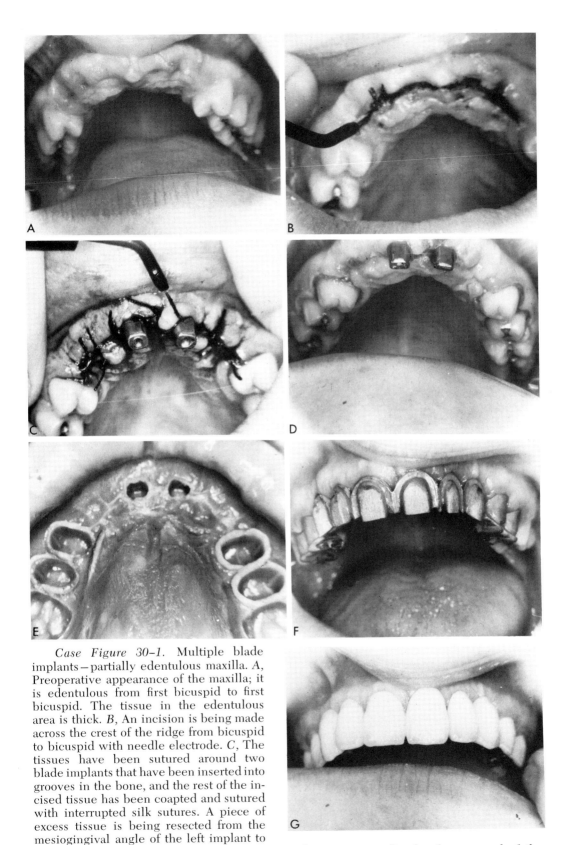

Case Figure 30–1. Multiple blade implants—partially edentulous maxilla. *A,* Preoperative appearance of the maxilla; it is edentulous from first bicuspid to first bicuspid. The tissue in the edentulous area is thick. *B,* An incision is being made across the crest of the ridge from bicuspid to bicuspid with needle electrode. *C,* The tissues have been sutured around two blade implants that have been inserted into grooves in the bone, and the rest of the incised tissue has been coapted and sutured with interrupted silk sutures. A piece of excess tissue is being resected from the mesiogingival angle of the left implant to eliminate a puckering bulge. *D,* Appearance of tissues immediately after removal of the structures, one week postoperatively. The posterior teeth are being prepared for full crown coverage. *E,* The hydrocolloid impression that has been taken of the maxilla. *F,* The cast metal framework for the prosthesis in position. *G,* The prosthesis has been inserted. Note the excellent tissue tone and aesthetics.

A

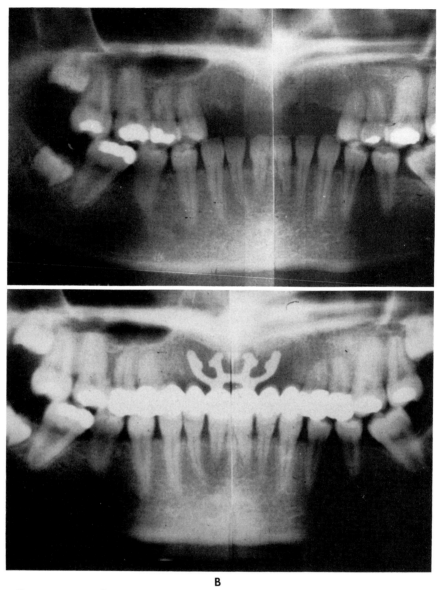

B

Case Figure 30–2.   This is a panographic view of the maxilla. *A*, This roentgenogram shows the edentulous anterior area of the maxilla where the implant will be inserted. *B*, This roentgenogram shows the blade implant that has been used to restore the missing teeth. Note that the blades have not involved the nasal fossa or the maxillary sinuses.

after each contact of the activated electrode, a "cooling off" period was permitted to elapse before again bringing the activated electrode into contact with the tissues and bone. Thus, although the tissue margins became somewhat charred from the reincisions, undesirable lateral heat penetration did not occur and damage to the adjacent soft tissues or to the bone adjacent to the groove that would be cut into the bone was avoided.

The mucoperiosteal tissue flaps created by the incision on the labial and palatal aspects were gently but firmly undermined with the blunt, broad end of a periosteal elevator and were displaced laterally to expose the denuded bone. A bur was used to cut a precise groove on either side of the midline, and the blade implants were inserted into the grooves into which they were lightly but firmly wedged. The margins of the incised mucosa were coapted and sutured, with the tissues sutured around each implant's coronal end that projected above the mucosa.

Since no space had been provided in the tissue flaps to accommodate the implant projections, the tissue puckered and bulged somewhat around each projection. These tissue bulges were easily reduced by dissecting away some of the tissue with the needle electrode.

Healing proceeded without incidence and the sutures were removed after five days. A slight amount of tissue was found bulging on the palatal aspect around the left implant and this bit of excess tissue was easily and quickly reduced by shaving with the electrode to normal dimension.

When healing was completed, the tissues were tightly adherent to the neck of the implant projections and normal in tone and texture. The permanent prosthesis was inserted and, after the occlusal harmony was established, it was cemented in permanently. The insertion of the two blade implant dummy abutments made it possible to provide firm stability around the entire arch, which would not have been possible if the length of the endentulous span had not been so markedly reduced by the presence of the implant abutments.

Unlike the two previous cases which demonstrated typical uses of blade implants to supplement the remaining natural dentition as functional abutments that make it possible to avoid cantilevered restorations and long unsupported pontic spans, the following case demonstrates typical use of blade implants to convert a totally edentulous alveolar ridge into an artificially dentulous state that permits restoration with a fixed prosthesis instead of a full denture.

If the implant restoration is to be functionally successful the edentulous alveolar ridge must be anatomically suited for implantology. When the blade type of implant is to be used it is necessary to have an alveolar ridge and jawbone of adequate physical dimension to permit cutting of the necessary grooves into the bone for insertion of the blade into the jawbone.

Total senile resorption of the alveolar ridges is by no means uncommon. In many such instances, the body of the jawbone itself also has undergone some degree of resorption. Such cases are anatomically unsuited for implantology. Blade implants in particular would be distinctly contraindicated.

The following case involved an edentulous mandibular alveolar ridge that was rather thin, and the crest of the alveolar bone was so irregular that about 2 to 3 mm. of vertical height had to be sacrificed to create a reasonably smooth, rounded alveolar crest. Despite this loss of vertical height there was sufficient bone left to permit the cutting of grooves deep enough to permit insertion of the blades of the implants.

CASE 31

PATIENT.   Details unknown.
HISTORY.   Details unknown.
CLINICAL EXAMINATION.   The mandibular alveolar ridge was edentulous. The

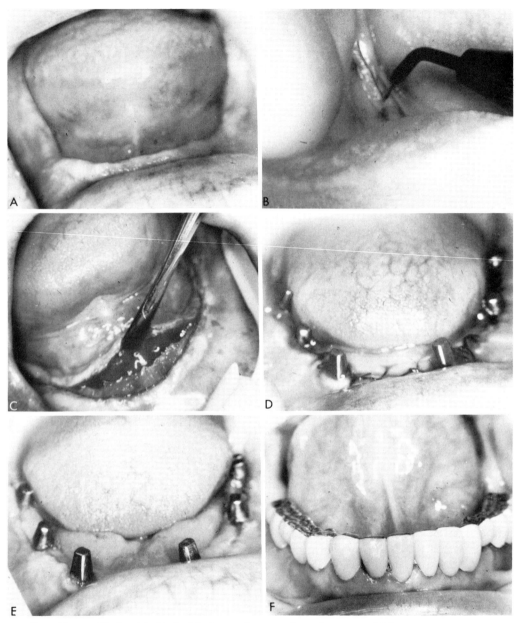

Case Figure 31–1. Multiple blade implants — edentulous mandible. *A,* Preoperative appearance of the edentulous mandible. *B,* Incision being made with a needle electrode for a mucoperiosteal flap that will extend from the retromolar pad on one side to the other side. *C,* The incised tissue has been reflected, revealing sharp irregular crestal bone. *D,* Appearance of the tissues one week after the blade implants have been inserted, just before the sutures are to be removed. *E,* Appearance of the tissues two weeks later. Note close adaptation around the implants and the almost invisible line of incision. *F,* Appearance of the completed case.

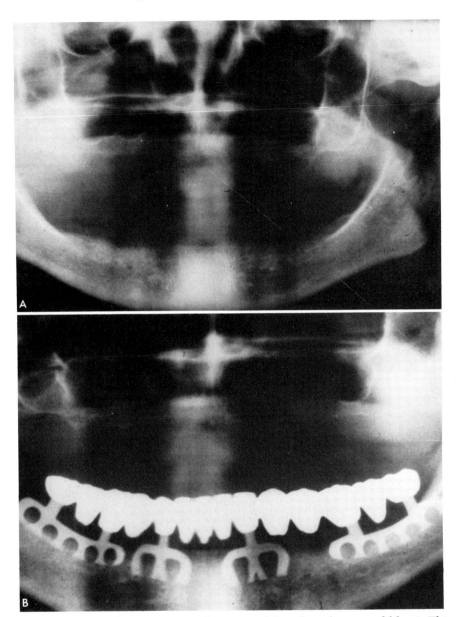

Case Figure 31–2. This is a panographic view of the edentulous mandible. *A,* This is the preoperative roentgenogram of the mandible. *B,* This roentgenogram shows the four blades that have been inserted, two anteriorly and two posteriorly, which are serving as the foundation for the fixed prosthesis that extends from second molar to second molar.

anterior part of the ridge from cuspid to cuspid area was normal in height but rather thin in labiolingual diameter. The ridge height in the two saddle areas had undergone some degree of resorption (Case Figs. 31–1 and 31–2).

TREATMENT.   The mouth was prepared and bilateral inferior alveolar-lingual nerve block anesthesia was administered. A line of incision was outlined on the crest of the ridge with indelible pencil, and the tissue was incised by electrosection with a 45-degree-angle needle electrode, as outlined.

The tissue on the labial aspect was carefully undermined and reflected from the bone with a periosteal elevator. The lingual flap was then partially reflected from the bone, fully exposing the entire alveolar ridge and part of the jawbone. No free bleeding had been caused by the flap incisions, and gentle, careful elevation of the mucoperiosteal flaps caused some oozing of blood, which was of short duration. Thereafter the surgical field was clearly visible, revealing a thin alveolar ridge that was sharply jagged at its superior surface.

Two to 3 mm. of the crestal bone was reduced and rounded off with a sterile diamond stone, creating a relatively smooth rounded ridge crest. A bur was then used to cut the grooves into the bone at intervals to create molar, bicuspid, cuspid, and anterior implant sites. When the grooves were completed, the blades were inserted. Each groove was narrow enough so that the blade was firmly wedged without any crushing of the bone and without lateral mobility that would traumatize the bone. The flaps were then restored to position, coapted, adapted around the implants, and sutured.

Healing progressed favorably, and one week postoperatively the sutures were removed. Clinical healing appeared complete within three weeks, and the fixed prosthesis that had been fabricated to restore the missing teeth was inserted. Functionally as well as aesthetically the restoration was gratifyingly satisfactory.

VII. CROWN AND BRIDGE FAILURES: REASONS AND CORRECTIONS

Introduction

Fixed partial prostheses, designed to restore missing teeth in the dental arch, or splints constructed to restore or create occlusal harmony often trigger unfavorable responses in their investing structures. The responses usually are inflammatory in nature and frequently deteriorate into iatrogenic periodontoclasia.

Improper functional occlusion and failure to restore occlusal harmony are a major cause for unfavorable tissue responses. Crowns that fail to provide adequate embrasure space due to poor mesiodistal contour, improper buccolingual contour, inefficient preparation of abutments, and slipshod subgingival adaptation and finish of the castings are other important factors.

However, the only factor that rivals occlusion as the major cause for unfavorable reaction to a restoration is the failure to provide and *maintain* sufficient subgingival space to accommodate the subgingival portion of the crowns without traumatic impingement against the periodontal structures. With the greatly increased use of full crown coverage for full mouth rehabilitation, the importance of this factor has increased proportionally.

Serviceable durability is an important factor in planning and designing a restoration. Durability is by no means the ultimate criterion of success, however. If a restoration triggers unfavorable reactions that lead to further loss of teeth, its durability becomes meaningless. Iatrogenic periodontoclasia often leads to loss of teeth. In such cases, regardless of how beautiful the aesthetics or how exquisite the occlusal contours, the restoration is a failure.

Iatrogenically induced periodontoclasia is in a sense reminiscent of Marc Anthony's funeral oration for Julius Caesar: "The evil that men do often lives after them; the good is interred with their bones." Man-made periodontal deterioration is in virtually every instance the end result of faulty restorative dentistry.

Of the many ways in which a fixed prosthesis can cause iatrogenic periodontoclasia, by far the most common is by impingement of the subgingival portion of the restoration against the subgingival structures. If the restoration projects into the tissues like a splinter under the thumb nail and impinges on the subgingival tissues, the groundwork for iatrogenic periodontoclasia is created.

Restorative Factors Responsible for Iatrogenic Periodontoclasia

In addition to improper occlusion, a number of structural factors involved in the art and science of restorative dentistry can become the direct trigger mechanisms for tissue irritation resulting in iatrogenic periodontoclasia.

Improper mesiodistal contour results in inadequate embrasure space, causing crowding of the interdental papillae. Inflammation, engorgement, hyperplasia, and partial or complete detachment of the papillae are likely aftermaths. This hazard is eliminated when a bullet-shaped mesiodistal contour is created.

Improper buccolingual crown contour, excessive thickness of the subgingival terminal end of the crown, and overextension of the subgingival end of a shoulderless crown are other important culprits. Each constitutes a source of irritation capable of producing severe inflammatory response in the gingival and subgingival tissues.

Perhaps the most irritating trigger source of all, however, is created by failure to provide and/or to maintain adequate subgingival space to assure atraumatic accommodation of the subgingival portion of the restoration. The following cases demonstrate various degrees of tissue response to irritation resulting from failure to create *and preserve* a subgingival trough around the crown preparation. They substantiate the fact that the major function of the subgingival trough is not merely to provide gingival retraction to permit impression material to flow into the crevicular space unimpeded, but to provide the subgingival accommodation to assure against inflammatory irritation and deterioration and to provide adequate space to permit atraumatic preparation of an impeccable shoulder preparation.

The degree of unfavorable tissue response, and the severity of the response that can be triggered by irritation from a fixed prosthesis runs the gamut from mild gingival or subgingival proliferation and gingival recession to extensive destruction of the jawbone.

The factors that create the triggering irritation also run the gamut from failure to provide adequate subgingival accommodation to faulty fabrication and poor clinical judgment that results in an unsuitable treatment plan.

A number of representative illustrative cases are being presented. They fall into two categories: One group will illustrate typical unfavorable sequelae, but the electrosurgical corrective procedures that were instituted will also be reviewed. The second presents visual examples of the various types of unfavorable sequelae, and what triggered the unfavorable reactions, without reviewing the corrective procedures they required to restore the tissues to normal health.

GROUP 1: ILLUSTRATIVE CASES AND THEIR TREATMENT

Simple Failures That Are Readily Corrected

CASE 32

This case demonstrates what is likely to happen when the subgingival tissue is retracted to facilitate impression-taking and is then permitted to return to its former dimension and tissue-tooth relation before the insertion of the restoration.

PATIENT.   A 69-year-old white male in normal health.

HISTORY.   The mandibular central and lateral incisors having been lost, the mandibular cuspids had been prepared for full crown coverage with porcelain veneer crowns to serve as abutments for a Chayes type of movable-removable bridge. By the time the crowns were ready for cementation the gingival tissue had become closely adherent to the teeth and the crowns had to be forced down to seat and cement them into place. The frictional pull created subsequently by frequent removal of the bridge would in all probability not have disturbed the cement adhesion, but when pressure from moderate proliferation of the marginal gingiva was superimposed, it proved sufficient to cause a loosening of the left cuspid crown, which permitted the tissue to flow under the subgingival portion of the crown and eventually caused its physical dislodgment. When he consulted his dentist, the latter was unable to reseat the crown, owing to the presence of the intervening tissue. He was referred for removal of the proliferated tissue and preparation of a subgingival trough around the shoulder of the preparation.

CLINICAL EXAMINATION.   The tissue tone of the marginal gingiva was relatively normal in all but the tissue edge in contact with the right crown and the edge in contact with the left cuspid preparation. The entire shoulder area of the crown was covered with tissue, so that the shoulder was completely obscured from view. Whereas the marginal edge of the marginal gingiva normally is feather edged, the marginal gingiva around the two abutment teeth, especially around the left cuspid preparation, was thick with a rounded blunt edge.

TREATMENT.   A 45-degree-angle medium-width loop electrode was selected, and current output was set at 4 on the power output control dial. The tissues around

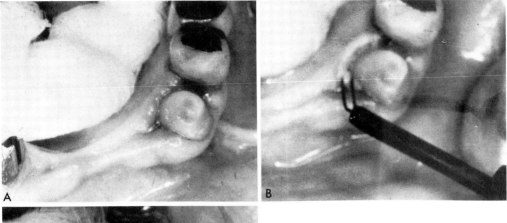

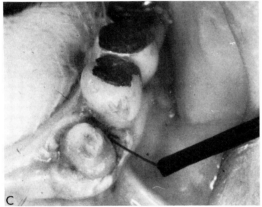

Case Figure 32–1. Removal of redundant tissue to re-expose shoulders of preparation. *A,* Preoperative: The shoulder area of the crown preparation is completely covered with redundant tissue. The tissue on the lingual aspect is inflamed and friable, and the tissue normally in the embrasure between two teeth has disintegrated in the cuspid-first bicuspid embrasure. The buccal interdental papilla between the two teeth is engorged, enlarged, and detached. *B,* The redundant tissue is being resected from the lingual with a medium-width 45-degree-angle U-shaped loop electrode. *C,* The buccal and lingual papillae between the cuspid and bicuspid have been recontoured to normal architecture, and the granulomatous tissue in the embrasure is being resected with a J-loop electrode.

the left cuspid were prepared and infiltration anesthesia administered. The loop was activated and used with short brushing strokes to clear away the lingual and mesial tissue until the shoulder became exposed to view (Case Fig. 32–1). The tissue in the interproximal space between the cuspid and bicuspid was then removed with a J-loop electrode and cutting current was set at 3.5, since the space between the two teeth was too narrow to permit use of the full loops. This loop was then used to create the subgingival troughs. Tincture of myrrh and benzoin was applied in air-dried layers, and the patient returned to his dentist for reinsertion and cementation of the displaced crown. Healing proceeded uneventfully.

CASE 33

This also is an example of the mildest form of unfavorable tissue reaction to subgingival impingement and irritation that resulted from failure to provide adequate subgingival space to accommodate the restoration without irritation after insertion. It differs from the previous case only in the fact that the narrow U-shaped electrode was used to reexpose the shoulders, and is included to demonstrate the instrumentation and also the rate and quality of the tissue repair which the previous case was unable to demonstrate.

PATIENT.   A 53-year-old white female.

HISTORY.   She had had a four-unit fixed bridge inserted in the mandibular left quadrant about six months previously. Several months later the temporary cement adhesion with which the restoration had been maintained loosened, and the restoration had to be recemented. The restoration loosened once more several weeks later, and again was recemented. A few days previously the bridge not only loosened but became physically displaced. When she returned to her dentist he found that it was not possible to reinsert and recement it because tissue had proliferated and covered the shoulders of the preparations so that the bridge could not be properly seated. He referred her to the author for reexposure of the shoulder areas.

CLINICAL EXAMINATION.   The bridge had been a cantilever type attached to the two bicuspids and first molar with veneer crowns and a second molar pontic cantilevered from the splinted crowns as a free distal end. The marginal gingivae had flowed over the shoulders of the preparations, completely covering them. There also appeared to be some slight proliferation of submucous tissue, especially in the embrasures. This tissue was much more friable and engorged than the gingival proliferative tissue.

TREATMENT.   The tissues were prepared and an inferior alveolar-lingual block injection was administered. A 7-mm. round loop electrode was selected, cutting cur-

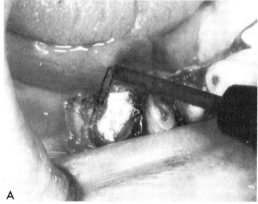

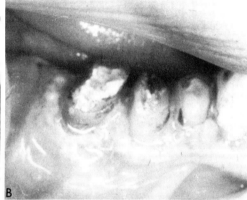

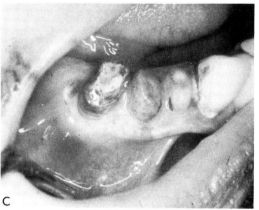

Case Figure 33–1. Removal of redundant tissue to re-expose shoulder preparation. *A,* The gross redundant tissue has been reduced to normal dimension with a 45-degree-angle wide U-shaped loop. The tissue covering the shoulder is being excised with a 90-degree-angle narrow U-shaped loop electrode. A proliferation of tissue distal to the tooth has been reduced by loop electrosection. *B,* Appearance of the tissues around the tooth on fifth postoperative day. Healing by granulation repair is progressing favorably and rapidly. There is no swelling, edema, inflammation, or engorgement. The surface of the tissue is covered with a thin film of coagulum. *C,* Appearance of the tissues 2 weeks later. The tissue is fully healed, and the surface epithelium appears to be undergoing normal maturation. The edentulous tissue distal to the tooth is no longer bulging upward, but is harmonious with the level of the rest of the tissue.

rent was set at 5, and the activated electrode was used to reduce the redundant tissue, especially at the distal aspect of the first molar, by loop planing that simultaneously recontoured the tissue, and also along the lingual aspect of the three teeth. The round loop was replaced with a right-angle narrow U-shaped loop electrode, current output was reduced to 3.5, and the redundant tissue that covered the shoulder areas was resected (Case Fig. 33–1A).

All the redundant tissue having been resected and the gingivae restored to normal contour, tincture of myrrh and benzoin was applied in air-dried layers, the sterilized bridge was reinserted, and a periodontal pack was applied around the gingivae and the restoration. The patient returned on the fifth postoperative day. The cement pack was removed, the tissues were cleansed by gentle irrigation, and the restoration was cleansed by vigorous brushing. The tincture of myrrh and benzoin was again applied, the bridge reinserted, a fresh cement pack was applied and the patient was instructed to return again in five days. When she returned and the bridge and pack were removed, the tissues appeared to be healing well and to be adapting themselves against the subgingival portions of the restoration (Case Fig. 33–1B), but a very thin layer of coagulum indicated that the healing process was as yet not complete.

Tincture of myrrh and benzoin was again applied to the tissues, care being taken to avoid covering the shoulder areas with it. The tissues and preparations having been thoroughly dried by the application of the medicament, the restoration was cemented with temporary cement and she was instructed to continue the saline lavage and other postoperative instructions for two more weeks. At the end of that period the tissues were fully healed and with the restoration removed the preservation of the space to accommodate the subgingival portion of the restoration could be seen (Case Fig. 33–1C). At this point the patient returned to her dentist for the permanent cementation. The bridge has not given her any trouble since.

Failures Requiring Extensive Corrective Treatment

The next case is an excellent example of iatrogenic periodontoclasia that was triggered by inadequate subgingival accommodation for the porcelain veneer crowns used to restore the occlusion. It also typifies the major reason why many dentists maintain permanent fixed prostheses in the mouth with temporary cementation for prolonged periods. Their reluctance to cement a restoration permanently stems from the fact that if the tissue response to the restoration should prove unfavorable, because of the temporary cementation the restoration can be quickly and easily removed without danger of fracturing the coronal portions of the preparations, as is likely to happen if the restoration has been inserted with permanent cement that has to be fractured to remove the prosthesis.

It is rather ironic that the patient involved was himself a dentist. He had undergone an occlusal rehabilitation to restore the vertical dimension which had been altered owing to coronal attrition resulting from bruxing. The loss of vertical dimension had apparently produced a mild but alarming temporomandibular joint syndrome. The occlusal reconstruction had been prescribed to restore the normal vertical dimension and thereby abort the TM joint deterioration.

Before the occlusal reconstruction was performed, the gingivae appeared to be healthy, and there was no clinical evidence of even incipient periodontal deterioration. Soon after the veneer crown splints were inserted the marginal gingivae around the crowns began to turn purplish red in color and to become hyperplastic and atonal. Despite conscientious oral hygiene and repeated attempts by the prosthodontist to relieve the condition by curettage, the gingivae continued to deteriorate and the splints began to become loosened and displaced by pressure from subgingival tissue proliferation. He therefore made arrangements for treatment by the author to eliminate the diseased tissue and also provide adequate subgingival space to accommodate the subgingival portions of the restorations without impingement.

CASE 34

PATIENT.   A 41-year-old white male.

HISTORY.   The patient was a dentist. He had had a "complete occlusal reconstruction" performed two years previously. Gingival retraction with chemically impregnated cords packed subgingivally had been used to facilitate impression-taking. The restorations were well designed, and an acceptable occlusal relationship was carefully established. The restorations were inserted and maintained under temporary cementation to the present time. Permanent cementation was repeatedly deferred because the gingival tissues deteriorated progressively despite frequent manual curettage and vigorous oral physiotherapy. The patient came to the author for consultation and treatment.

CLINICAL EXAMINATION.   All the teeth in both jaws had been restored with full porcelain and gold crowns. The gingivae, both marginal and alveolar, appeared inflamed, engorged, and hyperplastic. On closer inspection it became apparent that the marginal gingivae were partially detached from their underlying structures. When the restorations were removed, the marginal gingivae around the tooth preparations were found to have proliferated, so that the subgingival portions of the restoration were impinging and displacing them and covering the shoulders of the preparations completely (Case Fig. 34-1).

TREATMENT.   The best treatment plan appeared to be to start with a gingivoplasty to restore the gingivae to normal architecture, then to resect the tissues from the shoulder areas and create well-defined subgingival troughs around the preparations.

The mandible was treated first, since the greatest damage appeared to have occurred there. The right quadrant was anesthetized with an inferior alveolar-lingual nerve block. A flame-shaped loop electrode was bent to form a somewhat curved shape and the cutting current power output was set at 4.5 on the instrument panel dial. The bulging, somewhat bulbous tissue was resected with short brushing strokes, with a 10-second rest interval observed after 2 to 3 momentary brushing contacts of the activated electrode with the tissues. The surface tension of the tissues was restored during each rest interval and the excess saliva was removed immediately.

The electrode was replaced with a 45-degree-angle, medium-width loop electrode, and cutting current was increased to 5. The activated electrode was then used in a similar manner to perform the gingivoplasty on the lingual surface.

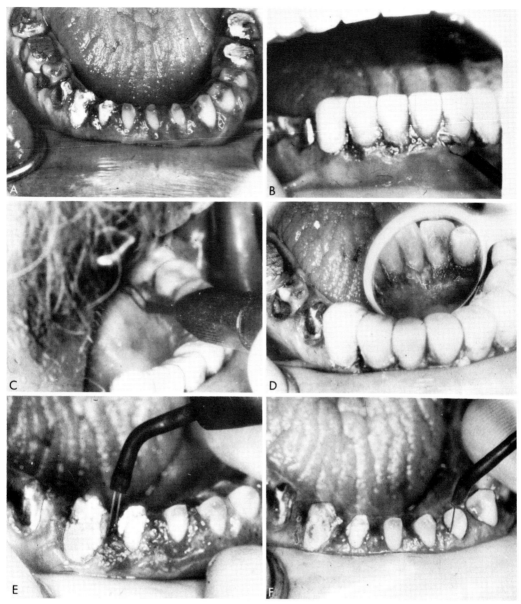

Case Figure 34–1. Iatrogenic periodontoclasia due to failure to provide subgingival accommodation. *A*, Appearance of the tissues with the "roundhouse" restoration of the mandibular dentition removed. From the right cuspid to left third molar the marginal gingivae are
severely engorged and so massively hypertrophied that the shoulders of the crown preparations
are completely covered with friable proliferative tissue. The tissues in the right quadrant from
first bicuspid to third molar offer a dramatic contrast. Surgical repreparation of these tissues,
similar to the procedure as seen in the remainder of the photographs in this series, had been
performed the previous week and provides visual evidence of the beneficial results that can
be achieved. The tissues in this quadrant are normal in tone and contour, and the shoulders of
the crown preparations are fully exposed and well defined. *B*, The restoration has been replaced, and the marginal gingivae are being recontoured externally with a flame-shaped loop
electrode to restore normal gingival contour and feather-edged gingival margins. *C*, The
gingivoplasty is being performed on the lingual aspect with a medium-width, 45-degree-angle
U-shaped loop electrode, which provides better tissue access and contact in that part of the
mouth. *D*, Mirror image of the lingual tissues after the loop planing. *E*, The redundant tissue
in the embrasures is reduced by resection with a narrow, 45-degree-angle U-shaped loop electrode. *F*, The subgingival troughs are being created around some of the teeth with a J-loop
electrode, especially where the shoulders of the crown preparations are very narrow.

487

The restoration was then removed, and the redundant tissue covering the shoulder preparations was resected with a 45-degree-angle, narrow U-shaped loop electrode. The instrumentation was continued in some areas to create subgingival troughs. In some other areas, the J-loop electrode was substituted and used to create the troughs, especially in the anterior embrasures.

Tincture of myrrh and benzoin was applied to the cut tissue surfaces, the restoration was reinserted, and a periodontal cement pack was applied to the area. The patient returned on the fifth postoperative day, the cement pack was removed, and the left quadrant was prepared for surgery. After regional block anesthesia was administered, the tissues were treated in the same manner as has been described. Cement packs were applied.

The cement packs were discarded on the tenth respective postoperative day, and the patient was advised to use a mouthwash of salt and alum to toughen and tan the tissues. This styptic mouthwash, consisting of one part powdered alum and three parts salt in powder form, of which 1 teaspoonful was dissolved in a glassful of water, was prescribed as a mouthwash to be used four times a day for one week. By the end of the third postoperative week the tissues were sufficiently healed to permit vigorous gingival massage with a toothbrush; at first, a very soft nylon bristle brush and, six weeks later, with an extra hard natural bristle brush.

As the tissue on the internal surface of the subgingival troughs healed, it adapted closely around the subgingival portion of the restoration, without any clinical evidence of irritation, inflammation, or proliferation. Ten weeks after the surgery, the restorations were cemented in permanently.

Iatrogenic periodontoclasia is not the only sequel to failure to create and preserve adequate subgingival space to assure irritation. Other sequelae are gingival recession, gingival proliferation, and tooth decay.

When gingival recession occurs it may expose the finish line where the artificial crown ends, and thus permit the cement to disintegrate. When that happens and food debris becomes entrapped in the space and disintegrates, decay is likely to set in. If the latter is asymptomatic, the decay may penetrate through the full thickness of the root and separate the crown from its roots. This occurred in the next case, which demonstrates the technique for removing the affected abutment tooth and converting the crown into a pontic without sacrificing or impairing the usefulness of the fixed prosthesis.

CASE 35

PATIENT. A 79-year-old white male.

HISTORY. The patient was the late William Coles, inventor of the fully rectified electrosurgical circuit. He had had a complete mouth reconstruction performed by one of the most eminent prosthodontists. All the necessary ingredients for success but one had been employed in the restoration. The mesiodistal and buccolingual contours were excellent. The preparations were thorough, and copper band impressions had assured an accurate reproduction of the subgingival areas for an accurate finish line. The occlusion was carefully determined, and the crowns were bullet-shaped to assure adequate space in the embrasures for the interdental papillae. But no subgingival troughs had been prepared, nor had subgingival space been preserved for introduction of the subgingival portions of the restoration. Despite excellent oral hygiene, the patient noticed a gradual recession of the gingivae and exposure of narrow gold bands at the necks of his teeth. About a year previously, he had noticed a dark line resembling a fine fissure or crack immediately beyond the gold band of his maxillary first bicuspids. A few months previously, he began to have a slight sensation in these teeth like a mild toothache, but it was so mild that he ignored it until it became severely painful for two days and then subsided again. Fearful of renewed increased pain, he came to the author for diagnosis and treatment.

CLINICAL EXAMINATION.   The tissues looked healthy and normal, despite recession of the marginal gingivae and exposure of the gold finish lines of the crown restorations. A periodontal probe was then inserted at the necks of the right and left first bicuspids, and the probes penetrated through from buccal to palatal without resistance (Case Fig. 35–1).

ROENTGENOGRAPHIC EXAMINATION.   X-rays confirmed the through and through decay of the roots of the bicuspids, which separated the coronal from the root portions of these teeth. The bone factor throughout was excellent.

TREATMENT.   The decay gap was slightly wider over the left bicuspid, so this tooth was treated first. Buccal and lingual subperiosteal infiltration anesthesia was administered, and a 45-degree-angle needle electrode was selected. Cutting current output was set at 3 on the instrument panel and the activated electrode was used with a wiping stroke to create a vertico-oblique incision from the junction of the areolar and alveolar mucosa to the mesiobuccal angle of the second bicuspid, then across the apex of the bicuspid interdental papilla to sever the apical attachment (Case Fig. 35–2). The flap was elevated and the retained roots were extracted. The entire coronal portion of the tooth had disintegrated, leaving a mushy residue in the crown. The debris in the crown was removed, and the crown was irrigated with a strong solution of Kasdenol. The internal area of the crown was carefully aspirated and then swabbed with a small pellet moistened with 70% alcohol, care being taken to avoid contact with the tissues in doing so. The internal area of the crown was then dried with air and filled with self-curing acrylic, which was polished as much as possible after it had set. This converted the crown into a pontic and preserved the restoration intact. The

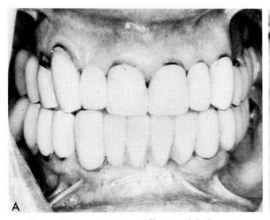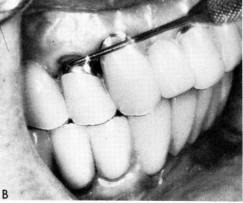

Case Figure 35–1.   Effects of failure to provide adequate subgingival accommodation. *A,* Preoperative: The entire dentition has been restored with full crown splints. The subgingival gold finish lines of the crowns and some of the root surfaces have been exposed, owing to gingival recession in both jaws, and the roots of the maxillary left second bicuspid and right first bicuspid have become separated from their crowns as a result of decay extending through from buccal to palatal aspects. *B,* A 10-mm. periodontal pocket probe has penetrated buccopalatally its full length in the right first bicuspid crown-root separation. Insertion into the left second bicuspid defect produced an identical result.

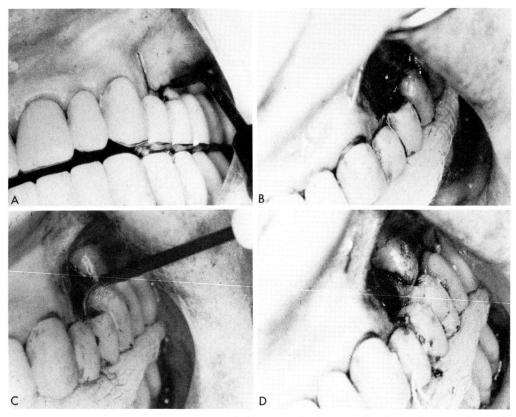

Case Figure 35-2.   A, Operative: A 45-degree-angle fine needle electrode is used to make an incision for a mucoperiosteal flap. A vertico-oblique incision on the buccal aspect of the left first bicuspid to within 3 mm. of the marginal gingiva over the pontic is being continued horizontally in a distal direction to the mesial aspect of the second bicuspid. Note the absence of free bleeding. *B,* The flap has been elevated and the retained root removed. The area has been thoroughly debrided, including the crown of the tooth which is now empty. The coronal portion of the tooth had decomposed and liquefied, and the crown had been cleansed by excavation and irrigation. *C,* The debrided crown is being sterilized by electrocoagulation with a cylindrical silver coagulating electrode. *D,* The crown has been filled with acrylic to convert it into a pontic.

flap was restored to position and sutured, and tincture of myrrh and benzoin was applied in air-dried layers.

The patient returned on the fifth postoperative day for removal of the sutures. The tissues appeared normal in tone and gave evidence of early primary repair (Case Fig. 35-3). Repair continued without incidence, the tissues having adapted themselves nicely to the acrylic in the crown. Several months later, the surgery was repeated on the right (Case Fig. 35-4). Here, however, the coronal portion, although separated from its roots by decay, was intact in the crown. It proved impossible to remove the coronal portion completely, so after having removed as much as could be removed, the remainder was sterilized in part by application of the 70% alcohol and also by fulguration. The self-curing acrylic flowed into the vacant part of the crown and was polished after it had set. The tissues were restored and sutured and healed without incidence. The last surgery was done approximately one and one half years before the patient's demise, and during that period he had no trouble from the pontic converted crowns.

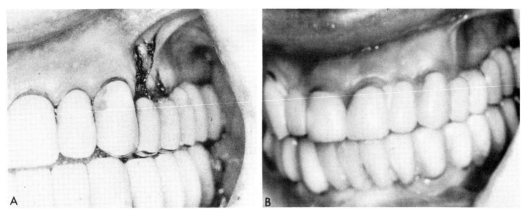

Case Figure 35–3. A, Fifth day postoperatively, the tissues that have been coapted and sutured with silk show evidence of initial primary repair. B, Postoperative: The line of incision is fully healed. The alveolar bone has filled the defect without much loss of convex contour and has adapted itself around the acrylic-filled crown, maintaining good aesthetics and function.

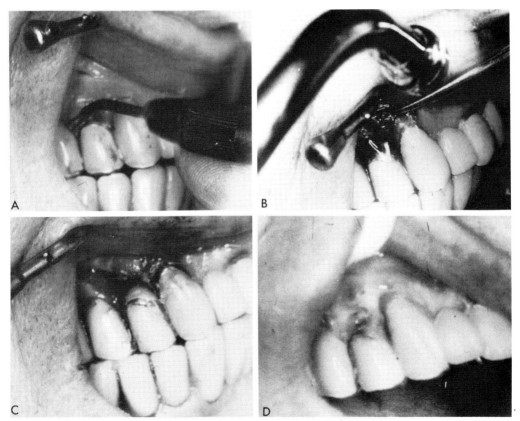

Case Figure 35–4. A, Treatment, right side: Proliferative tissue is being excised from the embrasures on either side of the maxillary right first bicuspid with a narrow U-shaped loop electrode. B, A vertico-oblique mucoperiosteal flap incision has been made with the needle electrode, the flap elevated, and retained roots removed. The natural tooth crown, intact, remained in the veneer and had to be cut out with burs and diamond stones. The hollow veneer and root sockets are being inspected with a transilluminating light to verify total debridement. C, The veneer crown, sterilized by electrocoagulation, has been filled with acrylic to convert it into a pontic. Absence of free bleeding made immediate conversion possible. D, Appearance of the wound one week later, immediately after suture removal. Healing progressed rapidly thereafter and the crown pontics successfully preserved the usefulness of the restoration.

Failure Due to Systemic Influence

CASE 36

This case demonstrates the influence of uncontrolled diabetes on rate and quality of tissue repair.

Faulty crown form, with inadequate embrasure space for the interdental papillae or improper buccolingual dimension; occlusal disharmony with traumatizing prematurities; and failure to create and preserve a subgingival trough around a full crown preparation are the major *mechanical factors* that are responsible for iatrogenic periodontoclasia and other restorative failures.

Systemic factors that impair the ability of the patient's tissues to repair properly can also result in untoward effects and failure. One of the most important of these is uncontrolled diabetes mellitus.

This case offers an excellent example of the cause and effect of the failure to have the tissues treated electrosurgically for favorable repair. It also serves to emphasize the importance of establishing conclusively whether a known diabetic is in a controlled or uncontrolled stage, and to avoid treatment in the latter event.

PATIENT. A middle-aged female.

HISTORY. She was a patient of the hospital's diabetic outpatient clinic. She convinced her physician that she was having difficulty eating and following her prescribed diet regimen because her old fixed bridge was causing her pain and difficulty. He referred her to the dental department for fabrication of a new restoration. The abutment teeth had short clinical crowns, and she was referred to the surgery department for the author to elongate them by electrosurgery.

CLINICAL EXAMINATION. The maxillary right central and lateral incisors were missing and had been restored by a fixed bridge with Steele's facing pontics. The bridge was anchored by a porcelain veneer crown on the right cuspid and a three-quarter crown on the left central incisor. The right first bicuspid had a large mesio-occlusal gold inlay, and the tissue had proliferated downward incisally so that almost half of the inlay was covered with tissue. The mesio-incisal angle of the left central had fractured, exposing the gold casting. Several patches of white materia alba plaque adhering to the gingival tissues gave evidence that her oral hygiene left much to be desired (Case Fig. 36–1A).

TREATMENT. Normally, blood sugar and glucose tolerance tests would have been ordered to determine whether the diabetes was under control, but in this case, since the patient had been referred for treatment by the diabetic clinic, the author assumed that she was under control and proceeded with the surgery without the preliminary tests.

The tissues were prepared and bilateral infraorbital block anesthesia was administered. A flame-shaped loop electrode was selected, and the activated loop was used to resect the marginal gingivae by electrosection to elongate the clinical crowns to the desired height (Case Fig. 36–1B). The right first bicuspid, which would also be utilized as an abutment in the new restoration, was then elongated with the same electrode, fully exposing the mesial surface of the inlay. The electrode was then used with a downward pulling motion to create a concave-contoured papilla between the two bicuspids (Case Fig. 36–1C). Tincture of myrrh and benzoin was applied to the tissues in air-dried layers, and the patient was reappointed for the following week.

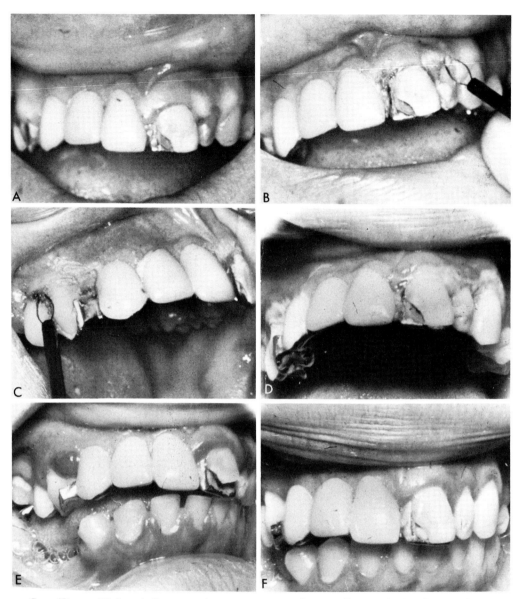

Case Figure 36–1.   A, Preoperative appearance. The maxillary right first bicuspid and left central, lateral, and cuspid are to be restored and require elongation of the clinical crowns. *B,* Elongation being performed by gingivectoplasty with a flame-shaped loop electrode. *C,* Right bicuspid crown is being elongated and redundant tissue in the cuspid-bicuspid embrasure that had grown down coronally and partially covered the proximal gold inlay has been resected. *D,* Appearance of the tissues one week postoperatively. Healing appears to be progressing favorably. *E,* Appearance of the tissues six weeks postoperatively. Instead of progressive healing there has been progressive deterioration. Patient is found to be an uncontrolled diabetic. *F,* Appearance of the tissues one month later, after institution of a rigid regimen of diabetic control. Without any assistance, the tissues have proceeded to heal by virtue of the patient's regained health.

When she returned, the tissue surfaces that had been treated were covered with a light layer of coagulum and appeared to be healing satisfactorily (Case Fig. 36–1D). She was instructed to continue the regimen of home care that had been prescribed and to return in two weeks. When she was seen again, the healing did not appear to be progressing normally, and she was asked to follow her diet and medication and perform her oral hygiene faithfully. However, instead of improving, the tissues continued to deteriorate, so that by the end of the sixth postoperative week the unmistakable conclusion was that the tissues lacked the ability to repair (Case Fig. 36–1E), because her diabetic condition was uncontrolled. On questioning, she denied this at first but eventually admitted that she had not been observing her diet or taking her insulin for almost a year. She was referred back to the diabetic clinic with instructions not to return until blood sugar and glucose tolerance were normal.

One month later she returned to the dental clinic. On examination, the tissues were found to be almost fully healed and appeared to have good tone (Case Fig. 36–1F). Her record of laxity in oral hygiene suggests that the improvement was not due to her efforts in that respect but solely due to the fact that the systemic condition had improved to the degree that her tissues now were capable of normal repair.

This case impressed upon the author the fact that at no time, and for no reason whatsoever, is it safe or justifiable to jump to conclusions. When a patient presents a history of systemic disease that is able to disrupt tissue healing, a medical evaluation and laboratory tests should always be performed prior to institution of electrosurgical therapy or, for that matter, any other surgical procedures, rather than to trust to chance that all is well.

Failure Due to Improper Treatment Plan

CASE 37

This case is being retained from the old edition to demonstrate how *not* to treat. Hopefully, much can be learned from examining failures as well as successes, and this case will stress the importance of a proper treatment plan based on sound clinical judgment and the undesirable aftermath of unsound planning. It involves the combined use of coronal elongation and subgingival troughs to achieve good aesthetic and functional results in difficult restorations. It also demonstrates the importance of local factors of health and tissue tone of the investing gingivae around the treated teeth and their relation to the quality and rate of tissue repair achieved.

PATIENT. A 28-year-old white female.

HISTORY. The patient was referred for elongation of the clinical crowns of six maxillary anterior teeth and creation of subgingival troughs around the centrals and laterals as a preliminary to their restoration with a unit-built porcelain bridge.

CLINICAL EXAMINATION. The following salient features were revealed: The crowns of the six anterior teeth appeared to be too short when compared with the coronal height of the rest of the teeth, all of which appeared to be normal in size. The left central and lateral incisors were restored with badly off-color porcelain jacket crowns. The mesio-incisal angle of the right central incisor was missing. The gingival mucosa dipped down slightly over the porcelain crowns. This plus the fact that both crowns were substantially shorter than their normal counterparts further exaggerated the lack of coronal height.

The tissue tone of the gingivae around these teeth was good except in the left

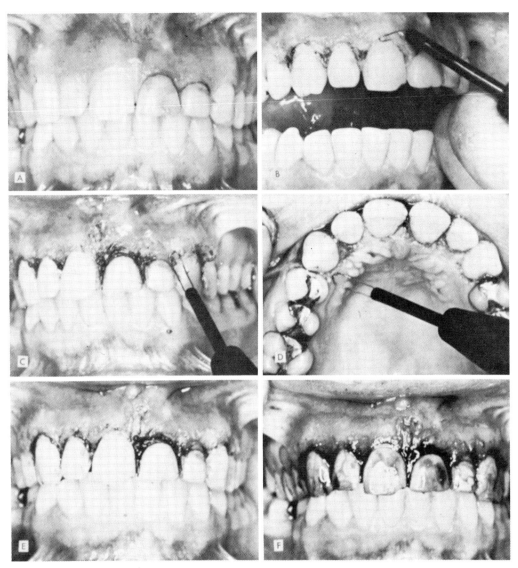

Case Figure 37–1.   Elongation of clinical crowns and preparation of subgingival troughs created for this patient in two separate stages. *A*, Clinical appearance of mouth. Left central and lateral incisors badly discolored. Mesio-incisal angle of right central missing. Crowns of the six anterior teeth short. A fistulous orifice present over left central incisor. *B*, Clinical crowns elongated. Elongation started with 50-degree-angle narrow U-shaped loop electrode. *C*, Convex interproximal papillae reduced to concave sluiceways with curved, straight U-shaped loop electrode. *D*, Palatal marginal mucosa reduced with same electrode. *E*, Elongation completed. Procedure virtually bloodless. *F*, Topical application of tincture of myrrh and benzoin, only obtundent dressing required.

central-lateral area. Here the mucosa was hyperemic, and a small, round protruding mass was present on the labial surface over the root of the central incisor. The mass, which had a fistulous orifice, was located about 1 cm. above the gingival margin over the distal part of the root of the central (Case Fig. 37–1). Roentgenographic examination confirmed the abnormal crown-root ratio of the six anteriors, and their roots substantially exceeded the normal 2 : 1 root-length ratio.

TREATMENT. The choice of treatment plan for this case had to be patterned to conform with the plans of the referring dentist, which left much to be desired. In order to do so, the procedure had to be divided into two separate treatment stages. The first stage was planned to consist of only the elongation of the clinical crowns of the six anteriors. After these tissues were fully healed, the dentist planned to prepare the right central and lateral for full-shoulder crown preparations, reprepare the left lateral, extract the left central, and then construct a temporary splint restoration to serve until the final restoration was completed. Subgingival troughs would not be constructed until the preparations were completed and ready for insertion of the permanent restoration.

The tissues were prepared for surgery and infiltration anesthesia was administered. A 50-degree-angle U-shaped narrow loop electrode was selected and current output was set at 4.5 for electrosection. The electrode was held at an acute angle to the mucosa with the loop directed downward and was used with short brushing strokes to reduce the marginal gingivae 2 to 3 mm., starting from the distoproximal papilla of the right cuspid.

The electrode was then replaced with a slightly wider straight U-shaped loop electrode which had been bent into a convexoconcave curve. Intensity of current output was increased to 5 because of the use of a larger electrode, and the latter was applied to the interproximal papillae with a downward motion to create slightly concave sluiceways. The palatal marginal gingivae were also reduced approximately 3 mm. with this electrode, and the interproximal papillae on the palatal aspect were reduced and recontoured with both types of electrode. Feather-edged margins were then created by beveling the new margins with the narrow 45-degree-angle loop electrode.

The entire procedure was relatively bloodless; even the hyperemic mucosa around the abscessed left central produced only slight surface oozing. Topical application of tincture of myrrh and benzoin appeared adequate to provide obtundent and hemostatic protection. A temporary dressing of adhesive ointment was applied to the operative field. The patient was instructed in postoperative care and reappointed.

She returned on the fifth postoperative day. The sequence of postoperative healing she presented was interesting and significant. The mucosa around the right central, lateral, and cuspid showed unmistakable evidence of early normal repair, but the mucosa around the two porcelain jacket crowns appeared hyperemic and hypertrophic. Persistent slight hypertrophy of the interproximal papilla was easily reduced by electrocoagulation with a small ball electrode and a narrow loop electrode (Case Fig. 37–2). Then a one tenth of one per cent dilution of chromic acid was applied to the tissues for 30 seconds and washed off. This was followed by application of tincture of myrrh and benzoin. The patient was instructed to continue the postoperative routine and home care and was reappointed.

At her next two visits, one week apart, this regimen of treatment was repeated. By the end of the third postoperative week the gingival mucosa was healed, but some hyperemia and hypertrophy was still in evidence around the two crowned teeth. At this point the patient was dismissed with instructions to return for further treatment after the preparations for the crown restorations were completed.

The patient returned one month later for creation of the subgingival troughs. The left central incisor had been extracted more than two weeks previously, but the socket and gingival mucosa was still incompletely healed. The right central and lateral incisors had been prepared for full crown coverage, and the left lateral incisor had been built up with a gold core.

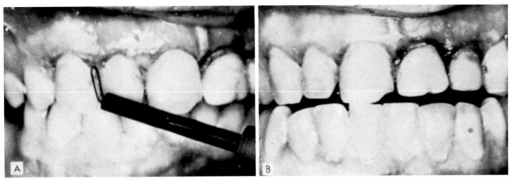

Case Figure 37–2.   Postoperative healing. *A,* Healing progress good except in left central-lateral area. Persistent slight hypertrophy of their interproximal papilla was easily reduced with a 45-degree-angle U-shaped loop electrode. *B,* Appearance at the end of third postoperative week. Hyperemia and some hypertrophy still persist around the left central and lateral.

The tissues were prepared for surgery and infiltration anesthesia was administered. Local factors created need for use of the three different types of electrode to prepare them. The shoulder for the lateral was narrow and the marginal-cemental gingival mucosa was thin around this tooth; the solid conical electrode would be best suited for use on this tooth. The central had a normal-sized shoulder and normal marginal gingiva; the cylindrical electrode would be well suited for that tooth. The nonvital left lateral was a poor risk. The mucosa in the lateral–extracted-central area was severely engorged and atonal. It appeared, therefore, that a loop electrode operated by electrosection, making momentary contact with these tissues to resect the trough, would be preferable and probably safer to use than the coagulating electrodes, which must be kept in contact with the tissues for several seconds. This treatment plan was followed.

A solid, conical or flame-shaped coagulating electrode was selected, and coagulating current was set at 2. This electrode was used to prepare the subgingival trough around the right lateral by rotating the electrode several times in the gingival crevice space (Case Fig. 37–3). A solid cylindrical coagulating electrode was substituted, inserted into the gingival crevice space of the right central, and employed in the same manner to prepare the subgingival trough around that tooth. A narrow loop electrode was then selected, substituted for the solid electrode, and used with coagulating current set at 4 to prepare the subgingival trough around the right lateral incisor. The electrode was inserted into the gingival crevice and rotated around the stump of the right lateral to deepen and widen the subgingival trough.

When all the subgingival troughs were completed they fully circumscribed the three teeth, exposing the shoulders to full view (looking rootward from below). Tincture of myrrh and benzoin was applied, and the temporary splint was inserted with a mixture of zinc oxide and petrolatum as the cementing medium. Normal healing ensued without further incident. Three weeks later she was dismissed from further treatments.

The patient was seen again almost five months later. The permanent restoration had not yet been completed, and the temporary splint was several millimeters short of the shoulders and gingival margins of the abutment teeth. Some of the mucosa had overgrown the unprotected shoulders with friable hypertrophic tissue. The mucosa was anesthetized by infiltration of several minims of solution, and the hypertrophic tissue was removed by electrocoagulation with the solid and narrow loop electrodes.

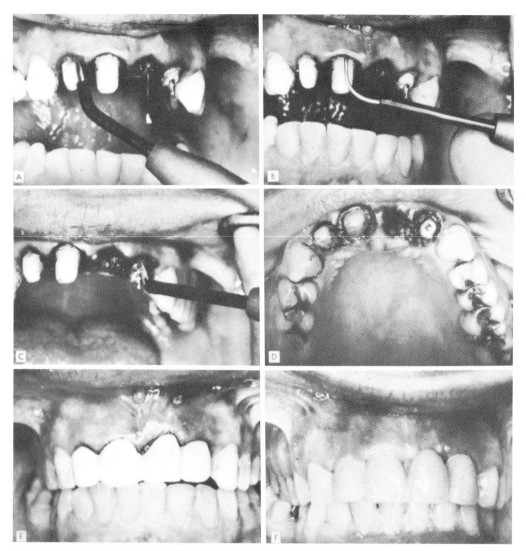

Case Figure 37–3. Second stage of treatment: creating subgingival troughs. *A,* Conical coagulating electrode used to create trough around right lateral incisor because tooth had narrow shoulder. *B,* Cylindrical electrode used to create subgingival trough around right central. This tooth had wider shoulder and thicker marginal gingiva. *C,* Because of engorged, inflamed looking tissue around the gold post in the left lateral, a narrow loop electrode was used to create the subgingival trough for this tooth by electrosection. *D,* Appearance of the gingivae around the prepared teeth looking upward. The gingival troughs are well defined. *E,* Temporary splint inserted with a cementing mixture of zinc oxide and eugenol mixed with petrolatum. *F,* Permanent restoration inserted. The crowns are all normal in size and present good gingival harmony. The inflammatory hyperemia in the left central-lateral incisor area still persists but is less severe.

The space between the gingival margins and the splint was filled in with surgical cement, and the splint was temporarily recemented. The permanent restoration was completed shortly thereafter. The temporary splint was discarded and the permanent restoration was inserted. The gingivae and subgingival tissues on the right side now appeared normal, but some inflammatory hyperemia still persisted in the left central-lateral incisor area.

A few months after the permanent restoration was permanently cemented the gingival mucosa over the labial aspect of the right lateral incisor suddenly became engorged and atonal. The patient was referred back for examination and treatment. The tissues were found smooth and shiny, and dark red in color. No pathologic condition was revealed in a roentgenogram of the area. Transillumination suggested deep-seated irritation and inflammation. The use of steroid ointment applied locally to inflammatory areas having proved successful in other cases, after application of direct-contact ultraviolet irradiation with a quartz applicator in order to stir up the blood circulation in the deep vascular bed of the area, Neomagnacort ointment (Pfizer) was rubbed gently into the affected tissue. The patient returned twice a week for two weeks, then once a week for three more weeks, for continuation of this therapy. At the end of that time the condition had subsided and the tissues again looked normal. They have remained normal since that time.

GROUP 2: VISUAL EXAMPLES OF TYPICAL AND ATYPICAL REASONS FOR CROWN AND BRIDGE FAILURES

CASE 38

This case demonstrates that despite excellent mechanical design with good mesiodistal and buccolingual contours and a balanced occlusion, the gingival tissues and supportive structures can undergo iatrogenic deterioration because no provision was made for subgingival accommodation with suitable subgingival troughs. It is being presented not to demonstrate electrosurgical therapy, but as an excellent visual example of iatrogenic periodontoclasia due to failure to provide subgingival accommodation.

PATIENT.   A 34-year-old white female in normal health.

HISTORY.   She had had maxillary full arch reconstruction to restore lost tooth structures and missing teeth and to provide a balanced occlusion. All the maxillary teeth were restored with unit-built porcelain crowns. The aesthetics was excellent. Each crown was properly contoured in all dimensions. The embrasure spaces were adequate to accommodate the interdental papillae without crowding. The occlusion was well balanced. Despite all this, the patient had developed an advanced case of periodontal disease, with deep infrabony pockets. She was referred for definitive periodontal therapy.

CLINICAL EXAMINATION.   The mouth looked quite healthy at a casual glance. Closer inspection revealed slightly hyperplastic interdental papillae and a slight thickening of the labial marginal gingiva around the maxillary right central incisor (Case Fig. 38–1).

Examination with a periodontal pocket probe revealed that almost every tooth in

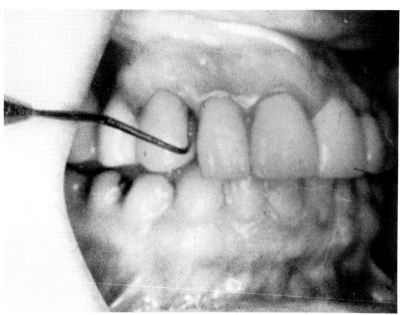

Case Figure 38-1.   A heavy periodontal pocket probe penetrating more than 6 mm. into an infrabony pocket. This case is an excellent example of iatrogenic periodontoclasia despite the supragingival excellence of the restoration. The mesiodistal and buccolingual diameters and bullet shapes of the crowns are excellent and help to assure against impingement against the interdental papillae in their embrasures. The unmistakable clinical evidence of advanced periodontal disease is directly attributable to failure to provide for adequate *subgingival* accommodation for the restoration by preparation of subgingival troughs around the crown preparations.

the maxillary arch had deep infrabony pockets along the mesial and/or distal aspects of the roots of the teeth. The pockets measured 5 to 11 mm. in depth. A full mouth x-ray series confirmed the extensiveness of the periodontal deterioration. There had been no history or clinical evidence of pre-existing periodontal disease prior to the full crown reconstruction. Gingival retraction had been performed prior to impression-taking of the crown preparations by packing chemically impregnated cord subgingivally around each preparation. The space created by the chemical retraction was transitory, and no comparable space was available to accommodate the subgingival portion of the restoration when it was inserted into the mouth. The subsequent physical displacement of the subgingival tissues violated a basic law of physics—two things cannot occupy the same space at the same time. Something had to give, and under such circumstances in all instances it is the gingival tissues that "give" or break down.

CASE 39

This case also is being reported not to demonstrate the electrosurgical procedure, but rather to demonstrate another typical cause for iatrogenic periodontoclasia.

In this case the irritation was triggered by improper buccolingual crown contours. The subgingival and gingival portions of the crowns were too thick so that even though the restorations were porcelain jacket crowns they created enough subgingival bulk to displace the marginal gingivae and trigger an inflammatory response.

PATIENT.   A 39-year-old white female.

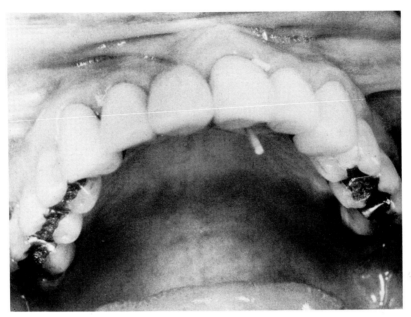

Case Figure 39–1.   Another case of iatrogenic periodontoclasia due to lack of subgingival accommodation. Large gutta percha points have been inserted at the distobuccal and disto-palatal of the left central and have penetrated almost to the apex of the tooth.

HISTORY.   She had had her maxillary six anterior teeth restored with porcelain jacket crowns. Subsequently the marginal gingivae began to become thickened and the interproximal papillae became enlarged, engorged, and, especially in one area, became detached from the teeth and bone. She was referred for restoration of a normal gingival architecture.

CLINICAL EXAMINATION.   The six porcelain crowns looked more like biscuit bakes than finished fully fire-glazed porcelain jackets. The crowns were thick at the gingival ends and physically displaced the marginal gingivae, especially on the labial aspect. The tissue in the right lateral area appeared dark red, and the papillae on either side of the tooth were detached. The centrals appeared to be impinging against the fibers of the labial frenum. The tissues on the palatal aspect also were partially detached and the papillae hypertrophied. There were numerous infrabony pockets. One at the distopalatal aspect of the left central was so deep a molar gutta percha point was inserted and penetrated almost to the apex of the tooth (Case Fig. 39–1).

This case is an example of deterioration that can result from inferior quality workmanship in fabricating the restoration and poor clinical judgment in attempting to use the fabrication as a restoration.

CASE 40

This is another of the group of cases being presented not for the purpose of reviewing electrosurgical procedure, but to demonstrate the reasons for failures and iatrogenic periodontoclasia.

PATIENT.   A 61-year-old white male.

HISTORY.   He had had his mouth restored by "full mouth rehabilitation" by

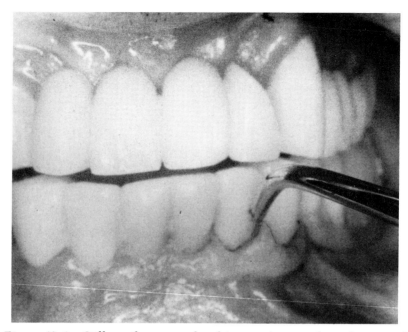

Case Figure 40–1. Still another example of iatrogenic periodontoclasia resulting from failure to provide subgingival accommodation without impingement. The marginal gingivae are hyperplastic, hyperemic, and detached from the teeth. A blast of air from an air syringe is seen to have detached the tissue from the embrasure.

three eminent prosthodontists, each of whom had found his predecessor's restoration unsuited, and remade the case. The patient, of very modest means, had spent practically his entire life savings on his dentistry and the repeated failures were having a psychological effect on him. He finally went to a neighborhood dentist, who found that he had an advanced case of periodontoclasia and referred him to the author for periodontal therapy.

CLINICAL EXAMINATION. The entire dentition had been restored with full crown roundhouse restorations. The occlusion was excellent, and the mesiodistal and buccolingual contours were as good as could be done. But the gingival tissues were grossly hyperplastic and totally detached from the teeth and bone, so much so that they could be flapped away from the underlying structures by simply blowing air into the sulcus spaces with an air syringe (Case Fig. 40–1).

It was obvious that despite all the skills involved in sophisticated occlusal registrations, transfer copings, incisal guidance and similar methods for achieving a balanced occlusion the case had failed because the need to provide and maintain the subgingival space to assure against subgingival impingement had been overlooked.

CASE 41

This is the final case that is being presented to demonstrate the ill effects due not to failure to provide subgingival accommodation but to faulty treatment and poor clinical judgment.

PATIENT. A 56-year-old Puerto Rican female.

HISTORY. She had had several missing teeth restored with a fixed bridge that extended from the right second bicuspid to the left first bicuspid. Approximately 6

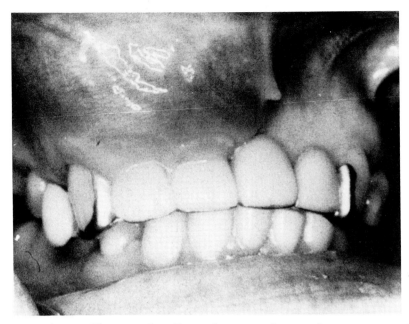

Case Figure 41–1. Illustrates the effects of severe subgingival impingement. The irritation has resulted in development of a huge cyst that involves the entire right half of the maxilla and caused a severe bulging of the labial alveolar plate; it has also caused some pressure against the ala of the nose; both combine to create considerable facial disfigurement.

months later she suddenly noticed a very large swelling in the anterior part of the mouth and consulted her dentist. He found the mass to be fluctuant and referred her to the author for the necessary surgery.

CLINICAL EXAMINATION. The bridge extended from the maxillary left cuspid to the right second bicuspid. The two cuspids and right second bicuspid were the abutments restoring the two centrals, the right lateral, and the right first bicuspid. The three anterior teeth were restored with Steele's facing pontics.

Apparently the latter had been butted to the gums and were receiving premature occlusal contact from the mandibular natural teeth, which were in almost tip-to-tip contact. There was a huge swelling involving the entire right side of the maxilla (Case Fig. 41–1). The mass was fluctuant, and the roentgenographic examination confirmed almost the entire right half of the maxilla was radiolucent; either an acute abscess or a huge cyst, and the only treatment possible was removal of the restoration and oral surgery to eliminate the pathologic condition.

In this case there were two major causes of failure; traumatic occlusion, and improper placement of the pontics so that they impinged severely against the mucous membranes and the alveolar bone. The tissue insult produced by the two triggered the acute reaction that had destroyed almost one half of the maxilla.

FOOTNOTE REFERENCES

1. A collection of Lederle newsletters for the dental profession. Lederle Laboratories Division, American Cyanamid Co. Pearl River, N.Y., 1956, pp. 1–8.
2. Tinker, H. A.: Some essentials of crown and bridge work. North-West Den., 28:29, Jan., 1949.
3. Bartlett, A. A.: Some principles of modern fixed bridge construction. J.A.D.A., 29:2166, Dec., 1942.

4. Dolan, W. W.: Verbal communications, scientific programs of the American Academy of Dental Electrosurgery and other programs.
5. Flocken, J. E.: Verbal communications to the author.
6. Harrison, J. D.: Verbal communications, scientific programs of the A.D.A. and the American Academy of Dental Electrosurgery.
7. Kelly, W. J., Jr., and Harrison, J. D.: Heat generation and penetration in gingival tissues using electrosurgery. (Kelly's M.Sc.D. degree thesis.) Verbal communications, scientific programs of A.D.A. and American Academy of Dental Electrosurgery.
8. Malone, W. F., Eisemann, D., and Kusek, J.: Electron microscope histologic evaluation of cold steel and fully rectified electrosurgical cutting. J. Prosth. Dent., 22:555, 1969.
9. Malone, W. F.: Verbal communications, scientific programs of A.D.A. and American Academy of Dental Electrosurgery.
10. Miller, C. J.: Verbal communications, American Academy of Dental Electrosurgery and other scientific meetings.
11. Miller, I. F.: Preparation of teeth for jackets for abutment purposes. First District (N.Y.) Dental Society (postgraduate course).
12. Pankey, L. D.: Verbal communications.
13. Stein, R. S.: Verbal communications, A.D.A. – American Academy of Dental Electrosurgery scientific program.
14. Thomas, P. K.: Verbal communications to the author.
15. Brecker, S. C.: Clinical Procedures in Occlusal Rehabilitation. Philadelphia, W. B. Saunders Co., 1958, 157–163.
16. Brecker, S. C.: Electronic surgery in restorative dentistry. New York J. Den., 25:10, 295–299, Oct., 1955.
17. Fox, L.: Verbal communications.
18. Glickman, I.: Verbal communication, at a scientific program of the First District Dental Society, New York.

ORTHODONTICS

As the electrosurgical aids to the various dental disciplines are reviewed, it will become apparent that a degree of overlapping of surgical procedures is inevitable. When judged solely as a surgical exercise, there can be but little difference between surgery instituted to expose or elongate a clinical crown for restorative purposes or in orthodontic therapy and the same surgery instituted in periodontal therapy. The real differences are created by the anatomic and pathologic handicaps encountered in the various branches of dentistry, which create unusual surgical problems requiring specific and special adaptations of the techniques.

In orthodontia, surgical problems result mostly from the handicaps imposed by anatomic abnormalities. The more complex the abnormality, the more marked the resultant surgical handicap. The simplest surgical assistance required in orthodontia deals with cases of tardy eruption in an otherwise normal permanent dentition. The most complex surgical aid usually must be rendered for complicated orthodontic problems that are created by severe abnormalities such as micrognathia and cleft palate.

Orthodontics consists primarily of arch expansion and tooth movement and realignment. Therefore, electrosurgery's contributions to this discipline are, of necessity, adjunctive rather than definitive. However, some orthodontic cases present anatomic obstacles that make treatment impossible unless preliminary surgical intervention is instituted prior to the orthodontic treatment. In some of these cases the complications are such that only electrosurgery, with its unique inherent characteristics, can make the necessary surgery feasible.

The value of the contributions electrosurgery offers orthodontia increases in proportion to the complexity of the case, especially when electrosurgery makes otherwise untreatable cases amenable to successful orthodontic treatment. Cases of marked anatomic abnormalities such as cleft palates, micrognathias, and comparable developmental defects are most likely to require preliminary electrosurgical intervention.

Orthodontists have as a rule been reluctant to have frenectomies performed prior to orthodontic treatment, even in cases of very broad frena creating wide diastemas between the maxillary central incisors. Their reluctance is not motivated by a wish to contend with frenal interference, but such interference is preferable to that created by the mass of avascular fibrous scar tissue that invariably replaces the frenum after a traditional cold-steel frenectomy has been performed.

The electrosurgical technique developed by the author that combines frenectomy of the attached alveolar frenal fibers and frenotomy of the areolar fibers that control lip movement eliminates the basis for the orthodontists' objections to frenectomy. The end result of the electrosurgical frenectomy-frenotomy procedure is the elimination of frenal interference with tooth movement, without the customary postoperative complication of more handicapping interference from the scar tissue adhesions and reduction in lip control, as will be seen in Chapter 16.

A question frequently asked about electrosurgery in relation to orthodontics is "What will happen if the activated electrode should make contact with a steel orthodontic band?" As is the case with electrode contact with bone, it is not the contact per se but the duration of contact that is the determining factor. If the electrode contact is just momentary and an adequate time interval is permitted to elapse before repeating the momentary contact, nothing untoward will result, no matter how many times the contact must be repeated to complete the surgical intervention. One of the clinical cases that will be reviewed in Chapter 17 was included because it admirably demonstrates the total absence of danger to tooth, bone, or tissue when contact of an activated electrode with metal orthodontic bands is properly made.

Chapter Sixteen

PREORTHODONTIC PROCEDURES

Orthodontic correction is usually a complex and difficult process even under optimal conditions. When orthodontic treatment is contemplated, all anatomic structures that will interfere with the movement of the teeth—nonpathologic, such as malposed or impacted teeth, or pathologic, such as cysts or supernumerary teeth—should be removed before the orthodontic treatment is begun.

Ideally the preliminary surgery should be concluded before the bands have been applied to the teeth, since bands often extend subgingivally and may interfere with repair and reattachment of the epithelial attachment.

The following cases demonstrate typical nonpathologic and pathologic impediments to orthodontic treatment and how electrosurgery simplifies and accelerates the surgical procedures involved.

Electrosurgical Exposure of Unerupted, Partially Erupted, Malposed, or Impacted Teeth

The surgical procedure for artificial exposure of unerupted malposed teeth consists of resection of overlying bone and/or mucosa, and destruction or resection of the coronal embryonal membrane. This procedure has been well documented by Thoma and many others.[1-5] Salzmann, in his "Principles of Orthodontics,"[6] ably describes Strock's electrosurgical technique for such exposures.[7] Local anatomic or pathologic factors, however, occasionally necessitate deviations from this routine treatment.

Coronal Exposure in Delayed Eruptions

BY ELECTROSECTION

In orthodontics as in all the other disciplines it is axiomatic that the value of electrosurgery's contribution to the efficacy of treatment and the significance of the advantages it offers in the treatment modus operandi become magnified with the magnitude of the degree of complexity and challenge the case presents.

In cases such as Case 1 that we are about to review, the simple matter of excising tissue to expose the incisal third of the tooth to permit its easy and rapid egress, it really matters little whether the tissue excision will be done manually with a steel scalpel or electrosurgically, as far as the end result is concerned. Yet even in such a simple procedure electrosurgery offers distinct advantages, not the least being the absence of free bleeding, since hemorrhage usually frightens the child, and the absence of scar tissue repair that can retard the speed of tooth eruption.

CASE 1

This case typifies the simplest surgical aid to orthodontics: exposing the crowns of teeth in cases of delayed eruption of the normal permanent dentition by electrosection.

PATIENT.   A 9-year-old white male.

HISTORY.   The patient was referred for exposure of the crown of the permanent right central incisor which had failed to erupt.

CLINICAL EXAMINATION. *Extraoral.* Negative.

Intraoral.   The right central and the two lateral incisors were fully erupted and in normal alignment in the dental arch. The crown of the left central incisor was not clinically visible. An expanse of gingival mucosa covered the crown of the tooth which bulged outward further labially than the contralateral teeth. The bulge stretched the tissue tightly, outlining the unerupted crown which appeared to be tilted labially and slightly distally (Case Fig. 1–1A).

Roentgenographic examination revealed that the unerupted tooth was in relatively normal alignment, tilted approximately 15 degrees from the vertical.

TREATMENT.   The mouth was prepared for surgery and infiltration anesthesia was administered. A flame-shaped loop electrode was selected and current intensity was set at 6 for electrosection. The electrode was applied to the overlying gingival mucosa at a 45 degree angle starting at the mesio-incisal angle of the unerupted crown. The overlying mucosa was resected to the level of the gingival margin of the fully erupted left central incisor, thereby exposing the incisal third of the unerupted tooth (Case Figs. 1–1B and C).

The entire procedure was bloodless. Postoperative dressing, therefore, was limited to topical application of air-dried layers of tincture of myrrh and benzoin. Postoperative instructions for home care were given and the patient was reappointed.

He returned two weeks later. The gingival mucosa appeared fully healed and the tooth had erupted about halfway down to the incisal level of the adjacent central incisor. The vertical alignment of the tooth was fairly good but it was rotated mesially. The patient was advised to press his tongue against his "new" tooth to help straighten it, and was told to return in three months for further postoperative observation.

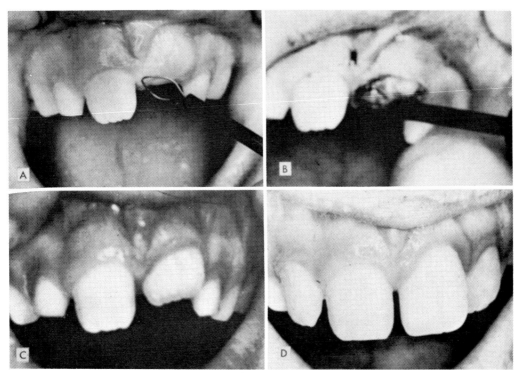

Case Figure 1–1. Exposing unerupted permanent central incisor. *A,* Loop in position at 45-degree angle to the tissues. *B,* Incisal third of the unerupted tooth crown exposed with loop. *C,* Postoperative appearance in two weeks. Tooth half erupted. *D,* Postoperative appearance three months later. Tooth fully erupted and in good alignment.

He returned as requested. The tooth was now in normal alignment and fully erupted. The gingival margin around the crown of the tooth was completely normal in all respects and gave no indication that it had recently undergone surgery (Case (Fig. 1–1*D*).

BY ELECTROCOAGULATION

In the overwhelming majority of instances the most effective way to elongate the clinical crowns of teeth is by simultaneous resection of the tissue and recontouring to restore a normal feather-edge, performed by loop electrosection.

Cases present themselves infrequently in which for some special reason it is imperative to avoid regeneration of the resected tissue and in which inadvertent exposure of an appreciably greater amount of the coronal portion of the tooth than planned will not be detrimental to the end result, as when the clinical crown is elongated to facilitate insertion of orthodontic bands that will not impinge on the gingival tissues.

For such cases, elongation of the clinical crown by means of electrocoagulation can be effective. The following case demonstrates this well.

CASE 2

PATIENT.   A 13-year-old white male.

HISTORY.   He was born with a developmental cleft in the left side of his maxilla, and the corresponding portion of his upper lip. The lateral incisor was congenitally missing in the line of cleft, and the cuspid was partially unerupted and slightly malposed. He was undergoing orthodontic treatment to bring the cuspid into normal alignment so that a fixed prosthesis could be made to span the gap and thereby provide aesthetic and functional improvement. Unless the cuspid were more fully exposed it would be impossible to use an orthodontic band on this tooth without causing substantial subgingival trauma. He was therefore referred for elongation of the clinical crown (Case Fig. 2–1).

CLINICAL EXAMINATION.   A scar in the anterior part of the left side of his upper lip where the cleft had been repaired surgically in infancy was visible. With the lip elevated, the cleft through the alveolar ridge became visible. The alveolar bone medial to the cleft was uneven and protruded slightly; the protrusion was exaggerated by

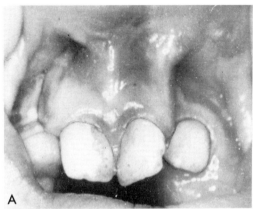
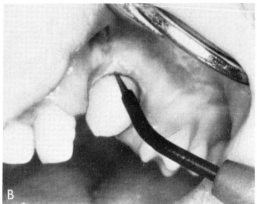
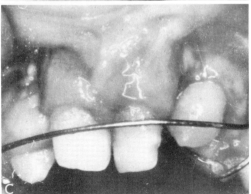

Case Figure 2–1. Electrocoagulation to elongate clinical crown for banding. *A,* Preoperative: There is a bilateral cleft of the maxilla in the area of the lateral incisors, both of which are missing from the dental arch. The permanent cuspid is partially erupted and occupies the place of the lateral in the left quadrant. The tooth lies in a postero-anterior direction, slanting across the line of cleft. There is a deep depression immediately anterior to the crown of the tooth, outlining the position of the cleft. The orthodontist plans to put a band on the tooth; it is therefore necessary to elongate the crown. *B,* Preferably, the tissue that will be removed should not regenerate. The elongation is therefore being performed by electrocoagulation. The current is being applied to the tissues with a solid point tapered conical electrode. The tip of the electrode is circumscribing the crown under the free gingival margin. *C,* Postoperative appearance of the tooth and tissues 19 days later. The coagulum has peeled away, and the crown has been exposed about 1 cm. The tissue around the crown has healed very well except the portion of marginal gingiva in the line of cleft, which is slightly puffy and atonal. The tooth is now ready for placement of an orthodontic band to be connected to the labial arch bar the patient is wearing.

the concave loss of contour in the cleft area. The lateral incisor was missing from the dental arch, and the cuspid was tilted approximately 30 degrees posteroanteriorly. This tooth was lying in superior version to the other teeth in the arch, and the apical third of the crown of the tooth was covered with gingival tissue. The marginal gingivae and interdental papillae of the anterior teeth were somewhat engorged and hyperplastic.

TREATMENT. A thorough prophylaxis initiated treatment, and the patient was instructed in simple methods of gingival massage. When the patient returned one week later the gingival tissue tone was considerably improved. The tissues were prepared and infiltration anesthesia was administered. A tapered conical coagulating electrode (Coles E–21–B) was selected and inserted into the coagulating handle. Coagulating current output was set at 2 on the power output rheostat dial, the circuit was activated, and the tip of the electrode was inserted under the free gingival margin and rotated around the tooth rapidly, care being taken to avoid making electrode contact with the tooth.

After a few applications of the activated electrode for one to two seconds followed by a rest interval of about 5 seconds, the marginal gingiva around this tooth began to turn white, evidence that the tissue had been adequately coagulated. When the rim of white paralleled the desired level of marginal gingiva visualized for this tooth, treatment was halted and tincture of myrrh and benzoin was applied in air-dried layers. Instructions were given for home care, stressing need to bathe the tissues frequently with salt water and to avoid injury to the tissues and coagulum by limiting food intake to liquids and semi-solids until his next visit.

He was seen again one week later, at which time the coagulum was no longer in evidence and the surface of the underlying tissue was only partially healed. Tincture of myrrh and benzoin was reapplied and the patient was instructed to continue with the regimen of home care until the tissues were fully healed and to return at weekly intervals for postoperative observation and control.

Six weeks postoperatively the tissues around this tooth were fully healed, and he was instructed to return to his orthodontist for insertion of the bands to institute active orthodontic treatment.

The level of the marginal gingiva at this time was about 2 to 3 mm. higher than had been intended, but unlike the problem in crown and bridge, where the additional irreversible recession would have exposed the finish line of the restoration, in this instance the recession created no disadvantage, but instead provided the advantage that the tissue did not regenerate downward and create subgingival irritation.

CASE 3

This case demonstrates judicious combined use of electronic cutting and coagulating currents to achieve a desirable postoperative result. It also provides an excellent basis of comparison between the type of tissue repair obtained with cold-steel surgery and that with electrosurery.

The case was treated in two separate stages. The first stage consisted of exposing an unerupted permanent anterior tooth by excising the overlying tissue with a steel scalpel. The second stage consisted of electrosurgical excision to eliminate and repair the unfavorable tissue response to the initial surgery.

Since the same patient was involved, the two surgical episodes were only one month apart and no physical changes or other variable factors were involved; the only difference was in the respective modalities used. Thus the drastic difference in the rate and quality of healing from the use of the respective modalities and immeasurable superiority of the results obtained with electrosurgery become conclusively significant.

HISTORY. The patient was a 20-year-old black girl undergoing treatment at the hospital orthodontia clinic for correction of an open bite. She was referred to the Oral Surgery Clinic for exposure of an unerupted maxillary central incisor.

CLINICAL EXAMINATION. *Extraoral.* Negative.

Intraoral. All her teeth except the maxillary right central incisor were fully erupted. The right central incisor area was edentulous and the left central and lateral incisors were tilted slightly toward each other, reducing the edentulous space at the incisal level (Case Fig. 3–1A). The gingival mucosa bulged over the area of the unerupted tooth and appeared fibrous in texture.

TREATMENT. The mouth was prepared for surgery and infiltration anesthesia with Xylocaine hydrochloride in 1:50,000 epinephrine concentration was administered for maximum hemostasis. The mucosa was incised with a No. 15 Bard-Parker scalpel blade. The incision was started high in the mucolabial fold (Case Fig. 3–1B); profuse bleeding ensued immediately. Two bleeder arterioles were clamped off with mosquito hemostats and the tissue excision was continued (Case Fig. 3–1C). Sufficient tissue was excised to expose the incisal third of the tooth, which was malposed in an oblique postero-anterior direction.

In lieu of the customary use of a celluloid form cemented over the crown of the tooth, or tying a ligature wire around the exposed tooth at its cemento-enamel junction, which would have necessitated resection of much additional tissue to provide access to the full crown, a ligature wire twisted into a double-end loop was cemented onto the labial aspect of the exposed portion of the crown in a manner that had recently been brought to my attention.[*,1,2] (This technique is especially advantageous when exposing impacted maxillary cuspids in cleft palate cases. These teeth usually lie at or very close to the line of cleft. In order to insert a celluloid crown-form or band over such a tooth for orthodontic movement, it is necessary to remove all the bone and tissue from around the crown, to eliminate impediments to the insertion. Removal of considerable tissue from around the crown of the tooth creates a distinct danger of traumatic perforation into the cleft. When the technique of cementation described above is utilized, it is not essential to remove impinging tissue from vulnerable areas, and danger of traumatic perforation is minimized.)

The exposed labial portion of the tooth was carefully dried with sterile sponges. A small strip of selvage gauze was then packed around the exposed crown of the tooth to help keep moisture seepage away from the labial surface. A drop of orthophosphoric acid cement liquid was applied to the dried exposed tooth surface for 30 seconds to lightly etch the enamel surface so that the cement would adhere to it.

The liquid was then carefully wiped away and a thin mix of oxyphosphate cement was placed on the etched area. One end of the double-end loop ligature was embedded into the cement and held in position until the cement set. This firmly attached the ligature to the exposed crown and left the free-end loop terminal available for attachment of elastic, spring or other suitable means of traction (Case Fig. 3–1D). When the cement was firmly set, a piece of adhesive dryfoil was adapted over the exposed coronal portion of the tooth and embedded ligature, to serve as a separating

---

*Riesner, S. E.: Personal communication.

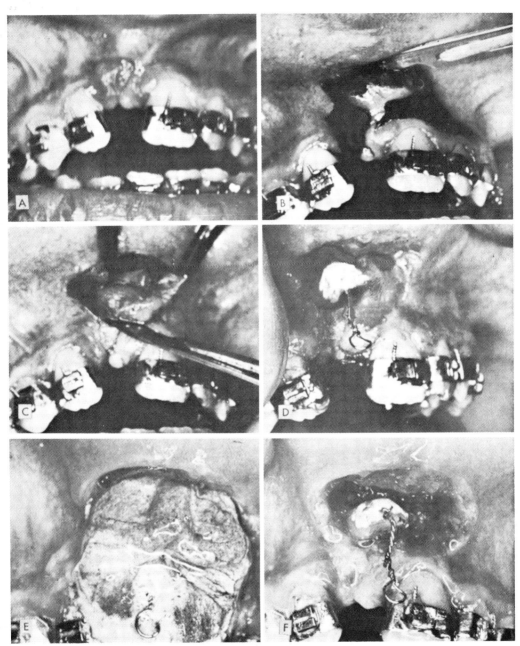

Case Figure 3–1.   Exposure of unerupted permanent central incisor with cold-steel instrumentation. *A*, Preoperative view shows prominent bulge over edentulous space in right central incisor area. *B*, Incision started high in labial vestibule with Bard-Parker scalpel. Note profuse bleeding. *C*, Two bleeders clamped off with mosquito hemostats to control hemorrhage. Dissection of overlying tissue continued. *D*, Crown of malposed tooth exposed. Surface etched lightly and double-end loop cemented to exposed incisal portion of tooth. *E*, Cement pack inserted into surgical defect (adhesive dryfoil insulation for separation cannot be seen). *F*, Postoperative appearance one week later. Tissues still raw; surface not covered with normal granulation tissue. Cemented loop is firmly attached.

medium to keep the surgical cement pack that was to be inserted over the operative field from adhering to the cemented ligature. The cement pack was then inserted (Case Fig. 3–1E) and the patient was instructed in postoperative care and reappointed.

She returned one week later. The cement pack, which had remained in place, was removed without disturbing the ligature. Although the latter was firmly attached and ready for use, the gingival tissue around the exposed crown was healing very slowly, with little evidence of normal granulation. The tissues were still far too raw to permit orthodontic movement to be instituted (Case Fig. 3–1F). Further protection for the area being indicated, a strip of selvage gauze was impregnated with B.I.P. ointment and packed around the crown. The patient was instructed to continue with the lavage and other postoperative care.

The patient was seen every week for one month. Healing continued to progress unsatisfactorily despite continued postoperative care. One month postoperatively an epuloid mass of proliferating hypertrophic tissue suddenly developed over the exposed crown, the mass jutting downward from the superior border of the gingiva over the crown (Case Fig. 3–2A). This tissue was so markedly hyperemic and friable that it bled at the slightest touch. In view of the poor healing and hypertrophy the patient was reappointed for electrosurgical removal of the tissue mass and coagulation of the incompletely healed mucosa.

She was seen at the author's office one week later. The mouth was prepared for surgery and infiltration anesthesia administered. The cemented ligature wire was removed and the surface of the crown thoroughly cleansed. A medium-sized round loop electrode was selected and current output set at 5 for electrocoagulation. The superfluous tissue mass was resected with a wiping motion of the round loop electrode (Case Fig. 3–2B).

The engorgement of the hypertrophic tissue was so great that despite use of biterminal coagulating current to resect the mass, profuse bleeding ensued. The bleeding could not be stopped by use of biterminal coagulating current within the safe limits necessary to avoid possible bone damage. A heavy, wire needle electrode was substituted, current output set at 9 for monoterminal application, and the bleeding site fulgurated. The electrode was kept in constant circular motion to prevent excessive concentration of heat. Fulguration was continued until the surface of the tissue was carbonized, which effectively checked the bleeding (Case Fig. 3–2C).

The exposed labial surface of the tooth was cleansed, dried and re-etched with orthophosphoric acid cementing liquid for 30 seconds. The etched area was thoroughly cleansed to remove orthophosphoric acid and thoroughly dried. Then one end of the double-end loop ligature was embedded into a small mound of thinly mixed oxyphosphate cement (Case Fig. 3–2D). When the cement solidified, it was coated with petrolatum to protect it until it was fully set. Kenalog ointment in Orabase was applied to the operative field as a postoperative dressing. Postoperative instructions were repeated and she was reappointed.

She returned on the fifth postoperative day. This time the tissues appeared to be healing satisfactorily. Tincture of myrrh and benzoin was applied in air-dried layers and she was instructed to continue her postoperative regimen. The following week the tissues appeared almost fully healed. Traction was applied to the tooth with a ligature wire tied to the free end of the cemented loop and to the archbar at the other end. The patient was seen again six months later. The tissues were fully healed, and the tooth, under elastic band traction, was almost fully descended and in good alignment (Case Fig. 3–2E).

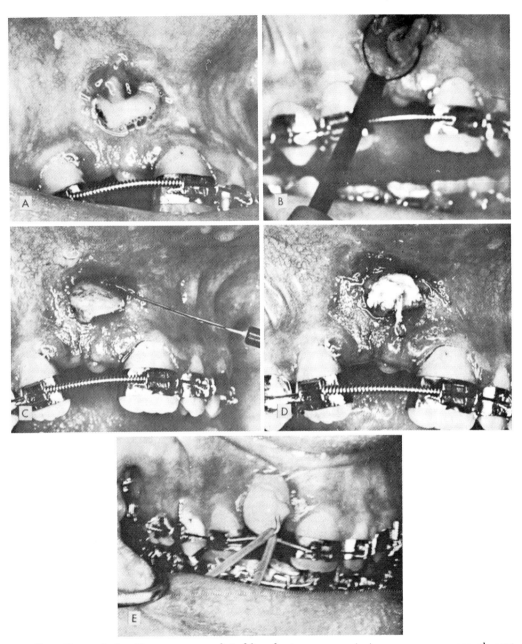

Case Figure 3–2. Exposure completed by electrosurgery. *A,* Appearance one month post-operatively. A large epuloid mass has developed on the gingival mucosa at the superior border of the exposed crown portion. *B,* Epuloid mass resected with round loop electrode. *C,* Bleeding point checked by fulguration. *D,* A double-end loop cemented onto labial incisal third of tooth. *E,* Postoperative view taken six months later. Tooth almost fully erupted in good alignment.

PLATE IV

Orthodontics

Figure 1a. Elongation of clinical crowns for insertion of orthodontic bands. Note the collapse of the palatal arch and dental arch owing to the abnormal traction created by the contractile cicatricial mass of scar tissue healing of a pharyngeal repair of a cleft palate. Note the subnormal condition of the marginal gingiva around the partially decayed left central or cuspid, and the fragment of decayed retained root of the deciduous cuspid on the right side, which will have to be removed. The gingival tissue around the other teeth is normal in tone.

Figure 1b. The elongation of the clinical crowns is being performed by loop resection with a flame-shaped loop electrode by electrosection. To provide space for the bands and to create a semblance of gingival harmony, a half centimeter of gingival tissue and more is being resected.

Figure 1c. Appearance of the tissues one week postoperatively. The tissue in the bed from which the fragment of retained root had been lifted with a surgical curet is still unhealed and raw looking. The tissue around the left cuspid which had been subnormal preoperatively is still somewhat atonal and subnormal. The tissues around the other teeth that had been treated are fully healed. Despite the remarkably rapid and favorable tissue repair of wounds created by electrosection, when the tissue tone is poor to begin with, the repair is much less favorable and slower than usual.

Figure 3a. Elongation of clinical crowns of teeth by resecting gingival tissue from metal orthodontic bands. The tissue must be cleared from these teeth to permit use of an obturator held in place by clasps. The tissue is being resected by electrosection with a medium-width U-shaped loop electrode that must contact the stainless steel bands in order to remove the tissue. The contact with the metal is only momentary, however, and a full 10-second interval is permitted to elapse between the contacts.

Figure 2a. Pushback to deepen the buccal vestibule to permit insertion of a labial arch bar. The anterior teeth and the molar have been banded. A low muscle attachment is traumatized when the arch bar is inserted into the molar buccal bracket. An incision to create a deepening of the buccal vestibule is necessary but creates danger of aspiration of blood into the lungs if free bleeding occurs because of a huge cleft of the hard and soft palates. (See case report.)

Figure 2b. Pushback being performed by incision by electrosection with a fine 45-degree-angle needle electrode. Note a slight trickle of blood resulting from performing a posterior superior alveolar nerve block injection, and total absence of free bleeding from the incision of this extremely vascular tissue.

Figure 2c. Appearance of the buccal vestibule 10 days postoperatively. Note that the tissue is fully healed, without closure from scar tissue adhesions, despite not having lined the area with a split-thickness skin graft, owing to the absence of scar tissue repair of the atraumatic wound.

Figure 3b. Appearance of the tissues five days later. The tissues are almost fully healed, and there is no clinical evidence of damage having occurred from the contact of the activated electrode with the metal bands and tooth structure.

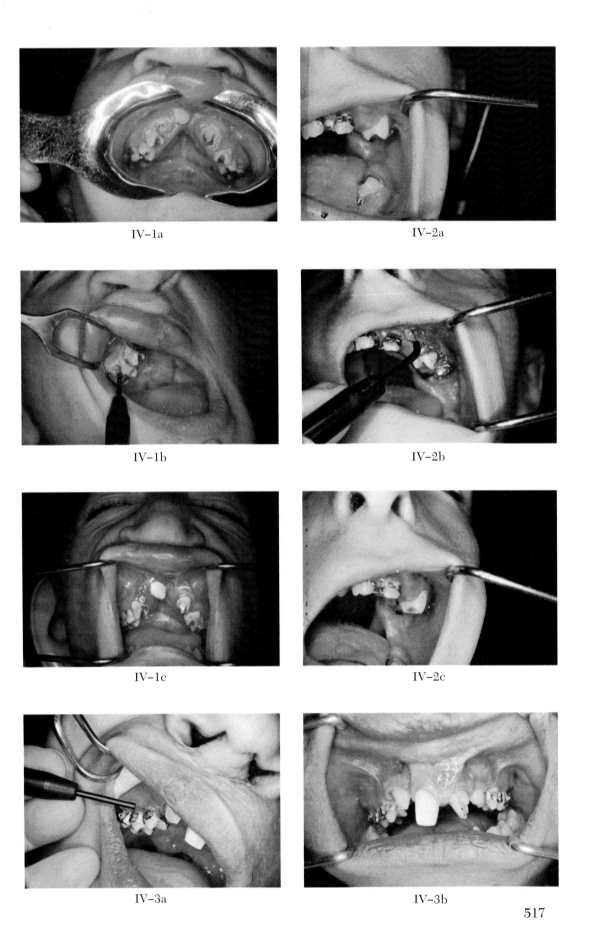

IV-1a

IV-2a

IV-1b

IV-2b

IV-1c

IV-2c

IV-3a

IV-3b

CASE 4

This case shows how combined use of loop and needle electrosection can minimize the surgery and accelerate and simplify it, in part by the greater efficiency in resecting tissue and in part by the elimination of persistent free bleeding that obscures the operative field and slows the surgical procedure.

PATIENT.   A 15-year-old white male in normal health.

HISTORY.   Due to irregular malposed dentition and unerupted teeth he was being prepared for orthodontia. He was referred for surgery to facilitate orthodontic movement of a rotated malposed maxillary cuspid and to create space between this tooth and the bicuspid so that they could be brought close together, thereby permitting the unerupted second bicuspid to come down.

CLINICAL EXAMINATION.   The maxillary right cuspid was elevated, so that the tip of the tooth cusp was at the midheight level of the lateral incisor (Case Fig. 4–1). There was a small space between the cuspid and first bicuspid and a wide space between the distal of the bicuspid and the mesial of the first molar. The second bicuspid was not present clinically in the dental arch.

ROENTGENOGRAPHIC EXAMINATION.   X-rays revealed that the cuspid was in postero-anterior version and that the first bicuspid had two incompletely formed roots. There was a 2-mm. space between the cuspid and first bicuspid which was filled with alveolar bone. The second bicuspid was in position in the dental arch at approximately 0.5 cm. elevation above the adjacent teeth.

TREATMENT.   The area was prepared for surgery and infiltration anesthesia was administered to both the labial and palatal mucosa. A flame-shaped (Coles E–6–A) loop electrode was selected and cutting current was set at 4.5 on the cutting current power output dial. The marginal gingival tissue around the cuspid was resected by shaving with short wiping strokes of the loop, applied for a fraction of a second and followed by a 10-second rest interval after each tissue contact.

When the entire crown of the tooth was fully exposed, the loop was used to resect all the soft tissue present between the cuspid and bicuspid. A 45-degree-angle needle electrode was substituted for the loop, and cutting current was reduced to 3 on the power dial. A vertico-oblique incision was made with this electrode. The incision was directed somewhat anteroposteriorly, and terminated at the mesiogingival angle of the cuspid. As the areolar mucosa was incised, the tissue margins parted and blood was released but there was no free bleeding. The blood was removed by aspiration, after which the labial gingival mucosa was elevated and reflected. This provided access to the interseptal bone that had to be removed between the cuspid and bicuspid to permit the cuspid to migrate downward. The intervening coronal part of this bone was removed by hand instrumentation with Weidelstadt chisels and sickle scalers. When the bone channeling was completed, the flap was restored and sutured with interrupted silk sutures.

The patient was seen again on the fifth postoperative day and reported a completely uneventful postoperative experience. The tissue tone was excellent, and the repair, although somewhat slower than usual owing to the combination of tissue planing and incision, was progressing favorably.

At this point the patient was referred back to his orthodontist for insertion of the orthodontic bands and arch bar for orthodontic realignment. Healing was reported to have progressed rapidly and uneventfully thereafter.

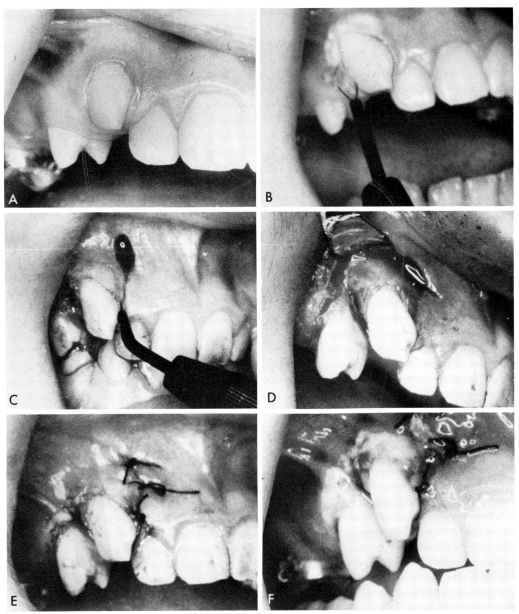

Case Figure 4–1.   Gingivoplasty and bone channeling for movement of a malposed partially erupted maxillary cuspid. *A,* Preoperative: The maxillary right cuspid is malposed labially, superiorly, and posteroanteriorly. Its cusp tip is at the level of the marginal gingivae of the adjacent teeth, and the gingival mucosa around the malposed crown is atonal, engorged, and proliferative. *B,* A gingivectoplasty is being performed with a flame-shaped loop electrode to expose the crown fully and simultaneously to recontour the gingival architecture. *C,* A mucoperiosteal incision is being made with a 45-degree-angle fine needle electrode. The almost vertical incision extends downward and slightly posteriorly from the top of the vestibule to the mesiogingival angle of the tooth. The areolar part of the incision has spread open and blood is present in it, but there is no free bleeding. *D,* The incised flap has been elevated and reflected upward, exposing the channel that had been cut in the 0.5 cm. of bone between the cuspid and first bicuspid to facilitate the orthodontic movement of the tooth. *E,* The flap has been restored and the coapted tissues have been sutured with interrupted silk sutures. Sutures have also been inserted through the mesial and distal embrasures. *F,* Five day postoperative appearance immediately prior to suture removal. The marginal gingiva, healing by secondary intention, is covered with a light layer of coagulum. Healing is progressing satisfactorily; the patient has had no facial swelling or postoperative pain.

519

CASE 5

This case is an example of the complications created by unfavorable local factors which necessiated two stage surgery, a deviation from the routine procedure of exposure of an unerupted, malposed, impacted maxillary cuspid for orthodontic movement. It also affords further evidence of the speed and quality of tissue repair following electronic electrosurgery.

PATIENT.   A 13-year-old white male.

HISTORY.   The patient had been undergoing active orthodontic treatment and was referred for removal of a retained deciduous maxillary cuspid and exposure of the permanent cuspid. The latter was impacted in an obliquely malposed position.

CLINICAL EXAMINATION.   *Extraoral.*   Negative.

Intraoral.   The left deciduous cuspid was retained in the maxillary dental arch. The tooth was firmly embedded and the gingival mucosa was normal.

Roentgenographic examination revealed the malposed tooth lying across the roots of the lateral and first bicuspid (Case Fig. 5–1). A large radiolucent area suggestive of a cyst surrounded the crown and coronal end of the root of the impacted tooth.

TREATMENT.   The large radiolucent area noted in the roentgenogram suggested the likelihood that the embryonal capsule around the crown of the impacted tooth had degenerated into a follicular cyst. If, as appeared likely, the cystic crypt formed a large defect in the investing bone around the crown of the impacted tooth, the most advantageous treatment plan would be to perform the exposure in two stages. The first stage would include extraction of the deciduous tooth and the channeling of the alveolar bone in order to provide an easy path of egress for the impacted tooth. Then, after the cystic space filled in with repair tissue, the final exposure of the crown would be performed to provide the means for orthodontic traction of the tooth in order to bring it down into the dental arch. It appeared likely that by following this treatment plan the danger of possible secondary infection being introduced deep into the body

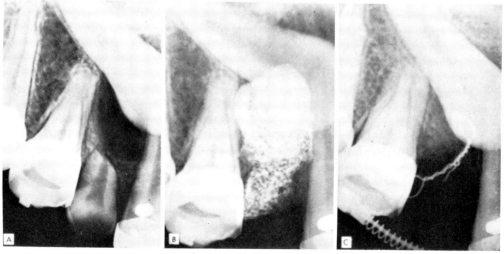

Case Figure 5–1.   Exposure of an obliquely impacted permanent cuspid, with large follicular cyst. *A,* Preoperative roentgenogram. Retained deciduous cuspid still in position. *B,* Roentgenogram showing B.I.P.-impregnated selvage gauze pack in channel. *C,* Postoperative appearance three months later; tooth being brought into alignment.

of the maxilla through the large cystic cavity present immediately following removal of the cyst would be eliminated.

The mouth was prepared for surgery and infiltration anesthesia was administered. A 60-degree-angle fine needle electrode was selected and current output set at 3.5 for electrosection. The electrode was used to perform a vertico-oblique incision (Case Fig. 5–2). The incision was started high in the mucolabial fold at a point over the center of the lateral incisor and carried downward to the distoproximal angle of the gingival margin of this tooth. The deciduous tooth was extracted. Then the incised tissue was elevated from the underlying bone and reflected in a distal direction, exposing the labial bone plate. The latter was removed with chisels and rongeur forceps until the crown of the malposed impacted tooth was fully exposed. The alveolar bone was channeled from the undersurface of the crown to the gingival margin to a depth of about 4 mm. The cystically degenerated embryonal sac was excised first, manually with curets; inaccessible adherent shreds were then removed by electrosection with a narrow U-shaped loop electrode. The latter was especially useful for removing tissue shreds that invaginated deeply between the tooth and the investing alveolar bone. Use of this electrode eliminated the need to remove sufficient additional bone to provide access to these shreds, as would have been necessary for other methods of instrumentation.

After all the cystic tissue was resected and the large bone cavity was thoroughly debrided the defect was alternately irrigated with Kasdenol and saline solutions and aspirated. Bleeding was induced, and a mixture of powdered medicated gelatin and "bone-growth inductor material" was introduced into the defect and incorporated with the blood present. The tissue flap was restored to position. The margins were coapted and sutured with 0000 interrupted silk sutures. A strip of selvage gauze impregnated with B.I.P. was inserted into the channel to keep the eruption pathway open. Postoperative instructions were given and the patient was reappointed.

He returned on the fifth postoperative day. The quality and rate of healing noted at this time was quite remarkable. The line of incision appeared fully healed by primary intention and the tissue tone was completely normal. The sutures and the selvage gauze pack were removed. The channel appeared fully open. Tincture of myrrh and benzoin was applied, and he was instructed to return in two weeks. At his next visit the line of incision was marked only by an almost imperceptibly slight depression in the gingival mucosa.

Six weeks later the second and final stage of surgery was performed. By that time the tissues were firm and the hollow created by the bone channeling was filled with normal but incompletely calcified repair tissue. The mouth was prepared for surgery and infiltration anesthesia administered. A flame-shaped loop electrode was selected and current output set at 6 for electrosection. The tissue over the crown of the impacted tooth was removed by shaving in layers with short brushing strokes (Case Fig. 5–3). Current output was reduced to 4.5 and a narrow 45-degree-angle U-shaped loop electrode was substituted. This electrode was used to excise the tissue surrounding the crown of the tooth. When the crown was sufficiently exposed it was thoroughly dried, the surface of the exposed enamel etched, and a double-end loop ligature was cemented onto the labial surface of the incisal third of the exposed crown. The entire procedure had been virtually bloodless with nothing more than a slight ooze of serum from the denuded surface of tissue. Tincture of myrrh and benzoin was applied to the exposed tissues. Then an adhesive ointment protective dressing was applied to the operative field. The patient was instructed to resume the postoperative routine and was reappointed.

He returned on the fifth postoperative day and reported that he had had neither

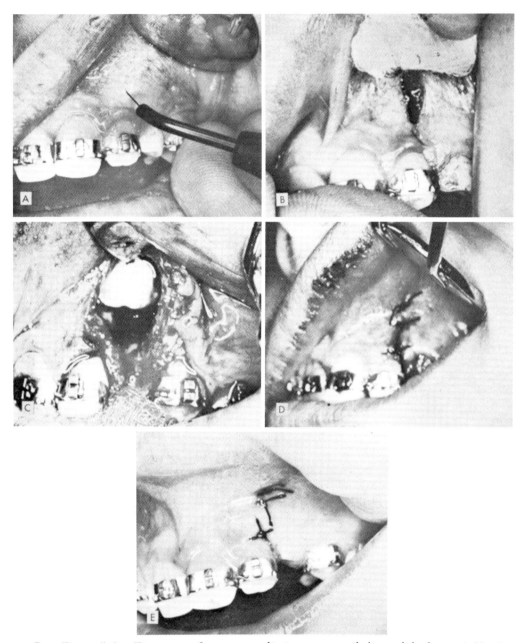

Case Figure 5–2.   First stage of surgery to eliminate cyst and channel the bone. *A*, Vertico-oblique incision with fine 45-degree-angle needle electrode made at distal of the lateral incisor. *B*, Incision completed and tissues spread. Deciduous tooth *in situ*. *C*, Tooth crown exposed; cyst enucleated from its cavity. Note deciduous tooth has been extracted, and bone channeled. *D*, Closure with interrupted braided silk sutures. *E*, Appearance on fifth postoperative day. Tissue healing rapidly by primary intention. Selvage gauze pack bulging slightly from socket.

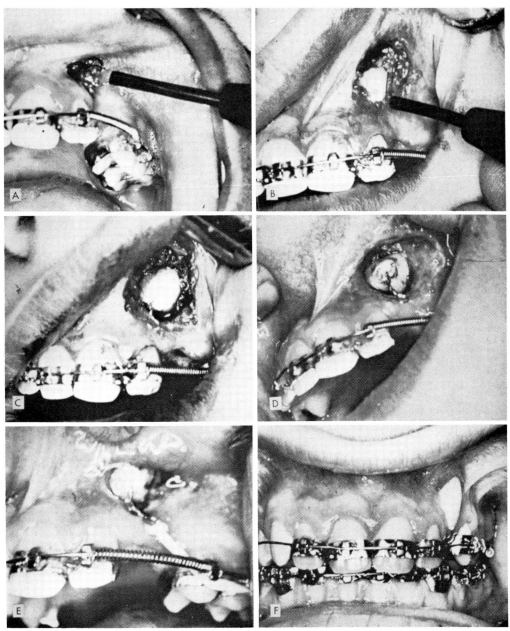

Case Figure 5–3.   Exposure of the crown for orthodontic movement. *A*, Mucosa overlying the crown of the tooth resected by shaving in layers with flame-shaped loop electrode. Procedure bloodless. *B*, Crown cleared of adherent mucosa with narrow U-shaped loop electrode. *C*, Ligature wire double-end loop cemented onto the exposed crown. *D*, Postoperative appearance on fifth postoperative day. Tissue healing rapidly. Only light coagulum remains on surface. *E*, Elastic-band traction being applied against malposed tooth. *F*, Final postoperative photograph taken almost one year after surgery shows complete healing without loss of normal alveolar contour. The tooth has been brought into normal alignment and is almost fully erupted.

pain nor swelling. The gingival mucosa was found to be healing very satisfactorily and the traction loop ligature was firmly attached to the tooth. He was seen again two weeks later, at which time the tissues appeared almost fully healed. His orthodontist had attached the loop ligature to the labial arch bar with a broad elastic band, and traction was being applied in a distal direction. Traction caused some mechanical trauma to the gingival mucosa at the distogingival angle of the tooth. The trauma was retarding the overall healing of the tissues to some degree. Topical anesthetic was applied for two minutes; then the surface of the tissue was shaved with a narrow loop electrode to clear it from contact with the ligature. Tincture of myrrh and benzoin was applied in air-dried layers and the patient was reappointed.

He returned one week later. The tissue was healing well and was covered with a thin layer of healthy coagulum. The area was irrigated and tincture of myrrh and benzoin applied. When he was seen again the following week the entire gingival mucosa appeared fully healed. He was told to use the salt-alum astringent mouthwash and to return again the following week. When he returned, the gingival mucosa was fully healed and its tissue tone was excellent. The tooth was gradually being brought down into the dental arch and the bone cavity was fully filled with normal bone.

Elimination of Cysts, Supernumerary Teeth, or Malposed Impacted Teeth That Cannot be Brought into Normal Alignment in the Dental Arch

There is no single all-pervading philosophy of orthodontic treatment. Thus there are many different orthodontic techniques and appliances, often very ingenious, that are suitable to the different techniques.

It is a fact, however, that no matter which technique is employed, or how ingenious the appliance used, if pathology is present in the jaws that would impede the movement and proper realignment of the dentition, successful treatment cannot be attained.

When the prospective orthodontic patient has a cyst, supernumerary teeth, or malposed impacted teeth that cannot be brought into the dental arch, these impediments must be eliminated before the orthodontic treatment is begun. The benefits that are derived from performing the preorthodontic surgery electrosurgically rather than by cold-steel manual instrumentation will be well demonstrated in the cases that follow.

CASE 6

This case is representative of pathologic obstructions to normal eruption that often make preliminary orthodontic surgery a prerequisite to successful orthodontic treatment. In this particular instance the obstruction consisted of a number of impacted supernumerary teeth in the mandible which prevented normal eruption of underlying permanent teeth.

PATIENT.   An 11-year-old white male.

HISTORY.   Roentgenographic examination prior to orthodontic treatment had revealed the presence of several supernumerary teeth impacted in the right mandibular lateral-cuspid region. The supernumerary teeth were preventing eruption of the underlying permanent teeth. He was referred for removal of the supernumeraries as a preliminary step in the orthodontic treatment.

CLINICAL EXAMINATION. *Extraoral.* Negative.

Intraoral. The mandibular right lateral was not present in the dental arch, and the deciduous cuspid was retained in the arch. An intraoral periapical roentgenogram revealed the permanent lateral and cuspid impacted in the mandible and presence of a supernumerary tooth. The two permanent teeth appeared to be in normal position for eruption but were locked in by the supernumerary tooth (Case Fig. 6–1).

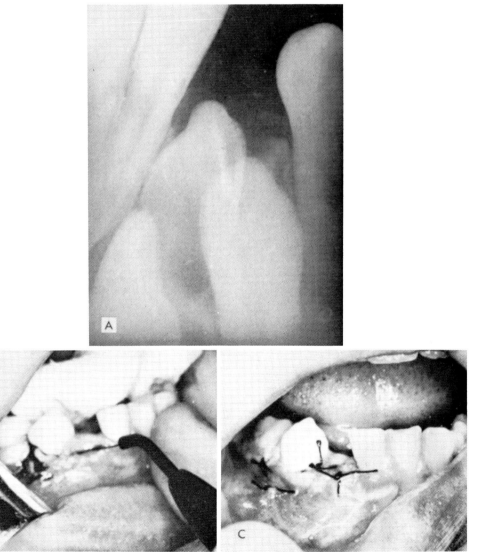

Case Figure 6–1. Removal of supernumerary tooth that prevents normal eruption of permanent teeth. *A,* Roentgenogram showing permanent teeth locked by supernumerary. *B,* Incision with fine 45-degree-angle needle electrode for flap. *C,* Postoperative appearance on fifth postoperative day shows excellent healing by primary union.

TREATMENT.   The mouth was prepared for surgery and infiltration anesthesia administered. A fine 45-degree-angle needle electrode was selected and current output set at 3.5 for electrosection. The electrode was used with a wiping motion to create a vertico-oblique incision distal to the deciduous cuspid which was extended downward and slightly backward to the areolar mucosa. A second incision was then made across the edentulous space between the central and deciduous cuspid. The flap was reflected and the supernumerary tooth extracted. Debridement was performed; the flap was then restored and the coapted margins sutured with 0000 braided silk interrupted sutures. The patient was given postoperative instructions and reappointed.

When he returned on the fifth postoperative day he reported that he had had no pain or marked discomfort. The lines of incision were almost fully healed by primary intention and the tissue tone was excellent. The patient was seen once more a week later, at which time healing appeared complete.

The deciduous cuspid was retained by request to help serve as a space maintainer until the unlocked permanent teeth erupted.

The rate and quality of healing noted is typical of what can be anticipated when tissue incised by electrosection is normally healthy. The lack of postoperative discomfort is also typical in such cases.

CASE 7

This case serves to demonstrate the remarkable rate and quality of tissue repair following electrosection properly performed with suitable current despite presence of metal orthodontic bands in the surgical field.

PATIENT.   A 16-year-old white male in normal health.

HISTORY.   Both maxillary permanent cuspids were impacted. They were so badly malposed that orthodontists considered it impossible to bring them into the dental arch without disrupting the entire dentition. He was therefore referred for surgical removal of the impacted teeth.

CLINICAL EXAMINATION.   All the teeth except the two maxillary cuspids were in the dental arches, and all were banded for orthodontic movement. Both impacted teeth were lying in labial version in the maxilla (Case Fig. 7–1).

Case Figure 7–1.   Bilateral labial impaction, maxillary cuspids. *A*, All the maxillary teeth have been banded. A vertico-oblique incision is being made slightly postero-anteriorly to the distobuccal angle of the first right bicuspid. The cuspids are not present in the dental arch. The incision, being created with a 45-degree-angle fine needle electrode, has caused no free bleeding. *B*, The apical attachments of the interdental papillae are being severed with the same electrode. Momentary contact with the metal bands in the process of severing the apical attachments is inevitable. *C*, The incised mucoperiosteal flap has been elevated, and the bone has been removed to expose the crown of the left cuspid. Note the absence of free bleeding that would obscure the surgical field. *D*, Both impacted teeth have been removed and debridement has been completed, without hindrance from hemorrhagic bleeding. *E*, The appearance on the fifth postoperative day, before the sutures were removed. There is evidence of early primary healing, and the tissue tone is excellent throughout. *F*, Appearance 2 weeks later. Healing is complete, and it is impossible to differentiate where the lines of incision had been except for a light pink color of the tissue surface owing to lack of surface keratin formation. The alveolar contour is normal, with no concavitation seen where the teeth had been removed. The interdental papillae have healed very well and are firmly reattached.

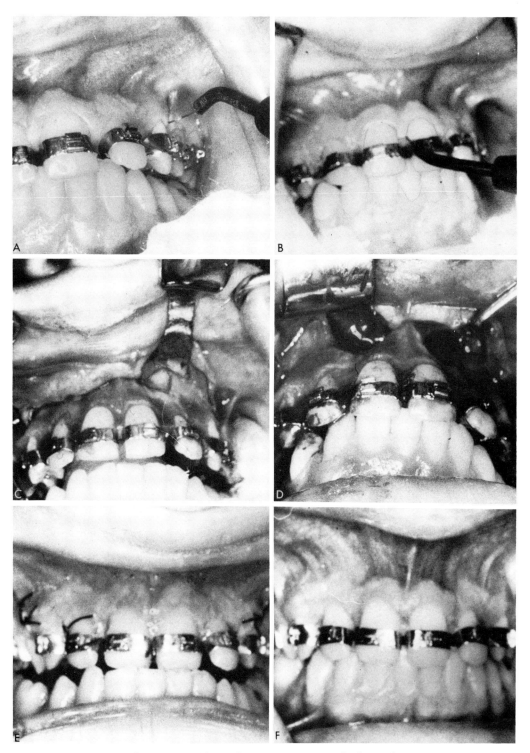

Case Figure 7–1. See opposite page for legend.

ROENTGENOGRAPHIC EXAMINATION. Periapical and occlusal x-ray views confirmed the presence of the impacted teeth high above the gingival level of the remaining teeth and rotated in postero-anterior version.

TREATMENT. The tissues were prepared for surgery and bilateral infraorbital block injections and palatal infiltration were administered. The mucogingival tissue was incised bilaterally with a 45-degree-angle fine needle electrode, with cutting current set at 3 on the instrument panel dial. The incisions were performed in a vertico-oblique direction and terminated postero-anteriorly at the distogingival angles of the first bicuspids. The apical attachments of the intervening interdental papillae were severed with the electrode to permit the entire labial gingival mucosa between the two incisions to be elevated and reflected and to expose the impaction sites. The exposed bone was removed with an automatic impactor chisel, revealing the coronal portions of the teeth. Both teeth were removed and debridement was completed, leaving two large cavities.

Powdered surgical gelatin was then introduced into the surgical defects and mixed with the blood present there to restore the defects to normal contour and help keep the tissue flap from sagging into the bone cavities. The flap was restored to position and sutured with interrupted silk sutures. First, the vertico-oblique incisions were sutured; then, sutures were inserted through the apices of the interdental papillae in their respective embrasures.

The patient returned on the fifth postoperative day for removal of the sutures. The healing progress was amazing; the tissue tone was excellent, the color was normal, there was no edema, and there was evidence of primary repair. He was seen again one week later. The incisions appeared fully healed, and there was no clinical evidence of the surgery that had been performed.

The quality and speed of repair was all the more remarkable in view of the fact that the activated electrode had to make momentary contact with the steel orthodontic bands as the incisions were performed.

Many orthodontists favor use of the Angle-edgewise technique to facilitate orthodontic realignment of malposed teeth. This technique is predicated on extraction of the four bicuspids to provide space in the dental arches and thereby reduce need for extensive arch expansion to realign the teeth and create optimal centric relations between the teeth in the respective arches.

In this case, however, the maxillary right first bicuspid was in normal alignment, and the second bicuspid was palatally malposed and impacted, so that the first molar was adjacent to the first bicuspid. The treatment plan for this case therefore had to be adjusted so that the malposed tooth would be sacrificed and the first bicuspid, which would otherwise be extracted, would have to be retained. Since the tooth was impacted as well as malposed, incision of a tissue flap and surgical removal of the tooth would be necessary. The Angle-edgewise technique also depends on banding all the remaining teeth in the two arches. Thus, this case provides an excellent example of the efficacy with which the palatal mucosa can be incised by electrosection to provide the advantages of reduced bleeding and scar-free nonfibrous tissue repair, and the fact that contact of an activated electrode with orthodontic metal bands is not inherently damaging if the contact is only momentary.

CASE 8

PATIENT. An 11-year-old white female.

HISTORY. Deciduous and permanent dentition had been somewhat slow in erupting, and when the permanent teeth did erupt, many were rotated or irregularly spaced in the dental arches. The patient was referred to an orthodontist for treatment, and treatment by the Angle-edgewise technique was instituted. The maxillary left first bicuspid and both mandibular first bicuspids were extracted, and bands were attached to all the remaining teeth. Since the second bicuspid, which is normally retained, had to be removed because it was impacted and malposed, the treatment plan had to be altered, and the first bicuspid, which would otherwise have been extracted, was retained in its normal site in the dental arch.

CLINICAL EXAMINATION. Orthodontic bands were present on all the teeth. The tooth alignment in the arches was irregular, and many teeth were rotated. The labial-buccal alveolar contours of both jaws were normal, but on the palate a round bulge was present in the right bicuspid-first molar area. The mass was hard, immobile, and resistant to pressure; measured approximately 0.7 cm. in diameter and 3 mm. in height; and was located immediately distal to the crown of the first bicuspid. The clinical impression that the bulge was due to presence of the crown of the missing second bicuspid was confirmed by intra-oral periapical x-rays, which revealed the presence of a well-formed, impacted bicuspid covered with a thin layer of bone, lying between the first bicuspid and first molar teeth (Case Fig. 8–1).

TREATMENT. The tissues were prepared and anesthetized by infiltration. A fine 45-degree-angle needle electrode was selected, and cutting current output was set at 4 on the instrument panel dial. The activated electrode was then used to make a vertical incision through the palatal mucosa approximately 2 cm. long, extending laterally in a straight line toward the marginal gingiva at the center of the crown of the first bicuspid, so that it bypassed the mesial aspect of the impacted tooth crown. A second incision was then made at right angles to the first, extending across the base of the interdental papilla between the bicuspid and molar and the space between the two teeth. This second incision was immediately anterior to the crown of the impacted tooth.

The incised tissue flap was detached from the bone with the broad end of a periosteal elevator and was reflected, exposing the bone-covered round bulge. The thin covering of palatal bone was removed with hand bone chisel and gouge, exposing the crown of the impacted tooth. The entire procedure to this point was virtually bloodless and the surgical field visibility unobscured, although the incised tissue margins were neither coagulated, seared, nor charred. The impacted tooth was removed with appropriate elevators, the bone edges were rounded smooth with a bone file, and some powdered Gelfoam was introduced into the socket and mixed with the blood present there. When the blood appeared partially clotted, the flap was replaced and sutured into position, with two interrupted silk sutures along the long palatal incision, one suture through the tissues of the second incision, and one suture through the interdental papilla between the first and second molars to secure the apex of the papilla, which had been severed to permit adequate flap reflection. A piece of thick Squibb Orahesive bandage material was cut to fit over the entire surgical field as a temporary protective bandage. The bandage material was held in place lightly but firmly, with finger pressure directed toward the edges to melt the waxy material to the tissues.

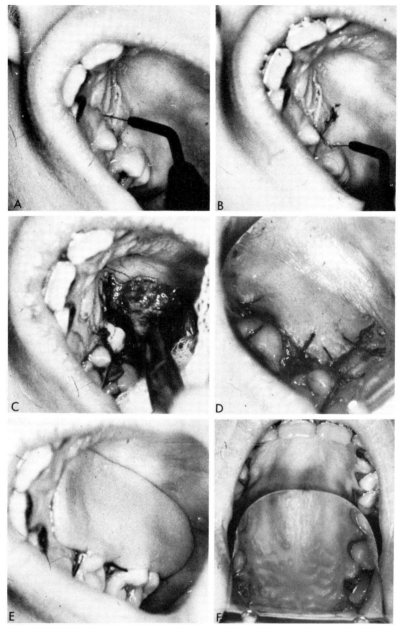

Case Figure 8–1. Removal of a horizontally impacted second maxillary bicuspid that is blocking eruption and orthodontic movement of the cuspid. *A*, The palatal right quadrant is seen from the ventral view. All the teeth bear orthodontic bands. The lateral is rotated mesio-palatally, and distal to the tooth, where the cuspid and first bicuspid should be, there is an edentulous area in the dental arch. An incision is being made parallel to the dental arch from the mesiopalatal aspect of the lateral to the distal of the second bicuspid, where it intersects with a vertical incision approximately 2.5 cm. long from near the midline of the palate. *B*, The horizontal incision is being extended with the same 45-degree-angle needle electrode across the palatal base of the embrasure between the bicuspid and first molar. *C*, The mucoperiosteal flap has been elevated and enough covering palatal bone has been removed to expose the crown of the first bicuspid, which is lying horizontally across the root of the cuspid, with its crown pointed palatally. The malposed impacted tooth is seen partially out of the jawbone as it is being removed. Note that there is no coagulation of the thick, tough palatal tissue, which is covered with a film of blood, but there is no free bleeding to obscure visibility and

(*Case Figure 8–1 continued on facing page*)

The patient returned on the fifth postoperative day for removal of the sutures. The tissue tone was excellent, and there was no evidence of edema. The incised margins appeared to be healing very well by primary intention. The sutures were removed and tincture of myrrh and benzoin was applied to the area. The patient was dismissed from further treatment and instructed to continue with the regimen of home care for two more weeks and to return for a final postoperative examination in three months. When she returned three months later, the palatal tissues were fully healed and the repair of the incised tissues was so completely free of scar tissue that there was no clinical evidence of the surgical site.

CORRECTION OF UNFAVORABLE TISSUE REACTIONS TO ORTHODONTIC TREATMENT

Up to this point we have considered typical electrosurgical techniques that make possible, or simplify, orthodontic treatment. In addition to the usefulness of electrosurgery for the cases cited, those requiring preparatory preliminary orthodontic surgery, this modality is ideally suited to the improvement or correction of a number of unfavorable tissue responses that are frequently manifested in the course of orthodontic treatment. Unfavorable tissue reactions are triggered by band irritation, excessively rapid tooth movement, and/or hormonal influences during puberty. Two typical tissue reactions are:

1. Interproximal papillae between orthodontically banded teeth often become severely irritated, particularly if the oral hygiene is poorly maintained. Such papillae tend to become markedly hyperemic, hypertrophic and partially detached. They bleed freely and may even become ulcerated.

Removal of the triggering mechanism (the bands) is of course impractical. Improvement of tissue tone under adverse conditions must become the substitute. This can be achieved best by a combination of electrosurgery and improved oral hygiene.

Hypertrophy can be reduced and tissue tone of the deteriorated papillae restored (if not for the full term of treatment, at least for considerable periods of time) by biterminal coagulation of the hypertrophied tissue. This can be accomplished in either of two ways:

a. Mass destruction of the bulging tissues by electrocoagulation applied with ball electrodes to destroy the superfluous tissue.

Case Figure 8–1. Continued.
hamper the surgery. *D*, The flap of palatal mucosa has been returned to position and secured with sutures across the vertical line of incision. There are also sutures through the bicuspid and molar embrasure and posteriorly to the molar, as seen in a mirror image view of the palate. *E*, A large bandage of Squibb Orahesive (thick) has been placed over the surgical field to serve as a pressure bandage and keep the palatal flap tight against the palatal bone. *F*, This is the final postoperative appearance of the maxilla, obtained three weeks later. There is only a slightly pinker color along the line of horizontal incision toward the midline, but the tissues are fully healed. The difference in color is due to a lack of mature surface keratin on the new epithelial surface tissue.

b. Use of loop electrodes to resect the epuloid excess tissue masses and create concave interproximal sluiceways.

If the electrosurgical treatment is supplemented with improved oral hygiene and daily saline lavage plus periodic use of an astringent salt-alum lavage, the newly acquired tissue integrity may be maintained for the extent of orthodontic treatment (if there are no complicating systemic involvements).

2. When orthodontic bands are cemented onto teeth whose clinical crowns have not been adequately exposed prior to insertion, the mesial and distal aspects of the bands are often forcibly pushed into—and sometimes even beyond—the bases of their gingival crevices and into the periodontal fibers.

The resultant injury resembles that produced when full-crown restorations are inserted without preliminary subgingival provision to accommodate their bulk: the circular fibers are irritated or traumatized, and severed. The usual tissue response is hyperemia, hypertrophy and loss of tissue tone. The hypertrophic tissue proliferates and tends to creep down over the bands and to bulge around their brackets, and sometimes against the archbars as well.

The proliferating hypertrophied tissue usually is spongy and often bleeds at the slightest provocation. It is almost impossible for the patient to maintain any semblance of good oral hygiene under such circumstances. The distressing taste of blood in the mouth, and poor hygiene, tend to make even the most cooperative patient cranky and difficult.

In such cases the friable hypertrophic tissue can be quickly and easily reduced to normal proportion with loop electrodes. This tissue should be removed with the loop energized by biterminal electrocoagulation instead of electrosection, and current output should be set at approximately the same potency as for cutting current instead of at the lowest current intensity possible, which is usually preferable for electrocoagulation.

CASE 9

This case is a typical example of proliferating hypertrophic tissue that develops in response to irritation of orthodontic bands that impinge deeply into the subgingival tissues. It demonstrates the technique for removal of the superfluous tissue by electrocoagulation with loop electrodes.

HISTORY.   The patient was a 14-year-old white boy. He had been under active orthodontic treatment for one year. All his teeth were banded. The gingival mucosa around a mandibular anterior tooth had begun to enlarge and bleed during tooth brushing and eating. He was referred for removal of the proliferating tissue.

CLINICAL EXAMINATION.   *Extraoral.*   Negative.

Intraoral.   An epuloid mass of proliferative gingival mucosa was present in the mandibular right lateral-cuspid interproximal embrasure, and additional proliferating tissue was also emerging from the labial free gingival margin. The oral hygiene was excellent.

TREATMENT.   The mouth was prepared and the tissues dried. Topical anesthetic was applied to the area for two minutes. A flame-shaped loop electrode was selected

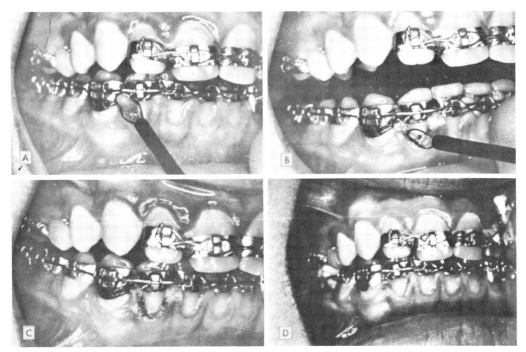

Case Figure 9–1. Removal of proliferating hypertrophic masses resulting from irritation to the gingivae from impingement of orthodontic bands. *A*, Flame-shaped loop electrode inserted under the mass to resect it by electrocoagulation. *B*, Hypertrophic tissue resected from marginal gingiva with the same loop. *C*, Appearance of gingival margin after light spot coagulation. *D*, Postoperative appearance of the tissues one week later. The tissues are fully and normally healed.

and current output set at 4 for electrocoagulation. The epuloid mass was elevated and the loop was inserted under it (Case Fig. 9–1*A*). The current was applied and the mass was removed with one lateral wiping motion of the loop.

After the large epuloid mass was removed, the tissue emerging from the free margin was removed with an upward scooping motion of the side of the loop electrode (Case Fig. 9–1*B*). Finally, the gingival margin was coagulated lightly with a small ball electrode to level off the tissue smoothly (Case Fig. 9–1*C*).

The entire procedure was virtually bloodless. Tincture of myrrh and benzoin was applied in air-dried layers. The patient was instructed in postoperative care and dismissed without applying a cement pack or other medication.

He was seen again one week later, and he reported that he had had no postoperative pain or swelling and little discomfort. The tissue was fully healed, normal in tone and contour (Case Fig. 9–1*D*), and the slightly concave interproximal papilla was tightly reattached.

It is interesting to note that postoperative requirements following orthodontic surgery are variable. If the surgery is limited to one or more isolated areas, surgical cement packs are usually unnecessary. But if the gingival proliferation is widespread and the surgery extensive, application of surgical cement packs is advantageous. Cement packs are especially useful when the gingivae are friable and bleed profusely even when surgery is performed with the electrocoagulating current.

Orthodontic appliances require protection from the cement packs to prevent damage or distortion when the cement is removed. If adhesive dryfoil is carefully adapted around the teeth, brackets and archwires, the cement will not adhere and can be removed easily. If the cement is stiffly mixed and tightly adapted and molded against the teeth and dryfoil it usually adheres well.

Orthodontic surgical procedures are usually remarkably free from postoperative pain and swelling and, as a rule, healing is rapid and without incident. After the initial tissue healing, use of the salt-alum astringent mouthwash helps to tan and toughen the tissues. Use of the toothbrush as a gum brush, and of the rubber stimulator, should be encouraged and prescribed to massage the gingivae and clean the teeth as an aid in maintaining the integrity of the gingivae against further degeneration.

FRENECTOMY — FRENOTOMY

The frenectomy is one of those surgical procedures that are entirely adjunctive to the needs and problems of the other disciplines. Thus the basic technique of the electrosurgical frenectomy-frenotomy developed by the author is the same no matter for which discipline it is being performed. But the problems the frenal fibers create in the various disciplines do vary, often substantially, and these problems often necessitate variations in the specific instrumentation they require.

Maxillary labial frenectomy for orthodontic purposes is no exception to this. Usually the frenum in these cases extends from the labial aspect through the median embrasure and terminates at the anterior border of the nasopalatine papilla, creating a diastema. If the frenum is in the form of a broad band, the diastema is usually quite wide. To remove the frenum for orthodontic purposes it is necessary to excise the fibers through the embrasure and from the nasopalatine papilla without injury to the latter. The surgical specifics involved in the frenectomy-frenotomy procedure will be reviewed in detail in the chapter on oral surgery and will not be elaborated here. However, the differences between this technique and the traditional steel scalpel excision are of special importance here. When the frenectomy is done with the steel scalpel, the cut tissue flares apart widely and there is profuse and persistent bleeding. When the electrosurgical excision is performed the tissues do not pull apart to the same extent, and there is little or no bleeding. But most important from the orthodontic standpoint is the electrosurgical healing with soft, supple tissue that is normal in all respects as contrasted to the mass of scar tissue that characterizes the repair tissue from the steel-scalpel surgery, which usually interferes with the orthodontic treatment and can disrupt the alignment of the teeth after the appliances are removed. The retention of control over lip movement with the electrosurgical procedure, which is usually lost or markedly impaired with the traditional steel-scalpel excision, is a very worthwhile additional benefit.

The following case offers an excellent demonstration of the advantages derived from orthodontic electrosurgical frenectomy.

CASE 10

PATIENT.   An 8-year-old white female child.

HISTORY.   She had a very wide frenum and a wide space between her upper centrals. Many of her teeth were badly aligned and her mother was informed by her dentist that she required orthodontic treatment. An orthodontist was consulted, and he came to the conclusion that unless it was removed the frenum would interfere with his treatment, particularly since he had had previous patients treated by the electrosurgical procedure and knew that no complicating postoperative scar tissue developed from this technique. He referred her to the author for the frenectomy.

CLINICAL EXAMINATION.   The maxillary teeth were incompletely erupted, and a very wide band of frenal fibers that extended through the embrasure, creating a wide diastema (Case Fig. 10–1A) coalesced with the nasopalatine papilla at its anterior border. The areolar portion of the frenum was particularly wide and flowed into the ventral surface of the lip.

TREATMENT.   Infiltration anesthesia was administered labially and palatally. The upper lip was lifted upward and outward. The frenal fibers were pulled into taut outline by this and clamped close to the ventral surface of the lip with a curved mosquito hemostat. A 45-degree-angle fine needle electrode was used to incise the frenum, following the outline of the fibers. The incision was extended to the junction with the nasopalatine papilla, where it was dissected away without invading the papilla. The tissue on the external part of the clamp was dissected away with the same

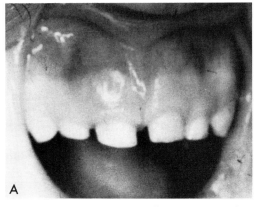 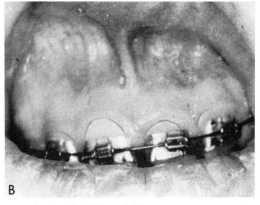

Case Figure 10–1.   A, Preoperative: A very wide band of frenal fibers is present in the maxilla between the two central incisors. The fibers extend around to the anterior border of the nasopalatine papilla, creating a wide diastema between the two teeth. B, Postoperative: Appearance two years later. The attached alveolar portion has been eliminated, without scar tissue repair, and the aureolar portion has been retained for control of lip movement. Orthodontic bands and a labial arch bar are present, for orthodontic realignment of the teeth.

electrode, which was then used rapidly to score the fibers in the median suture line by making momentary contact with the bone and following it with at least 5-second rest periods to prevent overheating the bone. Bleeding was induced in the alveolar portion of the wound after the areolar part was sutured with interrupted silk sutures. Tincture of myrrh and benzoin was applied and the patient was told to return on the fifth postoperative day. When she returned the tissues showed evidence of primary healing. The sutures were removed, and tincture of myrrh and benzoin was reapplied. Within three weeks complete healing was noted. The healed tissue was normal in all respects and there was no scar tissue present. The areolar portion of the frenum was present and also appeared to be healing well. The patient was instructed to return to the orthodontist. She was seen again periodically; the last photograph was taken two years postoperatively. At that time the teeth, fully erupted and banded, were in relatively normal alignment, and the diastema in the midline was closed. There was no clinical evidence of where the attached alveolar portion of the frenum had been, but the areolar portion was much in evidence and performing its function of controlling the lip movements (Case Fig. 10–1*B*).

FOOTNOTE REFERENCES

1. Thoma, K. H.: Oral Surgery. Vol. I, St. Louis, C. V. Mosby Co., 1948, pp. 332–336.
2. Gottlieb, B.: Timely removal of obstacles against the eruption of permanent teeth. Am. J. Orthodont. & Oral Surg., *31*:42–44, 1945.
3. Mershon, J. V., and Gunter, J. H.: Management of unerupted and impacted canines. J.A.D.A., *27*:1436–1439, 1940.
4. Taylor, K. E.: A safe and simple method of operating on and elevating impacted canines. Internat. J. Orthodont. & Den. Child., *20*:352–355, 1934.
5. Sippel, H. E.: Method of uncovering impacted canines and attachments used. Internat. J. Orthodont. & Den. Child., *19*:512–516, 1933.
6. Salzmann, J. A.: Principles of Orthodontics. 2nd ed. Philadelphia, J. B. Lippincott Co., 1950, pp. 671–675.
7. Strock, M. S.: A new approach to the unerupted tooth by surgery and orthodontics. Am. J. Orthodont. & Oral Surg., *24*:626–634, 1938.

Chapter Seventeen

TECHNIQUES ADJUNCTIVE TO TREATMENT IN CLEFT PALATE AND COMPARABLE ABNORMALITIES

Cleft palate surgeons are among the best trained personnel in the medical profession. Their skills are fully comparable to the skills of the cardiac surgeon, neurosurgeon, or vascular surgeon. Thus, the massive cicatricial scar tissue repair of their cleft palate surgery attests visually to the nature of the tissue repair that results from "traditional" cold-steel surgery, despite the skills of the surgeon, and offers a dramatic contrast to the soft, supple, normal tissue repair following electrosurgery.

The contrast will be especially dramatic in one of the cases that will be reviewed here. The author has designed a cheek-lip retractor that he has used in almost every case presented here (Fig. 17–1). It is made in three sizes: a child size, a medium adult size, and a large adult size. In this particular case, although the patient was a full grown 16-year-old youth, it was impossible to insert even the small child size retractor, which is used for 2- and 3-year-old patients, because of the constriction of the lips due to scar tissue adhesions. Needless to say, the inability to retract the lips and cheeks impaired the efficiency and speed of treatment substantially.

This case will also show, however, that the rate and quality of tissue repair is strongly influenced by the health of the tissues, even in electrosurgery. The retarded rate of repair of tissue that was preoperatively subnormal in tone as contrasted to the rate and quality of repair of tissue that was normal preoperatively attests to the need to improve the tissue tone as much as is possible before electrosurgery is instituted.

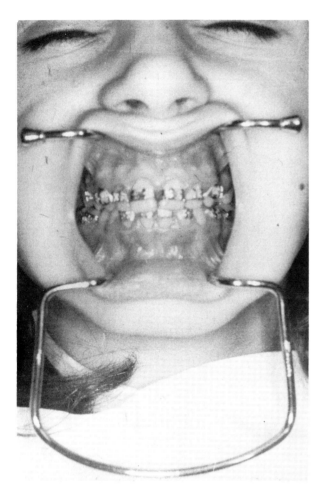

Figure 17-1. Self-retaining cheek-lip retractor designed by the author.

This next case demonstrates admirably the rapid and favorable tissue response to electrosection, despite adverse operating conditions. Much more important, however, is the clinical evidence it demonstrates of the influence of the preoperative tissue tone on the postoperative repair. This is evidenced by the contrast between the rate and quality of tissue repair of all the tissues that were relatively normal in tone preoperatively and that of the tissue around the maxillary left cuspid, which was inflamed and slightly proliferative preoperatively.

CASE 1

This case presented another example of the usefulness of electrosurgery in treatment of orthodontic problems created by cleft palate deformities. It is noteworthy that in many of the cleft palate patients the orthodontic treatment is not really definitive but merely a means to an end, the necessary preliminary that sets the stage for the ultimate definitive treatment—use of the orthodontically realigned teeth as anchor abutments for fixed prostheses that rehabilitate the dental handicaps and greatly improve the aesthetics.

In this case, the exposure and orthodontic movement of the unerupted tooth and realignment of the rotated central incisors served as the necessary preliminary step toward fabrication of an effective fixed prosthesis that created a functionally effective and aesthetically harmonious maxillary dental arch.

PATIENT. A 15-year-old white male.

HISTORY. The patient had had a cleft lip-palate surgical repair performed in infancy. The cosmetic result of the lip surgery was poor, and the functional result of the palatal repair was even more unsatisfactory. The posterior cleft of the soft palate had been only partially closed, and much of the palatal tissue was tough, fibrous, contractile white scar tissue. He was referred from the Cleft Palate Center for exposure of a cuspid tooth retained in the line of cleft, of which only the extreme tip was visible. The tooth had to be fully exposed to permit its movement orthodontically into the dental arch so that it could ultimately be used as an abutment for a fixed splint.

CLINICAL EXAMINATION. *Extraoral.* The lip was disfigured and off center due to a scar from the early repair.

Intraoral. An anterior cleft and a cleft in the soft palate were visible. The anterior cleft was unilateral and had not been subjected to surgical intervention. The cleft in the soft palate appeared as a rounded opening surrounded by very dense greyish white scar tissue. The tip of the cuspid was just visible at the disto-incisal angle of the anterior cleft (Case Fig. 1–1) and appeared partially decalcified and possibly slightly decayed.

The patient was wearing a removable appliance which fitted over the cleft and

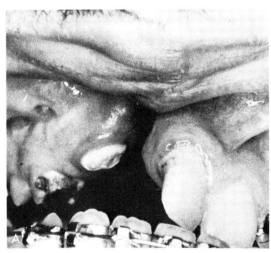 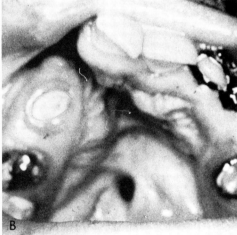

Case Figure 1–1. Exposure of an unerupted cuspid in the line of a maxillary cleft. *A*, Preoperative: only about 3 mm. of the decalcified tip of the maxillary right cuspid is visible. Between this tooth and the rotated central there is a wide cleft in the maxilla. The tissue in the cleft is atonal and appears somewhat engorged, and a similar thick roll of gingival tissue forms a band around the cusp. *B*, Ventral view of the palate reveals the extent of the cleft, and a remnant of cleft posteriorly where cleft palate surgery had been performed in infancy. The palatal mucosa is a mass of avascular scar tissue. It is obvious that free bleeding would cause a serious problem in this patient. The decalcified tip of the cuspid can be seen near the cleft.

the malposed unerupted tooth. The tissue immediately surrounding the tooth was hypertrophic and hyperemic and seemed to be deposited around it in concentric layers.

Orthodontic treatment had progressed to the stage of readiness to institute traction to bring the unerupted tooth into relatively normal alignment. This was to be done so that it could be utilized for the fixed prosthesis which was to bridge the cleft and lock the alveolar parts together.

TREATMENT. The mouth was prepared for surgery and infiltration anesthesia was administered. A flame-shaped loop electrode was selected and current output set at 6 for electrosection. The electrode was used with short brushing strokes to shave the mucosa in layers from around the exposed cuspid tip. When most of the crown was exposed, a medium-sized U-shaped loop electrode was substituted and used to bevel the newly created marginal gingiva to a feather edge. Then a small, narrow 45-degree-angle U-shaped loop electrode was substituted, cutting current reduced to 4, and the palatal, mesial and distal areas and gingival margin created around the newly exposed cuspid crown.

On the palatal aspect, in order to fully expose the crown and avoid creating a sharp undercut of gingival mucosa, a wide surface of the palatal mucosa had to be reduced gradually from approximately 1 cm. beyond the tooth and sloping gradually toward it. The entire operative procedure was performed without bleeding. After the crown of the tooth was fully exposed, a marginal crevice was created by electrocoagulation with a solid conical electrode, tincture of myrrh and benzoin was applied to the area in air-dried layers and the operative field was covered with a thin coating of the adhesive ointment dressing. The patient was instructed in postoperative care and reappointed.

He returned on the fifth postoperative day and reported that there had been no swelling and only slight discomfort on the first postoperative day. The tissues appeared to be healing very satisfactorily (Case Fig. 1–2), but a small area of the gingival mucosa appeared to be creeping down slightly on the medial aspect of the exposed crown. This regenerating excess was very superficial and confined to the area of the gingival crevice. The tissue was dried and anointed with topical anesthetic for 2 minutes. Then the excess was removed by electrocoagulation with a narrow U-shaped loop electrode and biterminal coagulating current intensity set at 4. Less than a 1 mm. rim of tissue was removed with the loop. Tincture of myrrh and benzoin was applied and the patient was told to return in a week. When he returned, the healing was much more advanced. He returned again for a final checkup two weeks later. When he was seen at that time, the gingival tissue around the tooth was fully healed and in excellent tone. The full crown of the tooth was normally exposed, and an orthodontic band had been cemented onto it.

The nature and location of the surgical area in this case created several special requirements. Due to the densely fibrous scarlike quality of most of the mucosa covering this tooth, a slightly higher than usual intensity of current output was required to assure that the electrosection would be performed cleanly. Cutting current output, therefore, was increased by 1 on the selector dial.

Due to the location of the unerupted tooth in the line of cleft and the amount and texture of the tissue that had to be removed in order to fully expose the crown of this tooth, it was far simpler to remove the undesirable tis-

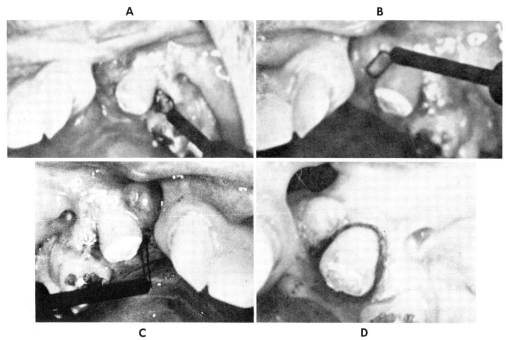

Case Figure 1–2.   Exposing an unerupted permanent cuspid, malposed and in the line of cleft of a unilateral anterior cleft palate, for use as an abutment for a fixed prosthesis to span the gap. *A,* Crown of the tooth exposed with flame-shaped loop electrode. *B,* Tough fibrous tissue on the medial aspect from the cleft planed with medium-sized U-shaped loop electrode by shaving the tissue in thin layers to bevel the tissue to a feather edge. *C,* The tissue has been resected to fully expose the entire crown of the tooth. A 90-degree-angle, narrow, U-shaped loop electrode is being used to create a sulcus around the tooth in a manner similar to that for creating a subgingival trough around a preparation. Note that the dissection is carried into the line of cleft with impunity. *D,* Gingival crevice completed around crown of fully exposed tooth. Note that the procedure was bloodless.

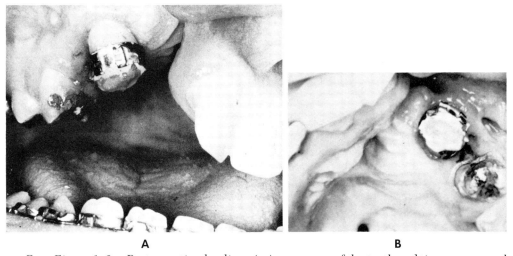

Case Figure 1–3.   Postoperative healing. *A,* Appearance of the tooth and tissues one week later, immediately after insertion of the orthodontic band. Note the normal gingival contour and the excellent tissue tone and degree of healing that has taken place. *B,* Palatal view of tissues at that time. Healing appears complete.

sue by shaving it off in layers by electrosection than to attempt its resection with cold-steel instrumentation. It also assured more harmonious contour of the gingival architecture around the tooth, and—probably most important of all—being bloodless, it eliminated the complication of having blood flow into the clefts, a potential complication when cold-steel surgery is performed in such an area.

CASE 2

This case is an example of the complex orthodontic problems created by cleft palate deformities and the usefulness of electrosurgery under adverse anatomic and orthodontic conditions.

PATIENT. A 16-year-old white male.

HISTORY. The patient had had a cleft lip-palate plastic repair performed in infancy. He had a floating premaxilla, and further plastic surgery at the Mt. Sinai Hospital Cleft Palate Center was planned for him.

A surgical splint was planned for immediate use to immobilize the parts preoperatively. It was necessary to elongate the clinical crowns of several banded and partially erupted teeth in order to provide sufficient space for the clasps of this splint. He was referred for electrosurgical elongation of these teeth.

CLINICAL EXAMINATION. *Extraoral.* There was a noticeable scar in the midline of his lip extending from the columella to the vermilion border.

Intraoral. There was a bilateral cleft with a wide diastema between the normally erupted left central incisor and the partially erupted, malformed, incompletely developed right central incisor. Both lateral incisors were missing and the cuspids were only partially erupted (Case Fig. 2–1). Orthodontic bands were present on all the fully erupted teeth except the left central.

Roentgenographic examination with an occlusal-view film revealed that the premaxilla was attached to the main body of the maxilla by a slender bony stem. His orthodontic problem was further complicated by an open bite with Class III prognathism.

TREATMENT. The mouth was prepared for surgery and infiltration anesthesia was administered. A narrow 45-degree-angle U-shaped loop electrode was selected and current output was set at 4.5 for electrosection. The surgery was begun at the left cuspid where approximately 3 mm. of the labial marginal gingiva was resected with short wiping strokes. Current output was increased to 5 and the labial marginal mucosa was resected from the three banded teeth with a slightly larger electrode of similar shape. The new marginal gingivae were then beveled to feather edges with a flame-shaped loop electrode and current intensity was set at 6.

The current intensity was then further increased to 7 and the same loop electrode was used to resect the palatal marginal mucosa from the teeth and bands and from the cuspid. After the height of the gingival margins had been raised approximately 3 mm. above the orthodontic bands, they were beveled to feather edges on the palatal aspect with the same electrode.

These tissues were dried and tincture of myrrh and benzoin was applied in air-dried layers as a protective coating. The electrosurgical procedure was then repeated on the right side. The narrow loop electrode was selected and current output reset at 4.5. After infiltration anesthesia was administered, 3 mm. of the marginal gingivae was removed from the labial aspects of the defective central, the bicuspids and first molar.

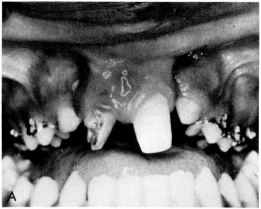
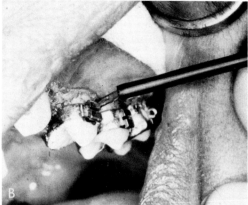
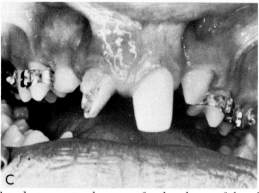

Case Figure 2–1. Resection of redundant tissue from orthodontic bands and teeth. *A,* Preoperative: There is a bilateral cleft palate with a floating premaxilla. The laterals are missing in the lines of cleft, and the incisal third of the crowns of the cuspids is exposed. The centrals diverge and the right central is rotated and badly decayed. All the posterior teeth bear orthodontic bands, and the gingival tissue has proliferated downward to cover most of the metal. *B,* The gingivae have been resected from the metal bands and the teeth beyond the bands to create clearance for the clasps of the obturator that is to be fabricated for this patient. The amount of tissue that has been removed is marked by the discoloration on the metal bands marking the former level of the tissue. The resection is being performed with a medium-width, straight, U-shaped loop electrode. Since contact of the activated electrode against the metal and teeth is only momentary, with a rapid brushing stroke, and adequate time is allowed between reapplications to prevent a cumulative heat effect, no damage is done to either teeth or investing structures. *C,* Appearance of the mouth one week later. Note the tissue tone and the degree of healing, both sure indications that no damage to teeth or tissues resulted from the instrumentation.

The flame-shaped electrode was substituted, current output increased to 6, and the new gingival margins were beveled to feather edges.

The right cuspid was a retained deciduous tooth and its root was considerably resorbed. The crown of this tooth was therefore not elongated. The palatal aspects of the teeth were treated in the same manner as on the right side. The entire electrosurgical procedure was virtually bloodless, and there did not appear to be need for protective surgical cement packs. Tincture of myrrh and benzoin applied in multiple air-dried layers was the only postoperative protection afforded the operative field. The patient was instructed in postoperative care and was reappointed.

He returned one week later, and healing was found to be progressing splendidly. Most of the thin surface coagulum had already peeled away and been replaced with normally epithelialized gingivae. The few isolated patches of coagulum still present were thin and healthy looking. The mouth was irrigated with Kasdenol solution and tincture of myrrh and benzoin was reapplied in air-dried layers. The patient was instructed to use the astringent salt-alum lavage and was reappointed. He returned again one week later, at which time the healing appeared virtually complete and the gingival re-epithelialization matured. The tissue tone was excellent.

Because contact of the activated electrode against metal tends to produce sparking, resection of marginal gingivae that encroach and overlap the typical orthodontic band creates a special challenge. Excessive sparking can be avoided in two ways. One is to avoid dehydrating the tissues, and the other is to exercise great care to make the initial electrode contact against only the tissue, and to continue the application with a very short light stroke so that if contact with the metal is inevitable it will be extremely slight and momentary.

In this case, resecting the tissue from around the partially erupted cuspid and deformed central created an additional hazard, since most of the tissue involved was a continuation of the fibrous scar tissue present in the bilateral clefts. It was necessary to remove some of this scar tissue right down to the bony margins of the clefts without injuring either the bone, teeth or tissues. In view of the densely fibrous nature of this tissue and its limited blood supply, the rate and quality of tissue repair obtained in this case was all the more remarkable.

CASE 3

PATIENT. A 16-year-old white male with marked disfigurement of the upper lip and deformity of the maxilla.

HISTORY. Plastic surgery had been performed for him in infancy for a columellar repair of midline cleft in the upper lip and a pharyngeal repair of an extensive cleft in the palate extending the full length of the hard palate and a considerable portion of the soft palate. The operation had failed to close the palatal defect completely.

CLINICAL EXAMINATION. The columellar repair had resulted in total obliteration of the labial vestibule in the anterior region caused by scar tissue adhesions. The avascular, fibrous, and cicatricial palatal repair had exerted so much tension on the palatal bone that it had caused a collapse of the hard palate, which was malformed into a V-shape with the apex of the V in the midline and inclined superiorly toward the base of the nose (Case Fig. 3–1).

A number of teeth were missing in the maxilla, apparently owing to anodontia, since no teeth had been extracted. These included the right third and second molars and cuspid, the left central and lateral incisors, and the second and third molars.

The right central was peg-shaped and malposed superiorly. A decayed fragment of retained root of the deciduous lateral incisor was present, but there was no evidence of a permanent lateral in the jaw, which was apparently congenitally missing. The left central and lateral incisors were also missing. The cuspid, peg-shaped, was malposed in the central incisor position in the arch and was displaced superiorly. The marginal gingiva around this tooth was puffy, inflamed in appearance, and slightly proliferative. The second and third molars were missing. The gingivae around all the other teeth in the maxilla were normal in tone.

TREATMENT. This was the only patient for whom the author's lip-cheek retractor could not be used, because the cicatricial contraction of the scar tissue adhesions of the upper lip and collapsed maxillary arch made the mouth opening too small and taut to permit insertion of the appliance.

Scar tissue adhesions of the lip to the gingival mucosa restricted the mouth opening and made instrumentation awkward and difficult to perform as rapidly as is con-

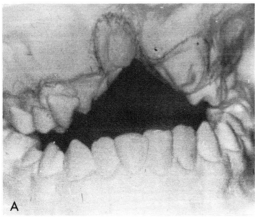

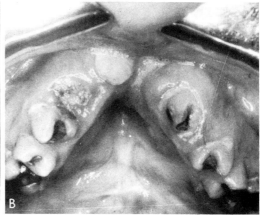

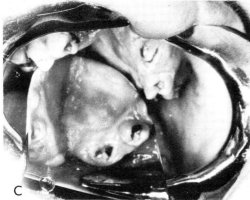

Case Figure 3–1. Elongation of clinical crowns for orthodontic banding in a deformed maxilla. *A,* Stone models of preoperative condition. The amount of tissue estimated to be excised is outlined on the maxilla. *B,* Preoperative: Cleft palate pharyngeal surgery had been performed in infancy. Scar tissue repair from the steel-scalpel surgery created so great a contractile traction that the maxilla is collapsed into a V shape, with the apex of the V facing outward. There is a fragment of retained root of a deciduous cuspid in the right quadrant and a malposed central-incisor. The left central and right and left laterals are missing from the dental arch, and the left cuspid is badly deformed. The gingival tissue around the retained cuspid deciduous root is engorged and proliferative, and so is that around the left cuspid to a slightly lesser degree. *C,* Mirror image view of the palatal deformity, a broad band of avascular scar tissue that appears dark and engorged in the black and white photograph.

sistent with good instrumentation. Very limited, inadequate lip and cheek retraction was obtained with two conventional half round retractors.

A flame-shaped loop electrode was selected, cutting current output was set at 4.5, and the activated electrode was used to elongate the clinical crowns and to create a relatively uniform gingival level in lieu of the very uneven gingival level present preoperatively.

The scar tissue adhesion of the inner aspect of the upper lip created the marginal labial tissue for the right central incisor, with a total absence of normal gingival mucosa. A J-loop electrode was used, with current reduced to 3.5, to create an equivalent of a normal crevicular sulcus to ease the tight attachment of the lip as much as possible without loop excision of the vestibular scar tissue, which was specifically ruled out by the Plastic Surgery Department.

The labial-buccal elongation having been completed, the instrumentation was reinstituted with the flame-shaped loop and current was set at 5 to elongate the palatal aspects, so that orthodontic bands could be inserted on all the teeth without impinging on their investing gingivae. The retained lateral root fragment was then extracted by lifting the shallow fragment from the tissues with a surgical curet, leaving a slightly depressed raw surface, with practically no free bleeding. Tincture of myrrh and benzoin was then applied to the surgical field in air-dried layers, and the patient was reappointed for the following week.

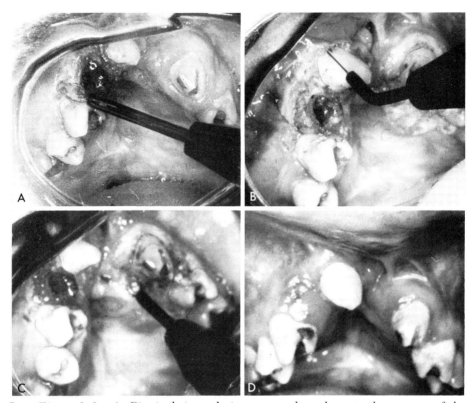

Case Figure 3–2. *A,* Gingival tissue being resected to elongate the crowns of the posterior teeth. Note the difference in color of the newly exposed tooth surfaces, which provide evidence of the 0.5 to 1.0 cm. of tissue that had to be removed. *B,* The scar tissue adhesions resulting from the columellar repair of the cleft lip have eliminated the vestibular space over the right central, and the internal mucosa of the upper lip is attached to the tooth, allowing no free movement of the upper lip. A subgingival trough is being created with a J-loop electrode to create a substitute gingival sulcus and free the tissues approximately 1.5 mm. by doing so. *C,* The retained root fragment of deciduous cuspid has been extracted. It was so shallow and frail that it really was not an extraction, but rather, the fragment was elevated and removed with a surgical-curet with no effort. The gingiva around the deformed left cuspid is being recontoured. The gingivoplasty is being performed with a flame-shaped loop electrode in an attempt to increase the clinical length of the crowns to a reasonably uniform level to improve aesthetics. *D,* Postoperative appearance one week later. Note the remarkable rate and quality of tissue repair around the posterior teeth and the right central incisor in contrast to the rate of repair of the very insignificant root fragment removal that is, nevertheless, a traumatic procedure. It is especially noteworthy that the only gingival tissue treated that is not healing as fast or as well as the marginal gingivae is the marginal gingiva of the left cuspid, *where the tissue tone was subnormal preoperatively.* The rate and quality of tissue repair around this tooth is much more comparable to that of the extraction site than to that of the gingivoplasty site. This underlines the importance of normal gingival tone when electrosurgery must be performed, especially for subgingival troughing in crown and bridge.

When the patient returned one week later, the gingival tissue around all the teeth except the right cuspid appeared fully healed and normal in tone. The extraction site was incompletely healed, and the tissue around the cuspid was also incompletely healed, with inflammatory proliferation on the mesial aspect, where the preoperative inflammation had been most notable.

This marked difference in healing between the normal and subnormal gingival tissues and the similarity between the rate and quality of repair of the subnormal tissue and that of a traumatic wound provide persuasive evidence of the atraumatic nature of electrosection and the importance of restoring the tissue tone to as close to normal as possible before instituting electrosurgery.

CASE 4

This case offers another example of anatomic deformities of the alveolar ridges and their soft tissue attachments which are so often concomitant to cleft palate incidence and complicate orthodontic therapy. It is also an excellent example of the usefulness of the pushback, a procedure usually associated with periodontal and prosthetic surgery. In this case a pushback was required in order to construct a buccal vestibule so that maxillary archbar traction could be instituted.

PATIENT. An 11-year-old white male.

HISTORY. The patient was under active treatment at the hospital Cleft Palate Center and Orthodontia Clinic. Attempts to insert a maxillary archbar were unsuccessful because of lack of vestibular space on the right side. Each time the bar was inserted it cut into the tissues and stimulated massive proliferation of hypertrophic tissue accompanied by massive edema and free bleeding. He was referred for vestibulotomy to deepen the buccal vestibule.

CLINICAL EXAMINATION. *Extraoral.* His face had a pinched, birdlike appearance.

Intraoral. There was a huge open defect involving most of the palatal vault (Case Fig. 4–1). There was some alveolar deformity and the alignment of his teeth was disrupted, with many teeth missing from the dental arch. Muscle bands and the buccal mucosa were attached to the gingival mucosa only 2 to 3 mm. beyond the necks of the teeth (Case Fig. 4–2). A large mound of hypertrophic tissue also partially obliterated the vestibular space. Since it covered a malposed unerupted tooth, resection of this mass would not increase the vestibular space.

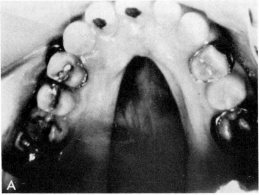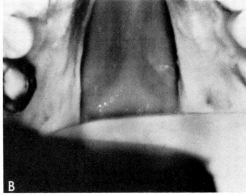

Case Figure 4–1. Palatal view of the enormous cleft of hard and soft palate. Note: the tongue blade being used to hold down the tongue blocks off the posterior extent of the cleft from view.

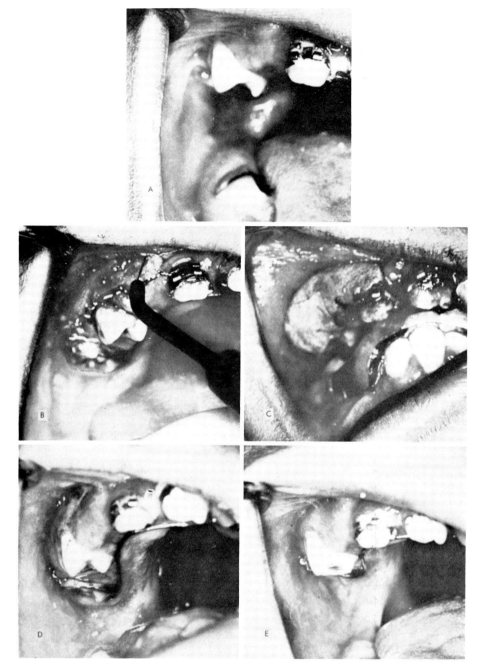

Case Figure 4–2. Pushback to increase height of vestibular fornix for insertion of maxillary archbar. *A*, Preoperative view. Vestibule obliterated by low muscle attachments and soft tissue mass. *B*, Incision posteroanteriorly with 45-degree-angle fine needle electrode. Note chain of stainless steel ligature wire loops for anchorage of cement pack. *C*, Cement pack inserted to serve as surgical stent. *D*, Appearance of tissue on fifth postoperative day immediately after removal of cement pack. Note well-defined vestibule. *E*, Appearance of tissue three weeks postoperatively. Note normal vestibular height. Tissue is fully healed and tone is excellent.

TREATMENT. The mouth was prepared and anesthetized by infiltration. A fine 45-degree-angle needle electrode was selected and current output set at 3 for electrosection. The incision to sever muscle attachments and low ridge of soft tissue was made close to the alveolar ridge and extended from the tuberosity to the lateral incisor area. The buccal mucosa was pushed upward by blunt dissection. Several fibrous strands required dissection with the needle electrode to free the tissue and complete its displacement. The incision was almost bloodless except for a surface ooze.

The vestibular space having been created, it would have to be maintained to keep the tissues from reattaching. Since no appliance was available for use as a stent, a surgical cement pack would have to serve in its place. In order to provide anchorage for the cement pack and prevent its displacement, a strand of stainless steel ligature wire was twisted to form a chain of loops. This had been preoperatively attached to the orthodontic bands on the molar and the lateral. A stiff mix of surgical cement was packed against this chain and up into the vestibular space, and the patient was given the usual postoperative instructions.

He returned on the sixth postoperative day and reported considerable edema, a trace of which was still present, but no pain. The cement pack was removed, the area irrigated, and the tissues inspected. Healing was progressing very well. All but a small round area was covered with a thin layer of coagulum, and the vestibular space was very well defined.

Chromic acid, 0.5 per cent, was applied for 30 seconds to the raw surface, washed away, and tincture of myrrh and benzoin was applied in air-dried layers. The vestibule was filled with Kenalog in Orabase in lieu of the cement pack. Healing progressed rapidly and uneventfully. In less than three weeks the tissues were fully healed; within six weeks, orthodontic treatment with a maxillary archbar was resumed without eliciting unfavorable reactions.

CASE 5

Abnormal growth of the face and anomalies of the teeth and oral structures often create local operative handicaps.[1-9] Anomalies particularly likely to create surgical handicaps are micrognathia and microglossia. This case is an example of inherent electrosurgical advantages that helped permit efficient orthodontic surgery despite the severe handicaps imposed by these anatomic abnormalities.

PATIENT. An 8-year-old black female.

HISTORY. The patient was at the Orthodontia Clinic of the Mt. Sinai Hospital in New York City. She was referred to the Oral Surgery Clinic for elongation of the clinical crowns of markedly malposed mandibular teeth in order to permit insertion of orthodontic bands, which were necessary to institute orthodontic movement for correction of the malocclusion and expansion of her mandibular arch.

It was the consensus of opinion of those concerned on the Orthodontia Clinic staff that her orthodontic problem had resulted from congenital micrognathia and microglossia.* These anatomic malformations created operative handicaps that made instrumentation with cold steel impractical and virtually impossible to perform effectively.

The Oral Surgery Clinic armamentarium did not include any electrosurgical equipment. Electrosurgical elongation of the clinical crowns of her teeth was performed at the author's office.

CLINICAL EXAMINATION. *Extraoral.* The patient had the classic bird-like face associated with micrognathia (Case Fig. 5–1).

Intraoral. The maxilla was normal in size, but owing to the micrognathia it appeared abnormally large. A mixed dentition was present in the dental arches. The tongue was a rudimentary, diminutive, prehensile organ and could not be thrust forward more than a few millimeters. She was unable to accomplish even that much without elevating the entire floor of the mouth. When the forward thrust was attempted the tongue deviated toward the left side. She was able also to drop the tongue backward to completely occlude the oropharynx without apparent discomfort (Case Fig. 5–2). Her speech was defective.

The mandibular teeth posterior to the cuspid bilaterally were tilted lingually at an approximate 30-degree angle toward the midline. As a result of the marked tilt the

---

*It is likely that the microglossia was the underlying cause. Lack of muscular tongue thrust against the mandibular alveolar ridges may have been the cause or a major factor in the failure of the mandible to develop normally, thus leading to collapse of the dental arch and tooth alignment.

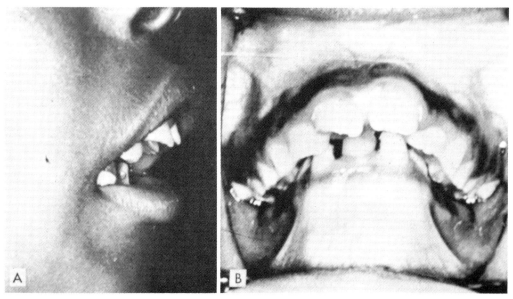

Case Figure 5–1. A, Micrognathia and microglossia. Extraoral photograph shows typical bird-like appearance of the face. B, Frontal view of closed mouth shows disproportion between respective sizes of normal-size maxilla and diminutive mandible.

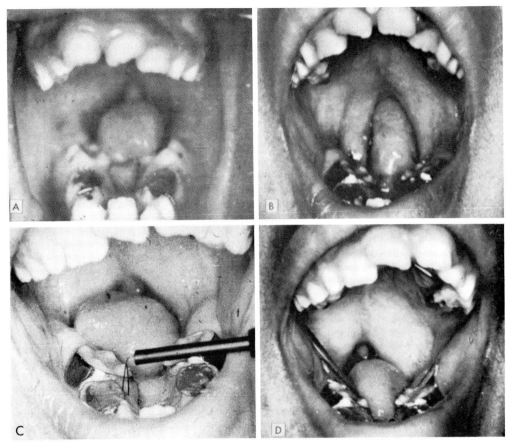

Case Figure 5–2. *A*, Intraoral view of mandibular teeth shows mixed dentition. Mandibular arch extremely narrow, and teeth tilted medially to further reduce the tongue space. Gingival mucosa reaches the occlusal surfaces of the molars on lingual aspect. *B*, Tongue drops back into oropharynx, causing the tissues of the floor of the mouth to be elevated almost to the occlusal surfaces of the teeth. *C*, Clinical crown of deciduous molar being elongated with long narrow loop electrode on lingual aspect. *D*, Orthodontic elastic band traction instituted after the teeth were banded.

gingival mucosa on the lingual aspects of these teeth virtually covered all but 1 to 2 mm. of the crowns. Furthermore, at the deciduous first molars, which were restored with large occlusal amalgam fillings, the gingival margins were flush with the occlusal surfaces of the teeth.

The deciduous molars were still firmly embedded. The treatment plan provided for utilization of all these teeth in the orthodontic movement. The surgical plan, therefore, was to elongate the permanent first molar crowns first, band them, and then elongate the crowns of the deciduous molars so that they could be banded and utilized pending eruption of the bicuspids and permanent cuspids.

TREATMENT.   The mouth was prepared for surgery and infiltration anesthesia administered. A narrow right-angle U-shaped loop electrode was selected and cutting current was set at 4.5 for electrosection. The electrode was applied to the mucosa around the two permanent molars with rotary brushing strokes until their crowns were fully exposed. The procedure was entirely bloodless. Tincture of myrrh and benzoin was applied in air-dried layers. Then the patient was given instructions in postoperative care and told to return after the orthodontic bands had been inserted.

She returned one week later. The mouth was prepared and anesthetized in the same manner as on the previous visit. The narrowest long, right-angle U-shaped loop electrode available was selected and used with the cutting current to loop off the marginal and cemental gingivae from the deciduous molars. Topical application of tincture of myrrh and benzoin was again the only medication or dressing applied, since the patient had reported that she had not had appreciable discomfort from the previous surgery. At this point the patient was referred back to the Orthodontia Clinic.

The newly elongated crowns were banded, as was the right central incisor, and orthodontic movement was begun. As the deciduous teeth were lost and the permanent teeth erupted, these too were fully exposed, banded, and intermaxillary elastic band traction was instituted.

Shortly thereafter the left cuspid became partially erupted, with approximately one third of the clinical crown of the tooth exposed (Case Fig. 5–3). Since this tooth was important to the orthodontic treatment, elongation of the clinical crown to permit banding was immediately instituted.

The mouth was prepared for surgery in the usual manner and infiltration anesthesia administered. A narrow U-shaped loop electrode similar to the one previously employed was selected and the cutting current set at 4.5. The gingival mucosa around the lingual aspect of the partially erupted tooth was removed in layers by shaving with short brushing strokes. In order to accomplish this in the narrow confines of the collapsed mandibular arch, the loop had to be held vertically parallel with the long axis of the tooth.

After the lingual portion of the crown was sufficiently elongated, the loop was applied to the new gingival margin at a 45-degree angle and used to bevel the tissue to a feather-edged margin. Cutting current output was increased to 6, and the labial aspect of the tooth was exposed with a flame-shaped loop electrode used in a similar manner, so that as the crown was being elongated the feather-edged margin was being created simultaneously. When the full clinical crown of the tooth was uniformly exposed, the mucosa was painted with tincture of myrrh and benzoin applied in air-dried layers, postoperative instructions were repeated, and the patient was reappointed for the following week.

When she returned the gingivae were found to be almost completely healed. The mouth was irrigated and tincture of myrrh and benzoin applied; she was told to return again in one week. At her next visit the tissues appeared fully healed and no further postoperative treatment was required.

Three years after her orthodontic treatment had been begun the patient was ready to enter the final phase of her treatment; the lateral movement of her mandibular second molars, which were now medial to the rest of her dentition.

Both teeth would have to have bands applied, but the distal half of the crown of each tooth was covered with a large mass of hyperplastic redundant tissue that resembled a greatly enlarged operculum of a third molar (Case Fig. 5–3D). This would have to be removed surgically in order to insert the bands.

The right molar was treated first. An inferior alveolar-lingual block was administered and a large guillotine type of loop electrode was selected. The tissue on this side appeared relatively normal in tone and texture and it was removed with this elec-

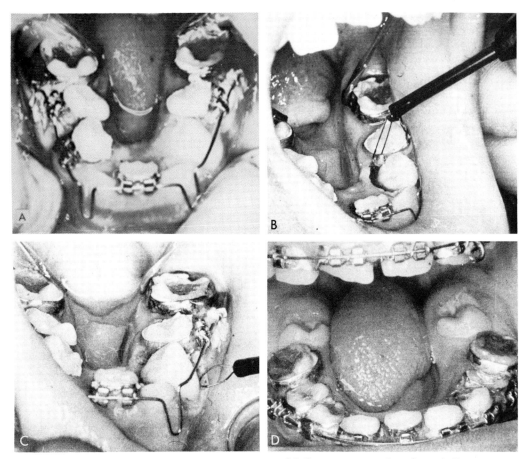

Case Figure 5–3. Exposing permanent cuspid fully to permit its banding. *A*, Preoperative view of tooth beginning to erupt. *B*, Lingual surface of tooth exposed with narrow U-shaped loop electrode. *C*, Buccal surface of tooth fully exposed with flame-shaped loop electrode. Crown of tooth is now fully exposed and ready for banding in less than one week. *D*, Appearance of the mouth prior to final treatment phase. In the three years that have passed since the initial electrosurgery was performed the mandibular arch was expanded by the orthodontic appliances and is now normal in maxillary-mandibular arch relation. The mandibular second molars are tilted medially and must be banded for final orthodontic movement. The distal half of each crown is covered with hyperplastic tissue that resembles the operculum over a third molar.

trode in two large sections. Cutting current was set at 8 on the Coles Radiosurg Scalpel IV unit and the activated electrode was used with a postero-anterior scooping motion that engaged about half of the gross tissue mass and removed it with a single stroke (Case Fig. 5–4*A*). This was repeated after a 10-second rest interval. A medium-size round loop electrode was substituted, cutting current was reduced to 5.5, and the cut tissue was recontoured to normal anatomic contour with this electrode, planing the tissue surface lightly to create a harmonious contour. This electrode was then replaced with a 45-degree-angle narrow U-shaped loop electrode, cutting current was again reduced to 3.5, and with the activated electrode a subgingival sulcus channel was excised (Case Fig. 5–4*B*). This instrumentation was similar to the preparation of the subgingival trough to some degree, and also to removal of the embryonal capsule

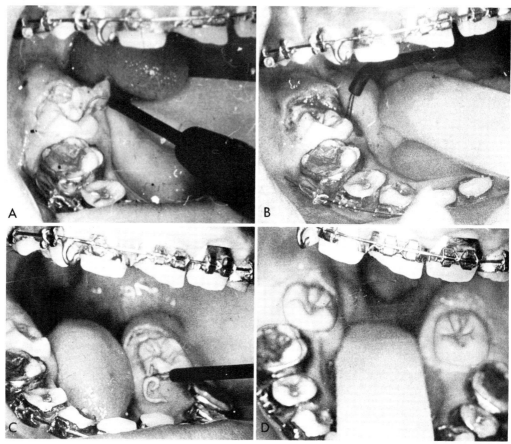

Case Figure 5–4.   *A,* The hyperplastic tissue mass is being resected with a guillotine type of electrode to fully expose the crown of the tooth. *B,* The 45-degree-angle narrow U-shaped loop electrode is being used to create a free gingival sulcus around the newly exposed distal half of the crown. *C,* The tissue around the left molar is being removed with a 45-degree-angle medium-width U-shaped loop electrode. Unlike the tissue on the right side, which was removed en masse with the guillotine loop, this tissue is being removed by planing to shave the tissue off in layers, owing to the denser, firmer texture of this tissue. Note the increase in the size of the tongue. While it still is far from a normal size tongue, it is filling the intra-arch space, and apparently as this space increased the tongue size increased proportionally. *D,* Appearance of the two teeth and their gingivae a week later. The tissue around the second molars appears to be healing rapidly and uneventfully. The tissue contour is normal, and the tissue tone is normal. The teeth are now sufficiently exposed to permit the orthodontic bands to be inserted without subgingival impingement.

around the third molar to a large degree. No periodontal pack was needed, since the tissue was normal, and neither bone nor periosteum had been involved. There was no free bleeding, so tincture of myrrh and benzoin was applied in air-dried layers.

    The left inferior alveolar-lingual block was administered, but for this side, owing to the fact that the tissue was somewhat avascular and denser than the tissue on the right side, it appeared advisable to reduce this mass by loop planing to shave it off in thin layers instead of attempting excision of a considerable bulk of tissue. A 45-degree-angle medium-size U-shaped loop electrode was selected, current output was set at 6, and thin layers of the redundant tissue were removed by planing (Case Fig. 5–4C) until the entire crown of the tooth was fully exposed. This electrode was replaced with the narrow U-shaped loop, and with current reduced to 3.5 the subgingival sulcus space was excised. Tincture of myrrh and benzoin was applied to the area and the patient was instructed to return in one week. When she returned the tissues around both teeth appeared to be healing very satisfactorily, and the contour of the tissues was normal (Case Fig. 5–4D). This completed the surgical interventions for this patient and she was told to return to the orthodontist to have the orthodontic bands inserted.

The molars responded to treatment as well as the other teeth had, and with the aid of the electrosurgical exposure of the teeth to make it possible to apply the orthodontic bands for the treatment the case was successfully concluded.

Orthodontic treatment of this case has been in progress approximately five years since it was initiated. Improvement has been encouraging and gratifying; slow but steady, and noteworthy if not spectacular. There has been a little improvement in the patient's ability to thrust her tongue forward; the floor of the mouth is still elevated somewhat by attempts to do so, but it does come straight forward almost 1 cm. instead of laterally as it originally had. Her mandibular arch has been expanded and the lingual tilt of the teeth has been completely corrected. As a result the position of the teeth in their respective arches has improved greatly, permitting relatively normal alignment of the erupting second molars.

As the tongue space has been increased it has facilitated and encouraged tongue movements which may stimulate further growth and development of that rudimentary organ. This has contributed to the success of the speech therapy she has been undergoing. As a result her speech has improved considerably.

The rapid progress of healing and virtually complete freedom from postoperative pain observed in this case is rather typical. As a rule, in cases where the gingivae are normally healthy and the patient's threshold of pain is also normal, tincture of myrrh and benzoin affords all the obtundent action and tissue protection required. Such patients do not usually require any analgesic medication or postoperative sedation.

Much of the improvement achieved must be attributed to the fact that orthodontic correction was instituted during the child's "golden age" for treatment, when bone growth could be most readily influenced and stimulated. Orthodontic correction was totally dependent upon proper banding of her teeth. The role played by electrosurgery in this particular case was important and should neither be underestimated nor overlooked. Ability to use the slender electrodes in narrow, confined areas with the tissues of the floor of the mouth almost reaching the lingual and occlusal surfaces of the teeth, and ability to resect the undesirable tissue without exerting pressure, to a great extent made early institution and efficiency of orthodontic therapy possible.

The following case demonstrates the fact that contact of an activated electrode with metal or vital teeth is not inherently and automatically harmful, but that damage, when it occurs, is due to faulty instrumentation and not to the fact that electrosurgery was used.

CASE 6

PATIENT.   A 14-year-old white male.

HISTORY.   He had had cleft palate surgery performed in infancy, with little beneficial success. The consensus of opinion among the personnel at the Cleft Palate Center was that an obturator should be constructed for him. Since he was under active orthodontic treatment, all his teeth had been banded. Since the obturator would have to be attached with clasps to the posterior teeth in the arch, he was referred to the author for resection of the marginal gingiva that had proliferated downward over the bands and brackets, to clear away the gingiva sufficiently to expose some of the teeth beyond the bands, and thus to make room for the clasps of the obturator.

CLINICAL EXAMINATION.   There was scar tissue evidence of the cleft palate surgery. All the teeth were banded, and the marginal gingivae extended downward several millimeters on the bands (Case Fig. 6–1).

TREATMENT.   The tissues were anesthetized by infiltration anesthesia. A medium-width, U-shaped loop electrode was selected, and cutting current set at 4 on the power rheostat dial. The tissues were then resected from the bands and brackets with short wiping strokes of the electrode (Case Fig. 6–2). Each contact with the activated electrode was for a brief fraction of a second, and was followed by a pause interval of 10 seconds to avoid any possibility of damage from cumulative heat, especially since metal is such an excellent conductor of heat. When enough of the tissue had been resected to expose 2 to 3 mm. of tooth structure beyond each band, tincture of myrrh and benzoin was applied to the tissues, and the patient was reappointed.

He was seen again one week later. The marginal gingivae were almost completely healed, and the tissue tone was excellent. The patient had not had postoperative pain or even notable discomfort in either the soft tissues or the teeth. It was obvious that although it had been physically impossible to resect the tissue without making contact with both the metal of the bands and the tooth structures, no ill effects had resulted therefrom.

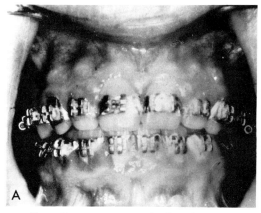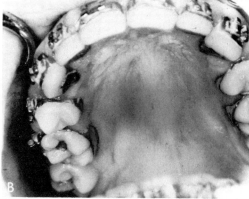

Case Figure 6–1. Labial. There is marked gingival hyperplasia, particularly of the interdental papillae in both the maxilla and the mandible. The orthodontic bands undoubtedly are producing subgingival irritation that has triggered the proliferation. All the bands in both arches extend considerably beyond the free gingival margins in the embrasures. *B,* Palatal. The bands can be seen projecting far beyond the gingival crevices, especially in the embrasures. The interdental papillae are massively enlarged in the cuspid to molar regions of the maxilla. The condition is comparable in the mandible.

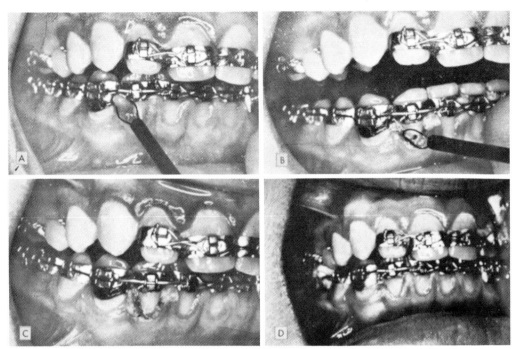

Case Figure 6–2. Removal of proliferating hypertrophic masses resulting from irritation to the gingivae from impingement of orthodontic bands. *A,* Flame-shaped loop electrode inserted under the mass to resect it by electrocoagulation. *B,* Hypertrophic tissue resected from marginal gingiva with the same loop. *C,* Appearance of gingival margin after light spot coagulation. *D,* Postoperative appearance of the tissues one week later. The tissues are fully and normally healed.

It is interesting to note that postoperative requirements following orthodontic surgery are variable. If the surgery is limited to one or more isolated areas, surgical cement packs are usually unnecessary. But if the gingival proliferation is widespread and the surgery extensive, application of surgical cement packs is advantageous. Cement packs are especially useful when the gingivae are friable and bleed profusely even when surgery is performed with the electrocoagulating current.

Orthodontic appliances require protection from the cement packs to prevent damage or distortion when the cement is removed. If adhesive dryfoil is carefully adapted around the teeth, brackets and archwires, the cement will not adhere and can be removed easily. If the cement is stiffly mixed and tightly adapted and molded against the teeth and dryfoil it usually adheres well.

Orthodontic surgical procedures are usually remarkably free from postoperative pain and swelling and, as a rule, healing is rapid and without incident. After the initial tissue healing, use of the salt-alum astringent mouthwash helps to tan and toughen the tissues. Use of the toothbrush as a gum brush, and of the rubber stimulator, should be encouraged and prescribed to massage the gingivae and clean the teeth as an aid in maintaining the integrity of the gingivae against further degeneration.

FOOTNOTE REFERENCES

1. Brash, J. C.: The growth of the alveolar bone and its relation to the movements of the teeth, including eruptions. D. Record, *46*:641, Dec., 1926.
2. Brash, J. C., and Keith, A.: The growth of the jaws, normal and abnormal, in health and disease. Dental Board of the United Kingdom, 1922.
3. Brodie, A. G.: Growth pattern of the human head from the third month to eight years of life. Am. J. Anat., *68*:209, Mar., 1941.
4. Brodie, A. G.: On the growth of the jaws and the eruption of the teeth. Angle Orthodont., *12*:109, 1942.
5. Hellman, M.: An introduction to growth of the human face from infancy to adulthood. Internat. J. Orthodont. 25:927, Oct, 1939.
6. Hellman, M.: Development of the face and dentition in its application to orthodontic treatment. Am. J. Orthodont., *26*:424, May, 1940.
7. Shafer, W. G., Hine, M. K., and Levy, B. M.: A Textbook of Oral Pathology. Philadelphia, W. B. Saunders Co., 1959, pp. 4–8.
8. Oringer, M. J.: Anomalies of human dentition. Oral Surg., Oral Med. & Oral Path., *1* (12):1119–1130, Dec., 1948.
9. Simon, P. W.: Diagnosis of Dental Anomalies. Boston, Stratford Co., 1926.

PART 3

PERIODONTICS

Chapter Eighteen

ELECTROSURGERY FOR DEFINITIVE CONSERVATIVE MODERN PERIODONTAL THERAPY

INTRODUCTION*

The single most significant feature of modern periodontal therapy is the lack of unanimity among periodontists not only as to methods of treatment but as to the objectives of treatment.

Some periodontists subscribe to the philosophy that the objectives of periodontal therapy should aim for (a) eradication of the diseased tissue, (b) reattachment of the marginal gingivae, and (c) maintenance of a zone of keratinized attached gingiva.[1] Others subscribe to the philosophy that in addition

---

*This introductory text originally appeared in an article by the author in *Dental Clinics of North America*, Philadelphia, W. B. Saunders Co., January, 1969.

to these essential objectives, the aim should be elevated to achieve an all-important fourth objective, the *regeneration of lost structures.*[2]

Naturally the respective exponents subscribe to substantially different concepts of treatment. The former subscribe to the formula of gingivectomy—resection of all the soft tissues down to the base of the periodontal pockets, and bone ramping extended to the base of the osseous defects.[3] Consequently root planing must be thorough enough to remove all the cementum, to assure smooth exposed denuded root surfaces in order to eliminate food debris adhering to rough cementum, and to avoid rapid and excessive calculus formation.

Exponents of the second theory subscribe to a much more conservative approach; resect only the diseased portion of the soft tissues, and retain as much of the bony wall of the pocket as possible to increase the chances for regeneration of the lost investing structures. Since regeneration is anticipated, root planing should be limited to removal of dead cementum to assure that some cementum will remain to which the regenerating periodontal fibers can invaginate and reattach.

I wholeheartedly subscribe to the latter school of thought. In the first edition of *Electrosurgery In Dentistry,* I emphasized that the periodontal structures and investing bone do not differ in their capacity for repair from any other organic structure of the body, if conditions conducive to repair are created and maintained for them. Hence, if the internal aspect of the periodontal pocket is denuded of its epithelial lining, the pocket thoroughly debrided of its granulomatous debris, and the external bony wall preserved instead of being ramped, a socket-like defect will be created. If the latter is irrigated and dried, and bleeding is induced, the defect will fill with blood that clots. The clot ultimately undergoes organization, and all components normal to the area will, under optimal conditions, regenerate.[4]

To assure optimal conditions, it is of course essential that traumatizing occlusal prematurities and all foreign matter, such as calculus and dead cementum, be removed from the root surfaces before surgery is instituted to prevent irritation or trauma during the reparative period.

Good oral hygiene can keep the normal mouth healthy. But once the periodontal tissues have undergone degeneration, good oral hygiene no longer is adequate; a high degree of oral *physiotherapy* must be instituted to maintain the health of these tissues.[5] And so, prior to surgery, the patient must be taught the proper use of manual and mechanical toothbrushes and the rubber tip, water jet, and even the fingertip massage, to assure maximum stimulation necessary for good physiotherapy. Even dietary supplements should be prescribed to increase the potential for regeneration of the lost structures.

Electrosurgical instrumentation for periodontal therapy does not alter either the objectives or the concept of treatment, but it does alter the method of treatment. When the necessary degree of skill in electrosurgical instrumentation is acquired, electronic periodontal surgery can be performed safely and efficiently, can greatly simplify treatment and can assure the maintenance of the marginal gingivae at, or nearly at, their original level.

Clinical experience has demonstrated that electronic cutting with fully rectified current produces a tendency for the tissues to regenerate toward their original level. Thus, in most instances periodontal therapy can be successfully achieved even in advanced disease with little or no alteration in the height of the marginal gingivae. This eliminates or dramatically minimizes the problem of exposed denuded roots with their aesthetic handicap and the concomitant problem of root hypersensitivity to thermal and chemical stimuli that accompany resection of the soft tissues and bone ramping of the conventional gingivectomy.

Opinions by some eminent periodontists to the contrary notwithstanding, nowhere in the entire realm of dental therapy does electronic electrosurgery make a more significant and valuable contribution than in the electrosurgical periodontal technique of gingivoplasty-intra-osseous pocket debridement for the conservative management of the definitive periodontal therapy developed by the author.

Some of the detractors of the usefulness of electrosurgery in periodontics have maintained that everything else being equal, electrosurgery would be acceptable, but, "our animal experimental investigations prove that tissues treated electrosurgically do not heal as well, or as rapidly, as tissues treated with conventional cold steel scalpel and curet surgery." And, from time to time, histologic studies comparing the effectiveness of cold steel and electrosurgical instrumentation have been offered in evidence. Most recent has been a report by Pope, Gargiulo, Staffileno, and Levy (1968).[6]

To be scientifically meaningful, an investigative comparative evaluation of modalities or techniques must fulfill two elementary fundamental requirements: (1) The proper modality or technique must be employed and must be accurately reported; and (2) the investigator must enjoy equal competency with both modalities or techniques being evaluated.

Let us consider the first requirement. Pope et al. reported that the investigators, in their investigation, used "a Cameron-Miller electrosurgical unit Model No. 26-255, built with power-vacuum-tube generators and mercury vapor tubes designed to deliver filtered, fully rectified current of undamped waveform."

According to the Cameron-Miller Surgical Instruments Company, manufacturer of the equipment in question, "Our model 26-255 delivers a partially rectified current."[7] Thus it appears that the current employed in their investigations was partially rectified, and not fully rectified as reported.

There is a highly significant difference in the respective self-limiting capacities of partially and fully rectified currents, as has been established in experiments by Harrison and other investigators.[*] Equally significant are the rate and quality of tissue healing with the respective currents. The results reported by Pope et al. are fully compatible with results obtainable with electrosection with partially rectified current, but not at all comparable with the results that can be obtained with electrosection with fully rectified current properly employed.

James D. Harrison of St. Louis University reported at the A.D.A. and

---

[*] The research investigations referred to here were comprehensively reported in Chapters 6 through 9 of this text.

American Academy of Dental Electrosurgery annual meetings in 1966 the results of his investigations on the amount of temperature rise and lateral heat dispersion into the adjacent tissues produced by partially and fully rectified currents. For the partially rectified current he used a Cameron-Miller Model No. 26-255 (similar to the one used by Pope et al.); for the fully rectified current he used a Coles Radiosurg Electronic Scalpel IV.

He reported that fully rectified undamped, surge-free cutting current produced a 13.5° F. rise in temperature at a distance of 3 mm. and a 31.2° F. rise at 1 mm. from the activated electrode. Lateral heat dispersion occurred over an area of 102 mμ beyond the site of application, a distance so minute as to be meaningless clinically, with no visible changes in the cells adjacent to the line of incision.

Partially rectified current used in an identical manner produced temperature rises of 16.2° F. at 3 mm. and 37.8° F. at 1 mm. but produced lateral heat dispersion over an area of 330 mμ beyond the site of application, more than enough to produce visible clinical evidence of destruction of several layers of adjacent cells, forming a thin layer of coagulum along the incised margins. His conclusions: "Most consistent results were obtained with the fully rectified current. It produced less temperature rise, least amount of lateral heat dispersion, and most rapid and uneventful healing."[8]

At the same meetings, his collaborator, William J. Kelly, Jr., reported the histologic findings produced by his two-year study of comparative electrosurgical subgingival surgery with partially and fully rectified currents. "Healing with the fully rectified current was almost complete within 8 days, with no evidence of vacuolation or lymphocyte concentration. Healing with the partially rectified current was notably slower. Vacuolation and some lymphocyte concentration [were] still in evidence on the 21st day."

It seems significant that Kelly and Richard Evans of the Temple University School of Dentistry, both equally well trained in the proper use of the modalities being evaluated, obtained results exactly opposite from those reported by Pope et al. in their comparative evaluations of the rate and quality of wound healing from electronic cutting with fully rectified current and from conventional cold-steel scalpel and curet surgery. Both investigators observed clinically and verified histologically (the former in animal experiments, the latter in human patients) that not only is the healing of electronic wounds as good as the healing from conventional cold-steel cutting, but it is appreciably superior and more rapid.[9, 10]

Despite excellent investigation the etiology of periodontal disease is still obscure. Moreover, practitioners of the discipline of periodontia have never been noted for agreement upon the rationale or actual techniques of periodontal therapy.

More than two decades ago Miller[11] claimed that an older patient will show a better response to periodontal therapy, while Burket[12] intimated that less favorable conditions exist when periodontal disease is seen in the aged.[13] More recently, sharply divergent concepts about periodontal therapy and the rationale for various techniques have been expressed by Glickman, Gold-man,[19] Schluger,[14] Fox,[15] Cohen,[19] and numerous other eminent periodontists.

In view of this lack of unanimity, it would be foolhardy to become embroiled in discussions of controversial concepts of etiology or therapy in a text that is not devoted exclusively to periodontal disease. This chapter, therefore, shall be limited to consideration of the advantages of electrosurgical techniques for periodontal therapy.

DETERIORATION OF THE PERIODONTIUM

Although our interst will be focused on surgical eradication of periodontoclasia by electrosurgical techniques, unfavorable local and systemic factors that predispose to deterioration of the periodontium shall not be ignored, since these usually exert profound influence on the prognosis of the ultimate surgical results.

Local Factors

These may be biomechanical, such as occlusal disharmonies; physiologic, such as deposits of serumnal and salivary calculus; or pathologic, ranging from simple inflammatory hyperemias of the gingivae to acute infections, such as necrotizing gingivitis or Vincent's stomatitis.

Unfavorable local factors as a rule are rather obvious and readily identified in the clinical evaluation of the patient. The importance of eradicating these factors or bringing them under control before surgery is instituted cannot be overemphasized. Occlusal disharmonies, gingival-subgingival erosions or caries, or presence of calcareous deposits are irritating to the local gingival tissues. Unless such irritants are quickly and thoroughly eliminated, they tend to produce inflammatory responses which trigger a chain reaction that usually degenerates into periodontal disease.

Inflammatory hyperemia creates a stasis of the local blood circulation. This usually leads to alteration in the cellular electrolyte and intra- and extracellular fluid balances of the affected tissues. Alteration of the pH of the local tissue fluids toward the acid side usually results and creates an unfavorable climate for good anesthetic or surgical results.

Acute infections such as Vincent's stomatitis create even more rapid and extensive deterioration of the periodontal tissues. In view of these facts it is essential that, wherever possible, all unfavorable local factors should be eradicated before periodontal surgery is instituted, in order to assure optimal results.

Except as otherwise specified, in the cases reported in the following chapter all known unfavorable local factors were eliminated preoperatively. It would serve no useful purpose to elaborate on the individual corrections instituted prior to surgery.

Systemic Factors

These may be physiologic, such as alterations in metabolism or in endocrine function during pregnancy, the menstrual cycle, or the menopause; or pathologic, such as diabetes insipidus or mellitus, the anemias or endocrine dysfunctions.

Unfavorable systemic factors are usually much more obscure than local factors and are therefore much more likely to be overlooked. Very often they remain unknown until they are brought to light by unfavorable postoperative results. As dentists our contribution to the control or eradication of unfavorable systemic factors is usually rather limited. It consists mostly of occasional early diagnosis, close cooperation with the patient's physician, and eradication of unfavorable oral factors.

When unfavorable local factors are eliminated and there are no complicating systemic factors to contend with, the prognosis is excellent for rapid normal healing following skillfully executed periodontal surgery. But when unfavorable systemic factors are superimposed upon local factors, eradication of the latter is not enough. The prognosis for the outcome of surgery under such conditions remains unfavorable irrespective of the skill and thoroughness with which the surgical intervention is performed.

If unfavorable systemic factors can neither be eliminated nor adequately controlled it is advisable to refrain from performing elective surgery.[17] Periodontal surgery usually falls into the latter category. If special considerations should make it necessary to institute periodontal surgery under such conditions as a calculated risk, possibility of failure must be anticipated and the patient advised of the doubtful prognosis.

PERIODONTAL ELECTROSURGERY

Should the results of surgery unexpectedly and inexplicably prove disappointing, it is imperative to refrain from jumping to the conclusion that either the technique or the modality must have been responsible. The operator who succumbs to such unwarranted reactions may render actual disservice to both the patient and himself by overlooking diagnostic investigations that might disclose other factors as the underlying cause of failure.

When a method such as electrosurgery has been employed, the temptation to jump to unsubstantiated conclusions is particularly great. This is not an unnatural reaction in view of the failures reported by many of the pioneers in periodontal electrosurgery. The fact that these failures almost invariably resulted from lack of electrosurgical training and/or from dependence in great measure on medical techniques of instrumentation often unsuited for application to the oral tissues[18] did not soften the impact of the failures on the profession, traces of which tend to persist to the present day even in the enlightened periodontal texts.

When periodontal electrosurgery is properly performed with modern electronic equipment by an operator who is adequately trained in both electrosurgical instrumentation and periodontal technique, it is unjustifiable to conclude that the modality, electrosurgery, is responsible for unsatisfactory end results.

If under such conditions a disappointing postoperative result is occasionally encountered it is far more realistic and scientifically sound to institute immediately a thorough diagnostic investigation in collaboration with the patient's physician (using laboratory and other modern diagnostic aids) in order to ascertain whether the failure may—as is highly likely—have been caused by interference from an obscure, previously undiagnosed systemic factor.

When periodontal electrosurgery is performed with good technique and under reasonably favorable conditions, the end results are exemplary and the probability of postoperative complications is greatly reduced. Periodontal electrosurgery can usually be performed with little or no bleeding. Direct benefits derived from this fact include clear visibility of the operative field and marked reduction in operating time and surgical shock. Use of suitably shaped loop electrodes makes harmonious recontouring of the gingival architecture relatively easy to achieve with minimal sacrifice of normal gingival tissue and minimal postoperative discomfort to the patient.

The techniques of periodontal electrosurgery that will be described in this chapter should prove particularly valuable to persons having had training in periodontal therapy and electrosurgical instrumentation.

Tissue Conservation

At this point, to avoid any possible misunderstanding, it is advisable to clarify the meaning and intent of the statement that periodontal electrosurgery permits minimal sacrifice of normal tissue.

Goldman, Schluger, Fox and Cohen, in their book, *Periodontal Therapy,* assert ".... it is the goal of the periodontist to conserve as much tissue as possible consistent with good health and with a long range favorable prognosis."[19] Although this is a fundamental tenet consistent with sound surgical procedure, many of the currently popular periodontal surgical techniques fail to comply with it; much normal gingival tissue is being sacrificed as a result.[15] The periodontal electrosurgical techniques that will be presented in this chapter are based upon this philosophy of effective therapy with maximum tissue conservation.

Instrumentation of Periodontal Pockets

Periodontal pocket formation may be either horizontal or vertical. *Horizontal* bone loss is usually quite regular in depth, creating bone loss and tissue detachment of uniform depth; it usually affects the entire circumference of the affected teeth. These defects contrast sharply with those that result when periodontal pockets are *vertical* instead of horizontal. Vertical pockets are usually deep and narrow and involve irregular bone loss, so that the pockets vary greatly in depth. A considerable amount of the investing alveolar bone around teeth with vertical pockets remains relatively normal and intact. With the exception of the tissue actually involved in pocket areas, the gingival mucosa usually remains normal and firmly attached to teeth and alveolar bone.

GINGIVAL STRIPPING. When mucogingival surgery is performed with cold-steel instruments the extent of periodontal involvement is customarily recorded by inserting a pocket marker down to the base of each pocket and piercing the mucosa at that point. This accurately represents the exact depth and extent of bone loss and pocket formation. The gingival punctures are finally linked together by scalpel incisions along a line drawn at the level of the deepest pockets. (This procedure is well demonstrated on a calf mandible in Figure 18–1). The incised strip of mucosa is then undermined, elevated and removed, leaving a wide expanse of denuded alveolar bone. The cut edge of the mucosa terminates in a sharp line angle. This surgical procedure has been described as "gingival stripping." When periodontal surgery is instituted to correct periodontal disease involving widespread horizontal bone loss, gingival stripping is practical and effective, since all the affected teeth have suffered uniform alveolar bone loss down to the base of the pockets along the full length of the dentition. Without alveolar bone the detached tissue cannot be permanently reattached. When the technique of gingival stripping is employed in treatment of such cases, all the tissue resected at the level of the base of the pockets is expendable, since it is detached, unsupported mucosa. In these cases no normal attached gingival mucosa is unnecessarily sacrificed, and little or no investing alveolar bone is denuded thereby.

But when the periodontal pockets are vertical, relatively narrow and irregular, gingival stripping creates an entirely different situation. In such cases practically all the gingival mucosa except the narrow portions that form the periodontal pockets is relatively normal and attached to the teeth and alveolar bone. When the mucosa is incised uniformly along the level of the base of the deepest pockets in order to obtain a harmoniously uniform line of resection and an even, new gingival margin, the normal attached portions of mucosa that are removed by such stripping are being unnecessarily sacrificed and considerable expanses of alveolar bone are unnecessarily denuded. Except in instances in which there is need for extensive osteoplasty, such extensive denuding of the alveolar bone has been condemned.[15]

ELECTROSURGICAL TECHNIQUES. When this type of periodontoclasia is treated electrosurgically, a technique can be employed that combines the

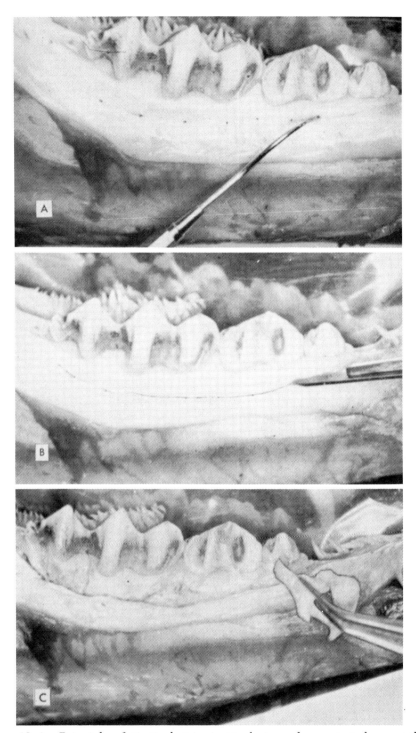

Figure 18–1. Principle of gingival stripping technique demonstrated on a calf jaw. *A,* Pocket depth registered by puncturing the gingivae with a pocket-marker device. *B,* Punctures joined into a continuous line by scalpel incision. *C,* Incised strip of mucosa excised. Note sharp line angle formed by the tissue incisions.

characteristics of gingivectomy and gingivoplasty with those of eradication of infrabony pockets, periodontal abscesses, and interradicular involvements. It differs greatly from earlier periodontal electrosurgical techniques that have previously been reported.[20-23]

Although there is a basic similarity, this electrosurgical technique also differs radically from the electrosurgical techniques mentioned by Beube,[24] Glickman,[25] Goldman *et al.*[19] and authors of some of the other modern periodontal texts. In the techniques described by them electrosurgery is purely adjunctive and relegated to a relatively minor accessory role (recontouring the gingival architecture) in the surgical treatment of periodontia. In the electrosurgical technique that will be described here, electrosurgery is not adjunctive, but is a primary, complete therapeutic measure. It also differs from the techniques described by Saghirian[26-29] in this and other respects.

With this technique, grossly detached *unsupported* gingivae can be resected easily with appropriate loop electrodes. Hypertrophic interproximal papillae can be reduced easily to self-cleansing concave sluiceways. Hypertrophic marginal gingivae can also be reduced to normal levels with appropriate loop electrodes.

Use of loop electrodes of suitable size and shape as periodontal curets simplifies thorough debridement of the pocket areas. Each individual pocket can be debrided with a thoroughness that would be difficult if not impossible to equal with cold-steel instrumentation. Necrotic debris and epithelial pocket linings are resected by inserting very narrow loop electrodes to the base of the pockets and manipulating them with rotary and push-pull motions in order to remove the debris. Tenaciously adherent shreds can be fulgurated *in situ.* Finally, with the use of appropriately shaped loops, the newly created gingival margins can be readily beveled for proper anatomic contour and feather-edge margins in order to restore normal gingival architecture.

By using this technique as described, unsightly gingival irregularities are avoided or minimized without need for resection of the healthy portions of attached gingivae. This is well demonstrated on a calf mandible (Fig. 18-2). Since this technique does not create large expanses of denuded alveolar bone, healing is likely to be more rapid, with minimal postoperative pain. Unnecessary exposure of sensitive root surfaces of teeth is avoided, a distinct aesthetic and physical advantage to the patient.

A variety of solid and powdered homologous and heterogenous graft materials have been implanted experimentally and clinically, with varying degrees of success, to help obliterate large periodontal pockets and accelerate regeneration of alveolar bone in order to immobilize loose teeth.[30-37] The use of cultured despeciated bone paste and/or gelatin in many of the cases reported in the first edition undoubtedly helped to accelerate repair and may have contributed to favorable outcome of the periodontal therapy.

Some of the surgical techniques used in periodontal therapy, such as gingivectomy and gingivoplasty and eradication of infrabony pockets, periodontal abscesses, and interradicular involvements, were developed to meet specific needs created by periodontal pathology. Some of the other surgical

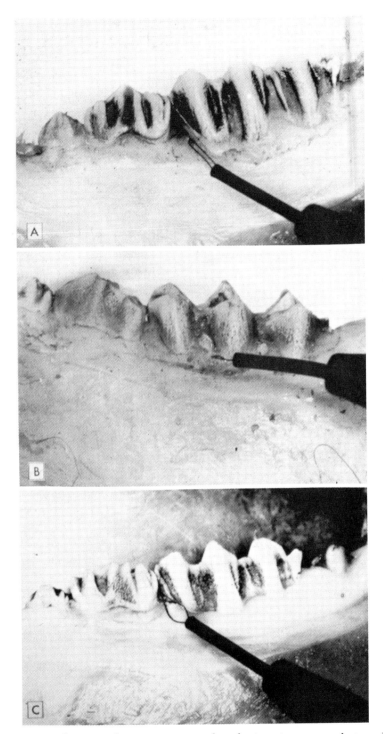

Figure 18–2. Technique of tissue resection by planing tissues, pocket eradication, and recontouring the gingival architecture with appropriate loop electrodes. *A*, Shaving gingivae with U-shaped loop electrodes. *B*, Eradicating an infrabony pocket with a bent loop electrode employed as a curet. *C*, Reducing an interproximal papilla to form a concave self-cleansing sluiceway with a flame-shaped loop electrode.

techniques that are used for periodontal therapy, such as repositioning gingival mucosa, push-backs, frenectomy or frenotomy, and muscle raising, are techniques that are also employed in oral surgery, prosthetic surgery and orthodontic surgery, and may be reviewed under any or all of these disciplines.

ELECTROSURGICAL TECHNIQUES FOR PERIODONTAL CURETTAGE

The late noted medical biographer and novelist, Paul deKruif, once made the penetrating but caustic observation that "there are many in the medical science[s] who appear to take a dark delight in destroying new ideas and methods, either by refusing to try them, or, by trying them improperly, and then condemning them."

This seems to describe the reaction of some in the periodontal discipline toward use of electrosurgery for definitive therapy. In part, the unfavorable attitude undoubtedly stems from the acceptance of myths and hearsay rather than from personal experiences. In many instances, however, the condemnation stems from unfavorable experiences resulting from improper electrosurgical instrumentation technique or from use of improper current, or from a combination of both. Under such circumstances, unfavorable results become inevitable sequelae through no fault of the modality.

President Goheen of Princeton University once said, "The mark of an educated man is his ability to change his mind when the evidence warrants it." Periodontists being educated men, the author presents these cases in the hope that they will provide the evidence that these techniques for definitive conservative electrosurgical periodontal therapy are not only acceptable but produce more desirable and effective results than can be achieved by other methods of instrumentation.

Although periodontal disease is essentially a disease of bone, its initial manifestation is gingival inflammation. As the disease progresses the gingival deterioration becomes much more marked, and the elimination of soft tissue disease constitutes the major portion of definitive periodontal therapy. The unique advantages electrosurgery offers can therefore be utilized by the therapist to achieve therapeutic results that cannot be equaled or duplicated by other methods of treatment.

Neither the concepts nor the techniques of periodontal therapy have been static. In fact, they have swung like a pendulum from extreme conservatism to extreme radicalism and are gradually approaching moderation. Periodontal therapy as conceived and practiced by McCall, Stillman, Box, and Gottlieb, the founding fathers of the discipline, consisted largely of occlusal equilibration to eliminate traumatizing occlusal prematurities, thorough scaling to remove all calculus, and manual curettage with special curets designed to resect the epithelial tissue lining the pockets and the friable soft tissue debris contained in them.

The key to treatment was resection of the epithelial lining from the pockets. Unless and until this tissue is removed, neither spontaneous repair nor repair following treatment of the defects is possible. When their regimen of treatment failed to produce consistently favorable results, these pioneers realized that the cause was failure to remove all the epithelial tissue by manual curettage. When McCall realized the limitations of manual curettage, he resorted to the use of a chemical solvent, sodium sulfite, to try to disintegrate and dissolve the epithelial tissue remaining after curettage, but this too failed to bring consistently successful results. Box, in Toronto, likewise began to use a chemical solvent, Antiformin, but this too was not consistently successful. Gottlieb, in Vienna, also recognized need for some means to supplement curettage to eliminate the epithelial debris, and he resorted to use of oxygen forcibly introduced into the periodontal defects, also without consistently uniform success.

The not infrequent failures resulting from the conservative curettage eventually led to a re-evaluation of the concept as well as methods of treatment which resulted in development of the surgical gingivectomy as the method of choice. The rationale for this method of treatment was that it would be most likely to fulfill the objectives of periodontal therapy, namely:

a. Eradication of the diseased tissue.

b. Reattachment of the marginal gingivae.

c. Regeneration of a zone of maturely keratinized attached gingiva.

The diamond stone maceration technique was a rather bizarre outgrowth of the gingivectomy philosophy of treatment.

The school of thought most recently developed subscribes to more than surgical elimination of diseased tissue. Subscribers to this concept seek a fourth, all-important objective to treatment—*regeneration of lost structure.* Obviously, if all the diseased tissue is resected, including all or most of the bony wall, regeneration of lost structure is not possible. Thus, those who subscribe to this school have refined a technique described by Zemsky in 1930 in which bilateral incisions are made in the gingival mucosa, a mucoperiosteal flap is reflected, the internal half of the flap tissue is dissected away, the friable soft tissue detritus from the bony defects is removed, the flap is restored to position, and the cut margins are reattached by suturing through the embrasures. The technique is known as the "split mucosal flap" procedure.[38]

This procedure makes it possible to achieve regeneration of the bone loss but is handicapped by many practical clinical factors. As soon as the tissue is elevated from its attachment to the underlying bone, it contracts, and it becomes very difficult to visualize accurately the diseased internal layer of tissue. It becomes far more difficult to try to dissect the tissue evenly and accurately owing to the extreme mobility of the tissue and the visual impairment due to the hemorrhagic bleeding that accompanies this method of treatment. Of course, postoperative surgical shock due to the blood loss is an additional handicap. Finally, since repair is by fibrous contractile scar tissue, and the flap is unsupported by bone in many areas, there very often is a lowering of the marginal gingival level, with subsequent concomitant problem created of hypersensitivity of the exposed root portions to thermal and chemical stimuli of the mouth.

The electrosurgical procedure developed by the author is similar in its objectives and concept to that of the split mucosal flap procedure. However, owing to the unique advantages inherent in electrosurgery, almost all the undesirable features inherent in the flap procedure are eliminated.

Unless a flap were incised and reflected, it would be impossible effectively to dissect out the lining epithelium and detritus with steel cutting instruments because their physical bulk and rigidity prevent them from being manipulated in the defects. For the same reasons it would be impossible to apply the pressure necessary to cut with cold steel. The electronic electrosurgical curet, on the other hand, is a hair-thin wire loop, 17 mm. in length, that has practically no physical bulk and is flexible enough to follow the contours of the internal surfaces of the periodontal defect. No pressure is required to cut efficiently with the loop curet, since neither the therapist nor the electrode really does the cutting. The latter results from disintegration of the tissue cells in the path of the concentrated heat generated as the RF (radiofrequency) current comes into contact with the tissues. Thus, the internal lining epithelium and soft tissue debris present in the pockets are effortlessly and efficiently resected with the loop electrodes (Fig. 18–3).

When the electronic curettage is properly performed no damage results from electrode contact with the bone and teeth. Safe, proper use consists of introducing the activated electrode into the defect for a fraction of a second at a time, with each application followed by a 10-second interval to allow dissipation of the heat and thereby prevent damage from cumulative heat. The electrode must be kept moving rapidly with an up and down and rotary motion, so that during each brief introduction into the defect it comes into contact with all the internal surfaces of the pocket.

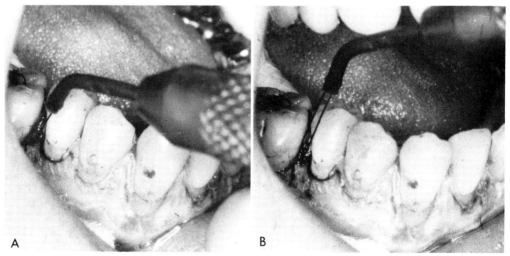

A   B

Figure 18–3. The 17 mm. electronic periodontal curet. *A,* The electrode is seen as it is being used with an up-down and rotary movement to debride a deep periodontal infrabony pocket. The electrode is penetrating toward the base of the defect and has penetrated approximately 11 mm. into the defect. *B,* The electrode is seen as it is emerging from the defect. Note the debris it is lifting out as it is being withdrawn from the pocket.

If the inactivated electrode is used to explore the defect, it reveals, by the tactile sensitivity every dentist develops, the internal topography of the defect in the same manner that the internal topography of a root canal is revealed when a fine reamer or file is introduced and used for exploration. Moreover, since the instrumentation is relatively bloodless, as far as persistent hemorrhagic bleeding is concerned, the defects can be cleared of blood by introducing a bit of selvage gauze under light finger pressure for one or two minutes, and then the defect can be illuminated or transilluminated for visual inspection even with loupe magnification. Since the tissue has not been detached from the bone, and especially since tissue cut by electrosection with fully rectified current tends to regenerate toward its original level, the marginal gingival level remains relatively unaltered, and there usually are no denuded root surfaces and thus there is no hypersensitivity.

Electrosurgical periodontal therapy is not a panacea. It requires skillful, knowledgeable use of treatment planning, instrumentation, preliminary customary preparation including thorough prophylaxis and planing to remove dead cementum from the root surfaces, elimination of all occlusal prematurities that would disrupt the repair process, and, perhaps most important of all, instruction of the patient in the most effective and efficient methods of oral *physiotherapy*, before the surgical treatment is instituted. It also involves conscientious postoperative maintenance care for several months and immobilization of mobile teeth to assure calcification of the regenerating bone.

When all these requirements are fulfilled, electrosurgery very often makes possible preservation of teeth that are considered "inoperable" by other methods of treatment. Pockets that extend to and even beyond the apices of the teeth can be treated effectively, and since the electronic energy sterilizes as it cuts, bacteria in the surgical field are destroyed, which substantially enhances the prospects for successful therapy.

The actual technique that will be described is a combination of both the gingivoplasty to recontour the gingivae to normal architecture and create concave self-cleansing sluiceways in the embrasures and the debridement of the individual infrabony defects that has just been described. The author has found the gingivoplasty desirable even when there is no gross deformity or disease of the marginal gingivae, since this resects the surface epithelium. He has found that the regenerating new surface epithelium appears to respond to postoperative care more than the original epithelium, so that in many instances a firm, well-defined zone of attached gingiva becomes clinically visible where no evidence of it was present preoperatively, even though the histologic elements undoubtedly are present in these cases.

PREOPERATIVE AND POSTOPERATIVE TREATMENT

The use of electrosurgery does not eliminate need for the preoperative preliminary procedures customarily instituted before performing surgery.

Should the patient be suffering from a systemic disease or deficiency, it must be cured, or at least arrested, before electrosurgical treatment can justifiably be instituted in *any* of the dental disciplines.

If biomechanical preparatory procedures are customarily instituted when other modalities are employed, these must also be utilized prior to electrosurgery. Thus, for endodontics, it is imperative that thorough reaming and filing of the canals to be obturated be performed before utilizing electrocoagulation to sterilize the canals. In crown and bridge fixed prosthodontics, it means thorough prophylaxis before completion of the full crown preparations and creation of subgingival troughs by electrosection. If incipient or mild gingivitis is present, thorough curettage must be instituted well in advance of the electrosurgery, and if periodontal disease is present, it must be eradicated prior to performing the restorative dentistry. In oral surgery and surgery adjunctive to needs of the other disciplines in addition to elimination of calcareous debris that could enter the surgical defect and disrupt healing, it is also necessary to eliminate or contain acute infection by judicious premedication for one to two days before instituting the surgical procedure.

In periodontia, the preliminaries of thorough prophylaxis, elimination of traumatizing occlusal prematurities, thorough patient instruction in proper methods of toothbrushing and other methods of massage to maintain a high degree of oral physiotherapy postoperatively are the ingredients for success.

Preparation of the Oral Cavity Prior to Periodontal Treatment

The customary essential preliminary preparation of the mouth should be fully and meticulously performed before periodontal treatment is instituted.

CALCULUS REMOVAL. Elimination of occlusal traumatizing prematurities and thorough scaling of the teeth to remove all salivary and serumnal calculus are the most important of these preliminaries. In many instances the occlusion is incapable of being "balanced" until after successful periodontal therapy, since a full mouth reconstruction may be required to achieve the balance. But traumatizing prematurities that would disrupt the repair process must be eliminated.

Removal of salivary calculus does not present any problems, since it is located on the external surface of the tooth and is superior to the periodontal pocket. It can be readily visualized optically and removed by hand scaling or with an efficient ultrasonic scaler. Serumnal calculus presents a considerable problem, since it is located subgingivally on the root surfaces, usually deep in the periodontal defect, where it cannot be readily seen by optical visualization. This does not mean, however, that serumnal calculus can be removed efficiently only by incising and reflecting a mucoperiosteal flap to expose it, any more than it would be necessary to split a root in order to visualize the internal topography of a root canal for endodontic therapy. It is possible to locate the serumnal calculus readily and efficiently by using the limber 17-mm. periodontal electronic loop electrode curet as the diagnostic instrument. The inactivated electrode is introduced into the pocket and slid along the surfaces of the root that can be contacted in the defect. If serumnal calculus is present on the root, the loop will engage it and transmit the information to the finger-tips as soon as contact is made, especially if the electrode handle is held with a very light grip, so that the least vibration is immediately transmitted. The calculus can also be visualized optically by directing the light beam of a trans-illuminating lamp through the alveolar investing structures. When serumnal calculus is present, it appears as a dark spot on the root surface when seen with direct vision and as a dark area in an otherwise brightly illuminated field when seen through the tissues by transillumination.

Serumnal calculus usually is in the shape of a flat, thin flake of dark calculus that is tenaciously adherent to the root surface. When a hoe or sickle scaler is used to attempt to remove it, especially with hand instrumentation, the scaler very often glides or skids over the flat surface without displacing it. The author has found that a half round explorer that has been bent open al-most completely, used with a jabbing motion like a spear, is far more effective for removing them. After the flake of calculus has been located, the tip of the explorer is placed against the superior edge, and with the instrument tip held at a slight angle to the root surface, the calcareous plaque is flicked off easily and cleanly with a slight jab, in most instances at the first attempt.

ROOT PLANING.   There have been reports by investigators to the effect that they have succeeded experimentally to achieve reattachment of the periodontal ligament and marginal gingivae after all the cementum had been planed off the roots of the teeth being treated experimentally. Perhaps this is possible to achieve in the laboratory with experimental animals. Clinically, the author has noted that when all the cementum is removed and the root sur-faces are planed smooth, regeneration of the periodontal fibers and reattach-ment of the marginal gingivae fails to occur. When only the dead cementum has been removed and the viable cementum has been retained on the root sur-faces, reattachment almost invariably occurs. For this reason, it is recom-mended that the prophylaxis be performed by either ultrasonic or hand in-strumentation; however, for root planing to remove only dead cementum, hand instrumentation appears to be preferable, because when the instrument is held lightly and used with light pressure against the tooth, the likelihood of inadvertently removing all the cementum is greatly reduced and retention of the viable cementum is enhanced.

Immobilization of Loose Teeth

It is an accepted fact that fractured long bones that are not effectively immobilized fail to knit properly, and repair is by fibrous malunion. It is also true that if mobile teeth are not effectively immobilized after the perio-dontal surgery, the bone defects also fail to heal properly, the teeth remain mobile, and continue to be functionally handicapped instead of becoming solidly immobilized by filling in of the defects with normal calcified alveolar bone.

Immobilization of loose teeth may be permanent or temporary, depending upon the clinical needs of the case. When irreversible horizontal circumscribing resorption of alveolar bone has occurred and the normal 1 to 2 crown-root ratio has been disrupted, permanent fixation is indicated to compensate for the crown-root ratio loss and thereby enable the mobile teeth to withstand the normal torques of function. There are two basic methods for providing permanent fixation. One method consists of locking the loose teeth together with a Whaledent type of non-parallel pin splint. The other is by locking the mobile teeth together with inlays and/or crowns into a fixed prosthesis. Other methods such as the internal "A" splint that was described in the first edition also have been used. Choice of method is determined by the clinical judgment of the therapist and the available techniques and material.

When the bone loss is reversible and temporary immobilization during the postoperative repair period is all that is required, it can be provided by any of the following methods. The loose teeth can be tied together with continuous loop wiring such as is used to immobilize fractured jaws. Or the loose teeth and, where feasible, the immediately adjacent firm teeth can be ligated to an appropriately contoured labial arch bar with stainless steel ligatures. Or the labial arch bar can be attached to the teeth with orthodontic bands and brackets, which is an excellent method, but often is neither feasible nor necessary.

The author has devised a simple but remarkably effective method for attaching the contoured labial arch bar to the teeth with cold cure quick setting acrylic such as is used for filling carious teeth (Fig. 18–4). The labial surfaces of the teeth to be ligated to the bar are dried thoroughly and a drop of liquid monomer is applied to each tooth's labial surface. A semi-fluid thin mix of acrylic is then applied to each tooth and the arch bar is brought into firm contact with the labial surfaces of the teeth so that it becomes imbedded into the acrylic. Additional acrylic is added, in a manner similar to the Neilon technique for inserting acrylic fillings. When the outer surface of the bar is covered on each tooth with the acrylic it is permitted to set. After the acrylic has hardened it is surprisingly strong and tenaciously adherent to the teeth, despite the fact that the tooth surfaces to which it has been applied were not etched preoperatively. After the splint has fulfilled its function it can easily be removed by prying it loose with a hand instrument such as a Wedelstadt chisel by directing the lifting force outward away from the teeth. The surface enamel of the teeth remains smooth and unaffected and this method does not create any problem of tooth decay such as often occurs under orthodontic bands.

When the mobile teeth have drifted apart owing to pathological migration and it is necessary to restore them to normal alignment in the dental arch before immobilizing them, the author has found they can usually be readily

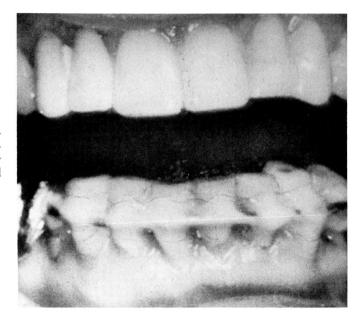

Figure 18–4. Immobilization of mobile teeth following periodontal therapy with an arch bar wire attached to the teeth with acrylic.

realigned by applying pressure very gradually with traction produced by a combination of Japanese grassline and elastic bands tied around the teeth to be moved. The grassline swells as the saliva of the mouth moistens it, causing it to contract. When the force of this contraction is combined with the pull of the elastic bands it produces a surprisingly effective amount of traction against the mobile teeth. Moreover, the therapist can direct the traction force by inserting soft stainless steel ligature wires through the embrasures and tying the ligatures around the combined elastic bands and grassline, then tightening the ligatures where additional traction is needed. Judicious utilization of this control of forces enables the therapist to move the teeth back into normal alignment in the dental arches efficiently and atraumatically.

After the realignment in their normal position in the dental arches has been achieved the mobile teeth can then be immobilized in their new position during the period of bone regeneration and maturation with the acrylic retained arch bar described above.

Postoperative Instructions to Patient Regarding Oral Physiotherapy

It is also necessary to instruct the patient in the method of toothbrushing preferred by the therapist. The author prefers the Stillman and Chartres methods of brushing. Since the advent of the soft nylon bristle brushes with polished rounded tips that will not cut and slash the tissues, the author instructs his patients to use this brush immediately after the second cement pack has been removed, and to use it for 4 to 6 weeks, until the tissues have matured and can tolerate the pressure from a hard brush. He then has the patient change to the double row, extra hard natural bristle type of brush and use it with vigor at least twice daily thereafter.

Other methods of massage are not overlooked. The patient is instructed in proper use of the rubber tip in the embrasures and of water jet spray used at not more than one half to two thirds power. He cautions the patient not to use the jet sprays at full power, since they can cause injury to the tissues and thereby actually stimulate periodontal deterioration. Even the ball of the fingertip is not overlooked. The patient is instructed to use the ball of the index finger with light rotary pressure high in the vestibules, so that even during the period when the cement packs are present, gentle but valuable fingertip massage to stimulate the blood supply can be instituted during the critically important initial healing period.

For postoperative care the patient is instructed to maintain a high protein intake even during the initial 10 days while on a liquid and semisolid diet. The author also prescribes ascorbic acid and multiple vitamins as dietary supplements and Meritene, Nutrament and Sustagen as balanced liquid meals. Before the periodontal electrosurgery is instituted, the patient is required to demonstrate to the author his mastery of the toothbrushing and other methods of massage of the gingivae.

Many people have difficulty manipulating the manual toothbrush with equal efficiency in all areas of the mouth. Right-handed individuals are prone to have difficulty managing the proper massage in the right quadrant, and left-handed individuals with the left quadrant. Under such circumstances the electrically operated automatic toothbrush can provide effective massage even in the areas awkward to manage manually.

There are two basic types of automatic toothbrushes. One type provides an up and down rotary movement of the brush head, the other, a side to side lateral movement of the brush head.

When the gingivae are completely healed and mature, and the interdental papillae are firmly attached in their embrasures, the up and down motion of the brush head is an acceptable and desirable means for providing tooth cleansing and gingival massage. But until the tissues are firmly reattached, such brushing may tear the interdental papillae loose from their embrasures. With the brush that provides a side to side motion, the Chartres or Stillman technique of brushing can be instituted, thereby avoiding the hazard of detaching the interdental papillae.

The General Electric Dual Motion toothbrush (Fig. 18–5) provides both the lateral and up and down movements. For this reason when an automatic toothbrush is indicated, the dual motion brush is recommended for lateral use with the side to side motion, with a very soft nylon brush for the first 2 to 3 months in accord with the Chartres or Stillman technique. After that initial period, the patient is given the option of continuing to use the brush in that manner, or to switch to the up and down stroke if preferred, but in either event to discontinue the soft nylon brush head and replace it with a hard brush head, preferably natural bristle rather than nylon.

Dual Motion Cordless Automatic Toothbrush
MODEL TB-9

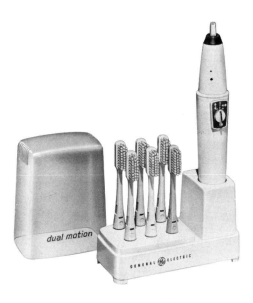

- Switch selects up and down or back and forth brushing action
- Cordless power handle may be rinsed for quick, easy cleaning
- Built-in recharging system has no metal contacts to corrode
- 6 Personal color-coded brushes
- Complete with bracket for wall mounting
- Replacement brushes easily available

Protective cover
helps keep brushes clean

DUAL MOTION CORDLESS AUTOMATIC TOOTHBRUSH   MODEL TB-9   A-1737

Figure 18–5. Electric toothbrush assembly with both horizontal and vertical stroke motions. (Courtesy of General Electric.)

President Hine of Indiana University stressed this need for oral physiotherapy during a Chicago Mid-Winter Dental Meeting panel symposium, which he moderated. He stated that when the mouth is healthy, all that is required to keep it healthy is good oral hygiene. But once periodontal disease has been manifested, oral hygiene alone is no longer adequate. Vigorous oral physiotherapy must thereafter be employed to maintain the health of the tissues after they have been restored to normal health by periodontal therapy.[5]

FOOTNOTE REFERENCES

1. Gargiulo, A. W.: Verbal communication. Symposium. Chicago Mid-Winter Meeting.
2. Hiatt, W.: Verbal communication. Symposium. Chicago Mid-Winter Meeting.
3. Prichard, J. F.: Verbal communication. Open Circuit T.V. Program, Chicago Mid-Winter Meeting.
4. Oringer, M. J.: Electrosurgery in Dentistry. Philadelphia, W. B. Saunders Company, 1962.
5. Hine, M. K.: Verbal communication. Symposium. Chicago Mid-Winter Meeting.
6. Pope, J. W., Gargiulo, A. W., Staffileno, H., and Levy, S.: Effects of electrosurgery on wound healing in dogs. Periodontics, 6:No. 1, 30–37, 1968.
7. Martin, J. W.: Written communication. Chicago, Ill., March 8, 1968.

8. Harrison, J. D.: Verbal communication. 1966 A.D.A. Meeting and 1966 American Academy of Dental Electrosurgery Meeting.

9. Kelly, W. J., Jr.: Verbal communication. 1966 A.D.A. Meeting, and 1966 American Academy of Dental Electrosurgery Meeting.

10. Evans, R.: Verbal communication. 1966 American Academy of Dental Electrosurgery Meeting. Also, Personal communication, 1968.

11. Miller, S. C.: Textbook of Periodontia. 3rd ed. Philadelphia, Blakiston Co., 1950.

12. Burket, L. W.: Oral Medicine. Philadelphia, J. B. Lippincott Co., 1946, p. 587.

13. Indications and contraindications for surgery in the treatment of periodontal disease, in Lederle Newsletters, A Collection for the Dental Profession, 1956, pp. 85–94.

14. Glickman, I., and Schluger, S.: Periodontia Symposium. Chicago Dental Society Midwinter Meeting, 1961.

15. Fox, L.: Communication to Dental Times (Periodontal surgery criticized). D. Times, 3:12, Jan., 1961.

16. Sugarman, S. S.: Verbal communication. Essay Before Greater New York Dental Meeting, 1959.

17. Shira, R. B.: Verbal communication. Essay Before Chicago Dental Society Midwinter Meeting, 1961.

18. Hyder, C. M.: Gingivectomy by electrodesiccation. D. Survey, Dec. 1958.

19. Goldman, H. M., Schluger, S., Fox, L. and Cohen, D. W.: Periodontal Therapy. 2nd ed. St. Louis, C. V. Mosby Co., 1960, pp. 250–261.

20. Ogus, W. I.: The elimination of the pyorrheal pocket by electrosurgery. Am. J. Orthodont. & Oral Surg., 27:135, 1941.

21. Orban, B.: Tissue healing following electrocoagulation of gingivae. J. Periodont., 15:17, 1944.

22. Webb, G. F.: Electro-surgical treatment of pyorrhea. D. Survey, Vol. 11, Aug., 1935.

23. Trotter, P. A.: Gingivectomy by short wave electrosurgery. Brit. D. J., 90:214, 1951.

24. Beube, F. E.: Periodontology: Diagnosis and Treatment. New York, The MacMillan Co., 1953, pp. 593–608.

25. Glickman, I.: Clinical Periodontology. Philadelphia, W. B. Saunders Co., 1953, pp. 877–880.

26. Saghirian, L. M.: Electrosurgical gingivoplasty. Oral Surg., Oral Med. & Oral Path., 2:1549, 1949.

27. Saghirian, L. M.: Pocket elimination by electrosurgery. D. Digest, Apr., 1949.

28. Saghirian, L. M.: Periodontosis: treatment by surgical and electrosurgical gingivoplasty. J.A.D.A., 38:67, 1949.

29. Saghirian, L. M.: Theory and practice of electrosurgery. New York J. Den., 22:390, 1952.

30. Beube, F. E., and Silvers, H. F.: Influence of devitalized heterogeneous bone-powder on regeneration of alveolar and maxillary bone of dogs. J. D. Res., 14:15, 1934.

31. Beube, F. E., and Silvers, H. F.: Further studies on bone generation with the use of boiled heterogeneous bone. J. Periodont., 7:17, 1936.

32. Cross, W. G.: Bone grafts in periodontal disease: A preliminary study. D. Practitioner, 6:98, Nov., 1955.

33. Cross, W. G.: Bone implants in periodontal disease—a further study. J. Periodont., 28:184, 1957.

34. Forsberg, H.: Transplantation of os purum and bone chips in the surgical treatment of periodontal disease (preliminary report). Acta Odont. Scandinav., 13:235, 1956.

35. Hegedüs, Z.: The rebuilding of the alveolar process by bone transplantation. D. Cosmos, 65:736, 1923.

36. Losee, F.: Bone treated with ethylene-diamine as a successful foundation material in cross-species bone grafts. Nature, 177:1032–1033, 1956.

37. Cross, W. G.: The use of bone implants in the treatment of periodontal pockets. Symposium on Practical Periodontal Therapy. D. Clin. North America, Mar., 1960.

38. Zemsky, J. I.: Oral Diseases. New York, Physicians and Surgeons Book Co., 1930, pp. 332–342.

Chapter Nineteen

CLINICAL TECHNIQUES IN PERIODONTAL ELECTROSURGERY

INTRODUCTION

The immortal Roger Bacon, by perceiving the need for differentiating between the abstract and the material, in a sense founded modern science at Oxford University many centuries ago.

Bacon risked burning at the stake for heresy by daring to proclaim that whereas *"credo quindi cognosco"* ... to believe is to know, to take things on faith, may be an acceptable tenet for theology and philosophy, for science it must be *"cognosco quindi credo"* ... to know is to believe.

The general practice of dentistry has gradually been divorcing itself more and more from involvement in the treatment of periodontal disease. As a result many general practitioners tend to take on faith the opinions of some periodontists that electrosurgery has no place in modern periodontal therapy. The following chapter is presented in the hope that it will rekindle for each reader Bacon's dictum "cognosco quindi credo," and that each will exercise his own judgment with regard to the merits of the following techniques and their rationale, rather than accept by default opinions that all too often are based on hearsay or lack of electrosurgical skill, know-how, and experience.

A large number of diverse factors are capable of triggering periodontal disease, and a considerable variety of specific electrosurgical techniques have been devised for the definitive treatment of periodontoclasia. Since both are conducive to confusion, this chapter has been subdivided into four major component parts to help facilitate orderly review of the typical clinical cases with which the various procedures will be demonstrated.

The four major components are
      I. Periodontal Disease Induced by Unfavorable Local Factors
     II. Periodontoclasia Attributable to Systemic Disease
   III. Management of the Individual Infrabony Pocket
   IV. Miscellaneous Periodontal Procedures
Each of these is in turn subdivided into subsections covering the respective periodontal conditions that constitute each category.

I. PERIODONTAL DISEASE INDUCED BY UNFAVORABLE LOCAL FACTORS

There are two major categories that can trigger periodontal deterioration:
    A. Mechanical Factors
    B. Biomechanical Factors
The most important of the purely mechanical factors are irritation produced by salivary and serumnal calculus that Gottlieb[1] characterized as "schmutzpyorrhea" (Fig. 19–1), irritation produced by traumatic occlusion, and irritation from overhanging margins of fillings and sharp rough edges of subgingival caries.

The biomechanical factors include pockets of hyperplastic gingivae created by rotated or malaligned teeth, irritation from rapid tooth movement, and subgingival impingement by orthodontic bands. By far the most important factors, however, which will be discussed and reviewed here, are the conditions called endodontic-periodontal pathology and iatrogenic periodontoclasia produced by unfavorable tissue reaction to irritations created by improper removable and fixed prostheses. Periodontal deterioration induced by

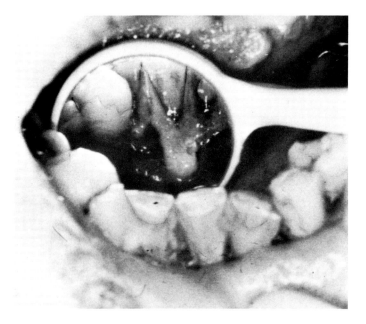

Figure 19–1. A classic example of Gottlieb's "schmutzpyorrhea" — periodontoclasia caused by massive calculus deposit irritation, a form seen less and less as the practice of toothbrushing becomes more universal.

excessive traction against the marginal gingivae by abnormal frenal ligaments and high muscle attachments also is biomechanical in nature, but this will be reviewed later in the chapter under the heading Miscellaneous Procedures.

Cases in which local factors are the principal cause for periodontal deterioration but are also complicated by minor secondary systemic factors are included in this part of the chapter.

Mechanical Factors

TRAUMATIC OCCLUSION

Traumatic occlusion is not a single entity. There are two distinctly different types of traumatic occlusion, each of which produces a totally different clinical reaction and requires different therapeutic measures.

One type is characteristically sudden in onset and is an acute localized response to disruption of a normal occlusal relation by a prematurity produced by a newly inserted restoration such as a filling, an inlay, or a crown. The acute pericementitis that ensues usually is so painful that unless the prematurity is promptly eliminated and the occlusion restored to normal, even devitalization of the tooth may fail to provide adequate relief from the pain, and the tooth may have to be extracted. If the prematurity is promptly eliminated, the pericementitis almost invariably subsides and no further trouble is experienced. This type of traumatic occlusion therefore rarely causes periodontoclasia.

The second type of traumatic occlusion invariably is a relatively chronic type produced by malocclusion of long duration that may involve two opposing teeth, or much or all of the dentition. Pain rarely is a factor with this type. Rather, it is characterized by a progressive breakdown of the investing alveolar bone of the affected teeth that results in a localized or generalized periodontoclasia. Both types will be reviewed and demonstrated.

CASE 1

This case is an excellent example of localized traumatic occlusion involving two opposing teeth and demonstrates the advantageous use of electrosurgery for definitive conservative treatment of the large periodontal defect.

It also offers an excellent example of the nature of alveolar destruction often seen in this type of case. Although a considerable amount of the labial cortical bone is destroyed, the destruction of the inner spongiosum is much more extensive and rapid and often extends to and beyond the level of the apex of the affected tooth. It is interesting to note that despite the extensive bone destruction the tooth usually remains vital, so that, although the roentgenographic appearance resembles the pathology of the endodontic-periodontal cases, the absence of a root canal filling provides positive differentiation.

PATIENT.   A 49-year-old white male.

HISTORY. He suddenly noticed that the gingival tissue appeared to have become detached from the maxillary left cuspid tooth and bled occasionally during toothbrushing. He also experienced tenderness in the tooth while eating. He consulted his dentist, who x-rayed the tooth and found a large amount of radiolucence in the periapical region and referred him for treatment.

CLINICAL EXAMINATION. The gingival tissue appeared reasonably normal in color and tone but was detached from the left cuspid on the labial aspect. A periodontal pocket probe was inserted under the gingiva and penetrated its full length without encountering resistance (Case Fig. 1-1). A sterile silver endodontic point was in-

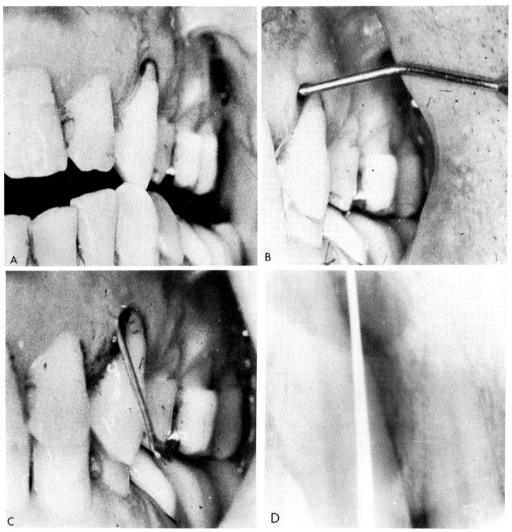

Case Figure 1-1. Traumatic occlusion. A, A preoperative view, showing the traumatic premature contact of the maxillary and mandibular cuspids and the detachment of the marginal gingiva. B, Depth of the defect can be seen as a regular periodontal pocket probe is inserted its full length without encountering resistance. C, A long sterile silver point has been inserted into the defect and advanced until it met resistance. The point is left in place to serve as a radiopaque periodontal pocket marker. D, X-ray with silver point in situ as a radiopaque marker. Note the penetration extends about 2 mm. beyond the apex of the tooth, and that the latter appears to be vital.

serted as a pocket marker, and a periapical x-ray film was taken with the point in situ. The silver point penetrated beyond the apical level of the tooth, but the penetration followed the medial surface of the root, and on the x-ray film the radiolucence appeared to be limited to that area, without involving the rest of the periapical region. The occlusal relationship of the teeth appeared normal in centric relation, but in the protrusive position the maxillary left cuspid came into contact so prematurely that the remaining teeth in the two arches stayed almost a centimeter apart. The marginal gingiva was discolored along its detached edge, creating a dark marginal line.

TREATMENT. A pulp vitalitest was performed on the cuspid, with normal response, confirming the lesion to be of periodontal rather than periapical origin. The occlusal prematurity was eliminated by grinding the palatal aspect of the maxillary cuspid cusp and the labial aspect of the mandibular cuspid cusp, without appreciably reducing the overall length of the two teeth. The tissues were then prepared for injection and infraorbital block and palatal infiltration anesthesia was administered.

A fine 45-degree-angle needle electrode was selected and cutting current was set at 3 on the power output dial. The electrode was activated and used to make a verticooblique incision for a mucoperiosteal flap, extending downward and slightly posteriorly from the areolar mucosa midway between the lateral and cuspid root apices to the mesiogingival angle of the cuspid (Case Fig. 1–2). The apical attachment of the papilla in the embrasure distal to the cuspid was then severed to permit adequate reflection of the tissue flap, which exposed the cuspid root fully denuded of its labial bone and the infrabony lesion.

A 0.7-cm. round loop electrode was substituted for the needle, and cutting current was increased to 5 on the power output dial. The mucoperiosteal flap was rotrated to expose the ventral surface, and the epithelialized lining of the defect was resected from the ventral surface of the flap with this loop electrode. The round loop was then replaced with a 17-mm. periodontal loop electrode and current output was reduced to 4.5. The loop was activated and used as an electronic curet to thoroughly debride the defect, which extended about 7 mm. beyond the apex of the cuspid. The activated electrode was introduced each time for a fraction of a second during which it was moved rapidly in an up and down and rotary direction, and withdrawn for 10 seconds, to permit the heat being generated to become totally dissipated. The completion of debridement was ascertained by digital inspection of the defect with the inactivated electrode and by transillumination. The *dead* cementum was then removed gently but thoroughly by manual curettage of the exposed root surfaces, with care to leave the remaining viable cementum still present undisturbed. At this point the coronal two thirds of the lateral-cuspid interseptal bone was intact, and the exposed root surfaces were relatively smooth, the infrabony defect extending superiorly beyond the remaining interseptal bone.

The activated loop curet was brushed rapidly over the exposed root surfaces to destroy any bacteria that might remain on the viable cementum. A steel periodontal curet was introduced into the infrabony defect and used to encourage bleeding. A small amount of powdered Gelfoam was introduced and mixed with the blood, the flap was restored to position, and the tissue margins were coapted and sutured with interrupted silk sutures. When the blood was clotted, tincture of myrrh and benzoin was applied, and a piece of Squibb Orahesive bandage large enough to cover the entire surgical field was prepared and attached to the tissues by gentle but firm digital pressure.

The patient was instructed in postoperative care and reappointed for removal of the sutures, which was performed on the fifth postoperative day. Healing progressed

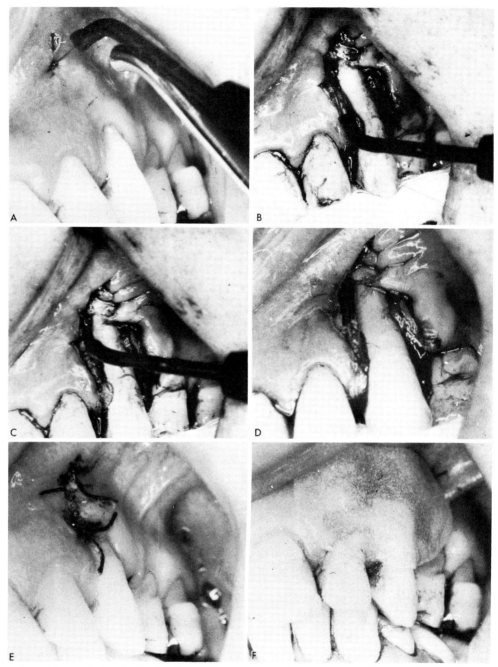

Case Figure 1–2. A, Beginning of the vertico-oblique incision for a mucoperiosteal flap. The incision is being made with a fine 45-degree-angle needle electrode, and the surgical site is being illuminated with a transilluminating lamp. *B*, The flap has been elevated, revealing total destruction of the labial bone plate and extensive destruction of the alveolar bone on the mesial aspect of the tooth. A 17-mm. periodontal electronic curet electrode has been activated to begin debridement of the defect. *C*, The electrode has penetrated approximately 12 mm. into the defect. *D*, The infrabony lesion has been thoroughly debrided. *E*, The flap has been restored to position and sutured. *F*, A piece of Squibb Orahesive Bandage material has been applied over the cuspid, and a large sheet of the bandage material has been superimposed over the lateral-cuspid-first bicuspid area.

rapidly and uneventfully. He was seen for the last time at the end of six months, at which time the bone as well as the soft tissues appeared normal, and the tooth responded normally to a pulp vitalitest.

The pioneers in modern periodontal therapy believed that traumatic occlusion, in particular, and irritation from salivary and serumnal calculus, to a lesser degree, were the main culprits responsible for periodontal deterioration. The accepted formula of periodontal therapy as a result consisted essentially of thorough prophylaxis and balancing of the occlusion, followed by manual curettage to resect the epithelial lining and debris from the pockets.

With the passage of time, knowledge about the etiology of the disease began to expand and in addition to traumatic occlusion and calculus, other factors began to emerge as important triggering agents. Although this brought about a shift in therapeutic focus, the importance of balancing the occlusion in the treatment of this disease has not diminished. To the contrary, it has contributed to the development of sophisticated philosophies of occlusion and complex anatomic articulators that help to achieve the balance.

CASE 2

This case is an excellent example of advanced periodontoclasia created by a generalized traumatic occlusion. A very atypical appearance of the gingival tissues challenged the diagnostic skill as much as the deep pocket formation resulting from extensive bone destruction challenged the surgical skill.

A particularly interesting aspect of this case is that it demonstrates the utter futility of attempting to "balance" the occlusion prior to instituting periodontal therapy, despite the availability of highly sophisticated instruments and philosophies of occlusion, when the occlusal imbalance is widespread with much rotation, elongation, and drifting of the teeth. All that can be achieved preoperatively in this type of case is elimination of traumatizing prematurities that would disrupt the tissue repair postoperatively, since meaningful balancing of the occlusion can be accomplished only by performing a complete occlusal reconstruction.

Since it would have been highly impractical to subject the patient to such extensive and expensive reconstruction until a favorable outcome of the periodontal therapy was assured, the actual "balancing" of the occlusion was not instituted in this case until after satisfactory completion of the periodontal therapy, whereupon she was referred back to her dentist for the reconstruction.

PATIENT.   A 33-year-old white female.

HISTORY.   As a result of advanced periodontoclasia, all the teeth were mobile. For the past three years several posterior teeth had been developing paradontal abscesses which regressed spontaneously. A periodontist recommended extraction of the posterior teeth and three anteriors and gingivectomy for the remaining teeth. She rejected this treatment plan. She was referred to the author for the more conservative electrosurgical therapy.

CLINICAL EXAMINATION

Extraoral.   Negative.

Intraoral.   She had almost a full complement of teeth. They were in marked malocclusion, particularly the maxillary left lateral and cuspid. Both teeth were rotated and the cuspid was greatly elongated, creating a locked bite. The marginal gingivae throughout the mouth appeared somewhat desquamated of their normal surface keratin. The gingivae were hyperemic and the interproximal papillae were hypertrophied. Every tooth was involved with one or more deep irregular pockets (Case Fig. 2–1).

Roentgenographic examination showed deep pockets and extensive bone loss throughout the mouth. The most severe loss had occurred in the interseptal and intraradicular bone. The molars showed bifurcation and trifurcation involvement. The maxillary right third molar appeared hopelessly involved. The remainder of the mouth appeared likely to respond to combined gingivectomy–infrabony pocket eradication. Extraction of the third molar and conservative electrosurgical pocket eradication – gingivectoplasty for the remainder of the mouth was recommended, and this treatment plan was accepted by the patient.

TREATMENT. The patient was premedicated with Panalba for three days prior to surgery, which was performed two days postmenstrual.

Owing to its extensiveness, surgery was planned in two stages five days apart. The maxilla was prepared for surgery and bilateral posterosuperior alveolar, infraorbital, nasopalatine and anterior palatine blocks were administered. A flame-shaped loop electrode was selected and current output set at 5 for electrosection. The hypertrophic hyperemic gingival mucosa on the labial aspect of the right lateral and its interproximal papilla were reduced with the activated electrode (Case Fig. 2–2). A persistent spurting bleeder in the distal interproximal embrasure was brought under control by fulguration with a straight heavy needle electrode.

The anterior marginal and cemental gingivae were reduced on the labial aspect with the flame-shaped loop electrode used with short wiping strokes. Current output was reduced to 4, and the deep mesial and distal infrabony pockets were debrided with a 17-mm. 45-degree-angle periodontal loop electrode. The electrode was inserted into and used with rotary and push-pull motions as a periodontal curet that resected the granulomatous debris and epithelial lining of each pocket to the base of the defect.

The buccal aspect of the bicuspids and molars were then planed with the flame-shaped loop, and interproximal pockets and trifurcation involvements were debrided in the manner described above. When the labial-buccal surgery was completed, the anterior palatal marginal mucosa was reduced with the flame-shaped loop electrode, with current increased to 6 because of the greater thickness and density of the palatal tissues. A flame-shaped electrode bent to a right angle was used to plane the posterior palatal tissues from around the bicuspids and molars. When the palatal surgery was completed the tissues were dried with sponges, tincture of myrrh and benzoin applied, and a stiffly mixed surgical cement pack inserted around the entire operative field. The condemned tooth was then extracted, debridement performed, and medicated gelatin deposited in the socket.

She returned on the fifth postoperative day and reported having had moderate discomfort the first two days. The cement pack was removed and the tissues were irrigated and inspected. They still looked rather raw. It was apparent that the healing was not progressing as rapidly as usual. Tincture of myrrh and benzoin was applied and a fresh cement pack inserted.

The mandible was prepared for surgery and anesthetized with bilateral inferior alveolar regional blocks. A tapered flame-shaped loop electrode was selected and current output set at 5 for electrosection. The interproximal papillae were reduced to concave sluiceways with pulling motion directed from the apex to the base (Case Fig. 2–3). Then the labial gingivae were reduced to normal level by shaving the tissue

(Text continued on page 592)

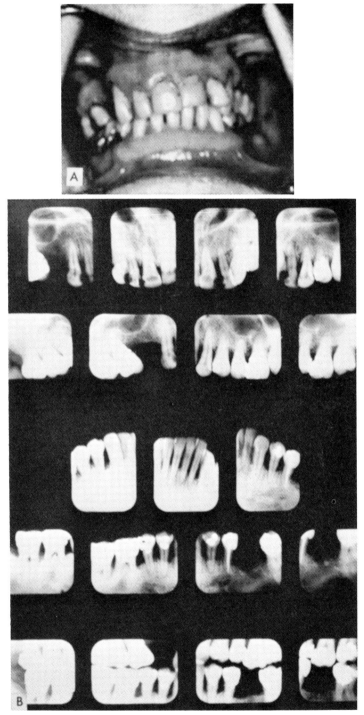

Case Figure 2–1. Full mouth gingivectoplasty. Treatment of extensive periodontal deterioration complicated by unfavorable systemic and local factors. *A*, Preoperative appearance, labial view. Note massively hypertrophied gingivae and rotated left lateral and cuspid. *B*, Full mouth series of roentgenograms reveals extensive bone loss, deep irregular pocket formation, bifurcation and trifurcation involvement of almost all the teeth.

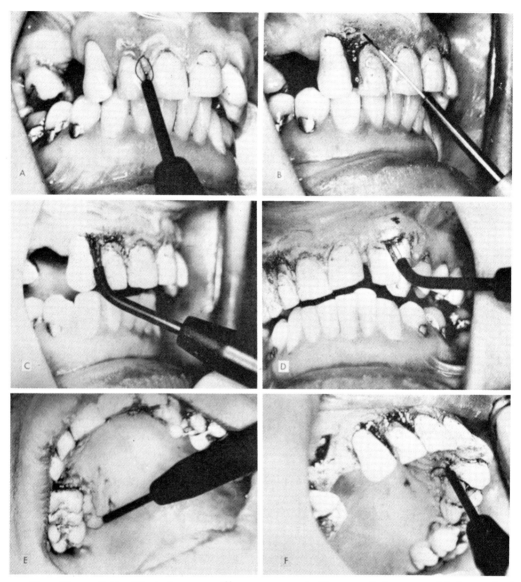

Case Figure 2–2. First stage: maxillary surgery. *A,* Hyperemic hypertrophied marginal gingivae and interproximal papilla in central-lateral embrasure reduced to normal contour by planing the tissues with a flame-shaped loop electrode. *B,* Persistent bleeding from a spurter vessel stopped by fulguration. (Note sparks arcing from the electrode tip to the tissue surface.) *C,* Debridement being performed in an infrabony pocket. *D,* Debridement of infrabony pocket on opposite side. *E,* Hypertrophic posterior palatal mucosa reduced to normal contour by planing with 90-degree-angle bent flame-shaped loop electrode. *F,* Anterior palatal mucosa treated in a similar manner.

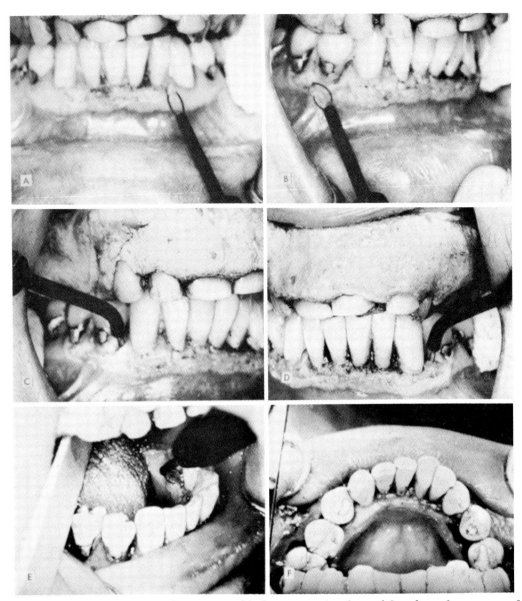

Case Figure 2–3.   Second stage: mandibular surgery (performed five days after surgery of maxillary tissues). *A*, A narrow flame-shaped loop electrode is used with a wiping motion directed from above downward to reduce a hypertrophic papilla to a concave sluiceway. *B*, Regular flame-shaped loop electrode is used to plane the hypertrophied labial gingivae to normal contour and simultaneously bevel the marginal tissue to a feather edge. *C*, A deep infrabony pocket being debrided with a narrow 45-degree-angle U-shaped loop electrode used with push-pull and rotary motions. *D*, An infrabony pocket on the opposite side used in a similar manner. *E*, Lingual gingivae and interproximal papillae are reduced to normal contour with a flame-shaped loop electrode that has been bent to a 90 degree angle to facilitate planing and shaving in layers. *F*, Mirror image of lingual tissues after surgery is completed. Note the evidence of infrabony pocket debridement (arrows).

with brushing strokes. A somewhat larger flame-shaped loop electrode was substituted and the posterior buccal gingivae reduced by shaving in layers.

The deep pockets were then debrided with a narrow 45-degree-angle U-shaped loop electrode and reduced current output. The debris was resected from these pockets, also with rotary and push-pull motions of the electrode.

The lingual gingivae were reduced in the same manner with the straight flame-shaped loop electrode in the anterior region, and with the bent right-angle flame-shaped loop electrode in the posterior region. The interproximal papillae on the lingual aspect were reduced to concave sluiceways. For better control and to avoid excessive reduction of the papillae, the loop was directed from the base upward to the apical attachments of the papillae. When the lingual surgery was completed, the tissues were dried, tincture of myrrh and benzoin was applied, and a stiffly mixed surgical cement pack was inserted. Antibiotic therapy was renewed for three days, and she was reappointed.

She returned five days later. The cement packs in both jaws were intact, and the socket of the molar was almost fully healed. The cement packs were removed, and the mouth irrigated. There was some improvement in the maxillary healing, but the mandibular gingival healing seemed somewhat more advanced than the maxillary, which had been done five days previously. It was reasonable to assume that the difference in the rate of healing might be due to the time element as it related to her menstrual cycle.

Tincture of myrrh and benzoin was applied to both operative fields in air-dried layers, then a fresh cement pack was inserted over the mandibular gingivae. She returned in five days and the cement pack was removed. The mandibular gingivae still appeared somewhat more advanced in healing than the maxillary. The occlusion had been balanced preoperatively as much as possible. The teeth were splinted with continuous loop intramaxillary wiring to reduce their mobility (Case Fig. 2–4). Elastic band traction was applied to the rotated lateral and cuspid to help bring them into better alignment and occlusal relationship.

She returned one week later. The mandibular gingival healing progress compared to the maxillary was more pronounced than ever. Irritation from the intramaxillary wiring had caused marked hypertrophy of the maxillary median papilla. It was treated with superficial spot coagulation under topical anesthesia. This failed to produce appreciable reduction of the hypertrophied papilla. At her next visit the papilla was reduced to normal level by fulguration performed under topical anesthesia.

Almost one month after the maxillary surgery a large paradontal abscess suddenly appeared on the palatal aspect of the maxillary left first-second molar area, and several other palatal and lingual posterior areas showed evidence of deterioration with tendency for proliferative granulation. Since the deterioration occurred during her menstrual period, and the maxillary surgery had failed to heal as well as the mandibular, which had been performed well after her menstrual period, it appeared likely that the latter might have some bearing on her healing and gingival health. D. W. Cohen has reported a number of cases that presented a similar syndrome of abscess formation in the posterior part of the mouth on the lingual and palatal aspects, which he classified as "cyclic neutropenias."[2] These cases showed sharp drop in neutrophils every four weeks, with spontaneous increase in neutrophil count and decrease in white cell count.

A complete blood count was ordered. Although she had a slight neutropenia, a white cell count of 11,800 appeared more significant, strongly suggestive of acute infection. A paradontal abscess on the palatal aspect of the maxillary left second molar

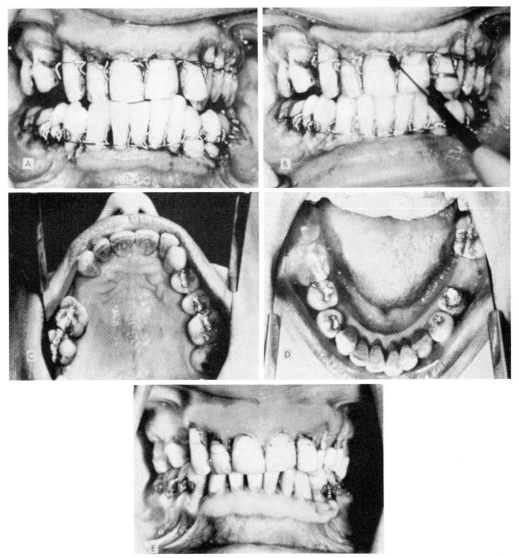

Case Figure 2–4. Postoperative sequence. *A*, Postoperative appearance of tissues 10 days after mandibular surgery. Note that healing appears more advanced in the mandible although the maxillary surgery preceded it by five days, and that all the teeth have been ligated with continuous loop intramaxillary wiring to immobilize the teeth. *B*, Granulation tissue proliferating slightly in response to irritation from the ligature wires in the median maxillary embrasure is destroyed by fulguration. Note elastic band traction has been instituted to reduce malposition of the rotated left lateral and cuspid. *C*, Postoperative appearance of the palatal tissues four months after surgery. *D*, Appearance of the lingual tissues at this time. *E*, Labial appearance of the gingivae at this time. Note the excellent tissue tone, concave self-cleansing sluiceways and improved alignment of the rotated teeth.

was incised and a smear of its contents made on a blood agar plate for culture. A sensitivity test was also ordered.

A pure strain of *S. aureus* was cultured, and Chloromycetin was ascertained to be the drug of choice. Chloromycetin was prescribed, but because of potential side effects of aplastic anemia, semiweekly blood counts were ordered. The first showed a reduction in white blood cells to 9600, and no evidence of side effects. The second one, taken one week after the drug was started, showed a drop in hemoglobin and red blood cells, and an increase in lymphocytes, with slight anisocytosis and occasional atypical lymphocytes. Although the paradontal abscesses responded to this drug, the white blood cell count still remained rather high. Because of the danger of aplastic anemia, this drug had to be discontinued.

Tetracycline was substituted. Healing continued to progress slowly in the maxilla and somewhat more favorably in the mandible. After one month the tissues were beginning to appear normally healed, but with the onset of another menstrual period, moderate regression again occurred. The elastic traction had to be discontinued because of hypertrophic granulation tissue which began to proliferate around these teeth. In those areas where the abscesses had been prone to develop, a tendency for proliferating granulation was manifested, particularly during the menstrual periods. The proliferation was controlled by spot coagulation.

After three months the intramaxillary wire splints were removed. All the teeth were notably more firm, although not all were completely immobile. Areas where the wiring had impinged against the tissues were somewhat hypertrophied, especially the interproximal papillae. These were treated with superficial spot coagulation.

Two weeks later the gingivae appeared fully healed. The tissue surface was fully matured and normally keratinized, and the tissue tone was normal. All the teeth except the left mandibular central and lateral and the two bicuspids were normally firm. The latter four teeth still showed class I mobility which persisted for approximately three more months. The alignment of the left lateral and cuspid was much improved. Except for a slightly purplish hue of the maxillary labial gingivae the mouth appeared normally healthy in all respects.

The postoperative healing sequence that occurred in this case appears to have been adversely influenced by a number of unrelated, unfavorable local and systemic factors. The advanced state of the disease and bone loss constituted one handicap. The marked malocclusion that could not be fully corrected or compensated was a further handicap. Superimposed on these local factors were two secondary systemic handicaps: marked periodic hormonal imbalance and chronic infection and reinfection from one of the most resistant strains of bacteria. Under such circumstances, the improved stability, eradication of the deep infrabony pockets, and termination of periodic abscess formation are gratifying. Tissue tone is excellent, the mouth is healthy, and the teeth are functionally useful.

CASE 3

This final case of this series has been included because it presents a number of interesting features. It demonstrates that the degree of periodontal deterioration which often accompanies the downward drift and elongation of maxillary molars resulting from failure to replace extracted opposing teeth is likely to be greater, owing to loss of occlusal function, than where occlusal function has been maintained. It also demonstrates the possibility of acceleration of the periodontal deterioration if such teeth are eventually utilized as abutments and are subjected to torque from non-parallel wrought wire clasps. It also offers evidence that the conservative attempt at treating extensive trifurcation lesions even when the prognosis appears unfavorable is worthwhile, since the resultant improvement in tissue tone and blood supply greatly increases the prospects for success of more radical follow-up surgery.

PATIENT.   A 63-year-old black female.

HISTORY.   Many years previously she had had multiple extractions in both jaws without having the missing teeth replaced. Approximately six months ago she had two lower molars extracted, and all the missing teeth were restored with a partial upper denture and a lower lingual bar denture, both retained with wire clasps.

Shortly after she began to wear the dentures the maxillary right and left first molars and the right first bicuspid, all of which were serving as abutments, began to feel sore and seemed to become slightly loose, especially when she wore the dentures for long periods without removing them. Several weeks later she noticed bleeding from the gingivae that persisted despite frequent salt water lavage, so she consulted her dentist. After several treatments of manual curettage failed to improve the situation he referred her to the author for periodontal surgery to try to preserve the abutment teeth for functional use.

CLINICAL EXAMINATION.   The denture clasps were unsurveyed, nonparallel wrought wire clasps. Clinically, the maxillary left third molar, first and second bicuspids, and central, and the right lateral, second bicuspid, and first molar were missing from the dental arch. The left first and second molars, second bicuspid, and right first and second bicuspid, and first, second, and third molars were missing in the mandibular arch. The alveolar ridges in all the edentulous areas except the left mandibular first and second molar area, the sites of the recent extractions, were rather thin and covered with considerable mobile tissue on the crests of the ridges. The recent extraction site had a well rounded ridge.

Visual examination and examination with a periodontal pocket probe revealed the presence of deep infrabony pockets along the palatal roots of the maxillary right first bicuspid and right and left first molars. Particularly deep pockets were present along the molar palatal roots; they obviously communicated with the trifurcations of these teeth. Pockets also were present along the distal surfaces of the mandibular right cuspid and left first bicuspid, also abutment teeth, but they were much shallower in depth. A 4 mm. pocket also was present on the distal aspect of the right lateral. The tissue tone was rather poor throughout the mouth but was especially poor on the palatal aspect of the right first molar, and the tissue appeared somewhat more detached than that of the left molar.

TREATMENT.   The mandibular periodontal surgery was routine and did not present a challenge comparable to that of the maxillary treatment. This review will therefore be limited to the maxillary therapy.

Treatment was begun in the left maxilla, which was anesthetized by local anesthesia of that quadrant plus infiltration in the right central-lateral area. A flame-shaped loop electrode was selected, cutting current output was set at 5, and the activated electrode was first used to resect the redundant mobile tissue on the crest of the alveolar ridges in the central-lateral edentulous areas (Case Fig. 3–1A). The electrode was then used to perform the gingivoplasty on the labial aspect of the anterior teeth (Case Fig. 3–1B). A 45-degree-angle medium-width U-shaped loop electrode was substituted for use on the mesial aspect of the left first molar, with power output increased to 5.5. since that electrode provided better access to the tissues in the edentulous area (Case Fig. 3–1C). The palatal gingivoplasty was then performed with a flame-shaped loop electrode that had been bent to form a curve for good tissue contact (Case Fig. 3–1D).

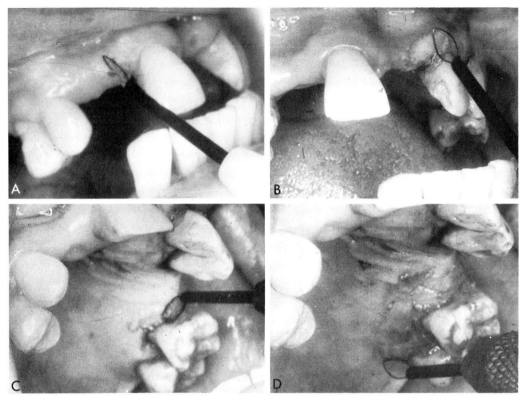

Case Figure 3–1. Electrosurgical management of periodontal disease due to traumatic occlusion and to loss of functional occlusion. *A,* Mobile redundant tissue is being resected from the crest of the edentulous space in the arch with a flame-shaped loop electrode. *B,* Gingivoplasty on labial aspect of maxillary left quadrant being started with the same electrode activated with cutting current. The marginal gingiva of the left lateral is being recontoured with the electrode. *C,* The gingivoplasty around the first molar is being performed on the mesial aspect with a 45-degree-angle medium-width U-shaped loop electrode, which provides better access to the tissues in that area. *D,* The gingivoplasty is resumed on the palatal aspect with the flame-shaped loop.

The gingivoplasty having been completed, a 45-degree-angle 17-mm. periodontal loop (vertical or hatchet-shaped type) was then used with current output reduced to 4.5 to debride the infrabony pockets present in that quadrant. The worst by far was the pocket along the palatal root of the first molar, which communicated with the trifurcation. The gross debridement was performed with the loop used with an up-down-rotary motion; the 90-degree-angle version of the loop (horizontal or hoe-shaped) was then substituted and used to resect the epithelial tissue lining the inner surface of the pocket mucosa (Case Fig. 3–2A). When debridement was completed, bleeding was induced, and powdered surgical gelatin was introduced into the defect and mixed with the blood, which proceeded to clot. Tincture of myrrh and benzoin was then applied and followed with a periodontal cement pack. The right quadrant was then anesthetized, and after the gingivoplasty was completed the right first molar infrabony pockets were debrided with the 17-mm. loop electrodes. The worst of these was along the palatal root of the right first molar, and this defect also communicated with the trifurcation of the tooth. When debridement of this defect was attempted with the cutting current, profuse hemorrhage was encountered despite the hemostasis normally inherent in the cutting modality and despite a considerable increase in power output. It

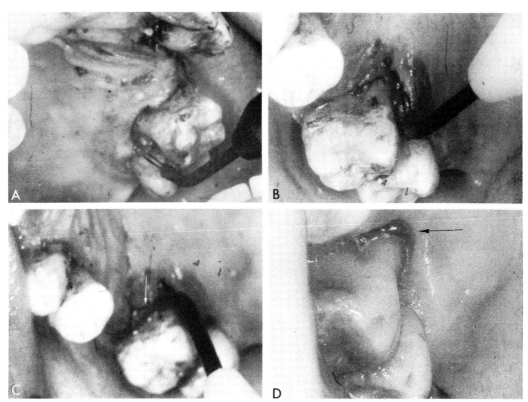

Case Figure 3–2. A, Debridement of a large, deep infrabony pocket on the palatal root of the first molar communicating with the trifurcation is being performed with a 17-mm. periodontal loop electrode. The 90-degree-angle (hoe-shaped) electrode is being used as an electronic curet to resect the epithelialized tissue from the inner surface of the gingival tissue of the infrabony lesion. B, Debridement of a similar infrabony lesion communicating with the trifurcation of the maxillary right first molar is being performed with a hatchet-shaped (vertical) 17-mm. periodontal loop electrode. Owing to profuse hemorrhage, the coagulating current is being used at a power output comparable to what would be required to perform it with cutting current. C, The debridement is being directed into the furca of the tooth. D, Postoperative appearance of the tissues on the palatal aspect of the right first molar. The attempt to treat the trifurcation definitively has failed, and proliferative tissue can be seen emerging from the defect.

thus became necessary to use the electrode with coagulating current set at the same power output setting as for cutting current to stop the bleeding and eliminate the pocket debris (Case Figs. 3–2B and C). A few shreds of tenaciously adherent tissue in the furca were destroyed in situ by sparking with the fulgurating current.

When debridement appeared to be completed bleeding was induced in the defect, and the powdered surgical gelatin was mixed with the blood. When the blood clotted, tincture of myrrh and benzoin was applied and followed with a cement pack. The primary packs were removed on the fifth postoperative day, the tissues were carefully cleansed, tincture of myrrh and benzoin was reapplied, and a fresh cement pack was applied for five more days. Healing progressed favorably everywhere but the right first molar trifurcation defect. Despite repeated postoperative treatments and spot coagulation, this defect failed to heal, the palatal gingiva failed to become reattached, and, instead, proliferative granulation tissue emerged from the defect (Case Fig. 3–2D). A second attempt at surgical correction therefore was attempted. The area was anesthetized with local anesthesia and a vertical incision was made into

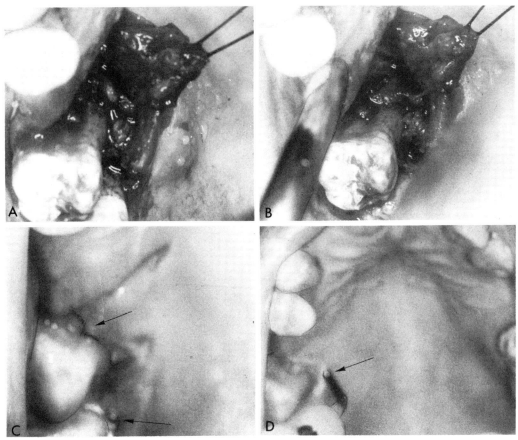

Case Figure 3–3. A, A second attempt to debride the trifurcation is being made. This time the palatal tissue was incised with a needle electrode to create a mucoperiosteal flap, which has been elevated and retracted to expose the trifurcation fully. The flap has been tied to a tooth on the opposite side of the jaw to eliminate need for manual retraction. Although there is no free bleeding, there is blood that was released as the tissues were cut still present on the tissue and tooth surfaces. *B,* The blood has been removed by sponging lightly with a 2×2 gauze sponge, giving an unobscured view of the surgical field. *C,* Appearance of the palatal mucosa on the fifth postoperative day, just before the sutures were removed. Primary healing appears to have started. *D,* Appearance of the tissues 10 weeks postoperatively. The palatal mucosa is fully healed, and the marginal gingival tissue on the palatal aspect has become re-attached to the tooth. An abrasion along the marginal edge of the tissue caused by the tooth-brush is being treated by spot coagulation with a small ball electrode (arrow) to abort any tendency for proliferation of the irritated tissue.

the palatal mucosa slightly anterior to the mesial aspect of the molar. The incision, made with a fine needle electrode and current output set at 4, was paralleled with a shorter incision slightly distal to but parallel with the first incision. Cutting power was reduced to 3, and the apical attachment of the first-second molar interdental papilla was severed to permit elevation and reflection of the mucoperiosteal flap that had been created. The flap was tied with a suture to a tooth in the left quadrant to eliminate need for manual retraction for full exposure of the trifurcation. Blood was present in the surgical field, but owing to the vastly improved tissue tone that had resulted from the previous attempt there was no free bleeding (Case Fig. 3–3A). The blood present on the surface of the defect was removed by gentle sponging with a sterile 2×2 gauze sponge to gain an unobstructed view of the surgical field (Case Fig. 3–3B).

The absence of free bleeding greatly facilitated meticulous debridement of the area. Gross debris was removed with U- and flame-shaped loops, and the furca was debrided with the 17-mm. periodontal loops. A few tissue fragments that were wedged between the roots in an area that was somewhat inaccessible to even the thin flexible 17-mm. loop were destroyed in situ by fulguration. When debridement was completed, bleeding was induced, surgical gelatin powder was mixed with the blood, the flap was restored to position, and the coapted margins and the papilla from the first-second molar embrasure were sutured with silk sutures to retain the tissues in their normal proper position.

Healing progressed uneventfully. On the fifth postoperative day the sutures were removed. The tissues showed evidence of the beginning of primary healing (Case Fig. 3–3C). By the end of the sixth postoperative week the palatal incisions appeared to be fully healed, and the trifurcation defect appeared to be healing well. The patient was seen every other week for six more weeks. By the end of the twelfth week the trifurcation defect appeared to be fully obliterated. The repair tissue was not yet maturely keratinized, but the palatal gingiva was tightly adherent to the tooth, despite an accidental abrasion created with the toothbrush that had occurred during the tenth postoperative week. Although the abrasion did not cause any unfavorable reaction, the abraded surface was treated prophylactically with superficial spot coagulation to minimize the possibility of proliferative reaction to the injury (Case Fig. 3–3D).

The marked contrast between the profuse hemorrhage from the original initial attempt at debridement of the trifurcation and the hemostasis enjoyed during the second surgical intervention merits comment, since it contributed materially to the end result obtained. The total absence of hemorrhage during the second, more radical procedure, in which all the cutting had been done with cutting current at normal current power output, offers excellent evidence of the benefit that was derived from the first attempt even though it failed to correct the defect. The benefit was a result of the tremendous improvement in tissue tone that occurred after the first surgical intervention. The improved tissue tone made possible the effective hemostasis that facilitated the debridement, made possible unimpaired visual inspection of the surgical field at all times, and thereby contributed substantially to the successful outcome of the second surgical procedure.

Biomechanical Factors

The biomechanical factors that will be reviewed and demonstrated with case reports fall into two categories:
1. Endodontic-periodontal disease.
2. Iatrogenic periodontal deterioration.

ENDODONTIC-PERIODONTAL DISEASE

Endodontic-periodontal disease qualifies fully as an excellent example of the age-old riddle—which came first, the chicken or the egg? Did the trouble start as a periapical lesion and then progress coronally, or did the periodontal lesion progress to and perhaps even beyond the apex of the tooth?

At best one can merely surmise or hypothesize about the pathologic sequence of events, and it is impossible to establish incontrovertibly whether the periapical disease contributed to the periodontal deterioration or vice versa. There is no need to surmise or hypothesize about one fact in these cases—the need for thorough eradication of both pathologic entities in order to effect a cure *is* incontrovertible.

CASE 4

Several years ago Hiatt demonstrated histologically the successful regeneration of labial alveolar bone that had been removed from a dog's canine tooth under surgically aseptic conditions. This case demonstrates that it is possible to achieve comparable results in the human patient, even when the bone loss is due to periodontal disease and the prognosis appears hopeless. It demonstrates that when debridement is thorough, and the involved tooth is immobilized during the postoperative reparative period, bone regeneration is so complete that the tooth regains normal firmness and functional usefulness without need for fixation to the adjacent teeth by permanent splinting.

It also provides examples of two invaluable inherent advantages electrosurgery offers the user: the ability to reshape electrodes to meet special needs of the case; and the ability to carbonize and destroy in situ by fulguration, undesirable tissue fragments in areas inaccessible to other methods of instrumentation.

PATIENT.   A 51-year-old white female.

HISTORY.   The maxillary left central which had been treated endodontically the previous year began to feel sore and loose, especially during eating or toothbrushing. The patient's dentist x-rayed the tooth, found evidence of extensive bone destruction, and referred her to the author for treatment.

CLINICAL EXAMINATION.   Three to 6 mm. of the labial root surfaces of the maxillary anterior teeth were denuded of bone. The marginal gingivae around the teeth were thick and round-edged, and the interdental papillae were hypertrophied. The left central was moderately mobile on palpation; the other teeth were firm. A periodontal probe inserted under the gingival margin of the loose tooth penetrated its full length without encountering resistance. A sterile endodontic silver point was substituted, inserted until it met resistance, and retained as a radiopaque pocket marker while the tooth was x-rayed. The roentgenogram revealed a huge amount of radiolucence around the apical two-thirds of the root. A 1-cm. elliptical area of more intense radiolucence midway along the mesial aspect of the root suggested extension of the bone destruction to the palatal aspect. Two mm. of gutta percha protruded beyond the resorbed apex of the tooth and the silver point extended 2 mm. beyond the root end (Case Fig. 4–1).

TREATMENT.   A smear was taken from the defect and colonies of staphylococcus and streptococcus were cultured. Sensitivity test established erythromycin as the antibiotic of choice. Ilosone was prescribed for 5 days. On the third day the area was anesthetized with a left infraorbital block, infiltration over the right central, and nasopalatine block. Cutting current was set at 3, and a 45-degree-angle fine needle electrode was activated and used to create a vertico-oblique mucoperiosteal incision extending from the mucogingival junction over the apex of the left cuspid anteriorly to the distogingival angle of the lateral. The apical attachment of the papilla in the left central-lateral embrasure was then severed to complete the flap incision (Case Fig. 4–2A).

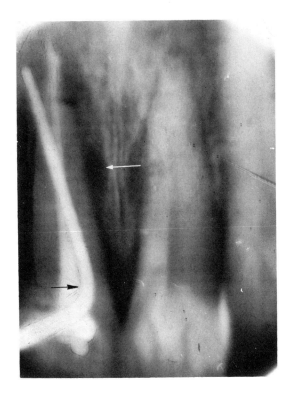

Case Figure 4-1. Preoperative periapical x-ray of affected tooth with silver endodontic point (black arrow) in situ, revealing a large amount of bone destruction. The radiolucence circumscribes the entire length of the root but appears to extend around to the palatal aspect of the maxillary central incisor (white arrow). Gutta percha extrudes through the apical foramen and radiolucence extends high beyond the apex of the tooth.

The flap was elevated and rotated, exposing its epithelial-lined ventral surface. The epithelial layer was removed by electrosection with a flame-shaped loop electrode; gross debridement was then performed by manual curettage, and followed by debridement by electrosection with a narrow 45-degree-angle U-shaped loop electrode. A 17-mm. periodontal loop electrode was then bent to curve around the root and used to debride the palatal part of the defect (Case Fig. 4–2B). Tissue fragments inaccessible to the loop resection were destroyed in situ by fulguration with a thick needle electrode that had been bent to direct the sparks between the root and palatal bone (Case Fig. 4–2 C). The rough apex was then reduced slightly and rounded with a diamond stone. The dead cementum was removed carefully by manual curettage to complete the debridement.

The debridement produced an area approximately 3.5 mm. wide around the mesial and two-thirds of the distal portions of the root devoid of bone (Case Fig. 4–2D). Bleeding was induced, powdered Gelfoam introduced into the defect and mixed with the blood. The flap was restored and secured in position with interrupted silk sutures inserted through the papillae and coapted incised margins (Case Fig. 4–2E).

The sutures were removed on the fifth postoperative day. Healing appeared to be progressing favorably. A stainless steel wire bar previously contoured to fit the labial aspect of the two centrals and left lateral was attached to the teeth with a thin mix of cold cure acrylic applied by the Neilon technique, to serve as an immobilizing splint. Healing progressed rapidly and uneventfully. By the end of the third month the defect was fully healed. The labial gingiva was firmly reattached and a periodontal pocket probe inserted under the free margin could not penetrate beyond the base of the gingival sulcus despite sufficient pressure to cause marked blanching of the tissues (Case Fig. 4–2F). When the splint was removed, the tooth proved to be normally firm.

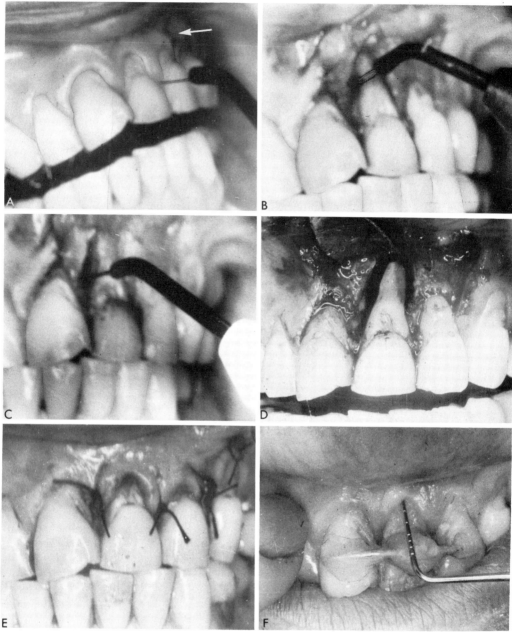

Case Figure 4–2. A, The vertico-oblique incision (arrow) through the gingival tissue extending from the junction of the alveolar and areolar mucosa downward and forward to the distogingival junction of the marginal gingiva of the lateral incisor has been incised with a fine 45-degree-angle needle electrode. The electrode can be seen in the act of severing the apical attachment of the central-lateral interdental papilla. B, The mucoperiosteal flap is reflected, revealing total destruction of the labial alevolar bone and extensive surrounding granulomatous debris. The 17-mm. periodontal loop electronic curet has been bent to conform to the curvature of the root and can be seen in the act of debriding the palatal extension of the destruction. C, Tenaciously adherent tissue shreds are being destroyed in situ by fulguration with a heavy needle electrode which has had the tip bent to form a right angle that makes it possible to direct the sparks of the fulgurating current to reach the palatal site. D, The debridement has been completed, the apex has been reduced, and the dead cementum has been planed from the denuded root surface. E, The mucoperiosteal flap has been restored to position and sutured

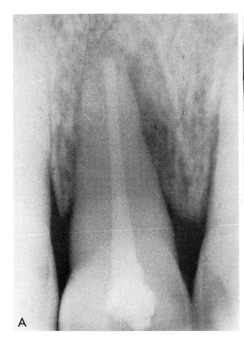

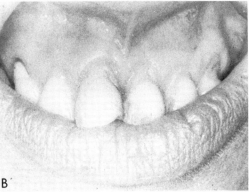

Case Figure 4–3. A, Appearance of the tooth one year later. The gingival tissue is normal and the tooth is as firm as the adjacent teeth, without fixation. *B,* Final postoperative x-ray one year later shows complete regeneration of the bone around the root of the tooth. Distinct evidence of trabeculation can be seen on the x-ray and the tooth has not been immobilized by splinting to the adjacent teeth.

The patient was seen for the last time one year postoperatively. A photograph taken a year after visit shows the gingival tissue and tooth to be normal (Case Fig. 4–3A). The final roentgenogram (Case Fig. 4–3B) at one year confirms the clinical evidence of complete regeneration of the investing alveolar bone and the absence of fixation to the adjacent teeth.

The huge amount of bone destruction in this case made the initial prognosis appear to be utterly hopeless. The favorable result obtained must be attributed to four unique advantages electrosurgery offers: the ability to eliminate all the diseased tissue, owing to the hemostasis which permits meticulous debridement under visual control; the ability to gain access to areas inaccessible to other methods of instrumentation without sacrificing additional bone; the ability to destroy in situ undesirable tissue in inaccessible areas; and the sterilizing effect of the currents on the surgical field. All these factors contributed materially to the successful outcome.

Iatrogenic periodontal deterioration

Iatrogenic periodontal deterioration is invariably triggered by irritation to the gingival and subgingival tissues by fixed or removable prostheses that are improperly designed or poorly fabricated.

Case Figure 4–2. Continued.
into position through the papillae in the embrasures. *F,* The appearance of the area three months postoperatively. The stainless steel labial arch bar that was used to immobilize the tooth is still in place. The line of incision has healed so completely that it is invisible. A periodontal pocket probe has been inserted under the gingival free margin to determine whether the gingiva is reattached. The tip of the probe is seen pushing against the base of the gingival sulcus, but cannot penetrate beyond despite pressure that causes marked blanching of the gingival tissue.

PLATE V

Periodontics

Figure 1a. Definitive treatment of massive bone destruction due to endodontic-periodontal deterioration. The x-ray has suggested that the entire labial plate of bone has been destroyed. A vertico-oblique incision has been made with a fine 45-degree-angle needle electrode to create a mucoperiosteal flap. The apical attachment of the papilla in the central-lateral embrasure is being severed to complete the flap incision.

Figure 1b. The tissue flap has been elevated and reflected, exposing the entire labial aspect of the root of the tooth which is completely denuded of bone. There is also a considerable amount of bone destruction around the apical two-thirds of the root. A 17-mm. periodontal loop electrode has been bent to create a curvature that will permit it to slide around the root and debride the palatal aspect without having to remove more bone. The activated electrode is seen being used to perform the debridement.

Figure 1c. Manual and electrosurgical debridement has been completed. The dead cementum has been carefully removed by manual curettage with appropriate scalers and curets. The necrotic debris and epithelial-lined tissue surfaces have been curetted by electronic curettage, and the apex of the root has been reduced, rounded, and resealed by electrocoagulation. The tissue flap can now be restored and sutured.

Figure 1d. Appearance of the tooth and tissue two years later. The tooth is firm, without having been splinted to the adjacent teeth. The tissue has reattached to the new bone that has regenerated. A periodontal pocket probe inserted under the free margin has penetrated to the base of the gingival sulcus and cannot penetrate further, despite enough pressure to cause marked tissue blanching.

Figure 2a. Definitive treatment of advanced periodontoclasia with pathological migration by combined gingivoplasty and electronic infrabony pocket debridement. The gingivoplasty is being performed by electrosection with a flame-shaped loop electrode. Note the diastemas and the absence of free bleeding.

Figure 2b. Five days later the second quadrant is being treated. The cement pack has been removed from the right quadrant; the gingivoplasty having been completed on the left side, the individual infrabony pockets are being debrided with the periodontal 17-mm. electronic curet. An 11-mm. pocket is being treated. Note absence of free bleeding.

Figure 2c. Mandibular right quadrant is being treated on the twentieth postoperative day. Note the chronological rate and quality of the tissue repair. The maxillary right quadrant 20 days postoperatively, and 10 days after removal of the cement packs, is almost completely healed. The left quadrant, 15 days postoperatively and 5 days after removal of the second cement pack is not nearly as far advanced in its healing. The gingivoplasty is being performed in the mandibular right quadrant. Very simple tooth movement with Japanese grassline and elastic band traction has been instituted to try to close the diastemas.

Figure 2d. Three month postoperative appearance of the tissues. The pathologically migrated teeth have been restored to their normal alignment in the dental arches. The gingival tissues are normal in tone and architecture, and the infrabony pockets have been obliterated. The patient is wearing a simple Hawley retainer with an elastic band that was prescribed for bedtime use for three months, until bone calcification is completed, to guard against any undetected tendency to brux that might interfere with and prevent complete bone repair.

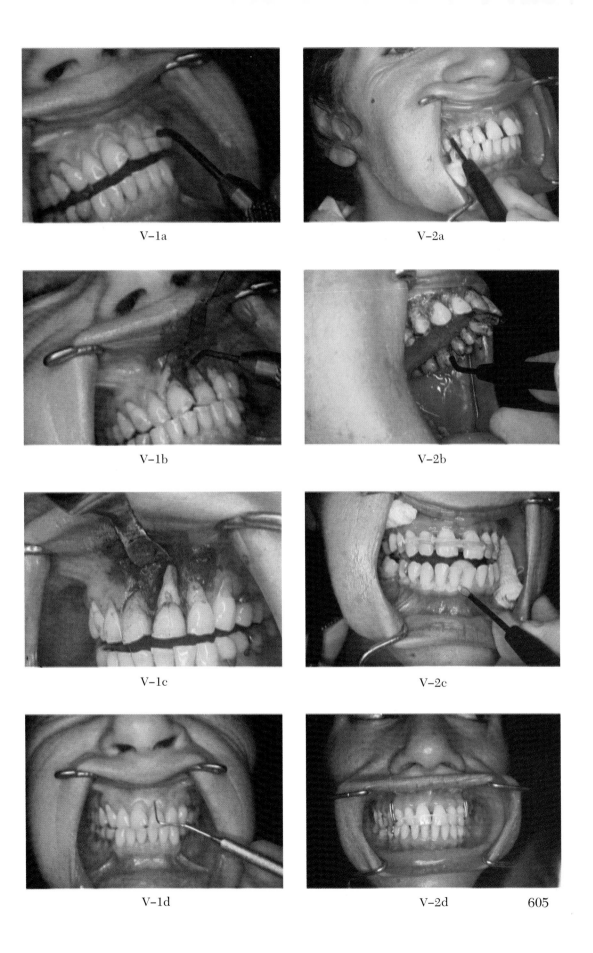

V-1a

V-2a

V-1b

V-2b

V-1c

V-2c

V-1d

V-2d

605

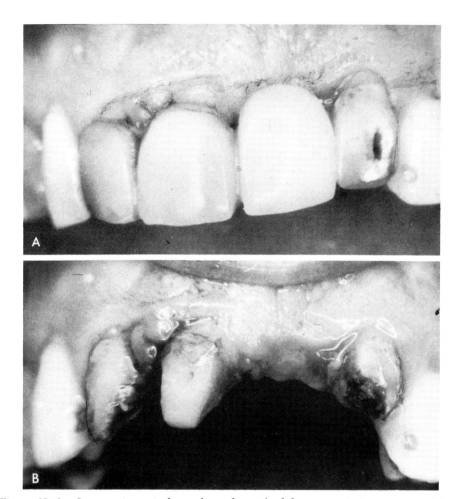

Figure 19–2. Iatrogenic periodontoclasia due to bad dentistry. *A*, Appearance of the teeth and gingivae, labial view. An acrylic bridge is present, extending from right to left lateral maxillary incisors. It consists of crowns on the right central and lateral and left lateral and a pontic restoring the left central. The crowns on the laterals are badly discolored and the left lateral has a large damage defect on the labial aspect. The marginal gingivae over the three crowns have receded, exposing 1.5 to 3 mm. of denuded roots. The tissue in the right central-lateral embrasure has proliferated into a bulbous mass. The interdental papilla in the left lateral-cuspid has also proliferated but to a slightly lesser degree. The gingival tissues around the restoration appear engorged, atonal, and hyperplastic. *B*, Appearance of the teeth and tissues with the bridge removed. The right and left lateral crown preparations are in a deplorable state of decay. There is extensive decay on the mesial aspect of the right lateral, and the incisal third of the left lateral has disintegrated. The two laterals have been prepared with uneven irregular partial shoulders and a fragmentary shoulder on the distal of the right central that has become covered with proliferative tissue. The tissue under the left central pontic is flabby and hyperplastic. A small ulcerated lesion is present at its distal (posterior) end. Periodontal pocket probe inspection reveals deep infrabony pockets in addition to a circumscribing horizontal bone loss except on the mesial aspect of the right central. In that area the periodontal probe can penetrate only about 4 mm., of which about 2 mm. is infrabony and 2 mm. the depth of the gingival sulcus. It is self-evident that the moderately severe periodontal deterioration around the three abutment teeth has been triggered by the inexcusably bad restoration.

The triggering mechanism is constant, but the nature and degree of impropriety of the prosthetic device are variable. It can range from deceptively innocuous looking restorations, which nevertheless cause serious tissue damage because of lack of subgingival accommodation for the restoration, to the deplorably bad dentistry depicted in Figure 19–2.

Secondary factors can influence the degree of tissue response to the irritant. The extent and severity of the periodontal deterioration therefore is not necessarily in direct ratio to the degree of irritation produced by the restoration. In the absence of secondary influencing factors, it is axiomatic that the more poorly conceived and executed the restoration, the greater the severity of the tissue reaction it will trigger. This is well demonstrated in Figure 19–2.

CASE 5

This case is an example of extensive periodontoclasia involving the entire dentition, with both typical and atypical characteristics encountered simultaneously. It presents a combination of typical extensive periodontal deterioration aggravated by traumatic injury from ill-fitting dentures, with atypical postoperative sequelae encountered in an isolated abutment tooth with a trifurcation involvement. The results obtained demonstrate that heroic measures are sometimes justifiable and necessary to preserve a functionally useful tooth.

PATIENT.   A 63-year-old white female in normal health.

HISTORY.   The patient was referred for gingivectomy and/or extractions.

CLINICAL EXAMINATION

Extraoral.   Negative.

Intraoral.   The patient wore an ill-fitting set of partial dentures. In the maxilla the six anteriors and left second molar remained in the dental arch. The centrals were separated by a diastema. In the mandible the six anteriors and first bicuspids remained (Case Fig. 5–1). There was much evidence of periodontal deterioration with alveolar resorption and deep pocket formation.

The maxillary denture impinged severely against the palatal mucosa and the mucosa at the distal aspects of the abutment teeth. The trauma had produced severe inflammatory reactions with marked hypertrophy and detachment of the marginal gingivae. The mandibular denture impinged against the distal gingivae of the terminal abutment teeth. This impingement had produced gingival recession of the distal half of each abutment and mesial hypertrophy.

TREATMENT.   The maxillary gingivae were treated first. The mouth was prepared for surgery; bilateral infraorbital block anesthesia and palatal infiltration was administered. A narrow 45-degree-angle U-shaped loop electrode was selected and current output was set at 4.5 for electrosection. The detached labial gingivae were resected in layers with short brushing strokes of the activated electrode (Case Fig. 5–2). A deep vertical pocket at the mesial aspect of the right cuspid was debrided of necrotic epithelial debris by inserting the loop electrode to the base of the pocket and manipulating it with rotary and push-pull movements.

The palatal hypertrophic mucosa was resected with a similarly shaped but larger electrode and current output increased to 6. A U-shaped electrode bent into a convexo-concave curve was substituted to plane the palatal mucosa in order to remove the

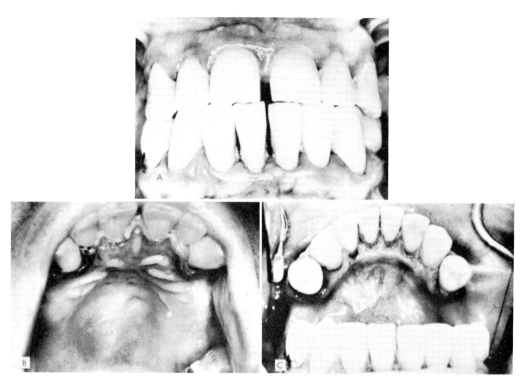

Case Figure 5–1. Gingivectomy of an entire mouth which has undergone severe periodontal deterioration as a result largely of irritation produced by a set of ill-fitting dentures.
A, Preoperative appearance. Labial view of the mouth showing clinical evidence of extensive
periodontal breakdown, with development of wide diastemas between the maxillary and mandibular centrals. *B,* Palatal view shows the extensive hypertrophy, ulceration and detachment
of the palatal gingivae. Deep pockets and trifurcation involvement of a key molar abutment can
be seen. *C,* Lingual view. Here too, deep pockets and hypertrophy, particularly marked around
the terminal abutment teeth, are clearly visible.

degenerated detached tissue and to restore the gingivae to normal contour with
feather-edged margins.

   Pockets at the distopalatal angles of both cuspids were debrided in the manner
described, with the same narrow loop electrode used previously but with a current
output of 5 instead of 4.5. This change was due to the greater thickness and density of
the palatal tissue. Because of massive engorgement there was a considerable ooze of
blood from the raw tissue surfaces, but no free bleeding. The oozing stopped when the
tissues were dried with sterile sponges. Tincture of myrrh and benzoin was applied.
Then a stiff mix of surgical cement was packed around the six anteriors.

   The isolated molar was treated next. The alveolar bone at the mesial aspect of this
tooth had resorbed beyond the trifurcation, creating a pocket partially covered with
detached mucosa. After the hypertrophic tissue around this tooth was removed by
shaving in layers, the narrow loop electrode was inserted into the trifurcation and manipulated with rotary and push-pull motions in order to resect the necrotic debris.
The new gingival margin around the tooth was beveled, and a separate cement pack
was inserted.

   The mandibular gingivae were then prepared and anesthetized with bilateral
mental block and lingual infiltration injections. The small narrow loop electrode was
applied to the labial tissues at a 60-degree angle and used to remove the detached

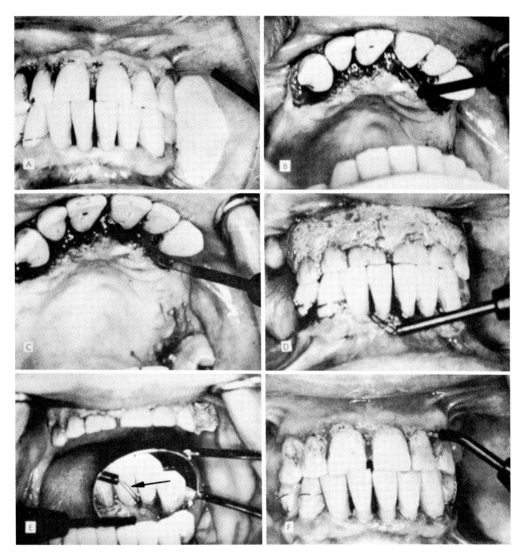

Case Figure 5–2. Operative procedure. *A,* Maxilla, labial. Resection of detached and hypertrophic tissue performed with a narrow U-shaped 45-degree-angle loop electrode by shaving the tissue in layers. An infrabony pocket in the right lateral-cuspid embrasure has been debrided with this loop. *B,* Palatal gingivae being reduced to normal contour and pockets eliminated with a similar but slightly larger loop.

C, Hypertrophied gingivae at the distal and palatal areas of the terminal abutment teeth are planed with a straight U-shaped loop electrode that has been bent to a gentle curve. *D,* Maxillary surgery has been completed and a cement pack inserted. The mandibular labial gingivae are being reduced to normal contour and the hypertrophied papillae reduced to concave sluiceways with a narrow 45-degree-angle U-shaped loop electrode. Note the stainless steel ligature splinting to immobilize the posterior teeth.

E, A lingual infrabony pocket is being debrided by inserting the loop (arrow) to the base of the pocket and manipulating it with push-pull and rotary movements until all the necrotic debris has been eradicated. *F,* Postoperative appearance on the 10th day when the second surgical cement pack has been removed. Healing is progressing satisfactorily. Mandibular healing appears particularly favorable. Marginal gingiva around the right central, and the central-lateral interproximal papilla, present some irregular tissue tabs, which are reduced by superficial spot coagulation with a ball electrode.

hypertrophic gingivae by shaving in layers with short brushing strokes. The interproximal papillae were then reduced to concave sluiceways with pulling strokes directed downward. The cutting current was increased from 4.5 to 5 and the convexoconcave bent U-shaped electrode was substituted. This loop electrode was used to resect the deteriorated lingual mucosa by shaving in layers with short brushing strokes. Current was reduced to 4.5. The narrow 45-degree-angle loop electrode was replaced and used to debride infrabony pockets and reduce the convexity of the lingual interproximal papillae. By applying the electrode to the papillae and pulling upward from their bases to their attachments, concave sluiceways were created. The new gingival margins were then beveled where necessary to create feather edges. When the gingival architecture was fully restored to normal the tissues were dried with sponges, and tincture of myrrh and benzoin was applied to the operative field. A surgical cement pack was inserted around the mandibular teeth and gingivae. Terramycin was prescribed for four days, and the patient was instructed in postoperative home care.

She returned on the fifth postoperative day and reported that most of the molar cement pack had come away a few hours after its insertion. Despite the exposure of a raw area of tissue she had had little discomfort.

The cement packs were removed and the mouth was irrigated. On inspection, the tissue healing appeared to be progressing satisfactorily, but several small hyperemic spots were present in the granulating tissue. Topical anesthesia was applied, and after two minutes the spots were treated by superficial spot coagulation. Areas on both the labial and palatal aspects of the maxilla were coagulated with the small ball electrode at a current output of 0.5. The mandibular mucosa was treated identically.

The mucosa around the molar was not as well healed as that of the rest of the mouth. The marginal gingiva on the palatal aspect in particular appeared laggard. Current output was increased to 2 and spot coagulation performed on this tissue. Then the tissues were dried and tincture of myrrh and benzoin was applied in air-dried layers. Fresh cement packs were inserted around the maxillary anterior teeth and the mandibular teeth. A length of stainless steel ligature wire was twisted to form a strand of closely linked loops; this strand was then wired around the molar to provide anchorage for retention of the cement pack which was then inserted.

The patient returned five days later. This time all the cement packs were intact and tightly adherent to teeth and tissues. The packs were removed and the mouth was thoroughly irrigated. The healing was further advanced, but the marginal gingivae of the mesioproximal surface of the right cuspid and around the left central, lateral and cuspid, and the palatal aspect of the molar still appeared somewhat hyperemic and were not yet completely epithelialized.

These areas were treated by superficial spot coagulation. Chromic acid, 0.1 per cent dilution, was applied for 30 seconds and washed off. Then tincture of myrrh and benzoin was applied in air-dried layers. The patient was instructed to use the astringent salt-alum mouthwash for intermittent five-day periods. She was also instructed to use the rubber stimulator tip of her toothbrush for gingival massage. Knox clear gelatin and ascorbic acid were prescribed as dietary supplements.

She was seen again two weeks later. Except for one small hypertrophic roll on the labial surface of the lower right central incisor and the palatal marginal gingiva around the denuded molar palatal root the tissue tone was excellent. Three minims of anesthetic solution were infiltrated around the molar root and 2 minims on the labial aspect of the mandibular central. The palatal gingiva around the molar was treated by spot coagulation, and the labial anterior hypertrophy was reduced with a small loop

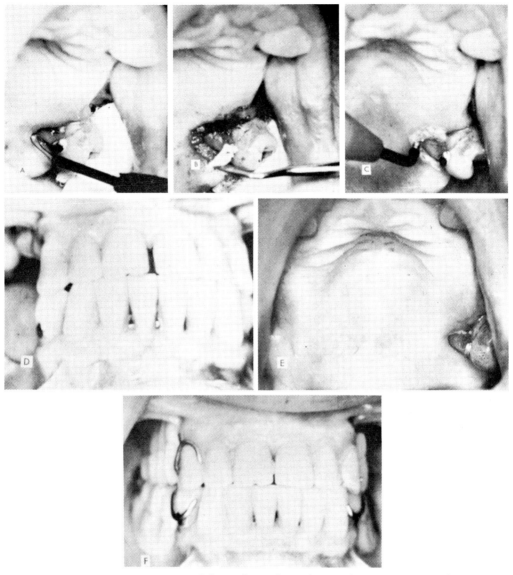

Case Figure 5–3. Treatment of the molar trifurcation involvement one year later. *A,* Hypertrophic, inflamed marginal gingiva around the palatal root and in the trifurcation pocket is resected with an appropriately curved, narrow, straight U-shaped loop, creating a channel all around the exposed portion of the palatal root (after the root had been planed to remove detritus). *B,* A mixture of medicated powdered surgical gelatin and cultured despeciated bone paste being gently tamped into the groove where it is mixed with blood present. When the blood clots this will be protected with a collodion dressing. *C,* Fifth postoperative day. A sharp tissue line angle is rounded by superficial spot coagulation. *D,* Labial appearance one year postoperatively. Note improvement in tissue tone and contour which is now quite normal. *E,* Palatal appearance one year postoperatively. The tissues are firm, well attached to the teeth and alveolar bone; the pockets have been eradicated, and the molar is firm and functionally useful. *F,* Final appearance four years postoperatively, labial view. Note the closure of the diastemas between the centrals. (The maxillary centrals have been permanently splinted with internal splints.)

electrode. Topical applications of chromic acid and tincture of myrrh and benzoin were applied; the two areas were covered with Kenalog in Orabase.

The patient was seen again two weeks later. This time the tissue tone throughout the entire mouth appeared excellent. Active treatment was discontinued and she was instructed to return in three months for follow-up postoperative observation.

She returned at the appointed time. The gingivae throughout the mouth except around the palatal root of the molar appeared firm and healthy, but the latter area was slightly hyperemic. It was so slight, however, that no treatment was indicated. She continued to return at three-month intervals. At the third visit it was apparent that the marginal gingiva around the molar palatal root was undergoing gradual deterioration. By the end of the year corrective measures became necessary. Further corrective treatment appeared warranted to preserve this tooth for continued use as an abutment.

The area was prepared and infiltration anesthesia administered around the molar palatal root. The marginal gingiva around this root was resected by electrosection with a narrow 45-degree-angle loop electrode to a depth of 2 to 3 mm., then the new margin was beveled to a feather edge with a narrow straight U-shaped loop electrode slightly curved (Case Fig. 5–3). The electrode was directed toward the trifurcation and used as a curet with a rotary motion to debride the area, then with pulling motion to create a slightly concave sluiceway. Light bleeding was induced in the trench around the root. A mixture of cultured bone paste and surgical gelatin was inserted and mixed with the blood. When the blood clotted a thick protective coating of collodion was applied.

She returned one week later and reported that the collodion dressing had peeled off on the third day. Inspection revealed that the tissue was healing very well but that the junction between the new and old gingival mucosa formed a sharp line angle. This was rounded by superficial spot coagulation under topical anesthesia. Tincture of myrrh and benzoin was applied and she was instructed to return.

She was seen again once a week for the next four weeks. During that period progressive maturation of this tissue was observed. Treatment was limited to applications of tincture of myrrh and benzoin, and intermittent use of the astringent salt-alum mouthwash for five-day periods was resumed. By the end of the month the tissue was fully healed and normally keratinized; the tissue tone was excellent.

The patient was recalled for semiannual postoperative observation for the next three years. Throughout that period the gingival mucosa remained healthy and tolerant of her new dentures, which had been constructed shortly after the original surgery had healed. The molar has remained firm, and the gingival mucosa around it healthy. The diastemas have disappeared and the centrals make contact.

Despite a number of regressions of the isolated molar that required repeated minor surgical interventions, a favorable result was finally obtained in this case, and the tooth is functionally useful.*

CASE 6

This case provides a typical example of complications created by the extensive fixed ceramic restorations in the dental arch when periodontal surgery is required.

---

*Fourteen years after the periodontal surgery that has been described a final surgical intervention was performed by the author to preserve the tooth for continued functional use as an abutment. The surgery was made necessary by total decay of the palatal root at the gingival level.

It demonstrates the advantages to be derived from careful electrosurgical instrumentation, through which it is possible to avoid potential undesirable effects.

One of the principal drawbacks of non-electrosurgical gingivectomy is the unfavorable cosmetic result achieved when the root portions of the teeth are exposed by the removal of diseased gingival mucosa. When gingivectomy is performed on gingival tissue around teeth that have been restored with porcelain jacket crowns or veneer crowns, double jeopardy results. In addition to the unfavorable cosmetic effect created by surgical exposure of the root shoulders and cementation lines, there is also the hazard that the cement may wash out and permit the onset of secondary decay which weakens the coronal preparation and root.

When cosmetic effects are unfavorable, regardless of the effectiveness of the surgical therapy and quality of tissue repair that ensues, the end results are usually unsatisfactory to fastidious, discriminating patients. Thus, the presence of extensive coronal restorations is not only an operative surgical handicap (and perhaps a retarding influence on healing) but a serious postoperative aesthetic handicap. The operator, therefore, must be as conservative of tissue as cold steel instrumentation permits. Electrosurgery permits conservation of much of the tissue that might otherwise have to be sacrificed to obtain a satisfactory periodontal result. It thereby offers the possibility of infinitely more desirable postoperative esthetic results.

PATIENT.   A 54-year-old white female.

HISTORY.   The patient had had extensive restorative dentistry performed. Subsequent conservative curettage of moderately advanced periodontoclasia proved ineffectual. She was referred for electrosurgical periodontal therapy.

CLINICAL EXAMINATION

Extraoral.   Negative.

Intraoral.   The maxillary anterior teeth had been restored with porcelain jacket crowns. The crowns looked natural and were perfectly adapted to their subgingival shoulders. They were permanently cemented.

The gingival mucosa in the anterior part of the mouth appeared atonal, hypertrophied and edematous. There were irregular deep pockets in the bicuspid-molar interproximal areas and some in the anterior region, especially in the right lateral-cuspid region. The maxillary posterior teeth were so mobile that her dentist had splinted them with wire ligatures before performing the periodontal curettage. The gingival mucosa around the mandibular posterior teeth appeared abraded, and some of the epithelial surfaces were denuded of their surface keratinization (Case Fig. 6–1A).

TREATMENT.   The mouth was prepared for surgery and the mandibular gingivae were anesthetized by infiltration. A medium-sized 45-degree-angle U-shaped loop electrode was selected and current output set at 5 for electrosection. Starting on the left side the labial marginal gingivae were reduced by shaving in layers with short brushing strokes (Case Fig. 6–1B). Hemostasis of a persistent bleeding point immediately beneath the left cuspid was quickly achieved by electrocoagulation with a small ball electrode and current output of 2 for biterminal application (Case Fig. 6–1C). The lingual gingivae were then reduced in the same manner. When the mandibular gingivectoplasty was completed, the tissues were sponged dry and a stiffly mixed surgical cement pack applied.

The maxillary mucosa was prepared and anesthetized with bilateral posterosuperior alveolar and infraorbital blocks and nasopalatine and anterior palatine blocks. The gingival mucosa of the buccal aspect of the posterior teeth on the left side was reduced to the bases of the pockets with a flame-shaped electrode. A narrow U-shaped

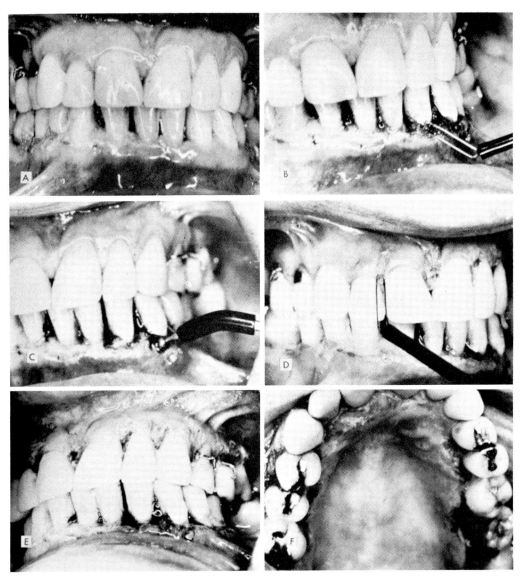

Case Figure 6–1. Gingivectomy of the entire mouth which is complicated by presence of extensive ceramic restorations.

A, Preoperative appearance, labial view. Tissues are atonal and there are extensive hypertrophy, engorgement and many deep pockets with loss of numerous papillary attachments. *B,* The mandibular labial marginal gingivae are reduced to normal contour by shaving in layers with a medium-sized 45-degree-angle U-shaped loop electrode. *C,* Bleeding from a small capillary controlled by coagulation with a small ball electrode. *D,* Hypertrophied maxillary interproximal papillae are reduced to form self-cleansing concave sluiceways with a narrow 45-degree-angle U-shaped loop electrode.

E, Appearance of the tissues on the fifth postoperative day after the cement pack has been removed. Granulation healing progressing well. *F,* Postoperative appearance of the palatal tissue at this time. Healing is progressing very well here too.

loop electrode was substituted, current output decreased, and the convexity of the anterior interproximal papillae reduced with wiping motions directed from above downward in order to create self-cleansing sluiceways (Case Fig. 6–1D).

The tissues on the right side were reduced in the same manner. The narrow loop electrode was then used to debride several narrow, deep pockets. The loop electrode was inserted into the deep pockets located at the mesial and distal aspects of the posterior teeth and used with rotary and push-pull motions to eradicate the debris. When this was completed, the narrow loop was replaced with a convexoconcave bent U-shaped loop electrode and current was increased to 7 to assure clean cutting. The hypertrophic and deteriorated portions of the palatal mucosa were reduced with this electrode to the level of the normal tissue by shaving in layers with short planing strokes. The new gingival margins were beveled to feather edges.

Most of the procedure had been remarkably free of bleeding, but one area on the palatal aspect of the second molar bled profusely. This bleeding was quickly controlled by electrocoagulation with a small ball electrode. The tissues were dried, tincture of myrrh and benzoin applied, and a stiffly mixed surgical cement pack inserted. The patient was instructed in postoperative care and reappointed.

She returned on the fifth postoperative day. The cement packs were intact except in the palatal maxillary left molar region where blood seepage apparently had interfered with the cement setting. In this area the cement had crumbled and left the area unprotected.

The cement packs were removed and the tissues were irrigated and inspected. Healing was progressing very satisfactorily and the tissues were covered with a thin healthy layer of surface coagulum. The palatal gingivae also were healing well (Case Fig. 6–1E and F). On the molar portion of the left palate where the tissues had remained exposed, the junction of old and new mucosa formed a sharp-line edge. This was eliminated by spot coagulation with a cylindrical coagulating electrode under topical anesthesia before the cement pack was replaced. Tincture of myrrh and benzoin was applied and fresh cement packs inserted.

She returned five days later. The cement packs were intact. They were removed, the mouth irrigated and the tissues inspected. The gingivae were healing very well except around the maxillary right lateral and the mandibular left cuspid, where the labial marginal gingivae appeared slightly hyperemic and hypertrophic. Both areas were brought under control by spot coagulation performed under topical anesthesia (Case Fig. 6–2A). Tincture of myrrh and benzoin was applied in air-dried layers; she was instructed to continue the regimen of postoperative care and return in two weeks.

At her next visit the tissues were almost fully healed, re-epithelialized, and keratinized. She was seen at weekly intervals for the next four weeks. At her last visit she was instructed to use her toothbrush for gingival massage. She returned for a final postoperative examination two months later. This time the tissues were fully healed and matured. Their tissue tone was excellent, and the tissues were firmly attached to the teeth and their investing alveolar bone. All the deep pockets were completely obliterated without loss of gingival harmony on palatal, lingual or labial aspects. The gingivae around the six porcelain jacket crowns were as healthy and firmly attached as those around the uncrowned teeth. The anterior interproximal pockets were obliterated without exposure of root surfaces, shoulders or subgingival cement lines (Case Fig. 6–2B to D).

The wire ligatures were removed from the posterior teeth, which were quite firm. All in all, except for the brownish stain resulting from repeated applications of tinc-

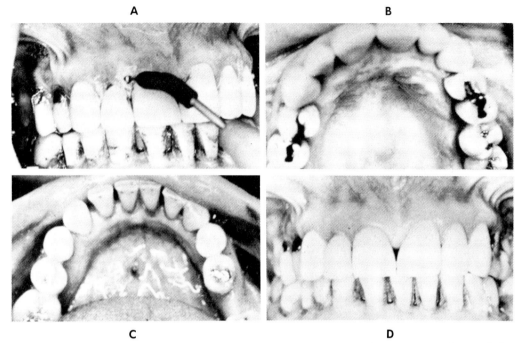

Case Figure 6-2.   Postoperative sequence. A, Appearance of the tissues on the tenth day after the second cement pack was removed. Hyperemic spots are coagulated with a small ball electrode. B to D, Palatal, lingual and labial views three months postoperatively.

ture of myrrh and benzoin (still present around the gingival thirds of the mandibular teeth), the esthetic result was fully comparable to that of the physical results of the gingival electrosurgery.

CASE 7

It is ironic that periodontal prostheses sometimes trigger, instead of prevent, further periodontal deterioration. This case is an excellent example of periodontal deterioration that was triggered by failure to provide adequate space to accommodate the subgingival portions of an extensive periodontal splint.

PATIENT.   A 42-year-old white female.

HISTORY.   The patient had been troubled almost half her life with periodontoclasia. A surgical gingivectomy had been performed several years previously in the conventional manner by cold-steel gingival stripping. Thereafter she had received periodic maintenance curettage. Despite this the periodontal deterioration continued. Finally, a complete mouth rehabilitation with fixed bridges to serve as periodontal splints to immobilize the teeth was prescribed. The splints had been inserted six months previously. In the maxilla all the teeth had been immobilized by splinting from molar to molar as a single unit. In the mandibular arch, bilateral fixed-bridge splints locked the teeth together from molars to the first bicuspids. From the outset the gingival tissues reacted unfavorably to the maxillary splint. The maxillary gingivae were badly compressed, and soon the papillae became greatly enlarged and detached. She was in considerable distress and had consulted a number of dentists both here and abroad. Their verdict was unanimous: the splint was creating severe periodontal deterioration and should be replaced. She was referred for periodontal surgery and a treatment plan.

CLINICAL EXAMINATION

Extraoral.   Negative.

Intraoral.   The gingival tissue tone was subnormal. The interproximal papillae were massively enlarged and appeared white from compression of the crowns against the subgingival tissues (Case Fig. 7–1). Practically every tooth had one or more periodontal pockets, and the molars had either bifurcation or trifurcation involvements. The anterior crowns were short and in tip-to-tip occlusion. When the splint was removed, the labial-proximal crown shoulders were found to be obliterated by hypertrophic tissue.

Roentgenographic examination confirmed the clinical findings. Periodontal deterioration was rampant, with marked bone loss and deep infrabony pockets and bifurcation-trifurcation involvements.

TREATMENT.   Two stages of treatment were planned: First, the periodontal surgery; second, when the gingival health had been restored, subgingival troughs would be created to prepare the mouth for a new restoration.

The mouth was prepared and a combination of maxillary regional and infiltration anesthesia was administered. Current output was set at 6 for electrosection, and a flame-shaped loop electrode was selected. With the splint in position the hypertrophic tissue was reduced to a normal level around the crowns by shaving in layers with short brushing strokes. Individual pockets were debrided with a narrow U-shaped loop electrode by inserting it to the base of the pockets and manipulating with push-pull and slightly rolling motions in order to resect necrotic debris.

When normal gingival contour was restored around the maxilla with the splint in situ, the latter was removed, and resection of detached tissue and hypertrophic tissue in the shoulder areas was completed. Intraseptal pockets inaccessible with splint in position were now thoroughly debrided. When the maxillary surgery was completed, a stiffly mixed cement pack was inserted.

Bilateral inferior alveolar blocks were administered and the mandibular gingivae were reduced in the same manner; since the mandibular bridges were permanently cemented, these were not disturbed. When surgery was completed a surgical cement pack was also inserted around these teeth and gingivae.

The patient's general physical condition was below par, so Ilosone, 250 mg. capsules, every six hours for three days, was prescribed and she was given the usual postoperative instructions. She returned on the sixth postoperative day and reported that a labial segment of the mandibular cement pack had broken away. She had been free of pain or severe discomfort.

The cement packs were removed and the mouth was irrigated. On examination the tissues appeared to be progressing splendidly. They were covered with a thin layer of normal coagulum, and there were but a few tiny areas of engorgement. A few of these tiny red spots, suggestive of superficial capillary regeneration, were coagulated with a small ball electrode.

The mouth was irrigated; 0.5 per cent chromic acid was applied to the coagulated areas for 30 seconds and then washed off with water. Tincture of myrrh and benzoin was applied to the entire operative field. The splint was reinserted and fresh cement packs were applied. She returned on the tenth postoperative day. The cement packs, intact, were removed and the mouth was irrigated. Tissue healing was gratifyingly advanced. The splint was removed and tincture of myrrh and benzoin applied in air-

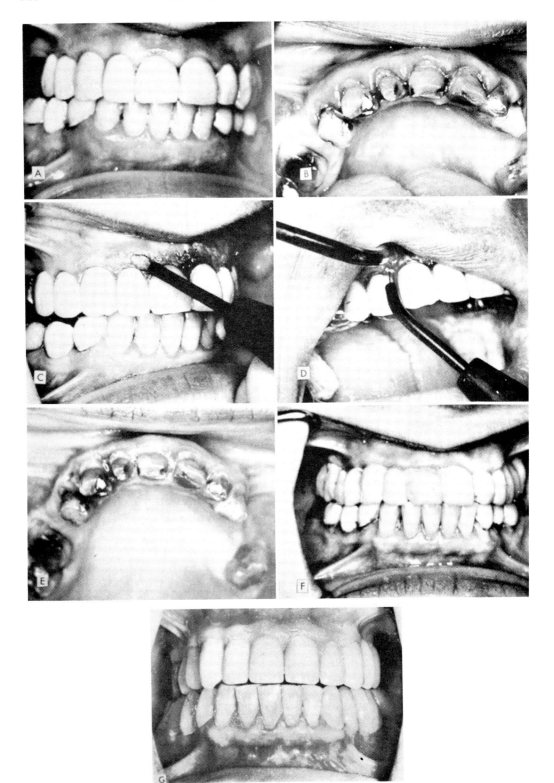

Case Figure 7–1.   See opposite page for legend.

dried layers. The splint was reinserted, and Kenalog in Orabase was applied to the tissues.

Thereafter, healing progressed uneventfully. Six weeks later the tissues were fully healed, and the patient was ready for the restorative dentistry and the subgingival troughs that would be required. The gingival tissues were normal in tone and contour but had receded from the old restoration which was being utilized as a temporary splint. After the subgingival troughs were created and the teeth prepared she had two maxillary fixed bridge unit-built porcelain crown restorations constructed in accordance with the treatment plan submitted to her dentist. When the new restorations were inserted, due to the space created for accommodation of the subgingival bulk, the integrity of the periodontal structures remained undisturbed. Note excellent gingival adaptation and tissue tone and concave self-cleansing interproximal sluiceways.

The following case demonstrates the importance of sound treatment plan and the need to vary it according to the specific clinical conditions that are encountered. It also serves to demonstrate the valuable contribution fulguration can make toward successful treatment of infrabony pockets that involve bifurcations and trifurcations.

CASE 8

As has been seen in the preceding cases, the author's gingivectoplasty-electronic pocket debridement technique normally eliminates need for incising and reflecting mucoperiosteal flaps, except for treatment of single isolated infrabony pockets.

However, no therapeutic procedure should ever be arbitrary and inflexible. In this case unusual clinical conditions dictated need to abandon the usual format and to create bilateral mucoperiosteal flap incisions. The deviation was necessitated by the fact that the patient's maxillary anterior teeth fixed splint prosthesis had been fabricated with a ledgelike palatal subgingival extension that made it impossible to perform efficient electronic curettage unless the tissue was reflected to provide free access to the periodontal defects.

Case Figure 7–1.   Periodontal deterioration triggered by periodontal splinting with a fixed bridge from molar to molar, without having provided subgingival space to accommodate the subgingival bulk of the restoration.

A, Preoperative appearance, labial view. The gingivae and especially the interproximal papillae are massively hypertrophied. The latter are so compressed that they are markedly blanched. B, The maxillary fixed-bridge splint has been removed, revealing almost total obliteration of the shoulders of the crown preparations by the hypertrophied tissues.

C, With the splint in position preliminary reduction of the gingival hypertrophy is performed by shaving in layers with a flame-shaped loop electrode. D, Individual infrabony pockets are thoroughly debrided with a narrow 45-degree-angle U-shaped loop electrode.

E, Appearance of the tissues on the sixth postoperative day. (Bird's-eye view of the maxilla with the splint removed, immediately after the first cement pack was removed.) F, Appearance of the tissues one month postoperatively. The gingivae are fully healed, the pockets have been eradicated, the tissue tone is excellent, the gingival architecture has been restored to normal, and the patient is ready for preparation of subgingival troughs and construction of new restorations. Note temporary cement filling the space between the new gingival margins and the old restoration.

G, Gingival adaptation, tissue tone and architecture now are normal. All infrabony pockets have been completely obliterated. Note concave self-cleansing interproximal sluiceways throughout the mouth except in lower anterior region where the four natural teeth are slightly crowded and the papillae have enlarged slightly.

In addition to demonstrating electrosurgical periodontal treatment technique, this case thus also demonstrates the importance of sound treatment plan and need for flexibility to vary treatment according to special conditions that may be encountered clinically. It also serves to demonstrate the invaluable contribution fulguration can make toward assuring successful debridement of molar infrabony pockets that communicate with their bifurcations and trifurcations.

PATIENT. A 59-year-old white male.

HISTORY. Approximately six months previously he had had his maxillary anterior teeth immobilized with a fixed prosthesis splint, and the molar teeth restored with crowns. Shortly after insertion of these restorations he noticed that the gingivae, which had responded to periodontal curettage prior to insertion, had begun to bleed again during tooth brushing, and that the palatal gingiva was tender and felt as though it was bulging slightly from under the splint. He returned to the dentist, who found extensive periodontal deterioration and referred him to the author for surgery.

CLINICAL EXAMINATION. The maxillary anterior teeth from cuspid to cuspid were locked into a fixed splint of porcelain veneer crowns. The right maxillary second molar was restored with a cast gold crown. The rest of the maxilla was edentulous. The mandible had a full complement of teeth. The second and third molars on each side had been restored with porcelain veneer crowns. The maxillary cuspid crowns had slots cut into their distal aspects into which the male attachments of a partial denture with Chayes type of attachments fitted. A similar slot was present in the mesio-occlusal surface of the molar crown. A deep periodontal pocket was present at the mesial aspect of the molar, and deep pockets also were present on the palatal aspect of the anterior maxillary teeth. The labial gingiva around these teeth was somewhat hyperplastic, and several pockets were also present on the labial aspect. The buccal gingivae in the mandibular molar areas also were slightly hyperplastic and partially detached, and there were multiple pockets present. Deep pockets also were present along the roots of the anterior teeth and the bicuspids. The anterior palatal tissue appeared to be proliferating and was somewhat engorged. Roentgenographic examination revealed extensive disease around the mesial root of the mandibular left second molar that appeared to involve the entire root. A second film taken with a gutta percha point inserted into the pocket as a radiopaque marker confirmed that the disease circumscribed the entire root. The roentgenographic examination also revealed communication of the periodontal disease with the trifurcation of the maxillary molar and with the bifurcation of the mandibular right second molar.

TREATMENT. The tissues were prepared and the maxillary molar was anesthetized with a posterior superior alveolar block and palatal infiltration. A flame-shaped loop was selected, cutting current was set at 5 on the instrument panel, and the marginal gingiva at the mesial aspect of the tooth was resected (Case Fig. 8–1A). The flame-shaped electrode was replaced with a 17-mm. right-angle periodontal loop electrode, cutting current was reduced to 4, and debris of the lining epithelium was resected from the defect, including the trifurcation (Case Fig. 8–1B). When the defect appeared to be fully debrided a heavy needle electrode was selected and used to fulgurate the trifurcation to eliminate tenaciously adherent fragments of tissue present there to complete the debridement. Bleeding was encouraged and powdered surgical gelatin was introduced and mixed with the blood which proceeded to clot, while treatment of the anterior area was initiated.

Bilateral infraorbital regional block and nasopalatine and anterior palatine anesthesia were administered, and the flame-shaped loop electrode was used to perform a gingivoplasty to recontour the labial gingiva to normal architecture, and to create self-

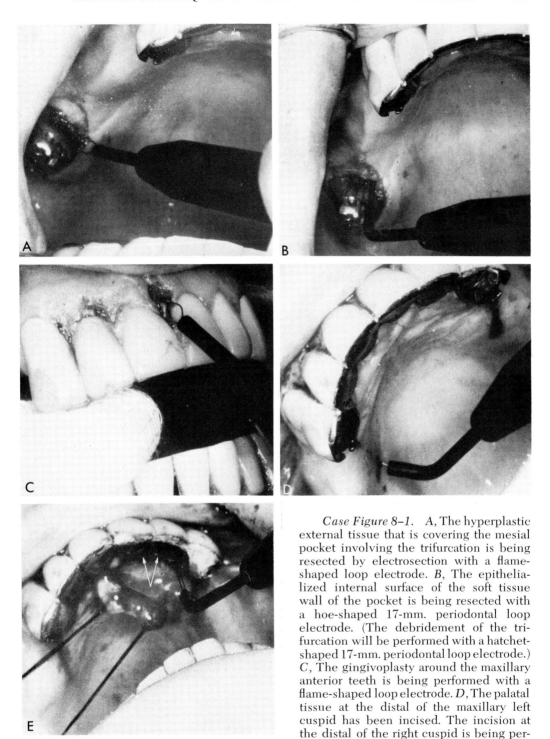

Case Figure 8–1. *A,* The hyperplastic external tissue that is covering the mesial pocket involving the trifurcation is being resected by electrosection with a flame-shaped loop electrode. *B,* The epithelialized internal surface of the soft tissue wall of the pocket is being resected with a hoe-shaped 17-mm. periodontal loop electrode. (The debridement of the trifurcation will be performed with a hatchet-shaped 17-mm. periodontal loop electrode.) *C,* The gingivoplasty around the maxillary anterior teeth is being performed with a flame-shaped loop electrode. *D,* The palatal tissue at the distal of the maxillary left cuspid has been incised. The incision at the distal of the right cuspid is being performed with a 45-degree-angle fine needle electrode, to create a mucoperiosteal palatal flap. *E,* The flap has been elevated and is being retracted with a 00 silk suture while the infrabony pocket debridement is being performed with the hatchet-shaped 17-mm. periodontal loop electrode. (The epithelialized ventral surface of the flap was resected with the hoe-shaped loop before the pocket debridement was instituted.)

cleansing sluiceways in the embrasures (Case Fig. 8–1C). A fine 45-degree-angle needle electrode was selected to replace the periodontal loop electrode and used to incise the palatal gingiva bilaterally (Case Fig. 8–1D). Each mucoperiosteal incision was made at the distal aspect of the cuspid and extended posteriorly and medially approximately 2 cm.; the apices of the interdental papillae on the palatal aspect were incised and the incised tissue flap was elevated and reflected. A length of 00 black silk suture was inserted first at the left half of the flap and used as a tissue retractor while the 17-mm. 45-degree-angle periodontal loop electrode was used to debride the defect, with current increased to 5 on the panel (Case Fig. 8–1E). This suture was removed, the right half of the flap was elevated and reflected, and another silk suture was inserted and used in an identical manner as a tissue retractor. When debridement was completed the flap was restored and secured into position by suturing through the interdental papilla. A pack of periodontal cement was applied to the two surgical fields, and the patient was instructed to return on the fifth postoperative day for further treatment.

When he returned the mandible was anesthetized by inferior alveolar regional block injections. A fistula on the labial gingiva midway between the right central and lateral was destroyed by fulguration (Case Fig. 8–2A). A flame-shaped loop electrode was selected and used to perform the gingivoplasty on the labial gingivae (Case Fig. 8–2B), in the right quadrant. A medium-width 45-degree-angle U-shaped loop electrode was chosen and used to perform the gingivoplasty on the lingual aspect (Case Fig. 8–2C). Debridement of the infrabony pockets was then performed with a 17-mm. 45-degree-angle periodontal loop electrode (Case Fig. 8–2D and E). Debridement of the diseased bifurcation of the right second molar was then performed with the right-angle 17-mm. periodontal loop electrode. When debridement appeared to be completed, bleeding was encouraged and powdered surgical gelatin was introduced and mixed with the blood in the defect.

The fine 45-degree-angle needle electrode was selected, and cutting current was reduced to 3 and used to incise the buccal gingiva at the mesiogingival angle of the mandibular left second molar. The incision was directed anteriorly and downward to the mucogingival junction, and the mucoperiosteal flap was elevated and retracted manually to expose the mesial root which was totally denuded of bone. The root was sectioned about 2.5 mm. beyond the furcation with a crosscut fissure bur. The cut edge of the root was rounded with a round diamond stone and the gutta percha resealed at the cut end with a medium-size round coagulating electrode. Debridement was performed in part with hand instrumentation and loop electrode curettage, and the furca was sprayed with fulgurating current to destroy any inaccessible fragments. Bleeding was induced, surgical gelatin was introduced into the defect and mixed with the blood, and the flap was restored and sutured; a postoperative x-ray was taken (Case Fig. 8–5B). (The surgical procedure will be adequately demonstrated in the chapter on surgery and therefore will not be illustrated here. The x-rays of the original defect and the progress of repair are included here as Case Fig. 8–5A to D). The cement pack on the maxilla was removed and replaced after the tissues had been cleansed and tincture of myrrh and benzoin was applied. A cement pack was then applied to the mandibular tissues.

Ten days later the second packs were removed. Healing was progressing favorably except for a surface layer of coagulum over the fulgurated site of the fistulous orifice and light layers of coagulum on the palatal tissue surface (Case Fig. 8–3A and B). Healing continued to progress favorably in all areas except the mandibular right second molar, where the buccal gingiva appeared to have failed to become reat-

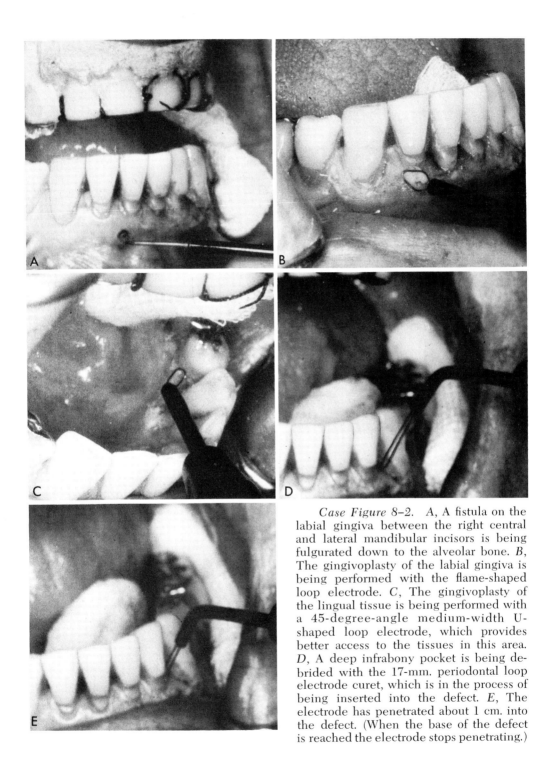

Case Figure 8–2. *A*, A fistula on the labial gingiva between the right central and lateral mandibular incisors is being fulgurated down to the alveolar bone. *B*, The gingivoplasty of the labial gingiva is being performed with the flame-shaped loop electrode. *C*, The gingivoplasty of the lingual tissue is being performed with a 45-degree-angle medium-width U-shaped loop electrode, which provides better access to the tissues in this area. *D*, A deep infrabony pocket is being debrided with the 17-mm. periodontal loop electrode curet, which is in the process of being inserted into the defect. *E*, The electrode has penetrated about 1 cm. into the defect. (When the base of the defect is reached the electrode stops penetrating.)

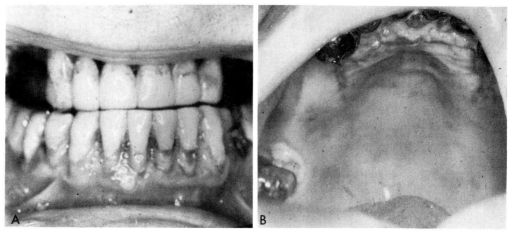

Case Figure 8–3. A, Appearance of the mandibular labial tissues after removal of the second cement pack on the tenth postoperative day. B, Appearance of the maxillary palatal tissues after removal of the second cement pack on the tenth postoperative day.

tached. The patient's cooperation in maintaining excellent postoperative physiotherapy contributed materially to the favorable rate and quality of tissue repair. The mandibular anterior teeth were slightly mobile during the early stage of postoperative repair. They were stabilized with a continuous stainless steel wire labial archwire that was discarded by the end of the fifth week.

Before the archwire was removed, the mandibular right second molar bifurcation lesion had to be re-treated. The quadrant was anesthetized and a mucoperiosteal incision was made with a 45-degree-angle fine needle electrode (Case Fig. 8–4A). The incision was started at the distogingival angle of the buccal gingiva of the first molar and directed anteriorly and downward to the mucogingival junction. The apex of the interdental papilla was then also severed and the mucoperiosteal flap was elevated and retracted. A 17-mm. periodontal loop electrode was substituted, current power was increased to 4.5, and the activated electrode was used to debride the defect (Case Fig. 8–4B). Debridement having been completed as much as could be determined grossly, the furca was sprayed with fulgurating current to destroy any inaccessible tissue fragments that might be wedged between the roots and bone (Case Fig. 8–4C). When debridement was completed bleeding was encouraged and the flap was restored and sutured with interrupted silk sutures (Case Fig. 8–4D).

The sutures were removed on the fifth postoperative day. Healing appeared to be progressing favorably. The patient was seen postoperatively at weekly intervals for three weeks, then bimonthly for the next two months. By the end of the twelfth week the tissues were completely normal in all respects, and the defects were totally obliterated (Case Fig. 8–4E and F).

It is interesting to note that the trifurcation responded superbly to treatment where the furca had been fulgurated; however, the bifurcation failed to respond to identical treatment (except for not having used fulguration in that defect) but did respond to the second attempt after the fulguration was used (Case Fig. 8–5A and B). Inasmuch as the only difference between the successful treatments and the treatment failure was the use or omission of fulguration it would seem that minute fragments of diseased tissue that defy efforts at removal with even the fine flexible loop electrodes can be destroyed in situ effectively by the sparks that can penetrate crevices where even the finest electrode cannot enter.

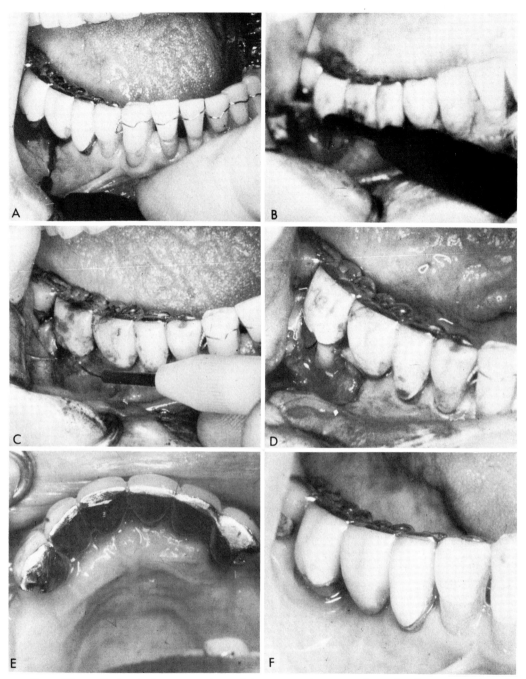

Case Figure 8–4. A, A mucoperiosteal incision is being made at the distogingival angle of the mandibular first molar down to the mucogingival junction with a 45-degree-angle fine needle electrode by electrosection. B, The mucoperiosteal flap has been reflected and the infrabony pocket into the bifurcation is debrided with a 17-mm. periodontal loop electrode. C, The bifurcation is being fulgurated to assure that fragments of tissue still wedged inaccessibly in the furca despite the loop debridement will be destroyed in situ. D, Appearance after completion of debridement. E, Postoperative appearance of the maxilla two weeks after removal of the second cement pack. The tissues appear fully healed except for lack of surface keratin along the lines of incision. Tissue tone is excellent, the gingival height has not receded from its original level, and there are no exposed denuded root surfaces present. F, Appearance of the tissues in the mandibular right quadrant one month after the second surgical debridement of the bifurcation. The gingival tissues appear fully healed, and the line of incision cannot be distinguished from the surrounding tissue. The gingival tissue appears firmly adherent to the tooth and bone in the bifurcation.

625

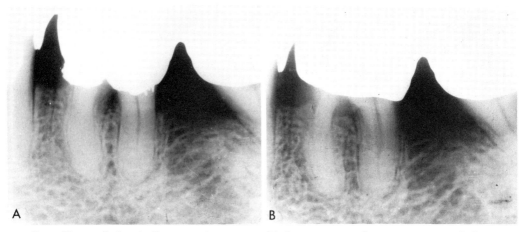

Case Figure 8–5. A, Preoperative x-ray of bifurcation involvement. Note radiolucence from destruction of crest of interseptal bone. B, Postoperative x-ray, six months later. Note regeneration of bone of interseptal crest. The bone has filled in and obliterated the bifurcation defect.

II. PERIODONTOCLASIA RELATED TO SYSTEMIC FACTORS

Periodontia Related to a Blood Dyscrasia

CASE 9

This case demonstrates two things: the unfavorable influence of a blood dyscrasia on the rate and quality of tissue repair, and the remarkable tendency of the tissue to regenerate toward its original level following electrosurgical gingivectoplasty, even under such a handicap.

This case also is an excellent example of how easily unfavorable local factors can mask the presence of systemic factors and the importance of looking beyond the local factors when inexplicable postoperative results occur.

PATIENT. A 58-year-old black female.

HISTORY. The author had performed an extensive preprosthodontic reduction of an abnormal tuberosity two years previously (see page 788), at which time the patient's postoperative reaction had been without untoward incident. She had had a gold crown inserted on the right maxillary cuspid and a partial upper denture restoration about six months previously. Soon thereafter the marginal gingiva around the crowned cuspid, which was serving as an abutment, became engorged and hypertrophied. Repeated curettage by her dentist failed to produce appreciable improvement. She therefore was referred to the author for a gingivectomy to try to preserve this key abutment tooth.

CLINICAL EXAMINATION

Extraoral. Negative.

Intraoral. The six maxillary anterior teeth were present and the two cuspids served as the abutments for a partial denture. The right cuspid was restored with a gold shell crown. The gingival mucosa around this tooth was hyperemic, hypertrophic, and partially detached from the tooth and alveolar bone (Case Fig. 9–1).

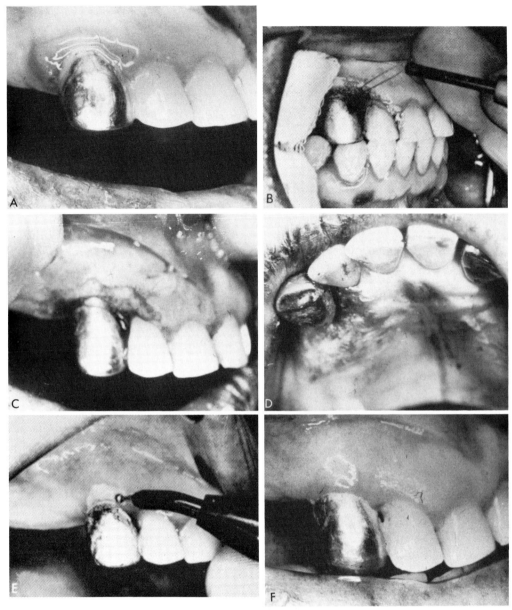

Case Figure 9–1.   Periodontia related to hematologic disease. Gingivectoplasty and infrabony pocket debridement of a key abutment tooth. *A*, Preoperative appearance. Gingiva around gold shell crown is hyperemic, hyperplastic, and partially detached. The tissue is severely engorged, and the marginal gingiva has receded slightly, the marginal edge forming a roll instead of a feather edge. *B*, The gingivectoplasty having been performed with a flame-shaped loop electrode, the infrabony pocket is being debrided with a 17-mm. periodontal loop electrode. *C*, Labial view, showing result of the gingivectoplasty. Normal gingival contour is restored and about 3 mm. of denuded root is exposed. *D*, Palatal view, showing extensiveness of area treated to bevel the tissue and avoid creating an undercut. *E*, Superficial spot coagulation with a small ball electrode applied along the edge of the marginal gingiva. *F*, Final postoperative result. After four months of postoperative treatment the gingival tissue has finally healed to an acceptable degree, although it is still well below the quality of tissue repair usually achieved. Note regeneration of marginal gingiva to its original level, covering the denuded root surface. The regeneration to or almost to its original level is a typical result when electrosection is used properly.

TREATMENT. The mouth was prepared for surgery and infiltration anesthesia administered. A flame-shaped loop electrode was selected and current output was set at 5.5 for electrosection. The activated electrode was applied to the tissue at a 45-degree angle, and with a wiping motion the detached roll of mucosa was resected.

A narrow 45-degree-angle U-shaped loop electrode was substituted and applied with a light wiping motion directed downward to reduce the mesial interproximal papilla into a concave self-cleansing sluiceway. Current output was increased to 6.5 and the palatal mucosa was reduced to normal contour by planing with the flame-shaped loop. In order to avoid creating an abrupt undercut it was necessary to plane the tissue (over an approximate 2 cm. area) into a gradual slope toward the palatal aspect of the tooth. When resection was completed, a 3 mm. space beyond the neck of the tooth was exposed. A protective surgical cement pack was applied to the entire operative field and the patient was given postoperative instructions.

She returned on the fifth postoperative day. The cement pack, intact and firmly in position, was removed and the area was irrigated. Healing by granulation appeared to be progressing satisfactorily. Tincture of myrrh and benzoin was applied and a fresh cement pack inserted. Inspection of the tissue on the tenth postoperative day revealed that the healing was inferior to that obtained two years previously. The repairing gingival tissue appeared atonal, hyperemic, and hypertrophic and appeared to be proliferating into unorganized granulation.

The area was dried and topical anesthetic ointment was applied for two minutes. Current output was set at 5 for biterminal electrocoagulation and the superfluous tissue was resected with a single wiping stroke of the flame-shaped electrode. Tincture of myrrh and benzoin was applied to the area in air-dried layers, and the patient was instructed to continue the postoperative home care.

She returned for treatment twice a week for the next three weeks. Despite the constant postoperative care, healing progressed slowly. By the end of the third week healing had progressed sufficiently to permit use of the salt-alum astringent mouthwash. By the end of the fourth week the tissue appeared healed but slightly hyperemic and not yet fully keratinized.

She continued to return at weekly intervals, and during the next six weeks a number of electrosurgical interventions were attempted in order to accelerate and improve the tissue maturation. At the first two of these visits superficial spot coagulation with a small ball electrode was performed under topical anesthesia. Some improvement resulted but not to the anticipated degree. The engorgement and tendency to hypertrophy still persisted, especially in the mesial interproximal area.

At the third visit deeper spot coagulation was performed under infiltration anesthesia. Then a narrow loop electrode was substituted for the ball electrode, coagulating current output was increased to 4, and the hyperemic mesial portion of the marginal gingiva was again reduced to normal level. Tincture of myrrh and benzoin was applied in air-dried layers and frequent saline lavage was prescribed.

At the following visit the tissue appeared considerably improved, but by the following week there was distinct evidence of regression. At this time it seemed logical to blame the recurrent deterioration on two local factors. First, the tooth was constantly subjected to considerable stress as the abutment for a large clasp-attached, tooth-and-tissue–borne partial denture. Moreover, the gold crown restoration was not perfectly adapted to the tooth; it extended upward, impinging into the marginal crevice space, especially in the mesial embrasure.

Two millimeters of the mesial hyperemic gingival margin adjoining the gingival end of the gold crown was therefore fulgurated under infiltration anesthesia. Tincture of myrrh and benzoin was applied and the tissue was further protected with Kenalog in Orabase. She was also instructed to leave the denture out for at least one week.

The final result obtained was reasonably satisfactory. The mucosa was completely healed and the tissue tone was normal except along the free margin and mesial embrasure. The tissue in these areas was darker red in color, owing to a slight amount of persisting hyperemia and incomplete keratinization of the tissue surface (Case Fig. 9–1).

The underlying reason for retarded rate, subnormal quality, and recurrent deterioration of tissue repair ultimately proved to be systemic in origin. The discovery that the patient had severe anemia occurred as a result of a third surgical procedure performed for this patient about two years later (see page 802).

This case presented two typical elements against which the operator must always be on guard. One, the danger of making diagnoses based on the assumption that obvious unfavorable local factors are the sole handicap to be overcome; the other, the insidious influence of hidden and usually systemic factors on the end result. A sound rule of thumb is that when normal tissue repair is not achieved despite treatment that customarily proves effective, hidden factors should be suspected.

Periodontal Disease Attributable to Nutritional-Hematologic Deficiencies

The patients in the next series of cases presented a unique combination of clinical abnormalities the author has not encountered in any other cases. Despite the limited number of cases in which the unusual manifestations were a common denominator they appear to be so intimately interrelated as to suggest that they constitute a syndrome rather than just an unusual coincidence.

In each of the cases the gingival tissues appeared desquamated of their normal keratinized layer of gingival epithelium. The alveolar (attached) gingivae were so atonal that there was no distinguishable clinical evidence of zones of attached gingivae and no visible demarcation between the alveolar and areolar gingivae.

Despite the atonal condition and extensiveness of periodontal deterioration, the gingivae in all three cases were pallid in color, in sharp contrast to the usual dark red engorged appearance of atonal tissues.

All these patients salivated profusely, and the saliva of all three was incredibly viscous in character. (The quality of the saliva and its copious flow has led the author to hypothesize that perhaps the constant tenacious adhesion of the viscous saliva to the tissues resulted in disintegration of the packed layers of dead cells that compose the keratinized epithelial surface, thereby producing the desquamation of the keratinized layer.)

All three patients had dietary deficiencies and all three were anemic. The fact that two of the patients had an almost identical dietary intake, and the third also had a marked dietary imbalance, strongly suggests that their anemias were nutritional in origin.

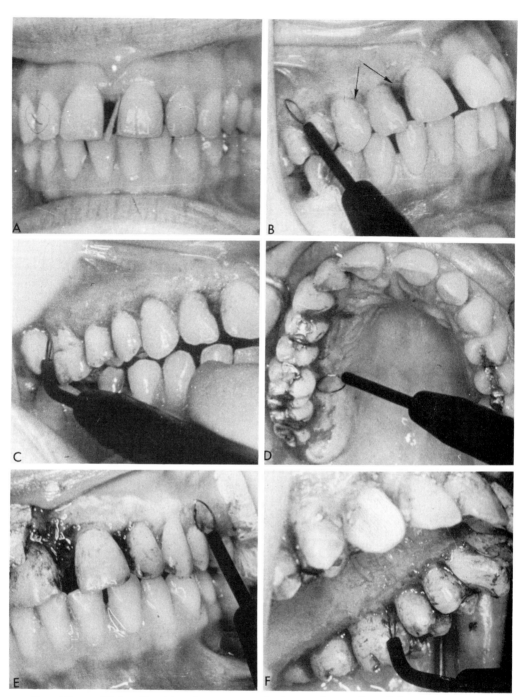

Case Figure 10–1. Combined treatment of advanced periodontal disease of nutritional and hematologic origin and simple tooth movement.

A, Preoperative appearance. The gingival tissues appear deceptively normal owing to absence of appreciable hyperplasia or detachment. Instead of the customary engorgement these tissues are pallid in color, and the surface of the tissues is smooth, shiny and translucently thin. There is a wide diastema between the maxillary centrals and between the maxillary laterals and centrals. There are also diastemas between the mandibular right central and lateral and between the two right bicuspids, and the right first molar is missing from the dental arch. The marginal gingiva on the labial of the left maxillary central is slightly thickened and a gutta percha point has been inserted into a deep infrabony pocket at the mesial of the tooth to serve as a radiopaque pocket marker. *B*, Despite the lack of need for architectural recontouring a flame-shaped loop electrode is being used to skim off the surface epithelium

The remarkable similarity in their nutritional and hematologic status and in the character of their periodontal disease lends credence to the concept that this combination of similarities adds up to a syndrome and is not merely accidental.

CASE 10

This case was characterized by a very extensive alveolar bone loss, creating marked pathological migration characterized by drifting of the anterior teeth labially out of the dental arch, and wide diastemas between the teeth. It was also characterized by an exceptionally copious flow of extremely viscous saliva that adhered tenaciously to the tissues and kept them constantly coated.

PATIENT. A 27-year-old white female.

CASE HISTORY. The patient had been under active folic acid-vitamin B complex therapy for treatment of a macrocytic anemia as well as a vitamin C deficiency for more than a year, and was reported to be responding favorably to the therapy.

CLINICAL EXAMINATION. The gingival mucosa was very pallid and was so atonal and edematous that light fingertip pressure produced indentations similar to those produced by light pressure against the skin of victims of decompensated heart disease.

The gingival surface was very shiny and appeared devoid of the normal keratinized surface layer of epithelium. There was no clinically visible evidence of a zone of attached gingiva. The gingival mucosa blended into the areolar mucosa with no visible line of demarcation between the two.

All the teeth were mobile; mobility ranged from moderately marked in the anterior to slight in a few of the posterior teeth. Probing with a periodontal pocket probe revealed that periodontal pockets were present along the roots of practically all the teeth in both dental arches. Pocket depth of probe penetration ranged from 3 to 9 mm. A molar gutta percha point used for x-ray visualization was easily inserted into a typical pocket located at the mesial aspect of the maxillary right central incisor (Case Fig. 10–1A).

TREATMENT. Treatment was performed in three stages: preoperative, operative, and postoperative.

Preoperative. The occlusion was checked and carefully balanced to eliminate traumatizing prematurities. The patient was instructed in the full routine of massage

---

Case Figure 10–1 Continued.
from the marginal gingivae in the maxillary right quadrant, exposing the infrabony defects (arrow). C, A 17-mm. periodontal loop electrode is being used as an electronic curet to debride an infrabony pocket at the mesial of the maxillary right second molar. D, An 8-mm. round loop electrode has been bent about 20 degrees to provide better tissue contact, and this electrode is being used to perform the gingivoplasty on the palatal aspect of the maxillary left quadrant. The cement pack has been removed from the right quadrant, and the tissues appear to be healing favorably. E, The gingivoplasty to remove the surface epithelium is being performed on the labial and buccal aspects of the maxillary left quadrant on the fifth postoperative day, while the cement pack that had been applied to the right quadrant is still in place. The heat penetration which normally is self-limiting to a remarkable degree is markedly greater owing to the lack of resistance of the frail edematous cells, and this is resulting in coagulation of the surface epithelium beyond the actual electrode contact with the tissues (arrow). F, The 17-mm. loop electrode is being used to debride an infrabony pocket on the mesiopalatal aspect of the maxillary left first molar effortlessly.

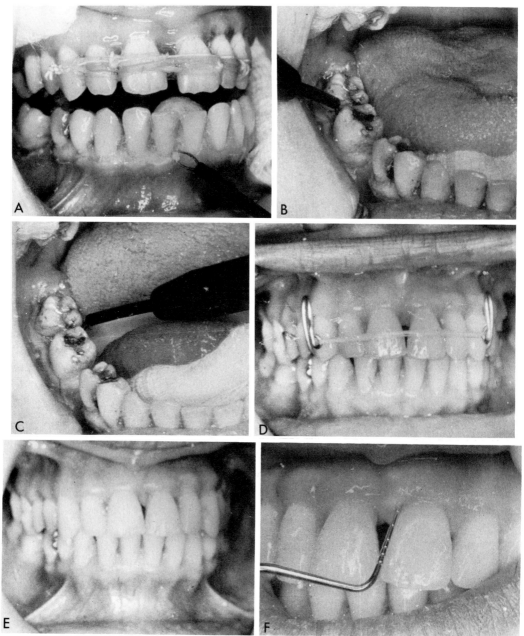

Case Figure 10–2.   A, The gingivoplasty is being performed with the flame-shaped loop electrode in the mandibular right quadrant. Elastic band-Japanese grassline traction has been applied to the maxillary anterior teeth to attempt repositioning of the teeth and closure of the diastemas. Note the clinical evidence of the chronological rate and quality of the tissue repair. The tissues in the right quadrant as seen 10 days after the second cement pack has been removed and the tissues in the left quadrant five days after the second cement pack has been removed show a marked difference in their respective degree of repair, indicating the rapid rate of repair progress in the five-day interval. *B,* The distobuccal infrabony pocket of the mandibular right third molar has been debrided, and the 17-mm. periodontal loop electrode is being used to debride the infrabony pocket at the mesiobuccal of the second molar. The electrode has penetrated approximately 14 mm. into the defect. *C,* The same electrode is being used to debride the distolingual infrabony pocket on the same tooth. This pocket is about 13 mm. deep. Both pockets are narrow, with a considerable amount of normal bone necessary to maintain good oral physiotherapy. Ths included instruction in use of the manual and the mechanical toothbrushes for the Charters method of brushing, proper use of the rubber tip, and even fingertip massage. A dietary supplement of clear gelatin and ascorbic acid was prescribed, to assure a high protein intake and to provide the catalyst necessary for maximum utilization of the protein. A thorough prophylaxis and root planing were performed the day of the surgery.

Operative.   Owing to the excessive salivation, which even premedication with an effective antisialogogue failed to reduce to normal dimension, and to the edematous condition of the tissues, quadrant surgery rather than surgery on the full arch was done.

Infraorbital, posterior superior alveolar, nasopalatine, and anterior palatine regional block anesthesia was administered in the upper right quadrant. An oral speculum retractor was inserted, and a flame-shaped loop electrode was used to plane the tissue surface (Case Fig. 10–1*B*). A minimal amount of recontouring was required, but the surface epithelium was removed by gingivoplasty to permit regeneration of a new surface epithelium. Pocket debridement was performed with a 17-mm. narrow U-shaped periodontal loop electrode (Case Fig. 10–1*C*).

Gingivoplasty and pocket debridement having been completed on both the labial and palatal aspects (Case Fig. 10–1*D*), bleeding was induced in the debrided pockets, and the blood permitted to clot firmly. A tincture of myrrh and benzoin dressing was applied to the operative field in air-dried layers. A hard mix of periodontal cement was carefully packed around the teeth. Care was exercised to direct pressure coronally to avoid displacing the blood clots and accidentally forcing the cement into the osseous defects.

On the fifth day, before the first pack was removed, the left quadrant was anesthetized in a similar manner and treatment instituted. Despite the remarkable self-limiting qualities of fully rectified cutting current and the normally clinically meaningless amount of lateral heat dispersion it produces here, the tissue surface 3 to 4 millimeters beyond the contact of the activated electrode turned white during the gingivoplasty, owing to the edema and lack of normal cellular wall resistance. A thin layer of surface coagulum, which could be peeled off, formed (Case Fig. 10–1*E*).

When the gingivoplasty had been completed on both buccal and palatal surfaces, individual periodontal pocket debridement with the periodontal electronic loop curet was performed. These pockets were present along the roots of practically all the teeth, and in many instances there were multiple pockets around the tooth. The pockets on the palatal aspect were just as easily accessible and effectively treated as the labial-buccally located ones (Case Fig. 10–1*F*).

Debridement having been completed, the debris was removed from the osseous

---

Case Figure 10–2   Continued.
remaining between them. *D,* Appearance of the teeth and tissues 3 months postoperatively. The teeth have been restored to normal alignment in the dental arches and the diastemas have been closed. The tissues are normal in tone and the pockets have been obliterated. The patient is seen wearing a Hawley retainer with an elastic band over the labial aspect of the anterior maxillary teeth which she wears at night to guard against the possibility of tooth movement should there be any bruxing while in the prone position during sleep, to maximize the potential for normal calcification of the repair bone in the defects. *E,* Appearance of the teeth and tissues 6 months postoperatively. The Hawley retainer has been discarded, as the bone is maturely calcified and the teeth are firmly retained in their new position. *F,* Close-up appearance of the tissues in *E.* The tissue tone is excellent, and the surface of the tissue has an orange-skin tippled appearance. A periodontal pocket probe has been inserted subgingivally at the site of the mesial defect into which the gutta percha point had been inserted as a radiopaque marker. The probe has penetrated to the base of the gingival sulcus and is unable to penetrate further despite pressure that is causing the tissue to blanch.

defects, bleeding encouraged, and the blood permitted to clot. A tincture of myrrh and benzoin dressing was applied, and the periodontal pack in the right quadrant, which had just been removed, was replaced at the same time that the initial pack was applied to the left quadrant.

Healing progressed without incident. After the second cement pack was removed from the left quadrant Japanese grassline and elastic band traction was applied to the maxillary teeth to try to bring them back into the dental arch and close the diastemas. The patient was seen again 5 days later, at which time an examination of the mouth revealed an excellent rate and quality of tissue repair (Case Fig. 10–2A). The right quadrant which had been operated on 20 days previously (10 days after the second cement pack was removed) appeared almost fully healed and normal. The tissues in the left quadrant, which had been operated on 5 days later, and from which the second cement pack had been removed 5 days previously, was not nearly as fully healed.

The mandibular right quadrant was prepared, anesthetized, and treated at this time. The gingivoplasty was performed with a flame-shaped loop electrode. To debride the lingual surface most efficiently a flame-shaped loop electrode was curved to form an approximate 45-degree angle, which gave better access to the tissues being planed and facilitated the gingivoplasty. When this was completed, the individual periodontal pockets were debrided in the manner described. A 17-mm. periodontal loop electrode was used with electrosection as an electronic curet to debride each pocket. Many of the pockets were 10 to 15 mm. deep. A 15-mm. pocket along the distal root of the mandibular right second molar was debrided (Case Fig. 10–2B) and a 13-mm. pocket along the mesiolingual aspect of the mesial root of the right third molar was debrided in an identical manner (Case Fig. 10–2C).

When all the pockets had been thoroughly debrided, which was ascertained by transillumination directly into the defects, and also by lightly probing in the pockets with a limber 17-mm. *inactivated* electrode, loose fragments of debris were removed by irrigation. This was followed with careful aspiration of all the fluid, and bleeding was induced in the osseous defects. After the blood had clotted the operative field was treated with a tincture of myrrh and benzoin dressing applied in air-dried layers. A hard mix of periodontal cement was then carefully packed against the teeth with the pressure directed coronally.

The patient returned on the fifth day postoperatively, at which time the last quadrant was treated in an identical manner, after which a cement pack was applied to the new surgical field and a fresh pack applied to the 5-day-old wound. Healing continued to progress rapidly and favorably.

Postoperative. The elastic band–grassline traction had succeeded in bringing the teeth back into normal alignment in the dental arch and had closed the diastemas. A stainless steel bar was applied to the teeth with acrylic to immobilize the anteriors during the reparative period. At the end of 3 months this bar was removed. Although all the teeth appeared normally firm, a Hawley retainer appliance was processed to which a heavy elastic band was attached so that it rested against the labial aspects of the anterior teeth to discourage any tendency toward labial rotation and drifting (Case Fig. 10–2D).

The Hawley retainer was used for 3 months. By the end of the sixth postoperative month the retainer was discarded. The clinical and roentgenographic evidence pointed to an eminently successful outcome. The patient was seen again at 6 month intervals for 2 years. When seen 2 years postoperatively, the tissues were healthy, the teeth were firm, and the pockets were permanently obliterated (Case Fig. 10–2E and F).

CASE 11

The saying that couples who have been married for a long time often begin to resemble each other applied aptly to the mouths of this patient and his wife, the patient in the preceding case, with one difference; the periodontal deterioration was much more profound in his case. In addition to loss of bone structure due to deep infrabony pockets, he also had lost more than half the investing alveolar bone because of horizontal circumscribing alveolar resorption, so that the infrabony pockets were extending beyond the level of the remaining bone almost to the apex of each tooth, resulting in marked pathologic migration of the teeth. Thus, unlike the preceding case, in which temporary splinting followed by temporary postoperative retention sufficed, in this case it would be necessary to have the teeth immobilized permanently if the condition responded favorably to the electrosurgery.

PATIENT.   A 31-year-old white male.

HISTORY.   He had noted a progressive development of spaces between his teeth and shrinking of the gingivae, exposing part of the roots of the teeth, and a marked loosening of the teeth. He also noted an occasional drop of pus oozing from under the gums. He consulted his dentist and was referred to several highly qualified periodontists who concurred that he would have to have all his maxillary teeth and most of the mandibular teeth extracted and replaced with dentures.

The patient had a morbid dread that his false teeth would drop out of his mouth while talking and rejected this treatment plan. Recalling that his wife had been advised to have many teeth extracted, and actually had had to have only one removed (a malposed maxillary third molar), he contacted the author for a consultation.

The clinical condition of his mouth was so obvious that he was told frankly that the prognosis for successful treatment was poor and the extensive, expensive procedure might well end in failure. He was so eager to try to save the teeth that he gladly acceded to the undertaking of treatment as a clinical experiment, and to the fact that if the treatment succeeded permanent fixation would be necessary for functional usefulness of the teeth.

CLINICAL EXAMINATION.   Diastemas measuring from 1 to 4 mm. in width were present between most of the maxillary anterior teeth. The two centrals were rotated labially, with the left central protruding outward most notably. The disease was clinically visible on the palatal aspect as well as the labial (Case Fig. 11–1A). A drop of purulent exudate was present on the tip of the papilla in the right central-lateral embrasure.

Owing to the absence of a keratinized layer of epithelium and the atonal puffy condition of the tissue it was impossible to differentiate the alveolar gingiva from the areolar gingiva. Deep pockets were present throughout the mouth. A typical pocket at the distal of the maxillary right central was penetrated 8 mm. with a blunt round type of periodontal pocket probe (Case Fig. 11–1B). Infrabony pockets that appeared to penetrate almost to the apices of the teeth were found on the palatal of the right central incisor and the lingual of the left mandibular first molar. All the other pockets were very deep, but not quite as deep as these.

TREATMENT.   It was obvious that the treatment plan would have to take into account the extensive bone loss if sharp thin marginal bone edges appeared to need ramping.

The maxilla was treated first. Bilateral posterior superior alveolar and infraorbital blocks on the labial-buccal surface, and nasopalatine and anterior palatine block injections were administered. Although it would be necessary to eliminate the flaps of

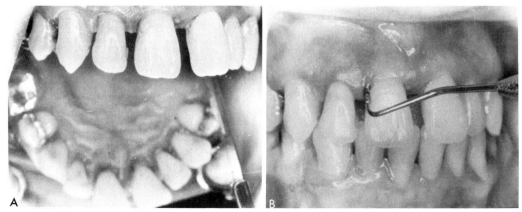

Case Figure 11–1. Combined horizontal and vertical bone loss and pathologic migration in both arches. *A*, Preoperative appearance of maxilla (palatal aspect seen as a mirror image). There are diastemas of varying widths between most of the anterior teeth. The tissues are completely atonal, and there is no clinical evidence of a zone of attached gingivae. A drop of purulent exudate is present at the mesial aspect of the right central. The marginal gingivae on the palatal aspect appear badly deteriorated. *B*, A periodontal pocket probe inserted under the gingival free margin at the distolabial angle of the right central penetrates approximately 7 mm. before encountering resistance. The pocket probe is a round, rather thick instrument of considerable bulk.

detached unsupported gingival tissue created by the horizontal bone loss, some gingival resorption that had accompanied the horizontal alveolar resorption minimized the amount of detached tissue materially. Instead of performing a gingivectomy and then recontouring the tissue margin, the undesirable portion of the tissue was resected by gingivectoplasty with a flame-shaped loop electrode used with cutting current set at 4.5 on the dial. The electrode was used with short brushing strokes for about 1 second and followed by a 2- to 3-second rest interval during which time the cut tissue surface was moistened with saliva and the excess wiped off to reconstitute a normal surface tension to the tissue. A medium-size round loop electrode was curved slightly and used in a similar manner to perform the gingivectoplasty on the palatal aspect (Case Fig. 11–2*A*).

When the redundant tissue was eliminated and a normal gingival architecture restored, the individual infrabony pockets were debrided with the 17-mm. periodontal loop electrodes. The pocket at the distal of the maxillary right central into which the blunt round pocket probe had penetrated 7 mm. was penetrated by the thin flexible electronic curet electrode to a depth of 13 mm. (Case Fig. 11–2*B*). (The absence of physical bulk permits the electrode to penetrate to the true base of the infrabony defect.)

The pockets along the roots of the posterior teeth were debrided as easily as the anterior ones (Case Fig. 11–2*D* and *E*). Considerable bleeding occurred during the electronic curettage, but this was readily controlled at will by applying pressure to the tissues with a sponge for 2 to 3 minutes. When the blood did not interfere with instrumentation it was permitted to remain on the tissues to keep them from becoming dried from exposure to the air.

The labial-buccal pockets having been debrided, those on the palatal aspect were treated with equal facility. The deep pocket on the palatal aspect of the maxillary right central was debrided first, and the electrode penetrated about 14 mm. before it met resistance (Case Fig. 11–2*D*). The posterior palatal pockets were debrided with com-

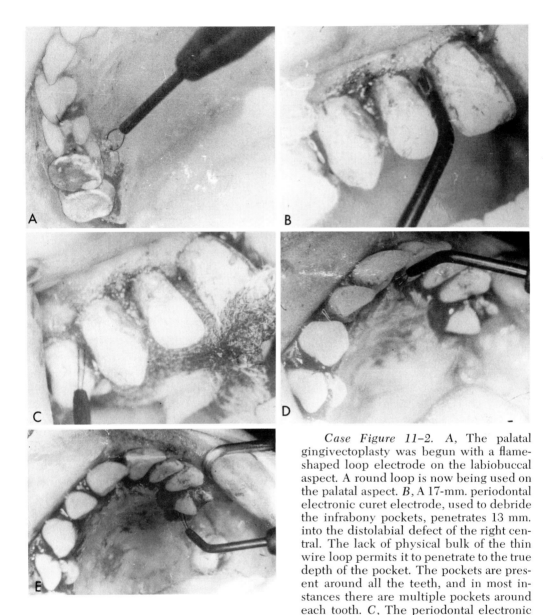

Case Figure 11-2. A, The palatal gingivectoplasty was begun with a flame-shaped loop electrode on the labiobuccal aspect. A round loop is now being used on the palatal aspect. B, A 17-mm. periodontal electronic curet electrode, used to debride the infrabony pockets, penetrates 13 mm. into the distolabial defect of the right central. The lack of physical bulk of the thin wire loop permits it to penetrate to the true depth of the pocket. The pockets are present around all the teeth, and in most instances there are multiple pockets around each tooth. C, The periodontal electronic probe electrode is being inserted into a pocket along the mesial aspect of the first bicuspid. Owing to the engorgement and atonal condition of the tissues there is considerable free bleeding despite the hemostasis of the cutting current. The bleeding can be staunched at will, however, by packing a strip of selvage gauze or a strip of the sterile surgical gauze sponge into the bleeding defect and holding it with moderate compressing finger pressure for 2 to 3 minutes. D, Deep pockets on the palatal aspect of the maxillary centrals are debrided as readily with the same 17-mm. periodontal electrode. E, Posterior palatal debridement is also readily accomplished.

parable ease. When debridement was completed, bleeding was induced in the infra-bony defects, and after applying tincture of myrrh and benzoin, a periodontal pack was applied. The patient was reminded of the regimen of home care he had been instructed about preoperatively and was reappointed.

There had been several areas where ramping of sharp labial-buccal bone edges would normally have been reduced somewhat. Because of the unusually large amount of bone loss the author was reluctant to remove even a millimeter of bone more than absolutely necessary, and it was impossible to tell precisely how much bone should be removed, so further reduction had been avoided on the basis that should it eventually prove essential to remove the bone it would be done when the exact amount of excess was apparent. This decision was also strengthened by the author's observation that when the spur of interseptal bone between the roots of a mandibular remains intact when the tooth is extracted, and it is not removed, the portion that projects beyond the surface of the blood clot in the socket sequesters, leaving a well-rounded normal bone covered with normal gingival mucosa, and that it was conceivable that a similar result might be obtained on the labial-buccal alveolar bone.

When the patient returned on the fifth postoperative day the mandible was anesthetized with bilateral inferior alveolar-lingual block injections and the gingivectoplasty performed with the flame-shaped loop electrode on the labial and the medium-width 45-degree-angle U-shaped loop on the lingual, with the cutting current output set at 4.5 and 5, respectively. The gingivectoplasty having been completed, the infrabony pockets were debrided with the 17-mm. periodontal loop electronic curet electrodes. A pocket at the distal of the right central that was 13 mm. deep and one at the distal of the left cuspid approximately 15 mm. deep were typical of the infrabony defects present along the roots of all the teeth (Case Fig. 11–3A and B). Similar pockets were also present on the lingual aspect. Most of the teeth had multiple pockets despite which considerable normal bone remained between them. The deepest pocket was at the lingual of the left first molar. This pocket was almost 16 mm. deep (Case Fig. 11–3C and D). It extended along the mesial aspect of the mesial root and was narrow despite its depth, so there was no bifurcation involvement, but a simple debridement of the relatively straight deep defect. When debridement was completed bleeding was induced in the defects, and surgical gelatin was introduced into the largest ones. The maxillary pack was removed while the blood was clotting, and after the mandibular pack was applied a fresh pack was applied to the maxilla.

On the tenth respective day the cement packs were removed, and the patient was seen twice a week for the next six weeks, during which time the tissue repair progress was distinctly unsatisfactory. By the end of the sixth week the condition of the tissues suggested a systemic factor (Case Fig. 11–4A). The patient also appeared somewhat pallid, and absence of normal blood supply in the lower eyelid and eyegrounds (Case Fig. 11–4B) confirmed the suspicion aroused by the poor healing that, in view of the similarity of clinical symptoms with his wife's condition and the fact that she had had anemia that had responded to treatment, he too might have anemia. He was referred to the hematologist who had treated his wife; the diagnosis of incipient pernicious anemia was confirmed and treatment begun. The response to this treatment was spectacular. About three weeks after the hematology treatment was instituted the tissue repair had progressed to the degree that simple tooth movement with elastic bands and Japanese grassline traction could be instituted (Case Fig. 11–4C). In the maxillary right central-lateral and lateral-cuspid embrasures fragments of bone sequestra appeared where the sharp alveolar edges had been. One week later the sequestered fragments were easily lifted away with a surgical curet under topical

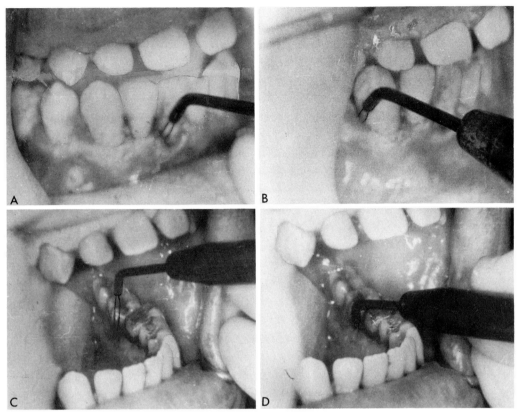

Case Figure 11-3. A, Mandibular gingivectoplasty having been completed, pocket debridement is being performed with the 17-mm. electrode. A pocket along the distal aspect of the left central, approximately 12 mm. deep, is being debrided. B, A 14-mm. pocket at distal of right cuspid is being debrided. C, The 17-mm. electrode is entering a deep pocket along the mesiolingual angle of the left mandibular second molar. The tip of the electrode has penetrated about 2 mm. into the defect. D, The electrode has penetrated approximately 15 mm. into the defect.

anesthesia, and the shallow craters filled with clotted blood. Within two weeks the craters were fully healed, and by the end of the twelfth week the gingivae were normal and healthy, and the infrabony defects were obliterated. The mobile teeth had responded admirably to the simple tooth movement and were in normal alignment (Case Fig. 11-4D). A slender pocket probe was inserted under the free margins to ascertain whether the gingivae had reattached. Pressure with the instrument against the bases of the gingival sulci determined whether the patient was ready for permanent fixation of the teeth. The probe was unable to penetrate beyond the base of the sulcus throughout the mouth. The patient was thereupon referred back to his dentist for insertion of the horizontal nonparallel Whaledent pin splinting that effectively replaced the internal A-splints.

The patient returned for postoperative observation semimonthly, monthly, and then quarterly for two years. Six months after the pin splinting the infrabony defect sites were again examined with a periodontal pocket probe. The probe was inserted under the free margin at the site of the 13 mm. pocket at the distal of the maxillary right central, and pressure was applied to try to penetrate into the defect site. The pressure was sufficient to cause blanching of the tissues (Case Fig. 11-5A). A similar

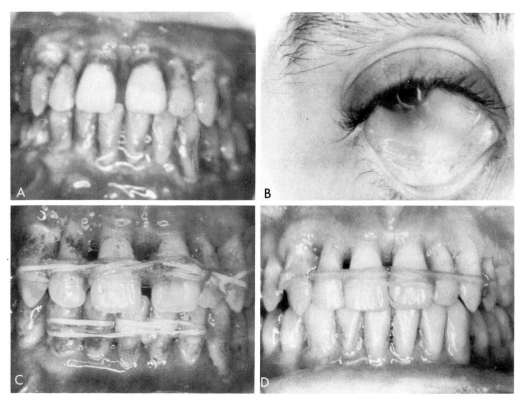

Case Figure 11–4. A, Appearance of the tissues 6 weeks postoperatively. The healing is disappointingly slow and poor. There are several areas in the maxillary right quadrant where there is evidence of excess bone that was not ramped at the time of surgery and is undergoing sequestration (as had been anticipated). *B,* Appearance of the patient's eye, which shows notable absence of normal blood supply in the lower lid and sclera, and strongly suggests the probability of anemia. *C,* Appearance of the tissues several weeks after hematologic therapy for anemia had been instituted. Note the tissues are now showing signs of normal healing as is customarily experienced under normal conditions when no systemic handicap is present. Simple elastic-band Japanese grassline tooth movement has been instituted to try to return the teeth to their normal places in the dental arch. Note the slight bone sequestra present in the maxillary right lateral and cuspid embrasures. *D,* Twelve weeks postoperatively, just before removal of elastic band traction and permanent fixation with a Whaledent pin splint. The tooth movement has restored the teeth into proper alignment in the dental arches. All the diastemas have been eliminated. The gingival tissues are completely healed and normal in color, tone, and contour.

result was obtained from an attempt to penetrate the former site of the infrabony pocket at the mesial of the first bicuspid (Case Fig. 11–5*B*).

Comparison was made between an x-ray of the teeth taken very soon after the permanent pin splint had been inserted (Case Fig. 11–5*C*) and one taken six months after the fixation (Case Fig. 11–5*D*). The latter shows the obliteration of the infrabony defects, and while it is impossible to get regeneration of the circumscribing bone that had been lost, there had been distinct regeneration of the apices of the interseptal bone.

The dentist had failed to cover the external surface of the pins for aesthetic improvement, but the patient was so delighted to have retained all his teeth that he did not mind the pinhead spots of dark color on the teeth.

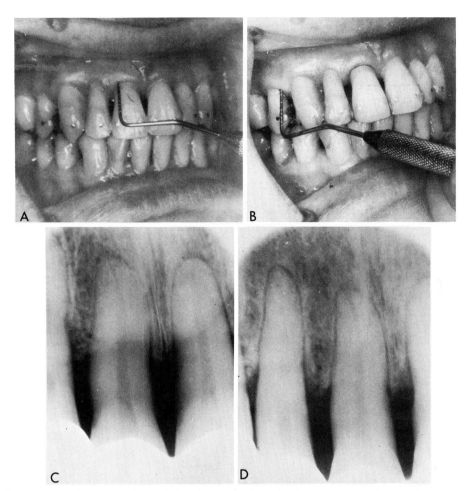

Case Figure 11–5. *A,* Site of infrabony pocket of 13 mm. at maxillary right central be-ing checked with pocket probe, which is unable to penetrate the gingival sulcus despite pressure sufficient to cause marked blanching of the tissue. *B,* The same test is applied to the mesial of the right first bicuspid. Note bleeding from sulcus of central, showing amount of pressure that had been exerted a moment before. *C,* Postoperative x-ray of maxillary an-teriors immediately following Whaledent pin splint fixation. *D,* Similar x-ray, 6 months later. Note evidence of slight bone regeneration at the tips of the interseptal bone.

CASE 12

This is the last of the three cases being reviewed as a series of unusual clinical features similar enough to suggest a syndrome.

The extent of alveolar destruction in this case was much less than had occurred in the two preceding cases, since definitive treatment was instituted at a much earlier stage of the disease. The gingival healing, however, was almost as troublesome as in the case that has just been reviewed, until the hematologic factor was eliminated. Prior to the normalization of his systemic condition, the gingivae, especially the inter-dental papillae, continued to proliferate despite continuous postoperative treatment and conscientious home care by the patient. Soon after the hematology medication was initiated, the proliferative tendency began to abate and was no longer in evi-

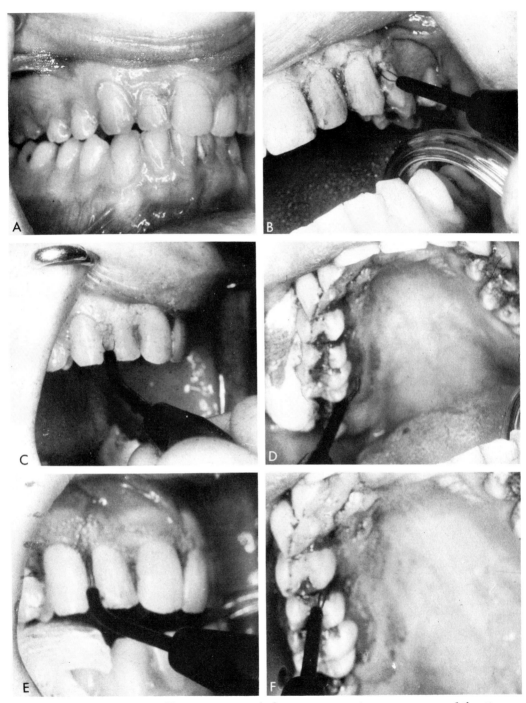

Case Figure 12–1. A, Close-up preprophylactic preoperative appearance of the tissues and teeth. The latter are covered with deposits of plaque and the enamel is stained (probably because of a carbohydrate-rich diet and poor oral hygiene). The gingival tissue surface is smooth and shiny and lacks the stippled evidence of keratinized epithelium. The tissue tone is very poor and the atonal tissues are hyperplastic. B, A flame-shaped loop electrode is being used with a downward wiping motion to resect some of the hyperplastic papillae by electro-section and thus recontour the tissues to create concave self-cleansing sluiceways in the embrasures. C, The gingivoplasty and reduction of bulbous papillae is being repeated in the dence by the time the anemia was cured. The time sequence of the improvement in tissue healing paralleled that of the elimination of the systemic factor.

PATIENT.   A 22-year-old white male.

HISTORY.   The patient was a sophomore medical student and had been living for the past year at a school dormitory and eating at the school cafeteria. A review of his typical daily diet revealed a marked dietary imbalance. His meals consisted mostly of carbohydrates, with few protein foods and even fewer fresh vegetables or fruits. Approximately six months earlier he began to notice bleeding from the gingivae during toothbrushing and occasionally while eating. He consulted his family dentist, and the latter referred him to the author for diagnosis and definitive treatment.

CLINICAL EXAMINATION.   He had a full complement of teeth, all fully erupted, but many were tilted palatally and lingually. The upper right lateral and the right bicuspids in both the upper and lower arches were tilted medially to a much greater degree than the left upper lateral and slightly more than the bicuspids (Case Fig. 12–1A).

The gingival mucosa appeared smooth, shiny, and apparently devoid of a normal keratinized tissue surface. Despite the obvious atonal condition of the alveolar gingivae they were rather pallid in color, in contrast to the usual dark red engorged appearance of atonal tissue. Only the apices of some of the interdental papillae, particularly on either side of the maxillary right lateral, appeared to be engorged.

TREATMENT.   Because of the innocuous appearance of the tissues and absence of extensive alveolar destruction and deep infrabony pocket defects, the condition was attributed primarily to a dietary deficiency, and a high protein diet plus ascorbic acid and mineral intake was prescribed before treatment was instituted. The maxillary left quadrant was treated first, under posterior superior alveolar and infraorbital blocks and anterior palatine and nasopalatine blocks. The flame-shaped electrode was selected, current output was set at 5, and the activated electrode was used with light wiping and brushing strokes to perform the gingivoplasty, starting with reduction of the redundant interdental papillae (Case Fig. 12–1A to F). The gingivoplasty of the maxillary left quadrant having been completed, tincture of myrrh and benzoin was applied to the surgical fields. The mandibular left quadrant was then anesthetized and treated in a similar manner (Case Fig. 12–2A). Several of the teeth had infrabony pockets 4 to 6 mm. in depth. These were debrided with the 17-mm. electronic periodontal curet electrodes. When the surgery was completed, tincture of myrrh and benzoin was applied, and periodontal cement packs were applied to both quadrants. The packs were removed on the fifth postoperative day, and the surgery of the right quadrants was performed under similar anesthesia. The flame-shaped and medium U-shaped loop electrodes again were used to perform the gingivoplasty (Case Fig. 12–2A to C); the 17-mm. periodontal loop electrode was then used to debride the infrabony pockets, some of them, in the maxillary right quadrant, 6 to 8 mm. in depth. When the gingivoplasty-infrabony pocket debridement was completed, tincture of

---

Case Figure 12–1   Continued.

maxillary right quadrant. Note how well suited the flame-shaped electrode fits into the interproximal embrasures. D, The labial-buccal gingivoplasty has been completed. The palatal gingivoplasty is being performed with the flame-shaped loop electrode. Note the facility with which areas usually relatively inaccessible to rigid steel instrumentation are accessible to treatment with the slender flexible electrodes. E, The gingivoplasty having been completed in the maxilla, a 17-mm. periodontal loop electrode is used to debride the buccal infrabony pockets. The electrode, used with up-down and rotary motions, is seen debriding a 9-mm. pocket along the distal surface of the root of the right lateral. F, The electrode is being used with equal facility to debride a deeper infrabony pocket on the palatal aspect.

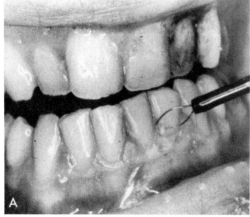
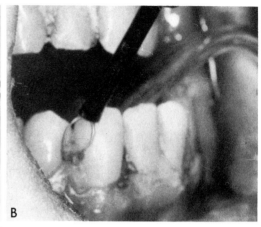
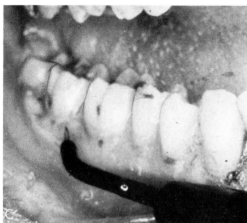

Case Figure 12–2. A, The gingivoplasty of the labial-buccal aspect of the mandible is being performed with a flame-shaped loop electrode. Note how the tissue is recontoured to a feather edge as the gingivoplasty is being performed. B, The same loop is being used to reduce the hyperplastic papilla and thus create the concave self-cleansing sluiceway in the embrasure. C, A 45-degree-angle medium-width U-shaped loop is being used to perform the gingivoplasty in the posterior buccal region by shaving the tissue in thin layers. This loop is also excellent for performing the gingivoplasty on the lingual aspect.

myrrh and benzoin was applied, and primary cement packs were applied to these quadrants and second packs applied to the left quadrants.

Healing progress was disappointingly atypical. The rate as well as the quality of the tissue repair was very slow and was characterized by a marked amount of proliferation (Case Fig. 12–3A to C). At this point, the author noted the similarity to the clinical symptoms and tissue response in the preceding case, before treatment for the anemia had been instituted; the patient was therefore referred to a hematologist. A mild anemia was diagnosed and treated. Healing began to improve as the hematologist's treatment progressed (Case Fig. 12–3D). About one month later the tissues were almost fully healed and beginning to show the characteristic stippled, orange-skin textured appearance of normal healthy attached gingivae (Case Fig. 12–3E). The hematologist discharged the patient as cured of the anemia after ten weeks of active therapy. Two weeks later, the gingivae now being in a normal healthy state throughout

---

Case Figure 12–3 Continued.
stained the teeth, but the stain will come off readily when a prophylaxis is performed. E, Appearance of the gingivae one month later. The tissue tone is greatly improved and the attached gingivae are beginning to assume a normal stippled appearance. F, Final postoperative appearance of the tissues. The hematologist has discontinued the medication and considers the patient cured of his anemia. The gingival tissues are now completely normal in all respects; the tone and color are excellent, and the zones of maturely keratinized attached gingivae are clearly defined.

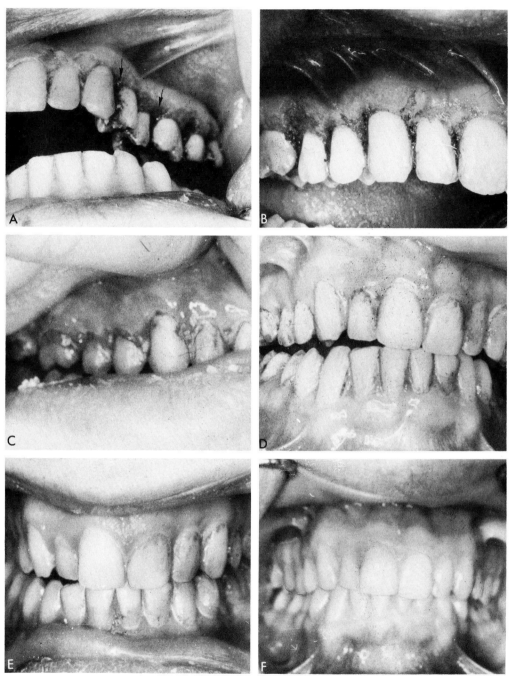

Case Figure 12–3. A, Immediate postsurgical appearance of the tissues in the maxillary left quadrant. Note the absence of free bleeding throughout the procedure. The tissue in this quadrant was easily resected and the tissue cleavage was clean-cut and precise. B, Immediate postsurgical appearance of the tissues in the maxillary right quadrant. This tissue had a rubbery consistency and could not be resected cleanly and precisely, since the tissue tended to shred, despite use of the proper amount of cutting current. C, Appearance of the tissue in this quadrant one week after the second cement pack was removed. The regenerating tissue is very friable and proliferative. D, Appearance of the gingivae soon after hematologic therapy was instituted. The proliferative tendency has ceased and the hyperplastic appearance of the tissues appears to be improving. Repeated applications of tincture of myrrh and benzoin have

(*Legend continued on p. 644*)

the mouth (Case Fig. 12–3F), he was discharged from active periodontal treatment. Although there had been no clinically discernible difference or demarcation between the appearance of the attached or alveolar gingivae and the areolar gingivae at the outset of treatment, there was now distinct visual evidence in both jaws of well-defined and differentiated zones of maturely keratinized attached gingivae that were readily distinguishable from the areolar gingivae. Significantly, no healing progress was achieved until the systemic health of the patient was restored.

Periodontia Related to Hormonal Influences

The term "periodontal disease" all too often evokes a mental image of a clinical picture of marked gingival engorgement or edema, hyperplasia, detached interdental papillae, exposed denuded roots, and pathologically migrated mobile teeth.

This mental image is particularly compatible with the clinical conditions in the type of case described by Gottlieb as "schmutzpyorrhea" (Fig. 19–1).[1] However, it is by no means typical. On casual inspection many cases of advanced periodontal disease present a deceptively innocuous appearance. The actual degree and extensiveness of periodontal deterioration in such cases does not become apparent until a thorough examination is performed with periodontal pocket probes and roentgenographic visualization.

The following case falls into this category. Throughout the mouth, with the exception of two localized areas, the gingival mucosa appeared normal in color and tone, but thorough examination revealed extensive periodontal disease with infrabony pockets throughout the mouth ranging from 3 to 12 mm. in depth.

In another respect, however, this case falls into a distinctly unique category. The author has from time to time encountered cases in which female patients who require periodontal therapy initially respond very favorably to treatment. Subsequently, however, starting a few days before each menstrual period, gingivae become engorged and somewhat atonal and tend to bleed during toothbrushing. This state persists until the menstrual period is terminated, whereupon the condition undergoes spontaneous regression and the gingivae return, without special treatment, to normal appearance and tone. This manifestation of periodic temporary hormonal imbalance was encountered in the case to be discussed (See Figure 19–3.)

This case also demonstrates the usefulness of transillumination in the debridement of infrabony pockets, a factor that is greatly enhanced by the absence of the hemorrhagic free bleeding characteristically encountered with "conventional" steel scalpel and periodontal curet instrumentation.

The next two cases demonstrate respectively the transitory influence of hormonal deficiency during the menstrual cycle and the more permanent influence of hormonal deficiency during the menopause.

In the first patient the gingival tone deteriorated for several days during each menstrual cycle and then returned to normal spontaneously after it was

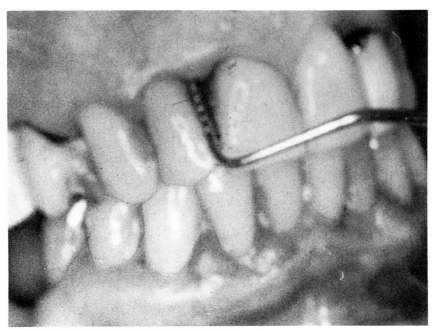

Figure 19–3. Periodontoclasia associated with menopausal estrogen deficiency. The condition of the gingivae around the maxillary fixed bridge is better than that around the mandibular natural dentition, indicating that the marked tissue deterioration and proliferation is not iatrogenic in origin. This type of condition usually responds favorably to estrogen therapy. If the hormonal imbalance is not corrected by administration of estrogens, the periodontoclasia usually does not respond optimally to periodontal therapy.

over. In the patient affected by hormonal imbalance during the menopause, the tissue tone was improved enormously after the periodontal surgery, and the infrabony pockets were successfully obliterated, but the gingival tone was not as good as it should have been in view of the favorable results of the surgery and the patient's conscientious oral physiotherapy. After the patient was discharged from postoperative observation she was placed on estrogen therapy and the gingival tone improved appreciably.

CASE 13

PATIENT.   A 34-year-old white female.

HISTORY.   Two years previously a space suddenly developed in the anterior part of her upper jaw. She was referred to a periodontist and treatment, consisting of manual curettage, was instituted. Instead of improving, however, the space gradually increased, and a few months after active treatment was completed she noted pus oozing from the open area. Despite renewed treatment, the purulent exudation persisted. A few weeks ago she suddenly became aware of a large swelling on the right side of her palate and an unpleasant sweet taste. She thereupon requested that her dentist refer her elsewhere for further diagnosis and treatment.

CLINICAL EXAMINATION.   The oral hygiene of her mouth was excellent. The

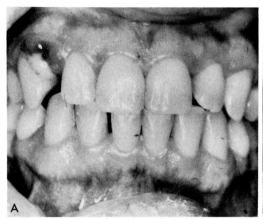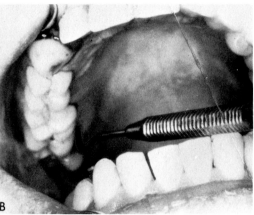

Case Figure 13–1. A, Preoperative view. Except for the marked deterioration of the gingival tissue in the diastema between the maxillary right lateral incisor and cuspid, and the large amount of purulent exudate exuding from the mesial aspect of the cuspid, the remaining gingivae appear deceptively normal. There is no notable hyperplasia, hyperemia, or recession, but the tissues are very atonal. B, There is a very large swelling on the palatal aspect over the maxillary right second molar. A periodontal pocket probe has advanced upward toward the apices of the tooth without encountering resistance.

maxillary right cuspid was rotated distobuccally, leaving a wide diastema between the lateral and cuspid. A globule of pus was present on the mesial aspect of the cuspid, and the marginal and alveolar gingivae between the two teeth were swollen, engorged, and ulcerated along the marginal edge. There was also a round fluctuant bulge on the palate over the right maxillary second molar. The gingivae throughout the remainder of the mouth appeared normal in color and tone, and there was a broad band of attached gingiva present (Case Fig. 13–1A).

A flat periodontal pocket probe was used to probe for infrabony pockets. Pockets were found throughout the mouth, ranging in depth from about 3 mm. in the lower anterior region to 12 mm. in the posterior areas. Upon insertion along the mesial aspect of the right cuspid the probe penetrated 8 mm. Upon insertion into the palatal fluctuant defect along the palatal root of the right second molar the probe penetrated its full length, without encountering any resistance (Case Fig. 13–1B).

ROENTGENOGRAPHIC EXAMINATION. X-rays confirmed the presence of the infrabony pockets. A sterile endodontic silver point was inserted into the second molar palatal defect and an x-ray film taken with the point in place as a radiopaque pocket marker. The film showed that the destruction involved the distobuccal as well as the palatal root, and that the destruction penetrated at one point beyond the level of the apex of the tooth.

TREATMENT. Before surgery was instituted all the essential preoperative preparation was concluded. This consisted of meticulous elimination of all occlusal prematurities, especially on the right cuspid, and thorough patient instruction in proper toothbrushing and other massaging so essential for postoperative oral physiotherapy. The day before surgery a thorough prophylaxis was performed, and root planing of the denuded roots to eliminate the dead cementum was performed by hand instrumentation. Smears for an agar plate and broth culture were obtained and a sensitivity test was requested. The tests, performed by the bacteriology laboratory of the Mt. Sinai Hospital in New York, revealed growths of *N. catarrhalis* and *S. viridans.* Erythrocin, 250 mg. every 6 hours for five days, was prescribed as the drug of choice.

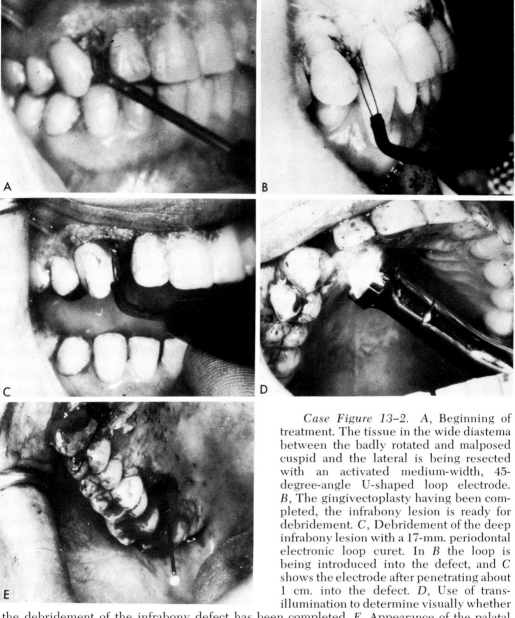

Case Figure 13-2. A, Beginning of treatment. The tissue in the wide diastema between the badly rotated and malposed cuspid and the lateral is being resected with an activated medium-width, 45-degree-angle U-shaped loop electrode. *B*, The gingivectoplasty having been completed, the infrabony lesion is ready for debridement. *C*, Debridement of the deep infrabony lesion with a 17-mm. periodontal electronic loop curet. In *B* the loop is being introduced into the defect, and *C* shows the electrode after penetrating about 1 cm. into the defect. *D*, Use of transillumination to determine visually whether the debridement of the infrabony defect has been completed. *E*, Appearance of the palatal lesion in the second molar area after the gingivoplasty has been performed in the maxillary right quadrant. A sterile silver point has been inserted into the defect to serve as a radiopaque marker on the intraoral periapical x-ray film that will be taken.

The antibiotic was then discontinued until the fourth preoperative day, at which time it was resumed and continued for four days postoperatively. The purulent exudation continued to persist, however, despite medication up until the time of surgery.

The involvement was too extensive to be treated in one session. The greatest amount of destruction being present on the right side, the right maxillary and mandibular quadrants were treated at the first surgical session.

First the maxillary tissues were prepared, and infraorbital and posterior superior

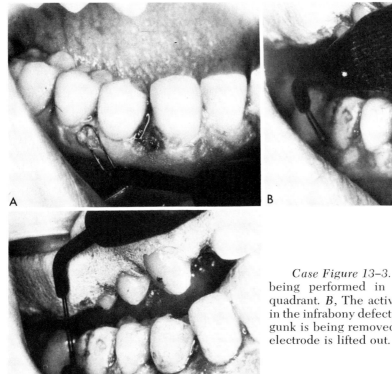

Case Figure 13–3. A, The gingivoplasty being performed in the mandibular right quadrant. B, The activated electrode is deep in the infrabony defect. C, The granulomatous gunk is being removed from the defect as the electrode is lifted out.

alveolar and palatine block anesthesia was administered. A 45-degree-angle loop electrode of medium width was selected for the initial gingivoplasty in the lateral-cuspid embrasure, cutting current was set at 6 owing to the engorgement, and the gingivoplasty was performed with short wiping strokes repeated at 10-second intervals (Case Fig. 13–2). The author's 17-mm., 45-degree-angle vertical loop electronic curet electrode was substituted and used to debride the large infrabony defect. The transilluminating light directed through the defect helped greatly to reveal remnants of debris that had to be removed. A few fragments that adhered tenaciously to the internal aspect of the labial gingiva were resected easily with the 17-mm. horizontal loop electronic curet electrode. When debridement was complete, bleeding was induced in the defect with a periodontal curet, powdered surgical gelatin was introduced, and the mixture of gelatin and blood was permitted to fill the defect and clot.

The remainder of the maxillary right gingival mucosa was treated in a similar manner. First the gingivoplasty was performed, followed by infrabony pocket debridement. After the palatal defect at the second molar was debrided, another sterile silver endodontic silver point was inserted and used as a pocket marker for x-ray visualization and transillumination. Powdered gelatin was also introduced into this defect and mixed with blood in it. Upon completion of the maxillary instrumentation, tincture of myrrh and benzoin was applied in air-dried layers, and a periodontal cement pack, consisting of the formula in this text, was mixed to as stiff a consistency as possible and was applied with care to avoid displacing the blood clots from the infrabony defects.

Inferior alveolar-lingual anesthesia was then administered, and identical surgery was instituted for the mandibular structures (Case Fig. 13–3), again using the medium-width, 45-degree-angle loop electrode for the gingivoplasty and the 45-degree-angle, 17-mm. loop electronic curet for the pocket debridement, assisted by transillumination to help determine completion of the necessary debridement. A similar cement pack was then applied to the mandibular surgical field, and the patient was instructed to return on the fifth postoperative day for surgery of the left quadrants.

When she returned on the fifth day, the patient reported a virtually total absence of pain, with only minimal discomfort which she felt was due more to the cement packs than to the surgery.

The left maxillary and mandibular tissues were anesthetized and treatment identical to that for the right side of the mouth was instituted. Cement packs were applied. The primary cement packs were then removed from the right side, the tissues were irrigated, and Peripak was applied as the secondary packing.

On the tenth day the secondary packs were removed and the tissues were found to be healing very favorably. Thereafter the patient was seen postoperatively at weekly intervals. By the end of the third month the tissue healing appeared complete

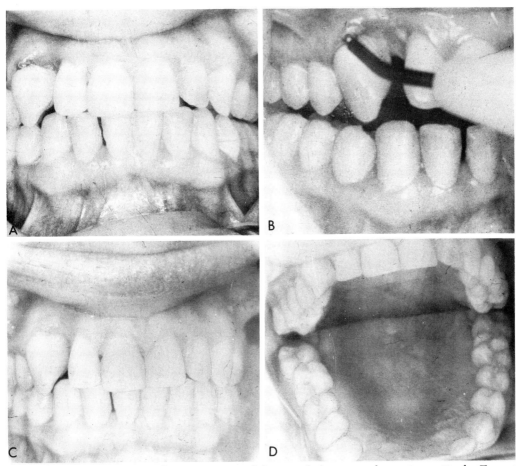

Case Figure 13–4. *A*, The appearance of the mouth three months postoperatively. Except for a slight proliferation along the edge of the marginal gingiva on the mesial aspect of the rotated cuspid, the tissues are fully healed, and the infrabony lesions appear to have been successfully obliterated. *B*, Superficial spot coagulation is performed to control the proliferation. *C*, The tooth is firm and totally asymptomatic, and the tissue is normal and firmly reattached. *D*, The palatal tissue has healed favorably.

and favorable except in the right lateral-cuspid embrasure, where the marginal edge of the repair tissue appeared slightly edematous, engorged, and proliferative. Superficial spot coagulation was performed to control the proliferative tendency. This succeeded in stopping the proliferation and greatly improved the tissue tone. The palatal tissue around the second molar was completely healed and tightly adherent to the tooth (Case Fig. 13–4). The patient has maintained a conscientious regimen of vigorous oral physiotherapy, and the gingival tissues have remained healthy.

This next and final case of this series presented an interesting contrast to the previous case in one respect. In the previous case, despite an almost total absence of clinically visible denuded roots, the teeth were very mobile and required temporary immobilization during the postoperative repair period. In this case, there was tangible clinical evidence of extensive bone loss, since 3 to 6 mm. of the roots of many teeth in both jaws were denuded of bone and gingivae and clinically exposed. Moreover, roentgenographic examination confirmed extensive horizontal alveolar resorption combined with vertical bone loss in deep infrabony pockets and multiple furca involvements. Nevertheless, the teeth were only moderately mobile, and there were only minor diastemas and no pathologic migrations. As a result, in this case neither temporary nor permanent splint fixation was required.

CASE 14

PATIENT. A 44-year-old white female.
HISTORY
Dental. For the past four years she had noted a progressive gingival recession and exposure of the roots and many of her teeth. The recession had begun in the maxillary and mandibular cuspid regions and the greatest amount of recession was present at those four sites. During the past year she had noted that her gums felt soggy and often bled during toothbrushing and, most recently, that the tissues over the maxillary left lateral incisor and mandibular right lateral incisor looked purplish red and swollen. She consulted her dentist, was referred for periodontal therapy, and was told that many of her teeth were hopelessly denuded of bone and would have to be extracted. She rejected this treatment plan, requesting another opinion, and was referred to the author.
Medical. Electrocardiograms showed nonspecific T-wave changes indicative of heart disease.
CLINICAL EXAMINATION. Upon casual inspection the tissues appeared normal in dimension and color except in the maxillary left lateral incisor and mandibular right lateral incisor labial areas. Careful examination revealed that the tissues were somewhat atonal, smooth and shiny, and devoid of the normal stippled orange-skin appearance of normal firm healthy gingival mucosa. Probing with a periodontal pocket probe revealed many deep infrabony pockets and furca involvements. The roots of most of the teeth were denuded of several millimeters of investing bone and tissue on their labial aspects and were clinically exposed (Case Fig. 14–1). X-rays revealed extensive horizontal bone resorption.
TREATMENT. The normal preliminary preparation of the patient was performed, consisting of elimination of traumatizing prematurities, instruction in proper postoperative maintenance of oral physiotherapy and dietary supplements, and prophy-

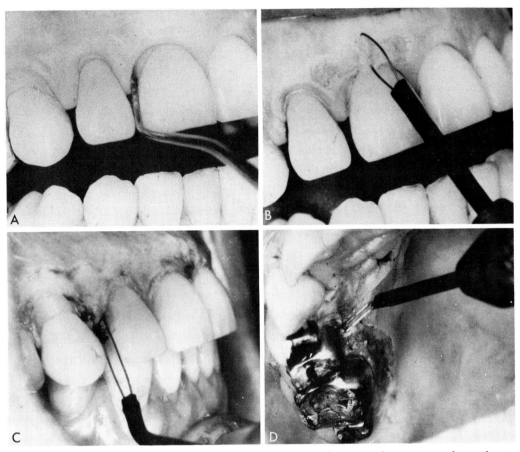

Case Figure 14–1. This figure demonstrates the technique of gingivectoplasty that is particularly useful where horizontal circumscribing alveolar resorption dictates need for resection of the detached unsupported gingival tissues and simultaneous recontouring of the remainder of the tissues as the resection is being performed, thereby creating immediately a normal gingival architecture.

A, A slight amount of gingival recession has occurred; most notably on the labial aspects of the maxillary cuspids. A round periodontal pocket probe has been inserted to measure the depth of the pocket at the distal aspect of the maxillary right central. The thickness of this probe allowed it to penetrate only 6 mm., but subsequent instrumentation proved the actual depth to be 9 mm. *B,* A long slender flame-shaped loop electrode is being used to perform the maxillary labial gingivectoplasty. *C,* The gingivectoplasty portion of the procedure having been completed, the individual infrabony pocket debridement is being performed with a 17-mm. periodontal loop electrode that serves as an electronic curet. The loop being used to resect the epithelial lining of the defect is the hoe-shaped type that is designed especially for this purpose. *D,* The gingivectoplasty is being performed on the palatal aspect with a 45-degree-angle medium-width U-shaped loop electrode that provides ready access to the palatal gingivae, particularly in the posterior areas.

laxis and root planing to remove dead cementum. Bilateral posterior superior alveolar, infraorbital, posterior palatine, and nasopalatine block anesthesia was administered.

A flame-shaped loop electrode was selected, cutting current was set at 4.5 on the power output rheostat, and the electrode was used with short wiping strokes to perform a gingivoplasty. In many areas this consisted of little more than skimming off the surface epithelium from the tissues; in other areas, unattached mucosa was partially resected and simultaneously recontoured to normal architecture. The electrode was

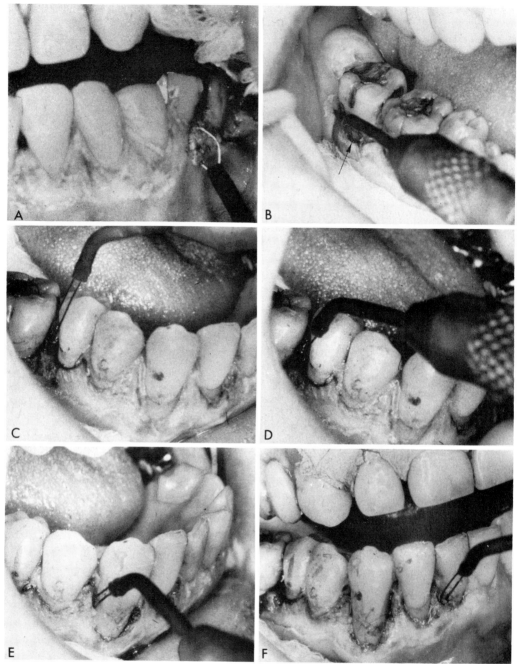

Case Figure 14–2. *A,* The flame-shaped loop electrode is being used to perform the gingivectoplasty on the labial mandibular gingivae. *B,* An infrabony pocket extending into the bifurcation of the right second molar is being debrided with a 17-mm. 90-degree-angle periodontal loop electrode. This electrde provides access to the furcas of the molar teeth; it has penetrated about 13 mm. into the defect. *C,* A hatchet-shaped 45-degree-angle periodontal loop electrode is being introduced into an infrabony pocket on the mesial surface of the mesial root of the first molar. *D,* The electrode has penetrated approximately 12 mm. and has reached the base of the defect. During the fraction of a second that the activated electrode has been in the defect it has been used with an up-and-down and rotary motion as an electronic curet. *E,* The same electrode is being used to debride a pocket along the distal surface of the right cuspid root. This defect is about 12 mm. deep. *F,* All the teeth have pockets along one or more surfaces of the roots. The electrode is seen debriding a 10 mm. pocket at the distal of the right central.

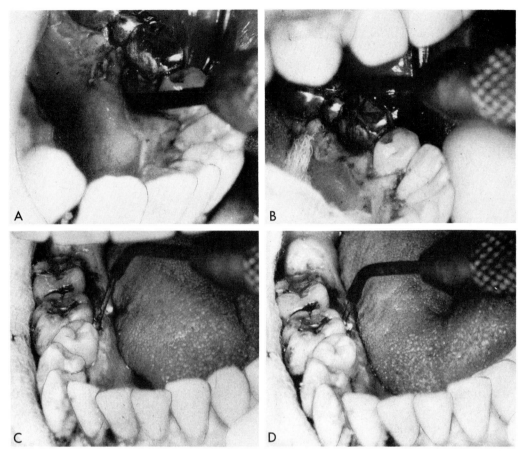

Case Figure 14–3. A, A gingivectoplasty of the mandibular lingual gingivae is being performed with an oval-shaped 90-degree-angle loop electrode which provides favorable access, particularly to the posterior lingual tissues that are difficult to reach using other methods of instrumentation. *B,* The 17-mm. 90-degree-angle periodontal loop electrode is being used to debride a pocket into the lingual furca of the left first molar. *C,* The 17-mm. 45-degree-angle periodontal loop electrode is being used to debride an infrabony pocket along the mesio-lingual aspect of the mesial root of the right first molar. The electrode has penetrated about 2 or 3 mm. into the defect. *D,* The electrode has penetrated about 12 mm. to the base of the defect.

then replaced with a medium-width, 45-degree-angle U-shaped loop electrode, and current output was set at 5.5 on the rheostat dial. The activated electrode was then used to perform the gingivoplasty on the palatal aspect (Case Fig. 14–1).

A 17-mm. electronic periodontal curet loop electrode was then substituted, cutting current was reduced to 4, and this electrode was used with up and down rotary strokes to debride the infrabony pockets. The electrode was in contact with the structures forming the infrabony pocket for only a fraction of a second at a time, with a 10-second rest interval before resuming the debridement. When all the maxillary pockets had been thoroughly debrided, bleeding was induced in the infrabony defects, and after the blood had clotted, the entire surgical field was painted with tincture of myrrh and benzoin in air-dried layers.* A very stiff mix of the periodontal pack formula was prepared and applied, care being taken to avoid displacing the blood clots from the infrabony pockets.

---

*The pharmacist had substituted compound tincture of benzoin for the tincture of benzoin, and the compound, being much darker in color, stained the teeth dark brown.

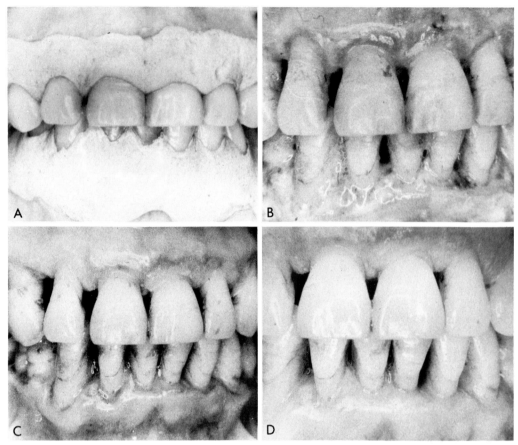

Case Figure 14–4.   *A,* Appearance of the cement packs; the second pack in the maxilla and the primary pack in the mandible. *B,* Postoperative appearance of the gingival tissues one week after the second cement pack was removed from the mandible. Note the healing progress; it is notably more advanced in the maxilla, which had been treated five days before the mandibular tissues. *C,* Healing progress; appearance of the tissues two weeks later. *D,* Appearance of the tissues ten weeks postoperatively. The healing is complete, and the tissue tone is excellent. Despite the exposure of considerable amounts of denuded roots each tooth has a normal gingival sulcus approximately 1 mm. deep, and an appreciable part of the interdental papillae has been preserved, reducing the aesthetic disharmony caused by the root exposures. The infrabony pockets have been obliterated, and the defects are filled with regenerated bone.

When the patient returned on the fifth postoperative day a patch of the pack was found to have broken away, exposing the tissues in the area. The tissue appeared to be healing satisfactorily previously. Bilateral inferior alveolar-lingual block anesthesia was administered, and the 45-degree-angle medium-width U-shaped loop was used with cutting current set at 4 to perform the gingivoplasty on the mandibular gingivae (Case Fig. 14–2).

The 17-mm. curet electrode was then used to debride the bifurcations and the infrabony pockets, many of which were 14 to 15 mm. deep. The 17-mm. curet electrode with the loop in the horizontal plane was used very effectively to perform resection of the internal portion of the soft tissue part of the pockets comparable to the internal bevel performed with the split mucosal flap procedures. When debridement was completed and blood clots were induced, tincture of myrrh and benzoin was applied, and the cement packs were applied to both upper and lower jaws. To avoid trauma to the healing tissues in the maxilla, Peripack was substituted for the regular pack. Postoperative healing was gradual but uneventful. New bone filled the infrabony defects without immobilization. The new marginal gingivae regenerated 1 to 2 mm. toward their original level, creating normal gingival sulci. The tissue tone was good and the maturation of the repairing surface tissue was almost complete three weeks after the cement packs had been discarded. The teeth were remarkably firm and did not require any fixation. There was, however, not much more improvement in the clinical appearance of the external gingival tissue surface, which failed to measure up fully to the usual quality of tissue repair despite the patient's conscientious efforts at oral physiotherapy. Almost a year after active treatment was discontinued, the patient's gynecologist prescribed estrogen hormone therapy and the quality of the tissue tone gradually improved. A particularly intriguing feature of this case was the contrast in the rate and quality of bone regeneration (Case Fig. 14–4D), which was excellent even before hormone therapy was begun.

Periodontia in Relation to Nonspecific Systemic Factors

Periodontoclasia related to nonspecific systemic factors often is characterized by marked horizontal circumscribing alveolar resorption. When the resorption exceeds half the length of the roots, this creates a reversal of the normal 1:2 crown-root ratio. The result is an abnormal torque that makes it impossible for the dentition to withstand the normal functional stresses, making it necessary to immobilize the teeth permanently so that they will be able to function normally, as was seen in Case 11 of this chapter.

When less than half the length of the roots become denuded by the horizontal alveolar resorption and no further collateral bone loss is incurred, the teeth are likely to remain reasonably firm. But when in addition to the horizontal bone loss there is also collateral bone loss from development of vertical infrabony pockets, the teeth usually do become quite mobile. The vertical bone loss permits the teeth to tilt, thereby creating pathologic migrations, particularly when there has also been a loss of normal tooth contacts.

Despite the fact that hypermobility of the dentition and pathologic migration are likely sequelae in these cases, there is no need for permanent immobilization of the teeth if the end result of treatment is obliteration of the infrabony defects through regeneration of the lost bone. Temporary immobilization during the postoperative repair period is essential, however, to permit the new bone to undergo normal maturation and calcification (Fig. 19–4). The specific techniques described in Chapter 18 fulfill this function efficiently.

If pathologic migration has occurred, it is necessary to institute tooth movement to restore the teeth to normal alignment in the dental arches before the temporary splinting is applied. Simple tooth movement to achieve the realignment can be accomplished efficiently and effectively through use of gradual traction applied with elastic bands and Japanese grassline.

CASE 15

This case is somewhat unusual in one respect. Whereas diastemas are often due to pathologic migration resulting from loss of alveolar bone support, in this case, despite considerable horizontal circumscribing bone loss and deep vertical infrabony pockets, the diastemas are unrelated to the advanced periodontal deterioration, since the patient related that she had had the spaces between her teeth all her life. It also demonstrates well a method of temporary splinting devised by the author that is easy to apply, highly efficient, and can be retained as long as necessary without replacement and without risk of damage to the teeth to which it has been attached (Fig. 19–4).

PATIENT.   A 39-year-old white female.

HISTORY.   Essentially negative. Several months previously she had begun to notice that the roots of her upper teeth were exposed but had done nothing about it until several sore spots developed, especially the lower right lateral and bicuspid areas, and the upper left lateral appeared to be getting loose. She consulted her dentist and after an x-ray examination was told she would have to have extensive periodontal treatment or extraction of many of her teeth. She was referred for periodontal consultation and was told she would have to have most of the posterior teeth and the left lateral extracted. She refused to have the teeth extracted and was referred to the author for possible electrosurgical periodontal therapy.

The patient was told very explicitly that the prognosis was uncertain for many of the teeth, owing to the extensive bone loss, but that many cases that had presented comparable or worse prognosis had responded in almost every instance to electrosurgical management of the condition, and that on the basis of past experience it appeared worthwhile to try to treat the apparently hopeless teeth, with their extraction as a last resort if they failed to respond to treatment.

CLINICAL EXAMINATION.   Dentition was complete except for the four third molars which were missing. There were diastemas between the maxillary centrals

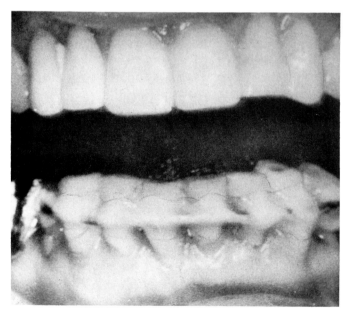

Figure 19–4.   A stainless steel bar, bent to adapt closely to the curvature of the dental arch, has been attached to the teeth with cold-cure acrylic in semi-liquid state applied to the bar and teeth by the Neilon technique. This arch bar fixation firmly immobilizes the teeth without causing any damage to the enamel. It remains firmly attached until time for its removal. This is accomplished by simply prying it away from the labial surface of the teeth with hand instrumentation. Unless mobile teeth are firmly immobilized during the period of bone regeneration to permit normal calcification, the latter will not occur; instead, repair will be by fibrous malunion identical to that resulting from improper or inadequate immobilization of a fractured long bone.

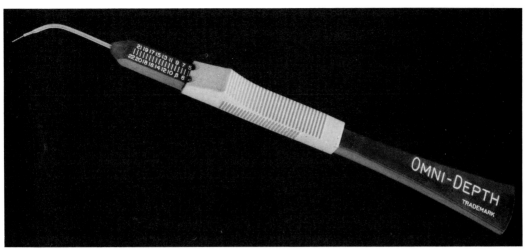

Figure 19–5. Whaledent Omni-Depth instrument for accurately measuring periodontal pockets.

and the right lateral and cuspid, and between the mandibular right central and lateral, lateral and cuspid, and cuspid and first bicuspid. The gingival tissues were normal in contour but atonal, with no well-defined zone of attached gingivae. The marginal gingiva over the maxillary left lateral was purplish red in color and extended over to the mesial half of the cuspid. There was also a purplish red discoloration of the marginal gingiva around the mandibular centrals and laterals, and the marginal edge of the gingiva of the right lateral was ulcerated. A smaller ulceration was also present at the marginal edge of the gingiva of the right first bicuspid. On digital palpation the maxillary left lateral presented class II mobility, and the mandibular four incisors class I mobility. The molars also gave class I mobility. From the x-ray evidence of bone loss the teeth proved firmer than anticipated. Examination confirmed the presence of many deep vertical infrabony pockets in addition to the horizontal bone loss. A sterile Whaledent Omni-Depth instrument, marked off at 1-mm. intervals and used to determine the depth of holes for insertion of pins, was substituted for the periodontal pocket probe (Fig. 19–5) and provided accurate measurement of the pocket. In this case, the instrument penetrated to a depth of 15 mm. before meeting resistance.

TREATMENT. The maxilla was prepared and anesthetized with bilateral posterior superior alveolar, infraorbital, anterior palatine, and nasopalatine regional block injections after the occlusion had been checked to eliminate traumatizing prematurities, and a thorough prophylaxis had been performed and the patient had received preoperative instructions in oral physiotherapy and postoperative home care and diet.

A medium-width, 45-degree-angle U-shaped loop electrode was selected and cutting current output on a Coles Radiosurg unit was set at 4.5 on the instrument panel power output rheostat. The activated electrode was used with a light brushing stroke to resect the detached unsupported gingival tissue beyond the receded bone (Case Fig. 15–1). This revealed 3 to 6 mm. of denuded root surfaces that had been planed.

When the gingivectoplasty was completed on the labial-buccal aspect it was continued on the palatal aspect with a slightly more rounded loop electrode which gave better planing contact in the posterior region. When the tissue planing was completed this electrode was discarded and replaced with a 17-mm. periodontal electronic loop

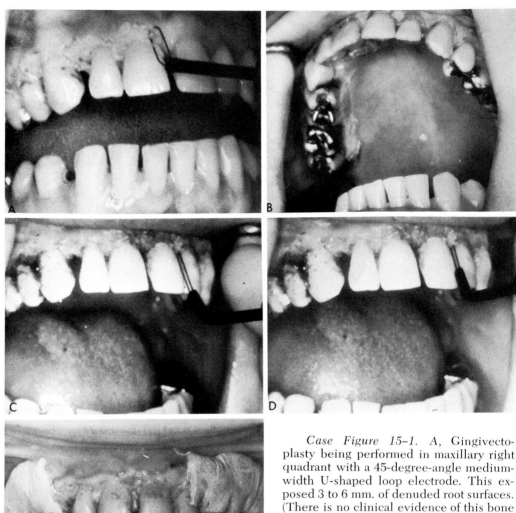

Case Figure 15–1. A, Gingivecto-plasty being performed in maxillary right quadrant with a 45-degree-angle medium-width U-shaped loop electrode. This exposed 3 to 6 mm. of denuded root surfaces. (There is no clinical evidence of this bone loss until the tissue is removed.) B, Gingivectoplasty being performed on the palatal aspect with a flame-shaped loop electrode. Even in the area of the tuberosity the visibility and access for treatment are excellent. C, Gingivectoplasty having been completed on the labial-buccal aspects of the maxilla, individual infrabony pockets are being debrided with a 17-mm. periodontal electronic curet electrode. The electrode is seen being inserted into the defect at the distal of the left central and has penetrated approximately 4 mm. D, The electrode has penetrated to the base of the pocket and is being used with an up and down, rotary motion to make contact momentarily with all the internal surfaces of the defect. The electrode has penetrated approximately 11 mm. into the pocket. E, Appearance of the tissues on fifth postoperative day, as the first cement pack is being removed. The tissue tone is excellent and the surface of the healing tissue is covered with a thin film of coagulum.

curet electrode (vertical plane type) and current output was decreased to 4. The activated electrode was used to debride the vertical infrabony pockets.

When all the infrabony pockets had been debrided, bleeding was induced in the defects, and once the blood had clotted, a periodontal cement pack mixed to as hard a consistency as possible was applied to the entire surgical field, and the patient was instructed to return on the fifth postoperative day. When she returned, the cement pack was removed and the tissues were cleansed with a water spray. The tissue tone of the gingivae was excellent. A thin film of coagulum was present on the cut tissue surfaces. Four air-dried layers of tincture of myrrh and benzoin were applied to the tissues, and the second cement pack, this time of Peripak, was applied to the entire arch.

The patient returned on the tenth day. The second cement pack was removed and the tissues were cleansed with the water spray. Healing was considerably advanced, and there was no evidence of the film of coagulum. Tincture of myrrh and benzoin was again applied, and mandibular regional block anesthesia was administered on the right side. The oval type of electrode used on the palate was used to perform the gingivectoplasty in an anteroposterior direction, starting at the midline and carried posteriorly around the distal of the second molar. The lingual tissues were treated similarly. When the gingivectoplasty was completed in this quadrant, the individual infrabony pockets were debrided with a 17-mm. periodontal curet electrode. Many of the pockets were 14 to 15 mm. deep. After the internal granulomatous debris had been cleaned out of the pockets, a hoe-shaped horizontal 17-mm. electrode was substituted and used to resect the internal epithelial tissue which the vertical electrode had failed to eliminate from the internal surface of the pocket tissue wall. Bleeding was then induced in the debrided pockets. After the blood had clotted, the left quadrant was anesthetized, and the electrosurgical procedure that has been described was repeated in this quadrant. When the surgery was completed, a stiffly mixed periodontal cement pack was applied to the entire arch and the patient was dismissed.

When she returned on the fifth postoperative day as instructed, the cement pack was removed. The tissues were cleansed with a water spray and dried. Tincture of myrrh and benzoin was applied in air-dried layers, and a fresh periodontal pack, this time of Peripak, was applied to the surgical field. The second pack was removed on the tenth day and tincture of myrrh and benzoin was applied. Two orthodontic stainless-steel wire labial arch bars were contoured to fit snugly around the maxillary and mandibular labial arches. The teeth in both arches were thoroughly dried, and the bars were attached to the teeth with a semifluid mix of self-curing acrylic. After the acrylic had set, the bars were firmly attached to the teeth, effectively immobilizing them (Case Fig. 15–2).

The patient was seen postoperatively on a weekly, then bi-weekly, basis for a total of 10 weeks during which time the tissues continued to heal rapidly and favorably. At the end of the tenth week the arch bars were ready for removal. The tissues were normal in texture and tone, and zones of maturely keratinized attached gingivae that had not been clinically evident preoperatively were present in both arches. The infrabony defects had filled with regenerating bone, and the periodontal pocket probe could not penetrate beyond the bases of the gingival sulci.

The arch bars were removed from the teeth, and the patient was instructed to return at monthly intervals. By the end of the sixth month the tissues were fully healed and the mouth was normal in all respects. The tissues were tightly adherent to the teeth, and each tooth had a gingival sulcus of 1.0 to 1.5 mm. in depth, owing to the regenerative tendency of the tissues cut by electrosection, a marked advantage over the zero degree sulci that result from typical steel scalpel gingivectomies. The only evidence of the periodontal condition that had been present was the 2- to 3-mm. ex-

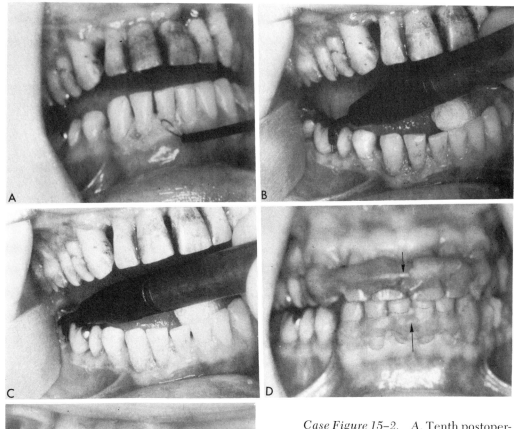

Case Figure 15–2. A, Tenth postoperative day. The second cement pack has been removed, tincture of myrrh and benzoin applied to the uncovered tissues; as a result, the teeth are badly discolored. Gingivectoplasty being performed in the mandible, and a 45-degree-angle oval loop electrode is being used to plane the tissues in the right quadrant. *B,* An infrabony pocket along the mesial aspect of the mesial root of the first molar is being debrided with a 17-mm. periodontal loop electrode. The electrode has penetrated 14 mm. into the defect before meeting resistance from bone. *C,* A similar pocket along the mesial aspect of the second molar is being debrided, with the electrode penetrating 15 mm. before reaching the base of the defect. *D,* Appearance of the mouth ten weeks postoperatively. A pair of labial stainless-steel arch bars that have been attached to the teeth in both arches with cold self-curing acrylic (arrows) are still firmly immobilizing the teeth. The gingivae are well healed, and there are distinct zones of maturely keratinized attached gingivae present. The marginal gingivae in both arches are normal in tone and architectural contour, and the deep infrabony pockets have been obliterated. By the time the splint is ready to be removed, the acrylic has become badly discolored from nicotine and food stains and applications of tincture of myrrh and benzoin, but it remains functionally useful. *E,* Six month postoperative appearance of the mouth. The teeth are firm, without having been splinted or otherwise immobilized except by bone regeneration. The tissues are firm and pink and tightly adherent to the teeth, with no evidence remaining of the infrabony pockets that had been present. Owing to the horizontal circumscribing bone loss that had occurred, 1 to 3 mm. of denuded roots are exposed, especially the two maxillary cuspids and the left lateral incisor which presented the 3-mm. gingival recession. The marginal gingivae had regenerated to provide normal gingival sulci approximately 1.0 to 1.5 mm. deep, instead of the zero-degree sulci that result from the typical steel scalpel gingivectomy.

662

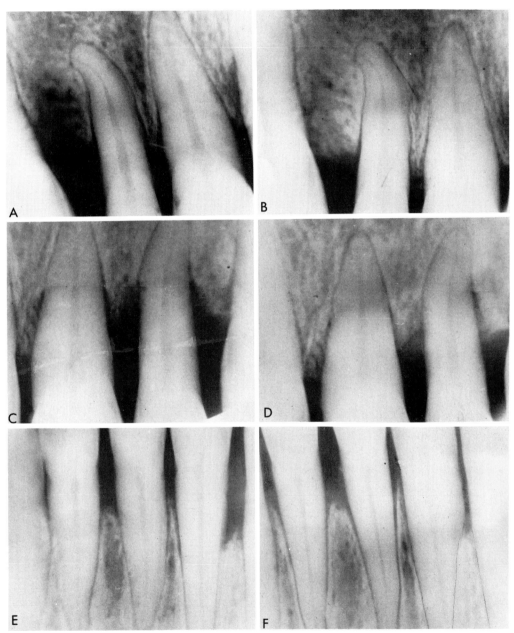

Case Figure 15–3. A, Preoperative x-ray of right maxillary anteriors. Note breakdown of interseptal bone and vertical pockets. B, Six month postoperative x-ray of teeth seen in A. Note bone regeneration. C, Preoperative x-ray of left maxillary anteriors. Note comparable bone destruction. D, Six month postoperative x-ray of teeth seen in C. Note bone regeneration. E, Preoperative x-ray of mandibular anteriors. Note trabeculation in interseptal bone. F, Six month postoperative x-ray of teeth seen in E. Note level of interseptal bone.

posure of denuded roots of the two maxillary cuspids and the left lateral and the 1-mm. root exposure of several other anterior teeth. The left lateral was surprisingly firm and did not require splinting to the adjacent teeth. None of the teeth had had to be extracted.

X-rays taken six months postoperatively compared with preoperative x-rays revealed solid repair of the infrabony defects and an increase in the crestal height of the interseptal bone (Case Fig. 15–3). A periodontal probe inserted into the sulci with pressure exerted at the former pocket sites produced blanching of the tissues without penetration beyond the bases of the sulci. From the clinical standpoint it would be proper to assume that a cure had been effected. However, the author must emphasize that a result such as this cannot be achieved through the efforts of the clinician alone but depends equally on the patient's conscientious maintenance of good oral physiotherapy postoperatively.

The next case is essentially similar in pathology and in treatment to the other cases that are being reviewed and, in common with them, is characterized by an innocuous, normal-looking appearance of the oral structures, despite advanced deterioration of the periodontal structures. It is being presented to suggest a means whereby it may be possible to accelerate bone regeneration by mechanically reducing the gap created by bone loss between teeth.

CASE 16

PATIENT.   A 43-year-old white female.

HISTORY.   She had consulted her dentist because she had been troubled by gingival tenderness and frequent bleeding during toothbrushing and eating. His examination revealed advanced periodontal disease. He referred her to the author for definitive treatment.

CLINICAL EXAMINATION.   All but the two third molars were present in the maxilla. The central incisors as well as the third molars were missing from the mandibular dental arch. The mandibular left first molar also was missing but had been replaced with a fixed bridge. The two centrals had been restored with a partial denture.

The gingival tissues throughout the mouth were normal in architecture except in the maxillary right lateral-cuspid embrasure, where the papilla was slightly hyperplastic. The tissues were normal in color, except for a dark red rim around the maxillary lateral incisors; this purplish red rim circumscribed the left lateral and was limited to the mesial half of the right lateral on the labial aspect but involved the entire palatal aspect of the tooth. Examination with a periodontal pocket probe revealed many infrabony pockets ranging from 4 to 12 mm. in depth.

TREATMENT.   The customary preliminary preparation of the mouth including instruction in oral physiotherapy, elimination of traumatizing prematurities, and thorough prophylaxis was completed. The maxillary arch was treated at the first surgical session. The tissues were prepared and anesthetized by bilateral infraorbital and posterior superior alveolar block and nasopalatine and anterior palatine block injections.

A medium-width, 60-degree-angle U-shaped loop electrode was selected, and cutting current output was set at 5 on the instrument panel rheostat. The activated electrode was used with a downward pulling motion to reduce the slightly hyperplastic interdental papillae in the embrasures of the two laterals to create slightly concave self-cleansing sluiceways (Case Fig. 16–1). The surface epithelium was then resected

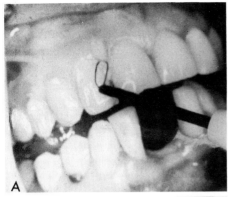

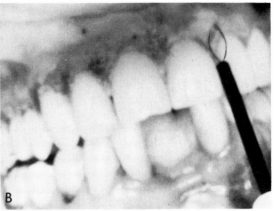

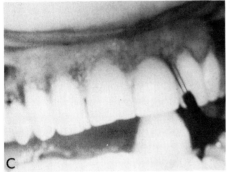

Case Figure 16-1. A, The gingival tissues throughout the mouth are deceptively normal in appearance. The mandibular central incisors are missing. The remaining dentition is present in the dental arches. The slightly hyperplastic right central-lateral interdental papilla is being recontoured to form a concave self-cleansing sluiceway by electrosection with a 90-degree-angle, medium-width U-shaped loop electrode. The electrode is being used with a downward slightly scooping motion toward the incisal edge. B, A gingivoplasty is being performed with a flame-shaped loop electrode. The loop is being applied to the tissue at an approximate 40-degree-angle, which automatically creates a beveled feather-edged marginal gingiva. C, A 17-mm. periodontal electronic curet electrode is being introduced into the infrabony pocket along the mesial of the left lateral incisor, where a 2-mm. wide diastema is present.

in a similar manner from all the other papillae. This electrode was replaced with a flame-shaped loop electrode, which was used to complete the gingivoplasty of the marginal gingivae on the labial-buccal aspects. The palatal marginal gingivae were then treated in a similar manner with the U-shaped electrode, with current increased to 5.5, owing to the greater density and keratinization of this tissue. A 17-mm. periodontal 45-degree-angle loop electrode was substituted and used to debride all the periodontal pockets. The activated electrode was applied for about one second with an up and down rotary motion to make contact with all the internal surfaces of the defects. The right second molar had a trifurcation involvement that was debrided with a right-angle 17-mm. loop electrode to create a clearance between the buccal roots.

When debridement was completed, bleeding was encouraged in the pockets. After the blood had clotted, tincture of myrrh and benzoin was applied to the tissues in air-dried layers. A very stiffly mixed periodontal pack was applied to the surgical field with care to avoid displacement of the blood clots when the cement was contoured into the embrasures.

On the fifth postoperative day the cement pack was removed. The tissues were found to be healing very well (Case Fig. 16-2). The tissues were cleansed by gentle irrigation with a solution of Kasdenol. Tincture of myrrh and benzoin was applied, and a second pack, this time using Peripak instead of the stiffly mixed cement pack to avoid crushing the healing tissue cells with the pressure necessary to apply a hard cement pack. Five days later this pack was also removed, and the tissues were not protected with any more packs. The patient was instructed to begin massaging the tis-

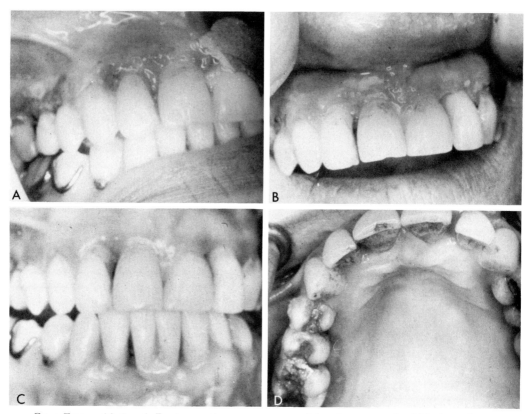

Case Figure 16–2. A, Postoperative appearance of the tissues on the fifth day, after some of the cement pack has been removed. Healing appears favorable. *B,* Appearance of the tissues on the tenth postoperative day, immediately after removal of the second cement pack. There is a 4-mm. recession of the marginal gingivae over the mesial halves of the two laterals, where the deep infrabony pocket debridement had been performed. *C,* Appearance of the labial gingivae two weeks later. The gingivae have healed well except in the two central-lateral embrasures. The tissue in these areas is still somewhat atonal and red, and infrabony defects approximately 3 mm. deep persist. *D,* A palatal view shows the tissues in the two embrasures are still immature. This view shows the dimension of the diastema on the left side. The tissue at the palatal aspect of the right bicuspid and molar is not yet fully re-epithelialized.

sues with gentle finger massage and with a very soft nylon toothbrush with rounded tips.

Healing progressed uneventfully, and two weeks later the gingival tissues appeared to be regenerating to their pre-surgical levels, but as maturation progressed and the tissues firmed up, the gingivae receded, exposing about 4 mm. of root at the mesial half of both lateral incisors by the time the mandibular surgery was instituted.

The left half of the mandible was treated first, after administration of an inferior alveolar-lingual nerve block injection. A flame-shaped loop electrode was selected, current output was set at 5, and the gingivoplasty was performed on the buccal and lingual surfaces (Case Fig. 16–3). A 17-mm. periodontal loop electrode was then substituted and used to debride the infrabony pockets that were present throughout the quadrant.

When debridement of the pockets was completed, bleeding was induced in the infrabony defects, clotting was permitted, and a cement pack was applied to that quadrant. The right quadrant was then treated in an identical manner and a cement pack was applied.

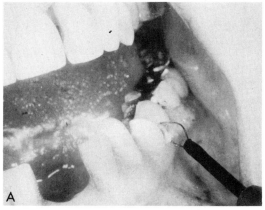
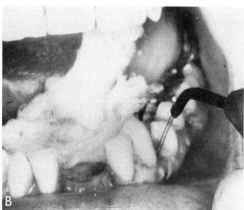
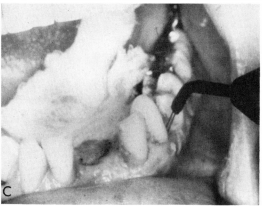

Case Figure 16–3.   *A*, A gingivoplasty is being performed in the mandibular left quadrant with a flame-shaped loop electrode. *B*, A deep infrabony pocket along the distal aspect of the left cuspid is being debrided with a 17-mm. periodontal electronic curet electrode. The activated electrode is beginning to penetrate into the defect. *C*, The electrode, being used with an up-down and rotary motion in the pocket, has penetrated about 1 cm. into the defect.

The pack was removed on the fifth postoperative day. The tissues, which appeared to be healing very favorably, were irrigated gently. Tincture of myrrh and benzoin was applied, and a second pack, of Peripak, was applied without pressure. The second pack was removed five days later, and healing appeared to be progressing so favorably that it was possible to resume treatment in the maxilla to try to close the slight diastema that had failed to close in the maxillary left central-lateral embrasure.

Although the diastema was very slight, there appeared to be a distinct likelihood that if the tooth could be moved by very gentle, almost imperceptible pressure, this not only would close the gap but also might stimulate further bone regeneration, particularly if this were supplemented with curettage to remove the surface of the tissues in the embrasures of the two laterals and centrals, so that blood clots would form and initiate the healing. To accomplish this, Japanese grassline and elastic bands were applied around the four incisors (Case Fig. 16–4), and the curettage was performed manually with steel periodontal curets. When this was completed, the blood was permitted to clot, and tincture of myrrh and benzoin was applied. The grassline-elastic band traction was maintained for three weeks. By the end of that period the diastema was closed, and about 2 mm. of tissue was regenerated in each embrasure. Owing to incomplete keratinization of the new tissue it was somewhat darker in color than the surrounding tissue but otherwise normal. The mandibular gingivae were firm and normal in tone. When a periodontal pocket probe was inserted into the two defects one month later, it penetrated 1 mm. beyond the marginal edge of the tissue.

The tissue tone was maintained in excellent condition by the patient's vigorous oral physiotherapy, and the diastema has remained closed. There has been no recur-

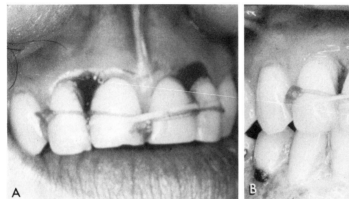
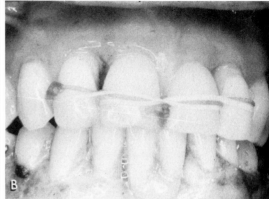

Case Figure 16–4. *A*, The mandibular tissues are beginning to heal very well, and the maxillary tissues are progressing well except in the two central-lateral embrasures. The teeth have been ligated with Japanese grassline and elastic bands to institute simple tooth movement to close the diastemas, and the tissue in the embrasures has been curetted manually with steel periodontal curets to create raw tissue surfaces and bleeding in the defects. *B*, The diastemas having been closed, 2 mm. of tissue has regenerated in each embrasure, and the infrabony pockets are obliterated to the level of the gingival sulci of the teeth. The marginal gingivae on the labial aspect of the teeth have grown downward slightly, reducing the root exposures to approximately 2.5 mm. over the right lateral and 3 mm. over the left lateral. The trifurcation has also filled in almost to the external level of the tissue.

rence of the periodontal deterioration in the 3½ years since the patient was dismissed from active treatment.

The use of slow simple tooth movement such as was instituted, combined with the curettage to induce bleeding and provide a raw surface of tissue to which the blood could adhere, appears to have been instrumental in stimulating further bone and tissue regeneration. In this type of case, the slight amount of tooth tilting needed to close the defect and the blood in the area may function in a manner similar to the fracture of the bone to close much wider diastemas between teeth, a technique that has been successful for several years.

THE INFLUENCE OF ORAL
HYGIENE ON PERIODONTOCLASIA

Good oral hygiene minimizes the severity of periodontal deterioration in two ways. It eliminates the irritating effect of calculus and plaque on the gingivae, both of which can trigger or increase the severity of periodontal deterioration. More importantly, it stimulates the blood flow, thus maintaining the supply of nourishment and oxygen to the tissues and carrying off the waste products. Stasis and engorgement that result from impairment of the blood supply are prevented, thus minimizing the severity and rate of periodontal deterioration.

Figure 19–6 provides an excellent demonstration of the beneficial role oral hygiene plays, even when the treatment of periodontoclasia of local origin is handicapped unsuspectingly by a secondary systemic factor that has a seriously retarding effect on tissue healing. Needless to say, when the presence of a secondary systemic factor is known, it is just as essential that it be brought under control as in the cases of systemic disease that is the primary

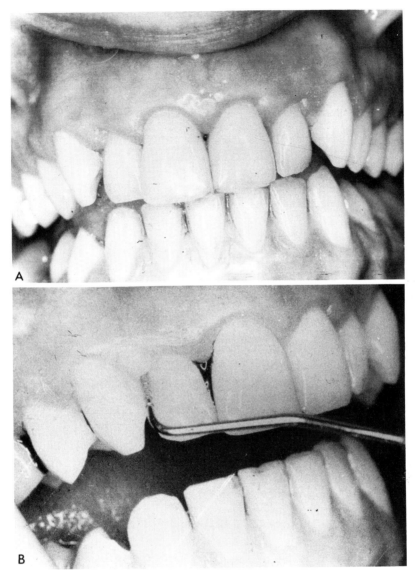

Figure 19–6. Periodontal deterioration minimized by good oral hygiene. *A*, Appearance of the teeth and gingivae with the jaws closed. The only teeth in functional occlusion are the maxillary centrals and the mandibular centrals and laterals. The rest of the teeth are in open bite relation. All the teeth are very clean, but those in functional occlusion are in traumatic occlusion. The gingivae are atonal. The surface of the gingival tissues is smooth and shiny, and they are moderately hyperplastic, but the dark red engorged appearance customarily seen in such tissues is not in evidence. These tissues are just as pink and normal in color as the normal healthy stippled orange-skin textured attached gingivae. *B*, A periodontal pocket probe is seen penetrating about 6 mm. into an infrabony pocket, which actually is 9 mm. deep. It is interesting to note that the periodontal deterioration is just as marked in the areas where there is no functional occlusion as it is where there is a traumatic occlusion.

factor. In this case, owing to medical and laboratory evaluations initiated to determine the reason for inexplicable unsatisfactory response to periodontal treatment, the existence of the disease was revealed. Such a finding is likely to render a far more important service to the patient than the treatment itself.

Periodontia Related to Cell Abnormalities

Abnormal cell pathogenesis may be internal in origin, owing to a derangement in the systemic mechanism of cell reproduction such as occurs in diffused gingival hyperplasia or increase in the number of *normal cells* in *normal arrangement* that is called generalized fibromatosis, or it may be external in origin, with intracellular changes triggered by the effects of drugs that result in abnormal change in the size and morphology of the individual cells, such as occurs in Dilantin hypertrophy.

Periodontal deterioration usually is associated with both types of cell abnormalities. The next two cases are examples of the two types of cell aberrations and the periodontal disease that may accompany them.

GENERALIZED GINGIVAL FIBROMATOSIS

CASE 17

This case characteristically presented massive hyperplasia of the gingival mucosa. The excess tissue was more dense and fibrotic than normal gingival tissue and bore a clinical resemblance to Dilantin hypertrophy, but only that portion of the gingiva directly involved with the periodontal pockets showed evidence of engorgement. The remainder of the hyperplastic tissue was normal in color and tissue tone.

The ease and simplicity with which the gingival architecture can be recontoured and restored to normal dimension by electrosurgical loop planing, without the profuse hemorrhage that is usually encountered with traditional cold steel gingivectomies, is well demonstrated by this case. It also exemplifies the increased efficiency and simplicity with which the periodontal pockets can be debrided when visibility is not obscured by free bleeding in the operative field.

PATIENT.   A 24-year-old white female.

CASE HISTORY.   The patient was referred for gingival surgery by her psychiatrist, who had diagnosed her emotional problem as stemming from two sources: disfiguring old acne scars that resembled smallpox scars, and the grotesque appearance of her mouth caused by the excess of gingival tissue.

CLINICAL EXAMINATION.   The gingival mucosa was very thick and appeared somewhat lobulated in the maxillary central incisor area. The tissue covered approximately one half the coronal portions of the teeth, which were normal in dimension, as verified by roentgenographic examination. There were diastemata between the anterior teeth. The teeth were firm, but the papillae appeared severely engorged (Case Fig. 17–1A). The left lateral incisor was rotated, and there was a marked overbite, which obscured two-thirds of the mandibular teeth. Probing with a periodontal pocket probe revealed pockets along most of the roots ranging in depth from 3 to 7 mm.

TREATMENT.   The tissues were prepared, and bilateral infraorbital, posterior superior alveolar, nasopalatine and anterior palatine regional block anesthesia was administered.

A flame-shaped loop electrode was selected and used to plane away the excess tissue with the cutting current (Case Fig. 17–1B). The loop, used with a light brushing stroke, dissected away the tissue, leaving a normal amount of coronal structure ex-

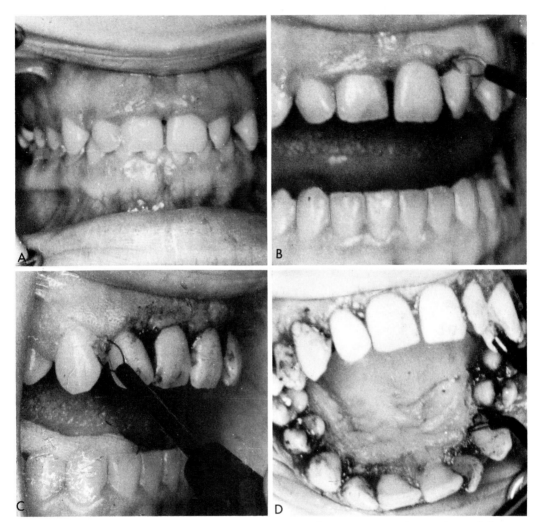

Case Figure 17–1. A, Preoperative appearance. There is massive hyperplasia of the gingival mucosa that covers approximately half the coronal portions of the teeth and resembles Dilantin hyperplasia clinically. Note the unmistakable evidence of periodontal deterioration despite the massive hyperplasia. B, Gingivoplasty being performed with flame-shaped loop electrode. The tissues are being recontoured as they are resected, creating a normal architecture without free bleeding. C, Crowns of teeth being fully exposed as the gingivoplasty continues. The bulging partially detached interdental papillae are being reduced by loop planing to form concave self-cleansing sluiceways. D, The gingivoplasty having been completed on the palatal as well as the labial aspects, the individual periodontal pockets are being debrided with a 15 millimeter periodontal loop electrode used with cutting current as an electronic curet. Arrows point to typical pockets that have been debrided.

posed and recontouring the gingival architecture to normal. The bulging interdental papillae were reduced to concave self-cleansing sluiceways with the loop electrode.

When all the crowns had been exposed to their normal size, the periodontal pockets were thoroughly debrided with a 17-mm. narrow U-shaped periodontal loop electrode (Case Fig. 17–1C to F). The pockets were easily visualized owing to the absence of free bleeding in the operative field, and with the aid of transillumination, the debris in the pockets was easily visualized and meticulously removed.

When the electrosurgical curettage was completed, the pockets were irrigated, the water carefully aspirated, and bleeding induced in the osseous defects. The blood was permitted to clot, the operative field was gently dried, and a dressing of tincture of myrrh and benzoin was applied in air-dried layers. A periodontal cement pack was carefully applied to the teeth, to avoid forcing the cement into the pockets. The patient returned on the fifth postoperative day. She reported complete freedom from postoperative pain or swelling. The pack was removed, the tissues irrigated and anointed with another dressing of tincture of myrrh and benzoin, and a fresh cement pack was reapplied for another 5 days. The second pack was removed, and the tissues proceeded to heal without incident (Case Fig. 17–2).

The patient was seen postoperatively twice a week for 4 weeks, then once weekly for the next 4 weeks. By the end of that time the gingival tissues were fully healed and appeared firm and healthy except at the mesial aspect of the maxillary left central incisor, where the tissue showed a slight tendency to proliferate. Careful examination revealed that the maxillary labial frenum, innocuous and flabby in appearance when relaxed, was exerting traction against the subnormal marginal gingiva when the lip was stretched taut and moved around.

A frenectomy was performed under infiltration anesthesia to eliminate the abnormal traction. The lip was extended to pull the frenal fibers taut. The frenum was then clamped as close to the ventral surface of the upper lip as possible with a curved mosquito hemostat, and the frenal tissue projecting from the beak of the hemostat was resected from the hemostat by electrosection with a needle electrode.

Frenectomy performed by dissection with a cold steel scalpel invariably is accompanied by profuse and often persistent free bleeding, with the margins of the wound tending to flare wide open and requiring suturing. In the electrosurgical frenectomy there was no free bleeding, and the tissues did not require suturing. Enough bleeding was induced to fill the surgical defect with a blood clot, and tincture of myrrh and benzoin was applied to the surgical field in air-dried layers.

Healing progressed without further incident. The abnormal traction having been eliminated, the tone of the marginal gingiva at the mesial of the central became normal, and there was no further evidence of proliferation. The frenal wound healed rapidly without forming scar tissue, and the objectives of the treatment were fully realized. The oral aesthetics were greatly improved (Case Fig. 17–2E and F), the tissue tone was excellent, and the periodontal pockets totally obliterated.

TYPICAL TISSUE RESPONSE TO
DILANTIN THERAPY

The case being reported here deals with treatment of Dilantin hypertrophy in a human subject. Electrosurgical and cold-steel gingivoplasty were performed on the gingivae in adjacent quadrants in the same mouth at the same surgical session under identical conditions by the same therapist, a

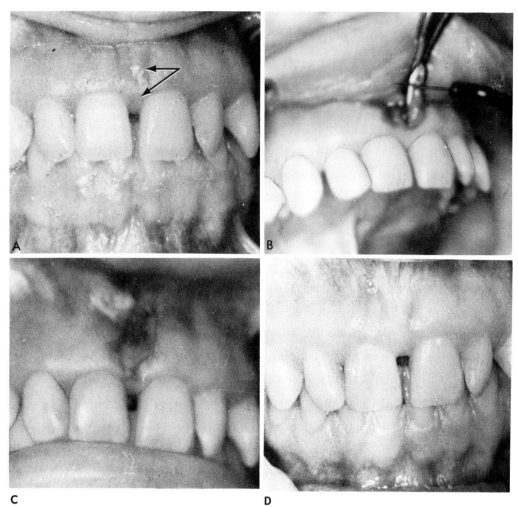

Case Figure 17-2. A, The appearance of the mouth 6 weeks postoperatively. The tissues have healed well throughout except at the mesial aspect of the maxillary left central incisor, where the labial frenum, which appears innocuous in repose, is exerting abnormal traction against the marginal gingiva. The tissue tone is somewhat subnormal, and there is a slight tendency for the tissue to proliferate. Arrows point to the frenum and the proliferating tissue. B, The lip has been extended, the frenal fibers pulled taut and clamped with a curved mosquito hemostat. The frenal tissue projecting from the beaks of the hemostat is being resected by electrosection with a needle electrode. C, The frenum having been resected, the mosquito hemostat is removed, leaving a smooth tissue bed with no free bleeding. No sutures are required. D, The appearance of the tissues 10 years later. The crowns of the teeth are fully exposed, the gingival architecture is normal, the tissue tone is excellent, there are well defined zones of attached gingiva, and the intraosseous defects have been obliterated.°

periodontist who was well trained in use of both modalities. It therefore provides an excellent opportunity for comparison and evaluation of the rate and quality of tissue healing of gingival tissue cut by electrosection and by cold-steel instrumentation under identical conditions, except that the quadrant presenting the *most extensive and pronounced amount of hypertrophy was treated by electrosection.*

°The patient was seen again 9 years later and the gingival tissues were still healthy and normal in appearance.

CASE 18

This case was reviewed in the chapter on research. It is being presented through the courtesy of Dr. Charles W. Conroy, Columbus, Ohio.

PATIENT.   A 23-year-old white female.

HISTORY.   She had been under treatment for grand mal seizures for many years and was being maintained on Dilantin medication to control the frequency and severity of her epileptic seizures. A moderate degree of Dilantin hypertrophy developed. More recently, the enlarged interdental papillae in several areas of the mouth became partially detached and caused some physical discomfort and interference with maintenance of good oral hygiene. Surgical reduction of these tissues therefore became necessary.

CLINICAL EXAMINATION.   The marginal and alveolar gingivae in both jaws appeared thickened and fibrotic. The interdental papillae in the mandible from first bicuspid to first bicuspid were enlarged and partially detached at their apical attachments. The papilla between the right lateral incisor and cuspid was greatly enlarged and engorged. The papilla on the contralateral side was much more normal in dimension and tone. The papillae in the maxilla were enlarged from first molar to first molar but were not as hypertrophic as their mandibular counterparts. The papillae on the right side were somewhat more enlarged than those on the left side (Case Fig. 18–1).

TREATMENT.   The decision was made to reduce the hypertrophied bulk of the tissue on the right side by electrosection and on the left side by Bard-Parker scalpel excision. The maxillary left quadrant was left untreated, since the hypertrophy in this quadrant was still minimal.

The surgery for both sides was performed under identical anesthesia. The tissue on the right side, in both the maxilla and mandible, was reduced by electrosection with a flame-shaped loop electrode. The gingivoplasties were performed without free bleeding but also without burning the tissues. The mandibular hypertrophy in the left quadrant was then reduced by gingivoplasty with the steel scalpel and was accompanied by free bleeding (Case Fig. 18–2).

When the bleeding stopped and the blood became clotted, protective periodontal cement packs were applied to the surgical fields, and the patient was reappointed. She was seen again one week later and the packs were removed. The tissues in the mandible provided an excellent opportunity for comparison of the tissue repair. The healing of the tissue in the right quadrant appeared slightly more advanced. The tissue of the right lateral still looked raw, but the tissue distal to the lateral-cuspid embrasure appeared surprisingly pink and partially healed. The tissues in the left quadrant appeared somewhat more red in color and less advanced in repair.

By the third week healing of the tissues on the right side was quite advanced except on the labial aspect of the lateral incisor, where the marginal gingiva still looked red and raw. The tissue on the left side was more uniform in color, but its healing did not appear as well advanced as that in the right quadrant other than the lateral area, and the tissue around the left lateral incisor showed some evidence of proliferative tendency (Case Fig. 18–3).

The healing progressed satisfactorily despite the fact that the patient continued Dilantin medication. The patient was seen again six months postoperatively. The tissue tone in the right lateral-cuspid embrasure and on the labial aspect of the lateral still looked red and engorged, but there was little evidence of renewed hypertrophy.

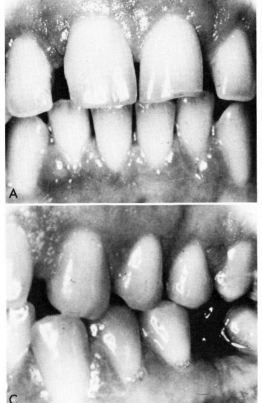

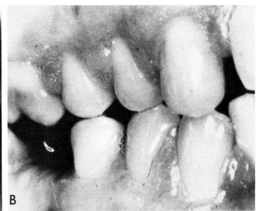

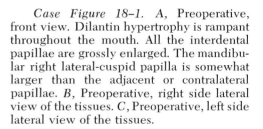

Case Figure 18–1. A, Preoperative, front view. Dilantin hypertrophy is rampant throughout the mouth. All the interdental papillae are grossly enlarged. The mandibular right lateral-cuspid papilla is somewhat larger than the adjacent or contralateral papillae. *B,* Preoperative, right side lateral view of the tissues. *C,* Preoperative, left side lateral view of the tissues.

The tissue in the left quadrant showed distinct proliferative activity in the interdental papillae.

Sixteen months later the hypertrophy was again rampant in both quadrants. However, the interdental papillae in the left quadrant were slightly more enlarged than those in the right quadrant. The papilla in the left lateral-cuspid embrasure was now largest of all, and the lateral incisor was being displaced lingually, creating a diastema about 3 mm. wide. The right lateral incisor was displaced lingually very slightly, and the space there was about 1 mm. wide.

This case offers several obvious deductions and conclusions.* First, that as long as the patient continues Dilantin therapy, regardless of the nature of the surgical intervention, the gingival hypertrophy will recur. Second, when the electrosurgical instrumentation is properly performed, the rate and quality of the tissue repair is not only as good as but actually better than comparable surgery performed by cold-steel instrumentation. Finally, although the hypertrophy will inevitably recur as long as the patient continues Dilantin medication, electrosection appears to tend to retard the rate and degree of recurrence.

---

*The author offers these deductions and conclusions. However, Dr. Conroy, the clinician who treated the patient, concurs with them.

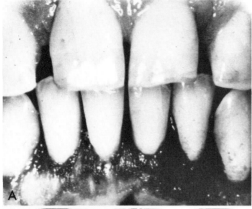
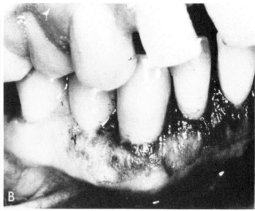
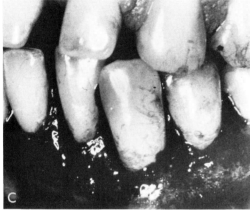

Case Figure 18–2. *A,* Operative appearance of the tissues that have just been treated by gingivoplasty. The tissues of the right central to first bicuspid have been reduced and recontoured by loop planing by electrosection. The tissues of the left central to left first bicuspid have been reduced by steel scalpel gingivoplasty. Note the free bleeding on the left side. *B,* Operative, a right lateral view of the operative field. *C,* Operative, a left lateral view of the operative field.

ATYPICAL TISSUE RESPONSE TO DILANTIN THERAPY

CASE 19

Victims of grand mal who have been on Dilantin therapy for long periods almost invariably experience aberrations in the morphology of the gingival tissue cells. These aberrations customarily are in the form of gross abnormal enlargement of the cells and their cellular components, manifested clinically as the massive customary overgrowth associated with this medication, called Dilantin hypertrophy.

This patient had been maintained on Dilantin therapy for many years. Nevertheless, the gingivae remained normal in dimension and architecture. The alveolar bone, however, as well as the texture and tone of the gingival mucosa, appeared to have been affected adversely by the Dilantin medication. As a result, an extremely extensive and severe deterioration of the periodontal structures had occurred, which required rather heroic therapeutic measures.

PATIENT. A middle-aged white male.

HISTORY. He developed grand mal in childhood and had been kept on Dilantin therapy for the past 18 years. The dimension and architecture of the gingival tissues remained normal, but the tissues became very spongy and engorged, and some of the

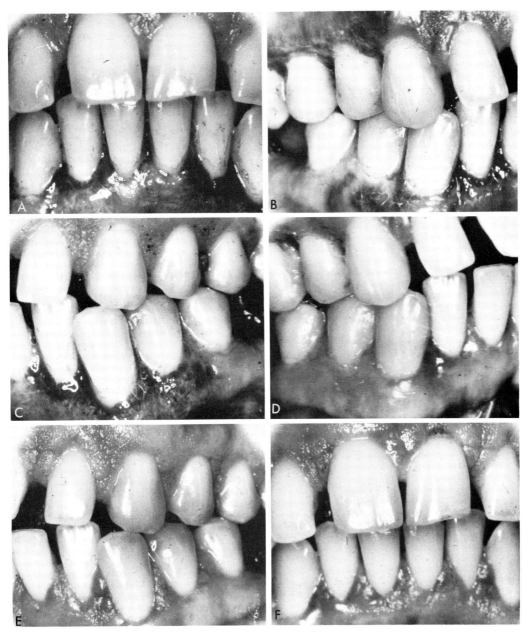

Case Figure 18–3. A, Postoperative appearance of the tissues, front view, one week later. The tissues on the right side, where the electrosurgery had been performed, are beginning to show definite evidence of healing. B, Postoperative appearance of the tissues, right lateral view, one week later. The tissues show unmistakable evidence of healing progress. C, Postoperative appearance of the tissues, left side, lateral view, one week later. The tissues here show very little clinical evidence of healing progress. D, Postoperative appearance of the tissues fourth postoperative week, right lateral view. The tissues in this area appear well healed and maturely re-epithelialized except in the lateral-cuspid embrasure, where the tissue healing appears slow and the tissue appears immature. E, Postoperative appearance of the tissues, fourth postoperative week, left lateral view; the tissues in this area appear to have healed to a lesser degree and appear not as maturely re-epithelialized as the right side. The tissue in the left central-lateral and lateral-cuspid embrasures appear to be beginning to reproliferate. F, Postoperative appearance one year later; the tissues have reproliferated throughout the mouth. However, the proliferation does not appear as marked on the right side where the electrosurgery had been performed.

677

anterior teeth drifted apart, creating a fairly wide diastema in the maxillary midline between the centrals. The marginal gingivae around several of the teeth seemed to have become ulcerated and the gingivae bled from toothbrushing and occasionally during mastication. The condition continued to deteriorate until he felt it necessary to consult his dentist, whereupon the latter referred him to the author for treatment.

CLINICAL EXAMINATION. The maxillary and mandibular gingivae were normal in dimension and architecture. The edge of the marginal gingiva on the labial aspect of the maxillary right central was markedly engorged, friable, and proliferative. A periodontal pocket probe inserted under the labial free margin of the maxillary right central, where the marginal edge of the tissue was ulcerated and proliferative, penetrated upward along the root surface its full length without encountering resistance (Case Fig. 19–1A). The mesio-incisal angle of this tooth had been fractured slightly and was slightly decayed. A 3 mm. diastema was present between the maxillary centrals and a 1.5 mm. diastema between the left central and lateral, and the maxillary labial frenum was a large wide ligament that formed an elevated V superimposed on the labial gingiva.

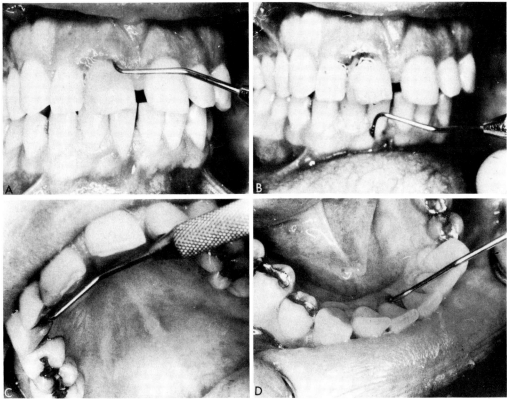

Case Figure 19–1. Atypical Dilantin periodontoclasia—Phase 1. *A,* Preoperative appearance. Maxillary and mandibular gingivae are normal in architecture. The marginal gingiva of the maxillary right central is engorged and the marginal edge of the gingiva is friable and proliferative. A periodontal pocket probe has penetrated its full length without meeting resistance from bone. The gingival tissue has receded about 0.5 cm. apically on the mandibular right central, and the tissue that is present over the facial aspect of the root of the tooth is severely engorged. *B,* The thick round probe has penetrated 7 mm. apically on the distolabial aspect of the mandibular right central. *C,* The pocket probe has penetrated its full length into a pocket at the distopalatal aspect of the maxillary right lateral incisor. *D,* The probe has penetrated 9 mm. into a pocket at the mesiolingual of the mandibular right lateral. The marginal gingiva has receded on the lingual aspect of this tooth about 3 mm. apically.

There was also a 1.5 mm. diastema between the mandibular centrals, and the labial marginal edge of the marginal gingiva of the right central also was friable and slightly ulcerated. The pocket probe penetrated almost 9 mm. when it was inserted along the labial surface of the root of the tooth (Case Fig. 19–1B). Despite the innocuous appearance of the gingival tissues, pockets of similar depth were present in many areas throughout the mouth, on the palatal and lingual surfaces as well as on the labial (Case Fig. 19–1C and D). The tissue on the lingual aspect of the mandibular centrals was considerably darker in color than the rest of the gingivae. Roentgenographic examination revealed extensive alveolar radiolucence.

TREATMENT. The maxilla was anesthetized with bilateral posterior superior alveolar and infraorbital blocks and nasopalatine and anterior palatine block injections, and a gingivoplasty was performed with a flame-shaped loop electrode (Case Fig. 19–2A). When this was completed, the 17-mm. periodontal loop electrode was substituted, current output was reduced from 5 to 4, and debridement of the infrabony pockets was performed by using the electrode with up-down and rotary motion for about one-half second at a time, with 5-second rest intervals between each application of the activated electrode. The electrode penetrated 14 mm. when used on the labial of the maxillary right central (Case Fig. 19–2B and C). In almost all the pockets the electrode penetrated from 9 to 14 mm. (Case Fig. 19–2D and E). The electrode penetrated 14 mm. into the defect on the palatal aspect of the maxillary right central (Case Fig. 19–3A) and about 9 mm. along the palatal root of the left second molar (Case Fig. 19–3B). Some of the debridement was accompanied by rather profuse bleeding at the outset, but this was readily brought under control by applying finger pressure for about 2 minutes, and increasing the current output to 4.5 and even to 5 when the initial bleeding was more profuse. Soon after the debridement was begun the bleeding ceased and the rest of the debridement concluded with unimpaired visibility in the surgical fields. When debridement was completed bleeding was induced in the infrabony defects and powdered surgical gelatin was introduced into most of them and mixed with the blood. When clotting was complete, a periodontal pack was applied and the patient was instructed to follow the regimen of postoperative home care that had been prescribed and was reappointed. He returned on the fifth postoperative day for removal of the cement pack. When it was removed a strange phenomenon was noted. A thick layer of coagulum covered the gingival surface and peeled off readily (Case Fig. 19–3C). When the coagulum was lifted away it exposed a somewhat raw tissue surface, but there was no exposed bone or evidence of sequestration. Healing progressed surprisingly well and rapidly especially after the mobile right central was temporarily immobilized by tying it and the right lateral together and ligating them to a small length of labial archbar wire.

Three weeks after the second cement pack was removed from the maxilla the mandibular surgery was performed under bilateral inferior alveolar block anesthesia. The gingivoplasty, performed with a flame-shaped loop electrode, was started in the right molar region and carried around the arch on the labial-buccal surface (Case Fig. 19–3D). The lingual gingivoplasty was performed with a 90-degree-angle medium-width U-shaped loop electrode (Case Fig. 19–3E) in the posterior regions, and with the 45-degree-angle version of this loop in the anterior region. Debridement of the individual infrabony pockets was then performed with the 17-mm. periodontal electronic loop curet electrodes. The gingival tissue, which had receded almost 0.5 cm. apically on the labial of the right mandibular central, was detached from the root surface almost to the apex of the tooth, and the electrode penetrated about 13 mm. beyond the receded gingival level (Case Fig. 19–3F). When debridement was completed, bleeding was induced in the defects, surgical gelatin was introduced into the larger ones, and a cement pack applied after the blood was clotted.

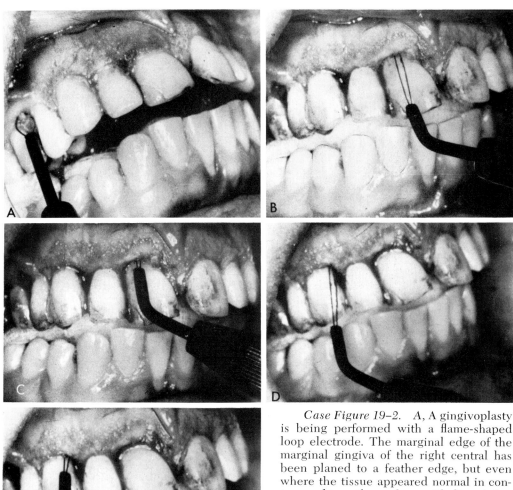

Case Figure 19–2. A, A gingivoplasty is being performed with a flame-shaped loop electrode. The marginal edge of the marginal gingiva of the right central has been planed to a feather edge, but even where the tissue appeared normal in contour and tone the surface epithelium is being planed to create a raw tissue surface. Note the low attachment of the labial frenum and the muscle attachment over the first bicuspid. B, Gingivoplasty having been completed throughout the maxilla, the infrabony pocket debridement is begun with a 17-mm. periodontal curet loop electrode. The electrode is being introduced into the deep defect on the labial aspect of the right central. C, The electrode has penetrated 15 mm. before meeting resistance from bone and is being used with an up and down, rotary motion. D, The electrode is being introduced into the pocket at the mesiolabial aspect of the right cuspid. E, The electrode has penetrated 13 mm. before meeting resistance. It is interesting to note that when the thick 10-mm. pocket probe was introduced into this defect it penetrated 7 mm. and stopped.

Healing progressed favorably, and by the end of the fourth week the healing was relatively complete. The patient was now ready for the second phase of treatment—permanent fixation of the maxillary right central, lateral, and cuspid, which were mobile, and repositioning of the marginal gingivae over the right maxillary and mandibular centrals for aesthetic improvement. After his dentist had inserted the Whaledent horizontal nonparallel pin splint, an infraorbital block was administered on the right side, and infiltration anesthesia was administered over the left central to block out anastomosing nerve innervation from that quadrant, and a few minims injected into

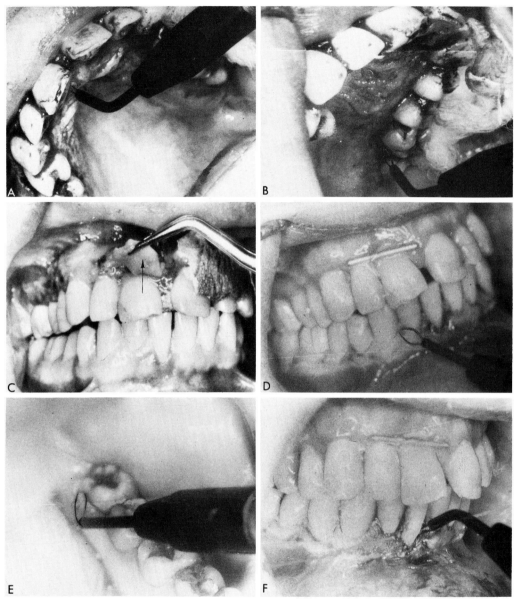

Case Figure 19–3. *A,* A 14-mm. pocket on the palatal aspect of the maxillary right central is being debrided. *B,* The electrode is seen penetrating the 11-mm. pocket at the distopalatal angle of the left second molar. The electrode had penetrated about 9 mm. when photographed. *C,* Appearance of the tissues on the fifth postoperative day as the first cement pack is being removed. The surface of the tissues in the surgical field is covered with a thick layer of coagulum, which is being lifted off with cotton pliers (arrow). The tissue under the coagulum appears relatively normal. *D,* The maxillary tissue healing is progressing favorably. The maxillary right central has been immobilized by ligation to a small labial wire bar that is also attached to the right lateral incisor. A gingivoplasty is being performed by planing the tissue with the flame-shaped loop electrode on the buccal-labial surface. *E,* The gingivoplasty is being continued on the lingual aspect with a 45-degree-angle, medium-width U-shaped loop electrode which provides better access and contact to the tissues in this area. *F,* The infrabony pocket debridement is being started in the mandible. The 17-mm. electronic curet electrode has been used on the labial aspect and can be seen in use on the mesial aspect where it has penetrated about 13 mm. into the defect.

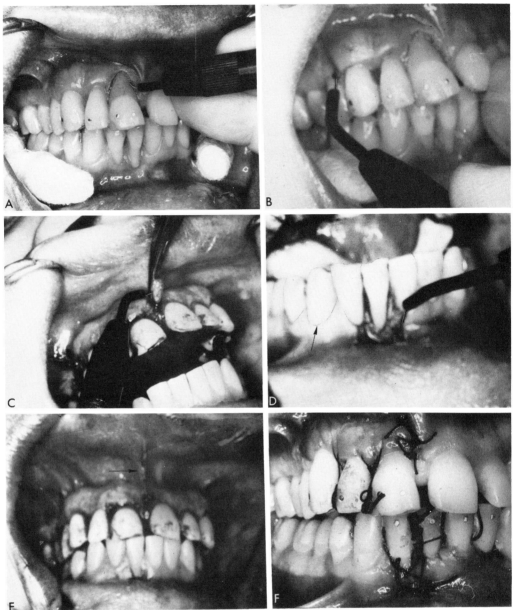

Case Figure 19–4. A, Phase 2 — Repositioning the marginal gingivae. To reduce the extent of root exposure and create a more harmonious gingival level, mucoperiosteal flaps will be created in the maxilla and mandible to reposition the gingivae. The marginal edge of the marginal gingiva on the labial aspect of the maxillary right central is being resected with a narrow 45-degree-angle U-shaped loop electrode to create the raw tissue surfaces that can be coapted and sutured for primary healing. B, The apices of the papillae between the central and cuspid have been severed with a fine 45-degree-angle needle electrode. The activated electrode is being used to create a vertico-oblique incision for a mucoperiosteal flap. The incision is directed postero-anteriorly and extends from the mucogingival junction to the distogingival angle of the cuspid. C, A frenectomy is being performed on the alveolar half of the maxillary frenum to eliminate unfavorable traction against the coapted tissues. D, The mandibular labial frenum has been removed to eliminate the traction that has contributed much to the gingival recession and denudation of the right mandibular central and lateral incisors. The electrode is being used to deepen the mandibular labial vestibule, so that the tissues can be coapted and sutured

(*Legend continued on p. 683.*)

the nasopalatine foramen. A short narrow 45-degree-angle U-shaped loop electrode was used to resect the marginal edge of the marginal gingiva and create a raw tissue surface (Case Fig. 19–4A).

A vertico-oblique incision was then made with a fine 45-degree-angle needle electrode from the mucogingival junction to the distogingival angle of the right cuspid into a postero-anterior direction (Case Fig. 19–4B), and the apices of the interdental papillae in the cuspid-lateral-central embrasures were severed. The large flabby labial frenum was clamped close to the ventral surface of the lip and excised with a V-Y incision with the needle electrode (Case Fig. 19–4C). The mucoperiosteal flap was elevated from the bone, the epithelialized tissue of the free margin of the central was resected, and the flap was shifted anteriorly to permit coaptation of the raw edges of the tissue over the right central. The coapted tissue was sutured with interrupted silk sutures, and the sutures were inserted labiopalatally through the embrasures.

The left quadrant of the mandible was anesthetized with an inferior alveolar block, and the tissues on the labial aspect over the right central and lateral were anesthetized with infiltration anesthesia. The labial gingiva over the right lower lateral was excised to the mucogingival junction (Case Fig. 19–4D) with the needle electrode, which was then used to create a vertico-oblique incision from the mesiogingival angle of the left cuspid downward and slightly anteriorly and to incise the intervening apices of interdental papillae. The more extensive excision of tissue from the mandibular central was necessary to eliminate traction from the mandibular labial frenum, which had submerged fibers that exerted considerable torque against the marginal gingiva.

The mucoperiosteal flap was elevated and the tissue was rotated anteriorly until the raw margins of the defect over the central were coapted. The coapted tissues were sutured with interrupted silk sutures, and sutures were inserted through the embrasures (Case Fig. 19–4E and F).

The sutures were removed on the fifth postoperative day (Case Fig. 19–5A). The tissues were still unhealed but gave evidence of primary union in its early stage. By the end of the third postoperative week the tissues were almost fully healed (Case Fig. 19–5B). A periodontal pocket probe inserted under the free margin of the maxillary central caused marked blanching without being able to penetrate beyond the base of the gingival sulcus (Case Fig. 19–5C). A similar result was obtained when the probe was inserted under the free margin of the mandibular central (Case Fig. 19–5D). By the end of the sixth week the marginal tissues were fully healed and maturely keratinized, and, although it was not possible to restore the marginal gingivae to the contralateral teeth, they did create a harmonious level with the adjacent teeth.

There is one interesting footnote to this case. The patient had not had an epileptic seizure for more than two years when he first came for treatment, but the Dilantin therapy had been continued. At the author's urgent request, this therapy had been halted for the surgical and immediate postsurgical periods to increase the chances for

---

Case Figure 19–4   Continued.
without obliterating it. *E*, Immediate postoperative appearance of the tissues. Note the absence of free bleeding throughout the procedure, and that the frenectomy has not caused the tissues to separate (arrow). *F*, Both mucoperiosteal flaps have been repositioned and the tissues coapted and sutured with interrupted silk sutures along the lines of coaptation and through the embrasures. An incision had been made from the distogingival angle of the left cuspid to the mucogingival junction and the intervening apices of interdental papillae had been severed to release the mucoperiosteal flap. In each jaw the rotation of the flap anteriorly resulted in a denuded area between the first bicuspids and cuspids, each of which filled with clotted blood after the tissues were repositioned and sutured.

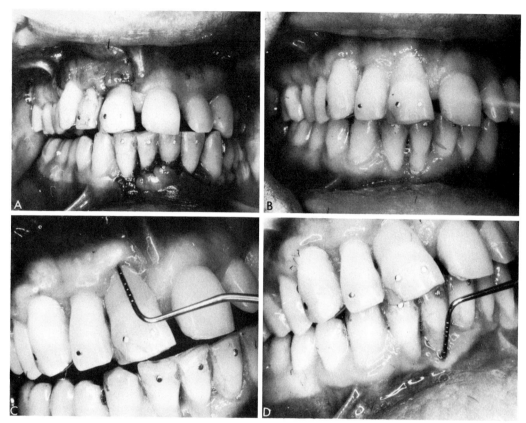

Case Figure 19–5. A, Appearance of the tissues immediately after removal of the sutures on the fifth postoperative day. Healing is very slow and at a very early initial stage, but sufficient to keep the flaps attached to the underlying tissues. The denuded areas are beginning to fill with immature granulation tissue as the blood clots are becoming organized. B, Three-week postoperative appearance of the tissues. Healing is almost complete, even in the denuded areas, but the marginal edges of the marginal gingivae over the two central incisors are slightly proliferative in contrast to the firm marginal gingivae over the other teeth. However, the tissues appear firmly attached to the underlying structures. C, A periodontal pocket probe has been inserted under the free gingival margin and is being forcefully pushed upward toward the apex of the tooth. The probe has penetrated less than 2 mm. and cannot penetrate further despite enough pressure to cause marked blanching of the tissues. D, The probe is being applied in a similar manner under the free gingival margin of the mandibular central, with the same result after penetrating only 1 mm. beyond the external marginal edge. Note that the pressure exerted against the maxillary tissue has caused a trace of blood to appear at that site, further evidence of the fact that pressure had been applied to try to establish whether tissue reattachment had occurred.

normal tissue healing, with the stipulation that if the epileptic seizures recurred, the Dilantin therapy would be resumed immediately. During that period the patient was maintained on phenobarbital and other drugs and remained free of attacks. He refused to resume the Dilantin therapy after the treatments were completed and has not had any epileptic seizures during the three year period of postoperative observation. There are undoubtedly many similar cases where the patient continues to be maintained on Dilantin medication as a prophylactic measure long after any real need for it exists.

Periodontoclasia Complicated by Unrelated Systemic Disease

This category differs in one major respect from the preceding categories. The latter had one common denominator; in every instance the periodontal disease was either directly attributable to or intimately interrelated with the systemic disease. In this category the periodontoclasia is neither attributable to nor interrelated with the systemic disease, but the systemic condition increases the complexity of treatment materially. It may also influence the ability of the tissue to heal and to regenerate.

In the case that is about to be reviewed, the influence of the disease on the treatment plan and on the surgical procedure itself was a known and predictable factor. But the matter of whether it would influence the tissue response to treatment was a totally unknown and unpredictable factor.

CASE 20

The degree and extent of periodontal deterioration, particularly the condition of the terminal abutment teeth of the patient's maxillary and mandibular fixed bridges, would have made the prognosis of treatment in this case unfavorable, even if her systemic health had been excellent. Superimposition of the handicaps created by the multiple sclerosis of which the patient was a victim would have been insurmountable and doomed the chances for successful treatment if only the "traditional" methods of treatment had been available. Thanks to the unique advantages electrosurgery offers the skilled therapist, all the extensively involved abutment teeth were treated successfully and were retained for continued functional use.

PATIENT. A 59-year-old white female.

HISTORY. She had been stricken with multiple sclerosis 29 years previously. The disease had incapacitated her from the neck down but had not impaired her mental functions at all. Although her muscles of mastication remained functional, she had difficulty moving her head and keeping her mouth open and was unable to expectorate.

Her brother, the referring dentist, had, under appalling operative handicaps, restored her dentition with a maxillary fixed bridge extending from molar to molar and bilateral mandibular bridges extending from cuspid to molar. The occlusion was excellent and the restoration was well fitted and properly fabricated, but the gingivae throughout the mouth underwent progressive deterioration that jeopardized the continuing usefulness of the terminal abutments for the bridges. She was referred for definitive treatment to try to preserve the dentition and avoid need for removal of and replacement of her prostheses.

CLINICAL EXAMINATION. The maxillary teeth had been splinted into a "roundhouse" unit extending from the maxillary left first molar to the right second bicuspid and continued as a cantilevered first molar pontic. The marginal gingiva had receded about 1 to 2 mm. from the abutment teeth, and the tissue was hyperplastic and atonal. The mandibular gingivae were in a similar condition, including the gingivae on the labial aspect of the anterior teeth that had not been restored with crowns (Case Fig. 20–1A).

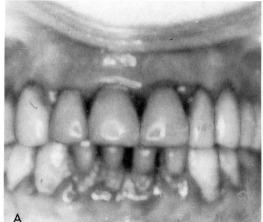

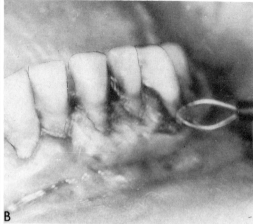

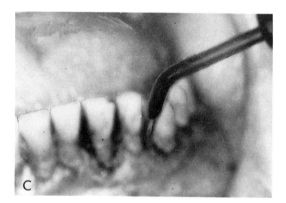

Case Figure 20–1. Periodontal therapy for a multiple sclerosis patient. A, Preoperative appearance. The gingival tissues in both mandible and maxilla are severely engorged and grossly hyperplastic; in the mandible, heavy accretion of salivary calculus detached the tissue from the teeth. In the maxilla there was proliferation of tissue under the free margins of the left central and lateral. There were diastemas between the mandibular centrals and between the left central and lateral incisors due to pathological migration of the central. B, Gingivoplasty being performed in the mandibular left quadrant with a flame-shaped loop electrode to reduce and recontour the tissues. C, Infrabony pockets being debrided with a 17-mm. periodontal electronic curet electrode.

Insertion of a periodontal pocket probe revealed many deep infrabony pockets, with a number of teeth having multiple pockets but an appreciable amount of healthy bone remaining between them. There was a deep pocket along the palatal root of the maxillary left first molar, and a deep pocket, an obvious trifurcation involvement, in the same tooth. The mandibular anterior teeth had moderately heavy deposits of calculus on the labial and lingual surfaces.

TREATMENT. The customary treatment routine was altered in two ways, since tissue repair in the multiple sclerosis patient is likely to be unusual. In periodontal therapy it is axiomatic to eliminate all unfavorable local factors, such as salivary or serumnal calculus, before surgery. Even when quadrant surgery is contemplated it is customary to perform complete prophylaxis. Under normal circumstances supplementary scaling poses no problems. But for this patient, who was unable to expectorate normally, a prophylaxis was a harrowing ordeal, although it was likely that additional prophylaxis would be required. The patient had to be transported in a special van with a ramp for her wheelchair, and the icy conditions at the time threatened to prevent continuity of treatment. Even if no interruptions occurred, by the time the third quadrant would be ready for surgery a supplementary prophylaxis would be required. Therefore, instead of performing a complete prophylaxis initially, an atypical treatment plan was formulated to perform a prophylaxis for each quadrant immediately prior to surgery.

Although the usual procedure would be to begin periodontal surgery in the maxillary right quadrant, there were two compelling reasons for beginning treatment in the mandibular left quadrant. The infrabony pockets in this quadrant were deeper and the teeth were more mobile, thus offering the least favorable prognosis. Should the end result prove unfavorable, or the systemic disease impair healing, the teeth in this quadrant would be more expendable. Since the response of the tissues to treatment was unpredictable, and to minimize the damage if poor healing resulted, this quadrant was chosen for the initial surgical procedure.

The quadrant was anesthetized with an inferior alveolar-lingual regional block injection. The salivary and serumnal calculus was removed. Upon completion of the partial prophylaxis a flame-shaped loop electrode was selected, and the cutting current output was set at 6 on the instrument panel. The edematous condition of the tissues suggested need for a current output more potent than the 4.5 to 5 that is usually adequate.

The activated electrode was used with a planing motion to reduce the labial and lingual gingivae to normal contour (Case Fig. 20–1B), without exposure of more root surfaces or lowering the gingival level. The flame-shaped loop was replaced with a 17-mm. hatchet-shaped periodontal loop electrode and cutting current output was reduced to 4. The activated electrode was used with an up-down and rotary motion to debride the pockets (Case Fig. 20–1C). This electrode was then replaced with the hoe-shaped 17-mm. periodontal loop, which was used along the inner surface of the gingival portion of the pockets to resect the epithelial lining uniformly and effectively. When all the loose fragments of tissue had been lifted out from the defects with an inactivated loop, the transilluminating lamp was used to verify that the debridement was complete. Bleeding was induced in each defect with periodontal curets and/or the tip of a half-round explorer that had been opened to almost a straight line. Powdered Gelfoam was deposited into the larger defects and mixed with the blood to form a spongy mass. When the blood had clotted, a cement pack, mixed to a hard consistency, was adapted around the surgical field, with care to avoid displacing the blood clots and forcing cement into the defects. The practical nurse who accompanied the patient was given instructions for her postoperative care.

The patient returned on the fifth postoperative day. Her nurse reported that there had been no need for postoperative sedation. The cement pack was removed, the tissues were gently irrigated and sponged dry, and tincture of myrrh and benzoin was applied in air-dried layers.

The maxillary left quadrant was anesthetized and a thorough prophylaxis was performed in the quadrant. A flame-shaped loop electrode was then used with cutting current set at 5 to perform the labial-buccal gingivoplasty. The proliferative tissue in the gingival sulci displaced the marginal gingivae away from the teeth. This would cause the marginal gingivae to become excessively thinned by the gingivoplasty. The loop was therefore first used to reduce the interdental papillae in the embrasures to concave sluiceways by planing the papillae in a coronal direction (Case Fig. 20–2A). This exaggerated the thickness and bulge of the labial marginal gingivae and thus helped to avoid excessive thinning of the marginal gingivae by the gingivoplasty.

The gingivoplasty having been completed on the labial aspect, a 17-mm., 90-degree-angle periodontal loop electrode was used with cutting current reduced to 4, to debride the trifurcation of the first molar. The involvement was extensive and required removal of the tissue to create a bucco-palatal tunnel (Case Fig. 20–2B). The trifurcation was inspected visually with a mouth mirror (Case Fig. 20–2C) and by

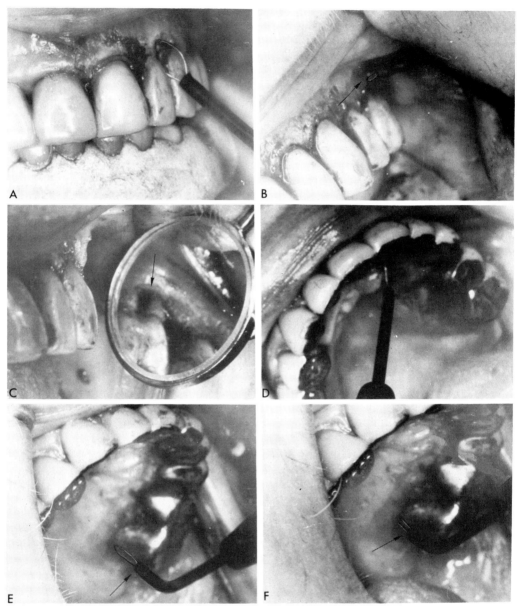

Case Figure 20–2. A, Gingivoplasty in maxillary left quadrant with a flame-shaped loop electrode. Because of subgingival proliferation and the thinness of the marginal gingivae exaggerated therefrom, the interdental papillae are being reduced to form concave self-cleansing sluiceways, thus bringing the labial gingivae into more pronounced contour that will help to recontour them with less hazard of resecting too much tissue. B, Labial and buccal gingivoplasty has been completed, and debridement of the trifurcation involvement of the first molar is being performed with a right-angle periodontal electronic loop curet. C, Mirror-image appearance of the trifurcation (arrow) after debridement has been completed and deep infrabony pockets at the distal of the molar and mesial of the molar have been thoroughly debrided. D, Gingivoplasty being performed on the palatal aspect with a flame-shaped loop electrode. E and F, Deep infrabony pocket along the palatal root of the molar being thoroughly debrided with the 17-mm. periodontal loop electrode. E shows the electrode after penetrating about 3 mm. into the defect. F shows the electrode has penetrated about 12 mm. into the defect.

transillumination to determine completion of the debridement. The flame-shaped loop electrode was then used with current output set at 6 to perform the palatal gingivoplasty (Case Fig. 20–2D). This electrode was replaced with a 17-mm. hatchet-shaped periodontal loop electrode that was used with current set at 4 to debride the infrabony pocket that extended along the palatal aspect of the palatal root almost to its apex (Case Fig. 20–2E and F). When this debridement was completed, bleeding was induced in the various defects and powdered Gelfoam introduced into the largest of them. A stiff mix of periodontal pack cement of sufficient quantity to cover the mandibular as well as the maxillary quadrant was prepared and applied to the two areas after tincture of myrrh and benzoin had been applied to the maxillary surgical field.

The patient was again brought in on the fifth postoperative day and the cement packs were removed from both areas. On inspection after gentle superficial irrigation the mandibular quadrant appeared to be healing satisfactorily and would need no further protection with cement packs. The maxillary quadrant also appeared to be healing satisfactorily. Tincture of myrrh and benzoin was applied to both areas. The prophylaxis was then performed in the mandibular right quadrant in preparation of the periodontal electrosurgery in that area, and the gingivoplasty and infrabony pocket debridement were performed in the manner previously described. Debridement of the defects was completed and bleeding was induced. After clotting occurred, cement packs were applied to this quadrant and the maxillary left quadrant. The patient was again brought in on the fifth postoperative day for removal of the packs and cleansing of the tissues. The maxillary quadrant was sufficiently healed to discard use of the cement pack, but a fresh pack was applied to the mandibular quadrant.

Five days later she was brought in for treatment of the fourth and final quadrant, but she asked that the surgery be deferred one week as she was feeling weak due to an upset stomach from the prolonged liquid-semisolid diet. The cement pack was removed from the mandibular quadrant and the cleansing by gentle irrigation was performed. The tissues in this quadrant also were healing rapidly and uneventfully, and did not require further cement pack protection.

Inclement weather prevented her return for almost three weeks. During the entire period since the surgery had begun her nurse had been laving the tissues and massaging them exactly as demonstrated to her before the treatment had been initiated, and even the untreated quadrant showed distinct clinical evidence of having benefited from the stimulation and improved blood supply. The tissue tone was improved and the gingival hyperplasia was less marked.

The quadrant was anesthetized with posterior superior alveolar, infraorbital, and palatal blocks. A flame-shaped loop electrode was activated with current set at 5 and was used first to create the interproximal concave sluiceways (Case Fig. 20–3A). The infrabony pocket debridement was performed with the 17-mm. periodontal loop electrodes; a gingivoplasty was performed on the palatal tissues with the flame-shaped loop (Case Fig. 20–3B). Upon completion of the debridement and clotting of the blood in the infrabony defects, a cement pack was applied, removed, and replaced on the fifth day and discontinued on the tenth day.

The patient was seen semimonthly for the next three months, and areas that required more efficient massage were brought to the attention of the patient's nurse. Examination of the mouth at the end of that period of postoperative observation disclosed excellent tissue tone throughout the mouth, normal gingival architecture (Case Fig. 20–3C), and remarkable immobility of the teeth. The posterior areas were examined with the aid of a mouth mirror. The examinations revealed that the trifurcation in the maxillary left quadrant was fully healed and the intraradicular tunnel

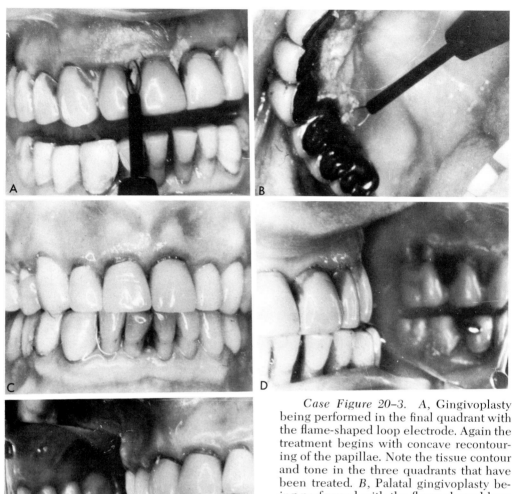

Case Figure 20–3. *A,* Gingivoplasty being performed in the final quadrant with the flame-shaped loop electrode. Again the treatment begins with concave recontouring of the papillae. Note the tissue contour and tone in the three quadrants that have been treated. *B,* Palatal gingivoplasty being performed with the flame-shaped loop electrode. *C,* Postoperative appearance of the gingival tissues. The tone is excellent, the gingival architecture is normal, and the teeth are firm. Despite the removal of the subgingival proliferative tissue from the maxillary teeth, only about 1.5 to 2 mm. of gold can be seen—the same amount as was visible preoperatively. *D,* Mirror image of the healed trifurcation. The tissues have healed, leaving a self-cleansing sluiceway between the roots of the tooth. The infrabony pockets along the mesial of the molar and distal of the bicuspid are completely filled and obliterated. Bubbles of saliva appear between the mandibular bicuspid and molar. *E,* Appearance of tissues in posterior on right side as seen in a mirror. Normal tone and contour and well-defined zones of attached gingivae, which had not been clinically discernible preoperatively, are present in both jaws. A large bubble of saliva is present at the mandibular first molar.

was self-cleansing (Case Fig. 20–3*D*). The infrabony defects were impenetrable; the periodontal pocket probe penetrated to the bases of the sulci (from 1 to 1.5 mm.), and the interdental papillae were firmly attached. Clinical inspection of the right side revealed similar evidence of complete repair and reattachment (Case Fig. 20–3*E*), and the patient was dismissed from active supervision, except for semi-annual inspections to detect and arrest any future incipient deteriorations. In the eight years that have elapsed the tissues have remained normal and, except for regular periodic prophylaxis, she has not required further treatment.

This case demonstrated that although multiple sclerosis is a tragic, totally incapacitating disease, it apparently does not impair the body's ability to repair. It also demonstrated that faithful vigorous oral physiotherapy can improve tissue tone, reduce edema and hyperplasia, and help to maintain normal gingival health.

III. TREATMENT OF INDIVIDUAL INFRABONY POCKETS

In the cases that have been reviewed, the infrabony pockets, including bifurcation and trifurcation involvements, have been treated, with few exceptions, by debridement with the electronic loop electrode curets, without reflecting flaps to accomplish it. (See Figure 19–7.)

When the entire mouth is being treated and there are infrabony pockets involving all or almost all the teeth, and often multiple pockets around a tooth, incising mucoperiosteal flaps to expose the defects is unnecessary. Because of the increased likelihood that the flap coaptation will be handicapped by lack of sound bony support when the infrabony defects are large, the author has found that reflection of the flap is unnecessary, since the internal surfaces of the defects can be visualized by transillumination or examined digitally with the same electrode, used inactivated. (See Figure 19–8.)

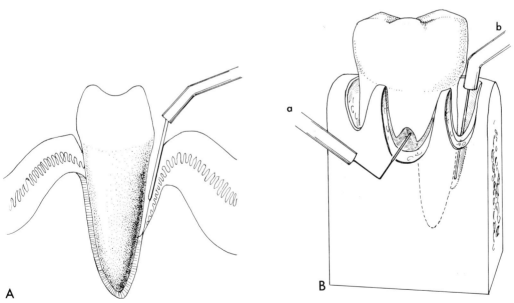

Figure 19–7.   A, The 45-degree-angle hoe-shaped loop electrode is being used to perform the internal bevel resection of the epithelial lining of the periodontal pocket of a single-rooted tooth. B, Cross-section of infrabony pockets of a double-rooted tooth; a right-angle hoe-shaped loop electrode is being used to debride the bifurcation (a) and a 45-degree-angle hatchet-shaped electrode is being used to debride the vertical infrabony pocket (b).

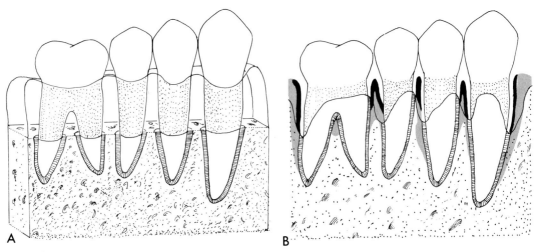

Figure 19–8. A, Cross-section of jaw showing uniform horizontal circumscribing periodontal destruction of investing alveolar bone. *B,* Cross-section of jaw showing the more common irregular vertical infrabony pockets, with much of the normal structure remaining intact.

When the infrabony pocket is limited to a single tooth or two adjacent teeth, and there will be no problem of lack of bony support for the flap when it is restored to position for suturing the coapted margins, reflection of the flap can facilitate the debridement of large defects without jeopardizing the outcome of the treatment. The treatment of the individual infrabony pockets in this series of cases will employ the mucoperiosteal flaps.

Single Root Involvement

CASE 21

This case presented seemingly hopeless periodontal deterioration of an infrabony pocket affecting a key abutment tooth. It demonstrates successful electrosurgical eradication of the pocket pathology and restoration of the tooth for functional usefulness.

PATIENT. A 62-year-old white male.

HISTORY. The patient was referred for electrosurgical treatment of an infrabony pocket of the mandibular second bicuspid, an abutment for a Chayes' bridge restoring the first molar, or, if the prognosis was deemed hopeless, extraction of the tooth.

CLINICAL EXAMINATION

Extraoral. Negative.

Intraoral. There was marked gingival hyperemia and edema on the buccal aspect of the mandibular right second bicuspid, extending around the distal angle of the tooth toward the lingual surface. The tooth was highly mobile and sensitive to percussion and lateral pressure. Pulp vitality test produced a somewhat hypersensitive response indicating probable hyperemia and inflammation of the pulp tissue. The marginal gingiva around the distobuccal half of the tooth was detached. A flexible silver probe was inserted into the marginal crevice after topical anesthetic had

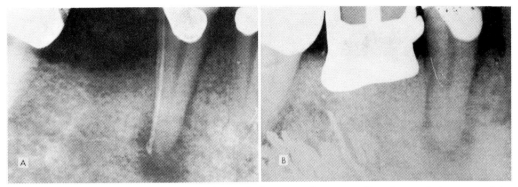

Case Figure 21–1. Eradication of an infrabony pocket extending beyond the apex of the tooth, a key abutment. *A,* Preoperative roentgenogram with a gutta-percha point inserted into the infrabony pocket as a marker shows the marker extending beyond the apex of the tooth. *B,* Postoperative roentgenogram taken four months postoperatively reveals evidence of complete alveolar regeneration, with calcification almost complete. The tooth is serving as a useful abutment for a small Chayes bridge.

been sprayed into it. The probe advanced toward the apex unimpeded. For maximum penetration a gutta-percha point was substituted for the probe, and a roentgenogram was taken with the point *in situ* as a radiopaque pocket marker to designate the exact depth of the destructive process.

The roentgenogram shows the gutta-percha point projecting down about 0.5 mm. beyond the apex of the tooth (Case Fig. 21–1).

TREATMENT. The affected bicuspid was an abutment for a small Chayes' bridge, and the patient was very anxious to retain it. He was warned that the prognosis was highly doubtful and that periodontal surgery must be considered as only an experiment in a case as advanced as his. He welcomed the risk so long as there was even a remote possibility that the tooth might be saved, and accepted full responsibility for the procedure.

The mouth was prepared and inferior alveolar block anesthesia administered. A 45-degree-angle fine needle electrode was selected and current output set at 3.5 for electrosection. A vertico-oblique incision was started at the distoproximal angle of the first bicuspid (Case Fig. 21–2) and carried downward and slightly posteriorly toward the apex of the second bicuspid. The incision was then extended along the edentulous alveolar ridge halfway to the molar. The incised tissue was undermined with a periosteal elevator and retracted. A small opening in the buccal alveolar margin between the bone and distal half of the root was revealed. The defect space was not large enough to permit introduction and manipulation of the electrode. It was therefore enlarged slightly by increasing the alveolar marginal space with a small fissure bur.

The needle electrode was replaced with a narrow 45-degree-angle U-shaped loop electrode and current output increased to 4.5 for electrosection. The activated electrode was introduced into the defect through the enlarged opening on the buccal surface and manipulated with push-pull and slightly rotary motions to remove the necrotic debris. A J-loop electrode with a small hook-like remnant of the loop remaining at the tip (see page 289) was substituted and used to complete debridement in areas at the base of the defect which the regular loop had been unable to reach.

Since the pulp of this tooth was vital and hypersensitive it was particularly impor-

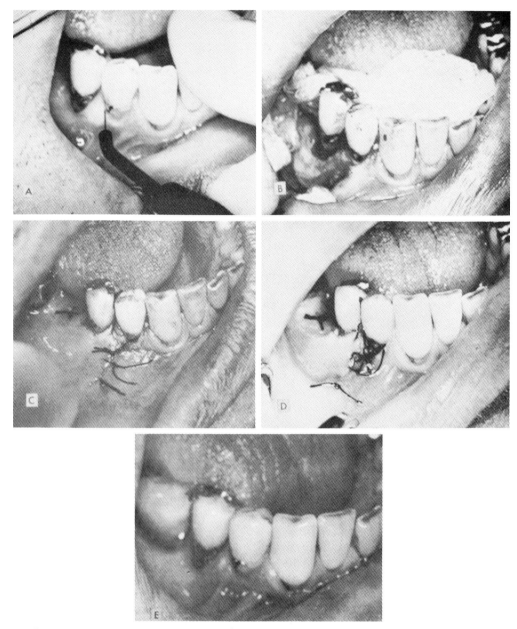

Case Figure 21–2. Operative procedure. *A,* A vertico-oblique incision from the gingival margin to the mucobuccal fold is started with a 45-degree-angle fine needle electrode. *B,* Flap is reflected and defect margin ramped to provide access for a narrow U-shaped loop electrode. *C,* Debridement having been completed, the flap is restored and sutured with buccal sutures and one on the crest of the alveolar ridge. *D,* Appearance of the tissues on the fifth postoperative day, with the sutures still in position. Primary healing of the incision is complete, and the tissue tone is excellent. *E,* Appearance of the tissues four months postoperatively. Soft tissue healing is complete. The tissues are firmly reattached to the necks of the teeth and alveolar bone. The pocket has been obliterated. The tissue tone is excellent, and the line of incision is invisible.

tant to avoid overheating the root and periapical bone during the manipulation. The broken loop electrode was ideal for this purpose. It could be manipulated rapidly and kept in constant motion for a few seconds at a time, and could be rotated almost as easily as a fine needle electrode in the confined area. Even the regular narrow loop electrode could be used safely by keeping it alternately activated for one to two seconds and deactivated for equal periods. Used in this manner it was not necessary to remove and reinsert the electrode every few seconds. (Since the vitality of such teeth has not been impaired by this procedure it is apparently a safe treatment formula.)

Debridement having been completed, a mixture of medicated, powdered surgical gelatin and cultured despeciated bone paste was inserted and mixed with blood present in the defect. The flap was restored and the margins were coapted and sutured with silk sutures on the buccal aspect, interproximally, and on the edentulous saddle area. Cosa-Tetrastatin was prescribed for three days and he was given complete postoperative instructions.

He returned on the fifth postoperative day. The area was irrigated and the sutures were removed. Healing was progressing very satisfactorily by primary intention and the tissues appeared to be firmly reattached to the necks of the teeth and the alveolar bone. Tincture of myrrh and benzoin was applied in air-dried layers, and vitamin B complex, ascorbic acid, and Knox clear gelatin were prescribed as dietary supplements.

The patient was seen postoperatively for the next four weeks at regular weekly intervals. During that period healing continued to progress rapidly and uneventfully and by the end of that time the soft-tissue healing appeared complete. A roentgenogram showed the defect area almost fully filled with regenerating bone which had begun to undergo normal calcification.

The patient was requested to return in three months for further postoperative observation. At his next visit tissue reattachment was so complete that the silver probe could not be introduced beyond the free margin. The gingivae appeared normal and the tissue tone was excellent. A final roentgenogram taken at that visit showed the original area of radiolucency completely obliterated. The area immediately adjacent to the tooth was fully filled with regenerating bone which appeared to have undergone almost complete maturation.

Clinically, the tooth was firm and was serving as a useful abutment for a Chayes' bridge restoration. Although he has not been seen again, he has reported periodically that the tooth has remained firm and asymptomatic.

CASE 22

The ultimate outcome of this case was distinctly atypical, but serves to demonstrate the success that can be achieved with electrosurgical debridement of a deep infrabony pocket. The rapid temporary regeneration of tissue obtained despite the handicap of unsuspected insurmountable local disease resulted solely from the efficacy of electrosurgical debridement.

PATIENT.   A 70-year-old white male.

HISTORY.   As a physician himself, the patient's oral hygiene was exemplary. Despite meticulous care and regular dental supervision he developed periodontoclasia. He had received periodic periodontal curettage for many years. His mandibular left second bicuspid had suddenly become quite painful and considerably looser than his other teeth. His dentist found a very deep infrabony pocket on the mesial aspect of this tooth. He was referred for possible gingivoplasty or, if necessary, extraction of the tooth.

CLINICAL EXAMINATION

Extraoral.   Negative. Personal and family histories: negative.

Intraoral.   The roots of all his mandibular anterior teeth and the left first bicuspid root were denuded of their investing alveolar bone and gingival mucosa to approximately 1 cm. beyond their cemento-enamel junctions. The left first bicuspid had a large disto-occlusal inlay and a buccal cavity filled with gutta-percha. The labial gingival margin around the gutta-percha was slightly irritated and engorged. The second bicuspid was restored with a cast veneer crown. This tooth was quite mobile and there was a wide, deep pocket along the mesial aspect of its root.

Roentgenographic examination revealed marked destruction of the interseptal bone, creating a deep infrabony pocket that extended along three fourths of the full length of the root.

TREATMENT.   The patient was informed that the prognosis was very doubtful. His reaction was that if there was even a slight hope that the tooth might be saved he preferred to have the periodontal surgery performed as a calculated risk.

The mouth was prepared for surgery and mental block anesthesia administered. A 45-degree-angle fine needle electrode was selected and current output set at 3.5 for electrosection. With the electrode held at right angles to the tissues, an incision was started at the distogingival margin of the cuspid and extended downward and about 10 degrees backward to the mucobuccal fold (Case Fig. 22–1). The incised tissue was undermined, reflected from the underlying bone and retracted posteriorly. A small adherent blood vessel was torn when the flap was elevated. The bleeder was clamped and coagulated off the beaks of a mosquito hemostat with a small ball electrode and

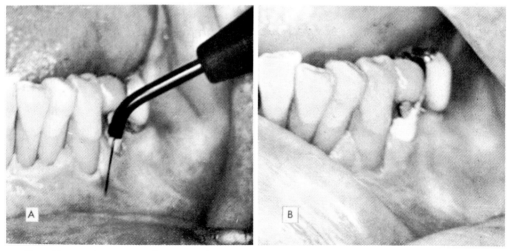

Case Figure 22–1.   Eradication of an infrabony pocket complicated by unsuspected presence of insurmountable local pathology.

A, A vertico-oblique incision is performed with a 60-degree-angle fine needle electrode, starting from the distogingival angle of the cuspid and extending from the gingival margin to the mucobuccal fold. Necrotic tissue fragments inaccessible to complete removal with the narrow loop electrode are destroyed *in situ* by fulguration. *B,* Appearance of the tissues three months postoperatively. The tissues appear healthy and are firmly reattached. Tooth mobility has been reduced to relatively normal limits.

current output set at 2 for biterminal electrocoagulation. The current was applied five times for two-second intervals with one-second intervening pauses to produce the desired hemostasis.

A narrow 45-degree-angle U-shaped loop electrode was substituted and current increased one degree. The electrode was inserted into the defect and used with rotary and push-pull motions to resect the necrotic contents of the pocket. Before the debridement could be completed, a small bleeder in a nutrient foramen first had to be coagulated with the small ball electrode. Debridement was resumed as soon as the bleeding was brought under control. Necrotic fragments in inaccessible areas were destroyed by fulguration *in situ*. Debridement was completed by trimming the sharp bone margin with a small bone file and curetting the proximal roots of the two teeth. The first bicuspid root surface was slightly rough. The detritus on the second bicuspid root surface seemed much rougher. Both root surfaces appeared much smoother after the planing.

A mixture of medicated surgical powdered gelatin and cultured bone paste was deposited into the defect and mixed with the blood present. The flap was restored and the marginal gingivae readapted to the teeth and bone. The incised margins were coapted and sutured with 0000 braided silk interrupted sutures. Then the detached interproximal papillae were sutured buccolingually. Tincture of myrrh and benzoin was applied topically and Cosa-Tetrastatin prescribed.

The patient returned on the fifth postoperative day and reported having had only moderate discomfort for the first two days. The line of incision was healing by primary union without cicatricial contraction. The gingival and interproximal tissues appeared firmly reattached to the alveolar bone and the necks of the teeth. The sutures were removed and tincture of myrrh and benzoin was applied.

He was seen again two weeks later. Healing was almost complete and the tissue tone was excellent. When he returned two weeks later the tissues were fully healed, with no gross visible evidence that any surgery had been performed in the area. He was discharged from active treatment and asked to return in three months for further postoperative observation and final roentgenograms.

The original roentgenogram had shown marked radiolucence along the medial surface of the second bicuspid root where bone destruction almost 3 mm. in width extended to within about 4 mm. of the apex of the second bicuspid. The first postoperative roentgenogram taken six weeks postoperatively, when he was discharged from treatment, showed noteworthy bone regeneration which had obliterated more than half of the length and width of the original defect area. The final roentgenogram taken when he returned three months later showed most of the defect obliterated by regenerating bone. The lower two thirds of the defect was fully obliterated but some radiolucence persisted in the upper portion nearest to the root surface (Case Fig. 22–2).

The tooth was firm and the gingival mucosa was healthy and firmly attached to the necks of the teeth and alveolar bone. The patient was seen semiannually for the next 1½ years, during which time the results remained highly gratifying.

Almost two years after the surgery was performed the gingival mucosa around the tooth suddenly deteriorated and the tooth became loose again. He returned immediately for consultation. The tissues were found to be almost identical with their original condition. They were hyperemic, hypertrophied, detached, and edematous; an infrabony pocket in the original area was again in evidence.

Roentgenographic examination confirmed the implications of the clinical appearance. The regenerated interseptal bone had deteriorated and was more radiolucent

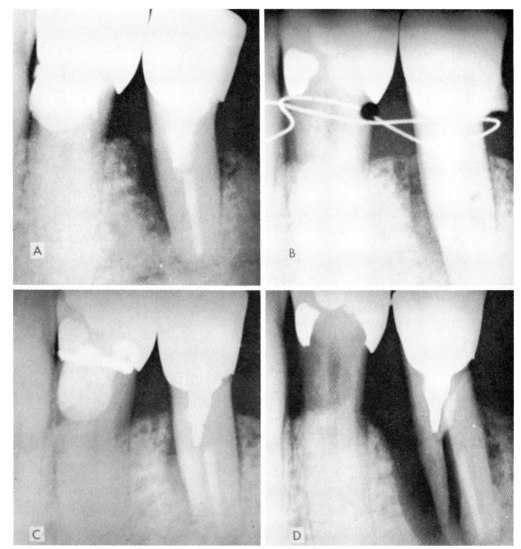

Case Figure 22–2. Roentgenographic record. *A*, Preoperative view shows marked destruction of interseptal bone that extends three quarters down the length of the root. The tooth is devitalized and has been restored with a veneer crown over a gold core which is inserted into the canal at an angle. *B*, Six weeks postoperative view. The teeth have been splinted, with stainless steel continuous loop wiring. There is marked reduction in the area and degree of radiolucency, indicating substantial alveolar repair. *C*, A view taken three months postoperatively shows the pocket almost fully obliterated by alveolar regeneration to the crest of the alveolar ridge. A small triangular area of moderate radiolucency is still noticeable immediately below the alveolar crest. *D*, Final view, almost two years later, reveals complete deterioration of the regenerated bone due to vertical fracture of the tooth.

than ever. He was not aware of any trauma or other logical reason for the sudden regression and was unable to account for it.

The area was prepared and anesthetized; the surgical debridement was performed exactly as previously described. The response to this treatment was very disappointing. Scarcely any improvement resulted. While checking the mobility of the tooth, pressure was inadvertently applied in a slightly lateral direction instead of anteroposteriorly. The tooth seemed to "give" with abrupt suddenness and became extremely loose. A roentgenogram taken at that time revealed that the root was fractured.

The tooth was immediately extracted. Examination showed that there had been a vertical fracture of the root, and that the fracture line was in an oblique direction and had remained unobserved on the previous films. Accidental palpation in the mesiodistal direction had caused a separation along the fracture line with enough rotation of the mesial fragment to show up clearly on the film. There was evidence of some attempt at repair and bridging with cementum which may have accounted for the marked roughness of the root noted during planing.

If, as is almost absolutely certain, the fracture was present when the infrabony pocket was first treated, the original deterioration may have been produced by a slight displacement of the fragments which then healed while the tooth was immobilized with wire splints. Under such circumstances it is surprising and very gratifying that the initial excellent result, which lasted for almost two years, was achieved at all.

Debridement of Extensive Bifurcation Involvement

There are many varieties of bifurcation involvement. One type, demonstrated in Case 14, extends far beyond the furca and involves all or a major portion of one of the roots, yet still remains amenable to treatment. Another type consists of considerable destruction of the coronal end of the investing bone around both roots, creating a tunnel-like defect directly under and through the furca. When the circumscribing bone loss is not so extensive as to upset the normal 1:2 crown-root ratio and cause excessive hypermobility, this type can be treated successfully by gingivectomy. When, as in the case to be reviewed, the disease has caused great destruction of the interseptal bone but the buccal cortical plate still is largely intact, treatment by cold-steel instrumentation creates a tunnel through the furca that remains open permanently and facilitates effective oral physiotherapy. But when the treatment is performed by electrosection, repair of the defect is by a fill-in of interseptal bone that is complete except for the original convexity of the alveolar contour. However, the slightly concave contour creates a natural self-cleansing sluiceway between the roots.

CASE 23

PATIENT. A 42-year-old white female.

HISTORY. The patient neglected to go to her dentist for her regular 6-month check-up for the past two years. A few weeks ago she noticed that toothbrushing caused some bleeding of her gums and some tenderness in the right side of her lower jaw, so she consulted her dentist. He found evidence of a periodontal lesion between the roots of her lower right second molar on the buccal aspect of the tooth. A periapical x-ray film of the right molar area revealed extensive radiolucence between the roots of the second molar, confirming the clinical evidence of a bifurcation involvement. He therefore referred the patient to the author for definitive treatment of the periodontal lesion or extraction of the tooth.

CLINICAL EXAMINATION. The marginal gingiva was detached from the buccal aspect of the mandibular right second molar. A periodontal pocket probe was inserted and penetrated its full 10-mm. length without encountering resistance. A large molar gutta percha point was inserted almost its full length before it met resistance (Case Fig. 23–1). A periapical x-ray film was taken with the gutta percha point in situ as a radiopaque marker. The film showed virtually total destruction of the intraradicular bone of the second molar. Despite the extensive bone loss in the furcation, the tooth was only slightly mobile even under rather vigorous digital palpation.

TREATMENT. The area was prepared for surgery and an inferior alveolar–lingual nerve block was administered. A 45-degree-angle fine needle electrode was selected, and cutting current output was set at 3 on the power rheostat dial. The electrode was activated and used to create a vertico-oblique incision for a mucoperiosteal flap. The incision was started at the mesiogingival angle of the first and second molar interdental papilla, with care to avoid splitting the apex of the papilla, and was extended downward to the mucobuccal fold. The apical attachments of the papillae on either side of the second molar were severed with the same electrode, and the incised tissue was elevated with the broad end of a periosteal elevator and reflected to reveal the underlying bone.

This exposed to view an elliptical defect in the superior part of the buccal cortical bone over the second molar and several millimeters of denuded roots, with the gutta percha point marker in situ in the defect.

The mucoperiosteal flap was reflected and pulled taut to expose to view the epithelialized ventral surface that had covered the defect, and a flame-shaped loop electrode was used with current output set at 4.5 to resect the tissue by shaving the tissue surface by loop planing. The granulomatous debris in the bifurcation was then resected with a 17-mm. periodontal loop curet used with current set at 4.5 and used for a fraction of a second each time with an up and down rotary movement to make contact with all the internal surfaces of the defect, followed by a 10-second pause interval to permit the heat to become fully dissipated before resuming the electronic curettage.

When complete debridement was verified by transillumination, the denuded root surfaces were carefully planed with steel periodontal curets to remove the *dead* cementum only. Bleeding was then encouraged by scraping the bone surfaces with a periodontal curet and a round explorer that had been opened so that it was almost a straight line to reopen the nutrient foramina. Powdered Gelfoam was introduced into the defect and mixed with the blood, and the mucoperiosteal flap was restored to position and sutured with interrupted silk sutures. A strip of adhesive dryfoil was applied over the sutures and a stiffly mixed periodontal pack was applied as a pressure pack to force the gingival tissue against the bone and tooth.

The patient was seen again on the fifth postoperative day, and the cement pack was removed. The line of incision showed evidence of beginning of primary repair. The patient, who had been instructed fully in the proper methods of massage to main-

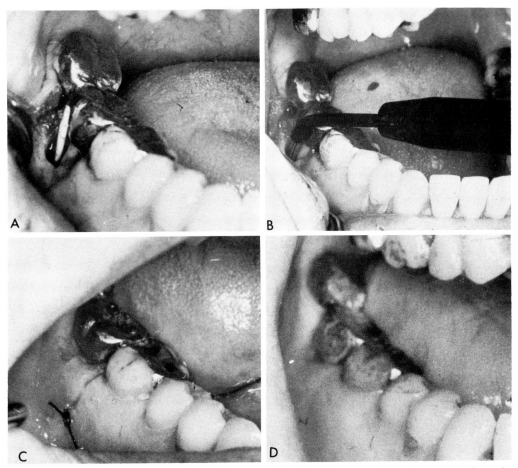

Case Figure 23–1. This case demonstrates the effectiveness of electrosurgical debridement of a large bifurcation infrabony pocket. It also demonstrates the use of a molar gutta percha point as a radiopaque x-ray marker. *A,* The mucoperiosteal flap having been incised, elevated, and reflected from the buccal aspect of the mandibular right first molar, a large defect into the bifurcation is fully exposed, as well as the large gutta percha point that had been inserted into the defect before the periapical x-ray of the tooth was taken. *B,* The bifurcation defect is being debrided by electrosection with a 17 mm. periodontal loop electrode being used as an electronic curet. *C,* Appearance of the tissues on the fifth postoperative day immediately after removal of the top suture and just prior to removal of the lower suture. *D,* Appearance of the gingival tissue three weeks postoperatively. The line of incision is just barely distinguishable due to incomplete surface keratinization. The tissue over the former opening into the bifurcation is firmly attached to the underlying tissues and the defect appears to be fully obliterated, without marked concavitation despite the large opening in the bone that had been present.

tain a high degree of oral physiotherapy, was instructed to institute the regimen of massage, beginning with an initial start of very gentle massage and increasing in vigor as the tissues matured. The patient was seen again two weeks later, at which time the tissue tone looked completely normal and healthy and, except for incomplete keratinization of the surface epithelium over the line of incision, the area was fully healed. The bone repair also was excellent but slightly concave, and about 2 mm. of the buccal aspect of the roots remained visible. The defect went on to complete repair and has not recurred.

CASE 24

This case is a typical example of intraradicular alveolar deterioration that extends to the buccal alveolar bone.

The bifurcation involvement in this type of case becomes relatively secondary in importance to the buccal extension, which may involve the entire investing bone around one root or even both roots. In the latter event the prognosis is usually hopeless and the tooth must be extracted. When only one root is involved, as in this instance, although the prognosis is very doubtful, it is not necessarily hopeless.

PATIENT.   A 43-year-old white male.

HISTORY.   The mandibular right second bicuspid and first molar had been extracted years previously. The right first bicuspid and second molar were devitalized teeth serving as abutments for a fixed bridge. Both teeth had been prepared for full crowns, and a temporary acrylic bridge had been constructed for use until the permanent bridge could be inserted.

While the permanent bridge was being processed, the buccal gingival mucosa suddenly became swollen, hyperemic and detached from the neck of the second molar. His dentist found marked roentgenographic evidence of intraradicular bone loss suggestive of a deep infrabony pocket. He was referred for gingivoplasty to eradicate the pocket and preserve the tooth for functional use as a key abutment.

CLINICAL EXAMINATION

Extraoral.   Negative.

Intraoral.   The acrylic bridge consisted of full acrylic crowns restoring the abutment teeth and a single molar pontic in the edentulous area. The bridge was firmly attached to the teeth although it was sealed with temporary cement.

The buccal gingival mucosa was edematous and detached from the second molar. A slight exudate was expressed by firm digital pressure against the swollen tissue. There was no palpable fluctuation. A silver probe inserted into the detached area advanced downward without resistance a distance of more than 1.5 cm. beyond the free margin.

Roentgenographic examination with the probe in situ showed the tip of the probe projecting 1.5 mm. beyond the apex of the distal root. There was a slight amount of radiolucence around the distal root suggestive of bone loss limited to the buccal aspect rather than circumferentially around the root.

TREATMENT.   The mouth was prepared for surgery and inferior alveolar block anesthesia administered. A 45-degree-angle fine needle electrode was selected and current output set at 3 for electrosection. A special wire frame cheek-lip retractor was inserted, and the four quadrants were blocked with gauze sponges to help keep the operative field free of saliva.

A vertical incision was started at the distal aspect of the first molar pontic, with a wiping motion, and extended from the crest of the alveolar ridge to the mucobuccal fold. A second horizontal incision was started 1 cm. distal to the distal surface of the second molar and carried anteriorly to the tooth (Case Fig. 24–1).

The incised tissue was reflected from the underlying bone, revealing a defect in the buccal marginal alveolar bone at the neck of the second molar. The flexible silver probe inserted through this defect readily advanced to the apical end of the tooth. The probe was removed, and a narrow 45-degree-angle long U-shaped loop electrode was inserted to the base of the defect. Current was increased to 4, and a considerable amount of necrotic debris was resected by using the activated electrode with push-pull and rotary motions.

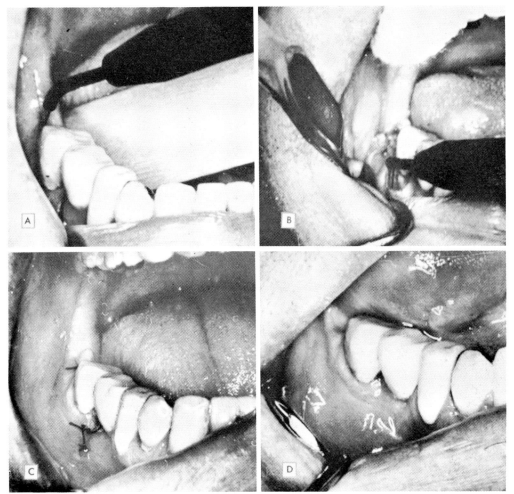

Case Figure 24–1.   Eradication of a bifurcation involvement, with destruction of the investing alveolar bone around one of the roots to and beyond the apex of the root. *A,* Incision made with a 45-degree-angle fine needle electrode in a vertical direction on the buccal aspect, and horizontally along the crest of the edentulous alveolar ridge. *B,* Flap reflected, debridement is performed with 90-degree-angle narrow U-shaped loop electrode. *C,* Appearance of the tissues on the fifth postoperative day. The sutures are still in position. Healing is progressing very favorably. *D,* Appearance of the tissues three months later. They are firmly reattached, their tone is excellent, and the line of incision is no longer visible.

Although the defect was large enough mesiodistally to permit insertion of a somewhat larger version of this loop electrode, the opening was too narrow to permit rotary use. In order to permit more rapid and rotary use of the electrode the superior margin of the buccal bone defect was ramped with a bone bur and bone file. The larger loop electrode was then inserted and used freely to thoroughly debride the root surfaces. Then the narrow loop electrode was replaced and used intraradicularly to curet debris from the bifurcation area by moving the loop in a postero-anterior direction with a scooping motion.

A few tenacious shreds of adherent necrotic tissue which could not be completely resected with the loop electrodes were destroyed *in situ* by fulguration with a heavy needle electrode and a current output of 9 for monoterminal application.

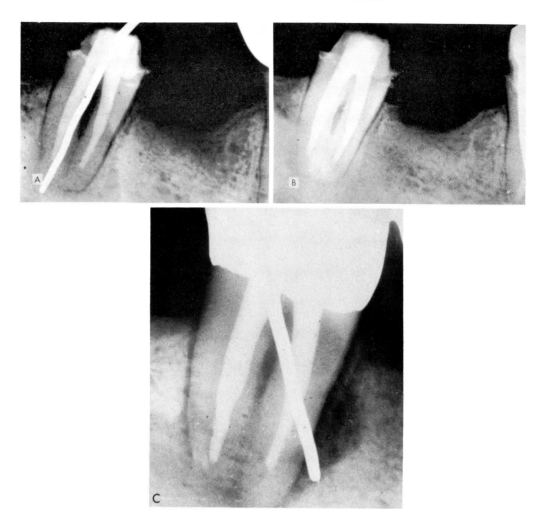

Case Figure 24–2. Roentgenographic record. *A,* Preoperative view shows the silver probe extending several millimeters beyond the apex of the molar. There is marked radiolucence. *B,* View taken three months postoperatively. The bone defect appears fully obliterated by regeneration of new alveolar bone which appears to be mature and well calcified. *C,* A 3-year postoperative x-ray of the same tooth. The regenerated bone has remained intact and normal despite the new pathologic condition that has developed on the mesial aspect of the tooth.

Debridement having been completed, bleeding was induced in the defect with a curet. A mixture of powdered surgical gelatin and cultured bone paste was inserted into the defect and mixed with the blood. The tissue flap was restored to position and sutured with two interrupted silk sutures inserted on the buccal aspect and a third suture inserted on the crest of the ridge near the distal aspect of the molar.

Three years postoperatively an infrabony pocket appeared that was identical in appearance to the original one. The silver probe was inserted into the new defect and an x-ray was taken. The film revealed that the original defect in the distal part of the tooth was fully healed, but a new infrabony defect had developed at the mesial part of the tooth. Despite the considerable breakdown of bone here, the area of bone regeneration at the distal aspect remains intact. Note the large area of internal resorption in the mesial root (Case Fig. 24–2*C*). The new periodontal lesion responded to treatment, but the internal resorption increased, and approximately two years after the periodontal lesion was treated successfully, the tooth had to be extracted owing to loss of the crown as a result of internal resorption.

Debridement of Extensive Trifurcation Involvement

CASE 25

The cases considered thus far have involved infrabony pockets resulting from deterioration of interseptal bone between teeth that originates on the buccal aspect and tends to remain confined to the medial surfaces of the involved teeth. This case presents another type of interseptal infrabony pocket. This type originates and points toward the palatal aspect of the interproximal embrasure, and tends to expand and destroy some of the investing alveolar bone around the palatal roots in addition to the interseptal bone. This case also serves to demonstrate the ease with which effective electrosurgical instrumentation can be performed in areas that are relatively inaccessible to controlled instrumentation by other methods.

PATIENT. A 56-year-old white female.

HISTORY. Sudden onset of pain in her maxillary right molar area and swelling of the palatal tissue around the molar teeth influenced her to consult her dentist. He found marked destruction of the interseptal bone between the first and second molars and a palatal paradontal abscess. She was referred for gingivoplasty or extraction of the teeth.

CLINICAL EXAMINATION

Extraoral. Negative.

Intraoral. The marginal mucosa on the palatal aspect of the two molars was detached from the teeth and alveolar bone. When the detached mucosa was gently retracted, considerable loss of investing alveolar bone and replacement with necrotic debris was plainly visible (Case Fig. 25–1A). Exploratory investigation under deeply sprayed topical anesthesia disclosed a deep infrabony pocket which extended almost to the apices of the two teeth and involved the distal aspect of the first molar palatal root and part of the mesial aspect of the palatal root of the second molar.

TREATMENT. The area was prepared for surgery and posterior superior alveolar and anterior palatine block anesthesia administered. A medium-sized 45-degree-angle U-shaped loop electrode was selected and current output set at 5.5 for electrosection. The detached tissue was retracted, and the electrode inserted into the defect and pulled with wiping motions against the inner surface of the gingival mucosa in order to scoop out the necrotic debris to the level of the alveolar bone.

A smaller version of this electrode was substituted and current output reduced to 4.5. This activated electrode was used with both push-pull and rotary motions to eradicate all the debris down to the base of the pocket and from the respective surfaces of the palatal roots of the two teeth (Case Fig. 25–1B).

When debridement was completed the surface bone margin of the defect was rounded with a slender bone file. A mixture of medicated powdered gelatin and cultured bone paste was inserted into the defect and mixed with blood in the area. The tissue was restored to normal position and secured by suturing the palatal interproximal papilla palatobuccally through the embrasure. A flame-shaped loop elec-

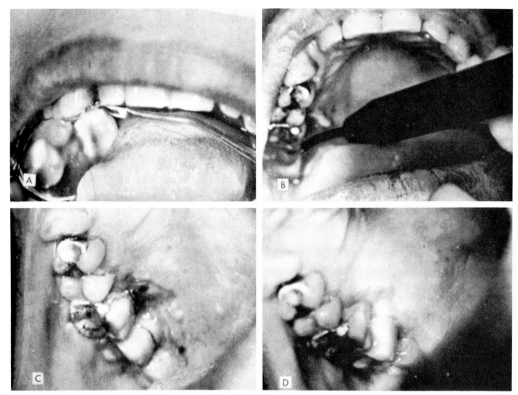

Case Figure 25–1.   Eradication of an infrabony pocket involving the palatal root of a maxillary molar. *A*, Mirror image of the pocket on the palatal aspect of the tooth. *B*, Necrotic tissue debrided with a narrow 45-degree-angle U-shaped loop electrode. *C*, Appearance of the tissues on the fifth postoperative day. The pocket is filled with normal reparative granulation tissue. The tissue is covered with a light surface layer of coagulum. The teeth have been immobilized by ligation with stainless steel wire. *D*, Appearance of the tissues seven weeks postoperatively. The area is fully healed, and the tissues are firmly reattached to the necks of the teeth and alveolar bone. The only evidence that surgery has been performed is the pinker color of the new tissue due to less keratinization of the surface epithelium.

trode was employed, with current output set at 6, to simultaneously resect the somewhat ulcerated marginal gingiva and restore it to normal contour and feather-edged margin. The molars were immobilized by ligating them with continuous-loop wiring. A surgical cement pack was then inserted over the operative field.

She returned on the fifth postoperative day and reported a completely uneventful postoperative period. The cement pack was removed and the area irrigated. Inspection revealed that the palatal gingiva was firm, granulating healthily, and snugly reattached to the necks of the two teeth (Case Fig. 25–1C). Tincture of myrrh and benzoin was applied and a fresh cement pack inserted.

The patient returned postoperatively at regular intervals for the next six weeks. Healing progressed steadily and uneventfully. By the end of that period the tissues were fully healed and normal in tone. There was complete tissue reattachment and obliteration of the infrabony pocket opening, and the interproximal papillae formed concave self-cleansing sluiceways. The only difference between the new tissue and the surrounding mucosa was the slightly lighter pink color due to less kera-tinization of the surface epithelium (Case Fig. 25–1D). After the wire ligature splints were removed, the teeth, which had been quite mobile, were normally firm.

She returned for observation once a month for the next three months. A roentgen-ogram taken at the third visit showed bone regeneration that matched the gingival repair in quality. She was seen thereafter semiannually for the next two years. During that period the teeth and their investing structures continued to remain normal and asymptomatic.

CASE 26

This case is a typical example of trifurcation involvement of a maxillary molar resulting from an intraradicular infrabony pocket originating on the palatal aspect. It also serves to demonstrate the effectiveness of electrosurgical debridement in an area that offers awkward access to cold-steel instrumentation.

PATIENT.   A 74-year-old white male in excellent health.

HISTORY.   The patient suddenly developed a localized swelling and tenderness on the palatal aspect of the maxillary left first molar, which served as a key abutment for a fixed bridge.

Ever since the bridge had been inserted he had been troubled with food impaction in an undercut created by the bridge in the affected area. He was referred for gingivoplasty as a means of preserving the tooth for continued functional use as a terminal abutment.

CLINICAL EXAMINATION

Extraoral.   Negative.

Intraoral.   The maxillary left cuspid and first molar were restored with cast-gold three-quarter crown inlay abutments for a fixed bridge carrying pontic restorations for the lateral and the two bicuspids. The pontics consisted of porcelain facings and cast gold backings. The junction of the second bicuspid pontic and the molar inlay created a deep undercut.

The palatal mucosa in the bicuspid-molar area was swollen, hyperemic and partially detached from the tooth. A deep infrabony pocket extending into the trifurcation was visible. The defect was filled with necrotic granulation tissue.

TREATMENT.   The area was prepared for surgery and posterior superior alveolar and anterior palatine block anesthesia administered. A 45-degree-angle fine needle electrode was selected and current output set at 4.5 for electrosection. An oblique incision was started at the distogingival angle of the first bicuspid pontic and extended 1.5 cm. medially on the palate (Case Fig. 26–1). The incision was carried across the attachment of the palatal interproximal papilla between the second bicuspid and first molar. The incised tissue was undermined and reflected from the underlying bone. A suture was inserted into the tip of the papilla and the flap was tied to the cuspid on the opposite side, out of the way.

The necrotic debris was resected with a narrow U-shaped loop electrode and current output set at 5; adherent fragments of tissue in the trifurcation were destroyed *in situ* by fulguration. An accretion of detritus on the medial aspects of the mesial and palatal roots was removed with McCall curets and a flat thin gold file.

When debridement was completed, some powdered medicated surgical gelatin was deposited and mixed with blood in the defect. The flap was then restored and

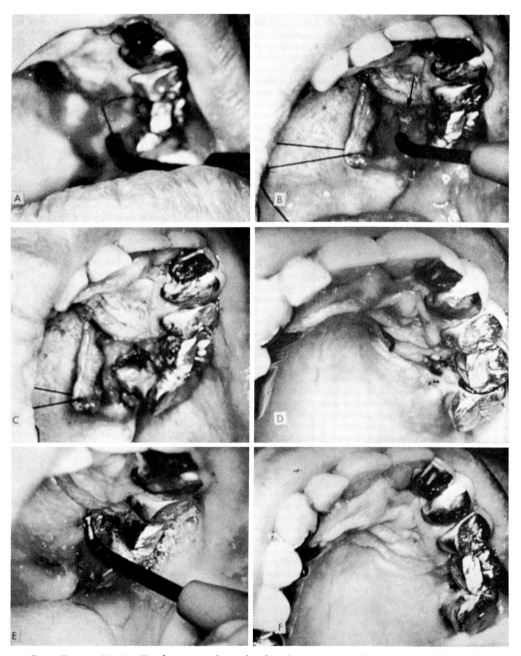

Case Figure 26–1.   Eradication of a palatal trifurcation involvement in a key abutment tooth. *A,* An oblique incision extending about 1.5 cm. from the gingival margin to the midline of the palate is made with a 45-degree-angle fine needle electrode. A moderate amount of bleeding results, which is brought under control by application of pressure. *B,* Flap is elevated and tied to the teeth on the opposite side to keep it out of the way. Debridement is completed by fulguration *in situ* (arrow). *C,* Appearance of the defect after debridement has been completed. *D,* Appearance of the tissues on the fifth postoperative day before the sutures have been removed. Healing by primary union is progressing very satisfactorily. *E,* Small retarded areas of healing and surface tissue irregularities are treated by coagulation with a small ball electrode. *F,* Appearance of the palatal tissues six weeks postoperatively. The tissue is fully reattached to the teeth and alveolar bone, the pocket site has been totally obliterated, and the tissue tone is excellent. Clinically the tooth is firm and asymptomatic.

secured in position with two palatal sutures and an interproximal suture. Panalba was prescribed for three days and postoperative instructions given.

He returned on the fifth postoperative day. Healing was progressing very satisfactorily. The·incision was healing by primary intention. The interproximal tissue was firmly reattached. The tissue tone was excellent and there was no edema. The sutures were removed. A slight bulge of tissue at the edge of the area of the defect, which had been planed to eliminate the undercut at the time of surgery, was reduced to normal level by superficial spot coagulation with a small ball electrode and current output set at 1 for biterminal electrocoagulation. Healing continued to progress satisfactorily and uneventfully, and the only postoperative treatment required was occasional spot coagulation in the undercut area and applications of tincture of myrrh and benzoin.

He was seen at weekly intervals for six weeks. At the end of that period healing was complete. This case has been completed too recently to report further postoperative observation at this time but the course of this case suggests a normal sequence with continued functional usefulness of the tooth.

IV. MISCELLANEOUS PERIODONTAL PROCEDURES

Relation of Abnormal Traction to Periodontoclasia

Maxillary labial frena, mandibular labial frena, and muscle attachments (especially broad-band attachments) that extend overly close to the gingival margins may tear loose the periodontal attachments to the alveolar bone and thereby trigger the onset of periodontal disease.

When a single slender muscle attachment exerts abnormal traction against marginal and cemental gingivae it should be resected or repositioned by frenectomy or frenotomy or their equivalent in order to eliminate or relieve the source of gingival trauma regardless of whether it is a frenum or another prominent muscle.

When the traction is exerted by a broad band of muscle attachment or by multiple individual slender strands of muscle so closely bunched that they function as a single unit, a pushback or combination of pushback and frenectomy may become necessary. Not infrequently, damage produced by abnormal traumatizing muscle attachments disrupts gingival harmony so badly that eliminating the cause may not suffice. Plastic repair of the defect for aesthetics and protection by repositioning the gingival mucosa may also be required.

FRENECTOMY-FRENOTOMY

The ideal frenectomy for periodontal therapy is one that eliminates the traumatizing effect on the periodontium of abnormal muscle pull against the gingivae without sacrificing control of lip movement by the upper portion of the frenum which blends with the mucosa of the inner aspect of the lip.

CASE 27

This case is an example of periodontal deterioration that may result from abnormal muscle pull against the marginal and cemental gingivae. In this instance an abnormally broad maxillary labial frenum not only extended around to the nasopalatine papilla and created a diastema between the teeth but also became superimposed on the labial marginal gingivae like a neoplasm and created additional traction against the tissues.

This case also affords an excellent demonstration of the efficacy of electrosurgery for eradication of abnormal gingival trauma without creating new stresses from cicatricial contraction.

PATIENT. A 28-year-old white female.

HISTORY. The patient was a dental hygienist and her oral hygiene was meticulous. The lower portion of her maxillary labial frenum and the labial marginal gingivae of the two centrals suddenly became inflamed. Traction of the frenum resulted in detachment of the proximal gingivae of the two teeth, with pocket formation. She was referred for frenectomy.

CLINICAL EXAMINATION

Extraoral. The columella of her nose dipped downward and the median line of her lip pulled upward. She had been informed by a plastic surgeon that the abnormal traction of her maxillary labial frenum was responsible.

Intraoral. The over-all condition of her mouth was excellent. There was a 3 mm. diastema between the maxillary centrals. A very broad prominent labial frenum extended down to the crest of the ridge, passed through the separation, and then blended into the nasopalatine papilla. The frenum fanned out near the crest of the ridge, and part of it became superimposed on the marginal gingivae (Case Fig. 27–1).

The proximal marginal gingivae were detached from the two centrals and the alveolar bone, creating moderately deep pockets on the medial surfaces of the two teeth. Purulent exudate could be expressed from the pockets.

Roentgenographic examination revealed radiolucence of the alveolar bone in the median line between the centrals, indicating some destruction of the bone forming

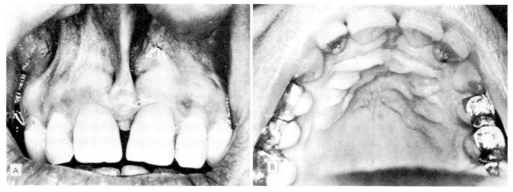

Case Figure 27–1. Frenectomy to eliminate abnormal traction against marginal and cemental gingivae which has resulted in formation of periodontal pockets. *A,* Intraoral view, labial aspect. There is a prominent labial frenum which fans out near the crest of the ridge, passes through a diastema between the centrals, and appears to be superimposed upon and merge into the marginal gingivae. *B,* Palatal view shows heavy band of tissue filling the diastema space, which may account for the diastema having developed.

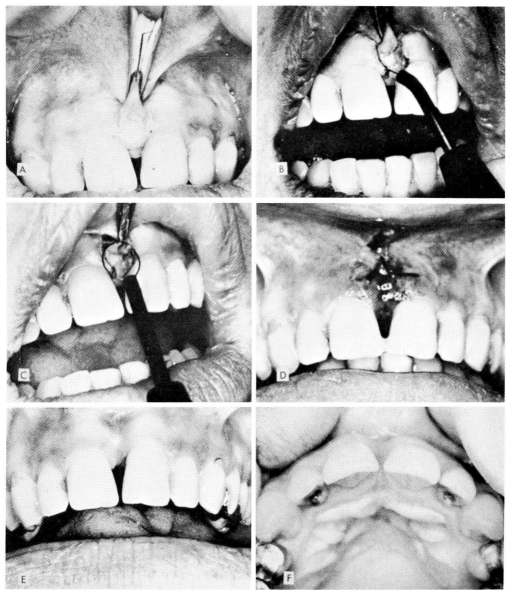

Case Figure 27–2. Operative procedure. *A*, A curved mosquito hemostat is clamped to the frenum close to the lip. Note the blanched appearance of the tissues, which has resulted from hemostasis of the anesthetic solution, and from clamping the frenum. *B*, Frenum is incised down to the bone with a 45-degree-angle fine needle electrode on both sides of the hemostat. *C*, Resection is completed by sliding a medium-sized round loop electrode along the beaks of the hemostat, removing projecting frenal tissue. *D*, Appearance of the tissues on the fifth postoperative day before the sutures have been removed. Healing is progressing normally, with a light surface layer of coagulum present. *E*, Appearance of the tissues six weeks postoperatively, labial view. Healing is complete. The pockets on the respective medial surfaces of the two centrals have been eliminated. The tissues are firm and supple. The upper half of the frenum is still functioning to control the movements of the lip, but is no longer exerting any traction against the gingivae. The gingival contour is normal and harmonious. *F*, Appearance of the palatal aspect at this time. The entire area extending to the nasopalatine papilla is fully healed and normal.

the crest of the alveolar ridge in the median line. The radiolucent area extended posteriorly almost to the incisive foramen.

TREATMENT. She had planned to have the frenectomy performed while on her vacation, for cosmetic reasons. When the gingivae suddenly swelled and became painful, frenectomy became an emergency measure instead of elective. The mouth was prepared and infiltration anesthesia administered. A 45-degree-angle fine needle electrode was selected and current output set at 3.5 for electrosection. The upper lip was pulled outward and upward until it was tautly distended. A curved mosquito hemostat was clamped to the frenum as closely as possible to the inner surface of the upper lip (Case Fig. 27–2). The lower half of the frenum, including the portion flatly attached on a broad base to the gingivae, was incised. The incision was then continued through the diastema to the palatal termination of the frenum at the nasopalatine papilla.

The incised tissue was undermined and reflected from its bony attachment. A round loop electrode was substituted and current output increased to 6. Resection of the frenum was completed by sliding the loop down along the concave surface of the hemostat beaks, thereby cleanly resecting the tissue projecting from them.

Adherent shreds of frenal fibers still embedded in the line of symphysis were removed with a fine ophthalmic tissue forceps. The upper half of the frenum was sutured, closing the Y half of the V-Y incision which had been created. Granulomatous epithelial debris was resected from the medial pockets with a narrow U-shaped loop electrode inserted flat against the proximal surfaces of the roots. These tooth surfaces were curetted to remove the accretions of detritus.

When debridement was completed, medicated powdered surgical gelatin was inserted into the crevice in the lower portion of the incised area and mixed with the blood. After the blood clotted, the area was dried and collodion was applied in thick layers as a protective dry dressing. She was given postoperative instructions and reappointed.

She returned on the fifth postoperative day and reported that the collodion dressing had peeled off on the third day but that she had had no difficulty from either pain or swelling. The mouth was irrigated and inspected. Healing was progressing very favorably. The lower half of the frenal area was filled with healthy granulating tissue and the sutured upper half was healing by primary union. The sutures were removed and tincture of myrrh and benzoin was applied in air-dried layers.

She was seen postoperatively at regular weekly intervals for the next six weeks. By the end of the third week the tissues appeared firmly reattached to the alveolar bone and almost fully healed. By the end of the sixth week the tissues were fully healed. The tissue tone was excellent, the tissues firm, in normal color and completely reattached to teeth and alveolar bone. The upper half of the frenum was maintaining normal functional control of lip movements, but it was no longer exerting abnormal traction against the marginal and cemental gingivae. There was no evidence of cicatricial contraction.

COMBINED FRENECTOMY
AND GINGIVAL REPOSITIONING

Abnormal mandibular frena or broad-band muscle attachments often create so much traumatic traction against the marginal and cemental gingivae that there is excessive resorption of alveolar bone and gingival mucosa.

Frenectomy in such cases removes the traumatic traction but does not restore the alveolar bone or gingival mucosa over the denuded roots. When this is very noticeable in the anterior part of the mouth it may be necessary to cover the defect by repositioning the gingivae for protection and aesthetics.[3-6]

CASE 28

This case is a typical example of the destructive forces that may be generated by abnormal traction from a broad mandibular labial frenum. The intrinsic fibers of the frenum in this case demonstrated an amazing capacity to regenerate. This created renewal of abnormal traction which in turn stimulated cicatricial fibrous scar tissue formation, such as is rarely encountered with electrosurgery, that tended to partially obliterate the desired surgical results.

This case required a combination of surgical procedures, including frenectomy, pushback, channeling the mandibular labial sulcus space, repositioning of the gingival mucosa and fulguration of the regenerating intrinsic fibers in the lip, in order to effect a satisfactory result.

PATIENT. A 45-year-old white female in normal health.

HISTORY. An unusually broad, prominent mandibular labial frenum exerted abnormal traction against the marginal gingivae of the central incisors and created deterioration of the periodontal structures of these teeth. She was referred for frenectomy and repositioning of the gingivae.

CLINICAL EXAMINATION

Extraoral. Negative.

Intraoral. The mandibular gingivae were normal except in the median area. There the gingivae were detached and appeared atonal, hyperemic, and slightly ulcerated (Case Fig. 28-1). The broad frenum appeared to consist of a number of slender muscle strands webbed together into a broad, strap-like mass which obliterated most of the labial sulcus. The root of the left central was exposed on the labial aspect about 6 mm. beyond the cemento-enamel junction. The edge of the labial gingival margin around this tooth was retracted into a ragged roll of hyperemic, hypertrophied tissue with an ulcerated edge.

TREATMENT. Since the frenum extended from the cemental gingiva into the intrinsic muscles of the lip, it seemed likely that neither frenectomy alone nor pushback alone, nor even the two combined, would prove adequate. A two-stage treatment plan was followed: the first stage, frenectomy and pushback; after primary healing, repositioning of the gingival mucosa with a sliding flap to cover the denuded root.

Stage I. The mouth was prepared and infiltration anesthesia administered. The lower lip was pulled outward and downward to pull the tissues taut. A curved mosquito hemostat was clamped to the frenum as closely to the inner surface of the lip as possible. A 45-degree-angle fine needle electrode was selected and current output was set at 3.5 for electrosection. Both sides of the frenum were incised. The incised tissue was then undermined and resected from the beaks of the hemostat by sliding the needle down along their concave surface after current output had been increased to 4.5 to overcome dissipation of energy.

Considerable bleeding ensued. The bleeders were clamped with mosquito hemostats and coagulated off their beaks. When bleeding stopped and the field was dried, numerous fine muscle fibers were plainly visible in the submucosa, which was

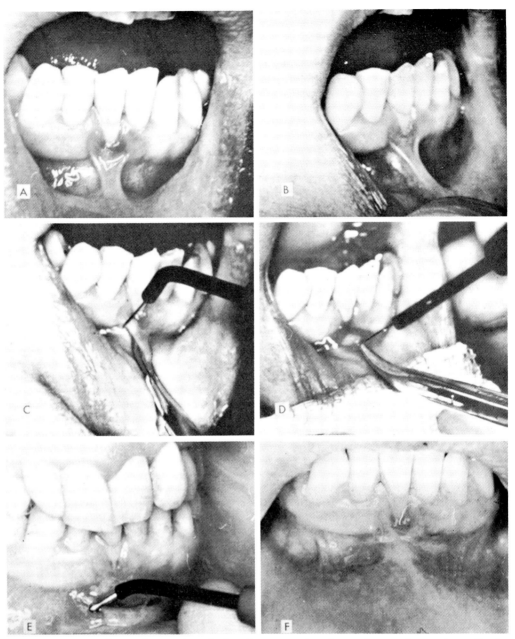

Case Figure 28–1. Gingival and alveolar resorption from abnormal muscle pull of a broad, highly attached mandibular labial frenum requiring combined frenectomy and gingival repositioning. First stage: Frenectomy. *A,* Preoperative view, full face. A broad flat frenum, attached high on the inner surface of the lip, extends and blends into the labial marginal gingiva of the mandibular centrals. The gingival tissue is engorged, hypertrophied, and ulcerated. *B,* Side view shows height of the frenal attachment and depth of the labial sulcus, which is separated into two sections by the frenal tissues. *C,* Operative procedure. The frenum, clamped close to the lip with a curved mosquito hemostat, is incised along each side of the clamp with a 45-degree-angle fine needle electrode. *D,* The incised tissue is resected off the beaks of the hemostat by sliding the electrode laterally along the beaks of the clamp. *E,* The sharp edges of a crater in the floor of the sulcus produced by irritation of the cement pack is reduced by spot coagulation. *F,* Appearance three weeks postoperatively. The tissues are healed but the sulcus space in the midline is partially obliterated by a dense mass of white scar tissue, probably produced by irritation of the surgical cement stent. The marginal gingiva of the right central is again engorged and proliferating.

714

firmly attached to the periosteum. These fibers were severed horizontally with the electrode. After the renewed bleeding was brought under control the severed tissue was pushed down to create a deeper sulcus space. A stiffly mixed surgical cement pack was inserted into the operative field to maintain the sulcus space during healing.

She returned on the fifth postoperative day and reported that the cement pack, although it had loosened and become detached the previous morning, had not caused any untoward postoperative reactions. She thought the sulcus space had refilled somewhat in the past 24 hours, although it had been asymptomatic. Inspection confirmed that the sulcus was partially obliterated and edematous, and that the surface was covered with a moderately thick layer of normal coagulum.

The outer periphery of the incised area was somewhat elevated and formed a sharp edge of tissue which was reduced to normal level by superficial spot coagulation with a small ball electrode under topical anesthesia. Tincture of myrrh and benzoin was applied to the entire area and a fresh cement pack inserted.

The patient returned for further postoperative care five days later. This time the cement pack had remained intact. It was removed, the mouth was irrigated, and the tissues were inspected. The marginal, cemental, and alveolar gingivae in the affected area were healing satisfactorily but the sulcus tissue was hyperemic and hypertrophied and showed evidence of marked irritation, especially the outer margin surrounding the cement pack. Tincture of myrrh and benzoin was applied and she was told to continue the home care.

She returned one week later. This time the labial gingiva was almost fully healed, but the sulcus space was partially filled with dense white scar tissue which contained some regenerated muscle fibers. Since the second stage of the procedure was to be done in about two weeks it appeared pointless to do any corrective surgery at this time. It was obvious, however, that an acrylic surgical splint would be required instead of a cement pack to protect the operative field and maintain the sulcus space without irritation. A colloid impression, therefore, was taken for a surgical splint which was processed.

Stage II. Two weeks later the second stage was performed. The acrylic splint was so closely adapted to the teeth that it stayed in place, but small holes were drilled in each embrasure area so that it could be wired to the teeth if necessary. The mouth was then prepared for surgery and infiltration anesthesia administered. A narrow 45-degree-angle U-shaped loop electrode was selected and current output was set at 4 for electrosection. One millimeter of the marginal gingiva on the labial surface of the denuded root was resected with the loop to freshen the margin (Case Fig. 28–2).

Current output was increased to 5, and a medium-sized loop electrode was substituted to resect the scar tissue from the anterior sulcus space by shaving in layers with short brushing strokes. A fine needle electrode was substituted, current output reduced to 3, and a vertical incision started at the mesio-incisal angle of the right cuspid and extended approximately 1 cm. downward toward the labiogingival fold. The incised tissue was undermined, reflected from the alveolar bone and swung across the denuded root. The flap tissue margin was then accurately coapted with the freshened distal margin of the gingival defect. The flap was sutured with 0000 braided silk interrupted sutures. The space created by swinging the flap laterally filled with blood, to which a small amount of powdered surgical gelatin was added. After the blood clotted, the acrylic surgical splint was inserted. The adaptation was so accurate that it was unnecessary to wire it to the teeth. Panalba was prescribed for three days, and ascorbic acid and Knox clear gelatin recommended as dietary supplements.

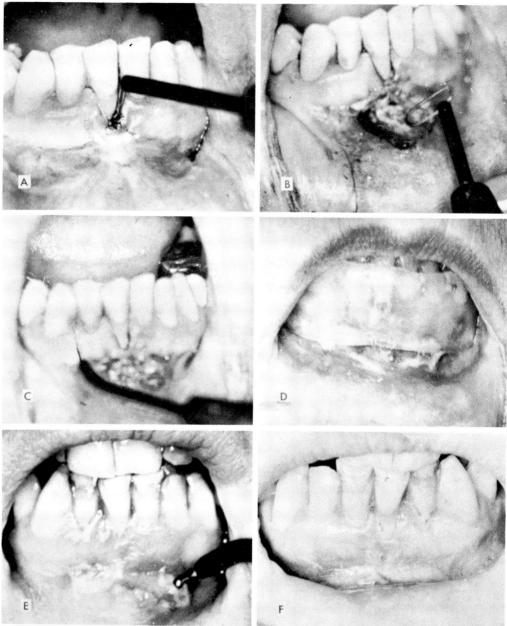

Case Figure 28–2. Second stage: repositioning the gingival tissue. *A,* One millimeter of the marginal gingiva around the neck of the central is resected with a narrow 45-degree-angle U-shaped loop electrode. *B,* The fibrous scar tissue in the floor of the sulcus space is resected with a large right-angle U-shaped loop electrode to restore the full sulcus space. *C,* A sliding flap is incised with a 45-degree-angle fine needle electrode. *D,* After the surgery has been completed and the margins coapted and sutured, an acrylic surgical stent is inserted and closely adapted to the teeth and tissues. *E,* Postoperatively, superficial spot coagulation is applied with a small ball electrode to level off raised irregular edges in the sulcus area and to coagulate a few tiny red spots which tend to bleed profusely when traumatized. *F,* Final postoperative appearance of the area. The tissues are fully healed and normal. The frenum has been completely eliminated, and there is no longer any abnormal traction against marginal gingivae. Although the gingival repositioning did not completely cover the denuded portion of the root of the central, it did cover more than half of the denuded area.

When the patient returned on the fifth postoperative day she reported two troublesome sore spots. Inspection showed the splint in position. When the stent was removed, a layer of healthy looking coagulum was seen lining the sulcus. The line of incision was healing by primary union except where the uppermost suture had torn away leaving a narrow V-shaped space approximately 2.5 mm. in length immediately below the mesial aspect of the crown of the right central incisor.

The splint had compressed the tissues at the inferior borders of its respective terminal ends, creating two raw ulcerated areas which were covered with a heavy layer of coagulum. The sulcus area was sprayed with a 0.1 per cent dilution of chromic acid. After 30 seconds this was washed away. The margins of the V-shaped gingival defect were scarified. After the blood clotted, tincture of myrrh and benzoin was applied. The terminal ends of the stent were trimmed; it was lined with Kenalog in Orabase and reinserted.

She returned the following week and reported that the ulcerated areas were almost completely healed. Inspection showed considerable progress, although there was still a layer of coagulum lining the sulcus area. Superficial spot coagulation was applied to a few tiny red spots and the elevated edge of the sulcus. Cordent was dusted into the stent and prescribed for home use. She returned once a week for the next three weeks. During this period healing progressed satisfactorily. By the end of the month the V-shaped defect was almost completely obliterated; the labial sulcus and gingival mucosa appeared almost fully healed and normally epithelialized.

At this time the patient left for an extended Florida vacation and discarded the stent. She returned one month later and reported that about one week after the stent had been omitted, the sulcus space had begun to fill with dense scar tissue. Examination showed the sulcus almost fully obliterated by dense fibrous scar tissue into which strands of muscle tissue from the lip and gingival mucosa extended and again exerted unfavorable traction.

Rechanneling the vestibule produced some improvement but the tendency to regenerate persisted. Finally, the fibrous scar tissue and muscle fibers were destroyed *in situ* by fulguration until the sulcus space was the proper depth and the base lightly carbonized. Use of the stent was resumed for the next two weeks and then discarded. The carbonized area underwent normal granulation, and healing progressed uneventfully to normal completion. The tension against the marginal gingivae having finally been eliminated, the gingival mucosa as well as the labial vestibular space were normal. In the few months since this case has been completed, these tissues have remained normal.*

Iatrogenic Periodontoclasia: the Mandibular Apically Repositioned Flap

When, as has been demonstrated, iatrogenic periodontoclasia develops in response to subgingival irritation by veneer crown splints, the condition responds very favorably to the combination of gingivoplasty and creation of adequate subgingival troughs around the crown preparations, so that the tissue will readapt itself around the subgingival portions of the restorations as it repairs, thereby eliminating the irritation that triggers inflammatory responses that lead to periodontal deterioration.

---

*The patient was seen again almost 10 years later. The labial vestibule looked the same as when she was dismissed from treatment.

However, when traction from these structures against the marginal gingivae contributes to the periodontal deterioration owing to unusually high mucogingival junction, high areolar gingivae, high mandibular labial frena, and/or high muscle attachments, this method of treatment becomes inadequate. In addition to the usual treatment, it becomes necessary to create a tissue flap that can be repositioned apically and thus recreate adequate vestibular space.

When the flap incisions are created by cutting with cold-steel scalpels and the flaps are displaced apically it is usually necessary to cover the surgical field with a split-thickness skin graft or other graft to protect the area and prevent obliteration of the vestibular space by cicatricial bands of scar tissue adhesions.

When the technique is performed electrosurgically with fully rectified cutting current, need for protective use of grafts to cover the surgical field is eliminated because of the atraumatic nature of the surgery and resultant splendid healing by secondary granulation repair that is totally free of fibrous scar tissue adhesions. The following case demonstrates the electrosurgical technique and its results.

CASE 29

This case presented an almost total absence of labial mandibular vestibular space owing to junction of the areolar gingiva with the labial marginal gingiva only about 3 mm. below the marginal crest, and insertion of the mandibular labial frenal fibers into the marginal gingiva in the median line, so that *clinically* the alveolar ridge was only 3 mm. high. There was no clinically discernible zone of attached gingiva.

PATIENT. A 67-year-old white male in good health.

HISTORY. All his maxillary and remaining mandibular teeth had been restored eight months earlier with acrylic veneer crown splints. A mandibular splint extending from cuspid to cuspid and the right third molar, the only teeth in the mandible, served as abutments for a lower lingual bar denture that restored the missing posterior teeth.

The permanent mandibular splint had been completed and inserted with temporary cementation about 10 weeks earlier. Temporary cementation had been continued during this period in preference to permanent cementation to permit easy removal of the appliance for periodic observation. Shortly after the splint was inserted the gingival tissues around the splint began to bulge and become partially detached from close adaptation to the splint. Despite palliative treatment by his dentist the condition deteriorated. He was therefore referred for surgical correction by electrosection.

CLINICAL EXAMINATION. The gingival tissues around the mandibular splint were grossly hyperplastic and partially detached. The splint was not cemented and was easily removed. The junction between the alveolar mucosa or zone of attached gingiva and the areolar mucosa was a mere 3 mm. below the gingival margin at its greatest dimension, and bilateral muscle attachments at the distal aspects of the two cuspids were only 2 mm. below the gingival margins of these teeth. The muscle attachment on the right side was slightly distal to the tooth and did not exert traction directly against the marginal gingiva of that tooth. The one on the left side, however, was attached almost exactly at the distogingival angle of the tooth and appeared to be producing a slight amount of traction against the gingival tissue of that tooth. The labial frenum in the midline was attached to the crest of the marginal gingiva between the central incisors.

The marginal gingivae were equally hyperplastic and detached on the lingual aspect. The gingivae around the maxillary teeth were slightly hyperplastic in several areas but comparatively normal by comparison with the mandibular gingivae. The referring dentist confirmed the patient's claim that the mandibular gingivae had been normal in dimension preoperatively.

TREATMENT. It was obvious that reduction of the external and subgingival redundant tissue and recontouring the architecture plus creation of adequate subgingival accommodation for the mandibular splint would not suffice, and that a pushback to increase the depth of the mandibular labial vestibule was the key to successful treatment of this case. A treatment plan to that effect was therefore consummated surgically.

The first step was reduction and recontouring of the external labial gingival tissue. A flame-shaped loop electrode was selected, cutting current output was set at 5 on the power output dial, and the activated electrode was used to reduce the bulging tissue to normal dimension after bilateral mental block-lingual infiltration anesthesia had been administered (Case Fig. 29–1).

When the recontouring was completed, the loop electrode was replaced with a 45-degree-angle fine needle electrode, and power output was reduced to 3 on the instrument panel. An incision was made with this electrode to but not through the periosteum at the level of the alveolar-areolar gingival junction. It was started just medial to the right muscle attachment and extended to and slightly beyond the left muscle attachment. The incised tissue was then carefully dissected downward approximately 0.5 cm. to separate it from the periosteum without injury to the latter.

The needle electrode was then replaced with a 45-degree-angle narrow U-shaped loop, and current output was increased to 3.5. The redundant subgingival tissue was resected and well-defined subgingival troughs were created around the respective crown preparations. The tissues were gently dried with a sterile sponge, and tincture of myrrh and benzoin was applied to the area in air-dried layers. The restoration was then replaced and a *hard* roll of periodontal pack cement was carefully adapted around the splint and extended into the pushback area, making certain that the base of the cement roll in the pushback was well rounded (Case Fig. 29–2). (It is imperative that the cement be firm enough to retain its shape despite pressure of the lip; otherwise, the vestibular contour will be diminished or lost [see text Figure 19–9].) While the cement was setting the patient was given instructions in home care and was reappointed.

He returned on the fifth postoperative day and reported a remarkably uneventful postoperative experience. The cement pack, which had remained intact, and the restoration were removed, and the tissues were gently sprayed to cleanse them. The tissues were healing splendidly by secondary intention and were covered with a very thin film of surface granulation. The restoration was replaced, the tissues were gently dried, tincture of myrrh and benzoin was applied, and a second pack, this time of Peripack, was adapted around the splint and into the pushback vestibular area. On the tenth day the second pack was removed, and thereafter the tissues remained open to the thermal and chemical stimuli of the mouth, but the patient was cautioned to stay on very soft food that would not injure the regenerating tissues.

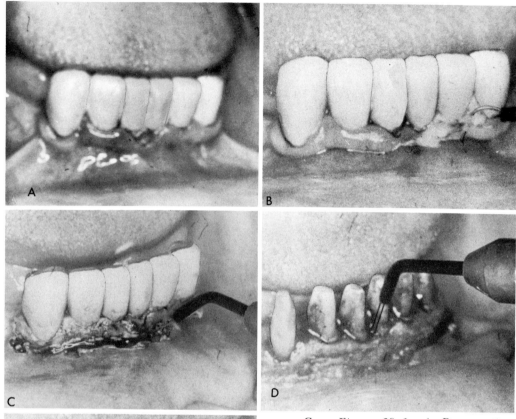

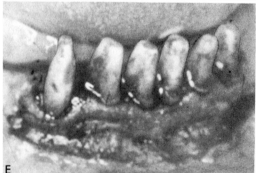

Case Figure 29–1. A, Preoperative view. The mandibular six anterior teeth have been restored with a full crown fixed prosthesis splint. The gingival tissues around the splint are massively hypertrophied and engorged, and are detached from the teeth and alveolar bone. There has been resorption of most of the labial gingiva in the midline area, and clinically the alveolar ridge is only about 3 mm. in height. There is no zone of attached gingiva and virtually no labial vestibule when the lip is extended anteriorly. *B*, Shows the beginning of the gingivoplasty to recontour the gingivae to normal architecture. The flame-shaped loop electrode is being used with the cutting current to perform the gingivoplasty. *C*, The gingivoplasty having been completed, a fine 45-degree-angle needle electrode is being used to incise the tissue at the junction of the alveolar and areolar mucosa of the lip. *D*, The areolar mucosa of the internal surface of the lip at the line of juncture has been displaced downward or apically. The gingivoplasty has been utilized to complete the recontouring of the marginal gingivae, and the infrabony lesions resulting from the faulty restoration are being debrided with the 17-mm. loop electronic curet. The shoulders of the crown preparations which had been completely covered with tissue are now fully exposed. *E*, Shows the appearance of the mouth immediately before the periodontal cement pack is inserted. Note that shoulders of the preparations are exposed and well defined.

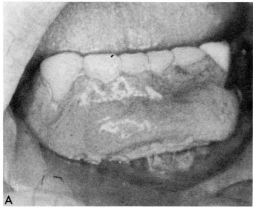

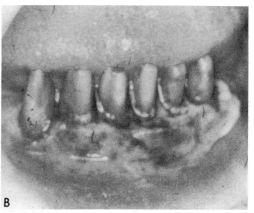

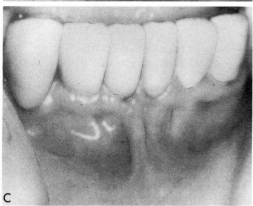

Case Figure 29–2. A, The cement pack, mixed to as hard a consistency as possible to help retain its shape despite the considerable pressure of the lip, has been inserted and packed down to keep the incised vermilion tissue displaced as desired, and to maintain as rounded a base as possible. This photograph shows the compression of the cement caused by the lip pressure, which necessitated addition of a small roll of extra-hard cement packed into the area. *B,* Appearance of the tissues immediately after the second cement pack has been removed, ten days postoperatively. The tissues appear to be repairing favorably by granulation repair. *C,* Shows the final outcome of treatment, three months postoperatively. The marginal gingivae are considerably improved in tone and in contour. There is a 3-mm. wide zone of attached gingiva present, and there is a well-defined, deep labial vestibule. Also present are fibers of the mandibular labial frenum which had caused the deterioration of the gingival tissue in the midline preoperatively. These fibers are now normally inserted into the lower edge of the attached gingiva, and no longer appear to be exerting destructive abnormal traction against the marginal gingivae.

By the end of the fourth postoperative week the tissues appeared fully healed and maturely keratinized, without loss of vestibular height due to cicatricial scar tissue adhesions and without need for a split-thickness skin graft. The mandibular labial frenum was attached about 3 mm. below the gingival margin and did not appear to be causing destructive traction. The vestibular space on either side of it was approximately 1 cm. deep and well rounded. The gingival contour was normal and the tissues appeared firmly and tightly adapted against the subgingival portions of the restoration.

Regeneration of Maturely Keratinized Zones of Attached Gingivae

During the span of more than two decades in which the author has been using electrosurgery for definitive periodontal therapy he observed that whenever the old surface epithelium was resected from the gingivae by loop

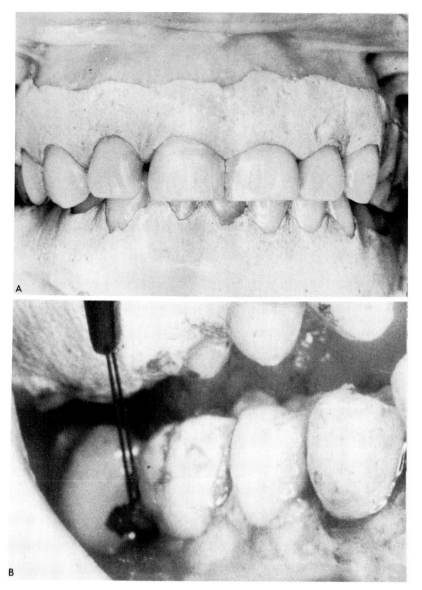

Figure 19–9.   A, A periodontal cement pack mixed to the proper consistency to be able to withstand pressure from lips and cheeks or tongue that would otherwise cause the cement to flow and become displaced. Note that only the gingival third of the crowns of the teeth are covered with the cement, and only about 1 to 1.5 cm. of gingival tissue is covered. The cement is closely contoured so that there is no disfiguring bulk, and it has been carefully moulded into the embrasures for retention, without displacing the blood that had been induced in the infrabony pockets. B, A poorly applied cement pack. It is obvious that the cement was too soft a mix to be able to withstand the pressure of the lips, cheeks, and tongue, and has flowed downward away from the tissues that it should be protecting and is covering the entire tooth crowns. The bulky mass interferes with eating and is quite uncomfortable, and has thinned out so much on the gingivae that it cannot perform its primary function of protecting them. This same photograph does, however, offer an example of the typical use of a 17-mm. periodontal loop electrode as an electronic curet. The activated electrode has resected some of the pocket debris, which is being lifted out of the defect as the electrode is rapidly moved around in it with an up and down rotary motion.

planing, well-defined zones of attached gingivae almost invariably regenerated, even in cases in which no comparable zones of attached gingivae were clinically discernible preoperatively.

Conversely, where the old epithelium had been permitted to remain undisturbed, zones of attached gingivae were not manifested postoperatively unless they had been present preoperatively. Moreover, where the old epithelium had remained undisturbed the postoperative zones of attached gingivae were neither as wide nor as well defined as those that regenerated after epithelial stripping.

In the case being reported here the referring dentist stated that in the 16 years he had been seeing the patient there had been no clinical evidence of zones of attached gingivae and that the areolar and alveolar gingivae in both arches had been indistinguishable in texture and color.

Following the periodontal surgery, which had included epithelial surface stripping, a few faintly white small areas that resembled nidi appeared on the surface of the regenerating gingivae. As the healing progressed and the patient began to follow a regimen of oral physiotherapy, these areas began to become more noticeable and appeared to be focal points where surface keratinization of the epithelium was beginning to develop. Eventually they began to coalesce and ultimately formed exceptionally well-developed and broadly defined zones of attached gingivae in both arches.

CASE 30

This case is being presented because it demonstrates the gradual development of the epithelial surface keratinization that characterizes well-defined zones of attached gingivae.

PATIENT.   A 47-year-old white male.

HISTORY.   Negative except that he had been receiving conservative (manual curettage) treatment for a generalized periodontal condition for two years, and despite this there has been a progressive worsening of the condition.

CLINICAL EXAMINATION.   The maxillary teeth had been restored with a fixed bridge from cuspid to cuspid, and also a fixed prosthesis restoring the right posterior quadrant. The left second bicuspid was missing. The mandibular right cuspid was restored with a cast veneer crown. The right first bicuspid also was restored with a cast veneer crown, and these crowns served as double abutments from which a second bicuspid pontic was cantilevered. The mandibular left posterior teeth also were restored with a fixed prosthesis.

The gingival tissues throughout the mouth were atonal and appeared to be partially detached from the necks of the teeth. Recession of the marginal gingivae had occurred in the upper anterior region and around the labial-buccal aspect of the mandibular left lateral and right cuspid and first bicuspid, exposing the gold finish lines of the crowns on these three teeth. There was no clinically discernible evidence of a zone of attached gingiva in either arch, and the mucosa from the marginal gingivae to the mucogingival junction were similar in appearance and texture. A 4-mm. infrabony pocket was present on the labial surface of the mandibular left lateral root (Case Fig. 30–1).

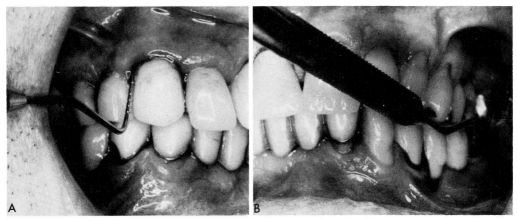

Case Figure 30-1. A, Preoperative appearance of the gingival mucosa. These tissues offer no clinically discernible evidence of any zones of attached gingivae. The tissues from the mucobuccal fold to the gingival margins appear identical in color, texture, and tone. The marginal gingivae are thick and rounded at the edges and appear engorged. A periodontal probe inserted under the free gingival margin of the maxillary right cuspid shows a typical partial detachment of the gingivae from the teeth and very shallow pockets. *B,* Similar conditions exist in the mandible.

TREATMENT.   As in all such procedures, the patient had been instructed previously in the proper methods for maintaining a high degree of oral physiotherapy postoperatively. To eliminate mechanical irritation as a factor, a thorough prophylaxis and elimination of occlusal disharmonies had been performed.

The first surgical session was devoted to treatment of the maxillary and mandibular right quadrants. The tissues were prepared and anesthetized by regional block and infiltration anesthesia. A flame-shaped loop electrode was selected, cutting current was set at 4.5 for the labial-buccal and lingual and 5.5 for the palatal, and a gingivoplasty was performed in each quadrant with the activated electrode. When the electrosurgery was completed and all the tissue debris removed, tincture of myrrh and benzoin was applied in air-dried layers. A very stiffly mixed periodontal cement pack was then applied to each quadrant, and the patient was reappointed.

He returned on the fifth postoperative day. The cement packs were removed, the tissues were irrigated, and tincture of myrrh and benzoin was applied, after which fresh cement packs were applied. Five days later both cement packs were removed, the tissues were cleansed by irrigation, and tincture of myrrh and benzoin was reapplied.

Due to an intervening business trip, the patient was unable to return for treatment of the remaining quadrants for two weeks. In the interim he maintained faithfully the regimen of home postoperative care that had been prescribed to provide effective oral physiotherapy.

At his next visit the left maxillary and mandibular quadrants were anesthetized, a narrow 45-degree-angle U-shaped loop electrode was selected, cutting current was set at 3.5, and the activated electrode was used to perform a gingivoplasty in the maxillary and mandibular quadrants.

To maintain a normal tissue architecture, the loose detached labial marginal gingival part of the pocket on the mandibular left lateral was removed by planing the tissue with a flame-shaped loop electrode with current set at 5. When the gingivoplasties were completed, tincture of myrrh and benzoin was applied and stiffly mixed cement packs were applied to the two quadrants.

Again he returned on the fifth postoperative day. The cement packs were removed and the tissues were cleansed by gentle irrigation with a solution of Kasdenol. At this time the tissues in the right quadrants offered a marked contrast. The tissues were almost completely healed and their tissue tone was excellent. The tissues in the left quadrants appeared to be healing favorably, but the color and tone of these tissues at the level beyond the surgical field of gingivoplasty were distinctly less favorable at this time. Several tiny white patches were present on the labial aspect of the anterior gingivae in both right quadrants (Case Fig. 30–2).

Healing progressed rapidly and favorably. Three weeks after the second cement

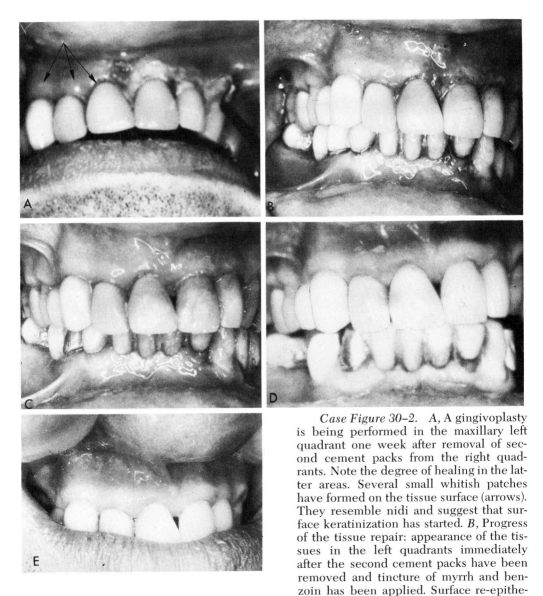

Case Figure 30–2. A, A gingivoplasty is being performed in the maxillary left quadrant one week after removal of second cement packs from the right quadrants. Note the degree of healing in the latter areas. Several small whitish patches have formed on the tissue surface (arrows). They resemble nidi and suggest that surface keratinization has started. B, Progress of the tissue repair: appearance of the tissues in the left quadrants immediately after the second cement packs have been removed and tincture of myrrh and benzoin has been applied. Surface re-epithelialization has started on the left side, and the maturation of the tissues on the right side has advanced substantially. C, One week later, healing has advanced appreciably in the left quadrants and the tissues in the right quadrants are fully healed. D, Appearance six months postoperatively. The marginal gingivae are tightly adherent to the teeth and normal in contour and tone. There are broad, well-defined zones of maturely keratinized attached gingivae in both the upper and lower jars and the mouth is in a normal healthy state. E, A close-up view of the maxillary gingivae.

packs were removed from the left quadrants the tissues began to show evidence of re-epithelialization, and the tissue around the left lateral incisor showed evidence of having regenerated slightly toward its original level on the mesial aspect of the tooth.

The patient was seen at regular intervals for six weeks thereafter and was instructed to return in six months for a semiannual checkup. When he returned, the tissues in both jaws were found to be in excellent condition. The marginal gingivae were tightly adherent to the necks of the teeth throughout the mouth, except for a 1-mm. gingival free margin. Bands of maturely keratinized zones of attached gingivae approximately 1 cm. wide in the maxilla and about 7 mm. wide in the mandible were present. The tissues had a stippled, orange-skin texture.

The patient returned semiannually for two years. Throughout that period the tissues remained firmly attached and in excellent tone. The role of vigorous oral physiotherapy in attaining and *retaining* maturely keratinized zones of attached gingivae in this type of case cannot be overemphasized. Optimal results cannot be achieved without the patient's contribution of vigorous oral physiotherapy. In cases in which favorable results have been achieved but patient cooperation ceases after a period of time, the tissue tone begins to deteriorate and eventually the zones of attached gingivae become ill-defined and atonal.

Nevertheless, the author feels certain that neither the electrosurgical treatment method nor the oral physiotherapy could produce the zones of attached gingivae such as were seen in this case, unless the necessary histologic elements are present in the tissues, even though they were not clinically discernible preoperatively.

An interesting collateral sequel to these cases has been the tendency of some individuals casually to dismiss the clinical results as interesting but incidental and distinctly secondary in importance to the cellular repair, with such comments as: "The clinical results are interesting, but what is the histologic nature of the repair? Are the teeth firm again because of bone and periodontal ligament regeneration, or is it merely because the gingivae have become firmly reattached? Is the periodontal probe unable to penetrate into the pocket sites because the defects have filled with bone and formed a new gingival sulcus, or is it fibrous repair and tight adhesion of the marginal gingivae that prevent penetration?" To the patients who have been told that their condition is untreatable and that all or nearly all the teeth will have to be extracted, the restoration of the dentition to normal functional usefulness is all that matters, and therefore such speculative academic questions are irrelevant. As a member of a scientific profession, the author does not consider the questions irrelevant from an academic standpoint. But as a clinician he cannot help but wonder whether the purist, in his zealous concern about the histologic characteristics of the repair tissue, does not tend to lose sight of the main objective of treatment—restoration of the oral structures to a healthy state and normal function, with minimal aesthetic impairment.

Some speculations about the histologic nature of the healing produced by electrosurgical periodontal techniques described here have no doubt been stimulated by the research reports of a few periodontists. In their comparative studies they found that electrosurgical instrumentation caused burn wounds in the gingival tissues, and that these wounds healed more slowly than comparable wounds created by steel scalpel and curet instrumentation. The author conducted experiments on animals and can attest that many unpredictable variables can influence, distort, or alter the results of such studies. All the unfavorable results had occurred in experiments with laboratory animals. At best, given the benefit of the doubt that their electrosurgical instrumentation technique had been adequately skillful, the variables factor should not be overlooked, especially since they were unable to maintain the postoperative control and lengthy periods of postoperative treatment that are possible with human patients, or the patient cooperation and postoperative physiotherapy, all of which contribute materially to the quality and character of the ultimate results of treatment. It is noteworthy that in all three experimental investigations conducted on human subjects reported in Chapter 9 of this text, electrosurgery produced highly favorable results. Therefore judgment of the efficacy of therapy based on animal experimentation alone is unjustified, and clinical evidence of optimal therapeutic results compiled over many years should not be casually disregarded.

Former President Goheen of Princeton University once said, "The mark of an educated man is his ability to change his mind when the evidence warrants it." The thoroughness and extensiveness of this review of clinical cases demonstrating the techniques of definitive conservative electrosurgical therapy was motivated by the hope that, being educated men, even those periodontists who formerly insisted that electrosurgery is unsuited for modern periodontal therapy will be persuaded to recognize that electrosurgical periodontal therapy not only is acceptable and has a place in modern periodontal therapy but in many instances is able to provide more desirable and effective results than can be obtained by other methods of instrumentation.

FOOTNOTE REFERENCES

1. Gottlieb, B.: Schmutzpyorrhoe, Paradentalpyorrhoe und Alveolartrophie. Urban & Schwarzenberg, Berlin, 1925.
2. Cohen, D. W.: Verbal communication. Periodontia Seminar. University of Pennsylvania School of Dentistry Postgraduate Division, May, 1961.
3. Grupe, H. E., and Warren, R. L.: Repair of gingiva by a sliding flap operation. J. Periodont., 27:92, 1956.
4. Grupe, H. E.: Horizontal sliding flap operation. Symposium on Practical Periodontal Therapy. Dent. Clin. N. Amer., March, 1960.
5. Hileman, A. C.: Surgical repositioning of vestibule and frenums in periodontal disease. J.A.D.A., 55:676, 1957.
6. Hileman, A. C.: Repositioning the vestibule and frenums as adjunctive periodontal treatment procedures. Symposium on Practical Periodontal Therapy. Dent. Clin. N. Amer., March, 1960.

READING REFERENCES

Carranza, F. A.: A technic for reattachment. J. Periodont., 25:272, 1954.
Fox, L.: Communication to *Dental Times*. (Periodontal surgery criticized.) Dent. Times, 3:12, Jan., 1961.
Goldman, H. M., and Cohen, D. W.: The infrabony pocket: Classification and treatment. J. Periodont., 29:272, 1958.
Goldman, H. M., Schluger, S., Fox, L., and Cohen, D. W.: Periodontal Therapy. 2nd ed. St. Louis, The C. V. Mosby Co., 1960, pp. 250–261.
Morris, M. L.: Healing of human periodontal tissues following surgical detachment from nonvital teeth. J. Periodont., 28:222, 1957.
Oringer, M. J.: Electrosurgery for definitive conservative modern periodontal therapy. Dent. Clin. N. Amer., Jan., 1969, pp. 53–73.
Pritchard, J.: Regeneration of bone following periodontal therapy. Oral Surg., Oral Med., Oral Path., 10:247, 1957.
Saghirian, L. M.: Electrosurgical gingivoplasty. Oral Surg., Oral Med., Oral Path., 2:1549, 1959.
Schaffer, E. M., and Zanders, H. A.: Histologic evidence of reattachment in periodontal pockets. Paradentologie, 7:101, 1953.
Zemsky, J. L.: Oral Diseases. New York, Physicians and Surgeons Book Co., 1930, pp. 332–342.

PART 4

PREPROSTHODONTIC ELECTROSURGERY

Denture failures still occur despite improved denture materials, impression materials, and impression techniques; complex, sophisticated articulators designed to fulfill modern concepts of occlusion, centric relation, rest position, retruded position, and freeway space; and similar significant influences on the art and science of denture construction.

Modern denture failures are attributable primarily to unfavorable physical factors and, to a much lesser degree, unfavorable psychosomatic factors. Our attention will be focused on the soft tissue abnormalities and bony anatomic abnormalities, deficiencies, and pathologic conditions that create physical handicaps. Special consideration will be given to the serious prosthetic problems created by geriatric resorption of the alveolar ridges.

From the dental standpoint, when a patient reaches the edentulous state he has reached the port of no recall. Unless a stable, functionally useful and aesthetically acceptable denture can be fabricated for him, the edentulous patient is doomed to considerable functional and social handicap.

The art and science of full denture prosthesis has improved spectacularly in the past half century. Nevertheless, full denture failures still occur. If the failures are the result of anatomic factors, preprosthodontic surgery often makes it possible to correct the anatomic defects. However, the fact that an anatomic abnormality or deformity is present in an edentulous jaw does not automatically create need for its surgical correction. The latter becomes necessary and justifiable only when the condition does not lend itself to correction in the denture without destroying its stability and functional and aesthetic usefulness. When preprosthodontic surgery is necessary electronic electrosurgery offers advantages unmatched by other modalities.

CRITERIA FOR SURGICAL INTERVENTION

Regardless of whether the anatomic defects are due to abnormal anatomy, deficiencies, or pathologic conditions, the following rule of thumb should be observed before we embark upon consideration of their surgical correction: *The mere presence of an anatomic defect does not create automatic need for surgical correction. Only when it is not possible to satisfactorily correct or compensate for the defect in the denture itself is surgical intervention indicated.*

The following constitute justifiable criteria for surgical preprosthodontic intervention:

1. When the defect would interfere with insertion and removal of the denture.
2. When it would impede the proper seating of the denture.
3. When it prevents fabrication of a labial flange for the denture.
4. When it prevents fabrication of an efficient peripheral seal for the denture.
5. When it would interfere with creating an effective postdam for the denture.
6. When it would impair or destroy the stability of the denture.
7. When it would cause the denture to impede speech.
8. When it would cause the denture to interfere with deglutition.
9. When compensation for the defect in the denture would cause tissue irritation that is likely to stimulate and accelerate alveolar bone resorption.
10. When creation of a denture accommodation for the defect would result in facial disharmony.

When any of these hazards are encountered, surgical intervention becomes a prerequisite for successful full denture construction.

Responsible Anatomic Defects

Anatomic defects are responsible for all the aforementioned disruptive results. In many instances more than one anatomic abnormality can produce a particular unfavorable result. For example:

Painful interference with denture insertion or removal most frequently results from bulging or undercut tuberosities, irregularities or undercuts in the alveolar ridge, sharp interseptal bone spurs, and similar defects that traumatize the tissues whenever the denture is inserted or removed.

Disruption of the peripheral seal can result from loss of vestibular space; abnormal muscle attachments or frena; degenerative tissue proliferation; senile resorption of the alveolar ridge, causing loss of vestibular space for the labial denture flange; neoplastic masses or cicatricial scar tissue adhesions that obliterate the vestibular space; and similar defects.

Postdam interference usually is created by palatal tori that extend to the junction of the hard and soft palates, clefts in the hard and soft palates, or neoplastic masses that extend to or beyond the junction of the hard and soft palates.

Denture stability loss usually is caused by hyperplasia or hypertrophy of the alveolar or palatal mucosa or the submucosa, or by shifting detached periosteum, knife-edge alveolar ridges, large compressible cysts, retained malposed impacted teeth, or high attachment of the mandibular lingual frenum.

Speech impairment is likely to occur when the tongue space is reduced by attempts to accommodate for mandibular or palatal tori in the denture.

Deglutition impairment may result from the presence of large neoplastic masses in the posterior part of the mouth, expanded maxillary tuberosities, or abnormally large palatal tori.

Seating of the denture is most likely impaired by bifid epulis fissuratum caused by denture irritation in the vestibular space of the mucolabial fold, or when the alveolar ridge has undergone such marked atrophy that the vestibular space for insertion of the denture's labial flange has disappeared.

Electrosurgical Techniques

The corrective surgical techniques vary greatly, and the specific electrosurgical techniques for the corrective surgery of many of these conditions will be reviewed here. Preprosthodontic electrosurgery can be used very advantageously for procedures ranging from simple removal of undesirable tissue tabs and routine uncomplicated alveoloplasty (alveolectomy) to sophisticated techniques for reconstructive plastic oral surgery and for removal and repair of gross pathologic lesions. Needless to say, the more complex and challenging the prosthetic problem, the greater the contribution electrosurgery makes to the successful outcome of the case.

Before reviewing clinical cases demonstrating most of these anatomic factors and the techniques for their correction, two procedural methods that will be described in the case reports require clarification.

1. In immediate denture cases it seems highly advisable that the person who will perform the surgery should trim and prepare the working model on which the denture will be fabricated. The model trimming becomes, in effect, a preview or trial-run of the surgical procedure, and the surgeon will, if he trims it himself, know precisely which and how much structure has been eliminated from the model and where. Thus, guesswork is eliminated, the surgical procedure is expedited, and the likelihood of achieving an accurate fit with minimal postoperative discomfort is greatly increased.

2. Use of a clear acrylic surgical template makes possible visual checking of the accuracy of denture fit. Need for additional bone trim as the alveoloplasty is being performed can be visualized through the clear acrylic, and the exact portion that should be removed is pinpointed. This further expedites and improves the prospect for a favorable surgical outcome. The template is fabricated on a duplicate of the trimmed working model before the surgery is instituted.

Chapter Twenty

REPAIR OF SOFT TISSUE DEFECTS

The wide variety of anatomic abnormalities and defects that require pre-prosthodontic surgical correction to prepare the mouth properly for dentures and the considerable number of specific electrosurgical techniques for performing the preprosthodontic corrections that have been developed by the author make it desirable to subdivide this chapter into the following parts:

    I. Minor and routine interventions
    II. Elimination of interference from frena (and muscle attachments)
    III. Correction of redundant mucous and submucous tissues
    IV. Mandibular and maxillary vestibulotomy for alveolar ridge extension
    V. Correction of abnormal tuberosities and other bone abnormalities and other defects
    VI. Influence of systemic and local factors on tissue repair

I. MINOR AND ROUTINE INTERVENTIONS

Preprosthodontic clinical electrosurgical techniques range in scope from the simple removal or destruction in situ of undesirable tissue tabs to elimination of gross pathologic tissue, and from the routine alveoloplasty to sophisticated reconstructive plastic oral surgery.

In this discipline, as in the others, it is axiomatic that the more complex the problem and the more challenging the clinical conditions, the greater and more significant is electrosurgery's contribution to the success of treatment. But even the minor, apparently insignificant problems provide excellent opportunities for electrosurgical intervention to facilitate and simplify the treatment.

Removal of Tissue Tabs

CASE 1

PATIENT.   A 65-year-old white male.

HISTORY.   He was referred for extraction of four mobile mandibular anterior teeth and insertion of an immediate denture.

CLINICAL EXAMINATION.   The mandibular central and lateral incisors were present. The rest of his mouth was edentulous. The three interproximal papillae between the four incisors were markedly hypertrophied.

TREATMENT.   The four remaining teeth were extracted for insertion of the immediate denture. After the teeth were extracted the interproximal papillae (especially the median one between the two centrals) projected about 3 to 4 mm. above the gingival margins of the sockets.

It appeared advisable to reduce the fleshy tips of the papillae to more harmonious level in order to avert future irritation and painful postoperative inflammation from pressure of the denture against soft tissue irregularities on the crest of the ridge.

A flame-shaped loop electrode was selected and current output set at 6 for electro-section. The activated electrode was wiped across each projecting tip at its marginal level in an anteroposterior direction. Each hypertrophied papilla came away with a single stroke of the loop without bleeding (Case Fig. 1–1). Healing ensued without incident.

Alveoloplasty (Alveolectomy)

When irregularities of the alveolar bone, particularly of the interseptal bone and the marginal labial edges of the tooth sockets, produce pain when the denture is seated, an alveoloplasty, properly and judiciously performed, will eliminate them as a factor and permit restoration of the dentition with a stable, comfortable, aesthetic and functionally useful denture. The alveoloplasty's objective should not be to make the alveolar bone as smooth as a

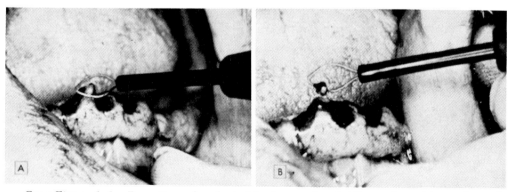

Case Figure 1–1.   Resection of undesirable tissue tabs. *A,* Flame-shaped loop electrode brought into position. *B,* Tissue tab resected to create harmonious tissue level.

billiard ball at the expense of the labial alveolar cortex. The bone reduction should be limited to elimination of irregularities that will interfere with the fit of the denture that cannot be taken care of in the denture.

The author has found it highly advantageous to retain irregularities that will not interfere with the functional usefulness and the fit of the denture. Thus, if there are bilateral undercuts that would abrade the tissues when the denture is inserted, only one side need be reduced, so that the denture can be inserted without causing abrasion, and the other side can be left undisturbed. Unnecessary, overzealous reduction of alveolar bone or tuberosities that results in tapering of the bone must be carefully avoided.

The author has found that when many teeth have to be extracted and considerable bone reduction will be required, it is highly advantageous to *predetermine* the exact amount of tissue that will become excess as a result of the bone reduction. Once this determination has been made, incision and excision of the amount of tissue that is expected to become redundant *before* extracting the teeth and elevating and reflecting the mucoperiosteum in order to perform bone reduction permits accuracy that cannot otherwise be achieved. It eliminates the guesswork that so often is inaccurate because the elevated tissue has contracted and therefore it is no longer possible to estimate how much of the contracted tissue will be redundant.

Excision of too much tissue makes it difficult if not impossible to coapt the tissue margins properly. The sutures often cut through the taut tissues and slough out, causing delayed healing by secondary intention. Inadequate excision results in formation of redundant submucous tissue that is mobile and incapable of providing a firm, stable base for the denture. The technique that is about to be described is invaluable because it eliminates the guesswork and assures precise, accurate excision of the excess tissue created by the alveoloplasty.

Predetermination of the exact amount of tissue that will become redundant is accomplished by measuring the study model after cutting the teeth off at the gingival level and remeasuring the model after trimming it exactly as it is anticipated the alveolar bone will be trimmed. (See Figure 20–3.) The difference between the two measurements is the precise amount of tissue that will become excess and should be removed. Incision and excision of this amount of tissue while it is in its normal attachment to periosteum and bone can be done far more expeditiously as well as precisely than could be achieved with mobile, contracted tissue that has been detached and elevated from the bone.

The following case demonstrates the reduction of tissue before extraction of the teeth, to assure the precise removal of redundant tissue that will be created by the alveolar bone reduction.

CASE 2

PATIENT. A 67-year-old white male.

HISTORY. All the teeth were periodontally involved. The disease was more advanced in the maxilla than the mandible; several of the maxillary teeth had become so painfully mobile that the referring dentist had had to remove them as emergency extractions a week or so previously. His treatment plan was to have the remaining maxillary teeth extracted and an alveoloplasty performed for an immediate denture insertion. He planned to retain the mandibular teeth as long as possible and had ligated them with a stainless steel ligature to try to stabilize them. The patient was referred for the immediate denture surgery.

CLINICAL EXAMINATION.   The maxillary left first bicuspid and cuspid, the right lateral, cuspid and first and second bicuspids were present in the dental arch. The area between the left cuspid and right lateral was edentulous. The mucosa in the edentulous area was incompletely healed from recent extractions. The posterior saddle areas and both tuberosities appeared normal.

The gingival mucosa throughout the maxilla and mandible appeared hyperemic. All the teeth were very mobile owing to advanced periodontoclasia and the mandibular teeth had been immobilized by ligation with continuous loop wiring.

TREATMENT.   The immediate denture and a clear acrylic template that had been processed for this case were immersed in cold sterilizing solution. The mouth was prepared for surgery and bilateral infraorbital and nasopalatine block anesthesia was administered.

A fine 45-degree-angle needle electrode was selected and current output set at 3.5 for electrosection. The interproximal papillae on the labial aspect were incised with the activated electrode across the highest level of the gingival margins (Case Fig. 2–1A). The teeth were extracted. Then the edentulous space was incised along the crest of the ridge with a wiping stroke (Case Fig. 2–1B). Current output was increased to 4.5 and the papillae were incised in an identical manner on the palatal aspect. The papillae were then excised.

The alveolar mucosa was undermined with a periosteal elevator and reflected from the underlying bone. The exposed bone was trimmed with rongeur forceps and a bone file in order to eliminate gross undercuts and sharp interseptal bone crests. When this was completed the area was thoroughly debrided, the mucosa restored and the coapted margins sutured with three interrupted silk sutures. One suture was inserted in the median line; then one on each side in the cuspid region (Case Fig. 2–1C).

The clear acrylic template was inserted to check whether the alveolar bone had been adequately and uniformly reduced. The template fitted accurately without any evidence of blanching of the tissues to indicate areas of compression that might require further bone reduction. The template was removed and three additional sutures were inserted to complete the accurate coaptation of the tissue margins. The mouth was cleansed and the sterilized immediate denture was inserted. Upon testing, the denture was found to fit well and seemed to be stable. It appeared to be adequately relieved for muscle trim and the labial frenum. The patient was instructed in postoperative care and reappointed.

He returned on the first postoperative day, however, because of marked postoperative edema and considerable pain. The denture was removed and the mouth irrigated with warm saline solution; then the tissues were inspected. Healing appeared to be progressing satisfactorily except for the edema and two areas of irritation which were tender to the touch. One of these was a fairly large area on the buccal aspect of the right cuspid—first bicuspid region. This area was covered with a layer of coagulum. The second was a small patch of irritation and coagulum in the left lateral incisor region. Both patches were apparently being caused by pressure of the denture.

The denture was relieved and a hydrocortisone acetate preparation, Cordent den-

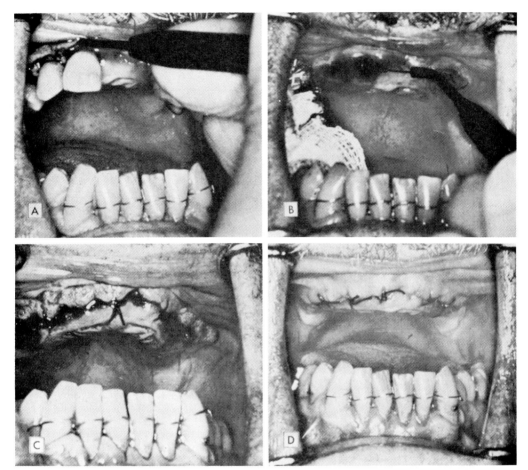

Case Figure 2–1. Routine alveoloplasty. *A*, Estimated excess tissue resulting from bone trim incised with a 45-degree-angle fine needle electrode before teeth are extracted. *B*, Edentulous area incised to excise strip of excess tissue after the teeth were extracted. *C*, Tissues coapted and sutured. *D*, Appearance of the tissues on fifth postoperative day before sutures are removed. Coapted margins have healed by primary union. The tissues are slightly edematous but firm, and the tone is good.

ture powder (Graham), was dusted over the two relieved areas in the denture. Tincture of myrrh and benzoin was applied to the entire operative field and the denture was reinserted. The patient returned on the fifth postoperative day for removal of the sutures. On inspection the tissues were found to be slightly edematous but otherwise healing satisfactorily (Case Fig. 2–1D). The sutures were removed, tincture of myrrh and benzoin applied in air-dried layers, and the patient instructed to continue the postoperative care and return in one week.

When he returned the tissues appeared almost completely normal. Tincture of myrrh and benzoin was applied and intermittent use of an astringent salt-alum mouthwash was prescribed; he was instructed to return in six weeks for further postoperative checkup. When he was seen at that time, the tissues were completely normal and fully healed and the tissue tone was excellent. The mouth and the denture were reported as being completely comfortable.

Control of Tissue Proliferation

A tendency for the repair tissue in a tooth socket to show proliferation is by no means rare. If the proliferative activity is permitted to continue undisturbed, the repair process is likely to be disrupted. Should the proliferation be occurring in a socket over which a denture has been inserted, it will interfere with the healing and also with the fit and the comfort of the restoration in contact with it. Judicious superficial spot electrocoagulation of the proliferating tissue can put a halt to the proliferation and accelerate the tissue healing. The following case demonstrates this.

CASE 3

This case is a typical example of the granulomatous type of proliferation that often occurs in a healing tooth socket, particularly when the latter has been covered and compressed by a restoration immediately after or soon after the extraction has been performed. It demonstrates the usefulness and simplicity of spot coagulation that is highly effective for control of such proliferative granulomatous repair.

PATIENT. A 68-year-old white female.

HISTORY. She had been referred for extraction of her remaining four mandibular teeth. The referring dentist had prepared her old denture for use as an immediate denture by adding comparable teeth to it.

CLINICAL EXAMINATION. The mandibular right and left central incisors and the right lateral incisor and cuspid were still present in the dental arch. The rest of her mouth was edentulous.

TREATMENT. The mouth was prepared for surgery, anesthetized by mental block and labial-lingual infiltration and the teeth extracted. The sharp interseptal bone crests were reduced, but a slight labial undercut that would not interfere with insertion or removal of the denture was left undisturbed in order to provide additional anchorage for the denture. The interproximal papillae had remained intact when the teeth were extracted, so that no suturing was required.

The patient returned on the fifth postoperative day for checkup. The mouth was irrigated and the tissues inspected. All the sockets of the recently extracted teeth were healing exceptionally well except that of the right cuspid, from which hypertrophic granulation tissue proliferated (Case Fig. 3–1A). Roentgenographic examination failed to reveal presence of any demonstrable pathology. In the absence of specific pathology, coagulation of the proliferative tissue rather than curettage appeared to be indicated.

A large ball electrode was selected and current output set at 1 for biterminal electrocoagulation. The electrode was applied for one second, removed for two seconds and reapplied for one second. This was repeated four times at the site of spot coagulation (Case Fig. 3–1B). After the electrocoagulation was completed, chromic acid, 0.05 per cent dilution, was applied to the area for 30 seconds, carefully washed away, and tincture of myrrh and benzoin applied in air-dried layers. The patient was instructed to use a saline mouthwash frequently and to return for a checkup in one week.

Instead of returning as requested she called to report that her mouth felt so good

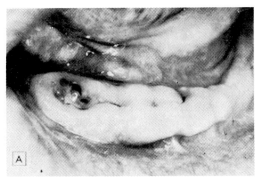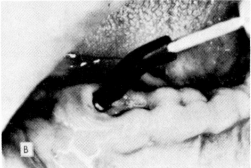

Case Figure 3-1. Control of proliferation of granulation tissue from a recent socket by electrocoagulation. *A,* Preoperative appearance. Three sockets have healed uneventfully. The right cuspid socket is filled with proliferating granulation tissue. *B,* Proliferating tissue contracted by coagulation to normal level.

that she did not think there was any point in coming back again unless she developed further trouble. Since nothing further has been heard from her it appears safe to assume that the treatment was successful and that satisfactory healing progressed uneventfully.

II. ELIMINATION OF INTERFERENCE FROM FRENA (AND MUSCLE ATTACHMENTS)

An effective peripheral seal is essential for success with a full denture. The maxillary labial frenum that extends down along the alveolar ridge toward the ridge crest and low muscle attachments are likely to require so much relief in the denture that the peripheral seal is lost. When such frena and muscle attachments are present, preprosthodontic surgery to eliminate them is the only means whereby the peripheral seal and resultant stability of the denture can be assured.

When these structures are removed by steel scalpel incision, the scar tissue repair and often loss of the vestibular height are likely to create more of a problem than the original condition. The absence of scar tissue when the surgery is performed by electrosection assures that the repair tissue will not prove to be a handicap. Low muscle attachments can often be corrected by simply incising the tissue horizontally and building up the denture flange with a hard roll of surgical cement to displace the tissue and act as a surgical stent (Fig. 20–1). When this is deemed inadequate, the muscle attachment can be resected in a manner similar to that for the frenum.

The next three cases demonstrate the difference in the kind of tissue repair that results from frenectomy by the respective methods of instrumentation and the advantages that are derived from the electrosurgical procedure.

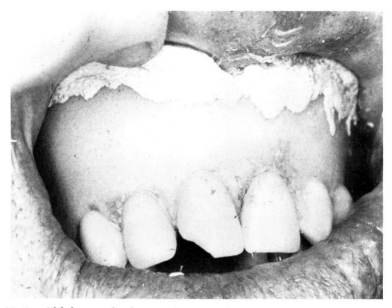

Figure 20–1. Old denture built up with surgical cement to displace the tissue and act as a surgical stent.

CASE 4*

PATIENT. A 48-year-old white female.

HISTORY. The patient had an edentulous maxilla and edentulous mandibular posterior saddle areas. She was referred to the Oral Surgery Clinic for frenectomy in preparation for prosthetic restorations.

CLINICAL EXAMINATION. Her maxillary labial frenum extended to within 2 to 3 mm. of the crest of the alveolar ridge. The oral mucosa appeared otherwise normal. It was obvious that relieving the denture sufficiently to accommodate the frenum properly would destroy the peripheral seal of the prosthesis. Surgery was therefore indicated.

TREATMENT. The mouth was prepared for surgery and infiltration anesthesia was administered. The upper lip was elevated and distended outward as far as possible. A mosquito hemostat was clamped to the frenum as closely as possible to the inner surface of the lip (Case Fig. 4–1A). The lower portion of the frenum, which extended below the beaks of the hemostat, was incised in a V-shaped manner with a No. 15 Bard-Parker scalpel blade.

The portion of the frenum that projected above the beaks of the hemostat was dissected from the concave surface of the hemostat beaks, completing the Y portion of the traditional V-Y incision. The incised tissue was elevated and excised. A moderate amount of bleeding ensued. The V-Y incision was converted into a straight line by pulling the tissues outward and upward and sutured with interrupted 0000 braided silk sutures (Case Fig. 4–1B). The patient was instructed in postoperative care and reappointed for removal of the sutures.

She returned one week later. The mouth was irrigated, the sutures removed and tincture of myrrh and benzoin applied to the area. She was seen for one month postoperatively at weekly intervals during which time healing progressed slowly. By the

---

*This case is presented solely for comparative purposes.

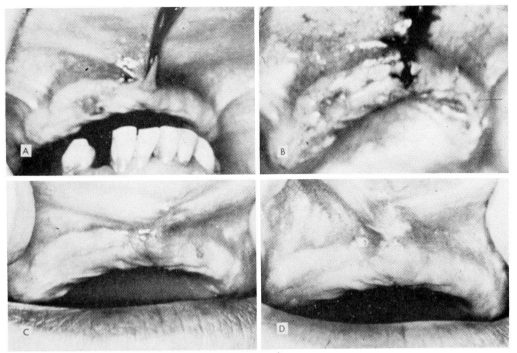

Case Figure 4–1. Frenectomy by cold steel instrumentation. *A*, Lip distended, the curved mosquito hemostat is clamped to the frenum as closely to the lip as possible. *B*, The V-Y incision resection completed, the incised tissues are pulled into a straight line and sutured with interrupted silk sutures. *C*, Postoperative appearance of the tissues one month later. A large mass of fibrous scar tissue has developed in the operative field. *D*, Appearance two months postoperatively. The mass of cicatricial scar tissue now partially obliterates the labial sulcus space and is much bulkier than the original frenum.

end of a month the tissues were well healed, but a cicatricial mass of scar tissue had formed in the midline where the suture line had been (Case Fig. 4–1*C*). By the end of a second month the cicatricial contraction had pulled the inner portion of the lip down toward the crest of the alveolar ridge sufficiently to obliterate more than half of the labial vestibular space (Case Fig. 4–1*D*).

Contraction by cicatricial bands of fibrous scar connective tissue, such as resulted in this case, is more or less typical of the type of tissue repair that is usually obtained with cold-steel incisions. In many respects the bulk of the reparative scar tissue which forms is likely to become much more of a hindrance than the original condition. The healing sequence in this case offers a decided contrast to the healing results usually obtained by similar incisions that are performed electrosurgically.

CASE 5

This case typifies the remarkable simplicity with which small nonfibrous frena can be resected by electrosurgery without bleeding or contractual scar tissue repair.

PATIENT. A 59-year-old white female.

HISTORY. The patient was referred for multiple extractions and alveoloplasty in preparation for immediate denture insertion.

CLINICAL EXAMINATION.   The maxillary left central, lateral and cuspid, and the right central and lateral incisors were still present in the dental arch. The rest of the maxilla was edentuloŭs. Between the centrals there was a soft pulpy mass of frenal tissue which dipped down between the two teeth low enough to create a problem with regard to peripheral seal of the denture. Resection of this mass was therefore planned as part of the preparation of the mouth for the immediate denture.

TREATMENT.   The mouth was prepared and bilateral infraorbital and nasopalatine block anesthesia was administered. The teeth were extracted. Then the upper lip was lifted upward and outward and grasped with the beaks of a mosquito hemostat in the manner previously described (Case Fig. 5–1A). A medium-sized round loop electrode was selected and current output set at 6 for electrosection. The loop was run down along the concave surface of the beaks of the hemostat with a wiping motion, resecting the tissue that hung down from the loop, leaving the beaks of the hemostat clean of tissue (Case Fig. 5–1B). When the hemostat was removed a light layer of

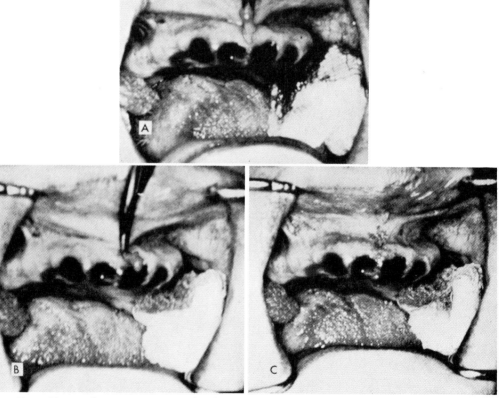

Case Figure 5–1. Frenectomy with a loop electrode. *A,* Curved mosquito hemostat clamped to the frenum. *B,* Projecting tissue, resected downward with loop electrode off the beaks of the hemostat, hangs down from its tip. *C,* Immediate postoperative appearance. Frenum removed bloodlessly and without distention of tissues or need for suturing.

coagulum marked where the frenum had been resected (Case Fig. 5–1C). There was no bleeding or open wound to suture. Tincture of myrrh and benzoin was applied to the area. The alveoloplasty was then completed and the immediate denture inserted. Healing progressed without incident.

Needless to say, frenectomies cannot always be performed electrosurgically with such dramatic simplicity. Even difficult frenectomies can, as will be seen, be performed with greater ease and simplicity by electrosurgery than with cold-steel cutting, and the postoperative results usually are functionally and aesthetically much more gratifying.

CASE 6

This case is an example of the usefulness of electrosurgery for performing difficult frenectomies in which the frenal fibers are deeply invaginated into the median suture line of the maxilla and must be fully resected if regeneration is to be averted.

PATIENT. A 59-year-old white female.

HISTORY. The patient had lost most of her maxillary and mandibular teeth by gradual extractions due to caries, abscess formation and periodontal deterioration. She was referred for frenectomy as a preliminary to prosthetic restoration of her mouth.

CLINICAL EXAMINATION. The maxillary labial frenum was very prominent and fibrous. It extended downward to within 3 mm. of the crest of the alveolar ridge. Several prominent muscle attachments were present on either side of the frenum. These also dipped down toward the crest of the ridge (Case Fig. 6–1A). The maxillary left second bicuspid and first molar, the right cuspid and second molar, and the mandibular six anterior teeth were still present in the dental arches. The edentulous areas in the maxilla appeared to be freshly healed sockets. The tissues were healthy and their tone normal.

TREATMENT. The mouth was prepared for surgery and infiltration anesthesia administered. The lip was lifted upward and outward, bringing the frenum into taut prominence. That portion of the frenum which projected outward beyond the alveolar mucosa was grasped between the beaks of a curved mosquito hemostat and clamped as closely as possible to the inner surface of the lip.

A 45-degree-angle fine needle electrode was selected and current output set at 3.5 for electrosection. The lower half of the frenum, which was flatly attached to the alveolar bone and adjacent mucosa, was incised with the activated electrode (Case Fig. 6–1B). These incisions formed two oblique lines which followed the outline of the frenum and converged to form a sharp V. The lower half of this incised tissue was undermined and elevated from the underlying bone. Adherent fibers invaginating into the median maxillary suture line were resected with the electrode until the loosened mass of tissue could be lifted from the bone freely. The upper half of the incised frenum, which extended from the alveolar mucosa into the areolar mucosa of the lip, was then resected by slicing the tissue off the beaks of the hemostat with the needle electrode (Case Fig. 6–1C), thus completing frenectomy.

A little blood oozed when the tissues were incised, but when the hemostat was removed the tissues remained tightly compressed so that there was no distention of the incised margins. The area was dried and tincture of myrrh and benzoin was applied in air-dried layers. Since the tissues did not gape open, no sutures were required.

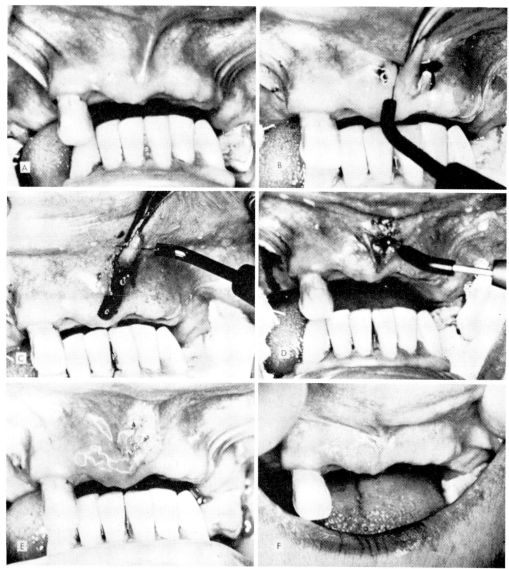

Case Figure 6–1. Electrosurgical frenectomy with V-Y incision. *A*, Preoperative appearance. Note prominent frenum and muscle attachment in bicuspid region attached low near crest of alveolar ridge. *B*, Clamped frenum is incised for V part of the V-Y incision with a 45-degree-angle fine needle electrode. *C*, Y part of the V-Y incision completed by resecting the frenal tissue off the beaks of the hemostat with the needle electrode. *D*, Bleeding controlled and irregular tissue tabs reduced by coagulating with a small ball electrode. Note bleeding from incised muscle. *E*, Appearance of the operative field on third postoperative day. Area is covered with healthy layer of coagulum. *F*, Appearance of tissues six weeks postoperatively. Healing is complete. Only a 1 mm. ridge of tissue is present in the frenal area. There is no bulk of tissue in, or cicatricial contraction of, the labial vestibule.

The prominent muscle attachment immediately distal to the left cuspid was then incised by nicking the taut fibers with the electrode just enough to relax the muscle tension. More bleeding resulted from this than from the frenectomy. Bleeding persisted despite applications of tincture of myrrh and benzoin and tannic acid powder.

This bleeding site was brought under control by electrocoagulation with a small ball electrode and current output of 1. Then a few ragged tissue tabs in the frenal area were reduced by spot coagulation (Case Fig. 6–1D). Tincture of myrrh and benzoin was reapplied and the operative sites were covered with Orabase adhesive ointment.

The patient returned on the third postoperative day and reported that although there had been initial edema of the lip and gingivae for the first 24 hours it had completely subsided by the second day. There had been no pain, merely mild discomfort. The tissue healing was progressing very satisfactorily except in one tiny area near the upper outer margin on the left side which still looked raw. The rest of the frenal area was covered with a light layer of healthy looking coagulum (Case Fig. 6–1E). The raw spot was treated by superficial spot coagulation. Chromic acid, 0.01 per cent dilution, was applied to the area for 30 seconds, washed off, and tincture of myrrh and benzoin applied.

She was seen again two weeks later. By that time the tissues were sufficiently healed and the tissue tone sufficiently improved to permit impression taking for her dentures; so active treatment was stopped. She returned for a final postoperative examination about one month after she had had her new dentures completed. This time the tissues were fully healed and the tissue tone was excellent. The only clinical evidence that surgery had recently been performed was a thin fibrous scar visible in the midline; the scar projected 1 mm. above the surface of the labial alveolar gingiva (Case Fig. 6–1F). Since it had no bulk and did not reduce the labial vestibule, it did not affect either the seating or peripheral seal of the denture. The incised muscle attachment in the cuspid region had also healed without contraction or interference with the peripheral seal.

III. CORRECTION OF REDUNDANT MUCOUS AND SUBMUCOUS TISSUES

Importance of Proper Maxillo-Mandibular Relations

For almost half a century, prevention has been dentistry's watchword and goal. As a result, much of dental research has been directed toward caries control and the etiology and prevention of periodontal disease.

In view of the stress on prevention, it seems ironic that dentistry's greatest advances have not been made in that area but rather in the art and science of restoration or replacement of the natural dentition.

The improvements in full denture techniques and materials have been particularly noteworthy. A brief comparison of present-day prosthodontics with that of a few decades ago reveals the magnitude of the improvements. Contrast the highly complex anatomic articulators in vogue today with the plane line articulators used universally, even in the leading dental schools, just a few decades ago. Equally dramatic are the influences of the sophisticated phenomena of occlusion and centric relation and of vertical dimension and freeway space on present-day prosthodontics in contrast to the utter lack of awareness of these factors in the past and the former total dependence of the prosthodontist on such primitive values as lip line measurements and the curve of Spee for achieving denture aesthetics and function.

When one considers in addition the improvements in modern impression materials and techniques over the plaster of Paris impressions and wax squash bites and development of the modern acrylic resin denture materials over the vulcanite dentures of a previous era, it becomes all the more remarkable and significant that despite the advances and advantages, the present-day prosthodontist still shares a common experience with his predecessors; he still encounters denture failures, and these are by no means infrequent, isolated phenomena.

Much attention has been drawn to the need for proper occlusion, and much time and effort have been devoted to discussion of improvements in impression techniques and of the benefits to be derived from cusped vs. cuspless teeth and many other aspects of full denture construction.

It is to be regretted that a paramount cause for denture failures and abnormal alveolar resorption tends to be overlooked by many, that is, the matter of the function and proper relation of the anterior dentition.

The posterior teeth are the grinders. The anterior teeth are the shearers; they normally function like a pair of scissors to cut the food. When the anterior teeth come into direct contacting impact with each other, they exert an enormous amount of traumatic force. When the teeth in one dental arch have been lost and artificially replaced with a full denture, and in the opposing jaw the natural teeth are intact, the impact of the relatively immobile natural teeth against a denture that is not firmly riveted to the jawbone but rests on a thin cushion of mucosa traumatizes the underlying bone and accelerates alveolar resorption.

The maxilla remains stationary during masticatory function, and only the mandible is the moving force. Thus, the damage from tooth impact instead of a shearing relation is greatly increased when the natural teeth are in the mandible and the maxillary teeth have been replaced with a full denture, since the natural dentition is delivering the blow, and the denture is the recipient of the forceful tilting impact. Thus, we shall see case after case in which this traumatic impact has literally disintegrated the maxillary alveolar bone and triggered proliferation or deterioration of the overlying mucosa.

When patients in this category are being treated in preparation for denture insertion, it is not enough to perform the necessary electrosurgery; it is equally important to be sure that the shearing action is restored by setting up the artificial teeth and beveling the natural ones to achieve it. Clinically we often see cases in which nature has tried to do the beveling, but too late or too incompletely to prevent the bone resorption.

Resection of Redundant Mucous-Submucous Tissues

The presence of excess mucous or submucous gingival tissue, scar tissue, epulis fissuratum (epulis granulomatosa; granuloma fissuratum) or similar areolar gingival hyperplasia[1-5] and/or alveolar atrophy interferes with denture seating and stability. It is rarely possible to compensate adequately for these defects in the denture itself without some risk of subsequent greater deformity resulting therefrom. As a rule, correction can be properly achieved only by means of surgery.

Kazanjian introduced a procedure called "ridge extension" (1924, 1935) which he recommended for cases of alveolar atrophy or obliteration of the normal mucolabial fold by scar tissue or muscle attachments at the level of the alveolar crest. The classic Kazanjian technique and modifications thereof for plastic restoration of alveolar ridges by means of extensive excisions, use of rubber tubing stents secured for the most part with button sutures or similar extraoral retaining devices, [6, 7] for many years served as the most effective methods for surgical improvement of the alveolar ridges and their gingival mucosa.

The simplicity and efficacy of the electrosurgical techniques that are about to be described for reduction or elimination of redundant tissue with appropriate electrodes makes these earlier techniques appear outmoded and unduly complicated for both the operator and the patient.

Although some of the corrective electrosurgery can be performed efficiently by incisional resection of the undesirable tissue, planing the mucosa by resection with appropriately shaped loop electrodes, unique to electrosurgery, is particularly effective. In many instances the best result is obtained by combining incisional with loop resection.

Incisional resection is preferable when the surface continuity of the tissue is broken by ulceration or necrotic degeneration. Loop resection is preferable to eliminate proliferative hypertrophy, as when the surface tissue is lobulated, or when the tissue is hyperplastic and atonal. When there is submucous hypertrophy combined with nonulcerated surface degeneration, the combination of incisional and loop resection is particularly effective.

Mucous and submucous dissection for hyperplasia due to trauma

Improper maxillo-mandibular relationship with traumatic impact of the anterior teeth instead of a shearing effect when there is a dentulous mandible and an edentulous maxilla is as has been mentioned extremely destructive.

In most instances, the destructive trauma results in disintegration of the alveolar bone, which is replaced by degenerative fibrous tissue. In some instances the victim is more fortunate, and the trauma stimulates massive hyperplastic proliferation without alveolar resorption.

The clinical appearance of the alveolar ridges and labial vestibules in such cases often is much worse than when there is bone resorption. In the latter cases the fibrous tissue merely replaces the bone, which retains its normal anatomic contour. But in cases in which there is no bone resorption the hyperplastic proliferation produces bulky, bulging distortions of the anatomic contour that are more disfiguring in appearance but more readily amenable to surgical repair by mucous and submucous dissection.

The next cases demonstrate the techniques for performing the mucous and submucous dissection and the advantages electrosurgery offers in facilitating and simplifying these surgical procedures.

CASE 7

This case is a typical example of necrotic degeneration of gingival alveolar mucosa which often results from traumatic impact of natural mandibular teeth against an ill-fitting maxillary full denture.

PATIENT.   A 69-year-old white male.

HISTORY.   Two years previously the patient had undergone surgery for carcinoma of the colon. Both the patient and his brother, the referring dentist, were concerned that the gingival deterioration and ulceration on the labial aspect of the maxilla might be a metastatic manifestation.

CLINICAL EXAMINATION.   *Extraoral.*   Negative.

Intraoral.   The right cuspid and left central, lateral, cuspid, and first bicuspid still remained in an otherwise edentulous mandible. The maxilla was edentulous. The patient wore a full upper and partial lower denture. His oral hygiene was deplorable. Two thirds of the crowns of the left lateral, cuspid, and first bicuspid were covered with massive deposits of calculus. The ridge between the right central and left cuspid was irregular and appeared incompletely healed from recent extractions (Case Fig. 7–1).

When the upper denture was removed, the gingival mucosa appeared atonal and degenerated. There was an oblong patch of necrotic slough present near the crest of the alveolar ridge in the left lateral-cuspid area. There were a number of ulcerated areas interspersed with irregular round masses of hypertrophied mucosa along the labial aspect about 3 mm. above the crest of the ridge. A number of keratotic patches marked the peripheral seal of the denture in the mucobuccal fold.

TREATMENT.   The mouth was prepared for surgery and bilateral infraorbital and nasopalatine block anesthesia was administered. A 45-degree-angle fine needle electrode was selected and current output set at 3.5 for electrosection. The full length of the ulcerated tissue was incised along two parallel lines of incision, joined together at the two terminal ends by horizontal V-shaped incisions with their apices directed distally. The incised strip of tissue was undermined, excised, and preserved in formalin solution for biopsy. The remaining labial alveolar mucosa was retracted and the alveolar bone examined for disease. The bone appeared intact and quite normal. Some hypertrophic submucous tissue was present in the area. This was partially removed by blunt dissection, but some of this tissue adhered and had to be resected with a small U-shaped loop electrode.

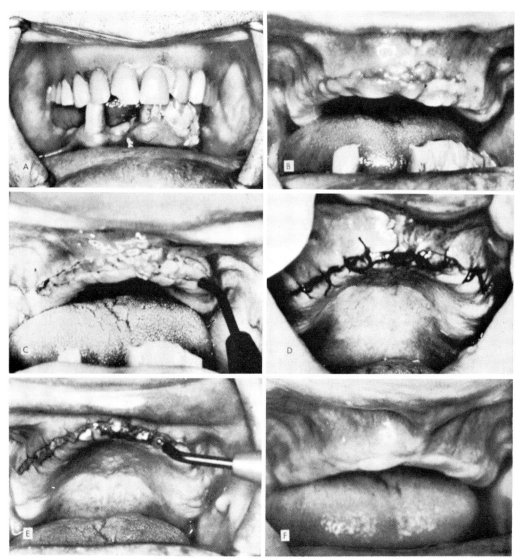

Case Figure 7–1. Resection of necrotic gingival mucosa degenerated due to denture irritation. *A,* Preoperative appearance of mouth with full upper denture occluding with natural mandibular dentition. Note calculus and other evidence of poor oral hygiene. *B,* Preoperative appearance of labial alveolar mucosa with denture out of mouth. Note lobulated appearance of degenerated tissue. *C,* Parallel horizontal incisions joined at the terminal ends performed with 45-degree-angle fine needle electrode. *D,* Debridement completed, the tissue margins are coapted and sutured with interrupted silk sutures. *E,* Fifth postoperative day. Sutures have been removed, and irregular tabs are reduced to normal level by coagulation with small ball electrode. *F,* Appearance in tenth postoperative week. Tissues fully healed. Tissue tone is excellent, and contour of alveolar ridge is good.

When debridement was completed the labial and palatal tissues were approximated and the coapted margins sutured with interrupted silk sutures. Tincture of myrrh and benzoin was applied to the operative field. A strip of adhesive dryfoil was placed over the sutures; then a surgical cement pack was inserted into the sterilized old denture which thus served as a surgical stent.

On the fifth postoperative day the patient reported no ill effects. The mouth was irrigated; the sutures were removed and the tissues inspected. Healing was progressing very satisfactorily by primary union. The suture line was covered with a thin layer of healthy looking coagulum. A few irregular tissue tabs were reduced by applying superficial spot coagulation with a small ball electrode and current output of 0.5 for split-second periods of momentary contact. Tincture of myrrh and benzoin was applied in air-dried layers.

He was seen at regular weekly intervals for the next 10 weeks. Steady improvement in healing and tissue tone was noted from the outset. The biopsy report was "benign inflammatory tissue with ulceration and necrosis." By the tenth week the tissues were fully healed, the alveolar ridge was firm and normal in contour, and the tissue tone was excellent.

The patient had received a prophylaxis during the postoperative interval and had had new dentures constructed. Fear of further complications impelled him to maintain a reasonable state of oral hygiene thereafter.

The author was kept informed of the patient's condition for more than 5 years postoperatively. During that period the gingival mucosa remained normally healthy and provided a stable base for the maxillary denture.

CORRECTION OF ANATOMIC HANDICAP DUE TO INJUDICIOUS ALVEOLOPLASTY

CASE 8

This case offers a classic example of the serious anatomic handicap that may be created when alveoloplasty is performed injudiciously and overzealously. The trauma of *normal functional stress* on these mutilated alveolar ridges produces excessive resorption, with subsequent mobility of the unsupported mucosa that destroys denture stability. In many ways this traumatic deformity resembles the deformity of senile resorption, in which the gingival mucosa as well as alveolar bone undergoes atrophic resorption that is likely to be unrelated to functional stress trauma. The two should not be confused.

The trauma in these cases of improper alveoloplasty results from the poor anatomic contour of the alveolar ridge. The latter, being tapered to a V-shaped crest instead of round, is incapable of providing a stable base for the denture. Denture instability creates traumatic irritation which stimulates and accelerates alveolar resorption.

In addition to eliminating the hypertrophic, mobile gingival tissue, corrective surgery should also restore adequate vertical dimension to the alveolar ridge to accommodate a denture with a functional labial flange and a peripheral seal.

PATIENT. A 56-year-old white female.

HISTORY. All the maxillary teeth had been extracted eight years previously, and a full upper and partial lower denture had been constructed. She reported that a con-

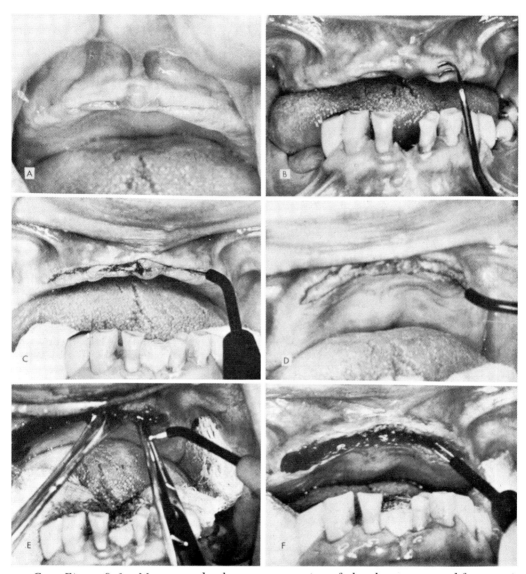

Case Figure 8-1. Mucous and submucous resection of alveolar mucosa and frenum. *A,* Preoperative appearance of crest of alveolar ridge. Note indentations due to degeneration and hypertrophy of the tissues. Note broad frenum attached low, and nasopalatine papilla on crest of ridge in midline. *B,* Mobility of hypertrophic soft tissue demonstrated by displacement with retractor. *C,* Horizontal incision with 45-degree-angle fine needle electrode along superior border of degenerated tissue. *D,* Paralleling palatal horizontal incision, joined to first incision by tapering to horizontal V's at the terminal ends. *E,* Incised strip excised. A bleeder is clamped with a mosquito hemostat and coagulated off beaks of the hemostat with a small ball electrode. *F,* Submucous tissue resected from channel with a narrow U-shaped loop electrode.

siderable amount of bone had been removed from the upper jaw but did not know why this had been done. The upper denture had been troublesome from the outset. In the previous year it had become so loose that she consulted a dentist about replacing it. His examination revealed that the prognosis for a new denture was very poor unless the alveolar ridge could be improved. She was referred for preliminary corrective surgery.

CLINICAL EXAMINATION. *Extraoral.* Negative.

Intraoral. The mandibular left first and second molars, first and second bicuspids, cuspid and lateral, and the right lateral, cuspid, and first bicuspid were present in the dental arch. The maxillary edentulous alveolar ridge was very thin, jutted forward at the crest, and was somewhat concave and very short on the labial aspect. Along the crest of the ridge there was a fibrous band of movable mucosa. A broad labial frenum extended downward to within 3 mm. of the ridge crest. In the midline about 1 mm. below the frenal attachment there was a round tissue bulge. This was the incisive papilla, which is normally located on the palatal aspect (Case Fig. 8–1).

TREATMENT. The surgery was performed in two steps.

Step I. The mouth was prepared for surgery and infiltration anesthesia administered. A 45-degree-angle fine needle electrode was selected and current output set at 3.5 for electrosection. An incision was made immediately superior to, and parallel with, the fibrous welt of mucosa along the crest of the alveolar ridge. A second paralleling incision was made immediately below the band of fibrous tissue along the palatal aspect of the ridge. The two paralleling incisions were joined at their respective terminal ends to form horizontal V's with their apices directed distally. Both incisions were bloodless. The incised strip of mucosa was undermined and excised. Some bleeding ensued; a small blood vessel apparently had been torn as the tissue was elevated from the periosteum and bled profusely. The bleeder was effectively controlled by clamping it with a mosquito hemostat and applying coagulating current to the beaks of the hemostat with a small ball electrode.

Adherent fibrous tissue shreds and submucous tissue were present in the groove formed by the tissue excision. This tissue was resected from the groove with a narrow U-shaped loop electrode. The incised tissue margins were coapted and sutured by inserting a central suture first and then suturing the tissues laterally on either side of the central suture (Case Fig. 8–2).

Step II. The alveolar gingival defect having been closed, the lip was elevated upward and outward and the taut frenum was clamped between the beaks of a curved mosquito hemostat as closely to the inner surface of the lip as possible. The frenum was then incised to form the V-Y incision and was excised off the beaks of the hemostat with a 45-degree-angle fine needle electrode in the manner previously described.

A periosteal elevator was inserted laterally through the incision, and the labial mucosa on either side of the frenal site was undermined to create slack in the tissues. The lip was then elevated to pull the V-Y incision into a straight line and sutured. A strip of adhesive dryfoil was applied to the sutured areas. A stiff mix of surgical cement was placed into the old denture which was then inserted to serve as a surgical stent.

She returned on the fifth postoperative day. The denture was removed, the mouth was irrigated, and the tissues were inspected. They appeared firm, the tissue tone was good, and healing was progressing satisfactorily by primary intention. The sutures were removed and tincture of myrrh and benzoin was applied. A small papillomatous tissue tab had been destroyed *in situ* by fulguration at the time of surgery. This area was healing by granulation, and was also painted with the myrrh and benzoin. Slight irregularities in the surface of the granulating tissue were reduced to harmonious level by superficial spot coagulation with a small ball electrode.

The patient was seen weekly thereafter. Four weeks postoperatively the tissues were firm, their tone was good, and the contour of the alveolar ridge was normal. The patient was informed that she was ready for a new denture; when made, it was stable and functionally useful.

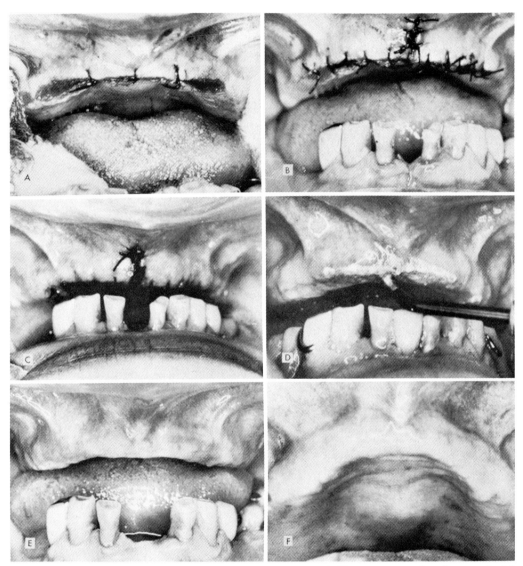

Case Figure 8-2. Operative-postoperative sequence. *A,* Tissues coapted and sutured with central and lateral guide sutures. *B,* Frenectomy completed, the suturing of alveolar ridge and frenal site is completed. *C,* Appearance of tissues on fifth postoperative day. Healing is progressing favorably. *D,* Sutures removed, tissue irregularities are reduced with small ball electrode by coagulation. *E,* Appearance four weeks postoperatively. Tissues are fully healed; the tissue tone is excellent, and the ridge is firm and normal in contour. *F,* Palatal view at same time. Note smooth round contour of the alveolar ridge, a good base for a stable denture.

CASE 9

PATIENT.   A 58-year-old black female.*

HISTORY.   Five years previously this patient's mandibular molars and all remaining maxillary teeth had been extracted, and a maxillary full upper denture and lower lingual-bar partial denture had been constructed. For the past year she had been noticing that the upper denture seemed to be loosening, and for the past few months she had difficulty retaining it in its position during speaking or eating. She noticed that the "gums in the front of the mouth seemed swollen" and she consulted her dentist. She was referred for the necessary reconstructive plastic oral surgery to restore the maxilla to normal dimension to enable him to fabricate a functionally useful and cosmetically acceptable new upper denture.

CLINICAL EXAMINATION.   With her upper denture in situ, twin bulges of tissue were visible, protruding above the superior border of the denture in the anterior region. The denture was unstable and tended to drop down when the patient opened her mouth.

When the denture was removed, two large bulging sessile masses on either side of the midline became visible, and an ovoid mass approximately 1.0 cm. in diameter and 0.5 cm. in thickness was located in the midline, separating the two lateral masses (Case Fig. 9–1).

TREATMENT.   The tissues were prepared, and bilateral infraorbital and nasopalatine regional block injections were administered to provide the anesthesia. A 45-degree-angle fine needle electrode was selected, cutting current output was set at 3 on the instrument panel dial, and the activated electrode was used with wiping motions to resect the central mass.

After the amount of excess tissue that would result following submucous redundant tissue resection was estimated, incisions were made to excise this excess. Since the outer surfaces of the lateral masses appeared intact, they would be preserved as protective flaps to cover the surgical field. Each flap was elevated with a tissue elevator, and the submucous tissue was resected with a medium-width U-shaped loop electrode used with current output set at 5.

When the redundant tissue had been removed, without disturbing the periosteum, the tissue flaps were sutured to close the wounds.

The entire surgical procedure, with only one exception, involved soft tissue resection. The exception was the reduction of the base of the naseous spine that was exposed when the median bulbous mass was resected. Its sharp bony pointed projection was reduced and rounded off with a rongeur forceps and a bone file.

After the suturing was completed, the old denture, which had been sterilized in a cold sterilizing solution, was washed and dried, and a roll of stiffly mixed surgical cement was inserted along the internal surface of the labial flange. A strip of adhesive dryfoil was carefully adapted to the labial mucosa to cover the sutures and prevent them from becoming embedded in the cement when the denture was inserted as a surgical stent to retain the tissues in their desired position. The dryfoil was secured to

---

*This case was photographed as one of the sequences in a motion picture film. As a result, this and the remaining figures in this case had to be enlarged from 16 mm. instead of 35 mm. slides. Owing to the greater amount of enlargement involved, there has been a slight loss of sharpness and depth of field in these photographs.

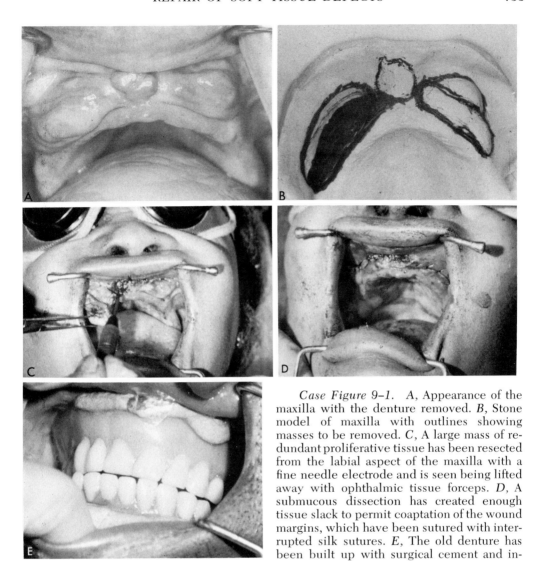

Case Figure 9–1. A, Appearance of the maxilla with the denture removed. B, Stone model of maxilla with outlines showing masses to be removed. C, A large mass of redundant proliferative tissue has been resected from the labial aspect of the maxilla with a fine needle electrode and is seen being lifted away with ophthalmic tissue forceps. D, A submucous dissection has created enough tissue slack to permit coaptation of the wound margins, which have been sutured with interrupted silk sutures. E, The old denture has been built up with surgical cement and inserted over the protected sutures to serve as a surgical stent and pressure pack.

the mucosa with flexible collodion painted over the dryfoil and the dry mucous membrane. When this was dry, the denture was carefully inserted and the cement molded into the vestibule to extend the denture flange and preserve the vestibular space in a similar manner to the muscle trimming of an impression.

Healing progressed uneventfully, and on the fifth postoperative day the sutures were removed. The tissue tone was good, and there was distinct evidence of initial primary repair (Case Fig. 9–2). Two weeks postoperatively the denture was rebased with acrylic, and 10 weeks postoperatively, the tissues being completely healed, impressions were taken and a new denture was made, with careful observance of proper anterior shearing action of the dentition.

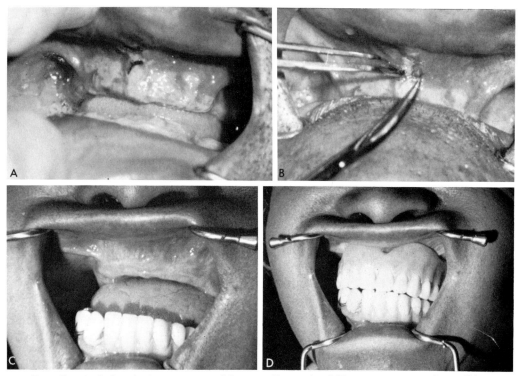

Case Figure 9–2. A, Appearance of the maxilla on the fifth postoperative day. All but one of the sutures have been removed. Note the excellent rate and quality of the tissue healing. B, The last suture is being removed. This photo shows the condition of the tissues more clearly to be almost fully healed and normal in tone. C, Appearance of the maxilla at the patient's final visit. The tissues are fully healed, their tone is normal, and the alveolar ridge is normal in contour. D, The patient's new denture is in place. It is stable and is a functionally efficient and aesthetically satisfactory restoration.

HYPERTROPHIC DEGENERATION FROM AN ILL-FITTING DENTURE

CASE 10

This case is an example of the huge amount of hypertrophic degeneration the gingival tissues may undergo when subjected for years to irritation from an ill-fitting denture superimposed on an anatomic handicap: in this instance, the collapsed palatal vault of the typical mouth breather.

PATIENT. A 39-year-old white male.

HISTORY. All the maxillary teeth and the posterior mandibular teeth had been extracted during his military service in World War II and been replaced with a full upper and partial lower denture. Both dentures had become unstable but he was still wearing them. He consulted a dentist about having them replaced. The maxillary alveolar gingivae had undergone such extensive deterioration and hypertrophy that it would have been impossible to construct a denture until the mouth had been suitably prepared. He was referred for the corrective surgery.

CLINICAL EXAMINATION. *Extraoral.* Negative.

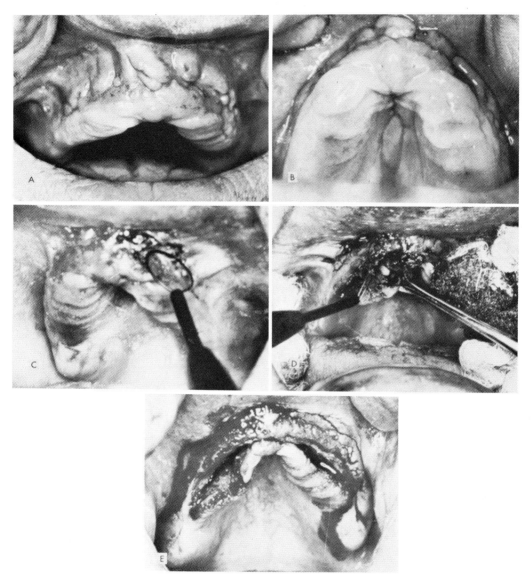

Case Figure 10–1. Resection of massive lobulated hypertrophic tissue and submucous resection of hypertrophic tissue. *A,* Preoperative appearance, labial view. The labial alveolar mucosa has undergone massive degenerative hypertrophy. The tissue is lobulated and one of the lobules is ulcerated. *B,* Preoperative palatal view. The labial hypertrophy can be seen partially obliterating the labial-buccal vestibule. The palatal vault is extremely narrow and the palatal mucosa is very thick. *C,* The labial hypertrophic tissue is resected with a large, round loop electrode. *D,* After the labial aspect was reduced to normal, the mucosa was incised on the palatal side of the crest of the ridge and the palatal mucosa was retracted. Massive submucous hypertrophic tissue is being resected from the palatal aspect with a narrow 45-degree-angle U-shaped loop electrode. *E,* Submucous resection is completed and the tissues are ready for coaptation and suturing. Note width of the palatal vault.

Intraoral. The entire maxillary mucosa was tremendously hypertrophied and had deteriorated into innumerable pendulous lobules. One large lobule was ulcerated. The ulceration had resisted routine treatment. This mass would be resected for biopsy. The palatal vault was very narrow owing to the thickness of the palatal mucosa (Case Fig. 10–1).*

TREATMENT. The mouth was prepared and was anesthetized by subperiosteal infiltration anesthesia with xylocaine (1:50,000). A medium-sized round loop electrode was selected and current output was set at 6 for electrosection. The lips and cheeks were uniformly retracted with the author's self-retaining retractor.

Before surgery could be started it became apparent that the patient was much too apprehensive to undergo surgery consciously. Anoci-association anesthesia would be required. Nitrous oxide–oxygen analgesia was therefore employed to supplement the local anesthesia. This provided excellent anesthesia for the procedure.

A fine ophthalmic tissue forceps was inserted through the loop electrode. The ulcerated lobule was grasped with the forceps, pulled taut, resected with a wiping stroke of the loop and preserved in formalin for biopsy. The remaining surface lobules were individually resected; then the remaining hypertrophic tissues on the labial surface were reduced to normal level by planing with short brushing strokes.

A 45-degree-angle fine needle electrode was substituted for the loop and current density was reduced proportionally to 3.5 for electrosection. An incision was made along the palatal aspect of the crest of the alveolar ridge. The palatal mucosa was undermined and retracted and clamped with an Allis forceps, and submucous dissection was performed. This was done in part by blunt dissection and then completed with a narrow 45-degree-angle U-shaped loop electrode used with current output increased to 4.5.

When the submucous dissection was completed, the palatal mucosa was normal in thickness and the palatal vault was much wider. The incised margins were coapted and sutured with interrupted silk sutures. The sutures were covered with a strip of adhesive dryfoil; the old denture was built up with surgical cement and inserted over the maxilla to serve as a surgical stent. Mysteclin was prescribed, and ascorbic acid–clear gelatin was recommended as a dietary supplement. The patient was instructed to leave the denture undisturbed for 24 hours and to return the following day.

Upon the patient's return, the denture was removed and the area was irrigated. The mucosa looked healthy and the sutured line of incision appeared to be healing satisfactorily. There was a little edema, and a thin layer of coagulum covered the labial portion of the alveolar ridge. Tincture of myrrh and benzoin was applied and the denture stent was reinserted.

The patient returned on the fifth postoperative day for removal of the sutures. The mouth was irrigated and the tissues were inspected. The mucosa appeared healthy and the line of incision almost fully healed. The labial alveolar surface in the anterior region, which had borne the brunt of resection, was covered with a moderately heavy layer of coagulum (Case Fig. 10–2). The coagulum appeared healthy, with no sign of necrosis. The palatal mucosa was slightly edematous, but otherwise it appeared in excellent condition. The sutures were removed and tincture of myrrh and benzoin was applied in air-dried layers.

Thereafter he was seen at regular weekly intervals. At his next visit healing appeared much further advanced. The coagulum had disappeared and the tissues seemed normal in tone and texture. By the end of the third week the buccal and palatal mucosa were superficially healed except for one small patch of coagulum which was still present in the right vestibule near the mucolabial fold in the median line.

---

*Differential diagnosis of submucous hypertrophy or palatal bone deformity can easily be established by inserting the anesthetic hypodermic needle into the palatal tissue and noting how deeply it penetrates.

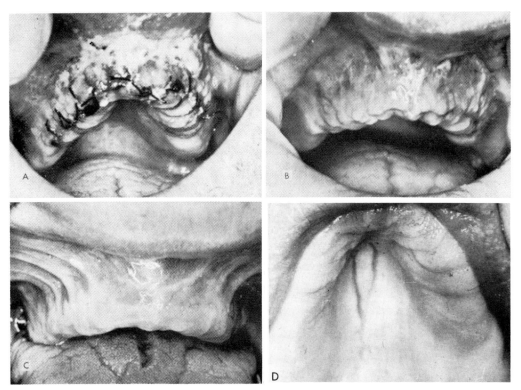

Case Figure 10–2. Postoperative sequence. *A,* Appearance of the tissues on fifth postoperative day. Line of incision is healing by primary intention. Labial surface where hypertrophic tissue was resected by shaving in layers is covered with a heavy layer of healthy coagulum. *B,* Appearance of the tissues three weeks postoperatively. Healing is almost complete. One small patch of coagulum is still present in the lateral incisor area at the labiogingival junction. The crest of the alveolar ridge is still somewhat uneven and ridged in appearance. *C,* Appearance of tissues in eighth postoperative week. The maxilla is completely normal in appearance. The labial mucosa is fully healed, smooth, and well epithelialized. The labial vestibule is high and well defined. The crest of the ridge is fully healed and even. *D,* Palatal view, 5 years postoperatively. The palatal tissues are firm and normal in thickness. The palatal vault is now at least twice as wide as it had been.

The old denture was relined in order to eliminate the surgical pack as the possible source of healing-retarding irritation in this area. Use of a salt-alum mouthwash was recommended, and ascorbic acid and clear gelatin added to supplement his diet. He was seen regularly every other week for the next 10 weeks. By the second of these visits the tissues appeared fairly well healed. At the fifth visit the mouth was fully healed and normal in all respects. The tissue tone was excellent and the alveolar contour was normal, with a full, well-rounded ridge. A palatal view shows that the mucosa there was firm, with no clinical evidence of hypertrophic submucosa. The palatal vault was much wider and the alveolar ridge was well defined. The labial vestibule was wider now that it was rid of the hypertrophic lobules.

The patient was referred back to his dentist for final impressions for new dentures, which were constructed. He has been seen postoperatively semiannually for the past two years. In that period the tissues have remained normal and have provided stable bases for the new dentures. The maxillary denture is functionally and aesthetically satisfactory.

It is very unlikely that the prosthetic surgery could have been performed in this case as efficiently by other methods of instrumentation. It is also unlikely that other methods would have produced a comparable rate and quality of tissue repair devoid of cicatricial contractions.

CASE 11

This case provides an example of anatomic deformity that can result from unsound denture design. Almost all of the labial flange of the patient's upper denture had been cut away by the dentist, to butt the anterior teeth against the alveolar ridge for aesthetic reasons. All that remained of the flange were two winglike extensions high in the vestibule that helped to retain the denture. The open space gradually filled with bulbous fibrotic tissue that made it impossible to wear the old denture or fabricate a new one. The patient was referred for the surgical correction. The case offers an excellent demonstration of the unique value of loop resection for elimination of undesirable hypertrophic tissues for prosthetic reasons.

PATIENT.   A 62-year-old white female.

HISTORY.   All her maxillary teeth and the mandibular posteriors had been extracted many years previously. An extensive alveoloplasty from tuberosity to tuberosity had been performed, and a prominent labial frenum had been resected by scalpel incision.

Apparently, too much labial and buccal alveolar bone had been removed, and excessive resorption ensued. A considerable bulk of fibrous scar tissue formed in the median line and extended laterally to the cuspid regions. As a result her denture had required ever-increasing relief until the peripheral seal was destroyed. As more of the denture had been cut away to provide relief, more cicatricial scar tissue developed in the area until the labial vestibule was entirely occluded by it, and her denture became useless. She sought the services of another dentist, who recognized the futility of attempting to construct a denture in the presence of such a severe anatomic handicap. She was referred for corrective surgery preliminary to the denture construction.

CLINICAL EXAMINATION. *Extraoral.*   Negative.

Intraoral.   The oral mucosa was somewhat hyperemic but the scar tissue mass was rather avascular. This mass partially occluded the labial vestibule from the mucolabial fold downward halfway to the crest of the alveolar ridge in the right central-lateral area and slightly less extensively in the corresponding left side. In the median line the scar tissue extended down to the crest of the ridge. The labial-buccal surface of the ridge was concave in shape instead of convex, so that the palatal portion of the ridge extended in a shelflike slope beyond it. The surface mucosa was abraded in the left cuspid region near the ridge crest. The left tuberosity tapered to a V-shaped heel which dipped downward (Case Fig. 11–1).

TREATMENT.   The mouth was prepared and bilateral infraorbital block anesthesia supplemented with palatal infiltration was administered. A round medium-sized loop electrode was selected and cutting current was set at 6. The fibrous mass was resected by shaving in layers with short brushing strokes until the labial mucosa was reduced to the level of the adjacent tissues.

Two small blood vessels were severed during the resection and bled profusely. One, in the right cuspid region, was brought under control by applying coagulating

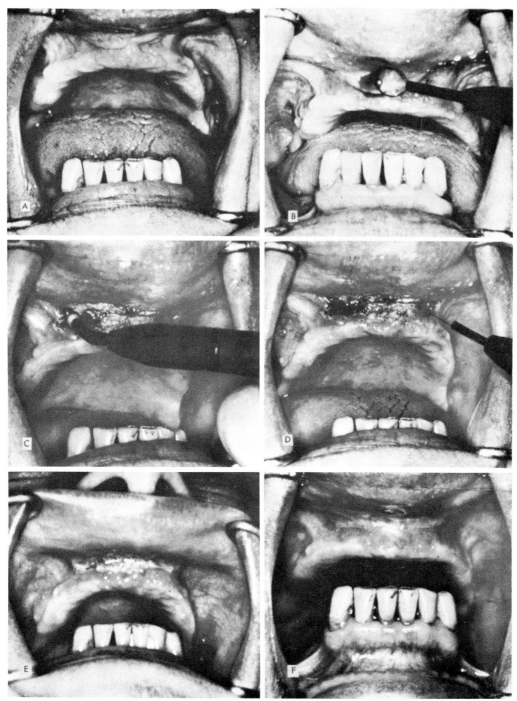

Case Figure 11-1. Resection of hypertrophic fibrous tissue obliterating the labial vestibule of the maxilla. *A*, Preoperative appearance. Note massive superimposition of fibrous scar connective tissue on the normal mucosa. *B*, Resection of fibrous hypertrophic mass performed with round loop. *C*, A persistent bleeding spot controlled by coagulation with ball electrode. *D*, A spurting bleeder controlled by fulguration. *E*, Appearance of tissues on fifth postoperative day. The operative field is covered with a layer of healthy coagulum. *F*, Appearance of the tissues one month postoperatively. The tissues are fully healed and mature. The tissue tone is good, and the labial vestibule is high and well defined.

current with current density set at 2 for the small ball electrode. The bleeder on the left side, a spurter, was not completely controlled by coagulation. A heavy needle electrode was substituted for the ball electrode and monoterminal current was set at 9 for fulguration. The carbonizing current was applied to the bleeding site for several seconds, with the electrode kept in constant rotary motion, until the tissue surface became carbonized and sealed off the bleeder.

The lip was then distended outward and upward, and the fibrous strip of scar tissue in the frenal line was grasped with a curved mosquito hemostat and resected from the beaks of the hemostat with a fine needle electrode and current output of 4 for electrosection. A pendulous mass of fibrous tissue on the crest of the alveolar ridge on the right side in the molar region was reduced to the level of the adjacent tissue with the loop electrode in the same manner as the labial mass. The buccal edge of the ridge close to the crest on the left side was also rounded with the loop to improve the ridge contour.

Surgery having been completed, the patient's old denture was inserted to check the amount of clearance which had been created. The labial flange of the denture had been cut down to within 2 mm. of the ridge crest to clear the mass. The missing anterior portion was built up with stiffly mixed surgical cement, and the denture was inserted to serve as a surgical stent. It was forced into position, and the cement was contoured into the newly created labial vestibular vault by lip manipulation. The patient was instructed in postoperative care and was advised to leave the denture undisturbed for 24 hours.

She returned on the fifth postoperative day. The denture was removed and the area was irrigated. Inspection showed excellent tissue healing with a thin layer of healthy looking coagulum covering the area. Chromic acid, 0.1 per cent dilution, was applied for 30 seconds and followed with tincture of myrrh and benzoin. Some rough spots on the anterior part of the labial cement wall were causing some irritation. These were eliminated, and adhesive dryfoil was adapted to the labial cement surface to create smooth surface contact.

She was seen once a week thereafter for the next month. By the end of the third week the tissues were sufficiently healed to permit impression-taking for a new denture. The mucosa was firm and smooth and the labial contour was quite normal. The vestibular space was clear and a denture could now be extended fully into the mucolabial fold.

She had a new denture made which was well adapted and very stable with excellent peripheral seal. For the past six years the gingival mucosa and denture stability have remained unimpaired.

Granuloma Fissuratum

When anatomic abnormalities or deformities prevent fabrication of a full denture with an effective peripheral seal or an efficient postdam and thereby make it impossible to produce a stable, functionally useful denture that is aesthetically acceptable, it becomes necessary to institute corrective or reconstructive preprosthodontic surgery before proceeding with the restorative work.

A wide variety of abnormalities and deformities may be encountered in an edentulous jaw. In some instances the deformity is created by proliferation of redundant tissue that will interfere with denture fabrication. In others, the abnormality results from the loss of anatomic structure due to disease or senile resorption. In many cases the deformity results from soft tissue proliferation; in others, however, as we shall see later on, the deformity results from bone proliferation, in which cases the proliferative tissue may be engorged and friable or fibrotic and avascular. It should be apparent that while the corrective preprosthetic surgery for these conditions will be similar to some degree, in many ways the surgical procedures will vary considerably, and the electrosurgical instrumentation will vary in accord with the anatomic variations.

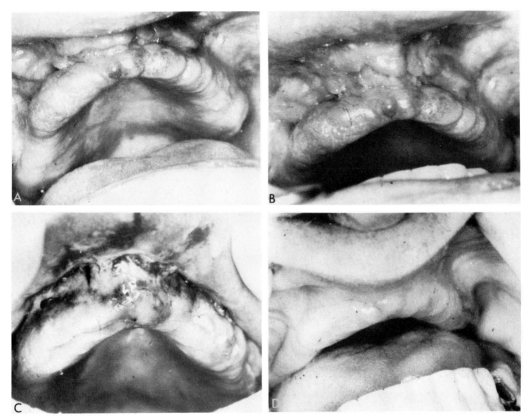

Figure 20–2. Restoration of a normal labial vestibule by elimination of proliferative tissue by loop planing electrosection. *A,* Preoperative appearance of maxilla. The alveolar ridge is normal in height and well contoured but the labial vestibule has become obliterated by superimposition of multiple proliferations of granulomata fissurata. The nasopalatine papilla, located on the crest of the alveolar ridge, is darker red in color and appears swollen and irritated. *B,* Appearance of maxilla and vestibular area, fully exposed by upward and outward elevation of the upper lip. The maxillary surface of the vestibular area is covered with large lobulated masses of degenerative tissue. Several of the masses are ulcerated, and two small patches of superficial ulceration are present on the alveolar mucosa, which is otherwise normal. *C,* Appearance of maxilla on the fifth postoperative day. Healing appears to be progressing favorably. The entire surgical field is covered with a layer of coagulum, which is compatible with normal healing by secondary intention after extensive loop resection such as had been performed to restore the vestibule to normal architecture. *D,* Final postoperative appearance three months later. The repair tissue is normal in all respects and indistinguishable from the surrounding tissues. The nasopalatine papilla is also normal in appearance. The labial vestibule is so well defined that there is ample room for a denture with a normal labial flange and effective peripheral seal to assure desirable aesthetics and function.

The most common cause for soft tissue abnormality in an edentulous jaw is irritation from an ill-fitting denture, and the second most common cause is improper occlusion.

When the maxillary labial denture flange is overextended, or when the prosthodontist has failed to provide adequate relief for the maxillary labial frenum, the irritation produced by compression of the tissues as the denture settles usually causes the type of tissue proliferation referred to as granuloma fissuratum.

Granuloma fissuratum may be the sole lesion that develops in response to the irritation, or it may develop in conjunction with other deformities. Granuloma fissuratum itself may appear in the form of a single mass, or it may form multiple lesions.

Sometimes the proliferation does not occur as granuloma fissuratum. Instead, the external surface of the tissue remains intact, and the redundant tissue is submucous. Figure 20–2 offers an excellent example of this type of lesion, and, like the next case, serves to demonstrate the technique for submucous dissection and preservation of the intact external gingival mucosa to serve as a protective flap covering the surgical field.

CASE 12

This case involved proliferation of the tissues, as did the preceding cases in which natural mandibular dentition was in contact with a full upper denture and caused much destruction. However, unlike the other cases, this case involved submucous rather than external mucous proliferation and there was no alveolar resorption. The surface mucosa was normal in texture except where it created a fold near the crest of the alveolar ridge. The only external effect was formation of a huge proliferative granuloma fissuratum. Treatment therefore differed in that the intact external tissue was utilized as a covering tissue flap instead of tissue resection. Healing was by primary intention instead of secondary granulation.

PATIENT.   A 61-year-old white female.

HISTORY.   All the maxillary teeth and several mandibular posterior teeth had been extracted several years ago, and the lost teeth were replaced with full upper and partial lower dentures.

The constant pounding of the natural mandibular dentition against the anterior teeth of the denture had apparently compressed and traumatized the labial maxillary gingival mucosa. The trauma had stimulated proliferation of submucous tissue that made it impossible for her to use her denture. She finally consulted a dentist, who told her she would have to have preprosthodontic surgery performed and referred her to the author.

CLINICAL EXAMINATION.   The mucosa on the labial aspect of the maxilla bulged outward more than 0.5 cm., and there was a large lesion, apparently a granuloma fissuratum, in the labial vestibule in the right cuspid-bicuspid region. A very large palatine torus was present but was sufficiently posterior that the denture could by-pass it without sacrificing an effective postdam. The mandibular teeth from first bicuspid to first bicuspid were present in normal alignment in the dental arch (Case Fig. 12–1A).

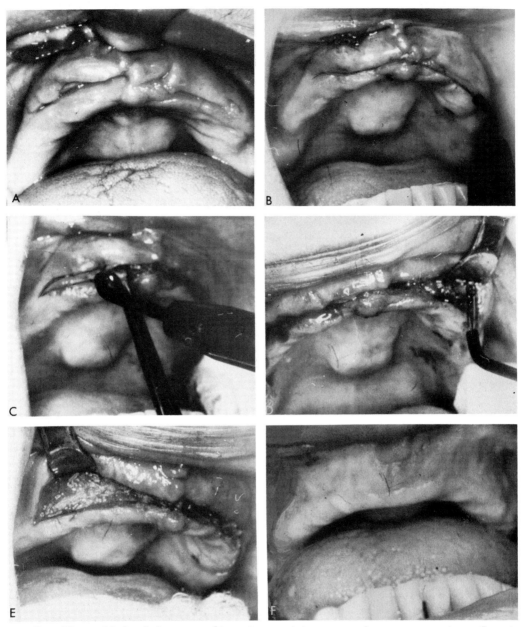

Case Figure 12–1. Submucous dissection retaining external mucosa as a tissue flap. *A,* Preoperative appearance of maxilla. There is a huge amount of redundant submucous tissue in the anterior region on the labial aspect of the edentulous maxilla. Submucous hyperplasia has produced a large bulge on the labial aspect of the maxilla, but the external mucosa is largely intact. There is a large bulging lesion in the right vestibule, apparently a granuloma fissuratum due to denture irritation. There is a fissure in the tissue on the base of the redundant mass in the right quadrant. *B,* Granuloma fissuratum has been resected by electrosection. An incision is being made along the inferior border of the redundant mass with a 45-degree-angle fine needle electrode. *C,* A second paralleling incision is being made to excise irregular tissue along the inferior aspect of the mass. The tissue is being grasped with an Allis forceps, and a strip of tissue (predetermined to become excess) is being excised. *D,* Redundant mucous tissue having been removed, the mass of submucous tissue is being resected with a 17-mm. periodontal right-angle loop electrode instead of by blunt dissection, to avoid cicatricial scar tissue repair. *E,* Submucous dissection has been completed on both sides, leaving a normal layer of submucosa attached to the periosteum for cushioning. *F,* Postoperative appearance. Tissues are fully healed; there is no clinical evidence of where the granuloma fissuratum had been. Wearing the denture with surgical cement as a stent for too long is causing irritation that resembles a callous formation. If the denture is not rebased or remade, breakdown of gingival mucosa could occur.

763

TREATMENT.   The lesion believed to be a granuloma fissuratum was located where it would interfere with administration of an infraorbital injection. This lesion was therefore resected for biopsy under circumferential infiltration anesthesia. The entire surgical area was then anesthetized by infiltration of the labial and palatal tissues. A 45-degree-angle fine needle electrode that had been used to perform the biopsy was used to incise across the inferior border of the distended tissue to create a straight line that could be coapted for suturing (Case Fig. 12–1B and C). The superior portion of the incised tissue was elevated to expose the submucous tissue, which was resected with a hoe-shaped 17-mm. periodontal loop electrode (Case Fig. 12–1D), care being taken to avoid resection of the periosteum. A small patch of periosteum measuring 2 mm. in width and about 7 mm. in length was accidentally resected, but no ill effects resulted because of the protective covering of the gingival tissue flap.

The submucous dissection having been completed, the intact gingival tissue flap was restored to position and the coapted margins sutured with interrupted silk sutures (Case Fig. 12–1E). The sutures were coated with flexible collodion, and the sterilized old denture, which had been built up with surgical cement to serve as a surgical stent to act as a pressure bandage and keep the flap in tight approximation to the underlying alveolar bone, was put in place.

The sutures were removed on the fifth postoperative day. Healing appeared to be progressing nicely by primary intention. The tissue repair where the granuloma fissuratum had been excised healed by granulation secondary intention and the sutured lines of incision by primary intention. By the end of the sixth week there was no visual clinical evidence of where the surgery had been performed. The only unusual effect was a slight blanching and callus-like toughening of the tissue in the left vestibule due to irritation from the surgical cement (Case Fig. 12–1F). At this point the referring dentist was persuaded that the tissues were ready and the denture could be rebased. Shortly after the rebasing was performed, the callus effect disappeared and the tissues regained a normal appearance.

CASE 13

This case is a typical example of marked mandibular alveolar resorption with accompanying tissue proliferation. Development of multiple granulomas fissurata in the mouth as occurred in this case is quite atypical, however.

In lieu of the customary single ridge of hypertrophic tissue created by the granuloma fissuratum, three distinctly separate soft tissue ridges, each much more prominent and better contoured than the actual alveolar ridge and larger in size, developed anterior to the alveolar ridge in tiers. The lingual tissue from the floor of the mouth bulged forward over the crest of the atrophied remnant of alveolar ridge, partially obliterating it and giving the appearance of a fourth soft tissue ridge. Treatment would therefore have to include reduction of the lingual tissue as well as of the labial hypertrophic masses in order to recontour the alveolar ridge to at least a semblance of normalcy.

PATIENT.   A 60-year-old white female.

HISTORY.   The patient had been wearing a full set of dentures for 12 years. Although they had initially been satisfactory, in the previous few years they had become unstable and eventually became so loose that the mandibular denture became functionally useless. Irritation caused by shifting of the denture produced ulceration in the labial vestibule and rapidly developed into a granuloma fissuratum. The denture was relieved on innumerable occasions, giving temporary relief followed by recurrence, until practically the entire labial denture flange was destroyed and the labial vestibule obliterated by hypertrophy. Even temporary relief could no longer be provided by grinding the denture. She was referred for resection of the hypertrophic masses.

CLINICAL EXAMINATION. *Extraoral.* Negative.

Intraoral. With the denture in position and the lips retracted, two folds of tissue were present anterior to the denture. With the denture out of the mouth a third prominent ridge of tissue anterior to the alveolar ridge became visible. Deep grooves between the ridges were partially ulcerated and keratinized. Most of the proliferative tissue was deeply engorged (Case Fig. 13–1). The alveolar ridge itself was almost completely resorbed in the median line, and on the right side the tissues of the floor of the mouth bulged over the crest of the diminutive ridge. There was an oval keratinized area in the center of this bulging area.

TREATMENT. The mouth was prepared for surgery and circumferential infiltra-

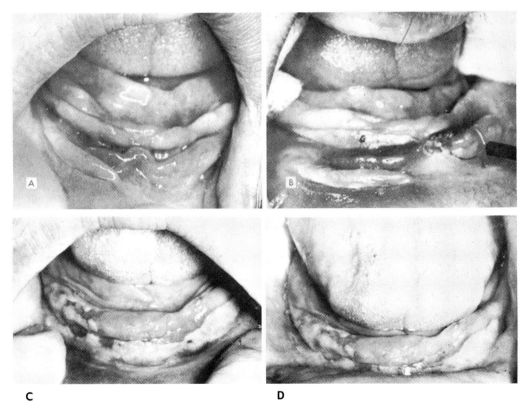

Case Figure 13–1. Mandibular granulomata fissurata resulting from denture irritation. A, Preoperative appearance. Note triple ridges of hypertrophic tissue on labial aspect and roll of hypertrophic tissue on lingual aspect (right side) with oval white patch of keratinization. B, Hypertrophic mass resected with medium round loop electrode. C, Appearance of tissues five days after the denture was built up with quick-curing acrylic to serve as a surgical stent. The ridge is well defined, and the surface is covered with a light layer of healthy coagulum. D, Final appearance six weeks postoperatively. The tissues are fully healed, and the ridge contour is normal and well defined. It is now a firm base for a stable, functionally useful denture.

tion anesthesia was administered. A medium-sized round loop electrode was selected and current output was set at 6 for electrosection. A segment of the hypertrophic mass on the left side was excised for biopsy. The remainder was reduced to normal level by shaving in layers with short wiping strokes. The other two tissue ridges were reduced in the same manner. A 45-degree-angle fine needle electrode was substituted and current output was reduced to 3. After the labial ridges were reduced to normal level and a bleeder was controlled by spot coagulation with a ball electrode, the bulge of lingual tissue on the crest of the ridge was resected. The excised tissue was preserved in formalin solution for possible biopsy evaluation in the event of adverse postoperative sequelae. The margins were coapted and sutured with silk sutures.

When the superfluous tissue was uniformly reduced to the level of the surrounding normal mucosa, a flame-shaped electrode was employed with current output of 5 to deepen the labial sulcus space by grooving the area with a wiping stroke. The denture was built up with surgical cement in the operative field to serve as a surgical stent, and the usual postoperative instructions were given.

The patient returned on the fifth postoperative day and reported no pain and only slight edema. Instead of having kept the denture in place undisturbed for 24 hours as instructed, she had removed it for several hours at a time because it caused discom-

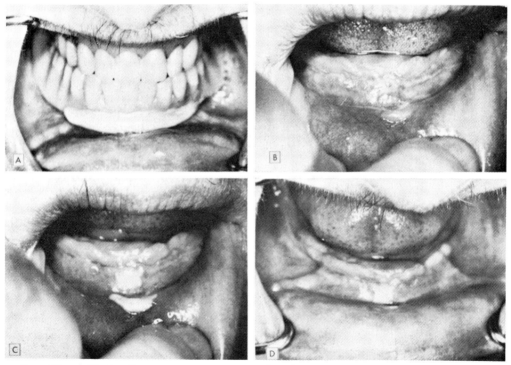

Case Figure 13–2.   Postoperative sequence of healing. *A,* Thick roll of quick-curing acrylic added to inferior border of anterior portion of denture to serve as a surgical stent and maintain the integrity of the newly created vestibular space. *B,* Appearance two weeks later. A new granuloma fissuratum is beginning to develop. *C,* The new hypertrophic tissue has been reduced to the level of the normal adjacent tissue by biterminal electrocoagulation. Note: topical anesthesia sufficed for this procedure. *D,* Appearance of mouth five weeks postoperatively. The labial sulcus tissue is fully healed and normally epithelialized. The alveolar ridge is well defined and provides a stable base for the lower denture.

fort. She had also disregarded dietary instructions and had attempted some moderately heavy mastication.

The denture was removed and the tissues examined. One of the sutures had been displaced and the tissue margins were partially reopened. There was also some evidence of regeneration at the distal end of the labial groove. The operative field was covered with a healthy layer of coagulum.

The mouth was prepared and infiltration anesthesia was administered in the two areas. A medium-sized round loop electrode was used with current output of 6 to reduce the excess tissue created by the reopening of the line of incision and the granulation tissue regenerating in the labial groove. The area was painted with tincture of myrrh and benzoin applied in air-dried layers, and a colloid impression of the mandible was obtained. The labial flange of the denture was restored in quick-curing acrylic. It was built up with a thick roll to fill the labial vestibule area in order for it to serve as a surgical stent (Case Fig. 13–2), since the cement pack in the denture appeared to be causing some irritation and to be stimulating proliferation of granulation tissue. The need for complete patient cooperation was impressed on the patient and she was reappointed.

When she returned one week later the condition of the mouth was greatly improved. The alveolar ridge was well defined and its height was considerably increased. The labial sulcus groove was also well defined and the entire area was covered with healthy coagulum. The denture was now stable and actually had suction. Healing progressed rapidly thereafter, but by the end of the second week a new granuloma fissuratum was beginning to develop. The hypertrophic tissue was reduced to normal level by coagulation with current output of 2 applied superficially and the denture labial extension was reduced slightly and polished smooth. Healing thereafter proceeded uneventfully and by the end of the fifth postoperative week the tissues were fully healed. The ridge contour was normal and well defined, and the tissue tone was excellent. The patient was now considered ready for construction of a new denture and required no further treatment.

IV. MANDIBULAR AND MAXILLARY VESTIBULOTOMY FOR ALVEOLAR RIDGE EXTENSION

Patients who have worn full dentures for many years usually undergo varying degrees of alveolar ridge resorption. Complete resorption of the entire alveolar ridge is by no means a rarity. Since the labial-buccal vestibules are created by the alveolar ridges and teeth, when the ridge becomes resorbed there is concurrent loss of the normal vestibular space into which the labial denture flange must fit if the denture is to be sufficiently stable to be functionally useful.

Implants do not appear to offer the ideal solution for the very advanced cases of ridge resorption. Thus, in the most extreme cases the best solution is achieved by surgically re-creating a vestibular space by performing a vestibulotomy, or a "pushback" procedure, so that the labial aspect of the jaw-

PLATE VI

Preprosthodontics

Figure 1a. Reduction of abnormal tuberosities to prepare for denture restoration. There has been an enormous bilateral expansion of the tuberosities owing to neoplastic degeneration of the normal cancellous bone into fibro-osteomas. The two masses extend far beyond the junction of the hard and soft palates.

Figure 1b. An incision through the mucoperiosteum being made with a fine 45-degree-angle needle electrode by electrosection to create a "pursemouth" incision for reduction of the mass. The incision is being made without free bleeding, although the tissues bled from the needle puncture to provide the anesthesia, as seen on the gauze sponge.

Figure 1c. The palate is almost fully healed from the surgery to reduce the neoplastic bone expansion, and incisions are being made for reduction of the height of the tuberosities. The contour of the tuberosity on the right side will require two parallel incisions for elimination of what will become redundant tissue. The twin incisions are being made with a bipolar needle electrode by electrosection.

Figure 1d. Final appearance of the palate and tuberosities. The tissues are fully healed, and their tone is excellent. The palate is now smooth, and the maxilla is ready for fabrication of a partial denture restoration.

Figure 2a. Pushback to create an artificial labial mandibular vestibule where senile resorption has caused total resorption of the alveolar ridge and some atrophy of the body of the mandible. The pushback is initiated by incising the tissue along the crest of the mandible with a fine 45-degree-angle needle electrode down to the periosteum. Note the absence of free bleeding and that the lingual aspect of the floor of the mouth is at a higher level than the crest of the mandible.

Figure 2b. The incised tissue has been carefully displaced downward and the submucous tissue is being removed down to the periosteum by electrosection with a 60-degree-angle medium-width U-shaped loop electrode. Note that the lingual frenum has been incised to eliminate displacement of a denture by its action.

Figure 2c. Appearance of the tissues on the fifth postoperative day, before removal of the sutures. The tissue tone is excellent, and healing is progressing favorably by secondary intention, without need for protection with a split-thickness skin graft over the surgical field. The sutures that have tied the inferior border of the gingival tissue flap to the periosteum are intact and ready to be removed.

Figure 2d. Final postoperative appearance; the body of the mandible is serving as a substitute alveolar ridge down to the symphysis. The tissue is devoid of scar tissue and normal in all respects.

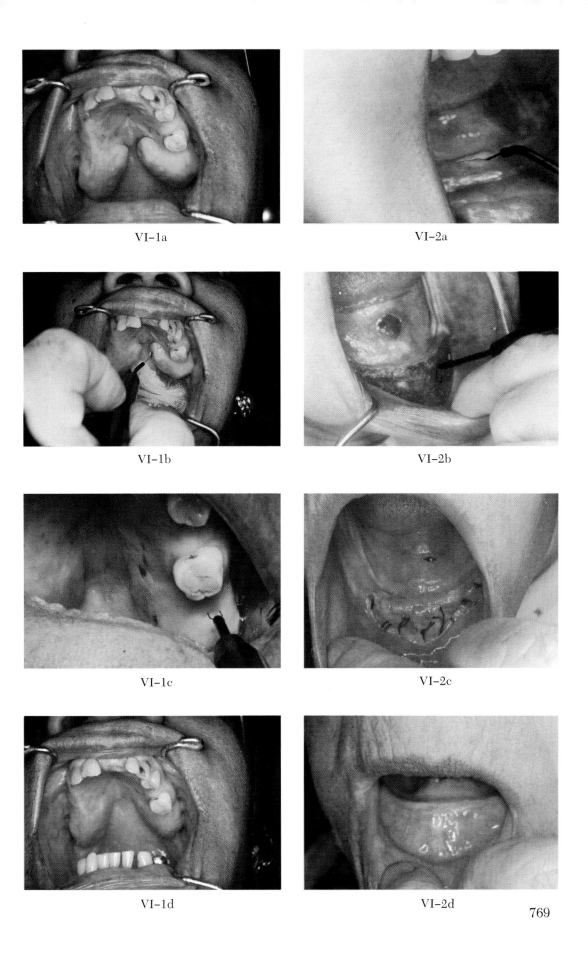

VI-1a

VI-2a

VI-1b

VI-2b

VI-1c

VI-2c

VI-1d

VI-2d

769

bone can be utilized as a substitute for the nonexistent alveolar ridge, thereby artificially creating the necessary vestibular space.

The pushback procedure consists of incising the tissues on the crest of the jawbone, following the outline of where the alveolar ridge had been, and displacing the alveolar mucosa downward or upward, as the case may be, to expose the labial aspect of the jawbone, being careful not to disturb or injure the periosteum which is permitted to remain in situ. The inferior margin of the incised tissue is then sutured to the periosteum. When the tissue healing is complete, the exposed portion of the jawbone substitutes for the missing alveolar ridge and provides the space for the labial flange of the denture with an effective peripheral seal to help provide stability.

When the incision is made with a cold-steel scalpel, it is necessary to cover the surgical field with a split-thickness skin graft in order to avoid obliteration of the artificially created vestibular space by fibrous scar tissue adhesions. This need for use of a split-thickness skin graft creates a Pandora's box of special problems.

The patients who suffer from total resorption usually are elderly. The patient must, as a rule, serve as autogenous donor for the skin graft. This subjects the geriatric patient to the hazard of physical and emotional stress from the plastic surgery required to obtain the graft. The more or less universal shortage of hospital bed space is especially acute for cases of elective surgery. This shortage can cause considerable delay in proceeding with the denture restoration. The plastic surgery to obtain the graft is an additional financial burden on the patient. Last, but far from least important, is the fact that the skin graft lacks the moist supple qualities of oral mucosa and does not provide a satisfactory tissue surface against which to obtain an effective peripheral seal, without which denture stability cannot be achieved. The denture must therefore be overextended to terminate against mucosa, which often contributes to poor aesthetics and jeopardizes the stability of the denture.

Owing to the soft supple nature of the tissue repair following an incision made by electrosection, the danger of the surgically created vestibular space being obliterated by scar tissue adhesions is eliminated. Since there is no need to cover the operative field with a split-thickness skin graft, the hazards associated with the skin graft also are eliminated.

The only protective covering of the operative field that is required is provided by adding a very hard mix of surgical cement to the patient's old denture and, after covering the sutures with a strip of adhesive dryfoil to keep them from becoming embedded into the cement, placing the denture into the mouth so as to displace forcibly the labial soft tissues and thereby to maintain the vestibular space that has been created. The labial alveolar mucosa undergoes granulation repair without incident if the periosteum has not been torn away from its attachment to the bone.

The following case demonstrates how well the tissues repair without adhesions even when the tissues must be displaced down to the symphysis to provide the substitute alveolar ridge and vestibular space for the denture.

Apically Repositioned Flap Pushback for Ridge Extension—Mandibular Vestibulotomy

CASE 14

Resorption of an edentulous alveolar ridge with its concomitant loss of vestibular space is a handicap to denture restoration that can sometimes be satisfactorily resolved by implant restoration.

Implantology has its distinct limitations, however. Blade implants, in particular, and subperiosteal implants, to a lesser degree, require a reasonably adequate amount of bone structure into or onto which to insert the implant. Thus, the greater the degree of bone resorption and the greater the handicap to satisfactory denture restoration with a full denture, the less likely is it that an implant can be utilized to resolve the problem.

The resorption in this case was so severe that not only the entire alveolar ridge but the superior part of the mandible proper had become resorbed. As a result, the tissues forming the floor of the mouth were at a higher level than the crest of the mandible. Roentgenographic examination revealed that the body of the mandible was approximately 1 cm. in diameter, and the dimension of the anterior part of the mandible was not much greater.

PATIENT. An 83-year-old white female.

HISTORY. She was edentulous for more than 20 years and during that span had had to have a number of new dentures made because of progressive loss of denture stability. Her most recent set of dentures had been made about two years previously. Until this time, large amounts of denture adhesive were necessary to keep the denture in place. But for the last few weeks even that did not help and the lower denture was completely unattached and was easily dislodged. She consulted her dentist and was told that perhaps surgery for an implant or a vestibulotomy to create space for a labial flange would help. He referred her to the author for a consultation and treatment.

CLINICAL EXAMINATION. The edentulous maxilla was normal in appearance. There was no clinical evidence of a mandibular alveolar ridge; the tissues from the floor of the mouth anteriorly to the base of the lip-gingival junction formed a straight line when the lip was pulled straight forward. The mucosa appeared normal in tone. Roentgenographic examination with intraoral periapical and occlusal views and extraoral lateral jaw views revealed that the body of the mandible in the bicuspid region was approximately 1 cm. in diameter and not much greater in the anterior region.

TREATMENT. It was obvious that this mandible was far too eroded to be restored with an implant, and that if any improvement could be attained it would have to be by means of a vestibulotomy to substitute the body of the mandible for the missing alveolar bone and thus create a labial vestibule. In performing the vestibulotomy it would be necessary to take care to avoid injury to the mental nerves.

The tissues were prepared and bilateral mental nerve block and lingual infiltration anesthesia was administered. A 45-degree-angle fine needle electrode was selected and cutting current was set at 3 on the panel dial. An incision was made with the activated electrode down to but not through the periosteum. This was accomplished by lifting the electrode slightly as soon as it met resistance from the bone. The incision was made along the crest of the mandible (Case Fig. 14–1A) and extended from first bicuspid to first bicuspid.

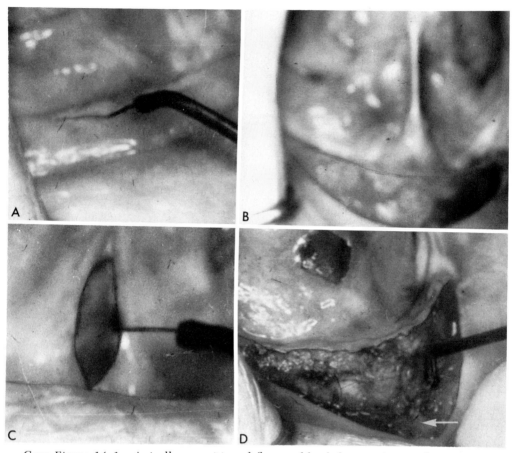

Case Figure 14–1. Apically repositioned flap pushback for creating a ridge extension —
mandible. *A,* An incision is being made along the crest of the mandible with a 45-degree-angle
fine needle electrode, since the alveolar ridge has been completely resorbed and the body of
the mandible is about 1 cm. in diameter. The floor of the mouth is at a higher level than the
crest of the mandible being incised. The lip extended outward creates an almost straight line
from the floor of the mouth outward. *B,* The inferior border of the incision has been displaced
downward toward the bottom of the jaw, exposing the submucous tissue covering the periosteum and bone. The tongue elevated reveals a short powerful lingual frenum that will, if permitted to remain intact, tend to displace the denture in function. *C,* The lingual frenum is
severed at approximately the midway point, and the thrust of the tongue pulls the horizontal
incision into a vertical straight line. The incision has been made with the same fine needle
electrode as the other incision, and care was exercised to incise only the frenal ligament, and to
avoid cutting into the ventral surface of the tongue, which has remained intact. *D,* The facial
aspect of the mandible has been exposed by displacing the mucogingival flap downward. The
submucous tissue is being resected carefully from the facial aspect of the mandible by electrosection with a round loop that has been squeezed to form an oval-shaped instrument for most
suitable contact with the structure. Note the symphysis of the mandible in the midline (arrow).
A small patch of periosteum has accidentally been resected in the right cuspid area, despite
careful instrumentation. This area will heal more slowly and will be the only area that is painfully uncomfortable during the postoperative healing period.

The lower incised tissue margin was lifted gently and pushed downward with a
periosteal elevator, revealing the anterior body of the mandible down to the symphysis (Case Fig. 14–1*B*). When the patient lifted her tongue it became obvious that
her lingual frenum, which proved to be very large and prominent, would have a bow
and arrow effect to displace her denture. The ligament was therefore incised horizon-

tally with the electrode (Case Fig. 14–1C), care being taken not to invade the body of the ventral surface of the tongue.

The needle electrode was replaced with a medium-width U-shaped loop electrode and cutting current was increased to 4. The activated electrode was used to resect the submucous tissue from the periosteum without resecting the periosteum (Case Fig. 14–1D). (The periosteum was accidentally resected in one very small area (arrow); this was the only area that caused postoperative discomfort and it healed much more slowly than the rest of the surgical field.)

The submucous dissection having been completed, the edge of the incised inferior tissue margin was sutured to the periosteum with 5-0 silk suture attached to an atraunic needle. Tincture of myrrh and benzoin was applied to the surgical field in air-dried layers, and flexible collodion was painted over the sutures to protect them from becoming imbedded into the surgical cement used to build up the old denture so that it would serve as a surgical stent to keep the tissues properly immobilized. The denture, which had been sterilized in cold sterilizing solution, was built up with a very hard roll of surgical cement and inserted. The cement was molded into the vestibule in a manner similar to muscle trimming an impression, making certain that it provided a thick well-rounded roll that would not flow under pressure from the lip and be displaced.

On the fifth postoperative day she returned for removal of the sutures. There was no swelling and no ecchymosis. When the denture was removed the surgical field was

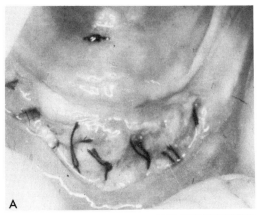

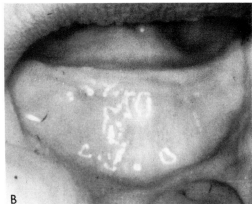

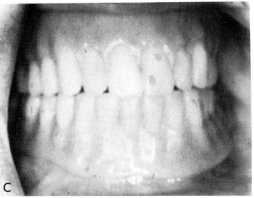

Case Figure 14–2. A, Appearance of the surgical field on the fifth postoperative day before the sutures were removed. Note the excellent tissue tone. There is no swelling, no edema, no inflammation. The entire surgical field is covered with a thin layer of coagulum, and the old denture, built up with a stiff mix of surgical cement to serve as a surgical stent, is maintaining the rounded contour at the base of the simulated labial vestibule that is so essential. B, Three month postoperative appearance of the mandible. The tissue has healed magnificently and is fully matured. Note the higher level of the tissues of the floor of the mouth. Also note the normal texture of the mucosa that had repaired by secondary granulation without the need for a split-thickness skin graft to protect the surgical field. C, Appearance of the mouth with a new denture in use. Note that there has been enough space created so that the denture with a full labial flange and effective peripheral seal does not come to the base of the new vestibule.

well defined down to the symphysis and covered with a light layer of normal coagu-lum (Case Fig. 14–2A). The sutures were removed, tincture of myrrh and benzoin was applied, and she was cautioned to continue following the postoperative regimen she had been observing faithfully.

She returned at weekly intervals for postoperative observation, and, except for the tiny area where the periosteum had been resected, healing by secondary granulation progressed favorably. By the end of the sixth week the tissues were almost fully healed, and by the end of the third month, when she was last seen, the tissues were completely normal (Case Fig. 14–2B). She had had a new set of dentures made, and the mandibular denture, which now had a full normal labial flange, was stable and functionally and aesthetically very acceptable (Case Fig. 14–2C).

There does not appear to be any other method by which a comparable result could have been attained. Had the surgery been performed by steel scalpel in-cision and the submucous dissection performed by scraping with a periosteal ele-vator, the scar tissue adhesions would have obliterated the vestibular space that had been created, unless the surgical field were covered with a split-thickness skin graft. In the latter event, in addition to the other disadvantages that have been mentioned elsewhere, the denture would have had to be so overextended to obtain a peripheral seal in mucous membrane that the functional and aesthetic usefulness of the denture would have been seriously compromised. If the mucosa of the cheek were used, as has been recommended by Shira, the steel scalpel mucosal excision would produce contractile scar tissue repair of the graft donor site. The totally normal repair by sec-ondary granulation is a welcome advantage that only electrosurgery can offer.

Mandibular Vestibulotomy

CASE 15

This case also involves a vestibulotomy to create a substitute alveolar ridge and labial vestibule. It was so similar to the previous case in clinical appearance and in surgical need that it would be redundant to review it here if it were not for the fact that in one very important respect the treatment and surgical procedure plan were just the opposite of those in the previous case. Whereas in that case it was necessary to do a submucous dissection to remove the submucous tissue from the periosteum to ob-tain a desirable result, in this case it was necessary to preserve the submucous tissue.

PATIENT.   A 60-year-old white female.

HISTORY.   The patient had lost all her teeth and sustained a fracture of the man-dibular alveolar ridge and numerous other injuries in an automobile accident 8 years previously. Treatment to reduce the maxillary and mandibular fractures and preserve what was left of the dentition was instituted but met with only partial success. The maxillary fracture repaired uneventfully, but the teeth in both jaws failed to respond to treatment and were lost, and with them, most of the mandibular alveolar ridge. A set of full dentures was made for her. The maxillary denture was aesthetically and functionally satisfactory, but the mandibular denture was unstable from the outset. The instability increased progressively until the denture virtually floated around in her mouth and interfered with her ability to eat solid foods or to speak. This in addi-tion to the physical discomfort and embarrassment forced her to consult her dentist for relief. He found that due to anatomic inadequacy it would be impossible to restore her mouth unless and until a vestibulotomy were performed, so that a labial flange could be accommodated and an effective peripheral seal created. She was referred to the author for surgery.

Case Figure 15–1. Mandibular vestibulotomy. The mandibular full denture has been relieved in the anterior region, leaving very little of the labial flange, which is partially covered with a bulging proliferation of vestibular tissue (arrow).

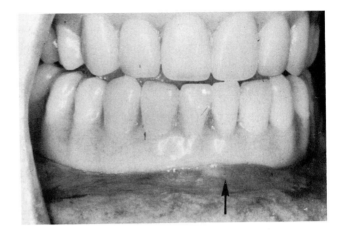

CLINICAL EXAMINATION. The edentulous maxilla had a functionally useful alveolar ridge, and the denture was reasonably stable. The mandibular denture was totally unstable. When the denture was removed, the tissues were seen as a straight line extending from the junction with the base of the tongue anteriorly to the vermilion border of the lip except for a 2-mm. elevation where the alveolar ridge is supposed to be (Case Figs. 15–1 and 15–2).

TREATMENT. The tissues were prepared and anesthetized with bilateral mental block anesthesia. A 45-degree-angle fine needle electrode was selected, cutting current was set at 3 on the power output dial, and an incision was made with the activated electrode along the crest of the 2-mm. elevation.

The incised mucoperiosteum was reflected after the tissue was carefully elevated to avoid displacing the periosteum from the bone. The incised labial mucogingival tissue was displaced downward toward the inferior border of the mandible. This revealed a bony rounded elevation in the midline, the symphysis of the mandible, which extended to within about 0.5 cm. of the crest of the mandible. The facial aspect of the mandible on either side of the symphysis was covered with submucous tissue that helped to maintain a harmonious mandibular contour instead of a pronounced bulging projection from the bony eminence. The 2-mm. elevation noted preoperatively proved to be mostly a fibrous ridge of tissue along the crest of the mandible, and there was no evidence of any alveolar ridge remaining.

If the surrounding submucous tissue were resected (as was done in the preceding case), the prominent bony bulge created by the symphysis would act as a fulcrum and disrupt the stability of the denture. In this case the tissue was therefore preserved to act as a contouring support for the denture. The margin of the tissue flap was then sutured to the periosteum close to the inferior border of the mandible, and two retaining sutures were inserted through the tissue on the crest of the mandible and the periosteum to keep that tissue from elevating and being displaced. Tincture of myrrh and benzoin was applied to the surgical field after the blood on the surface was clotted, a strip of adhesive dryfoil was placed over the sutures to keep them from becoming embedded in the cement used to line the old denture which would serve as a surgical stent, and the latter was inserted into position.

The patient returned the following day and the dryfoil was removed. The healing of surgical field looked favorable. Tincture of myrrh and benzoin was applied, and the patient was reappointed for removal of the sutures on the fifth postoperative day. When she returned the surgical field was covered with a light layer of coagulum (Case Fig. 15–3). There was no edema, inflammation, or pain, and healing appeared to be

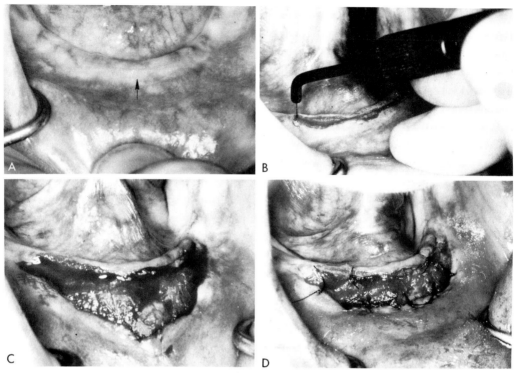

Case Figure 15–2. *A*, Presurgical appearance of the mandible with the denture removed. The alveolar ridge is completely resorbed. The tissue level is relatively uniform from the floor of the mouth postero-anteriorly to the ventral surface of the lip. There is no labial vestibule and a large mass of redundant tissue bulges upward on the labial mucogingival junction from right to left bicuspid (arrow). *B*, The mucosa along the crest of the ridge is being incised by electrosection with a 45-degree-angle fine needle electrode. *C*, The anterior portion of the mucogingival flap has been displaced downward, exposing the body of the mandible. This reveals that the 2-mm. elevation was not alveolar bone but a ridge of fibrous tissue along the crest of the mandible. The latter is so severely resorbed that the mandibular symphysis extends to within 6 mm. of the crest of the bone. The symphysis creates a convex bulge in the midline and a seeming concavitation of the surrounding adjacent labial aspect of the mandible. Submucous tissue covers the periosteum and fills in the hollow, thereby minimizing the bulge and maintaining a harmonious contour. Note the absence of free bleeding in the surgical field. *D*, The mucogingival flap has been sutured to the periosteum to keep the tissues displaced downward. Two sutures, one near each terminal end of the incision, have been inserted to keep the tissues along the crest of the mandible from being displaced lingually.

progressing very favorably. The sutures were removed, and tincture of myrrh and benzoin was applied in air-dried layers. She returned on the tenth day, and the healing was notably improved, but there was a 1.2 cm. slitlike separation of the tissues at the left terminal end of the surgical field. The inferior portion of tissue forming the slit was swollen, and the swelling appeared to be a small lumplike mass in the cheek rather than in the gingival tissue. A slightly darker pigmentation of the tissue around the slit area suggested a mild inflammation. The reason for this reaction remains unknown; there was no buried suture or other tangible reason for it. The swelling persisted and there was no evidence of improvement over the next 2 weeks, so the area was anesthetized and the swollen tissue was planed to normal dimension with a flame-shaped loop electrode and electrocoagulation to assure that this tissue would not regenerate redundantly; a coagulating power output of 5 was used to remove the tissue by tearing off the coagulated tissue efficiently. Tincture of myrrh and benzoin was applied, and a small amount of Peripak was added to the denture stent to act as a pressure pack against the cut tissue.

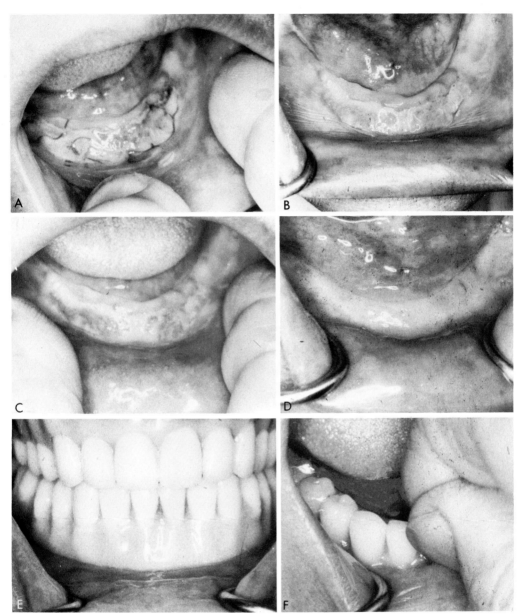

Case Figure 15–3. A, Appearance of the surgical field on the fifth postoperative day before the sutures were removed. There is a normal layer of coagulum covering the area which
had not been covered with a split-thickness skin graft. Healing appears to be progressing
rapidly and uneventfully. B, Appearance on the tenth day. Healing is progressing favorably
except in the left terminal area where there is a 1.2 cm. slit in the mucosa. C, Healing progress
by the end of the third week. The alveolar ridge is well rounded and well defined. The mucosa
is almost fully and maturely healed. D, Appearance at the end of two months. The alveolar gingiva is normal in all respects. The ridge is well defined and there is a 5- to 6-mm. labial vestibule. E, The patient is wearing a new set of dentures. The mandibular denture has a labial
flange 0.5 cm. in height. The denture is stable and is functionally and aesthetically acceptable.
F, Properly seated, the denture requires considerable lifting effort to remove it, and when it is
lifted makes a sound suggestive of suction.

Healing progressed rapidly and uneventfully thereafter, and by the end of the eighth week the tissues were fully healed and normal in all respects. With the lower lip extended, a 5- to 6-mm. labial vestibule could be clearly seen, and the old denture, which had been relined the previous week, had an effective labial flange. The denture now had an efficient peripheral seal, and when an attempt was made to elevate it from the new ridge, it remained firmly in place. A peripheral seal is effective if lifting the denture by exerting a distinct effort results in a sound of suction, and if placing the finger tips on the incisal edge of the anterior teeth and tilting the denture outward requires a considerable effort to displace it and there is again a sound of suction.

Had the submucous tissue been resected in this case, however, the bulging eminence created by the symphysis would have had a rocking-chair effect on the denture and destroyed the stability. Thus, despite clinical similarity, treatment plan and treatment must be predicated on clinical requirements and not on a blueprint.

Combined Alveoloplasty and Pushback for Vestibular Correction

Although most alveoloplasties are of the routine variety, consisting of reduction of sharp apices of interseptal and marginal socket bone and elimination of undercuts, alveoloplasty occasionally involves much more extensive surgical reduction combined with other surgery.

CASE 16

In this case, as in the case that follows, the maxilla had become severely deformed, with the anterior half of the maxilla projecting forward about 0.5 cm. and downward almost 1.5 cm. The downward dip had not resulted from elongated growth of the alveolar ridge alone, and the mucolabial junction dipped down in the anterior region proportionally to the bone deformity. Thus, it would be necessary not only to reduce the anterior height of the maxilla to restore it to normal dimension, but also to perform a pushback to elevate the mucolabial fold proportionally.

PATIENT. A 71-year-old white female.

HISTORY. She had had all but a few anterior teeth extracted many years previously and had worn a very unsophisticated partial upper denture with wrought-wire clasps. The latter apparently had not had occlusal rests. The anterior teeth gradually began to splay outward and downward, and she now had only two teeth remaining in the maxilla, which exaggerated the deformity. She was referred for surgical preparation of the mouth for a functional and aesthetically acceptable full upper denture.

CLINICAL EXAMINATION. The right central and lateral incisor teeth remained in the maxilla; the rest of the jaw was edentulous. The anterior half of the maxilla projected downward approximately 1.5 cm. and forward approximately 0.5 cm., but the alveolar ridge was not elongated since the mucolabial tissue junction also dipped down to within approximately 1.0 cm. of the alveolar ridge crest (Case Fig. 16–1).

TREATMENT. The tissues were prepared and bilateral infraorbital and nasopalatine block anesthesia was administered. The amount of mucosa that would become excess when the alveolar ridge was reduced to normal dimension was carefully deter-

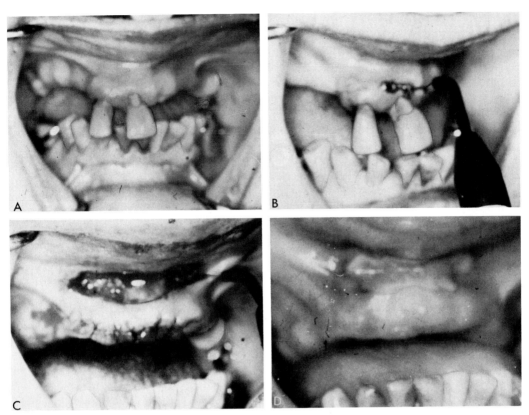

Case Figure 16–1. Combined maxillary alveoloplasty and vestibulotomy. *A*, Preoperative condition of maxilla. The maxillary right central and lateral incisors are the only teeth remaining in the maxilla. The anterior half of the maxilla projects downward and forward. The downward projection elongates the anterior part of the maxilla approximately 1.5 cm. toward the mandible. The junction of labial and gingival mucosa to form the mucolabial fold dips downward in the anterior part of the maxilla in proportion to the alveolar dip. *B*, The predetermined amount of excess tissue that will result from reduction of the alveolar height is being incised for excision by electrosection with a 45-degree-angle fine needle electrode. *C*, The alveoloplasty having been completed and the tissue margins coapted and sutured, a second incision is being made at the alveolar-areolar tissue junction to create a pushback elevation of the mucolabial fold. *D*, Appearance of maxilla two weeks after removal of sutures. The incision along the crest of the alveolar ridge is fully healed. The healing in the mucolabial fold has progressed considerably but the surface of the pushback area is still covered with a layer of coagulum. Irritation from the surgical cement that had been added to the old denture to convert it into a surgical stent is at least partly responsible for the somewhat retarded healing. The contour and dimension of the alveolar ridge are now acceptable and there is ample space for a labial flange with good peripheral seal.

mined, and a horizontal incision was made to eliminate the predetermined excess before the two teeth were extracted. The incision by electrosection was made with a 45-degree-angle fine needle electrode and cutting current was set at 3 on the power output dial. Current output was increased to 4.5 for the palatal continuation of the incision.

The incised tissue was removed, the teeth were extracted, and the excess alveolar bone was removed with rongeur forceps to a level harmonious with that of the posterior half of the maxilla. The alveoloplasty having been completed, the incised tissue margins were coapted and sutured along the newly formed ridge crest. The upper lip was then elevated upward and outward to pull the tissues taut and to delineate sharply the mucolabial junction. The needle electrode was then wiped across the line of junction with a single stroke, separating the areolar labial tissue from the attached alveolar tissue. As the tissue was incised, blood appeared on the tissue surface, but there was no free bleeding. The blood was sponged off with a gauze sponge, exposing submucous tissue on the surface of the periosteum. The submucous tissue was carefully resected with a flame-shaped loop electrode which was curved slightly to provide better tissue access and avoid injury to the periosteum. The absence of bleeding resulted in a clear surgical field that greatly facilitated the submucous resection without damage to the periosteum.

The old denture had previously been sterilized and dried. A very stiff mix of surgical cement (the periodontal pack formula) was inserted into the anterior part of the denture against the labial flange and extended upward to form a round roll on the upper edge of the flange. When the blood had clotted, tincture of myrrh and benzoin was applied in air-dried layers, and flexible collodion was applied over the sutures to prevent their becoming embedded in the cement. The denture was inserted and the cement was packed up into the pushback area and molded like a muscle-trimmed impression with compound, to serve as a surgical stent. When the cement was set the patient was reappointed and dismissed, with instructions to follow the directions given for home care.

She returned on the fifth postoperative day for removal of the sutures. The tissue tone was excellent, and the healing appeared to be progressing well. A thin layer of coagulum covered the surgical field. The sutures were removed, care being taken not to disturb or displace the coagulum. Tincture of myrrh and benzoin was reapplied, and she was instructed to continue the regimen of home care. She was seen at weekly intervals postoperatively. Two weeks later the line of incision was fully healed, and the tissue tone was excellent, but a layer of coagulum still covered the pushback area, and the distal edge of the coagulum had torn slightly loose from the tissue on the right side. The cement along the superior margin of the labial flange had begun to become somewhat porous and appeared to be contributing substantially to the slower rate of healing. The patient's dentist was persuaded to rebase the denture at this time, and very soon thereafter the healing was completed.

This case reemphasized the importance of not prolonging the period for use of the surgical cement as a surgical stent but replacing it with a rebased denture 10 to 14 days postoperatively.

Resection of Maxillary Ridge Redundant Tissue

CASE 17

This case demonstrates the problem created by total resorption of maxillary alveolar ridge with degenerative redundant mucosa replacing the bone, creating a total loss of denture stability, so often seen when natural mandibular dentition and a maxillary full denture are present. To re-create a labial vestibule that will be lost when the redundant tissue is resected, it is necessary to do a pushback and submucous dissection to utilize the facial aspect of the maxilla as a substitute for the missing alveolar bone. Absence of free bleeding during the surgery simplifies and accelerates the procedure. The soft tissue repair, devoid of fibrous cicatricial scar characteristics, eliminates the problem of postoperative loss of vestibular space due to scar adhesions.

PATIENT. A 61-year-old white male.

HISTORY. The edentulous maxilla had been restored with a full upper denture. The impact of the natural mandibular dentition had gradually disintegrated the maxillary alveolar ridge, with redundant mucosa replacing the lost bone and subsequent loss of denture stability, a great handicap to the patient, who was often called upon to deliver lectures. Since the denture shifted and dropped when the patient spoke, despite the use of adhesive denture powders, he consulted a dentist about rebasing or remaking the case, and was referred to the author for corrective preprosthodontic surgery.

CLINICAL EXAMINATION. What had apparently been an excellent alveolar ridge now consisted of a mass of degenerative fibrous tissue that moved freely under pressure. On palpation the base of the nasal spine was felt as a sharp projection superiorly in the midline. It appeared obvious from the clinical examination that it would be necessary to reduce the base of the nasal spine in order to extend the vestibular space that would be created high enough to permit construction of an effective labial flange and peripheral seal that would be essential for the success of a new denture (Case Fig. 17–1).

TREATMENT. Local anesthesia—bilateral posterior superior alveolar and infraorbital blocks, and nasopalatine and anterior palatine blocks—was administered to anesthetize the entire maxilla.

A 45-degree-angle fine needle electrode was used to resect the mass of redundant tissue by electrosection, with cutting power output set at 3 on the dial setting. The small amount of areolar tissue remaining on the labial aspect was elevated to expose the remainder of the alveolar ridge and the base of the nasal spine. A razor-thin ridge of bone 2 to 4 mm. in height was all that remained of the original alveolar ridge. Since the knife edge of bone would not provide a suitable surface on which to compress the mucosa, and since the base of the nasal spine would interfere with creation of the vestibular space, both were reduced with a rongeur forceps and bone file. A submucous dissection was then performed with the 17-mm. 25-degree-angle periodontal loop electrode to create the tissue slack necessary to re-position the tissues superiorly and thereby create a labial-buccal vestibule. The cut tissue margins were then coapted and sutured with interrupted silk sutures. A high muscle attachment was noted on the right side after the tissues were sutured. The tension of this muscle attachment was relieved by simply incising with a small horizontal incision by electrosection with the needle electrode.

A very hard mix of the zinc-oxide surgical cement formula used by the author (listed in the chapter on armamentarium) was then inserted into the anterior part of the old denture which had been sterilized by immersion in a cold sterilizing solution. A strip of adhesive dryfoil was placed over the sutures to keep them from becoming embedded in the cement, and the denture was inserted under pressure. As the cement was forced out of the denture anteriorly, it was displaced upward and molded against the facial aspect of the maxilla in a manner similar to molding compound for a muscle-trimmed impression.

The patient was instructed to leave the denture in place for the rest of that day and to start lavage with a saline solution when he removed the denture. He returned for removal of the sutures on the fifth postoperative day. The tissues appeared to be healing well, except for a small spot over the base of the nasal spine, where the underlying bone appeared to be retarding the repair owing to pressure. The sutures

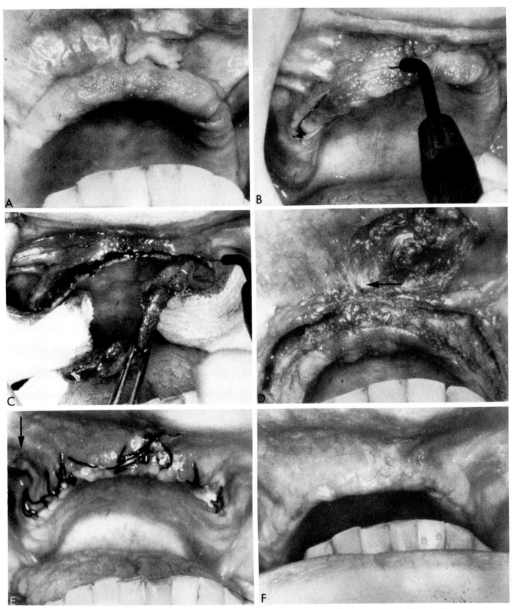

Case Figure 17–1. Maxillary ridge extension to re-create labial vestibule. *A,* Preoperative appearance. The maxillary alveolar ridge has been replaced by degenerative fibrous tissue owing to traumatic impact of natural mandibular dentition against the maxillary full denture. There is a large proliferative mass of redundant tissue, probably a granuloma fissuratum, filling the labial vestibule immediately left of the labial frenum. *B,* The major portion of the "alveolar ridge" is being excised by electrosection with a 45-degree-angle fine needle electrode. The incision, started on the palatal aspect, is being carried around to the labial. There is no free bleeding. *C,* The huge chunk of tissue is being resected at its left terminal end, leaving no meaningful alveolar ridge. Note the absence of free bleeding, and also of coagulation. There is blood present but no free bleeding. *D,* The submucous tissue has been removed from the facial aspect of the maxilla which will substitute for the resorbed alveolar ridge. The granuloma fissuratum has also been resected. The base of the nasal spine has been reduced and its sharp point rounded (arrow). *E,* Appearance of the maxilla on the fifth postoperative day, before suture removal. The tissues are healing favorably. Note where a low muscle attachment had been released by a small horizontal incision in the right bicuspid area (arrow). *F,* Two week postoperative appearance. The surgical cement pack that has been inserted into the denture to act as a surgical stent has kept the tissues displaced superiorly as desired. The body of the maxilla is substituting well for the missing alveolar ridge, and there is ample vestibular space for good labial flanges with effective peripheral seal to provide denture stability.

782

were removed and a slight amount of cement immediately over the nasal spine was removed with a small round bur to provide relief.

The patient was seen again on the tenth postoperative day, and the body of the maxilla substituted well for the alveolar ridge, the surgical cement pact having acted as a stent. The facial aspect of the maxilla appeared well defined, with ample space for a good labial flange and an effective peripheral seal. At this time the patient decided to return to his home in England to have the denture made, so that he could not be followed postoperatively except by periodic reports by mail. He had a new denture made, and the dentist followed the suggestion to create a proper shearing relationship between the artificial maxillary and natural mandibular teeth partly by beveling the incisal edges of the natural dentition and partly by the manner in which the artificial teeth were set up in the dental arch. The results, according to the patient's periodic communications, were a stable, functionally useful, and aesthetically acceptable denture, with no evidence of further bone resorption.

V. CORRECTION OF ABNORMAL TUBEROSITIES AND OTHER BONE ABNORMALITIES AND DEFECTS

Correction of Abnormal Tuberosities

An abnormal maxillary tuberosity is one of the more common varieties of anatomic handicaps to successful denture construction. They may interfere with denture construction in three major ways.

1. The tuberosity may project downward toward an opposing edentulous mandibular alveolar ridge and prevent restoration of the missing posterior teeth. This is more likely to happen when the teeth are lost at a relatively early age and are not restored for a long time.

2. The tuberosity may become expanded or otherwise distorted from normal contour by neoplastic degeneration. Most commonly the distortion is due to osteofibroma or fibroma durum. Expanded or distorted tuberosities create undercuts or occlude the normal buccal vestibular space and thereby interfere with seating of the denture.

3. A dense ledge or knob of sclerotic bone may project laterally from the buccal aspect of the cortical plate of the tuberosity, creating an undercut which will traumatize the tissues when the denture is inserted or removed.

A fourth anatomic defect, acquired, is the tapered, narrow, V-shaped tuberosity. It usually results from injudicious removal of the buccal alveolar plate when performing posterior alveoloplasty. This type is the opposite of the three types listed above. It cannot be corrected by reduction, although some benefit may be derived from rounding the crest of the ridge to eliminate excessive sharpness. The acquired type will not be included in this review.

When an abnormal tuberosity must be reduced or otherwise reshaped, extraction of teeth and reduction of excess bone to normal level is usually a relatively simple surgical procedure. But accurate reduction of the excess soft tissue that results is far from simple, and in many respects is actually the most important part of the surgical procedure. If the precise amount of tissue that becomes superfluous is not accurately estimated and excised it becomes impossible to coapt the tissues accurately to assure good healing by primary intention.

Should an excess amount of tissue be retained it remains slack when the margins are sutured. This permits formation of hypertrophic submucous tissue. If, on the other hand, an excessive amount of tissue is excised, it prevents the tissue margins from being coapted without undue tension. Tension usually results in the sutures cutting through the tissues as they become slightly edematous postoperatively. The margins of the wound then tend to separate, permitting hypertrophic granulation to proliferate between the separated margins.

The difficulty encountered in attempting to estimate the precise amount of tissue to excise arises from two related factors. The first factor is associated with the phenomenon that occurs when gingival mucosa that is firmly attached to its underlying bone is incised and elevated from its bony base. Normal mucous membrane of this type is highly resilient. When it is lifted from its attachment it immediately contracts. Contraction makes it difficult to estimate accurately the proper amount of tissue to be removed. The second factor is that resilient tissue that has been elevated and has undergone contraction is extremely difficult to cut cleanly and precisely. The tissue can no longer be incised with a scalpel as it could when it was stretched tightly over bone. It tends to skid between the beaks of tissue-cutting rongeur forceps or the cutting blades of scissors, even the surgical scissors with serrated cutting edges.

On the other hand, if the operator is able to visualize and estimate accurately the amount of excess tissue that will result when the excess bone is removed, it is easy to incise the tissue cleanly and precisely while it is still attached to the underlying bone, then to resect the incised tissue and expose the excess bone. Despite the fact that the retracted tissue also becomes contracted, if the bone is accurately reduced to predetermined dimension this tissue contraction will not interfere with accurate coaptation of the incised margins. The contracted tissue readily stretches back to its original size when it is drawn together and immobilized with sutures. If the amount of tissue resected was accurately predetermined, the coapted margins should meet without tension or slack and should heal by primary intention without incident.

It is possible to achieve consistent accuracy by combining thorough treatment planning (based upon painstaking preoperative survey of the mouth and preparation and measurement of study models) with sound surgical judgment, which is acquired with clinical experience. When these ingredients are combined with skillful use of electrosurgery, accurate atraumatic incisions and excision of superfluous tissue can easily and speedily be performed even in awkward, relatively inaccessible parts of the mouth.

The technique for predetermining the precise amount of tissue that will

Figure 20–3. Diagram of technique for accurate predetermination of tissue excess. *A*, Measurement of original tuberosity bulge on study model from point a to point b. Line a–b depicts the result of this measurement. *B*, Measurement of the reduced tuberosity on the study model from point a′ to point b′. The difference in length from b′ to b equals the exact amount of tissue that will become excess when the bone bulge is reduced as planned on model *B*.

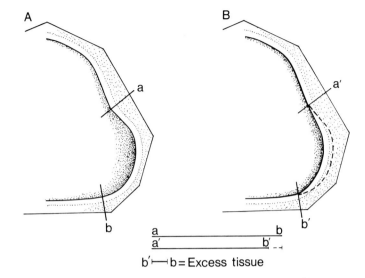

b′⊢──┤b = Excess tissue

become redundant when a bulbous undercut tuberosity is reduced to normal dimension is predicated on the same broad principle as for predetermining the excess in an alveoloplasty, but the specific technique for ascertaining the determination of the excess varies owing to the anatomic locale.

The study model of the maxilla is marked off at the respective terminal ends of the reduction site as points a and b. A measurement is taken from the widest dimension of the area between a and b (Figure 20–3A). The study model is then trimmed to the exact dimension anticipated to be created in the mouth by the bone reduction which extends from a to b; these now become a′ and b′. A new measurement is taken from a′ to b′ (Figure 20–3B). The difference between the two measurements (b′–b) is the predetermined precise amount of tissue excess that will result from the bone reduction.

In the mouth the procedure is performed in the following manner: Two incisions are made in the tissue on the crestal part of the tuberosity. The incisions, separated the exact distance of the difference between the two measurements of the study model, are made parallel to each other (1) and are joined together at their respective terminal ends (2). The junction of the two is in the form of an inverted V at the anterior terminal end and a V at the posterior or distal terminal end (Fig. 20–4A).

The incised tissue is excised, and the tissue on the buccal aspect of the excision is elevated and reflected from the bone to expose the bulging tuberosity (Fig. 20–4B). The external cortical plate of the bulge is removed and as much of the cancellous portion as is necessary to eliminate the undercut created by the bulge. The reflected tissue flap is replaced and coapted to the adjacent undisturbed tissue and sutured with interrupted silk sutures (Fig. 20–4C).

If the measurements that had been taken were accurate, and the bone reduction had been checked by use of a clear acrylic stent to assure that the proper amount of bone had been removed, the two tissue margins will come into perfect apposition and can be sutured without tension and without sub-

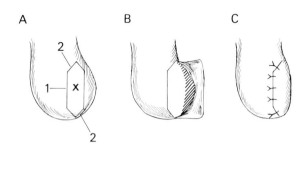

Figure 20–4. Diagrammatic visualization of the technique for incising and excising the tissue that has been predetermined to become excess. A, Two parallel incisions (1) are made on the crest of the bulbous tuberosity. The two incisions are joined at the anterior end with an inverted **V** incision and at the posterior end with a **V** incision (2). The incised hexagon of tissue (×) is undermined and removed. B, The tissue covering the bone bulge is elevated and reflected to expose the bone. C, The tuberosity has been reduced to normal dimension, the mucoperiosteal flap has been restored and the coapted margins have been sutured with interrupted sutures.

sequent displacement by pressure of blood that would clot and result in the formation of submucous redundant tissue.

The following series of case reports not only will demonstrate electrosurgical techniques for correction of abnormal tuberosities but will also cover the technique for predetermining the proper amount of excess tissue to resect.

CASE 18

This case is a typical example of the elongated tuberosity that results when posterior teeth are lost at an early age and are not restored, permitting the opposing teeth to drift downward toward the opposing alveolar ridge. Correction is achieved by horizontal alveolectomy to reduce the vertical dimension.[1, 2]

PATIENT. A 35-year-old white female.

HISTORY. The patient was referred for extraction of the maxillary left second bicuspid and first molar, and alveoloplasty to reduce the alveolar ridge to normal height.

CLINICAL EXAMINATION. *Extraoral.* Negative.

Intraoral. A considerable number of maxillary and mandibular teeth were missing. The maxillary right lateral and first bicuspid were abutments for a fixed bridge restoring the cuspid. The maxillary left second and third molars were missing. The mandibular left first, second, and third molars had been extracted long before and had not been restored. The maxillary left second bicuspid and first molar dipped down so that their buccal cusps came into contact with the edentulous mandibular ridge with the mouth in centric relation (Case Fig. 18–1). Their investing alveolar bone was proportionately elongated. The oral hygiene and tissue tone were excellent.

TREATMENT. A working study model was obtained and prepared in three steps.

1. The teeth were cut off at the gingival margins.
2. The resultant alveolar ridge was measured.
3. The alveolar ridge on the model was trimmed to proper height and contour, and the new ridge was measured.

The difference between the two measurements represented the pre- and postoperative difference in bulk. This determined the amount of superfluous tissue that would result when the bone was reduced in the mouth. In this instance it was established that there would be 4 mm. of excess tissue created in the anterior half of the tuberosity and 5 mm. in the posterior half of the newly created ridge. Thus it would

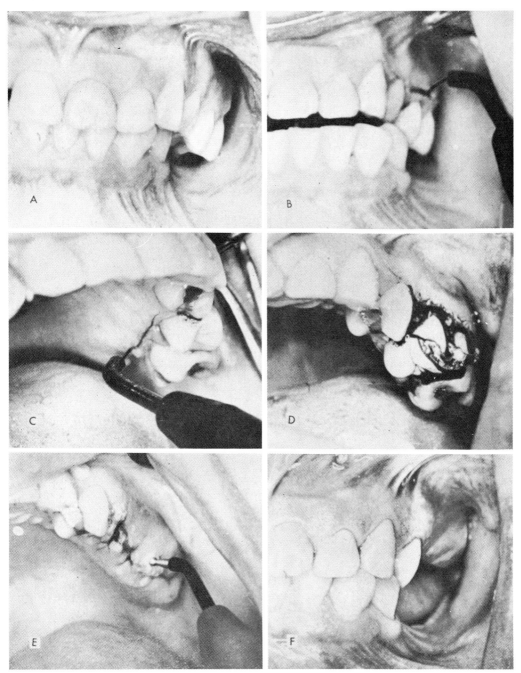

Case Figure 18–1. Reduction of elongated tuberosity and alveolar ridge to permit restoration of edentulous areas with normal-sized teeth. *A,* Preoperative view. The maxillary left second bicuspid and first molar are elongated. With the mouth in centric relation the buccal cusps of the molar are in contact with the edentulous mandibular alveolar ridge. *B,* Incision for resection of excess tissue is performed on buccal aspect with 45-degree-angle fine needle electrode at predetermined level. *C,* Incision for resection of excess tissue performed on palatal aspect. *D,* Incised strips of tissue are excised before the teeth are extracted. *E,* Appearance of tissues on fifth postoperative day. Healing has progressed by primary intention. One bulging spot where the suture caused a tissue pucker is reduced to normal level by spot coagulation with a small ball electrode. *F,* Final postoperative appearance. The tuberosity is normal in shape. With the mouth closed in centric relation there is sufficient space between the two ridges for restoration with normal-sized teeth.

787

be necessary to excise 2 mm. from the buccal and palatal mucosa in the anterior half and 2.5 mm. in the posterior half. Both incisions were to be made before the teeth were extracted.

The mouth was prepared and posterior superior alveolar and anterior palatine block anesthesia administered. A 45-degree-angle fine needle electrode was selected and current output set at 3.5 for electrosection. To put the treatment plan into operation the buccal incision was started 2 mm. above the gingival margin of the second bicuspid (which coincided with the level of the gingival margin of the normally aligned first bicuspid) and was carried in a posterior direction. Current output was increased to 4.5, and the mucosa on the palatal aspect was incised in the same manner. Both incised strips of mucosa were excised.

The two teeth were then extracted, the interseptal bone reduced, and the buccal and palatal alveolar cortical plates reduced with rongeur forceps to the predetermined height. Both bone margins were rounded to proper contour with bone files. The area was thoroughly debrided and medicated gelatin powder inserted into the two sockets; then the tissue margins were brought into normal coaptation and sutured with 0000 braided silk interrupted sutures. The sutures were tied firmly but without tension. The posterior end of the heel of the tuberosity still projected downward forming a sharp V. The projecting tissue was dense and fibrous. Its sharp point was reduced and rounded by looping it off with a round loop electrode and current output was increased to 6 for electrosection. Tincture of myrrh and benzoin was applied, a gauze pressure pack was inserted, and the usual postoperative instructions were given.

The patient returned on the fifth postoperative day. The area was irrigated and the tissues were inspected. The tissue tone was excellent and the line of incision was healing by primary union. One bulging irregular spot was reduced by coagulation. The sutures were removed and tincture of myrrh and benzoin was applied.

The patient was seen again one week later, at which time the tissues were almost fully healed. The space created between the two alveolar ridges was now adequate to permit restoration of the edentulous saddle areas with normal-sized teeth. The fibrous area at the extreme heel of the tuberosity still dipped down slightly beyond the level of the rest of the ridge but not enough to interfere with the planned prosthetic restoration.

CASE 19

This case is a typical example of the anatomic handicap that expanded tuberosities that form deep undercuts and occlude the mucobuccal vestibule pose to prosthetic restoration.[3, 4]

PATIENT.   A 58-year-old black female.

HISTORY.   This was the first of three surgical procedures. She was referred for reduction of an abnormally expanded maxillary tuberosity so that a partial denture could be constructed.

CLINICAL EXAMINATION.   *Extraoral.*   Negative.

Intraoral.   The maxillary left central was restored with an open-face gold crown, and a fixed bridge from the lateral to the first bicuspid restored the cuspid. The right maxillary alveolar ridge was edentulous from the cuspid posteriorly. The right tuberosity was expanded to such a degree that it completely occluded the buccal vestibule (Case Fig. 19–1). The left third molar was also missing, but the tuberosity on that side appeared normal. The mandibular ridge on the right side was edentulous from the first bicuspid posteriorly, and the left second and third molars were missing.

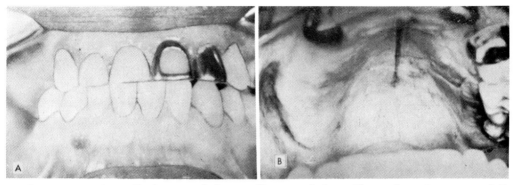

Case Figure 19–1. Reduction of abnormally expanded maxillary tuberosity to normal dimension. *A,* Preoperative appearance. The right tuberosity is tremendously expanded and completely fills the buccal vestibular space. *B,* Final postoperative appearance of tuberosity, which is now normal in size and width. The buccal vestibular space is normal.

TREATMENT. Accurate preoperative estimate of the amount of excess tissue to be excised was the first step in the surgical correction.

The mouth was prepared for surgery and posterior superior alveolar block and palatal infiltration anesthesia was administered. A 45-degree-angle fine needle electrode was selected and current output set at 3.5 for electrosection. An incision was started 2 mm. palatal to the center of the crest of the ridge and extended the full length of the edentulous ridge and tuberosity. A second paralleling incision 2 mm. buccal to the center of the ridge was then created. The two incisions were united by tapering their terminal ends into horizontal V's with apices directed distally. The incised strip of tissue was undermined and excised; then the buccal mucosa was retracted upward, exposing the round bulge of the expanded tuberosity.

Careful instrumentation is essential for reduction of expanded osteofibromatous tuberosities. Their outer cortex usually is thinned out but densely sclerotic and resis-

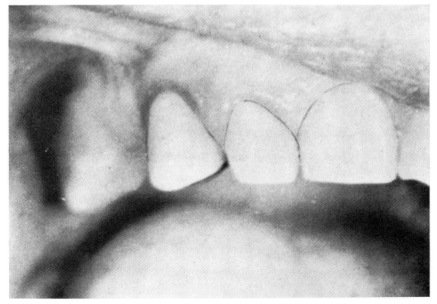

Figure 20–5. Preoperative appearance of fibroma which has elongated the tuberosity. The tissue is so dense and avascular that it resembles a tooth at first glance.

tant to cutting. The inner spongiosum undergoes the neoplastic degeneration. When the outer cortex is penetrated, the friable inner portion tends to disintegrate under instrumentation, like shredded wheat. Thus, if care is not exercised much more structure may be destroyed than had been planned. Use of chisels was therefore avoided.

The outer cortex was pierced with a Crane pick, reduced with regular and side-cutting rongeurs, and rounded smooth with bone files. Although the spongiosum tended to crumble under the instrumentation it was reduced to preplanned dimension. When debridement was completed the tissue margins were coapted without difficulty and sutured without tension with 0000 interrupted silk sutures. An initial dose of Crysticillin, 600,000 units intramuscularly, was administered and three similar daily doses were prescribed.

She returned on the fifth postoperative day for removal of sutures. The mouth was irrigated and the tissues were inspected. Healing was progressing normally by primary intention. There was no pain or edema. The sutures were removed and tincture of myrrh and benzoin was applied. She returned at regular weekly intervals for one month, then every other week for another month. Healing progressed normally throughout this period and by the end of the second month the tuberosity was fully healed. The tissue was firm, the tissue tone was excellent, and the ridge and tuberosity were normally contoured. The alveolar bone appeared fully regenerated.

The rate and quality of healing that resulted following this surgical episode differed dramatically from the unsatisfactory healing that followed two

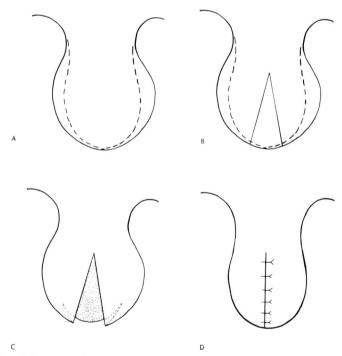

Figure 20–6. Schematic drawings of technique for restoring normal contour and dimension to the deformed tuberosity. *A*, Dotted line denotes desired size of the tuberosity. *B*, Triangular incision into the tuberosity from crest of ridge. (Bulbous tuberosities are incised as depicted here. For elongated triangular-shaped tuberosities the incisions should form a shorter equilateral triangle.) *C*, Shaded triangle indicates area of excised tissue. Lateral dotted lines indicate incisions to undermine the tissues to create slack. *D*, Incised margins coapted and sutured. Tuberosity now is the desired dimension, which had been predetermined.

other surgical experiences. This case offers striking evidence of the tremendous importance systemic factors exercise in the rate and quality of postoperative repair.

Figure 20-5 is an example of anatomic abnormality created when a tuberosity undergoes neoplastic degeneration into fibroma durum—fibromatosis that usually causes alteration of normal anatomic contour.[5, 6] Biopsy confirmed the clinical diagnosis in this case.

The technique for restoring normal contour and dimension to a tuberosity deformed by degenerative fibromatous expansion is well demonstrated in Figure 20-6.

Reduction of Bilateral Osteofibromas of the Hard Palate

CASE 20

This case offers an excellent example of the advantage of hemostasis in performing surgery on the posterior part of the hard and/or soft palate. It also offers an excellent example of postoperative tissue breakdown due to mechanical irritation and how this contrasts with necrosis of tissue postoperatively due to systemic factors that impair the ability of the tissues to repair such as existed in the preceding case.

PATIENT. A 73-year-old black female.

HISTORY. The patient had a lengthy history of cardiac therapy on an outpatient basis. The Prosthodontia Clinic had referred her for surgical preparation of the mouth for dentures.

CLINICAL EXAMINATION. The hard palate was markedly elongated posteriorly. The elongation was due in large measure to the presence of two huge hard masses projecting outward about 1.5 cm. beyond the surface of the palate bilaterally. Both masses projected posteriorly well beyond the junction of hard and soft palates. The tuberosities were somewhat expanded, creating undercuts, and dipped downward almost to the level of the mandibular alveolar ridges (Case Fig. 20-1).

TREATMENT. Since this patient was a poor surgical risk, surgical procedures for each of the masses, then each of the tuberosities, were performed separately at staggered intervals rather than all at once. Owing to the cardiac condition, an antibiotic, Crysticillin, was administered daily in 1,000,000 unit doses intramuscularly for four days, beginning one day preoperatively and continuing daily thereafter, for each of the surgical procedures.

Because there was a small ulcerated lesion on the tissue covering the mass on the right side of the palate, this mass was treated first. A combination of posterior superior block and palatal infiltration and anterior palatine block anesthesia was administered. A 2 × 2 sterile sponge was placed across the oropharynx to prevent seepage of blood down the throat.

A 45-degree-angle fine needle electrode was used to make two incisions forming a football-shaped oval ellipse, with the intersecting lines of incision extended beyond their points of intersection, for resection of the amount of tissue that had been predetermined as excess when the bone mass was reduced to normal dimension. This type of incision creates what the author feels is best described as a purse-mouth, since it

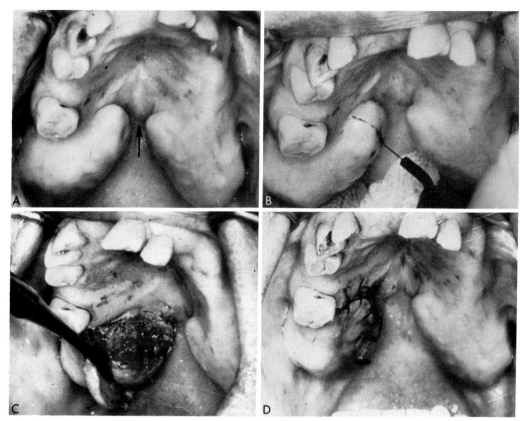

Case Figure 20–1. Reduction of bilateral osteofibromas. *A,* Preoperative appearance. Maxilla is tremendously elongated in the respective tuberosity areas. The tuberosities not only are elongated and enlarged but continue toward the midline of the palate. The junction of the hard and soft palates (arrow) gives a better idea of how great the enlargement is. The palatal extensions almost close the oropharynx, and make swallowing and other normal functions difficult. There are six teeth remaining in the maxilla: right first molar, first bicuspid, cuspid and lateral, left central and lateral. The cuspid has a large mesial cavity. There is an ulcerated lesion on the right palatal extension of the tuberosity near its tip at the midline. *B,* A mucoperiosteal incision is being made with a 45-degree-angle fine needle electrode and cutting current is set at 4, to begin the excision of what has been predetermined will be the amount of excess tissue when the osteofibroma has been eliminated. Note that the needle puncture for infiltration anesthesia produced bleeding that was absorbed by the gauze sponge, but the incision by electrosection is not producing any free bleeding. *C,* The predetermined tissue excess has been excised, and the mucoperiosteum has been elevated with the broad end of a periosteal elevator and peeled back to expose the deformed bone. The extremely dense external cortex of the bone has been removed, and the palatal bulge of bone has been reduced to the level of the surrounding bone. The internal cancellous portion of the bone has been largely replaced by neoplastic fibrous tissue, leaving myriad needle-like sharp spicules of bone now exposed. *D,* The mucoperiosteal flap has been restored to its site and the coapted margins have been sutured with interrupted silk sutures. Note that the tissue flap is neither too loose nor too taut.

permits the tissue to be elevated much as a purse is opened wide, without tearing at the terminal ends of the incisions. The incised segment of tissue was excised.

The mucoperiosteal flap was elevated and reflected exposing a sclerotic mass of bone. The osteofibroma is a true neoplasm which is characterized by replacement of the cancellous spongiosum by degenerative neoplastic fibrous tissue. The fragments of cancellous bone that remain are extremely fine needle-sharp spicules that are crushed as easily as shredded wheat. The cortical bone, however, becomes extremely dense and sclerotic because the calcium is not excreted but displaced outward toward the cortical bone. After the outer cortex has been removed great care must be exercised in reducing the spicules to avoid accidental loss. The mass having been reduced to the desired dimension the cut tissue margins were coapted and sutured with interrupted silk sutures, and normal instructions for home care were given.

The patient was seen on the fifth day postoperatively (Case Fig. 20–2). The entire flap of mucoperiosteum had disintegrated, with just one of the sutures still in situ. The entire operative field was covered, however, with healthy-looking granulation tissue, evidence that the tissue flap had disintegrated in response to the irritation of myriad needle-like sharp bone spicules and not to inability of the tissue to repair. The granulation repair progressed without incident and without appreciable discomfort to the patient.

Two weeks later the surgical procedure was repeated on the left side, and again the mucoperiosteal flap disintegrated and repaired spontaneously by secondary

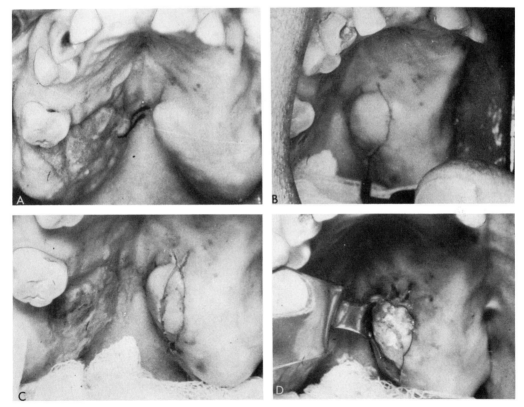

Case Figure 20–2. *A,* Appearance of the palate on fifth postoperative day, before removal of the remaining suture. The entire tissue flap has disintegrated and sloughed away, but unlike slough due to disease, in this instance there is no inflammation or edema; the color and tone are normal, and spontaneous repair by secondary granulation is taking place. There is no pain, and no distress is felt. *B,* The first half of a "purse-mouth" incision is being made with the needle electrode. *C,* The purse-mouth incision has been completed for excision of the predetermined tissue excess that will result from reduction of the bone mass. Note the V at the superior end and inverted V at the inferior end of the incisions. When the tissue is peeled back to expose the bone fully, the tissues open like a purse on hinges, so that the terminal ends will not tear traumatically. *D,* The mucoperiosteum has been peeled back, fully exposing the extremely dense sclerotic outer bone cortex. Note the coagulation and absence of free bleeding.

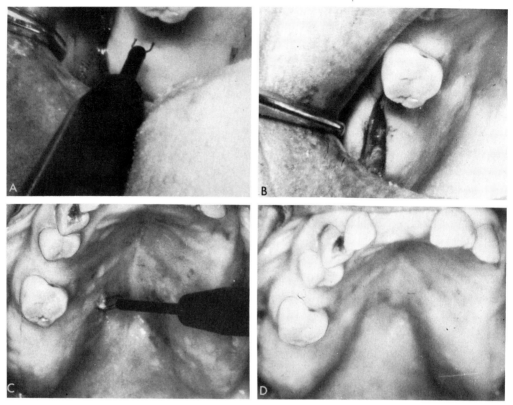

Case Figure 20–3. *A,* Simultaneous parallel incisions are being created with a bipolar electrode made from a medium-width U-shaped loop electrode that was broken, leaving enough wire to be serviceable as a bipolar cutting instrument. *B,* The tissue has been excised after the parallel incisions were joined by extending them to intersect into an inverted V at the anterior end, and a V at the posterior end of the excision. Note that the abnormal height of the tuberosity has been due to hypertrophy of the submucous tissues and not bone. *C,* Loop planing the junction of hard and soft palate mucosa to eliminate a slight wrinkle of tissue excess. The very superficial tissue planing has been performed on the left side, and now is being performed on the right side, using a 7-mm. round loop electrode and cutting current set at 6 on the instrument panel. The loop is permitted to barely graze over the surface of the tissue as it is moved rapidly with a light wiping motion. *D,* Final postoperative appearance of the mouth. The palatal obstruction has been eliminated and the tuberosities have been reduced to reasonably normal dimension. The patient is now ready for operative dentistry and fabrication of a functionally useful partial upper denture.

granulation repair. Six weeks thereafter the palate was fully healed, and the right tuberosity was anesthetized for surgery. The contour of this tuberosity permitted use of two parallel incisions the width of the amount of excess that would result from reduction of the tuberosity to normal dimension. A bipolar needle electrode made from a U-shaped loop electrode that had been broken, leaving twin usable needle projections, was used to simultaneously make the paralleling incisions (Case Fig. 20–3). The tuberosities had appeared to be of bony consistency, but upon incision and excision it was found that the excess mass of the tuberosity consisted of fibrous submucous tissue. A wedge of this tissue was resected, the remainder was undermined, and the cut margins were coapted and sutured with interrupted silk sutures. The following week, since the patient had appeared to take this surgery in stride, the second tuberosity was reduced in a similar manner. Again the mass consisted of fibrous submucosa rather than bone and was easily reduced to normal dimension by electrosection, with the current output increased to 6 on the power output dial of the Coles Radiosurg electrosurgical unit being used. Tissue repair again was rapid and favorable.

One week later the patient was ready to be referred back to the Prosthodontia Clinic, except for a slight wrinkle of excess tissue at the junction of the hard and soft palates. A medium-size round loop electrode was selected, cutting current output was set at 5, and the surface layers of tissue were skimmed off very superficially, removing just a few layers of cells, but enough to provide a smooth palatal surface. The following week the palate was fully healed and normal looking, as were the tuberosities. The patient was referred back to the Prosthodontia Clinic for the denture restoration.

Correction of Deformed Maxilla from Transverse Fracture

CASE 21

All the preceding cases involved preparation of the mouth for full dentures; this case involves preparation of a partially dentulous jaw. It is being included because it offers an excellent example of another of the many preprosthodontic uses for which electrosurgery is so invaluable.

PATIENT. A 34-year-old white female.

HISTORY. While horseback riding the previous year she was thrown by her mount and was accidentally kicked in the face. The maxillary anterior teeth were knocked out bodily or so badly loosened that they had to be removed, and the maxilla sustained a transverse fracture. The fracture was poorly realigned and resulted in marked deformity of the anterior alveolar bone that made it difficult to construct an aesthetically acceptable restoration of the missing teeth. She was referred to the author for preprosthodontic surgery.

CLINICAL EXAMINATION. There was a marked bulge of bone extending from the right lateral to the left first bicuspid. The missing teeth had been restored with a temporary partial denture that left much to be desired from the aesthetic standpoint. The bone bulge was most marked in the midline of the maxilla where it extended from the nasal spine to the crest of the ridge. The mandibular central incisors and several posterior teeth were missing and had been restored with a poorly fitting temporary lower partial denture. The gingival tissue on the mesial aspect of the right maxillary cuspid and left first bicuspid had proliferated downward, partially covering the coronal portions of the teeth (Case Fig. 21–1A).

TREATMENT. The tissues were prepared and bilateral infraorbital and nasopalatine block injections were administered. A 45-degree-angle fine needle electrode was selected, cutting current was set at 3, and the activated electrode was used to make two vertico-oblique incisions immediately anterior to the two abutment teeth. The incisions, extending from the base of the buccal vestibule to the crest of the alveolar ridge, were connected with an incision extending along the crest of the ridge (Case Fig. 21–1B). The mucoperiosteal flap was elevated from the bone and reflected upward, exposing the bony bulge, which was reduced with a rongeur forceps and bone

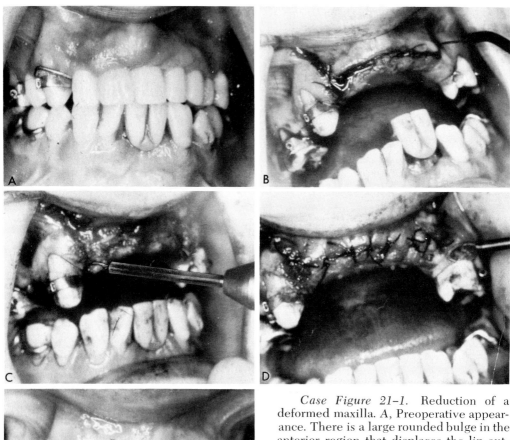

Case Figure 21-1. Reduction of a deformed maxilla. *A,* Preoperative appearance. There is a large rounded bulge in the anterior region that displaces the lip outward. The patient is wearing a temporary partial denture, with the anterior teeth butted against the alveolar ridge, and a lower lingual bar denture restoring the mandibular centrals. *B,* A mucoperiosteal flap is being incised with a 45-degree-angle fine needle electrode. Blood is present on the cut tissue surfaces, but there is no free bleeding. The tissue in the edentulous saddle area has extended downward along the mesial aspects of the two terminal abutment teeth. *C,* The proliferated tissue at the mesial of the right cuspid is being reduced by loop electrosection to make room for a proper clasp. The labial bone bulge has been reduced restoring the maxilla to normal dimension. *D,* The mucoperiosteal flap has been restored and sutured in position. The redundant tissue is being cleared away by loop resection from the mesial of the left bicuspid. *E,* Appearance of the maxilla after initial tissue healing with the repaired old partial in position. Note the space for the clasp and that the slowest healing area is where there is *no* occlusal contact, in the left cuspid-bicuspid area.

bur and a bone file. When the reduction was completed the redundant tissue along the mesial aspect of the two terminal teeth was resected with a flame-shaped loop electrode. The right cuspid was treated before the flap was restored to position and sutured (Case Fig. 21–1C), and the left bicuspid was treated after the flap had been sutured into position (Case Fig. 21–1D).

The patient was seen again on the fifth postoperative day and the sutures were removed. Healing was progressing very favorably. She was seen again the following week; by that time the teeth on the old denture had been built up with acrylic to fill the space created by the bone reduction, and the tissues were almost fully healed (Case Fig. 21–1E). The two abutment teeth were fully exposed and ready for preparation for full crown coverage to serve as abutments for a more sophisticated and aesthetically acceptable permanent restoration.

VI. INFLUENCE OF SYSTEMIC AND LOCAL FACTORS ON TISSUE REPAIR

CASE 22

This case involves two preprosthodontic surgical procedures, the second of which was performed 18 months after the first; the physical condition of the patient at the time of the second procedure was markedly different from what it had been earlier. The physical and emotional status of the patient as well as the difference in the respective local conditions that existed at the time of the two procedures is significant in this case, and the influence of these various factors on the ability of the tissues to heal and on the rate and quality of healing is amply demonstrated.

The postoperative results of the two surgical procedures were dominated by totally different unrelated factors. In the first surgical procedure the factors were systemic in nature; in the second procedure, local. Thus, this case admirably demonstrates the influence of systemic factors on the rate and quality of tissue repair and the influence of local impairment of blood supply to the surgical field on the rate and quality of subsequent tissue healing.

PART A. MAXILLA.

PATIENT. A 49-year-old white female.

HISTORY. Her physician reported that she had very recently undergone a series of 17 shock therapy treatments for morbid depression and severe emotional instability and was under active psychiatric guidance.

CLINICAL EXAMINATION. *Extraoral.* She was visibly extremely apprehensive about the prospect of having to undergo oral surgery.

Intraoral. The gingival mucosa throughout the mouth was atonal. The maxillary mucosa was hypertrophic and fiery red. A thick roll of hypertrophic mucosa formed a flabby mobile ridge crest which extended to the labial aspect. Where the roll joined the tissue on the labial aspect of the alveolar ridge near the lower border of the mucobuccal fold, it created a deep linear indentation. This tissue roll appeared to be an extension of palatal mucosa carried over to the labial aspect in a previous alveoloplasty (Case Fig. 22–1).

There were a number of lacy, milk-white patches on the surface of the mucosa. The mucosa of the mandibular alveolar ridge appeared equally deteriorated. The mandible was edentulous except for the right cuspid and retained roots of the left cuspid and first bicuspid which projected about 1 mm. above the mucosa.

TREATMENT. In view of the patient's neuropsychogenic background the white

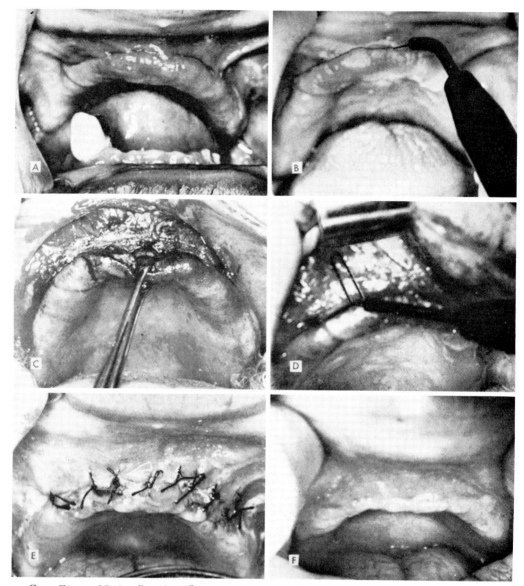

Case Figure 22–1. Part I. Influence of unfavorable local and systemic factors on healing following mucous and submucous resection. *A,* Preoperative appearance of maxilla. Note engorgement, hypertrophy, deep labial groove and numerous areas of lichen planus. *B,* Incision paralleling tissue groove, made with 45-degree-angle fine needle electrode. *C,* Degenerated tissue resected, palatal mucosa retracted to expose alveolar ridge. *D,* Labial and palatal submucosa resected with 45-degree-angle loop electrode. *E,* Appearance of tissues on fifth postoperative day before sutures were removed. Note white patches of lichen planus around the sutures and throughout the maxilla. *F,* Appearance of tissues two months postoperatively. Although the tissues are healed, the tissue tone is still subnormal and the contour of the alveolar ridge is poor.

patches were clinically diagnosed as lichen planus. Patients in her physical condition are also vulnerable to moniliasis, however. Since the antimicrobial antibiotics destroy the vitamin B-forming bacteria in the gastrointestinal tract, Mysteclin was selected as the drug of choice for preoperative prophylaxis because of its antifungicidal properties. In addition to Mysteclin for three days, Kasdenol, ascorbic acid, and clear gelatin were also prescribed.

On the fourth day the mouth was prepared for surgery and infiltration anesthesia administered.* A 45-degree-angle fine needle electrode was selected and cutting current was set at 4 for electrosection. The labial tissue was incised along the indented line, undermined, and retracted upward. The palatal mucosa was grasped with an Allis forceps and pulled downward and posteriorly, fully exposing the alveolar ridge. A considerable amount of submucous tissue was present and firmly adherent to the periosteum. A narrow 45-degree-angle, U-shaped loop electrode was substituted for the needle, and current density was increased to 6. The submucous tissue was resected from the ridge with the short brushing strokes of this electrode.

When the labial aspect was fully cleared of submucosa, submucous tissue was resected from the undersurface of the palatal tissue roll with the loop electrode until this tissue was thinned to a thickness comparable with that of the remainder of the labial alveolar mucosa.

The tissue margins were coapted and sutured with interrupted silk sutures. The sutures were covered with a strip of adhesive dryfoil and a stiff mix of surgical cement was inserted into the sterilized old denture, converting it into a surgical stent. The cement was packed high in the anterior area to help maintain the desired tissue relations and to increase the vestibular height. She was given instructions in postoperative care, and the preoperative medication was continued postoperatively.

She returned on the fifth postoperative day. The mouth was irrigated and the tissues inspected. Healing did not appear to be progressing as favorably as could be desired but not as badly as might be anticipated from the condition of her mouth. The line of incision was healing by primary intention, but it had a number of indentations and was covered with a superficial layer of coagulum. Some atonal hypertrophic tissue had regenerated on the crest of the ridge, and milky-white patches were present around the sutures.

The sutures were removed, the area was irrigated, and chromic acid, 0.5 per cent dilution, was applied for 30 seconds. The chromic acid was washed off and tincture of myrrh and benzoin was applied. The operating field was then covered with a protective coating of adhesive steroid (Kenalog) ointment. She returned one week later. This time the tissues showed some improvement but were still far from satisfactory, and the milky-white patches were more prevalent than ever. The use of an astringent salt-alum mouthwash was recommended to try to improve the tissue tone.

The patient was seen thereafter at regular weekly intervals. It was not until the seventh visit that the tissues were sufficiently healed and the tissue tone sufficiently improved to permit impression-taking. Even at this time the tissues were far from being in ideal condition, but she was dismissed from active treatment since it was apparent that further delay in obtaining new dentures would increase her handicap and be of doubtful value. After her new dentures were processed she returned for postoperative observation bimonthly for six months. During that period the gingiva did not deteriorate but neither did it improve materially.

PART B. MANDIBLE.

Approximately one year after the original maxillary surgery the patient was referred for a pushback procedure to increase the height of the mandibular alveolar ridge and to eliminate undesirable high muscle attachments.

At this time the patient's emotional status was quite well stabilized, and her oral hygiene was satisfactory.

CLINICAL EXAMINATION. The oral tissue tone appeared relatively normal and there was no longer any evidence of lichen planus. The cuspid and retained roots had

---

*Owing to the patient's emotional status, the more desirable infraorbital block anesthesia was omitted to reduce manipulation.

been extracted and their sockets were well healed. The mandibular alveolar ridge was to all intents and purposes completely resorbed. There was just a roll of mucosa forming a soft tissue ridge about 3 mm. high which was undercut and created a noticeable labial bulge. A number of prominent muscle attachments present on both sides of the median line were attached to the lower border of the ridge crest (Case Fig. 22–2).

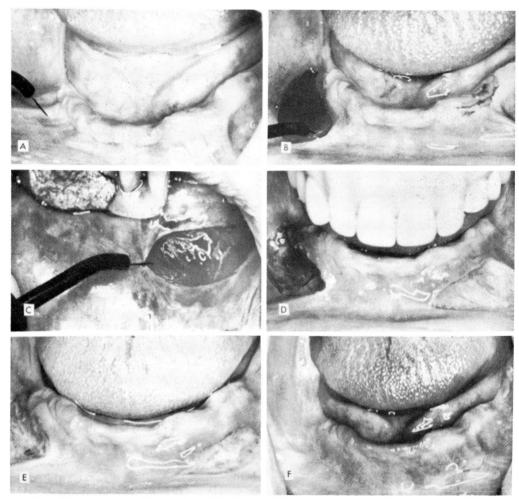

Case Figure 22–2. Part B. Mandibular pushback. *A,* Preoperative appearance of mandibular alveolar ridge prior to incision. Muscle attachments come to within less than 0.5 cm. of the crest of the alveolar ridge. *B,* Muscle attachment on right side incised. Profuse bleeding ensued. *C,* Muscle attachment on left side incised. Bleeding nominal, a mere ooze. Note old partial denture in use as a surgical stent. *D,* Appearance of incised areas 24 hours postoperatively. Note difference in rate of healing in the two areas. Right side, site of profuse bleeding, has scarcely begun to heal. Left side, where bleeding was very slight, is well healed with a layer of normal coagulum over it. *E,* Appearance on fifth postoperative day. Healing has progressed considerably, but right side is now approximately as far progressed as the left side was after 24 hours. *F,* Final postoperative appearance one month later. Healing is complete. The ridge is well defined, without hindrance from muscle attachments. The height of the alveolar ridge has been increased by deepening the labial sulcus space. The tissue tone is normal, and there is no evidence of the lichen planus that was prevalent in the maxilla one year previously.

Lateral jaw roentgenograms confirmed the atrophy of the alveolar ridge.

TREATMENT. The mouth was prepared for surgery and bilateral mental block and lingual infiltration anesthesia was administered. A 45-degree-angle fine needle electrode was selected and current output was set at 3.5 for electrosection. The muscle attachment on the right side was incised first. The incision was directed posteroanteriorly in a horizontal line with a single wiping stroke across the highest point of attachment.

A small aberrant blood vessel was severed by the incision and considerable bleeding ensued. It was brought under control by pressure and clamping with a mosquito hemostat; then the incised tissue was pushed downward by blunt dissection toward the mucobuccal fold. The patient's old partial denture had to be utilized as an emergency surgical stent by building up the right saddle area with a thick roll of stiffly mixed surgical cement in order to help keep the tissues retracted downward.

The left side was incised in the manner described above. This incision was virtually bloodless. The incised tissue was retracted by blunt dissection which produced a slight amount of oozing, but this was quickly halted and the area dried by pressure with a sponge. The partial denture was removed, and the left side was also built up with surgical cement. The denture-stent was reinserted and the two saddle areas closely adapted to the tissues by gentle pressure and manipulation of the cheeks. She was instructed to leave the denture undisturbed until her return in 24 hours.

The following day the denture was removed, the mouth was irrigated, and the tissues were inspected. An interesting phenomenon was observed which did not alter as healing progressed. On the left side, where the pushback had been performed bloodlessly, the pushback was granulating remarkably well. On the right side, where the blood vessel had been severed, the blood clot was beginning to organize but at a much slower rate and not as uniformly.

The two operative sites were painted with tincture of myrrh and benzoin, and Cordent powder was dusted over the right saddle area. The patient returned on the fifth postoperative day and healing was observed to be progressing very well. The left side was healing very rapidly. It was covered with a thin layer of healthy coagulum which peeled off like sunburned skin when healing was complete. The right side was also beginning to granulate, but at this stage it was not much further advanced than the left side had been on the first postoperative day.

Two tiny pinpoint spots of blood were coagulated using a small ball electrode with current output of 0.5. Chromic acid, 0.5 per cent dilution, was applied for 30 seconds. Tincture of myrrh and benzoin was then applied in air-dried layers, the steroid powder was dusted over the right saddle area, and the patient was instructed to return weekly.

By the end of the month the tissues were fully healed and normal in color and tone, and the alveolar ridge height had increased to useful dimension. There was no longer interference from high muscle attachments. Two weeks later it was advised that construction of a new lower denture be undertaken.

This case presented two unusual features. The first, relation of emotional factors to oral health and ability of tissues to repair, has been explored. The second, and perhaps even more significant, is the influence of bleeding and impaired blood supply on tissue repair. Impairment of blood supply to the severed area until a collateral blood supply developed appears to be the most valid explanation for the difference in rate of tissue repair that occurred in this case.

This would partially account for the remarkable rate and quality of tissue repair noted when electrosurgery is properly employed under normal physical conditions, when the procedures can be performed more or less bloodlessly.

CASE 23

This case is an excellent example of the influence of unfavorable systemic factors upon the rate and quality of tissue regeneration. It also serves to demonstrate the difficulty of inducing regeneration of tissue to span large denuded areas of dense cortical bone.

PATIENT.   This is the same patient reported in Case 7 of Chapter 19 and Case 2 of Chapter 22.

HISTORY.   Approximately two years had elapsed since she had been treated for periodontoclasia of the abutment maxillary cuspid. Her complaint this time was that a recently constructed lingual-bar denture cut into her gums so badly on the right side that she was unable to wear it. Attempts to relieve the traumatic pressure by grinding in order to clear a mandibular torus and provide relief proved ineffectual. She was referred for surgical reduction of the torus.

CLINICAL EXAMINATION. *Extraoral.* Negative.

Intraoral. She had prominent bilateral mandibular tori, cauliflower in shape. The mass on the left side was the larger, but since it was located close to the floor of the mouth, the upper edge of the torus had been successfully bypassed with the lingual bar. The mass on the right side was smaller and less prominent but located closer to the crest of the alveolar ridge. As a result there was not enough space between the top of the torus and the gingival margins for the lingual bar to bypass it. A deep ulcerated groove had been cut by the bar into the upper edge of the left torus (Case Fig. 23–1).

TREATMENT.   The mouth was prepared for surgery and inferior alveolar regional block anesthesia was administered. A 45-degree-angle fine needle electrode was selected and current output was set at 3.5 for electrosection. The gingival mucosa was incised 1 mm. beyond the upper edge of the left torus with a wiping stroke of the activated electrode. The gently arc-shaped incision was extended 1 cm. beyond the anterior and posterior ends of the torus. A second paralleling incision was made about 1 mm. below the inferior border of the ulcerated groove. The two incisions were joined at their terminal ends with horizontal V-shaped intersections and the incised strip of tissue was excised.

The mucosa was reflected from the torus with a periosteal elevator and retracted downward, exposing the bulging mass of sclerotic bone which had a large nutrient foramen in its center. To avoid burning or burnishing the lingual cortex and to minimize trauma the torus was reduced with impactor chisels and bone files. When the bulge was fully reduced to the level of the surrounding bone, debridement was performed, and the flap was restored to position. The margins were coapted and sutured with 0000 braided silk interrupted sutures. The coaptation was achieved without slack from excess tissue or undue tension. The patient was given postoperative instructions and Mysteclin was prescribed for three days.

She returned on the fifth postoperative day for removal of the sutures. The mouth was irrigated and the operative area inspected. Instead of finding the usual normal

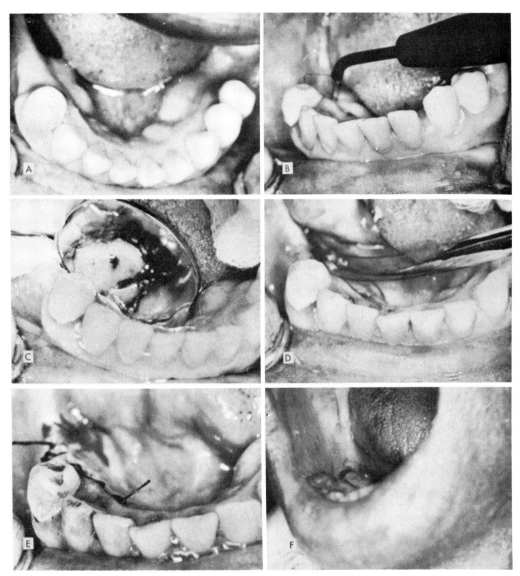

Case Figure 23–1. Mucous membrane graft following reduction of mandibular torus. *A*, Preoperative appearance. Bilateral mandibular tori present. Large left torus located deep, close to the floor of the mouth. Slightly smaller right torus, located high near crest of the ridge, presents a deep groove on its superior border, resulting from pressure of lingual bar. *B*, Incision of lingual mucosa with a fine 45-degree-angle needle electrode. *C*, Reflection of flap reveals a bulging sclerotic torus with a nutrient foramen in its center (mirror image). *D*, Torus reduced to normal level with impactor chisel to avoid overheating or burnishing the bone. *E*, Reduction complete, the flap is restored and sutured without slack or tension of the tissues. *F*, Postoperative appearance five days later. The flap mucosa has sloughed off, exposing the lingual alveolar cortex.

healing by primary intention, most of the flap tissue was sloughed away leaving the mandibular lingual cortex exposed. The exposed bone was a dirty gray and looked necrotic.

The sloughing remainder of the deteriorated flap was removed, the bone was freshened, and bleeding was induced to cover the denuded area with blood into which a small amount of medicated surgical gelatin powder was incorporated. After the blood clotted, the area was painted with two per cent aqueous solution of acriviolet and the patient was instructed to continue the postoperative regimen.

This postoperative treatment routine was repeated twice a week for the next two weeks to no avail. At the next visit antibiotic therapy was reinstituted. Next day the area was prepared and anesthetized, and the tissue margins were freshened; a piece of the cultured mucous membrane soaked in Terramycin solution was sprinkled with sulfathiazole crystals[1] and sutured into position. The graft was protected with clear collodion applied in air-dried layers and she was reappointed.

She was seen again five days later. The graft was still in position but it had not "taken"; instead, it was undergoing liquefaction necrosis. It was removed, the site was thoroughly irrigated, and acriviolet was painted over the area.

Obviously, something was disrupting the healing process. There was no evidence of local infection: no pus, no fever or malaise, and no fetid odor. Local trauma and overheating of the bone had been meticulously avoided. There had been neither excess tissue slack nor undue tension on the tissue margins. This led to the inescapable conclusion that some systemic factor must be responsible.

The patient had mentioned a constantly tired feeling and her behavior had been listless. Her skin, normally a rich chocolate brown and lustrous, was yellowish and murky. Examination of her eye grounds revealed a pale bluish sclera with no evidence of the normal blood vessel pattern, and the inner aspect of her lower eyelids was very pale (Case Fig. 23–2). These physical symptoms strongly suggested an anemia or other hematologic disturbance to be the underlying disruptive factor.

She was referred to her physician for a thorough hematology work-up, and a moderately severe anemia was revealed. After three weeks of intensive therapy the anemia appeared to have been brought under control. Her skin appeared normal again, with good color and lustrous tone, and both eye grounds and lower lids were

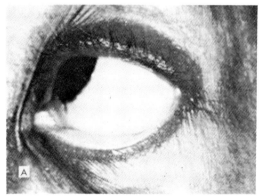 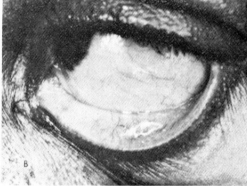

Case Figure 23–2. Clinical evidence of anemia. *A,* Eye: grounds pale and bloodless, sclera watery bluish in color. Skin: pale, almost jaundiced in color, lusterless (before treatment). *B,* After hematology work-up and treatment. Eye: grounds and sclera both normal in color and generously supplied with rich blood circulation.

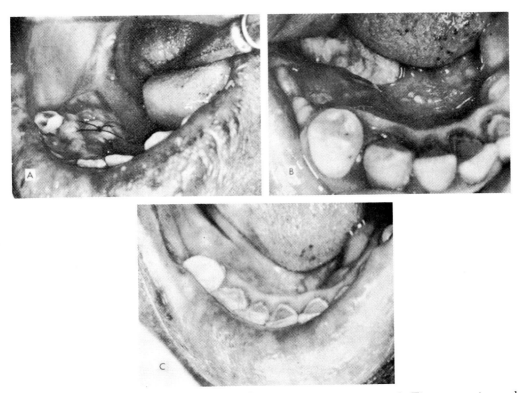

Case Figure 23–3. Final operative and postoperative sequence. *A,* Tissue margins and bone surface having been freshened, graft of Gelfoam moistened with growth inductor material sutured into position. *B,* Sutured graft protected with thick dressing of clear collodion. *C,* Appearance of mucosa one month postoperatively. Healing is complete. The mucosa is intact and normal in color, texture, and tone.

richly endowed with a normal blood supply. Her overall vitality was greatly improved.

As soon as she was pronounced a reasonably normal risk, reparative surgery was reinstituted. Antibiotic premedication was prescribed for three days and supplemented with regular use of a bactericidal mouthwash. On the fourth day the mouth was prepared for surgery and inferior alveolar block anesthesia was administered.

The tissue margin around the defect was freshened with a curet. The surface of the denuded bone was then freshened in a similar manner. Debridement was completed by spraying the area under pressure with Kasdenol solution. A piece of Gelfoam sponge was saturated in a solution of experimental "bone growth inductor" which had recently become available. Excess moisture was expressed and the sponge was used as a substitute for the mucous membrane graft. The substitute graft was inserted into the defect and secured to the surrounding mucosa with three sutures (Case Fig. 23–3). It quickly absorbed and became impregnated with blood in the area. It was air-dried for several minutes until the blood clotted and then covered with a heavy protective coating of clear collodion.

The patient continued the antibiotic therapy for three more days and continued the prescribed postoperative regimen. She returned on the fifth postoperative day. The collodion dressing was intact. It was removed, and this time the graft was found to have "taken" successfully. All but approximately 3 mm. in the center of the defect was covered with normal-looking granulating tissue. The bone in the denuded area appeared healthy. The area was irrigated and the margin of the remaining defect freshened; a suitable piece of Gelfoam moistened with the growth inductor material was inserted and covered with a protective collodion dressing.

The patient returned five days later. The collodion dressing was removed, and this time the defect was completely obliterated with healthy looking tissue. The patient was seen once a week thereafter. Healing continued to progress rapidly and uneventfully, and within one month the lingual mucosa was fully healed with normal-looking, healthy tissue which was undistinguishable from the surrounding mucosa.

This case presents a number of unusually interesting features. Probably the most important is that when systemic handicaps are eliminated the human body is capable of rapidly resuming its normal functions. Of comparable importance is that it emphasizes the need for thorough diagnosis when patients whose healing has been normal suddenly encounter unexpected, unaccountable postoperative complications.

It seems that when electrosurgery has been used there has been an almost instinctive tendency to blame the modality for any untoward result rather than to look for remote systemic factors. It is easy to succumb to this natural but dangerous temptation. Such snap judgments, based on hasty, unwarranted conclusions, are unscientific and may result in a disservice to the patient as well as to the operator's professional skill.

FOOTNOTE REFERENCES

1. Bernier, J. L.: The Management of Oral Disease. 2nd ed. St. Louis, The C. V. Mosby Co., 1959, pp. 418–420.
2. Shafer, W. G., Hine, M. K., and Levy, B. M.: A Textbook of Oral Pathology. 3rd ed. Philadelphia, W. B. Saunders Co., 1974.
3. Color Atlas of Oral Pathology. U.S. Navy Dental School of the National Medical Center. Philadelphia, J. B. Lippincott Co., 1956, pp. 88–89.
4. Thoma, K. H.: Oral Diagnosis. Philadelphia, W. B. Saunders Co., 1946, pp. 256–257.
5. Thoma, K. H., and Goldman, H. M.: Oral Pathology. 5th ed. St. Louis, The C. V. Mosby Co., 1960.
6. Thoma, K. H.: Oral Surgery. 3rd ed. St. Louis, The C. V. Mosby Co., 1958, pp. 229, 285–289, 294–309.
7. Archer, W. H.: A Manual of Oral Surgery. 2nd ed. Philadelphia, W. B. Saunders Co., 1956, pp. 190–196.
8. Thoma, K. H.: Oral Surgery. 3rd ed. St. Louis, The C. V. Mosby Co., 1958, p. 229.
9. Archer, W. H.: A Manual of Oral Surgery. 2nd ed. Philadelphia, W. B. Saunders Co., 1956, p. 196.
10. Thoma, *op. cit.*, pp. 285–287.
11. Archer, *op. cit.*

PART 5

ORAL SURGERY

Man, collectively, as the species *homo sapiens*, is a creature of habit. He characteristically tends to cling to the traditional or "conventional" way of doing things.

Oral surgeons are no exception to this universal behavioral pattern. Thus, many oral surgeons continue to cling to the use of the traditional steel scalpel despite its many limiting handicaps. By doing so they continue to deprive themselves and their patients of the innumerable truly remarkable advantages that modern electronic electrosurgery offers the surgeon and that eliminate the unfavorable factors traditionally associated with oral surgery.

Factors that Plague the Oral Surgeon

In enumerating the factors that plague the oral surgeon most, a representative list would feature the following:
1. Bleeding that obscures the operative field.
2. Patient shock due to blood loss during surgery.
3. The customary unfavorable postoperative sequelae:
   a. Pain
   b. Edema
   c. Trismus
   d. Swelling
   e. Tenderness in the submaxillary triangle
4. Difficulty in reducing redundant tissue accurately to retain normal anatomic architecture by block dissection.
5. Danger of surgical or mechanical metastasis of malignant tumor emboli during biopsy and oncological surgery.
6. The contractile nature of the fibrous scar tissue repair of cold-steel surgery that often causes functional and aesthetic cicatricial impairment.
7. Necessity for use of split-thickness skin grafts to protect the operative field in alveolar ridge extension and similar surgical reconstructive procedures to prevent obliteration of vestibular spaces by scar tissue adhesions.
8. The hazards to geriatric patients resulting from the physical and emo-

tional stresses created by the need to submit to hospitalization and additional surgery in order to be donors for autogenous skin grafts.

9. The hazard of transient bacteremia.

10. Vulnerability to secondary infection of wounds created by a steel scalpel, particularly when incisions are made in contaminated areas.

Each of these potential hazards is inherent in conventional cold-steel scalpel surgery. When electrosection with fully rectified cutting current is substituted for the steel scalpel instrumentation, its unique inherent characteristics allow for the elimination of these factors as potential hazards.

Specifically why and how this happens is readily revealed by review of the respective inherent characteristics of the two modalities. The steel scalpel blade appears very thin and smooth when viewed with the naked eye. But when the blade is viewed edge uppermost under the microscope, it no longer looks thin or smooth. The width of the cutting blade is much greater than the diameter of a single tissue cell. It becomes readily apparent that when the blade is forced against the tissues to create an incision it will crush many tissue cells in its path. Tissue that has been traumatized in this manner heals by fibrous scar tissue repair that is contractile in character.

The victims of cleft palate plastic surgery offer eloquent testimony to the traumatic nature of cold steel cutting and the cicatricial character of the repair of the traumatized wound. The plastic surgeon is as well trained, and matches the skill and competency of neurosurgeons, cardiovascular surgeons, tumor surgeons, and comparable surgical disciplines. The end result of cleft palate surgery, despite the plastic surgeon's skill, is a mass of cicatricial palatal scar tissue that is not only functionally useless but often disabling as a result of tension-induced partial or total collapse of the maxillary arch. Several of the cases in Chapter 17, Orthodontics, show typical examples of such unfavorable results, the responsibility for which rests in the inherent traumatic nature of steel scalpel cutting.

Since the steel scalpel blade incises tissue by manual pressure, all blood vessels in its path are severed in a like manner. Thus, cutting with the steel blade causes bleeding, often profuse and persistent in nature. Blood vessels severed by the scalpel remain open unless they are tied off, and these may become avenues for direct invasion into the bloodstream by bacteria or by malignant tumor emboli.

Blood loss incurred during extensive oral surgery often causes considerable postoperative shock. Because of the traumatic nature of the wound, pain, edema, trismus, swelling, and submaxillary tenderness are commonplace postoperative sequelae to steel scalpel surgery. It is necessary to protect the surgical field with split-thickness skin grafts to prevent obliteration of vestibular spaces by scar tissue adhesions. Since the steel scalpel lacks self-sterilizing capabilities, the hazard of secondary infection of the operative field is magnified.

Cutting by electrosection offers a dramatic contrast. Neither the surgeon nor the electrode actually does the cutting. As described earlier in the text, the latter results from conversion of the high-frequency radio (RF) current into heat energy at the site of contact of the activated electrode with the tissues. The heat conversion results from the resistance offered by the tissues to passage of the current. Thus, the tissue cells in the line of cleavage are disintegrated by the heat energy, undergo molecular dissolution, and are volatilized. This causes the tissue to split apart as though cut with an incredibly sharp knife, although no pressure has been applied.[1] Needless to say, bacteria present in the operative field, no matter how virulent they may be, undergo similar disintegration and volatilization. Thus, electrosection sterilizes as it cuts. This helps to sterilize contaminated wounds, and reduces greatly the vulnerability to secondary infection of the surgical field.

Wound Healing

When tissue is cut by electrosection, if the proper type and potency of cutting energy is used, and it is properly employed, the margins of the cut tissue will look exactly the same as those cut with a very sharp surgical scalpel, with neither coagulation nor searing of the tissue. Unless the atraumatic electrosurgical wound is traumatized postoperatively, the wound heals with repair tissue that is soft, supple, and totally indistinguishable in color, texture, or function from the surrounding tissues. This characteristic quality of electrosurgical wound repair must be attributed to the totally atraumatic nature of the surgery, in view of the fact that when such a wound is traumatized postoperatively the subsequent repair is by fibrous cicatricial scar tissue repair identical to the repair of a steel scalpel wound (see Case Fig. 11–1 in Chapter 24, Biopsy).

Since the repair of an electrosurgical wound results in tissue totally devoid of fibrous contractile scar tissue characteristics, there is no tendency for scar adhesions to develop. Thus, there is no need to protect the surgical field with split-thickness skin grafts to prevent scar adhesions and obliteration of vestibular spaces, even for repair by secondary intention.

The atraumatic nature of electronic surgery also accounts for the amazing absence of the unfavorable postoperative sequelae usually experienced after steel scalpel surgery. When the electronic energy is used skillfully and sound surgical and clinical judgment have been exercised, electrosurgery is characterized by a virtually total absence of postoperative pain, swelling, trismus, or bleeding, and transitory bacteremias.

When unsuitable current is used, the modality is used improperly, or poor surgical technique or clinical judgment has been used, such optimal results cannot be expected. Untrained or inadequately trained operators who misuse electrosurgery are responsible for the occasional reports in the literature of undesirable postoperative sequelae. Such reports help to perpetuate the myths and misinformation about electrosurgery and tend to discourage its use.

Electrosurgical Hemostasis — Why and How

With respect to the question of whether the tissues bleed when cut electronically, hemostasis is inherent in electrosurgery to the extent that when tissue that is normal in tone is cut electronically with fully rectified current or modified continuous wave current there is no *free* bleeding, despite the absence of tissue searing or coagulation. A small amount of blood escapes as the capillaries are severed in the process of incising the tissue. But these capillaries, if normal in size and not engorged, are sealed off as they are severed, so that there is no free or hemorrhagic bleeding. The sealing process that provides the hemostasis is believed to result from plugging of the open ends with the atomic carbon that is the end-product of the disintegration and volatilization of the tissue cells and a submicroscopic degree of coagulation of the cut cells. The inherent hemostasis enjoyed with fully rectified or modified continuous wave electrosection greatly reduces the dangers of metastasis during surgery, and the hemostasis and sterilization achieved while the tissues are cut greatly reduce vulnerability to secondary infection.

When blood released from the tissues at the time of incision is wiped away gently with a sterile gauze sponge, the wound remains free of bleeding. However, when the tissue tone is subnormal and the capillaries being severed are dilated to the size of arterioles by engorgement and stasis, incision by electrosection produces free bleeding identical to that encountered with steel scalpel incisions, since the lumina of the vessels are too large to be effectively sealed off by the electrosection-released carbon.

Effects of Electrosection on Bone

Now let us examine the myth that it is inherently dangerous to contact viable bone with an activated electrode. This too is predicated upon a half-truth. The mere act of making physical contact with the activated electrode against viable bone is not *inherently* dangerous. Rather, it is a matter of how, and more specifically, for how long, the contact is maintained. If the activated electrode is permitted to linger in contact with the bone, it certainly will cause severe damage. But if the contact is momentary, and never permitted to exceed 1 second of total contact along the line of incision, during which time the electrode is moved as rapidly as possible along the bone surface, and a 10-second interval is permitted to elapse before contact is repeated, there is no more danger of damage than there is from contact of the steel scalpel blade with the bone.

Clinically, one of the most advantageous uses for electrosection is for incising mucoperiosteal flaps. This of course necessitates incising through the periosteum down to the bone. Obviously such incisions could not be performed safely if the mere physical contact of the activated electrode against the bone were inherently and automatically dangerous.

The importance of the full 10-second pause interval before the activated electrode is reapplied to the tissues cannot be overemphasized. This is just as important as the rigid limitation of contact for no more than 1 second (with the activated electrode in rapid motion during contact). It has been established experimentally that the lateral heat penetration of fully rectified current is so infinitesimal as to be meaningless clinically. Nevertheless, unless adequate time is permitted to elapse between applications there will be a cumulative build-up of retained heat in the tissues that is likely to become destructive, despite skillful instrumentation and suitable cutting current.

As the reader may have surmised by this time, electrosurgery is an exact and an exacting procedure. The necessary skill and know-how to use this discipline successfully cannot be achieved by wishful thinking or by trial and error. One cannot reasonably expect to become a self-made expert and acquire the necessary expertise merely by purchasing the equipment and working with it. As with all other disciplines, instruction and diligent practice are necessary to develop the skills that make it possible to enjoy the invaluable advantages it offers.

For the edification of those readers who may have turned directly to this part of the text without having read the earlier chapters, among the advantages electrosurgery offers the oral surgeon specifically are as follows: the ability to bend the electrodes and literally manufacture, at a moment's notice, the instrument best shaped to afford maximum access and visibility and efficiency; the ability to reduce redundant tissue by shaving it in layers by loop planing to restore a normal architecture accurately; the ability to destroy necrotic or cystic tissue shreds in situ in inaccessible areas for curettage; the ability to destroy fistulae and their tracts without use of caustics or escharotics; the ability to control soft tissue bleeding by coagulating the bleeder off the beaks of a mosquito hemostat, with a special coagulating forceps designed by the author or by direct contact of a ball electrode; the ability to control bleeding deep in a bony crypt by use of a special combination aspirating-coagulating instrument; and the ability to incise highly vascular, mobile tissues, such as the lip and tissues of the floor of the mouth, precisely, without hemorrhage that may obscure the operative field. This makes it possible to perform definitive intraoral surgery electronically for procedures formerly considered impossible to do via the intraoral route.

ARMAMENTARIUM

Sutures and Suture Needles

Oral wound closure involves the suturing of gingival or other mucous tissues, gingivae to periosteum, or extraoral skin incisions. The more delicate the tissues the greater the dependence of suturing success on use of a combination of good suturing technique and appropriate suture materials and needles.

The ideal suture material is one that provides strength without bulk, limp flexibility, and ability to tie firm knots that do not slip from stretching of the suture material. The ideal suture needle provides efficient cutting penetration of the tissues with minimal diameter thickness and appropriate shape to engage and penetrate the tissues with minimal effort.

Excessively thick sutures are frequently used in oral surgery. When incised palatal mucosa must be pulled together forcefully for closure, or when the tissues will be subjected to considerable postoperative functional stress, the breaking strength of a 3-0 suture is needed, but for most other suturing of oral mucosa 3-0 suture is undesirably thick and unnecessarily strong; 4-0 and often 5-0 sutures usually are much more suitable. The author has found the J & J 4-0 black braided silk suture (#2766) with atraunic FS-2 cutting needle usually is strong enough to provide optimal suturing. The J & J 5-0 black braided silk suture (#682) with atraunic FS-2 cutting needle often is also strong enough when the tissues are not subjected to functional stress. The latter suture is especially suitable for closure of incised vermilion lip tissues.

When it is necessary to suture the gingival mucosa to the periosteum, as in performing a "pushback" to provide ridge extension, or to apically reposition the marginal gingivae, the suturing problem is greatly complicated owing to the delicate texture of the periosteum and its tenacious adherence to underlying bone. Being firmly attached to the bone, the periosteum cannot provide slack to permit the suture needle to slide between it and the bone. As a result the needle tends to tear through and shred the periosteum. Even when the suturing is accomplished without such shredding, the thin delicate texture of the periosteum greatly increases the likelihood that the sutures will tear free postoperatively under even minimal functional stress.

Needless to say the hazard of shredding the periosteum is increased greatly if the suture needle is too thick, or unsuitably shaped. Likewise, when the suture material is too thick or lacks limp flexibility the hazard of postoperative tearing free of the sutures is greatly increased.

Johnson & Johnson's relatively new Ethiflex 5-0 green braided suture #6870 with atraunic tapered cutting V-5 needle attached is superbly suited for suturing mucoperiosteal flaps to periosteum, and for suturing free gingival grafts to the surrounding tissues. When extraoral incisions make closure of skin wounds necessary, the J. A. Deknatel & Sons Deknatel 4-0 green braided (Tevdek) skin suture #79–812 with atraunic ³⁄₈ circle K needle attached is ideally suitable.

Suturing Accessories

The suture needle will penetrate through the tissue margins most readily and efficiently if the tissue is tautly immobilized. When the Allis forcep or rat-tooth forcep is used to grasp the tissue margins to immobilize them, these instruments tend to crush and perforate a considerable amount of the marginal tissue. The ophthalmic tissue forceps, a miniaturized rat-tooth forceps used extensively by ophthalmic surgeons for cataract and other eye surgery, is ideally suited for grasping the tissue margins, since the beaks are so tiny that they will not crush an appreciable amount of tissue and will not interfere with placement of the sutures where desired, yet they grasp the tissues firmly and thereby facilitate penetration of the needle. When the suturing is performed in an area that offers poor access, and when suturing to periosteum, it is a simple matter to grasp the tip of the needle as soon as it emerges through the tissue surface and complete pulling it through with the ophthalmic forceps, instead of trying to complete the penetration by rotating the needle holder or hemostat that is holding the needle, which often results in the needle tearing through the tissues.

Another important accessory for good suturing is *sharp* scissors that are suitably shaped. Many times sutures are torn through delicate or fragile tissue while one attempts to cut the suture with dull scissors or one that offers poor access to the site.

One other instrument that is an excellent and universally useful device is the oral speculum designed by the author for use as a self-retaining lip-cheek retractor that eliminates need for manual retraction by the assistant and releases her to be free to perform other duties.

This retractor exerts uniform, evenly distributed traction against the lips and cheeks. It is therefore almost totally atraumatic since it does not exert forceful traction in one direction that often crushes the delicate tissue cells and causes marked postoperative swelling and pain when manual retraction is employed. Because of the lack of trauma, it is possible to use the retraction for prolonged operative procedures with the mouth open or closed, without appreciable discomfort. Since it can be obtained with pins that permit use of the rubber dam without need to remove the retractor, it is equally useful for operative and restorative dentistry and for clinical photography.

When cutting instruments such as the safeside disc, the knife-edge diamond stone disc, or high-speed carbide bur are used in the mandibular region, it is necessary to guard against accidental injury to the tongue, the lips, and cheeks; in the maxilla, the lips and cheeks must be guarded. The same precautions hold true when electrosurgery is to be used, with one important difference. Whereas it is permissible to use metal retractors with the former, it is not permissible to use them with electrosurgery, since they are excellent conductors, and accidental contact of an activated electrode would burn the tissue that the retractor happens to be contacting.

Two items commonly found in the dental office can serve as excellent retractors, especially for use with electrosurgery, since both are nonconductive. One is the fiberglass mirror; the other, the ordinary wooden tongue blade.

When the fiberglass mirror is used for retraction it is advisable to place the mirror surface against the tissues, particularly when the metallic rhodium-coated Dixson type of mirror is used, since the metallic coating is extremely thin and contact of the activated electrode will melt the plating and permanently mar the mirror.

The tongue, despite its size, is reputed to be the second strongest muscle in the human body. When wooden tongue blades are used to retract the tongue, the saliva moistens the blade and the pressure of the tongue usually becomes great enough to bend it out of shape and destroy its effectiveness for retraction. To overcome this, one can tie two blades together with Dermicel or Scotch Tape and use the doubled blade as the retractor. This makes the device strong enough to resist the pressure of the tongue even when moistened by the saliva, and does not materially add to the bulk, so it will not interfere with ease of instrumentation.

TRANSILLUMINATION

Transillumination is the use of an intensely bright light that is directed to shine through the tissues instead of into them to illuminate them by direct vision. When the light is directed to penetrate through the tissues (soft tissues and bone), areas of infection, and areas of inflammation and engorgement, the presence of foreign debris such as pus in a maxillary antrum or granulomatous debris in a periodontal pocket impairs the penetration of the light and these appear as dark areas that contrast diagnostically with the normal structures through which the light passes unimpeded.

The transilluminating lamp was the major instrument for establishing a differential diagnosis and was used extensively by dentists and EENT specialists before x-ray equipment became universally available. Soon after roentgenographic examination became commonplace transillumination became more or less a lost art. The author has found it extraordinarily useful for clinical visual examination of periodontal pockets and similar oral defects. Inasmuch as the Coles Electronic Radiosurg Scalpel units the author has used for many years provided facilities for use of the transilluminating lamp with the electrosurgical unit acting as the power rheostat for the light, he found it particularly useful for instantaneous visual examination of infrabony pockets being debrided by electrosurgical electronic curettage.

Since most of the other brands of electrosurgical equipment do not provide comparable facilities for use of the transilluminator in conjunction with the electrosurgery, when the fiberoptic lights became available the author purchased one and tried to use it as a substitute for, or improvement over, the traditional transilluminating lamp. It soon became apparent, however, that the much more intensely brilliant light produced by fiberoptics was self-defeating for direct vision illumination as well as for transillumination. The intense brilliance of the fiberoptic light produces a black "blind spot" at the base of the defect when the light is directed into it for direct vision. When it is used for transillumination, the brilliance tends to wash out the dark appearance of the pathologic areas that are essential for visual differential diagnosis.

The author recently found a disposable pocket-sized fiberoptic unit that provides a somewhat less intensely brilliant light than the large electrically powered fiberoptic units, and can therefore be used satisfactorily as a substi-

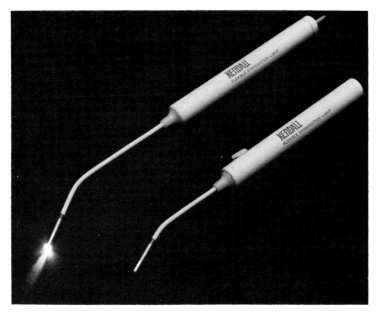

Pocket portable fiberoptic light that can be used for transillumination.

tute for the transilluminating light in conjunction with electrosurgical units that do not provide transilluminating lamp facilities.

This disposable fiberoptic unit is powered by an internally sealed battery which the manufacturer claims will last 6 to 12 months. The unit is relatively inexpensive and when the battery becomes exhausted it is discarded and replaced with a new unit. It is in the form of a cylindrical plastic body with a long slender flexible gooseneck extension that can be bent in any direction to facilitate directing the light into all parts of the oral cavity. The light emanates from the tip of the gooseneck and there are no exposed metal parts in it, so accidental contact of an activated electrode will not produce sparking or cause tissue burns. The light is more intensely brilliant than that of the transilluminating lamp, and does not eliminate completely the "blind spot" and washing out of dark differential coloring, but is sufficiently less intensely brilliant to make it a reasonably satisfactory substitute for the traditional transilluminating lamp.

Chapter Twenty-One

MINOR ORAL SURGERY

Oral surgery ranges in scope from incisions for drainage of acute infection to sophisticated complex techniques for eradication of disease, reparative traumatic surgery, and reconstructive plastic surgery.[2-12]

The most significant difference between this chapter and the next one is that most of the techniques reviewed here are within the capabilities of the general practitioner who has had clinical experience with minor oral surgery. The large variety and complexity of conditions that fit into the category of minor oral surgery and the large number of specific electrosurgical techniques that have been developed by the author for their treatment make it advisable to subdivide the contents of the chapter into representative component entities. These include the following:

1. Miscellaneous minor surgical interventions
2. Electrosurgical techniques for exodontia
3. Frenectomy, operculotomy, and similar soft tissue surgery
4. Subtotal radectomy (root amputation)

I. MISCELLANEOUS MINOR SURGICAL INTERVENTIONS

Incisions for Drainage of Acute Abscesses Using Needle Electrode

The incision for drainage of acute abscesses (I and D) is so simple a surgical procedure that a 6 year old could perform it. However, the I and D creates problems for most general practitioners.

Needless to say, the surgery involved in making an incision for drainage rarely is the problem. Rather it is the inability to use local anesthesia for this procedure, since there is no area into which an injection could be made safely.

816

But why should anesthesia be a problem? The nerve supply to the area has been destroyed at the site of infection, and topical anesthesia is quite adequate for anesthetizing the anastomosing surface innervations. Pressure is the factor that makes more profound anesthesia necessary. When a steel scalpel is used to make an incision, pressure must be applied to cut through the distended tissue. The pressure compresses the fluctuant mass and forcibly displaces the purulent contents against the nerves in the immediate adjacent surrounding tissue and triggers a pain response. Thus, since local anesthesia cannot be safely employed, intravenous inhalation anesthesia must be administered. Most general practitioners are not equipped to employ these agents.

When the I and D is performed by electrosection, the incision can be made without applying pressure to the fluctuant mass. If an adequate amount of current is used, the electrode literally floats through the distended mucosa effortlessly, releasing the purulent exudate. An effective topical anesthetic applied to the external tissue surface for 2 minutes is all that is required for a painless incision.

The patient's reaction to the incision is an accurate yardstick of pain or lack of it. If there is pain and the patient's eyes are open, there will be a telltale pupil reflex from even very phlegmatic patients with high pain thresholds. If the eyes are closed, the most phlegmatic patient will evince a facial response and wince. If the incision is created without evincing either response, it is conclusive evidence that no pain was felt.

CASE 1

The patient kept her eyes closed while the incision was made. The lack of facial response as the tissue was incised is indicative of a painless procedure.

PATIENT. A 19-year-old white female.

HISTORY. She suddenly developed a painful swelling under her upper lip. She consulted her dentist and was found to have an acute abscess requiring drainage and either endodontics and a root end resection or extraction of the tooth. She was referred for treatment.

CLINICAL EXAMINATION. There was a large fluctuant bulge in the mucobuccal fold over the left lateral incisor, involving an area about 1.5 cm. horizontally and 1 cm. vertically, and bulging outward convexly about 7 mm. The gingival tissue over the tooth appeared inflamed and atonal.

TREATMENT. The surface of the fluctuant area was carefully and gently dried with a sponge, and topical anesthetic in an oil base was applied for 2 minutes and the excess was wiped off without drying the tissue.

A 45-degree-angle fine needle electrode was activated with cutting current set at 3 and was used to incise horizontally along the center of the bulge. There was no evidence of a pain reaction as the electrode began to incise (Case Fig. 1–1A and B). As the tissue was incised, the purulent exudate gushed out (Case Fig. 1–1C and D). The exudate was aspirated with care to avoid traumatizing the incised tissue with the aspirator tip. A centipede rubber dam drain was then gently inserted after a second

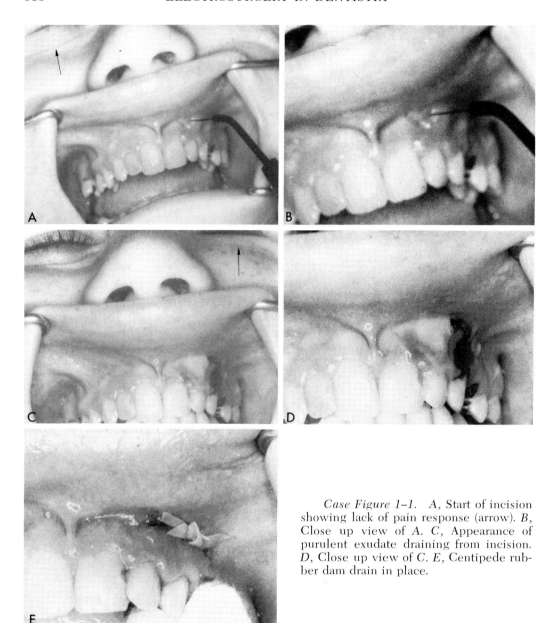

Case Figure 1–1. *A*, Start of incision showing lack of pain response (arrow). *B*, Close up view of *A*. *C*, Appearance of purulent exudate draining from incision. *D*, Close up view of *C*. *E*, Centipede rubber dam drain in place.

application of the topical anesthetic (Case Fig. 1–1*E*), and the patient was instructed to return the following day.

The next day the drain was removed and discarded, since there was no evidence of further exudation. Two weeks later, the incision having healed uneventfully with antibiotic therapy, endodontics was performed. The canal was overfilled after sterilization by electrocoagulation, and a successful root end resection was performed, completing the treatment begun with the I and D.

There is a sound rationale for use of rubber dam drains in preference to gauze drains. Rubber dam drains are easy to prepare and are much more ef-

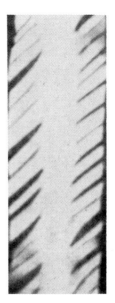

Figure 21–1. Appearance of a typical fenestrated centipede rubber dam drain.

ficient. They do not become saturated and encrusted with the purulent or mucopurulent exudates as do gauze drains. Therefore, they do not act as plugs to prevent free drainage from the incised area as gauze drains have a tendency to do. They do not absorb odors, and, since rubber becomes very slippery when wet (it does not adhere to the tissues), rubber dam drains can be removed easily and painlessly.

To make fenestrated rubber dam drains a sheet of rubber dam is cut into strips approximately 1 cm. wide. Each strip is then slit obliquely on the bias with a suture scissors. The slits are directed so that they slant upward on one side and downward along the other, creating finger-like projections approximately 1 mm. wide and 3 mm. long along both sides of the strip that give it a ciliated or centipede-like appearance (Fig. 21–1). Each finger-like projection provides additional drainage surface by capillary attraction, which adds materially to the efficiency of the drain.

CASE 2

This case demonstrates a somewhat unusual type of acute pericoronitis that developed into an acute abscess. The tissue around the distal of the mandibular third molar and on the lingual aspect as far anteriorly as the middle of the first molar was ballooned out almost 2 cm. beyond the lingual alveolar plate. The treatment, like the condition itself, was atypical. Instead of the usual operculotomy to resect the pericoronal flap that covers all or part of the third molar, treatment in this case was an incision for drainage.

PATIENT. A 19-year-old white male.

HISTORY. The mandibular right third molar had erupted in normal alignment without causing appreciable distress, but after the tooth had erupted the gingival tis-

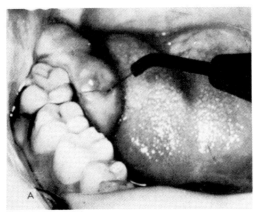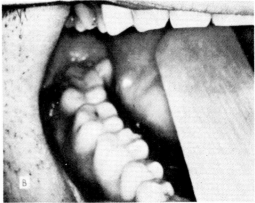

Case Figure 2–1.   Acute pericoronitis simulating an acute alveolar abscess. *A*, Pericoronal and lingual mucosa, tremendously distended with pus, is incised with a 45-degree-angle fine needle electrode for drainage. *B*, Drainage completed, the swelling has subsided considerably. The pericoronal tissue is still edematous and engorged, but the crown of the third molar is almost fully exposed along its distal aspect.

sue behind the tooth appeared to be detached from the tooth. This tissue felt sore, and food packing into the crypt between the tooth and tissue increased the tenderness, but within tolerable limits. He suddenly felt a huge bulge in his mouth, and tenderness in the submaxillary area. He consulted his dentist and was referred for surgery.

CLINICAL EXAMINATION.   The patient had a partial trismus and was unable to open his mouth fully. Opening his jaws as much as he could was quite painful, and he had some pain on swallowing. The tissue was enormously expanded from a point 2 cm. posterior to the crown of the third molar anteriorly to the center of the first molar, and 2 cm. medially toward the midline of the mouth. The swelling was fluctuant. His temperature was 101.2° F. on the oral thermometer. The tooth was firm and normal in all respects.

TREATMENT.   An intramuscular injection of 600,000 units of Crysticillin was administered. Topical anesthetic was applied for 2 minutes, then gently removed with a gauze sponge. A 45-degree-angle fine needle electrode was selected, cutting current was set at 3 on the dial, and the activated electrode was used with a wiping motion to make a horizontal incision from the alveolar edge of the swelling medially to the edge adjacent to the tongue (Case Fig. 2–1A).

Despite the fluctuance the purulent exudate did not gush out until the lips of the incision were spread apart with a curved mosquito hemostat. The remainder of the purulent contents was gently aspirated, and the defect was very gently irrigated with isotonic saline solution at body temperature. A centipede type rubber dam drain was inserted and the patient was instructed to return the following day. When he was seen 24 hours later the drain was removed, the area was again irrigated, and a second injection of Crysticillin was administered. The swelling was greatly reduced.

He returned 24 hours later and was given another injection of Crysticillin. The tissues were now normal except around the distal of the third molar (Case Fig. 2–1B). Saline lavage was maintained for another week. By the end of that period the tissue around the distal of the third molar was normal in dimension, and the epithelialized lining of the tissue in contact with the tooth was resected with a 45-degree-angle narrow U-shaped loop electrode under inferior alveolar regional block injection. Healing progressed uneventfully and the tissue around the tooth when fully healed was tightly adherent to the distal of the tooth and was firm, with excellent tissue tone.

The keys to the successful conservative treatment of this case, in addition to the initial incision for drainage, were the total evacuation of the gelatinously viscous purulent exudate and resection of the epithelial lining (Naismith's membrane).

Loop Excision for Debridement of the Socket

Extraction of teeth without debridement of their sockets often results in retarded or unsatisfactory healing. This is just as likely to happen either when degenerative sulcus epithelial tissue and periodontal pocket epithelial linings are not resected or when sharp spurs of interseptal bone are ignored.

Epithelial lining tissue prevents the blood clot from adhering to the marginal tissue just as it prevents reattachment of the gingival tissue in a periodontal pocket. As a result the blood clot fails to fill the socket to the surface. The epithelial debris can be resected with rongeur forceps or scissors, or with curets, but this frequently increases bleeding and the potential for prolonged postoperative marginal oozing.

Resection of this tissue with suitably shaped loop electrodes by electrosection is simple to perform, is not time consuming, and virtually eliminates postoperative bleeding as a significant factor.

CASE 3

PATIENT.   A 47-year-old black female.

HISTORY.   She required extraction of the mandibular left second molar.

CLINICAL EXAMINATION.   The two bicuspids and the two molars in the left mandibular quadrant were rotated in various directions. The second molar had extensive

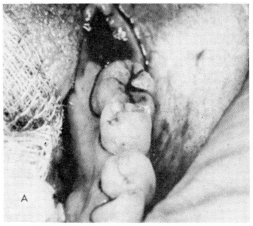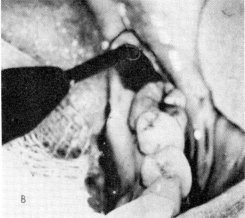

Case Figure 3–1.   Electrosurgical debridement of marginal gingivae around fresh sockets. *A,* Hypertrophied marginal epithelial debris around a fresh socket. *B,* Debridement performed with a flame-shaped loop electrode.

caries that extended below the level of the marginal gingiva on the buccal aspect, and some of the marginal gingiva had proliferated into the huge cavity.

TREATMENT. The tooth was extracted under inferior alveolar block anesthesia. The proliferative buccal gingival tissue would interfere with the healing of the socket unless it was eliminated surgically. A flame-shaped loop electrode was selected, current output was set at 5, and the activated electrode was used with a light brushing motion to skim off the redundant tissue from the internal surface of the marginal gingiva of the socket (Case Fig. 3–1). The blood completely filled the socket and after it had clotted the patient was dismissed with instructions for home care. The healing proceeded rapidly and uneventfully, leaving a normal rounded alveolar contour.

Electrocoagulation

One of the more prosaic uses for electrosurgery — superficial electrocoagulation — is invaluable as an aid to control of granulation repair of fresh wounds or sockets and to accelerate healing. Superficial spot coagulation helps to maintain control over any healing area.

CASE 4

This case is an excellent example of the usefulness of electrocoagulation and the simplicity of its application. In tooth sockets that communicate with the antrum, if a perforation occurs, as happened in this case, control exercised over the repair process may mean the difference between uneventful primary healing and need for plastic repair of an oro-antral fistula.

PATIENT. A 42-year-old white male.

HISTORY. A maxillary molar had become abscessed and was extracted. One of its roots communicated with a low-dipping antrum. When the tooth was removed an oro-antral perforation resulted. The socket was carefully debrided, partially filled

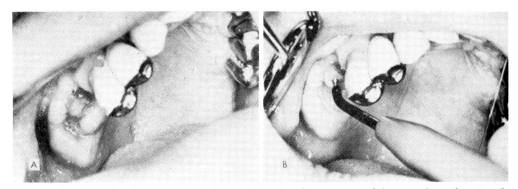

Case Figure 4–1. Electrocoagulation of hypertrophic tissue proliferating from the site of a recent extraction communicating with the antrum. *A*, Preoperative appearance of socket. Granulation tissue resembling polypoid tissue proliferates from mesiobuccal socket. *B*, Tissue is contracted and reduced to normal level by coagulation with the small ball electrode.

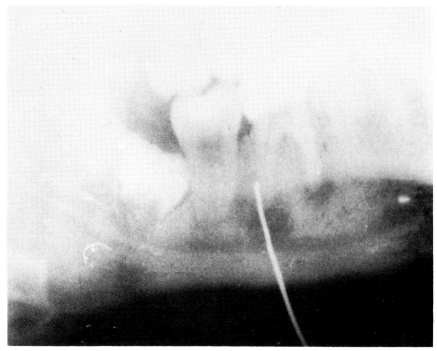

Figure 21–2.   Occlusal view x-ray of a submaxillary calculus with the flexible silver lachrymal probe in the duct in contact with the calcareous mass.

with a small plug of Gelfoam sponge and filled with medicated surgical gelatin powder. These became saturated with blood in the socket, which clotted.

Subsequent healing showed a slight tendency for tissue proliferation and slow granulation repair. Polypoid proliferation was aborted and healing control was maintained by superficial application of electrocoagulation, with current output of 0.5, applied with a small ball electrode (Case Fig. 4–1). Normal healing resulted in two weeks with no clinical evidence of oro-antral communication.

Fulguration

DESTRUCTION OF FISTULAE

Fulguration is *not* suitable for destruction of fistulous tracts through soft tissues. For such cases, insertion of a flexible silver probe through the fistula and application of coagulating current to the probe is best suited (Fig. 21–2).

CASE 5

This case demonstrates the advantageous use of fulguration to destroy a fistulous orifice and tract down to alveolar bone.

PATIENT.   A 48-year-old white female.

HISTORY.   A lesion suddenly developed on the labial gingiva in the anterior part of her mouth. She consulted her dentist, the tooth was x-rayed, and a considerable amount of radiolucence was found around a maxillary lateral. She was referred for the necessary surgical treatment.

CLINICAL EXAMINATION. The right first bicuspid and left lateral were missing from the maxillary dental arch. An oval bulging lesion measuring approximately 6 mm. in length and 4 mm. in width was present on the labial gingiva on the mesial side of the root of the right lateral about 1 cm. above the marginal gingiva (Case Fig. 5–1A). There was no other evidence clinically of any other disease. A periapical roentgenogram confirmed the radiolucence over the mesial portion of the root of the lateral and the embrasure space almost to the mesial aspect of the right central.

TREATMENT. It appeared reasonably possible that the lesion could be destroyed in situ by thorough fulguration without having to extract the tooth. The patient and the referring dentist were informed of the possibility that this would fail to effect a cure and that the tooth might eventually have to be extracted. Both were delighted with the possibility of successfully avoiding need to extract the tooth, and eagerly concurred in choice of treatment.

The tissues were prepared and an infraorbital block injection was administered. Fulgurating current output was set at 8, and the activated electrode was used with a rotary motion to destroy the external orifice, followed by a short jabbing motion toward, but not to, the bone (Case Fig. 5–1B). The fulguration created a carbonized tissue perforation down to the alveolar bone. The debris was carefully removed by scraping it out lightly with a flexible 17-mm. periodontal loop electrode that was used inactivated as a curet to lift out the debris, then to inspect the defect to feel whether there was any more debris still adhering in the area. When all the debris was removed the wound was irrigated with saline solution, bleeding was stimulated, and after the blood clotted, tincture of myrrh and benzoin was applied.

The patient was followed postoperatively for several weeks during which time healing appeared to be progressing favorably. There was no specific need for the patient to be seen further by the author, but he was kept informed about the progress of the case, and healing was complete and satisfactory.

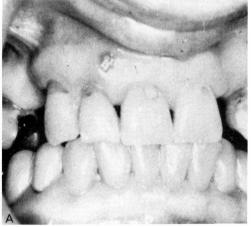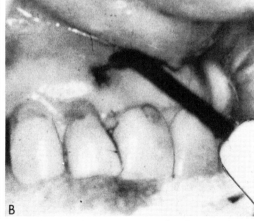

Case Figure 5–1.   Destruction of an alveolar fistula by fulguration. *A,* A fistulous orifice is present in the maxillary alveolar gingiva between the right central and lateral incisors. *B,* The fistula is being fulgurated down to the alveolar bone. The electrode is being used with a circular movement and the fistulous tissue is being carbonized without damage to the bone.

DESTRUCTION OF CYSTIC AND NECROTIC TISSUE IN SITU

CASE 6

A variety of cases have been reviewed that demonstrated fulguration's contributions to preservation of teeth through the ability to destroy disease in areas inaccessible to other methods of instrumentation. This case demonstrates fulguration's contributions toward effecting a cure for osteomyelitis and accelerating its healing.

Prior to the advent of sulfonamides and antibiotics osteomyelitis was one of the most hopeless and dreaded bone diseases. There was no cure, only an endless treadmill of sequestration, incision, and drainage. With the advent of the "wonder drugs," cure became attainable. But even these drugs cannot assure a cure if all the pathologic tissue is not thoroughly debrided. Failure to remove even minute fragments of diseased tissue will prevent a cure.

Bone destruction in osteomyelitis is extensive, and perforation of the cortical bone occurs frequently. Fistulization and purulent exudation usually accompany perforation. If this occurs, it is essential to destroy the fistulas in addition to debriding the bone defect. This case demonstrates use of fulguration to destroy multiple fistulas and complete total debridement of the bone defect, which facilitated regenerative healing.

PATIENT.   A 58-year-old white male.

HISTORY.   The patient developed a dull ache in his lower jaw and noted a peculiar sweet taste that persisted despite frequent use of mouthwashes.

CLINICAL EXAMINATION.   This patient's oral hygiene had been sadly neglected, and most of the teeth that remained were facet eroded from severe bruxing. The left mandibular quadrant was edentulous distal to the cuspid. The mucosa on the buccal aspect was red and atonal. Three fistulas were visible in the bicuspid region. Palpation elicited fluctuance and purulent exudation from the fistulas (Case Fig. 6–1A). Intraoral x-rays revealed two large sequestra of cortical bone above a diffused radiolucent area (Case Fig. 6–1B). A clinical diagnosis of localized osteomyelitis of the mandible was confirmed by biopsy.

TREATMENT.   Panalba was prescribed for one week. On the third day the left quadrant was anesthetized by regional block injection. A 90-degree-angle long needle electrode was activated with fulgurating current set at 7 and was used to destroy the fistulas (Case Fig. 6–1C and D). A 45-degree-angle fine needle electrode was then activated and used to create an incision extending from the second molar anteriorly to the cuspid. A copious flow of purulent exudate escaped as the tissue was incised. The incised tissue was displaced downward and outward, and the two large sequestra were removed and preserved for biopsy. Smaller sequestra and the remainder of the purulent exudate were removed, exposing the alveolar bone which appeared parchment-thin with a 3-mm. perforation in the bicuspid area, and brownish discoloration on the ventral surface of the corresponding tissue. The discolored tissue was planed with a round loop electrode, and the planed surface was lightly fulgurated to assure destruction of any remaining diseased tissue. The perforation was enlarged with a rongeur forceps to create an 8-mm. circular opening through which tissue debris and several additional small sequestra were removed with surgical curets. The defect was irrigated, aspirated, and inspected. A number of tenaciously adherent shreds were removed by electrosection with a U-shaped loop. A few fragments that resisted loop resection were destroyed in situ by fulguration. Bleeding was induced in the defect and some surgical gelatin was introduced and mixed with the blood, creating a spongy mass that served as a support for the tissue flap which was restored and sutured in position.

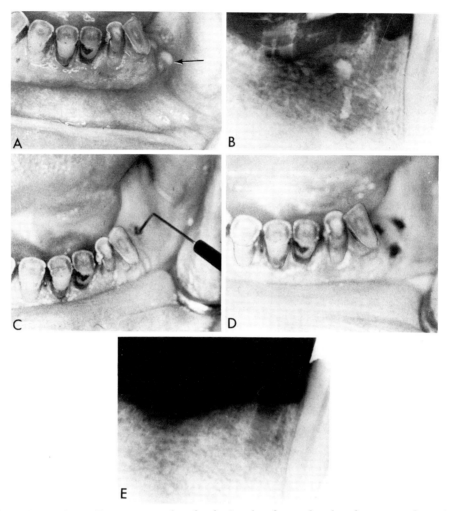

Case Figure 6–1. Destruction of multiple fistulas due to localized osteomyelitis. *A,* Preoperative appearance. The left mandibular quadrant is edentulous distal to the cuspid. Three fistulous orifices are present in the edentulous first-second bicuspid region. Purulent exudate has been expressed by gentle palpation (arrow). The anterior teeth have been eroded by bruxing so extensively that the calcified pulp chambers are visible. *B,* Roentgenographic appearance of the lesion. There is a large area of diffused radiolucence, with a 3 mm. area where the bone appears to have been perforated. Two large and several small sequestra are separated from the alveolar bone. One large elongated sequestrum looks like cortical bone. *C,* One of the fistulas is being fulgurated with a long thick needle electrode. *D,* Appearance of the area immediately after the three fistulas have been fulgurated. *E,* Six month postoperative appearance of the roentgenographic alveolar ridge. The pathologic area has been completely eradicated and the destroyed bone has been replaced with normal, maturely calcified new bone.

Healing progressed steadily and uneventfully. On the fifth day the sutures were removed. By the end of one month the gingival tissue was healed but slightly atonal. By the end of the sixth month the tissue was completely normal and the bone defect was obliterated with maturely calcifying bone (Case Fig. 6–1*E*).

DESTRUCTION OF ULCERATED LESION

CASE 7

This case is an example of the need for resection or excision of extensively diseased tissue by preliminary use of electrosurgical fulguration and electrodessication.

PATIENT. A 63-year-old white female.

HISTORY. The patient, the sister of a dentist, suddenly developed an ulcerated swelling on the labial mucosa in the maxillary right central-lateral region, accompanied by a strong taste of pus. She was referred for extraction of the central incisor.

CLINICAL EXAMINATION. *Extraoral.* The right side of her upper lip was slightly swollen.

Intraoral. There was a swelling of the gingival mucosa between the right central and lateral incisors that extended into the mucolabial fold. There was a small fistulous orifice present at the level of the root apex from which purulent exudate was readily expressed by light pressure. At the lower end of the swelling there was a circular area of ulceration about 4 mm. in diameter (Case Fig. 7–1A). The rest of the gingival mucosa appeared normal. The central was extremely mobile. The lateral was normally firm.

Roentgenographic examination revealed extensive radiolucence which extended around the full length of the root of the central. The bone around the lateral appeared normal.

TREATMENT. The mouth was prepared for surgery and infraorbital block, nasopalatine block and infiltration anesthesia were administered. A flexible silver probe inserted into the fistulous tract penetrated well beyond the labial surface without encountering resistance. When the probe was inserted through the ulcerated lesion it met resistance from the root surface.

Fulguration of the surface ulceration followed by fulguration of the fistulous orifice, desiccation of the fistulous tract before the tooth was extracted, then electrosurgical debridement of the socket, would eliminate need for extensive curettage, which should minimize bone loss and help preserve the labial alveolar contour.

A long, thick needle electrode was selected, current output set at 9 for fulguration and the ulcerated lesion thoroughly carbonized, with the electrode kept in constant rotary motion (Case Fig. 7–1B). The tooth was extracted and the orifice of the fistula fulgurated. Then the electrode was inserted until it met resistance and used to thoroughly desiccate the necrotic tissue. The tooth was extracted and the socket thoroughly debrided with a narrow beak rongeur forceps and a flame-shaped loop electrode used with current set at 6 for electrosection. Although the entire labial bone plate and part of the palatal bone had undergone necrotic degeneration the necrotic debris was resected with relatively little instrumentation. Adherent shreds that remained were removed with a long, narrow 45-degree-angle U-shaped loop electrode used with electrocoagulating current set at 4 for biterminal application.

When debridement was completed, the defect was filled with a mixture of cultured despeciated bone paste, medicated surgical gelatin and sulfathiazole crystals[14] which was thoroughly mixed with the blood in the socket (Case Fig. 7–1C). A dryfoil insulated gauze bitepack was inserted over the operative field, and Achromycin was prescribed for three days. She was given postoperative instructions and reappointed.

She returned on the fifth postoperative day. Healing was found to be progressing favorably. Both the ulcerated area and the fistulous orifice were covered with a layer of healthy coagulum (Case Fig. 7–1D). Superficial spot coagulation was applied to a small red spot and tincture of myrrh and benzoin was applied. She was instructed to continue the postoperative care and return in one week. When she was seen again the site of the fistulous tract appeared almost fully healed, but the large circular defect near the gingival margin had partially deteriorated, and some of the granulating tissue was decomposed, creating an indentation extending from the labial surface to the palatal aspect of the socket.

The depressed area was irrigated; then topical anesthetic was applied. After two

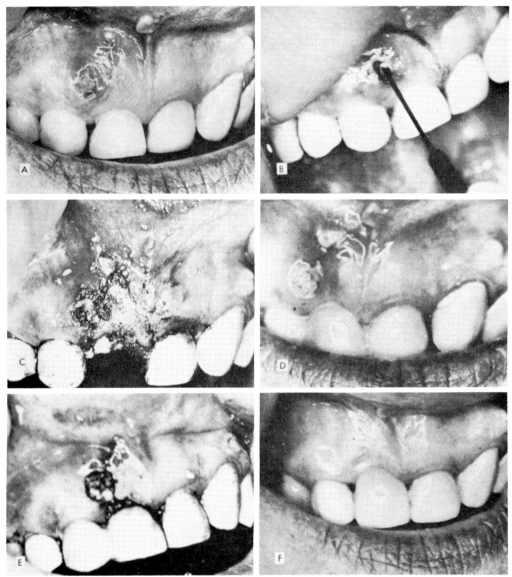

Case Figure 7–1. Use of fulguration: desiccation to debride extensive necrotic degenerative tissue around a tooth to conserve alveolar contour. *A*, Preoperative appearance clinically of maxillary right central incisor. There is a large area of ulceration extending from the labiogingival fold to within 3 mm. of the gingival margin and a fistulous orifice close to the fold midway between the lateral and central. *B*, Fulguration of the ulcerated area. Note sparking against the tissue. *C*, Debridement completed after extraction, the defect is filled with a mixture of cultured despeciated bone paste and medicated powdered surgical gelatin. *D*, Appearance on the fifth postoperative day. Both the ulcerated area and the fistulous orifice covered with a layer of healthy coagulum. *E*, Small graft of cultured mucous membrane inserted into residual defect. *F*, Final postoperative appearance of the healed area. Normal contour of the alveolar ridge has been retained. Healing is complete, and only a very slight, almost imperceptible shallow depression marks the site.

minutes the lining tissue was lightly curetted to induce bleeding and create a raw tissue surface. The outer perimeter of the defect was scarified; then medicated surgical gelatin powder was deposited into the area and mixed with the blood. Antibiotic therapy was renewed and postoperative instructions were continued.

She returned one week later, at which time the defect was found unimproved. The area was prepared and infiltration anesthesia administered. The periphery of the defect was freshened by electrosection with a flame-shaped loop electrode. The center of the defect was freshened by curettage. A small piece of despeciated mucous membrane was cut to fit the defect. The defect was then partially filled with a mixture of bone paste and surgical gelatin which combined with the blood present. The mucous membrane graft was inserted to fill the remainder of the defect to the level of the surrounding mucosa (Case Fig. 7–1E). The area was dried and a piece of adhesive dryfoil was carefully adapted over the site and sealed to the tissues with a heavy layer of collodion to afford some protection to the graft.

The patient returned on the fifth postoperative day. The defect was found almost fully healed but a small residual defect remained which persisted for a considerable time. After three months of periodic scarification and insertion of surgical gelatin, the regenerative obliteration of the alveolar defect was complete. The maxillary alveolar contour was normal. The only remaining evidence of the extensive alveolar destruction was a very shallow, small dimpling depression on the surface of the gingival mucosa (Case Fig. 7–1F). Roentgenographic examination revealed comparable bone repair.

As a rule, when both the labial and palatal cortical plates have been perforated and partially destroyed by alveolar necrosis, marked concavitation with permanent loss of normal convex contour results. When the destruction is as extensive as in this case, the concavitation is usually so pronounced that artificial recontouring with porcelain gum-block or similar prosthetic device is required to re-create satisfactory esthetics. The normal regeneration and favorable cosmetic result achieved in this case was gratifying.

Use of fulgurating and desiccating currents permitted destruction in situ and total resection of the necrotic tissue with minimal loss of normal tissue and bone. This helped to reduce the loss of alveolar contour. It also helped to provide an additional matrix for alveolar regeneration, which is often sacrificed when considerable amounts of normal tissue and bone must be resected to effect satisfactory debridement. While the use of the graft materials helped to obliterate the defect, it is more than likely that conservation of the tissues made possible by electrosurgery played the more important role in influencing tissue repair.

DESTRUCTION IN SITU OF TUMOR MASSES

Fulguration is also very useful for destruction of neoplasia. When the nature of a lesion or neoplasm has been established and there is no need to preserve any of the tissue for biopsy, destruction of the mass in situ assures that there will not be any regeneration of the tumor tissue. When the electrode is kept in constant rotary motion while fulguration is performed in order to prevent overheating injury to the underlying structures, satisfactory uneventful healing may be anticipated.

CASE 8

This case is an example of the efficacy of total destruction in situ of a soft tissue neoplasm by fulguration.

PATIENT. A 58-year-old white male.

HISTORY. In the previous two years a number of soft tissue masses similar in appearance and identical in texture developed in various parts of his mouth. They were asymptomatic. Two months previously one of them was resected for biopsy. It was reported to be a soft fibroma.*

CLINICAL EXAMINATION. *Extraoral.* Negative.

Intraoral. The mandibular bicuspids and molars were missing bilaterally. A large mass approximately 1.5 cm. in diameter was located on the tip of his tongue on the right side of the midline. A small round tissue bulb about 6 mm. in diameter projected above the surface of the tissue at the edentulous site of the second bicuspid

---

* He had been advised to have the neoplasm on the tip of the tongue removed, but since it was asymptomatic he was reluctant to do so.

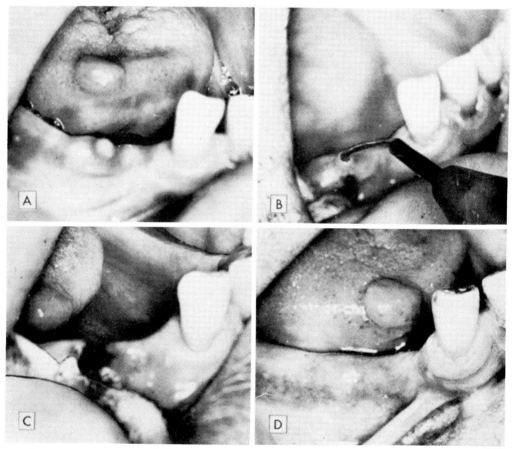

Case Figure 8–1. Total destruction in situ of a soft tissue neoplasm by fulguration. *A*, Preoperative appearance of the lesion. *B*, Mass being fulgurated. *C*, Mass totally destroyed and underlying tissues carbonized. *D*, Postoperative appearance one month later. The defect has filled with normal healthy gingival tissue that is identical with the surrounding mucosa.

(Case Fig. 8–1A). Biopsy appeared unnecessary, so destruction of the mass in situ was chosen as the treatment of choice.

TREATMENT.   The mouth was prepared and anesthesia administered by circumferential infiltration. A heavy-gauge, straight needle electrode was bent to a 45 degree angle and monoterminal current set at 9 for fulguration. With the electrode kept in constant motion, the mass was totally destroyed and the immediate underlying structures carbonized by fulguration (Case Fig. 8–1B and C). Bleeding was then induced in the area, and a small amount of medicated powdered surgical gelatin was deposited into the surgical defect and mixed with the blood. The operative field was then protected with a thick coating of clear collodion.

Healing progressed rapidly and uneventfully. The area filled with normal granulation tissue which was covered with a moderately thick layer of healthy coagulum. By the end of the first postoperative month the area was fully healed with mature normal tissue and the site of fulguration was no longer distinguishable from the surrounding tissue (Case Fig. 8–1D).

Obliteration of Hemangiomas

In Chapter 1 (page 37) it was emphasized that there are only three justifiable uses for electrodesiccation in dentistry. One of these is obliteration of hemangiomas, particularly the cavernous type. The hemangioma is a benign tumor of blood vessels. This vascular lesion is not encapsulated and frequently extends far beyond its apparent clinical base. Thus when this tumor is treated by surgical excision there is an ever-attendant danger of profuse, persistent hemorrhage, especially with the cavernous type, which is characterized by very large blood spaces.

The surgical risk of hemorrhage accounts for the preferential treatment of the hemangiomas by injection of sclerosing solutions or by electrodesiccation. By and large, both methods have proved effective. But both methods require considerable skill and expertise for favorable efficient use, since neither is self-limiting in its destructiveness, and can therefore cause damage to the surrounding normal tissues. Because it is possible to see when the tissue dehydration has penetrated beyond the confines of the tumor, indicating it has been destroyed, it is possible to control the destruction better with the desiccating current than with the sclerosing solution.

According to the pathology textbooks, hemangiomas are blue, purple, or purplish red in color and usually blanch when pressure is applied.[13, 14] When their clinical appearance fits this description, the advantages gained from elimination of the hazard of severe hemorrhage more than justify use of sclerosing solutions or electrodesiccation despite the difficulty of controlling their destructiveness.

But when an atypical cavernous hemangioma is encountered which does not resemble the typical lesion in any way, and the lesion is surgically excised and severe persistent hemorrhage ensues, electrocoagulation may prove more effective than electrodesiccation.

II. EXODONTIA

Exposure of Retained Roots

It is axiomatic that good surgical technique includes minimal instrumentation and sacrifice of normal tissue. The less alveolar bone sacrificed to perform the oral surgery, the less the likelihood of creating anatomic deformity, and the greater the likelihood for normal, rapid, uneventful repair.

When retained roots are submerged and covered by mucosa, unless they can be removed atraumatically without soft tissue laceration or bone damage it becomes necessary to incise a flap and expose and remove the buccal alveolar bone so that the roots can be removed without lacerating the tissue or mutilating the bone.

If the overlying mucosa is removed, exposing the roots to view, it often becomes possible to elevate them without the need to incise a flap. When this is not feasible it is often possible to eliminate need to remove the overlying alveolar bone by drilling a perforation through the bone plate and into the root with a small round bur so that the root can be engaged with an exolever, apical elevator or Crane pick. The feasibility of removing retained roots by simple elevation cannot be determined until the overlying mucosa is removed to provide good visibility and access to the submerged roots. One of the simplest uses of electrosurgery in exodontia is to facilitate removal of submerged retained roots by resecting covering gingiva to expose them to view. This often eliminates need for their surgical removal (Fig. 21–3).

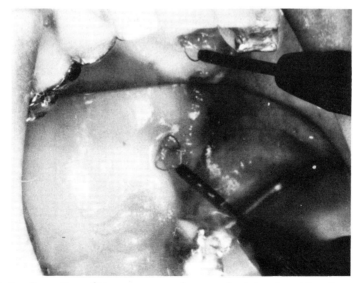

Figure 21–3. Resection of tissue over a submerged retained root by electrosection with a round loop electrode that has been bent to a curvature that facilitates the excision with a scooping motion of the loop. The mirror image reflection shows the loop very clearly as it is being applied.

CASE 9

This case demonstrates the usefulness of electrosurgery to expose retained roots that are completely submerged beneath the surface mucosa, thereby facilitating conservative removal.

PATIENT. A 47-year-old black female.

HISTORY. The coronal portion of her mandibular right first molar had disintegrated, leaving retained roots completely submerged under the surface mucosa. An acute abscess developed. She was referred for extraction of the offending roots.

CLINICAL EXAMINATION. *Extraoral.* There was a moderate amount of swelling of the lower third of her face and the submaxillary triangle on the right side.

Intraoral. A sac-like swelling was present in the first molar area of the mucobuccal fold. The distended tissue was fluctuant. The mucosa over the edentulous first molar area was intact except at one small point near its mesiobuccal angle. At that point a tiny spur of root projected very slightly beyond the surface.

TREATMENT. The mouth was prepared for surgery and inferior alveolar regional block anesthesia was administered. A 45-degree-angle fine needle electrode was selected and current output set at 3.5 for electrosection. The abscess was incised with

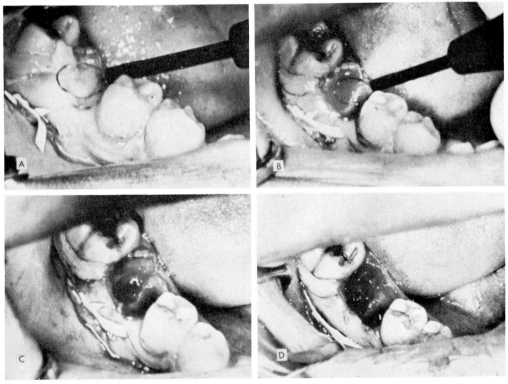

Case Figure 9–1. Exposure of retained roots by resection of overlying mucosa to permit conservative removal without incising a flap or removing the buccal alveolar bone plate to expose the roots. *A*, Retained roots covered with mucosa; loop in position. *B*, Overlying mucosa resected with the loop electrode, exposing the roots. *C*, Distal root removed from its socket by conservative elevation. *D*, Mesial root removed from its socket in identical manner.

a single wiping stroke of the activated electrode. A profuse flow of purulent exudate was aspirated, and a fenestrated rubber dam drain was inserted.

A medium-sized round loop electrode was then substituted for the needle electrode, with current output increased to 6, and used to resect the overlying mucosa with a scooping motion (Case Fig. 9–1A and B). This exposed the retained roots to full view. The distal root was loosened with a straight gouge elevator, then elevated from its socket with a Stout A elevator (Case Fig. 9–1C). The mesial root was loosened in the same manner and elevated with an East-West elevator. The result was a normal, intact socket (Case Fig. 9–1D) which healed without incident.

Surgical Removal of Impacted Teeth

No discussion of oral surgery techniques would be complete without a review of techniques for surgical removal of impacted teeth.

The mandibular third molars, maxillary cuspids and maxillary third molars — in that order of frequency — are the teeth that most often remain impacted in the human jaws. In most instances impacted teeth are malposed in mesioangular, distoangular or horizontal version.[15] Occasionally, although in normal alignment, teeth remain vertically impacted deep in the jaw bone. Marked deviations from these classic malpositions are rare. The author has encountered only three marked deviations in all his years of practice. One was an inverted maxillary third molar lying upside down with its root apices near the crest of the alveolar ridge in the tuberosity. The second, a mandibular cuspid, was horizontally embedded in the symphysis with its root apex pointed labially and the crown in contact with the lingual plate. The third involved mandibular second and third molars horizontally impacted, with their crowns in cusp to cusp contact.

Due to infrequence of deviations, surgical techniques for removal of impacted teeth are distinctly stylized.[16-24] Nevertheless, surgical removal of impacted teeth is not devoid of hazards. Anatomic deformities and location contribute a number of hazards. Notable are: extreme dilaceration of the roots; ankylosis of roots to investing bone; physical contact of the roots with the mandibular canal or the inferior border of the mandible; projection of roots into, or ankylosis with, the bony floor of the nasal fossa or maxillary antrum. Pathology also contributes hazards, especially that of pathologic fracture of a jaw due to cystic destruction of bone.

By far the most common hazard, however, is faulty technique. In addition to unnecessary laceration of tissue and mutilation of bone, faulty technique may result in displacement of a maxillary third molar into the sphenomaxillary fossa, or of a mandibular third molar into the pterygomandibular space; fracture of the mandible, fracture of the maxillary tuberosity, and fracture of instruments with impaction of metallic fragments into the jaw bone.[25]

Three factors govern most faulty technique hazards: first, lack of surgical training and experience; second, poor access and visibility in the operative field; third, careless or faulty instrumentation. Without good access and visibility, careful instrumentation is almost impossible even for the trained, experienced operator.

All the surgical procedures for removal of impacted teeth have one common denominator: the need for incisions to create tissue flaps. If the flaps are properly designed, the hemostatic action inherent in the electrosurgical cutting current insures good visibility in the operative field. The cases to be presented demonstrate advantageous flap designs, and techniques for performing the incisions electrosurgically. The desired incisions can be easily performed with suitably shaped electrodes by electrosection, even in relatively inaccessible areas, with little or no bleeding to obscure the field of vision. Each case reported is included because it presents a somewhat different yet typical surgical problem or an atypical variation that required special planning and technique modification.

MANDIBULAR THIRD MOLARS

Hemorrhage is always a serious handicap to efficient removal of the impacted tooth and the subsequent debridement of the socket. Electrosurgery with its inherent hemostasis facilitates delivery of the impacted tooth and assures thorough debridement after its removal.

CASE 10

This is the first of a series of cases involving electrosurgical flap incisions for the surgical removal of malposed impacted mandibular third molars. Although the basic technique is the same in all cases, individual factors that influenced the treatment plan or the postoperative repair vary greatly. This case offers an interesting contrast in the rate of healing of healthy tissue and diseased tissue in the same mouth.

PATIENT. A 24-year-old white female.

HISTORY. All four third molars were impacted and malposed. Several of the teeth had been affected by transitory episodes of subacute pericoronitis. Since she was a concert singer on tour almost constantly, she was advised to have them removed without delay. She was referred for their removal.

CLINICAL EXAMINATION. *Extraoral.* Negative.

Intraoral. The patient's oral hygiene was excellent. The tissue tone was normal throughout the mouth except in the four respective third molar areas. The mandibular third molar areas, especially the one on the right side, were rather atonal, hyperemic and hypertrophied. Slight breaks in the surface continuity of the mucosa immediately distal to the distobuccal aspects of both mandibular second molars were visible.

There was some tenderness in the right submaxillary triangle and a feeling of tenderness on swallowing. It therefore appeared desirable to remove the impacted teeth on the right side in one sitting and to remove the remaining two teeth after the right side was fully healed.

TREATMENT. The mouth was prepared for surgery and inferior alveolar regional

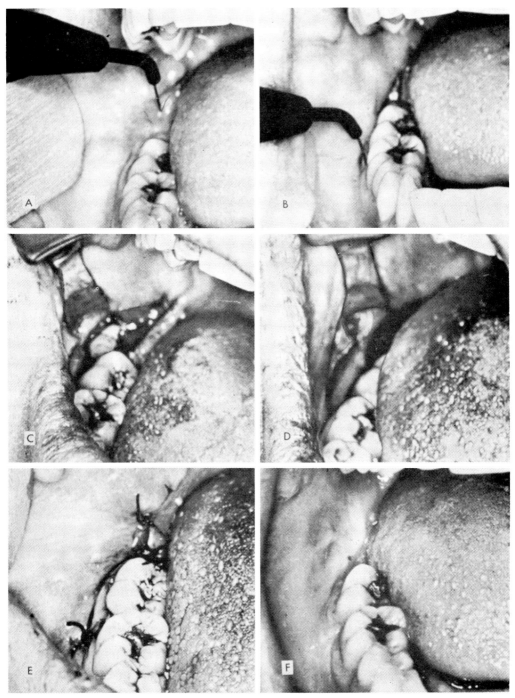

Case Figure 10–1. Surgical removal of impacted mandibular third molar. *A,* Incision through retromolar pad along crest of ridge directed postero-anteriorly to distal of second molar performed with 45-degree-angle fine needle electrode. *B,* Second incision on buccal aspect, vertico-oblique, extends from the distogingival angle of first molar down to the mucobuccal fold. *C,* Tissue retracted, overlying bone removed, exposing crown of impacted tooth. *D,* Tooth has been sectioned and removed, and debridement of socket has been completed. *E,* Flap has been restored and sutured along both lines of incision. *F,* Clinical appearance of fully healed tissues.

block anesthesia was administered. A 45-degree-angle fine needle electrode was selected and current output set at 3.5 for electrosection. An incision with the activated electrode was started at the most posterior part of the mandible and carried forward in a postero-anterior direction. The incision was carried across the center of the retromolar pad and the mucosa over the third molar with a continuous sweeping motion until the electrode made contact with the distal surface of the second molar (Case Fig. 10–1A). A second incision was then started at the mesiobuccal angle of the second molar and extended downward and slightly anteriorly from the gingival margin to the mucobuccal fold (Case Fig. 10–1B).

The incised tissue was elevated from its alveolar base and retracted with a periosteal elevator to expose the overlying alveolar bone and the mesiobuccal cusp of the impacted malposed tooth. The bone was removed with automatic impactor chisels until the crown of the tooth was sufficiently exposed. The tooth was lying in mesioangular version in a vertico-oblique position and tilted medially (Case Fig. 10–1C). The tooth was sectioned and removed in three segments. After debridement was completed, a mixture of cultured despeciated bone paste and medicated surgical gelatin was deposited into the defect and mixed with the blood. The incised margins were coapted and sutured with 0000 braided silk interrupted sutures (Case Fig. 10–1D and E). Removal of the maxillary third molar, which will be described in Case 13, was then performed. Achromycin was prescribed for four days to control the bacteremia that could be anticipated in view of the history of low-grade infection, and she was given postoperative instructions.

She returned on the fifth postoperative day for removal of the sutures. After their removal the mouth was irrigated and examined. Healing by primary intention appeared to be progressing satisfactorily. Tincture of myrrh and benzoin was applied and she was told to continue the home care. She returned for postoperative treatment at weekly intervals for the next six weeks. Gingival healing was very gradual and the tissue was not fully healed until the end of that period. By that time the tissue tone was normal and there was no visible evidence of cicatricial contraction or scar tissue formation in the area (Case Fig. 10–1F).

Two months after the initial surgery the patient was ready for removal of the left molars. The mouth was prepared and inferior alveolar block anesthesia was administered. The incisions on the crest of the ridge and on the buccal aspect were performed in the same manner as on the right side (Case Fig. 10–2A and B). The flap was retracted and overlying bone exposed; the crown was exposed, sectioned and removed (Case Fig. 10–2C). Debridement completed, the margins were coapted and sutured after bone paste and surgical gelatin were deposited into the surgical defect.

Since this side had been asymptomatic, no antibiotic therapy was prescribed. Kasdenol lavage, saline lavage and postoperative home care were prescribed. The sutures were removed on the fifth postoperative day. Healing by primary intention was progressing very satisfactorily (Case Fig. 10–2D). Within three weeks the tissues were well healed. The condition of the tissues on this side after three weeks was fully comparable to that of the tissues on the right side which had been healing for two months (Case Fig. 10–2E).

It is significant that the left side, which had been very slightly affected by pericoronal deterioration, healed much more rapidly than the right side, which had been subjected to repeated subacute episodes of active pericoronal infection. This affords an excellent demonstration of the significant role played by unfavorable local conditions in influencing the repair process.

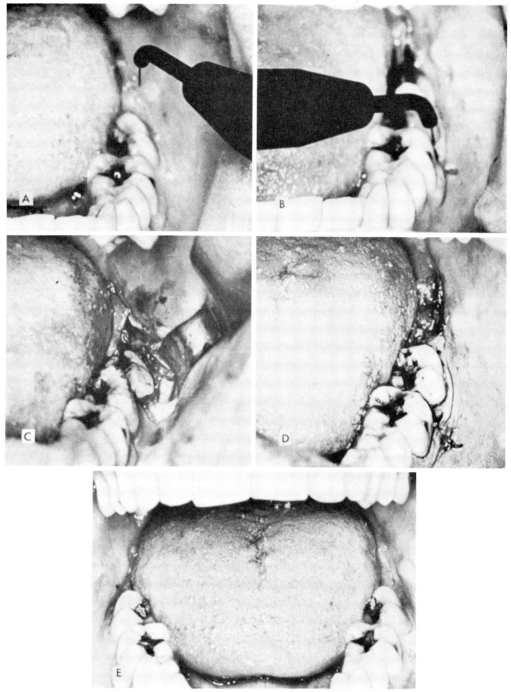

Case Figure 10–2. Surgical removal of impacted molar on opposite side. *A,* Posterior incision along crest of alveolar ridge. *B,* Anterior incision on buccal aspect (directed upward). *C,* Flap retracted exposing crown of impacted tooth and considerable submucous tissue including hypertrophied embryonal capsule. *D,* Tooth sectioned and removed, debridement of socket completed, the flap has been restored and the incised margins coapted and sutured. *E,* Appearance of the mouth two months postoperatively. Note that the healing on this side is quite comparable to that of the first side.

CASE 11

This case is an example of an acute type of pericoronal infection that leaves the surface mucosa over the impacted tooth intact but produces marked submucous hyperplasia, inflammation and suppuration. In this type of case the infection often penetrates deeply into the investing structures. Severe postoperative edema and trismus are characteristic postoperative sequelae.

PATIENT. A 25-year-old white female.

HISTORY. The patient, an airline stewardess, was troubled with periodically recurring episodes of subacute pericoronitis. When these occurred during flights, her symptoms were much more severe and interfered with her efficiency. She was referred for removal of all four molars, which were malposed and impacted.

CLINICAL EXAMINATION. The patient was seen during one of her subacute episodes.

Extraoral. There was moderate swelling in the lower third of her left cheek and some induration and tenderness in the left submaxillary triangle. She was unable to open her mouth wide.

Intraoral. The left third molar area was so swollen that the retromolar pad could not be differentiated from the alveolar mucosa, which was detached from the distal aspect of the second molar. Submucous hyperplasia and hypertrophy were so pronounced that some of this tissue bulged along the anterior border against the tooth. Light pressure caused severe pain and produced a copious flow of purulent exudate.

TREATMENT. Surgery was deferred for one day to permit preliminary treatment and premedication. A throat pack was inserted to block off the oropharynx and the area was vigorously irrigated. The pack was discarded and a fenestrated rubber dam drain inserted into the pocket behind the second molar. Panalba was prescribed for four days. She was given instructions in home care and reappointed.

She returned the following day and reported that all the acute symptoms had subsided. When the rubber dam drain was removed no exudate could be expressed by manipulation or pressure. The mouth was prepared for surgery and inferior alveolar block anesthesia was administered. A 45-degree-angle fine needle electrode was selected and current output set at 4.5 for electrosection to provide sufficient heat energy to efficiently incise the hypertrophic, hyperplastic tissue.

An incision was made with the activated electrode along the crest of the ridge, extending from the angle of the ascending ramus anteriorly to the distal of the second molar (Case Fig. 11–1A). A second incision was made on the buccal aspect, starting at the distoproximal angle of the first molar and extending downward and slightly anteriorly from the gingival margin to the mucobuccal fold.

The incised tissue was undermined with a periosteal elevator, reflected from the bone and retracted, exposing the mesiobuccal cusp of the impacted tooth and a considerable mass of submucous tissue (Case Fig. 11–1B). The needle electrode was replaced with a flame-shaped loop electrode which was used to resect the submucous tissue from the under surface of the mucosa. Overlying bone was removed to expose the crown, which was sectioned with impactor chisels and removed. Thus the degenerated embryonal capsule became exposed. The main bulk of the capsule was removed with a curet. Adherent shreds were resected with a narrow loop electrode. A few tenaciously adherent shreds in the distolingual area could not be resected even with the loop electrode but had to be destroyed in situ by fulguration.

Debridement having been completed, the defect was filled with medicated surgical gelatin, the incised margins coapted and sutured with 0000 braided silk su-

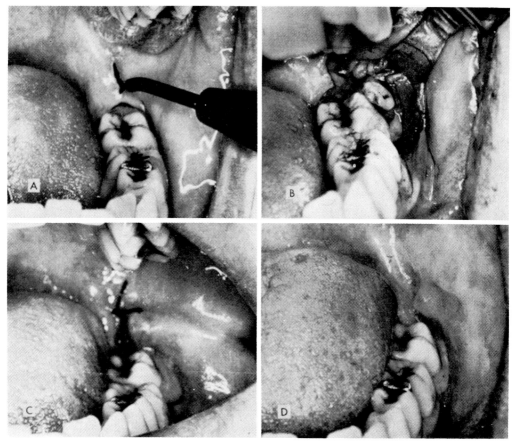

Case Figure 11–1. Surgical removal of a mandibular impacted third molar complicated by acute pericoronitis. *A,* Typical incision along crest of alveolar ridge through distended retromolar tissue with 45-degree-angle fine needle electrode. *B,* Incisions completed, flap is retracted exposing crown of impacted tooth and hypertrophic, hyperplastic submucous tissues. *C,* Appearance of operative field on fifth postoperative day before the sutures were removed. Note extensive edema and hyperemia. *D,* Final postoperative appearance, tenth postoperative week.

tures. The maxillary impacted third molar was then removed and she was instructed to continue the regimen of home care and antibiotic therapy begun preoperatively.

She returned on the fifth postoperative day for removal of the sutures. She was unable to open her mouth more than 2 cm. due to trismus, and opening even that limited distance caused much discomfort. There was little extraoral swelling but marked intraoral edema and hyperemia (Case Fig. 11–1C). The mouth was irrigated and tincture of myrrh and benzoin was applied in air-dried layers.

She returned once a week thereafter for regular postoperative observation and treatment. Healing progressed slowly during the first three weeks; then it suddenly accelerated. During the next three weeks healing progressed very satisfactorily; by the end of that time healing was complete and the impacted teeth on the left side could be removed. The healing after both of these teeth were extracted progressed rapidly and uneventfully. By the end of the tenth week both sides were so well healed that there no longer was any clinical evidence that surgery had been performed. The tissue tone was excellent throughout and the alveolar contour was normal (Case Fig. 11–1D).

CASE 12

This case is an example of the challenge to treatment planning ability and operative skill that is occasionally created by atypical mandibular third molar impactions. Atypical cases are usually created by anatomic abnormalities and/or pathology. When atypical abnormalities affect impacted malposed mandibular third molars they usually exercise a strong influence on the nature and extent of the surgical intervention required. In this case the abnormality made conservative management mandatory.

PATIENT.   A 19-year-old white male.

HISTORY.   The patient suddenly began to experience acute discomfort in his lower jaw while home from college on a brief holiday. He was referred for consultation and necessary surgery.

CLINICAL EXAMINATION.   *Extraoral.*   Negative.

Intraoral.   Clinically his mandibular right second and third molar area was edentulous. The gingival mucosa in this area appeared normal in tone, but the ridge abnormally wide. Digital pressure on the buccal and lingual cortical plates produced a slight amount of crepitus.

Intraoral periapical and occlusal view roentgenograms revealed that the second molar was vertically impacted. Its roots were extremely dilacerated, and the inferior surface of the curved mesial root was only 1 mm. from the inferior border of the mandible. The crown of this tooth was locked under an exaggeratedly bell-shaped undercut on the distal of the first molar. The third molar was horizontally impacted and wedged against the crown of the impacted second molar. A wide areola of radiolucence around the crown of the third molar suggested cystic degeneration of the embryonal capsule (Case Fig. 12–1A). The occlusal view revealed that the cyst enveloped the crown of the second molar as well as the third molar and had expanded the buccal alveolar bone plate (Case Fig. 12–1B).

It was clearly evident that an attempt to remove the second molar must inevitably result in pathologic fracture of the mandible. Joint consultation with his dentist and orthodontist resulted in the decision to expose the crown of the second molar, remove the third molar and try to thoroughly enucleate the cyst. Orthodontic movement of the second molar would be attempted postoperatively either to permit the tooth to erupt or to at least rotate and elevate it sufficiently to permit its ultimate extraction with less risk of a fracture.

TREATMENT.   The mouth was prepared for surgery and inferior alveolar block anesthesia administered. A medium-sized round loop electrode was selected and current output set at 5 for electrosection. The mucosa over the crown of the impacted second molar was resected with the activated loop electrode by shaving the tissue in layers with short brushing strokes (Case Fig. 12–2A) until the occlusal aspect of the crown was exposed.

The loop electrode was replaced with a fine 45-degree-angle needle electrode, current output reduced to 3.5 and the mucosa on the alveolar ridge incised from the retromolar fossa to the distal aspect of the first molar. A second buccal incision was then made from the distogingival angle of the first molar downward and anteriorly to the mucobuccal fold in the second bicuspid region.

The incised tissue was undermined with a periosteal elevator, reflected from the bone and retracted to expose the mandibular external oblique line and the alveolar bone overlying the third molar (Case Fig. 12–2B). The overlying bone was removed with impactor chisels; the tooth was split into two segments and removed (Case Fig. 12–2C). The cystic sac was disengaged from its bony crypt by blunt dissection,

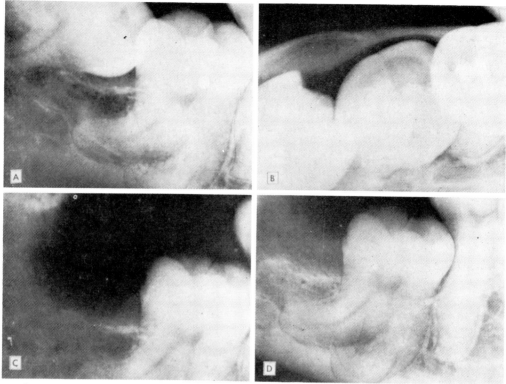

Case Figure 12–1. Roentgenographic sequence. *A*, Preoperative, periapical. The second molar is impacted vertically; the third molar, horizontally, with radiolucence between the two. *B*, Occlusal view reveals that cystic involvement extends to the first molar. *C*, Immediate postsurgical view reveals extent of bone loss. *D*, Four month postoperative view: bone regeneration is complete and normal. Slight distal rotation of the second molar has elevated the mesial root to 2 mm. above the external edge of the mandible.

grasped with an Allis forceps and removed from the third molar socket. The blunt dissection was then continued around the crown of the second molar. A major portion of the cystic mass was resected in this manner; but in several tightly wedged areas it could not be resected even with fine McCall curets and a narrow U-shaped loop electrode — even after the bone margin was ramped to provide better access. These shreds were destroyed in situ by fulguration.

Thorough debridement having been completed, the defect was filled with a mixture of cultured despeciated bone paste, bone chips and medicated surgical gelatin (Case Fig. 12–2D). The incised margins were coapted and sutured with 0000 braided silk interrupted sutures. Postoperative instructions were given and 600,000 units of Crysticillin, the first of three daily doses, was administered by intramuscular injection.

He was seen daily for the next three days. Each day the area was irrigated and tincture of myrrh and benzoin applied. He had remarkably little postoperative reaction: no trismus, pain, edema or adenopathy. On the fifth postoperative day the sutures were removed and the tissues inspected. The tissues appeared to be almost fully healed but the marginal gingiva on the lingual aspect of the newly exposed second molar crown was hyperemic and somewhat hypertrophied so that the tissue again reached the level of the occlusal surface of the tooth. Topical anesthetic was applied

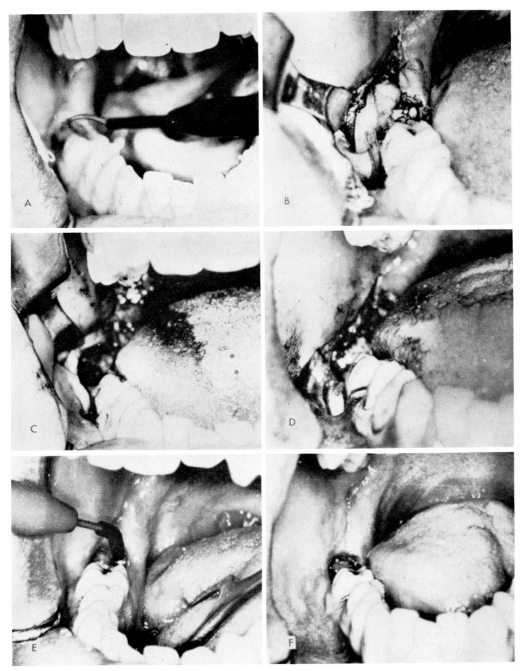

Case Figure 12-2 Clinical sequence. Removal of horizontally impacted mandibular third molar and extensive follicular cyst, and exposure of the vertically impacted second molar with a dilacerated root less than 1 mm. from inferior border of the mandible. *A*, Gingival mucosa over crown of impacted second molar resected with a large round loop electrode to expose occlusal surface of tooth. *B*, Flap retracted, exposing buccal alveolar bone and part of tooth crown. *C*, Tooth sectioned and removed from its socket, cyst enucleated. *D*, Debridement completed, bone-gelatin mixture deposited into defect. *E*, Marginal gingiva, lingual aspect, of exposed crown of second molar reduced to normal level by spot coagulation with large ball electrode. *F*, Appearance four months postoperatively. Top of impacted second molar visible. Note brass ligature wire between second bicuspid and first molar inserted for orthodontic movement.

and the upper rim of this tissue was coagulated lightly with a large ball electrode (Case Fig. 12–2*E*). Chromic acid, 0.05 per cent dilution, was applied for 30 seconds, washed away, and tincture of myrrh and benzoin applied in air-dried layers.

Roentgenographic examination indicated that the bone repair appeared to be keeping pace with the rapid rate of soft tissue repair. An immediate postoperative view (Case Fig. 12–1*C*) revealed the extent of bone destruction from cystic pressure. A film taken one week later revealed some reduction in the degree of radiolucency, which was compatible with the physical presence of the bone mixture in the defect.

The patient returned to school and was not seen again for four months. When he returned, examination revealed complete soft tissue healing and normal alveolar ridge contour; the dilacerated second molar appeared to be responding slightly to orthodontic movement. A brass ligature wire had been inserted between the first and second molars to create pressure in a distal direction. As a result, the second molar now was slightly elevated and tilted posteriorly, and the mesial half of its crown was visible above the gingival margin (Case Fig. 12–2*F*). A roentgenogram taken at this time showed comparable alveolar repair. The new bone appeared almost fully calcified, and homogenous with the older bone (Case Fig. 12–1, *D*). In the seven years since surgery was performed there has been no sign of cystic regeneration.

Two features of this case appear noteworthy. First, it is unlikely that with the second molar remaining in position total debridement of the cystic mass could have been performed effectively if the inaccessible cystic fragments had not been destroyed in situ by fulguration. Second, the bone paste, bone chips and surgical gelatin proved thoroughly compatible with their host bone and appeared to accelerate osteogenic regeneration.

MAXILLARY IMPACTED THIRD MOLARS

Two factors are essential to guard against accidental displacement of impacted maxillary third molars into the sphenomaxillary fossa. One is good access to and visibility in the operative field; the other, careful instrumentation. Obscured visibility from bleeding in the operative field increases the operative hazards enormously.

To provide good access and visibility it is necessary to create a flap that will expose, when reflected, the buccal cortical plate and most of the crest of the alveolar ridge of the tuberosity. Such incisions are awkward and difficult to perform with cold-steel instrumentation under pressure and are usually accompanied by profuse bleeding. They are easily performed by electrosection with acute-angle fine needle electrodes, without pressure and with little or no bleeding to obscure the visibility in the operative field.

Occasionally a previously undetected impacted maxillary third molar may, under pressure from a denture, suddenly begin to erupt in an edentulous area and require extraction. This type of impaction does not present the same surgical hazard or handicapping inaccessibility that is customarily encountered in removal of teeth impacted in dentulous mouths.

Unless there are special complicating features, surgery for removal of teeth impacted in edentulous areas is simple and does not require special techniques. It involves merely routine incision of the overlying tissue and does not merit detailed review. A technique for surgical removal of typical impacted malposed maxillary third molars from dentulous mouths will therefore be presented.

CASE 13

This case is a typical example of the surgical technique and electrosurgical incisions involved in removal of impacted malposed maxillary third molars from dentulous mouths.

The customary case history and clinical findings will be omitted from this report since the patient was the same young woman described in Case 10.

TREATMENT. The area was prepared for surgery and anesthetized with posterior superior alveolar block and palatal infiltration. A 45-degree-angle fine needle electrode was selected and current output set at 3.5 for electrosection. An incision was started high in the mucobuccal fold and directed downward toward the distobuccal gingival margin of the first molar (Case Fig. 13–1A). The electrode was replaced with an acute-angle fine needle electrode, and a second incision was started at the posterior heel of the tuberosity and carried along the crest of the ridge to the distal aspect of the second molar (Case Fig. 13–1B and C; mirror image).

The incised tissue was undermined, reflected from the bone and retracted, exposing the thin alveolar plate which was easily pierced with a Crane-pick elevator. A rongeur forceps was then used to remove the thin bone covering the crown of the impacted tooth (Case Fig. 13–1D). The latter was elevated from its crypt and extracted. The socket was debrided; then it was filled with a mixture of bone paste and medicated surgical gelatin which was incorporated with the blood. The incised tissue margins were coapted and sutured with 0000 braided silk sutures.

When she returned for removal of the mandibular and maxillary sutures on the fifth postoperative day, the rate of healing by primary union noted in the maxilla was highly gratifying. Despite a thick coating of food debris the tissue was firm and its tone excellent. A photograph taken at her final visit revealed complete healing with visible evidence that surgery had been performed (Case Fig. 13–1E and F). Healing in this area, uncomplicated by pericoronitis or other infection, proceeded much more rapidly than the mandibular healing on this side.

PALATALLY IMPACTED CUSPIDS

It is often far more difficult to bring palatally impacted cuspids into normal alignment in the dental arch by orthodontic movement than labially inclined impacted cuspids. Not infrequently, unfavorable malposition necessitates extraction of palatally impacted cuspids that are not amenable to orthodontic movement.

Electrosurgery not only facilitates and simplifies exposure of impacted cuspids but also can be used advantageously to facilitate extraction of the unmanageable teeth.

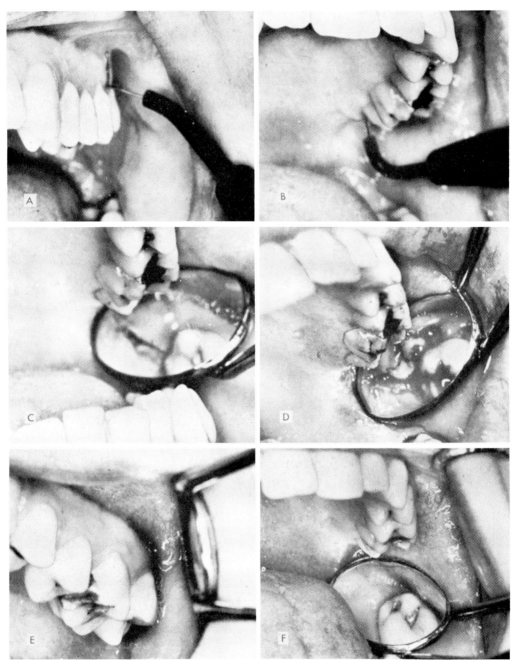

Case Figure 13–1.   Surgical removal of a typical maxillary impacted third molar. *A,* Buccal incision with 45-degree-angle fine needle electrode started high in mucobuccal fold and extended obliquely downward to distobuccal angle of the first molar. *B,* Second incision along crest of ridge from distal of tuberosity to distal of second molar. *C,* Mirror image of incision across tuberosity. *D,* Flap retracted, overlying bone removed, exposing crown of impacted tooth (mirror image). *E,* Final postoperative appearance, buccal aspect. Healing complete. *F,* Final postoperative appearance, heel of tuberosity (mirror image). Healing complete; tissue tone excellent; lines of incision invisible; alveolar contour normal.

CASE 14

This case demonstrates techniques for both procedures in the same patient; namely, exposure of an unerupted labially inclined cuspid and removal of an unfavorably malposed palatally impacted cuspid on the opposite side.

PATIENT. A 13-year-old white female.

HISTORY. The patient was under active orthodontic treatment and was referred for surgical exposure of a labially inclined unerupted cuspid on one side and removal of its palatally impacted counterpart.

CLINICAL EXAMINATION. *Extraoral.* Negative.

Intraoral. Both deciduous cuspids were present in the dental arch. The entire oral mucosa appeared normal. There was a slight bulge present in the right buccal vestibule in the cuspid–first bicuspid area, and a bulge on the palatal surface near the midline in the left cuspid region. Both elevated areas were firm and gave no evidence of either fluctuance or crepitus on palpation.

Roentgenographic examination with periapical and occlusal views revealed the right cuspid located high on the labial aspect of the alveolar ridge in a vertico-oblique position, with its cusp in contact with the apex of the retained deciduous tooth. The left permanent cuspid was malposed in a horizonto-oblique position on the palate. The cusp of the crown of this tooth was located at the midline behind the central incisor and incisive foramen.

TREATMENT. The retained left deciduous cuspid root was well developed and unresorbed. The coronal portion was equally well developed and filled the cuspid space in the dental arch. Retention of this tooth and extraction of its right counterpart to clear a pathway for eruption of the permanent tooth was clearly indicated.

The mouth was prepared for surgery and bilateral infraorbital and nasopalatine block anesthesia was administered. The deciduous right cuspid was extracted. A flame-shaped loop electrode was selected and current output set at 5.5 for electrosection. The mucosa was resected from over the crown of the impacted tooth by shaving in layers with short brushing strokes of the activated electrode until the outline of the crown of the impacted tooth was clearly delineated. Overlying bone was removed to fully expose the crown, then the mesial and distal interseptal bone reduced to create a channel to serve as a pathway for unimpeded eruption of the impacted tooth. The exposed crown and the bone channel were covered with a stiffly mixed surgical cement pack.

Then the palatal mucosa at the distogingival angle of the left second bicuspid was incised with a 45-degree-angle needle electrode and current output increased to 4.5, instead of the 3.5 usually necessary on the labial surface, due to the thickness and density of the palatal tissue. The incision was extended from the gingival margin 1 cm. medially toward the midline. Then the attachments of the interproximal papillae were incised along the palatal aspect as far anteriorly as the median papilla between the two centrals. The incisions were virtually bloodless; only a minute trickle of blood oozed from the incised papillae.

The incised palatal tissue was undermined with a periosteal elevator and retracted posteriorly. The flap was retained in the retracted position with a suture inserted into the flap and tied to the first molar on the opposite side. The palatal bone was removed from around the crown of the impacted tooth with impactor chisels, fully exposing the crown (Case Fig. 14–1A). The embryonal sac was removed from around the crown and the tooth was elevated and extracted. When debridement was completed, medicated powdered surgical gelatin was introduced into the defect and

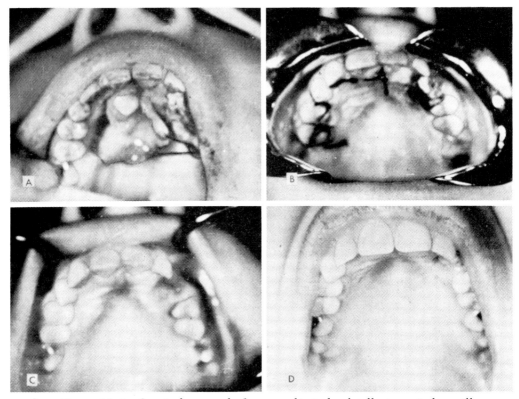

Case Figure 14–1. Surgical removal of uncomplicated palatally impacted maxillary cuspid. *A*, Incised palatal flap retracted with suture tied to opposite side. *B*, Appearance on fifth postoperative day before sutures were removed. *C*, Clinical appearance of palatal tissues on the tenth postoperative day. Note rapid progress of healing. *D*, Appearance two weeks later. Tissues fully healed without scar tissue or cicatricial contraction are perfectly attached to the teeth.

mixed with the blood. The flap was restored to position and reattached with sutures inserted through the interproximal embrasures and the labial and buccal papillae. This restored their palatal counterparts to normal contact with the teeth and the alveolar bone. One suture was also inserted at the marginal end of the palatal incision. A gauze bitepack was placed against the palatal mucosa to maintain firm tissue-bone contact and reduce postoperative edema. Aureomycin was prescribed for three days, and instructions for home care were given.

She returned on the fifth postoperative day for removal of the sutures. Healing appeared to be progressing favorably. The incised papillae were reattached to the teeth and bone and there was practically no edema except in the immediate region of the palatal incision from the molar to the cuspid region. In this area the tissue was slightly swollen (Case Fig. 14–1*B*).

The cement pack was removed from the right cuspid area, the tissues were irrigated and a fresh cement pack was inserted. The sutures were removed and tincture of myrrh and benzoin was applied. The patient was instructed to substitute the astringent salt-alum one week postoperatively and to return for further postoperative treatment on the tenth postoperative day.

When she returned the cement pack was removed from the right cuspid. The tissue underneath it was found to be granulating healthily, but, since it was not yet fully epithelialized it was a deeper red in color. The palatal mucosa was almost fully healed (Case Fig. 14–1C). Two weeks later the palatal mucosa was fully healed; the mucosa around the exposed crown was almost fully healed and in good tone (Case Fig. 14–1D).

This case afforded an excellent demonstration of the remarkable rate and quality of palatal healing following electrosurgery when no complicating factors are present and the patient is in normal health.

CASE 15

This case, the removal of a palatally impacted cuspid, affords an excellent demonstration of the malign influence that unfavorable local (or systemic) factors can have on the rate and quality of healing.

PATIENT. A 58-year-old white female.

HISTORY. The patient required extraction of a number of teeth, because of advanced periodontoclasia, in order to prepare her mouth for partial-denture restorations. Her dentist planned to extract these teeth, but he referred her for removal of a palatally impacted cuspid disclosed by roentgenographic examination.

CLINICAL EXAMINATION. *Extraoral.* Negative.

Intraoral. There were only four sound, firmly embedded teeth in the maxilla: the right bicuspids and cuspid and the left second bicuspid. The remaining teeth were very mobile, their gingivae partially detached and involved with deep periodontal pockets. The right molars and the remaining left molar showed marked alveolar resorption, and the latter was extruded and showed extensive trifurcation involvement. There was an ulcerated lesion on the palatal mucosa behind the left central. The gingival tissues were hyperemic and atonal. Although the left cuspid was missing, there was no vacant space for it in the dental arch.

Roentgenographic examination with periapical and intraoral occlusal views revealed that the impacted tooth was lying along a horizontal plane in palatolabial version. The apical end of the root of the impacted tooth was locked between the roots of the lateral incisor and the first bicuspid.

TREATMENT. The mouth was prepared for surgery and labial-buccal infiltration, nasopalatine and anterior palatine block anesthesia administered. A fine 45-degree-angle needle electrode was selected and current output set at 5 for electrosection. The palatal mucosa was incised at the mesial aspect of the left molar with a wiping stroke. The incision was carried about 1 cm. toward the midline in a horizontal plane. The incision was followed by profuse, persistent bleeding (Case Fig. 15–1A). The interproximal papillae from the molar on the left side to the cuspid on the right side were incised at their points of attachment (Case Fig. 15–1B).

The incised mucosa was undermined with a periosteal elevator. It was reflected from the underlying bone, retracted and secured in the retracted position with a suture tied to the right molar (Case Fig. 15–1C). The bone over the coronal end of the impacted tooth was removed with impactor chisels and bone burs, and extraction of the tooth was attempted. It resisted elevation, and pressure applied to it caused the lateral and first bicuspid to move as the impacted tooth was manipulated. Since these teeth were eventually to be extracted, they were extracted at this time to facilitate removal of the impacted tooth and prevent trauma to the palatal bone.

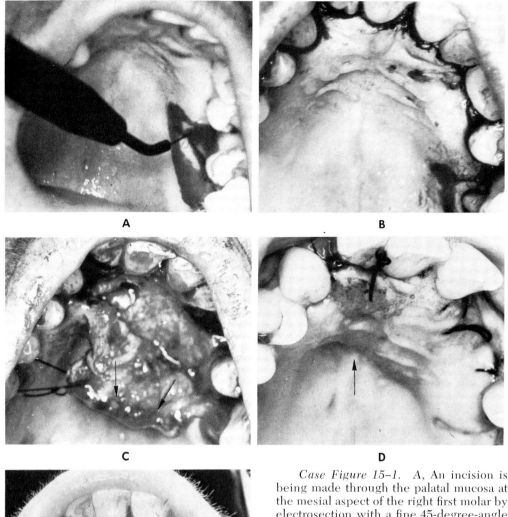

A

B

C

D

E

Case Figure 15–1. *A,* An incision is being made through the palatal mucosa at the mesial aspect of the right first molar by electrosection with a fine 45-degree-angle needle electrode. The incision is directed horizontally approximately 1.5 cm. toward the midline. The molar has a trifurcation involvement and all the maxillary teeth, particularly the anteriors, have deep periodontal pockets on the palatal aspect. Despite the hemostasis inherent in electrosection there is profuse free bleeding from the incision. *B,* The apices of the interdental papillae on the palatal aspect have been severed to permit the palatal mucosa to be elevated and reflected, providing access to the impacted tooth. There is profuse persistent free bleeding from this minimal cutting, owing to the advanced periodontal condition with engorgement and stasis of the blood supply. *C,* The flap has been elevated, rotated, and tied with silk suture to the teeth on the left side to keep it retracted during the surgical removal of the tooth. Note that the nasopalatine nerve and blood vessel emerging from the foramen have not been injured. Note the epithelial lining of the periodontal pockets that should have been resected from the flap tissue before restoring the tissue and suturing it into position (arrows). *D,* Postoperative appearance on the fifth postoperative day. The flap tissue in contact with the palatal aspect of the centrals and laterals appears to be sloughing, and there is an angry red degenerative extension to the left of the median line directed posteriorly that suggests that necrosis is extending posteriorly toward

(Legend continued on opposite page.)

850

The impacted tooth was elevated and removed, and debridement of the socket completed. A mixture of cultured bone paste and medicated surgical gelatin was deposited into the palatal cavity and mixed with the blood. Resection of the periodontal pocket epithelial linings from the ventral surface of the flap was inadvertently overlooked. The flap was restored to normal position and reattached with interproximal sutures carried through the embrasures and interproximal papillae and tied on the labial-buccal aspect. A pressure bitepack was inserted against the palatal vault and the patient was given instructions for postoperative care. Mysteclin was prescribed for three days and she was reappointed.

She returned on the fifth postoperative day and reported that for the first three days she had had severe pain, considerable swelling, and soreness in the anterior part of her palate. Examination revealed that a considerable amount of edema was still present; the gingival mucosa around the centrals and right lateral appeared necrotic, with considerable slough present on the palatal aspect (Case Fig. 15–1D).

The mouth was irrigated with warm Kasdenol solution and the sutures were removed. Tincture of myrrh and benzoin was applied topically to the necrotic tissue surface; then the affected tissues were covered with a protective coating of Kenalog-prototype adhesive ointment into which sulfathiazole and benzocaine powders were incorporated for obtundant and bactericidal effect.

This treatment was repeated twice a week for one month, then once a week for another month. The slough peeled away after the second week of treatment, and from that time on the area began to heal by granulating repair. By the end of the first month this tissue was normally epithelialized. By the end of the tenth postoperative week the tissues were fully healed, firmly reattached to the alveolar bone and the teeth, and the tissue tone was normal (Case Fig. 15–1E).

It is interesting to note that most of the teeth appeared to be much less mobile than preoperatively, and most of the periodontal pockets on the palatal aspect had been obliterated.

It appears reasonable to assume that the necrotic deterioration and sloughing in this case resulted from failure to resect the periodontal pocket epithelial linings from the flap, and from bacterial contamination from the organisms in the deep periodontal pockets. Impaired blood supply, abundance of virulent organisms, lowered local resistance of the tissues, and presence of epithelial lining on the inner surface of pocket-forming mucosa create handicaps that are not compatible with rapid normal healing.

Removal of Supernumerary Teeth

TREATMENT OF A CYSTIC ODONTOMA — MAXILLA

The cystic odontoma is a cyst that contains supernumerary teeth and toothlike structures. The surgical problem therefore consists of removal of the teeth and/or toothlike structures and also of the cystic sac in which they were contained. Should any of the sac remain, the tumor will recur.

The hemostasis provided by electrosurgery helps to facilitate the surgery and to assure that all the cystic tissue has been removed. The following case demonstrates one effective method for utilizing electrosection in these cases.

Case Figure 15–1. Continued.

the soft palate (arrow). *E*, Final postoperative appearance of the palate. The necrosis has eliminated the periodontal pockets, with the tissue slough having fulfilled the function of a gingivectomy. The tissues are fully healed and normal in appearance and tone, and the mobility of the teeth has been eliminated.

PLATE VII

Oral Surgery

Figure 1a. Removal of a ranula from floor of the mouth. Preoperative appearance: a previous attempt at marsupialization had been unsuccessful, since the contents of the retention cyst were semi-solid instead of liquid.

Figure 2a. Removal of a sialolith from the submaxillary duct. Preoperative appearance of the tissues of the floor of the mouth. The tissues in the left half of the floor of the mouth are swollen and severely engorged, and indurated. The tissues in the right half are normal.

Figure 1b. An incision is being made into the tissues of the floor of the mouth by electrosection with a 45 degree angle fine needle electrode, after the surface epithelium had been removed from the earlier surgical site. Despite the great vascularity of the tissues of the floor of the mouth there is no free bleeding.

Figure 2b. An incision is being made into the submaxillary duct by electrosection with a fine 45 degree angle needle electrode. The vascular tissues do not hemorrhage as they are incised.

Figure 1c. The debris from the ventral half of the cyst has been removed. Due to the absence of bleeding the submaxillary duct can readily be visualized, and grasped with an ophthalmic tissue forceps to pull the tissue taut. This makes it possible to visualize all important anatomic structures in the area and carefully guard against injury to them. It also facilitates the thorough removal of the cystic debris.

Figure 2c. The large sialolith has been expelled from the duct through the incision, and expelled into the floor of the mouth. A slight amount of blood has been released by this, but there is no free bleeding.

Figure 1d. Postoperative appearance of the floor of the mouth three weeks later. The tissues are fully healed, and the right and left halves of the floor of the mouth are identical in all respects. The tissues in the surgical field are normal in texture and color and completely devoid of scar tissue contraction.

Figure 2d. Appearance of the tissues of the floor of the mouth one month postoperatively. The tissue that had been incised is identical in all respects with the tissue on the other side of the floor of the mouth. The incised wound is fully healed, and the duct has remained patent.

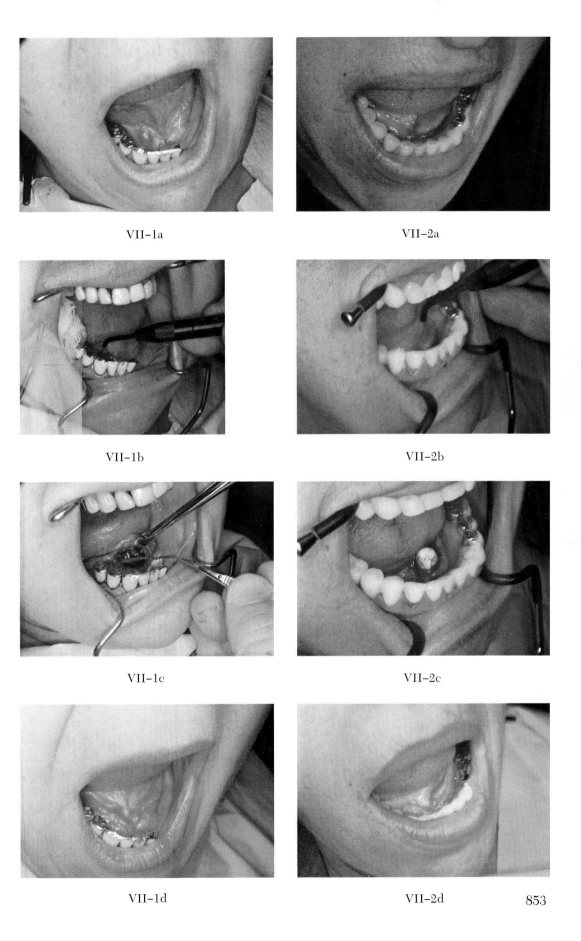

VII–1a

VII–2a

VII–1b

VII–2b

VII–1c

VII–2c

VII–1d

VII–2d

CASE 16

PATIENT.   A 13-year-old white female.

HISTORY.   She had begun to feel discomfort in the upper right jaw a few months ago. As time passed the discomfort began to become more pronounced. She consulted her dentist and described the feeling as one of pressure rather than sharp pain. He saw no clinical reason for the sensation but a periapical x-ray film revealed a radiolucent area containing several dense toothlike small structures in the space between the right second bicuspid and first molar. She was referred to the author for surgical removal of the lesion.

CLINICAL EXAMINATION.   The x-ray diagnosis was a cystic odontoma. There was no visible deformity of the alveolar bone, or other clinical indication of the pathologic condition, except a slight compressible "give" to the alveolar structure in that area on firm digital pressure that did not resemble typical crepitus.

TREATMENT.   The treatment plan was to make a mucoperiosteal incision on the buccal aspect to reflect the flap, expose the lesion, and remove it. A fine 45-degree-angle needle electrode was selected, and cutting current was set at 3 on the instrument panel dial. A vertico-oblique incision was made for a mucoperiosteal flap of the buccal gingival mucosa with the activated electrode after infraorbital regional block and palatal infiltration anesthesia was administered. The incision was started in the aureolar gingiva over the center of the root of the maxillary right second bicuspid, and extended downward and slightly anteriorly to the mesiogingival angle of the tooth (Case Fig. 16–1A). The apical attachment of the papilla in the embrasure between the bicuspid and first molar was then severed to permit adequate reflection of the mucoperiosteal flap. The incised tissue was elevated with a periosteal elevator and reflected posteriorly, exposing a defect between the bicuspid and molar from which five rudimentary diminutive toothlike structures and cystic debris were removed by manual instrumentation with a small surgical curet. This method of instrumentation was adequate for gross debridement of the hard structures and some of the soft debris in the defect, but was unable to complete the debridement of the cystic tissue in the defect without sacrificing a considerable amount of the buccal cortical bone to gain access. The needle electrode was therefore replaced at this point with a 17-mm. periodontal loop curet electrode, which was used to complete the debridement (Case Fig. 16–1B and C). When debridement appeared to have been completed the inactivated electrode was used to explore around in the defect to feel for any retained fragments. The transilluminating lamp was used (Case Fig. 16–1D) to illuminate the interior of the defect and inspect it visually. Since the debridement was performed relatively bloodlessly, the visual inspection was easily and clearly achieved. The complete debridement having been verified, bleeding was stimulated in the defect by scraping the internal bone surface with the curet to open the nutrient vessels. Powdered Gelfoam was introduced into the defect and mixed with the blood. The flap was restored to normal position and sutured with interrupted silk sutures (Case Fig. 16–2A). A section of the heavy-gauge Squibb Orahesive bandage material was cut and shaped to create clearance for free movement of a low muscle attachment, and applied to the surgical field (Case Fig. 16–2B). The patient was instructed in postoperative home care and reappointed for removal of the sutures.

She returned on the fifth postoperative day. The sutures were intact, and the tissue tone appeared normal, with evidence of favorable primary repair along the line of incision. Healing continued uneventfully. She was seen again six months postoperatively, at which time the tissues were fully healed and the periapical x-ray showed

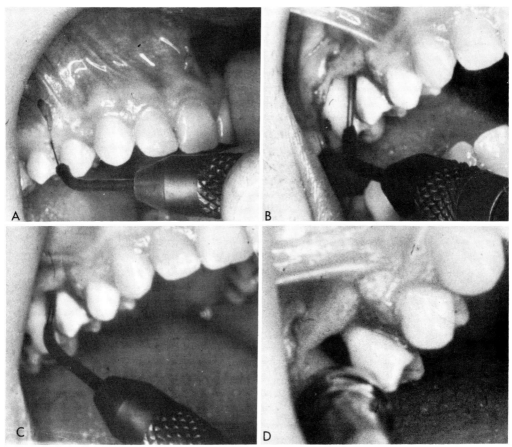

Case Figure 16–1. A, A vertico-oblique incision is being made to lift a mucoperiosteal flap. The incision, with a fine 45-degree-angle needle electrode, is being directed downward in a slightly postero-anterior direction from beyond the mucogingival junction to the mesiogingival angle of the maxillary right second bicuspid. B, The flap has been elevated and reflected, and the debridement of the cystic tissue is being performed with a 17-mm. periodontal loop electrode. C, The loop has penetrated about 9 mm. into the defect. D, The cyst and the tooth-like structure having been cleaned out of the defect, the area is being inspected visually with a transilluminating light to assure that debridement is completed.

comparable repair of the bone defect. Clinically there was no scar or other evidence to reveal the surgical site (Case Fig. 16–2C).

When the internal portion of a bone defect is to be examined to ascertain whether complete debridement has been achieved, the limber 17-mm. loop electrode is especially useful. The loop is sufficiently flexible to transmit to the fingers vibrations that are created when it encounters foreign debris, if the electrode is held very lightly so that the vibrations are immediately sensed. The usefulness of such manual examination is increased greatly by supplementing the digital examination with transillumination for visual examination. Directing the light through the structure rather than into the defect creates internal illumination that is far more revealing than directing the light into the defect. The latter often proves ineffective because the light directed into the defect creates a black blind spot. The hemostasis provided by electrosection makes the visual examination possible.

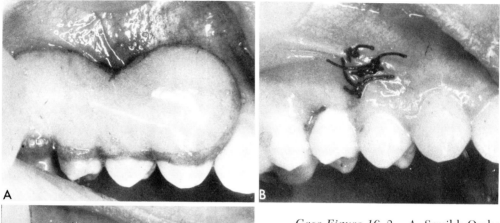

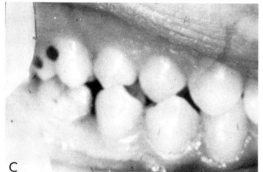

Case Figure 16–2. *A*, Squibb Orahesive bandage has been applied over the sutures to cover the surgical field. A double thickness has been applied and notched midway on the superior border for clearance of a muscle attachment. *B*, Appearance of the tissues on the fifth postoperative day before the sutures were removed. Note the excellent tissue tone and speed of repair. *C*, Final postoperative appearance. The tissues are fully healed, and except for the slightly pinker color of the tissue along the line of incision which has not yet become covered with a maturely keratinized epithelial surface, there would be no clinical evidence of the surgical procedure.

TREATMENT OF A CYSTIC ODONTOMA — MANDIBLE

CASE 17

This case also involved supernumerary teeth in cystic odontomas. It differed from the previous case in two respects. First, because it was bilateral instead of unilateral as the previous one was, and second, because they occurred in the mandible, where the cortical bone is very thick and dense, making it more difficult to debride thoroughly if much bone must be removed to do so. Both were in near proximity to the mental foramina and their contents. Electrosurgical debridement made it possible to avoid need for such excessive bone removal in order to perform the debridement efficiently.

PATIENT. A 14-year-old white male.

HISTORY. The presence of the previously unsuspected supernumerary teeth was discovered in a routine x-ray examination. The patient was referred for their surgical removal.

CLINICAL EXAMINATION. There was nothing present in the oral cavity to suggest the presence of the two defects. The tissues, teeth and alveolar bone all appeared entirely normal. Roentgenographic examination with periapical and occlusal view films revealed two radiolucent areas in which there appeared to be toothlike structures. Both areas were in the vicinity of the respective mental foramina.

TREATMENT. An inferior alevolar block was administered in the left quadrant. A

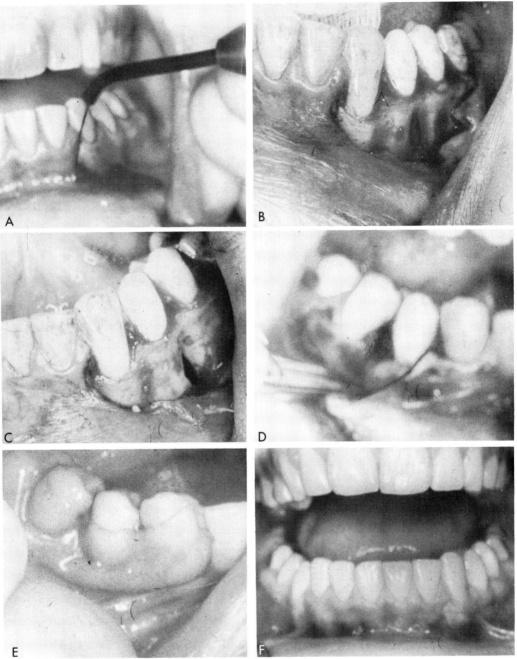

Case Figure 17–1. *A,* A vertico-oblique incision is being made with a 45-degree-angle fine needle electrode in an antero-posterior direction from the junction of areolar and alveolar mucosa midway between the lateral and cuspid to the mesiogingival angle of the cuspid on the left side of the mandible. A small vessel has been severed, and a small pool of blood has accumulated in the buccal vestibule. *B,* The incisions had been continued across the apices of the interdental papillae, and the mucoperiosteal flap has been reflected. The bleeding has been brought under control by coagulating off the beaks of a mosquito hemostat. The alveolar bone between the two bicuspids has been thinned out by the cyst to a thin translucency. *C,* The cystic sac and its contents, including miniature toothlike structures, have been removed. *D,* A similar mucoperiosteal flap has been incised and reflected on the side of the mandible, and the cystic contents of the defect have been removed. A bleeder in the cut tissue margin of the mucoperiosteal flap is being clamped with a mosquito hemostat prior to application of electrocoagulation with a ball electrode. *E,* The flap has been restored to position and sutured, and a piece of Squibb Orahesive bandage has been applied to the surgical site. *F,* Final postoperative appearance of the mouth about 3 months later. The incised tissues have healed and are practically invisible. The buccal contour of the alveolar ridges are normally convex.

45-degree-angle fine needle electrode was selected and activated with cutting current set at 3. The activated electrode was used with a wiping motion to create an incision starting at the mesiogingival angle of the cuspid and arcing downward and slightly anteriorly at the beginning and curving posteriorly as it passed the mucogingival junction (Case Fig. 17–1A). The mucoperiosteal flap was very carefully elevated from the bone and displaced posteriorly, revealing an elliptical spot in vertical position that appeared darker than the surrounding bone. The absence of free bleeding made it possible to notice this difference in the color of the bone and thus locate the site of the lesion (Case Fig. 17–1B).

A bone bur was used to cut out the discolored patch of bone, creating an access window into the defect (Case Fig. 17–1C). The contents, several small toothlike structures and the cystic sac, were removed with a small surgical curet. Fragments of cystic tissue that resisted removal with the curet were removed with an activated 17-mm. periodontal loop electrode used as an electronic curet. The thoroughness of the debridement was verified with transillumination. Some powdered surgical gelatin was deposited into the defect and mixed with the small amount of blood present there. The tissue flap was then restored to position and the coapted margins were sutured.

The right quadrant was then anesthetized with an inferior alveolar block, and a similar flap was incised and reflected, revealing a similar discolored spot and also a break in the continuity of the bone on the buccal aspect of the two bicuspids. A bleeder in the margin of the incised tissue was clamped with a mosquito hemostat and bleeding was stopped by coagulating off the beak of the hemostat (Case Fig. 17–1D).

The debridement was performed in the same way as on the left side, and when debridement was completed the tissue flap was restored to position and sutured. Patches of Squibb Orahesive bandage were applied to the two areas (Case Fig. 17–1E). The patient was instructed in home care, and told to return on the fifth postoperative day for removal of the sutures. Healing progressed very favorably and uneventfully. By the end of the third month the tissues were fully healed and there was no visible clinical evidence of where the incisions were made (Case Fig. 17–1F). Six months postoperatively the bone repair was equally complete.

The incision anterior to the cuspid and curving anteriorly convexly downward before proceeding somewhat posteriorly avoids injury to the mental nerve plexus in the area that was involved.

III. SOFT TISSUE SURGERY

Exposure of Unerupted Tooth by Cold Steel Excision of Tissue

CASE 18*

This case does not demonstrate an electrosurgical procedure. It is presented to demonstrate the typical result of incising gingival tissue with a steel scalpel. It em-

---

*This case is included for the purpose of comparison.

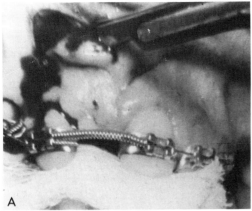
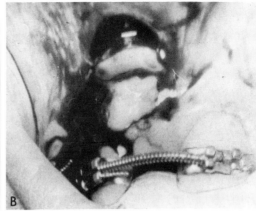
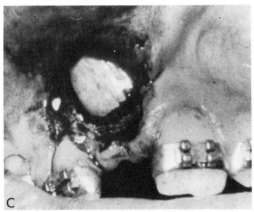

Case Figure 18–1. A typical example of gingival excision with a steel scalpel. *A,* The tissue covering an unerupted malposed maxillary central is being incised for excision with a Bard-Parker scalpel. Hemorrhagic free bleeding accompanies the initial incision. *B,* The incised tissue is ready for excision; the bleeding remains profuse and persistent. *C,* The labial aspect of the tooth has been uncovered, but owing to continued oozing of blood attachment of an appliance for orthodontic movement of the tooth must be deferred.

phasizes that the advantage of the hemostasis enjoyed with electrosurgery contrasted with the free bleeding that occurs with steel scalpel cutting is as great as the advantage of the absence of the typical postoperative sequelae of pain, swelling, and the other unfavorable postoperative reactions that usually accompany steel scalpel surgery.

PATIENT. A 13-year-old patient of the Orthodontia Clinic.

HISTORY. The maxillary right central incisor was unerupted. It was in relatively normal alignment but tilted slightly toward the midline. It was high up on the alveolar ridge, with a thick layer of mucosa covering it. He was referred to surgery for exposure of the unerupted tooth.

CLINICAL EXAMINATION. All the maxillary teeth were banded with orthodontic bands and brackets, and he was wearing a labial archbar. The crown of the unerupted tooth bulged outward, making it somewhat easy to locate it precisely. The overlying tissue was thick but normal in texture and tone.

TREATMENT. The area was anesthetized by infiltration and the overlying tissue was incised with a new Bard-Parker steel scalpel (Case Fig. 18–1A). Profuse, persistent bleeding ensued (Case Fig. 18–1B). The excision of the overlying tissue exposed the crown of the unerupted tooth, which proved to be tilted more acutely toward the midline than it had appeared on the x-ray film (Case Fig. 18–1C). The free bleeding, inherent in steel scalpel cutting, would have made it very difficult, if not impossible, to attach a ligature to the tooth surface with oxyphosphate cement or acrylic, such as have been described in preceding chapters.

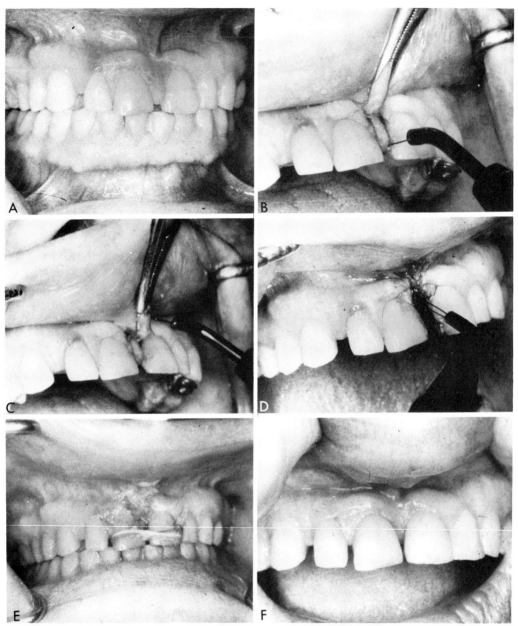

Case Figure 19–1. *A,* A considerable amount of fibromatosis is present in the alveolar portions of both arches, and a lesion, oval in shape, approximately 4 mm. in the horizontal dimension and 3 mm. in the vertical dimension, is present on the marginal gingiva of the maxillary right lateral incisor. A long frenum is present and appears clinically divided into two distinct portions: a broad band of fibers that appear somewhat superimposed onto the normal mucosa as well as attached to it laterally, extending around to the anterior junction with the nasopalatine papilla, and a second portion consisting of the upper half in the form of a prominent band of fibers that extend into the upper lip. *B,* The areolar portion has been clamped with a curved mosquito hemostat as close to the ventral surface of the lip as possible. The attached alveolar portion is being incised with a fine 45-degree-angle needle electrode along its lateral borders and through the diastema to the junction with the nasopalatine papilla, care being taken not to invade it. *C,* The remaining upper half of the frenum is being dissected from the *external* surface of the beaks of the hemostat. *D,* The frenal fibers having been removed, the

(Legend continued on opposite page)

Frenectomy-Frenotomy of Maxillary Labial Frenum

TREATMENT OF ADULT

CASE 19

This case demonstrates the advantageous features of the electrosurgical technique the author has developed for the "ectomy," the total removal of the attached alveolar fibers that usually are the sole source of interference that requires surgical intervention with an "otomy," partial removal of the areolar fibers of this ligament.

An interesting but puzzling sidelight was the presence of a small but persistent lesion at the labial marginal gingival edge of the maxillary right lateral incisor that underwent spontaneous regression in response to this treatment and thus eliminated need for biopsy.

PATIENT.   A 42-year-old white female.

HISTORY.   She had long been annoyed about spaces between some of her anterior maxillary teeth. Finally her dentist was persuaded to eliminate the spacing by making a fixed bridge restoration for her. She also complained about the presence of a very persistent small blister-like lesion at the gingival edge of one of the teeth, and he decided to have a biopsy performed that would serve to provide a diagnosis and also the treatment. There was a very wide diastema between the maxillary centrals that would have to be closed in order to be able to make the prosthesis. He referred her to the author for the two surgical procedures. He also asked that the author institute the simple Japanese grassline–elastic band traction for simple tooth movement to try to close the gap between the two centrals.

CLINICAL EXAMINATION.   The gingivae in both arches were fibrotic; it appeared to be an innocuous case of fibromatosis. There was a wide diastema between the right maxillary cuspid and lateral, and one between the two centrals. A broad frenum filled the space between the two teeth, and continued through to terminate at the anterior border of the nasopalatine papilla. The attached alveolar portion and the areolar portion looked like two separate structures. An elevated round lesion measuring 4 mm. mesiodistally, 2 mm. in width, and 2 mm. in thickness was present at the marginal gingiva of the right lateral (Case Fig. 19–1A). The lesion was dark red in color, and the

---

Case Figure 19–1.   Continued.
fibers that invaginate into the median suture line are being destroyed by scoring, i.e., rapidly running the activated electrode over the suture line. In this instance the suture line was found to be slightly open, so that the needle electrode failed to make contact with both surfaces simultaneously. A narrow U-shaped loop electrode has been substituted, rotated to an approximate 5- to 10-degree angle so that both sides of the suture line would be contacted simultaneously, and used several times by running down very rapidly and then waiting 10 seconds before repeating the stroke. *Note:* Use of the loop electrode as seen here is atypical; almost invariably the needle electrode can be used most effectively. *E,* Appearance on the fifth postoperative day. Japanese grassline and elastic band traction has been applied to the two centrals to try to bring them together. The surgical field is covered with a light layer of coagulum. The lesion of the marginal gingiva of the right lateral appears to be diminished in size and less red in color. *F,* Appearance of the surgical site three weeks later. The diastema is almost completely closed. The tissue on the alveolar surface is healed and smooth, without scar tissue formation. The areolar fibers are also healing and are controlling the movement of the lip without regenerating downward. The gingival lesion of the right lateral has undergone spontaneous regression.

tissue above it toward the vestibule also was dark red in contrast to the surrounding rather pallid tissues.

TREATMENT.   Normally the biopsy would have been performed first. The patient was rather apprehensive and it was decided that it might be best to defer the biopsy and the extensive case history questioning it requires until the patient had been given an opportunity to overcome her apprehension. The tissues were therefore prepared for infiltration anesthesia of the labial and palatal portions of the frenum. The lip was extended as far forward as possible and the areolar part of the frenum was clamped with a curved mosquito hemostat as close to the ventral surface of the lip as possible. A 45-degree-angle fine needle electrode was activated with cutting current set at 3 on the dial, and the activated electrode was used to follow the outline of the attached frenal fibers and incised to the bone (Case Fig. 19–1B). The incision was extended through the diastema and the frenal fibers were resected at their junction with the nasopalatine papilla. The incised tissue was elevated with a periosteal elevator, then the areolar portion that was firmly clamped by the hemostat was resected from the external surface of the hemostat (Case Fig. 19–1C).

The attached alveolar fibers that invaginate into the median suture line were then destroyed by running the activated electrode down over the suture line as rapidly as possible, and repeating 4 to 5 times with 10-second pause intervals to prevent damage from cumulative heat retention. In this case the suture line was not contacted with the needle electrode and seemed to be slightly open, so a narrow 45-degree-angle U-shaped electrode was substituted for the needle electrode, current output was increased to 3.5, and the electrode was tilted to create an approximate 10-degree angle and used to destroy the invaginating fibers (Case Fig. 19–1D).

There was no free bleeding, and the tissues had not flared apart widely, so no sutures were inserted. Tincture of myrrh and benzoin and a strip of Squibb's adhesive oral bandage were applied, after the two centrals were ligated with Japanese grassline and elastic bands. She was seen again on the fifth postoperative day and reported she had had no distress postoperatively. The two teeth appeared to have moved together slightly and there was a normal healthy layer of coagulum covering the surgical field (Case Fig. 19–1E). The grassline and elastic bands were intact and appeared to be somewhat effective. The lesion of the marginal gingiva of the lateral was notably reduced in size and almost normal in color. Fresh grassline and elastics were applied to the teeth, and the patient was asked to return the following week. Healing progressed very rapidly and by the third of these visits the tissue was fully healed and the gingival lesion had undergone complete spontaneous regression (Case Fig. 19–1F).

Aside from the interesting spontaneous regression of the lesion, this case presented with unusual visual clarity the two portions of the maxillary labial frenum that led the author to develop the technique of frenectomy-frenotomy, which eliminates the undesirable fibers and retains the desirable ones.

FRENOTOMY OF MANDIBULAR LABIAL FRENUM

Abnormalities of the mandibular labial frenum occur much less frequently than its maxillary counterpart. However, when they do occur, they are likely to cause more serious problems: periodontal deterioration with gingival clefts in the dentulous mouth and impairment of the peripheral seal,

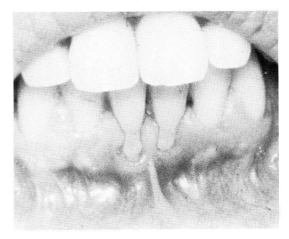

Figure 21–4. This is an excellent example of the destructive influence of abnormal traction from a single mandibular ligament that is inserted superiorly into the marginal gingivae of the central incisors. Note the marked recession of the labial marginal and alveolar gingivae that will require repair by surgical repositioning to close the defects.

with loss of denture stability in the edentulous mouth. The surgical intervention also is often more complex, as was seen in Case 28 of Chapter 19.

The mandibular labial frenum may be a single strand of ligamental fibers, as seen in Figure 21–4, or a broad band of multiple ligamental fibers such as those in Case Figure 28–1A, p. 718.

Treatment of the mandibular labial frenum varies greatly, depending on the severity of the abnormality. Although it often is far more troublesome than its maxillary counterpart both in the extent and severity of the disease it may cause and in its surgical management, there are many instances in which future problems can be averted through the simple expedient of incising and severing the frenal fibers. Then, either the latter may be sutured to their underlying tissues, or a cement pack surgical stent may be applied over the incised tissue. The former is indicated when the frenal fibers are very taut and exert marked irritating traction against the marginal gingivae, and the latter when the irritation is minimal.

CASE 20

PATIENT. A 20-year-old white female.

HISTORY. The patient had a maxillary labial frenum that was causing irritating traction of the marginal gingivae of the central incisors which would undoubtedly lead to periodontal deterioration unless it was eliminated, and a mandibular labial frenum that was also causing traction, but to a lesser degree, of the gingivae of the mandibular centrals. She was referred for frenectomy of both ligaments.

CLINICAL EXAMINATION. The author had excised the frenal fibers of the attached alveolar portion by the combined frenectomy-frenotomy technique the previous week (Case Fig. 20–1A). The area was healing nicely and the sutures were being removed at this visit (Case Fig. 20–1B). The mandibular labial frenum was a short, taut, single strand of ligamental fibers that was attached superiorly to the marginal gingiva.

TREATMENT. The mandibular frenum seemed to require minimal surgical intervention. A simple horizontal incision across the fibers and separating displacement of the cut margins with a surgical stent would suffice.

Topical anesthesia was applied, then a few minims of anesthetic solution were infiltrated very slowly into the tissues lateral to the frenum to prevent distorting

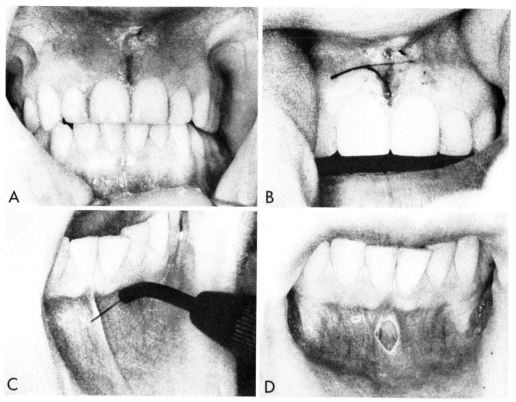

Case Figure 20–1. A, Postsurgical appearance of the surgical site after resection of the attached alveolar portion of the maxillary labial frenum by the combined frenectomy-frenotomy technique. B, Appearance one week later, before removal of the sutures. C, The mandibular labial frenum is about to be severed by incision with a 45-degree-angle fine needle electrode activated with cutting current. D, Appearance of the incised tissue immediately after incision. Note the absence of free bleeding, the intact condition of the submucous tissues, and the elimination of tension against the alveolar gingivae, denoted by the wide separation of the incised margins.

ballooning. The lower lip was pulled outward and downward to bring the ligament into taut relief. Cutting current was set at 3 and a 45-degree-angle fine needle electrode was activated and used with a single rapid motion to incise the taut fibers (Case Fig. 20–1C). The depth of penetration of the electrode as it severed the ligament was carefully controlled to prevent penetration and incision into the submucous tissues of the floor of the mouth. As a result, the procedure was virtually bloodless. Release of the traction of the gingivae resulted in spontaneous wide separation of the incised tissue margins (Case Fig. 20–1D). There was no need to suture the cut tissue to keep the margins apart. A very hard roll of periodontal pack cement was inserted over the incision site and attached to the teeth by packing into the interdental embrasures. The patient was seen again one week later; the tissues were almost fully healed, and there was no evidence of traction of the gingivae.

Frenotomy of the Lingual Frenum in Ankyloglossia

As a rule when we think of a frenum we think of the maxillary labial frenum. The mandibular labial frenum usually is overlooked except when it is a broad band that is exerting abnormal traction against the marginal gingiva and creating a periodontal lesion. As for the third type of frenum, the mandibular lingual frenum, this is almost invariably overlooked except when it interferes with the seating of a denture and displaces it, or when it interferes with the ability of the tongue to thrust forward enough to make contact with the palatal aspect of the maxillary anterior teeth and thereby causes the speech defect of lisping. This latter condition is known as ankyloglossia. Both the ankyloglossia and the speech defect it causes can very easily be corrected by simple surgical intervention—a simple incision.

When the incision is made with a steel scalpel two difficulties are encountered. First, the profuse hemorrhagic bleeding, and second, the tendency for the scar tissue repair to contract the tissues and thereby continue to prevent the tongue from thrusting forward enough to correct the speech defect. But when the incision is performed with a needle electrode by electrosection, both difficulties are averted as a result of the inherent hemostasis of electrosurgery and the soft, supple nature of the repair tissue. All that is required is a simple horizontal incision to sever the frenal fibers. Since no pressure is required to cut these fibers, the depth of the incision can easily be controlled, so that the fibers are severed without bleeding or invading the ventral surface of the tongue. The impediment having been eliminated, the tongue can now be thrust forward easily. This pulls the horizontal incision into a vertical line, and the incised tissues are sutured in the vertical plane. The soft, supple repair does not impede the tongue's mobility or ability to thrust forward until it makes contact with the palatal aspect of the maxillary anterior teeth. The tissue repair usually is complete within one week to 10 days, and with proper tongue exercise and speech practice the lisping is overcome shortly thereafter.

The choice of the most advantageous site for incising the frenum is very important. Even more important is the need to guard against secondary infection, since the proximity to the floor of the mouth increases the danger of infection along the fascial planes to the anterior or posterior mediastinum, which can prove fatal. Figure 21–5 is an example of the danger inherent in lingual frenotomy performed with a steel scalpel that becomes infected. The fact that the electrosurgical current sterilizes as it cuts helps greatly to prevent such unhappy results.

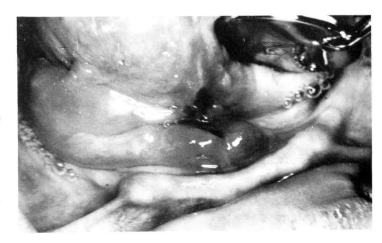

Figure 21–5. The appearance of the tissues of the floor of the mouth following a procedure to correct ankyloglossia by an operator who used a steel scalpel. There are massive edema and congestion, with the orifices of the salivary ducts greatly swollen. The inflammation extends into the ventral surface of the tongue and the tongue is partially immobilized. The patient has fever and malaise and requires antibiotic therapy.

The following case is an excellent example of the ankyloglossia caused by an abnormal lingual frenum and the simplicity with which it can be corrected by electrosection.

CASE 21

This case shows the effectiveness of the electrosurgical lingual frenotomy when sound treatment plan is combined with good electrosurgical technique.

PATIENT.   A 14-year-old white male.

HISTORY.   He was under treatment by a speech therapist for correction of a lisping speech defect. The therapist was aware that the defect could not be corrected sufficiently by nonsurgical means. She therefore referred him to the author for a lingual frenotomy.

CLINICAL EXAMINATION.   With the tongue extended forward and upward the lingual frenum was tautly outlined from the floor of the mouth to within 1 cm. of the tip of the tongue. He was unable to reach the palatal surface of his maxillary anterior teeth with the tongue.

TREATMENT.   The frenal tissues were anesthetized by infiltration anesthesia injected very slowly, a minim at a time, to avoid undue distention of the tissues. The tongue, one of the most powerful muscles of the human body for its size, contracted so forcefully that it was not possible to keep the organ fully extended. A few drops of anesthetic were injected into the tip of the tongue and a 000 silk suture was inserted through the tip of the tongue to serve as a tissue retractor. A 45-degree-angle fine needle electrode was selected, activated with cutting current set at 3, and used to create a horizontal incision across the taut frenal fibers (Case Fig. 21–1A).

Before the electrode lost contact with the incised tissue, the traction on the tip of the tongue pulled the horizontal incision into the vertical plane (Case Fig. 21–1B). The margins of the wound, now elongated, were sutured with interrupted silk sutures in the vertical plane (Case Fig. 21–1C). When the patient returned on the fifth postoperative day for removal of the sutures, the tongue was found to be normal in movement and quite supple. The line of incision was coated with a layer of coagulum that was compatible with the areolar nature of the tissues, and the tissues were perfectly healthy. The patient was now able to place the tongue against the palatal surfaces of the anterior teeth without difficulty (Case Fig. 21–1D).

Two weeks later the tongue was so fully healed, without scar repair, that it was impossible to tell that any surgery had been performed. The tongue could now be placed effortlessly against the palatal aspect of the maxillary anterior teeth (Case Fig. 21–1E) and within another two weeks of practice with the speech exercises that had been prescribed for him, the therapist was able to discharge him from further speech therapy.

Operculotomy (For Resection of Pericoronal Flaps)

Pericoronitis is one of the more common manifestations of oral pathologic conditions that require surgical intervention. When the mucosa and embryonal capsule around incompletely erupted mandibular third molars become inflamed and infected, their ultimate fate is usually determined by their alignment in the dental arch. If alignment of the teeth is faulty, resection of overlying pericoronal tissue fails to solve the problem and such teeth must be extracted.

If alignment and occlusion are good, surgical intervention often makes it

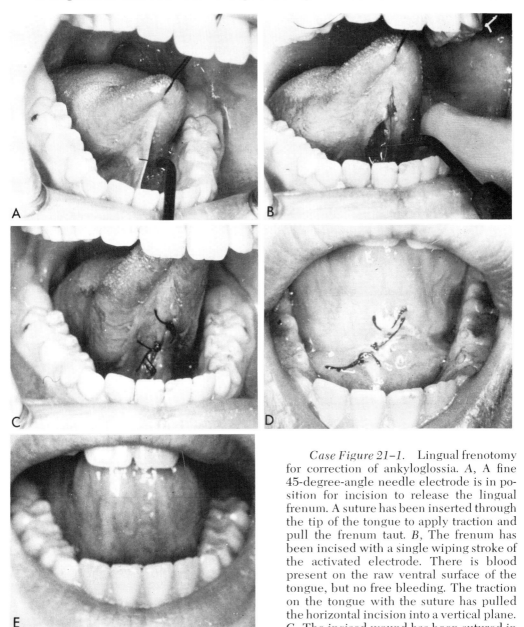

Case Figure 21–1. Lingual frenotomy for correction of ankyloglossia. *A,* A fine 45-degree-angle needle electrode is in position for incision to release the lingual frenum. A suture has been inserted through the tip of the tongue to apply traction and pull the frenum taut. *B,* The frenum has been incised with a single wiping stroke of the activated electrode. There is blood present on the raw ventral surface of the tongue, but no free bleeding. The traction on the tongue with the suture has pulled the horizontal incision into a vertical plane. *C,* The incised wound has been sutured in the vertical plane. Note that the tongue is now able to advance forward enough to be able to touch the palatal surfaces of the upper teeth. *D,* Postoperative appearance on fifth postoperative day, before the sutures are removed. There is no edema or swelling, and no inflammation. The tongue is supple and can now be placed against the palatal surfaces of the anterior teeth with no effort. Owing to the very delicate texture of the tissues of the floor of the mouth there is a light layer of coagulum along the line of incision, but otherwise the mouth is quite normal. *E,* Two weeks later the tissue on the ventral surface of the tongue is completely healed without a trace of the incision. The tongue is supple and can be placed against the teeth as desired without impediment.

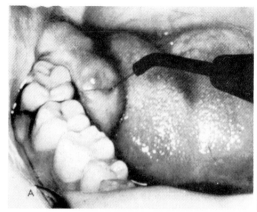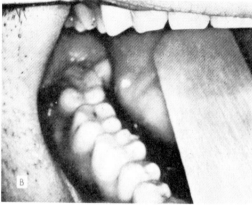

Figure 21–6.   Acute pericoronitis that has developed into an acute alveolar abscess. *A,* Pericoronal and lingual mucosa, tremendously distended with pus, is incised with a 45-degree-angle fine needle electrode for drainage. *B,* Drainage completed, the swelling has subsided and the crown of the third molar is almost fully exposed along its distal aspect.

possible to retain the teeth as functionally useful members. When pericoronitis develops into acute alveolar abscess, simple incision for drainage may suffice (Fig. 21–6). As a rule, however, even resection of the overlying diseased tissue alone will not suffice. In addition, resection of the deeply embedded deteriorated or cystically degenerated embryonal capsule is essential for success.

When, because of poor alignment, excessively deep impaction or lack of opposing occlusion, the teeth must be extracted, this alone is usually inadequate. Thorough resection of all the diseased tissue, internal and external, is essential for rapid healing.

Electrosurgery is uniquely useful in treatment of pericoronal involvements. Thoma, in describing removal of the operculum, states: "The electric wire loop is the ideal instrument for the removal of the operculum or gingival tissue. The operculum is removed first and then the gingiva around the crown is removed in a similar fashion until the entire crown is exposed.... The coagulating effect of the loop arrests bleeding and sterilizes the tissue at the same time. Healing takes place in a few days unless coagulation was excessive due to too strong a current or too slow cutting with the electrode. There is very little aftercare needed."[26] In addition to facilitating resection of the external superficial diseased tissue, electrosurgery makes resection of the deeply embedded embryonal capsule tissue equally simple. Electrosection, without coagulation, also eliminates or sharply reduces bleeding, which is usually profuse when these tissues are resected with scalpels, guillotines or other cold-steel instruments. In isolated rare instances under special conditions this technique can also be utilized to preserve horizontally impacted teeth. The operculotomy in the preceding case was atypical in that it did not result in the preservation of the tooth but merely facilitated its removal.

The operculotomy offers unique opportunities to put to good advantage the ability to bend and reshape electrodes to meet the special needs of a given case. Figure 21–7 demonstrates how an ordinary round loop electrode can be

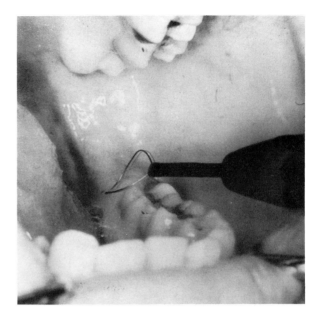

Figure 21-7. Reshaping of an electrode provides better tissue contact for operculotomy.

reshaped in a matter of seconds into a modified guillotine-shaped electrode that affords ideal tissue contact for maximum efficiency of the tissue resection.

TO FACILITATE REMOVAL OF A TOOTH

The operculotomy normally is performed to try to preserve the mandibular third molar by removing the overlying pericoronal flap, thereby exposing the crown of the third molar.

When the tooth is in normal alignment that is all that is needed. When the third molar is obliquely impacted and unable to erupt normally, removal of the operculum will not resolve the problem; however, if it is not removed, the tissue mass will complicate the surgical removal of the impacted tooth and will interfere with the healing of the wound by primary intention. It is therefore necessary to perform the operculotomy before proceeding with the surgical delivery of the impacted tooth. The first case of this series offers an excellent example of the need for such a procedure.

CASE 22

PATIENT.   A 24-year-old white female.

HISTORY.   She began to find chewing or clenching her jaws together painful and noticed on inspection in her mirror that the gingival tissue behind the last tooth in her lower jaw on the right side was swollen and darker red than the other tissues. She also noticed a break in the continuity of the tissue. She consulted her dentist and was referred to the author for surgery.

CLINICAL EXAMINATION.   A partial trismus prevented the patient from opening her mouth fully. There was a large pericoronal flap covering the third molar of which the mesiobuccal cusp was barely visible (Case Fig. 22–1A). Her temperature was 99.4° Fahrenheit. Her teeth and gingivae were normal except for the buccal rotation of the mandibular right first bicuspid.

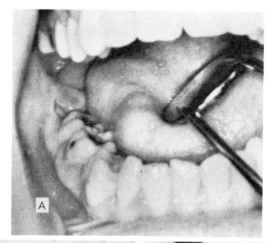

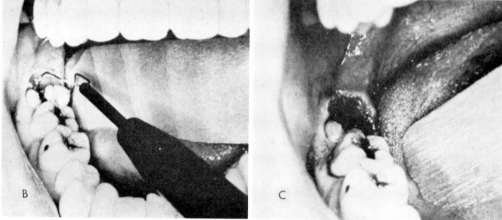

Case Figure 22–1. Subacute pericoronitis; tooth too malposed to be retained. *A*, Preoperative appearance. All but the mesiobuccal angle of the unerupted third molar is covered with a thick pericoronal flap. *B*, Inflamed flap resected with a guillotine loop electrode. *C*, Immediate postoperative appearance. The molar is tilted acutely and is too deeply embedded to be fully exposed and utilized.

TREATMENT. A 600,000 unit intramuscular injection of Crysticillin was administered. The pericoronal flap was lifted gently and, after a gauze sponge was placed across the oropharynx, irrigation with normal saline solution under the flap and simultaneous aspiration were followed by insertion of a centipede type of rubber dam drain under the flap. The patient was instructed to use very frequent lavage (every half hour), as warm as she could comfortably tolerate it; to apply ice packs extraorally, 15 minutes on, 45 minutes off, five or six times that day; and to return in 24 hours.

When she returned, the tissue flap was less swollen and was somewhat more normal in color, but she still was unable to open her mouth normally. A second injection of Crysticillin was administered, and an inferior alveolar regional block injection was administered. A large guillotine type of loop electrode was selected, cutting current was set at 8 on the dial, and the activated electrode was used with a scooping motion in a postero-anterior direction to resect the tissue mass (Case Fig. 22–1*B*).

When the tissue was removed, blood was released but there was no free flow of blood. The mesiobuccal cusp was now plainly visible (Case Fig. 21–1*C*), and it was obvious that the tooth, which was not only obliquely impacted but also slightly rotated so that the mesiolingual cusp was wedged tightly against the second molar, could not possibly erupt but would have to be removed.

The surgical removal was then performed and the defect closed in the usual manner with interrupted silk sutures for primary repair. Healing proceeded without incident. Had the diseased operculum not been removed before proceeding with the removal of the tooth, healing by primary intention could not have ensued, and the postoperative sequence undoubtedly would have been complicated.

TYPICAL OPERCULOTOMY FOR ELIMINATION OF PERICORONITIS

CASE 23

This case presents a typical example of the unique facility and efficiency of this modality for resection of degenerated hypertrophic pericoronal flaps from incompletely erupted mandibular third molars, and resection of the embryonal (Nasmyth's) membrane which also frequently undergoes hypertrophic and hyperplastic degeneration. It demonstrates a technique for reclaiming such teeth for functional use.

PATIENT. A 19-year-old white male.

HISTORY. His mandibular left third molar was incompletely erupted after three years and the posterior part of the crown remained covered with a loose hypertrophic mass of tissue. The latter periodically became acutely inflamed. During these acute episodes the loose pericoronal flap, the retromolar pad and the anterior pillar of the fauces swelled, making it difficult for him to swallow and painful to chew.

Submaxillary tenderness usually accompanied these symptoms. On each previous occasion the symptoms subsided after diligent use of antiseptic mouthwashes for a few days. About one week previously these symptoms recurred more acutely than on previous occasions, accompanied by fever and generalized malaise, and persisted despite frequent lavage. He was referred for resection of the pericoronal flap or extraction of the tooth.

CLINICAL EXAMINATION. *Extraoral.* There was a noticeable amount of swelling in the left cheek and angle of the jaw and in the submaxillary triangle. The latter area was tender to palpation.

Intraoral. The areolar lingual mucosa around the third molar was severely inflamed and engorged, and the posterior two-thirds of the tooth crown was covered with a loose flap of pericoronal tissue. This tissue also was swollen and engorged and appeared to have undergone necrotic degeneration along its anterior margin (Case Fig. 23–1A). Even light pressure proved very painful and produced a copious flow of viscous purulent exudate.

Roentgenographic examination revealed an area of radiolucence about 4 mm. wide around the posterior aspect of the crown of the tooth, extending posteriorly into the ascending ramus.

TREATMENT. A pharyngeal throatpack* was placed lightly across the posterior part of the mouth to block off the oropharynx. The pericoronal flap was elevated gently and warm Kasdenol solution vigorously sprayed under it and simultaneously

---

*The pharyngeal throatpack helps to reduce possible accidental dissemination of the infection into the pharynx or larynx during forceful irrigation under pressure.

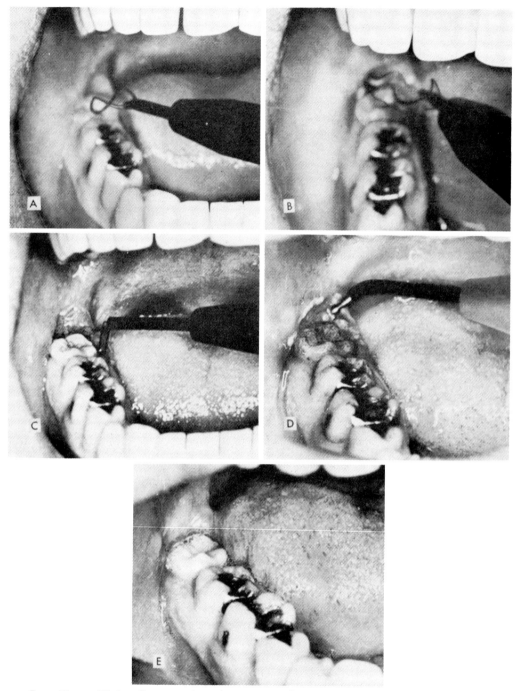

Case Figure 23–1. Conservative electrosurgical management of subacute pericoronitis. *A,* Preoperative clinical appearance of the affected third molar area prior to resection of the pericoronal flap. *B,* Inflamed hypertrophic mass being resected with a guillotine loop electrode. *C,* Embryonal capsule around crown of the tooth is resected with a narrow U-shaped loop electrode. *D,* Postoperative superficial spot coagulation to control healing. *E,* Final postoperative appearance. The tissues are healed, and the tooth is fully exposed and functionally useful.

aspirated. Some topical anesthetic solution was then sprayed under the flap, and two minutes later a fenestrated rubber dam drain, partially moistened with two per cent aqueous acriviolet solution, was inserted under the flap. Achromycin was prescribed for three days and frequent lavage recommended; he was instructed to return on the following day.

When he was seen again 24 hours later, marked improvement was noted. There was no longer any suppuration, the fever and malaise were eliminated, and the adenopathy was reduced. The mouth was prepared for surgery, and inferior alveolar regional block anesthesia was administered.

A specially designed guillotine loop electrode was selected and current output set at 8 for electrosection. The activated loop was applied to the distal part of the hypertrophic pericoronal flap and used with a postero-anterior scooping motion to resect the occlusal tissue mass and the lingual hypertrophic tissue (Case Fig. 23–1B).

The crown of the tooth was soon fully exposed. Cutting current was reduced to 5. A flame-shaped loop electrode was substituted and used to bevel and recontour the marginal gingiva to a feather edge. Current output was reduced to 4, a narrow 45-degree-angle U-shaped loop electrode was selected, and with this activated electrode the embryonal capsule was resected from the posterior and posterolingual areas of the tooth (Case Fig. 23–1C).

The resection having been completed, chromic acid, 0.05 per cent dilution, was applied to the raw tissue surfaces for 30 seconds, washed off, and tincture of myrrh and benzoin applied in air-dried layers. A surgical cement pack into which sulfathiazole and benzocaine powders had been incorporated was inserted over the operative field. The patient was instructed to continue the lavage and antibiotic therapy.

He returned on the fourth postoperative day. The cement pack was removed, the area irrigated, and tincture of myrrh and benzoin applied: then a fresh cement pack was inserted. He was seen again five days later. The cement pack was removed, the area irrigated and the tissues inspected. Healing was progressing very favorably, and normal granulation was marred only by presence of a sharp line of demarcation along the buccal aspect which delineated the junction between the old mucosa and the newly granulating tissue. The sharp edge was reduced to normal contour by spot coagulation with the small ball electrode used with current output of 0.5 (Case Fig. 23–1D). Use of an astringent salt-alum mouthwash was recommended, and he was told to return in two weeks for further observation.

When he was seen again the tissues were found to be fully healed and in excellent tone. The crown of the third molar was fully exposed. The gingival margin was normal and the tooth was functionally useful (Case Fig. 23–1E).

OPERCULOTOMY FOR EXPOSURE AND ERUPTION OF VERTICALLY IMPACTED MANDIBULAR THIRD MOLAR

CASE 24

This operculotomy differs from the usual cases of pericoronitis that require operculotomy to fully expose the erupting mandibular molar. In this case the third molar was vertically impacted and the operculotomy made it possible to release it so that it could erupt normally.

PATIENT. A 19-year-old white male.

HISTORY. He was home on a short school vacation and consulted his family dentist about a pain in his lower jaw. An x-ray was taken, and a vertically impacted third molar appeared to be the cause of the pain. He was referred to the author for removal of the impacted tooth.

CLINICAL EXAMINATION. All the mandibular teeth were present in normal alignment in the dental arch except the two third molars. The tissue covering the left third molar was thick and elevated slightly above the level of the occlusal surface of the second molar. A periapical x-ray of the molar area revealed the third molar in normal vertical position and alignment but unerupted, with the top of the crown of the tooth approximately 6 mm. below the superior edge of the alveolar bone. The appearance of the tooth suggested the likelihood that two small bone spurs in the embrasure between the second and third molar teeth were locking the tooth and preventing it from erupting. It also appeared likely that these bone spurs could easily be removed if the overlying tissue were resected to provide access to them. The dentist and the pa-

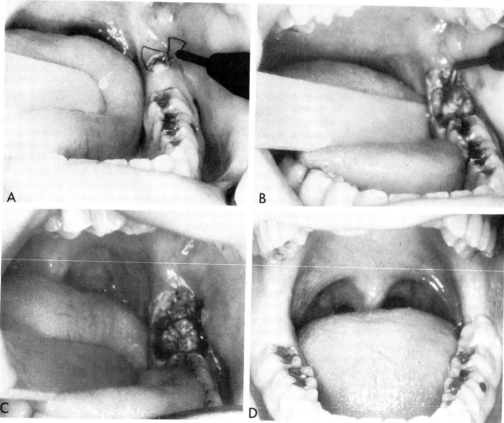

Case Figure 24–1. Operculotomy for exposure and eruption of vertically impacted mandibular third molar. *A,* The overlying tissue is being resected with a large guillotine loop electrode. *B,* The submerged tooth crown has been exposed and the tissues around it have been recontoured. The 45-degree-angle narrow U-shaped loop electrode is being used to resect the Nasmyth's membrane embryonal capsule from the lingual and distal surfaces of the crown. *C,* Appearance after the embryonal capsule has been eliminated. The area is now ready for application of the surgical cement pack. *D,* Postoperative appearance of the molar several months later. The tooth is now fully erupted, in normal alignment, and functionally useful.

tient were delighted that there appeared to be an excellent likelihood that the hazardous removal of a vertically impacted tooth could be avoided, and the tooth preserved for functional use.

TREATMENT. The tissues were prepared and an inferior alveolar block was administered. A guillotine-shaped electrode was selected and cutting current set at 9 on the power output dial. The activated electrode was used with a forward pulling motion to resect the overlying tissue (Case Fig. 24–1A). When the entire occlusal surface of the crown of the tooth was exposed, the marginal gingiva was beveled smooth. A 45-degree-angle narrow U-shaped loop was substituted, cutting current was reduced to 3.5, and all subgingival soft tissue around the crown was resected with it (Case Fig. 24–1B).

The entire procedure was performed without free bleeding. The blood that was produced was easily removed with a gauze sponge, so that there was excellent visibility in the surgical field all the time. A small McCall type sickle-shaped prophylaxis scaler was used to chip out the small bone spurs, a procedure that required little effort.

The area was debrided of all tissue and bone fragments, and tincture of myrrh and benzoin was applied in air-dried layers. A hard mix of surgical cement was packed over the surgical area, and the occlusion was checked to assure that the pack would not readily be displaced. The patient returned on the fifth postoperative day and the cement pack was removed. The area was healing very well. The patient was seen the following week, and healing appeared to have progressed gratifyingly. At this time he had to return to school. Several months later he was seen again, and the tooth was found to be fully erupted, in normal alignment, and functionally useful (Case Fig. 24–1D).

The combination of sound treatment plan and advantageous use of electrosurgery made it possible to avoid the need for surgical removal of a vertically impacted mandibular third molar with the ever-present hazard of accidental fracture of the jaw.

PALLIATIVE EXPOSURE TO RETAIN A HORIZONTALLY IMPACTED THIRD MOLAR

Normally, when a mandibular third molar is impacted in horizontal version, the tooth usually is causing discomfort, and there is no possibility of moving the tooth into normal alignment, it is necessary to remove it surgically.

Occasionally, however, a combination of special circumstances may make it advisable to compromise and treat the case palliatively, in order to avoid extensive traumatic surgery for removal of the impacted tooth and prevent elongation of the opposing tooth.

When conditions justify palliative treatment, electrosurgery, owing to its inherent advantages of sterilizing the tissues to which it is applied and of healing without contractile scar tissue repair, not only simplifies and accelerates treatment but also greatly increases the likelihood of a favorable result.

The unusual combination of conditions encountered in the next case made palliative treatment preferable to surgical removal of the impacted tooth. The case demonstrates a simple but effective method of palliative treatment.

CASE 25

PATIENT.   A 14-year-old white female.

HISTORY.   She had a moderately severe congenital cardiac defect and was under the care of a cardiologist. She began to have considerable discomfort while eating, owing to tissue trauma in the posterior part of the left side of her mouth. A dental examination revealed some irritation of the tissue immediately posterior to the second molar, and a periapical x-ray revealed that the third molar was impacted in horizontal version, with the crown of the impacted tooth in contact with the distal surface of the crown of the second molar. She was referred to the author for the surgery.

CLINICAL EXAMINATION.   *Extraoral.*   The mouth opening formed by the lips was so small that it was necessary to use the author's child-size cheek-lip retractor instead of the medium-size retractor that usually is well suited for a 14-year-old.

INTRAORAL.   The mandibular left third molar was horizontally impacted, and also rotated postero-anteriorly, so that the distobuccal cusp of the impacted tooth projected outward beyond the distobuccal angle of the second molar, toward the cheek. All but the distobuccal cusp of the impacted tooth was covered with tissue, which appeared to have been abraded traumatically by the maxillary opposing molar (Case Fig. 25–1A). The rest of the mouth appeared normal.

TREATMENT.   The patient's cardiologist advised against performing extensive traumatic elective surgery or use of prolonged general anesthesia. If surgical removal of the impacted tooth were to be performed, it would be necessary to use a mechanical mouth prop, which, in view of her very small mouth, would greatly increase the hazard of traumatic injury to her temporomandibular joint. The limited mouth access would also increase the hazard of accidental damage to the second molar. As a result of this combination of factors, palliative treatment appeared to be logical and justifiable.

The tissues were prepared, a topical anesthetic was applied, and anesthesia was administered by jet injection with a Sterijet syringe and 1:100,000 Xylocaine. Infiltration by jet injection was chosen partly because of the patient's fear of the regular hypodermic needle, but especially because this would make it possible to administer a precisely measured and controlled minimal dose of anesthetic and would thereby provide an additional safety factor that was desired by the cardiologist.

A round loop electrode 1 cm. in diameter was selected and bent to provide the most desirable tissue contact (Case Fig. 25–1B). The cutting current was set at 7.5 on the instrument panel rheostat and the activated electrode was used with a wiping, scooping motion in a postero-anterior direction to resect that portion of the overlying tissue that had been traumatized by the opposing molar. When the resection was completed, the loop was used to bevel the tissue margins to restore normal tissue architecture. Tincture of myrrh and benzoin was applied to the surgical field in air-dried layers. A stiffly mixed cement pack was applied but quickly became displaced and was replaced with a dressing of Squibb's Orahesive bandage. The patient was given instructions in home postoperative care and was reappointed.

She returned on the fifth postoperative day and reported she had had no pain, trismus, bleeding, or swelling. She had no difficulty opening her mouth maximally, and the tissues were carefully inspected. The tissue tone was excellent. There was no evidence of redness or edema, and the tissues appeared to be healing by secondary intention. The tissue surface was covered with a very thin film of coagulum, and there was no sign of proliferation. The area was cleansed by gentle irrigation with Kasdenol, and tincture of myrrh and benzoin was applied (Case Fig. 25–1C). She was in-

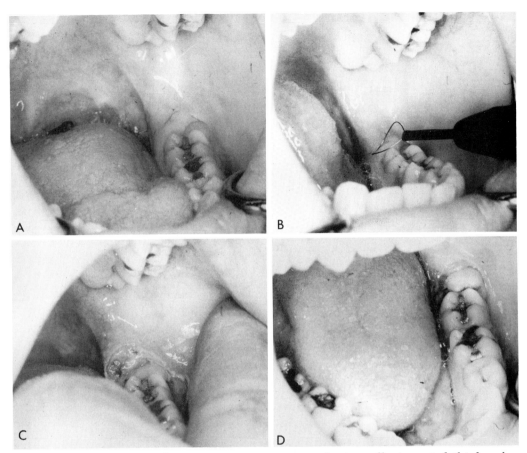

Case Figure 25-1. Palliative exposure to retain a horizontally impacted third molar. *A*, Preoperative appearance: the mandibular left third molar is malposed and impacted. The tooth is in a horizontal plane, with the distobuccal portion of the impacted tooth projecting buccally beyond the second molar, and only that portion of the crown of the tooth is exposed. The rest of the distal surface of the impacted tooth is covered with hyperplastic gingival tissue. The overlying tissue shows evidence of having been traumatized by the opposing molar tooth. *B*, A 12-mm. round loop electrode has been bent to form a curve that will provide a more efficient scooping effect for removal of the tissue. The reshaped loop has been activated and is being brought into contact with the tissues for the resection. *C*, The redundant overlying tissue has been removed, and the margins of the surrounding tissue have been recontoured to create beveled edges that eliminate tissue undercuts. *D*, Two week postoperative appearance of the tooth and tissues. The distal portion of the impacted crown has been exposed and provides continuity of the dental arch. The surrounding tissues are healed and almost fully matured. The opposing tooth makes normal contact with the exposed coronal surface without causing any tissue trauma. It is noteworthy that not only the occlusal surface has been cleared of tissue, but also the part that comes into contact with the buccal mucosa of the cheek has been exposed and cleared of tissue.

structed to continue the regimen of home care until further notice and to return once a week for further postoperative care and supervision. The following week there was a slight amount of proliferative tissue along the lingual marginal edge of the tissue. The proliferative tissue was destroyed by superficial spot coagulation with a small ball coagulating electrode and current output was set at 2. Tincture of myrrh and benzoin was applied in air-dried layers, and the patient was cautioned to continue to stay on a soft diet for a while longer. When she returned the following week the tissue was almost completely healed (Case Fig. 25-1*D*), but owing to the lack of surface epithelium the lingual marginal edge of the tissue was slightly darker red in color than the remaining tissue. Healing progressed uneventfully, and by the end of the fifth postoperative week the tissues were fully healed, and she was dismissed from further treatment.

The patient has had no further difficulties with this tooth, and there appears to be an excellent probability that, barring some future unforeseen complications, she will not have to have this tooth removed.

In addition to the advantages electrosurgery offers in unusual cases such as has been described, in this particular case it offered several additional important advantages. Due to the hemostasis inherent in electrosection, there was no surgical or postoperative hemorrhage, hence, no surgical shock. This patient's serious cardiac condition made this a very important factor. There was also a very helpful *indirect* advantage. Her obsessive preoperative apprehension had been due as much to the fear of being put to sleep as to the fear of having the tooth "chiseled" out of her mouth. When she was reassured that because of the nature of the treatment that would be performed she would not have to be put to sleep, would have no hemorrhagic bleeding, and would not have to have an injection, she became receptive to treatment and there was no need to premedicate her with a potent tranquilizer or narcotic.

IV. SUBTOTAL RADECTOMY (MULTIROOTED TEETH)

Introduction

The excellent results that have been achieved with the apicoectomy—the surgical resection of periapically diseased tissue and the affected apex of an endodontically treated tooth[27, 28]—eventually led to attempts to remove not only the diseased apex of a tooth but the involved roots of multirooted teeth, in order to preserve part of the teeth for functional use.

This technique of hemisection, consisting of the sectioning of the affected multirooted tooth by cutting through the crown of the tooth and extracting the coronal half with the affected root and then using the remainder as a bicuspid instead of a molar, was developed some time ago and has served a useful purpose. However, when the affected tooth is functioning as an abutment for a fixed restoration, and the coronal portion of the tooth is covered with a full cast or veneer cast crown, this procedure becomes impractical. Thus, when retention of the tooth is most important, this technique cannot be used.

The technique of subtotal radectomy developed by the author and reviewed in the first edition eliminates the need to sacrifice half of the crown of the tooth in addition to the offending root. Subtotal radectomy without hemisection can be achieved effectively when periapical debridement and especially interradicular debridement in the furcation between the roots are performed by electrosection. Should similar debridement be attempted with rigid steel instruments, the limitations inherent in this method of instrumentation make it physically impossible to debride the pathologic debris in the furcation thoroughly and effectively. Because of the flexibility and lack of physical bulk of the surgical electrodes, and the fact that no pressure is required to perform the debridement, even the furca are readily accessible to the necessary instrumentation, without need to remove additional bone to gain access. Moreover, should it prove difficult or impossible to effect total debridement by loop resection, the remaining tenaciously adherent tissue fragments can be destroyed in situ without hazard, thereby assuring total debridement.

The effectiveness of this method of treatment to preserve multirooted teeth for functional use is well demonstrated in the following series of cases.

The clinician often wishes, in vain, that it were possible to be able to reopen a surgical site to be able to visualize clinically the extent of regeneration that resulted, and to observe the character of the repair tissue, a wish that unfortunately cannot be fulfilled except in rare isolated instances where the patient had consented to experimental treatment.

The first case of this series is of special interest for two reasons: first, because it presents an excellent demonstration of the technique for sub-total radectomy, and second, and perhaps most important, because it subsequently required re-incision of the original surgical site, thus inadvertently making possible postoperative clinical visualization of the degree and quality of bone regeneration that had occurred.

Buccal Roots

CASE 26

PART I

PATIENT.   A 47-year-old white female.

HISTORY.   Approximately one year earlier she had had endodontic treatment for a maxillary first bicuspid that was to serve as the anterior abutment for a fixed bridge. The tooth had then been prepared and restored with a cast veneer crown that served as the anterior anchor for the bridge. One year later, she suddenly developed a large ulceration on the labiobuccal gingiva between the cuspid and bicuspid abutment. She consulted her dentist who x-rayed the area and found extensive periapical translucence. He referred her to the author with the request that if at all possible the tooth be treated conservatively to try to preserve it for functional use.

CLINICAL EXAMINATION.   A large oval-shaped ulcerated lesion was present on the labiobuccal gingiva at the level of the apex of the maxillary right first bicuspid and extended anteriorly downward in an oblique direction toward the center of the cuspid root, midway between the apex and cemento-enamel junction of that tooth. The first bicuspid was restored with a veneer crown that served as the anterior abutment for a fixed restoration that extended posteriorly to the second molar. With the exception of the ulcerated lesion the gingival tissues throughout the remainder of the mouth appeared normal in tone and texture.

TREATMENT.   The tissues were prepared for an infraorbital block and palatal infiltration anesthesia, which was then administered. A 45-degree-angle fine needle

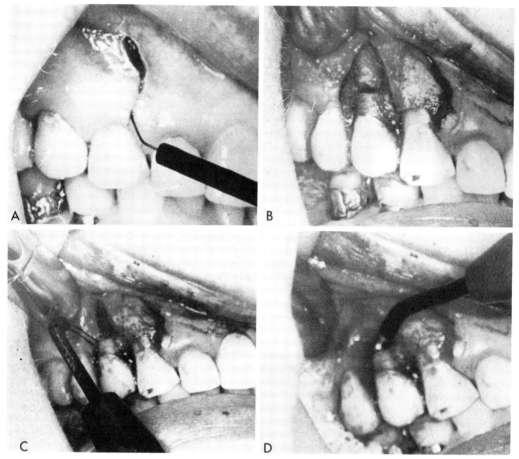

Case Figure 26-1. Subtotal radectomy of buccal root of maxillary first bicuspid
Part I. *A,* An incision is being made with a fine 45-degree-angle needle electrode to create a mucoperiosteal flap. There is a large ulcerated area in the vestibular areolar mucosa between the maxillary right cuspid and first bicuspid. The lesion is shaped like a football and slants downward and forward at a 45-degree-angle, and the incision is being made immediately anterior to and parallel with the anterior-most edge of the ulceration. The incision then is being carried downward and slightly posteriorly and terminates at the marginal edge of the gingiva about 3 mm. mesial to the center of the cuspid. *B,* A second, slightly vertico-oblique incision has been made at the distobuccal angle of the first molar. The apical attachments of the papillae in the molar-second bicuspid embrasure and the cuspid-first bicuspid embrasure have been severed to create a mucoperiosteal flap. The latter has been elevated, exposing the buccal root of the first bicuspid which is totally denuded of its buccal bone. The denuded root has been severed with a fissure bur at a level of 3 mm. above the furca between the buccal and palatal roots of the tooth. *C,* The severed root has been removed from the socket and debridement performed. Fragments of granulomatous tissue wedged between the buccal root stump and the distal bone and palatal root are being excised with a 17-mm. periodontal loop electrode with the loop bent to form an angle offering favorable access to the furcation. *D,* Debridement having been completed, the cut end of the buccal root stump has been rounded, and the gutta percha is being resealed with a ball coagulating electrode to assure a hermetic seal at the new apex of the root stump.

electrode was selected and cutting power was set at 3 on the power output dial of the instrument panel.

Inasmuch as it would be necessary to resect the ulcerated tissue, it was necessary to deviate from the usual vertico-oblique incision and to create two incisions, one anteriorly and the other posteriorly, for a Z-plasty repair. The activated electrode was therefore used to create a Z-shaped vertico-oblique incision for a mucoperiosteal flap, starting slightly superior to and immediately adjacent to the anterior edge of the ulceration and directed downward toward the mesiogingival angle of the cuspid marginal gingiva (Case Fig. 26–1A). The ulcerated tissue was then resected by circumferential incisional excision with the needle electrode. Then the second incision, which extended from the junction of alveolar and areolar gingiva over the mesiobuccal root of the first molar downward and anteriorly to the distogingival angle of the marginal gingiva of the second bicuspid, was created with the same electrode, after which the intervening apical attachments of the interdental papillae were severed, so that the mucoperiosteal flap could be reflected.

The tissue was elevated and reflected with the broad end of a periosteal elevator, exposing the buccal aspect of the first bicuspid fully. The entire length of the first bicuspid buccal root, from cemento-enamel junction to apex, was denuded of its overlying alveolar bone. Approximately 0.5 cm. of the cuspid root was also denuded at its coronal end.

The exposed bicuspid buccal root was severed with a fissure bur 3 mm. above the furcation (Case Fig. 26–1B). The severed root was then elevated and removed. The defect from which the root had been removed was grossly debrided with small steel

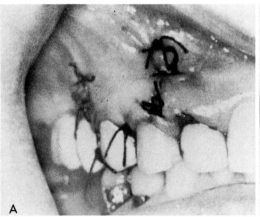
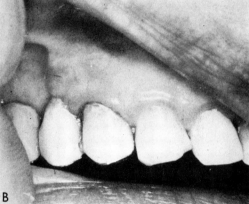

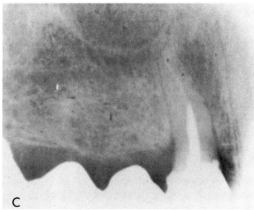

Case Figure 26–2. A, The posterior mucoperiosteal flap has been elevated and rotated anteriorly to provide slack, so that the anterior tissue margins will be coapted and make up for the loss of ulcerated tissue. The coapted margins have been sutured with interrupted silk sutures, and sutures have been inserted through the papillae and embrasures to secure the flaps firmly. *B,* Appearance of the tissues six months postoperatively. The tissues are normal in all respects, and the contour over the first bicuspid is as convex as that of the contralateral teeth. There is no scar tissue and the incision lines are not visible. *C,* Periapical x-ray taken at this time reveals excellent healing around the root stump. The bone appears to have almost completely filled the original defect.

surgical curets. Debridement of the furca and surrounding defect was then completed with a narrow U-shaped loop electrode, and cutting current output was increased to 4 on the power output dial. The tip of the loop was curved to provide easy access to the furcation and curved undercuts in the defect area (Case Fig. 26–1C).

The apical end of the buccal root stump was rounded with a diamond stone. The gutta percha at the top of the root stump was resealed by electrocoagulation with a small round ball coagulating electrode and power output was set at 2 on the coagulating power output dial, to assure a perfect seal in the event that severance of the root with the fissure bur had detached the gutta percha that was adhering to the internal walls of the canal (Case Fig. 26–1D).

Bleeding was then induced in the debrided defect, and some powdered Gelfoam was introduced into the defect and mixed with the blood. As soon as the gelatinous blood mass began to show signs of early clotting, the flap was restored to position, the cut tissue margins were coapted to compensate for the tissue lost in resecting the ulcerated lesion and were sutured with interrupted silk sutures. The interdental papillae were then secured in their embrasures by suturing bucco-palatally through the embrasures (Case Fig. 26–2A). Tincture of myrrh and benzoin was applied to the surgical field in air-dried layers, and the patient was given postoperative instructions and reappointed for removal of the sutures.

When she returned on the fifth postoperative day, there was evidence of early primary healing, and the tissue tone appeared excellent. The sutures were removed, tincture of myrrh and benzoin was applied in air-dried layers, and she was instructed to continue the prescribed home care and to return at weekly intervals until further notice.

Gingival repair continued without incident, and by the end of the third week it was complete. The marginal gingiva that had rested on the root stump appeared firmly attached to the underlying reparative tissues, and the buccal alveolar contour was normally convex in contour. She was dismissed from further active treatment, but asked to return in six months for a final postoperative check-up. She returned as instructed. The tissues appeared fully healed and maturely keratinized, so that the original lines of incision could not be distinguished from the surrounding tissues (Case Fig. 26–2B). A periodontal probe introduced subgingivally at the first bicuspid could not penetrate beyond the base of the gingival sulcus. A periapical x-ray of the area revealed apparent complete bone repair down to and including the furcation, although the x-ray suggested that the calcification of the new bone was not quite as dense as the old surrounding bone (Case Fig. 26–2C).

Thereafter almost two years elapsed without incident until she suddenly noted that the edge of the gingival tissue on the buccal aspect of the first bicuspid seemed slightly detached and darker than the surrounding tissue, and particles of food seemed to become trapped in a slight depression caused by the detachment. She also found an occasional trace of blood on her toothbrush after use in that area. She therefore arranged to return for re-examination.

PART II

CLINICAL EVALUATION. The marginal gingiva over the first bicuspid was detached on the buccal aspect, and gave a dark appearance to the tissue (Case Fig. 26–3A). A periodontal probe introduced subgingivally at that point penetrated about 3.5 mm. superiorly before it met solid resistance. It also penetrated approximately the

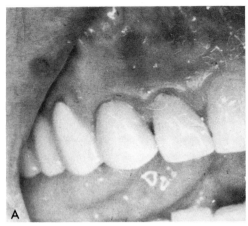
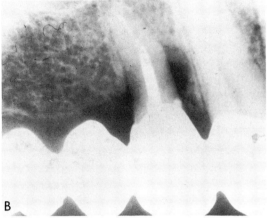

Case Figure 26–3. Part II. *A,* Appearance of the mouth 7 years later. The marginal gingiva has receded slightly from the neck of the first bicuspid, and there is a slightly cavernous recess there. *B,* A periapical x-ray of the tooth reveals a large area of radiolucence along the mesial half of the coronal end of the bicuspid root. The bone loss appears to be circumferential and extends around to the distal aspect too.

same distance when directed buccopalatally. A periapical x-ray revealed an oval area of radiolucence in the vicinity of the buccal root stump (Case Fig. 26–3*B*).

These findings led to the clinical diagnosis of incomplete bone regeneration or pathologic deterioration of the bone due to unknown causes. In either event it was apparent that it would be necessary to incise and reflect the mucoperiosteum over the bicuspid to visualize and treat the present defect.

TREATMENT. A 45-degree-angle fine needle electrode was selected and cutting current was set at 3 on the power output dial. The electrode was activated and the apical attachments of the cuspid and bicuspid interdental papillae were severed. The electrode was then used to make a vertico-oblique mucoperiosteal incision (Case Fig. 26–4*A* and *B*). The incised tissue was elevated and reflected. This revealed that the buccal alveolar bone over the original site of the subtotal root amputation had fully repaired except at the coronal end, where approximately 3 mm. of bone had not repaired, leaving a cavernous defect partially filled with granulomatous tissue (Case Fig. 26–4*C*). As much superficial soft tissue debris in the defect as possible was removed with a small steel curet. A medium-width U-shaped loop electrode was then selected, cutting current was set at 5 on the power output dial, and the activated electrode was used to remove the remaining accessible debris. A narrow U-shaped loop was substituted, current output was set at 4, and this electrode, curved to provide better access to concave contoured parts of the defect, was used to complete the debridement (Case Fig. 26–4*D*).

The buccal root stump was not fully visible. The top of the root stump was dark, rough, and somewhat pitted. The pits were eliminated and the root end made smooth by grinding the end of the root stump lightly with a long slender conical tapered diamond stone (Case Fig. 26–4*E*). A round bone bur was then used to freshen the marginal edge of the bone defect, following which debridement was completed by electronic curettage with a narrow U-shaped loop electrode, bent to a curvature that made it accessible to all parts of the internal aspect of the defect, and by fulguration, directing the sparks into the furca and along the anterior surface of the palatal root, to assure that no fragments of debris remained in the furca undetected. The gutta percha at the freshened end of the root stump was then resealed by electrocoagulation with a

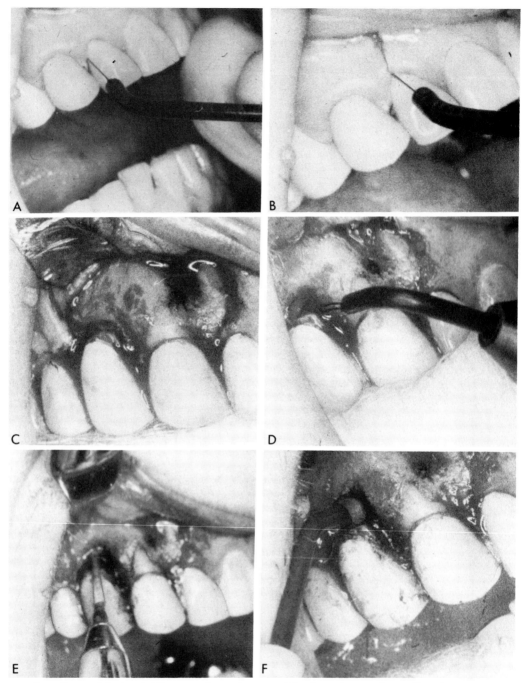

Case Figure 26-4. A, The apical attachment of the lateral-cuspid papilla is being severed with a fine 45-degree-angle needle electrode. B, A vertico-oblique incision is being made anteroposteriorly from the mucogingival junction to the distogingival angle of the lateral. The apex of the cuspid-first bicuspid papilla attachment has also been severed. C, The mucoperiosteal flap has been elevated and retracted, exposing an inverted crescent-shaped opening over the bicuspid crown and the anterior part of the buccal root stump. The entire buccal plate of bone has regenerated except for this 3-mm. opening. D, Granulomatous debris in the cavelike recess is being resected with a U-shaped loop electrode that has been bent to an angle that offers favorable access to the area. E, The buccal root stump is being reduced and rounded with a tapered diamond stone, to remove the pitted surface and facilitate complete debridement. F, The gutta percha at the end of the now 1-mm. root stump is being resealed by electrocoagulation with a large ball electrode.

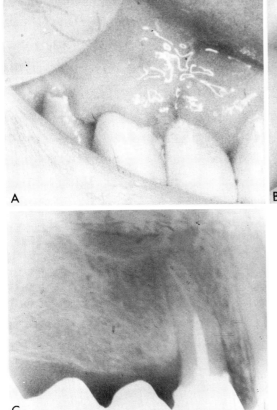

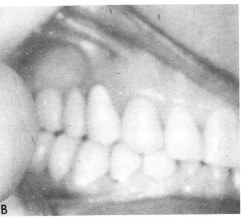

Case Figure 26–5. A, Appearance of tissues on the fifth postoperative day. Primary healing has begun. A small apron of marginal gingiva that had been pulled down over the external edge of the first bicuspid crown is still intact. *B,* Final postoperative photograph six months later. The tissues are fully healed and normal. The contour around the buccal of the first bicuspid is normal convex, and the marginal gingiva is tightly adapted around the top of the crown. *C,* A periapical x-ray of the area reveals complete regeneration of the interseptal bone on the mesial aspect. The bone has filled in completely in the vicinity of the remnant of root canal, filling in the buccal root stump. It also appears to have filled in around to the distal of the root stump, and the roentgenographic evidence confirms the clinical evidence of complete and favorable repair of the defect.

large ball electrode (Case Fig. 26–4F). The internal surface of the marginal edge of the marginal gingiva over the root stump was freshened by superficial loop planing to remove epithelialized tissue with the medium-width loop electrode.

Debridement having been completed, bleeding was induced in the defect and powdered Gelfoam was introduced and mixed with the blood. The tissue flap was restored to position, the coapted margins were sutured with interrupted silk sutures, and the papillae were secured in their respective embrasures by suturing buccopalatally through the embrasures. The occlusion had been checked preoperatively and was found to be normal. It was rechecked at this point and was still found normal. The patient was reappointed after a bandage of Squibb Orahesive was applied to the surgical field.

The patient returned on the fifth postoperative day for removal of the sutures. Soft tissue healing by primary intention appeared to be progressing very favorably. The sutures were removed and tincture of myrrh and benzoin was applied in air-dried layers. She was seen again one week later, at which time healing was considerably further advanced (Case Fig. 26–5A). She was seen again for two successive weeks and then asked to return in one year, or sooner if necessary. One year later she returned for a final postoperative examination. The tissues were fully healed and the alveolar repair appeared complete (Case Fig. 26–5B), since the periodontal probe could not be advanced subgingivally beyond the base of the gingival sulcus. A periapical x-ray confirmed the clinical impression of complete healing (Case Fig. 26–5C).

Two conclusions can be made with respect to this case: First, despite extensive bone deterioration and loss of alveolar contour that occur when all the diseased area has been removed atraumatically, regeneration does occur, including normal cortical surface density of the reparative bone. Second, failure of the regeneration to continue to fill in around the root stump in all probability resulted from failure to totally debride the furca. When the surgery was first performed, the author determined the complete debridement by feeling around with the inactive electrode for presence of tissue fragments. When this failed to reveal retained debris the debridement was considered complete, and the area was not fulgurated to destroy any contaminated tissue shreds that might still be present. Thus, although the debridement appeared complete after the second surgical and electrosurgical curettage, the author completed the debridement by sparking with the fulgurating current to assure that any undetected fragments that might still be present in the furca would be destroyed in situ, and thereby assure that debridement really was complete. The subsequent total repair of the defect appears to substantiate this belief. Thus, this case also provides a clue as to why, despite identical or seemingly identical treatment, some cases fail to respond to treatment that is successful for many others.

CASE 27

This case is an example of the practicality of total amputation of a badly abscessed root of a maxillary molar with trifurcation involvement, which ordinarily would be condemned to extraction.

PATIENT.   A 60-year-old white female.

HISTORY.   The buccal gingival mucosa and alveolar bone of the maxillary first molar had been undergoing gradual resorption. The tooth suddenly became very sensitive, and chewing on it caused throbbing pain. The patient and her dentist were keenly anxious to retain the tooth if at all possible. She was referred for consultation regarding possible root amputation and the necessary surgery if feasible.

CLINICAL EXAMINATION. *Extraoral.*   Negative.

Intraoral.   The buccal alveolar bone and gingival mucosa over the maxillary right first molar were resorbed from the mesiobuccal root, exposing about 6 mm. of denuded root.

Roentgenographic examination revealed that the first molar was devitalized and that there was marked radiolucence around the full length of the mesiobuccal root which extended into the trifurcation (Case Fig. 27–2A).

TREATMENT.   The mouth was prepared for surgery and the area was anesthetized by buccal-palatal infiltration. A 45-degree-angle fine needle electrode was selected and current output set at 3.5 for electrosection. An incision was made in the buccal mucosa, extending from the mucobuccal fold downward and anteriorly to the mesiobuccal angle of the second bicuspid (Case Fig. 27–1A). The interproximal attachments of the papillae were then severed in their respective embrasures, pos-

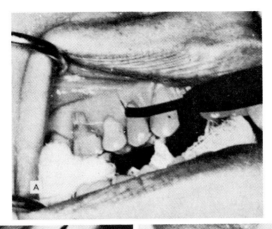

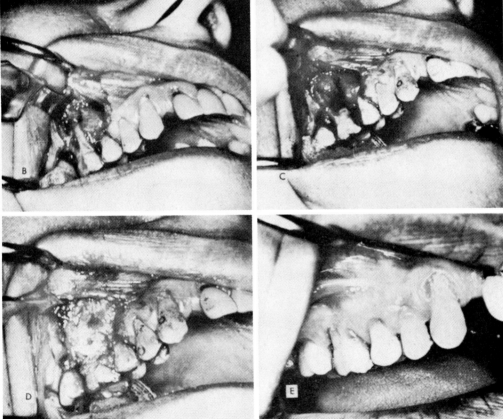

Case Figure 27–1. Total amputation of one root of a multirooted tooth; maxillary first molar mesiobuccal root and trifurcation involved. *A*, Vertico-oblique incision of buccal mucosa from mucobuccal fold downward to mesiobuccal angle of the second bicuspid. Note 6 mm. re-sorption of buccal gingiva and bone over mesiobuccal molar root. *B*, Flap retracted, reveals mesiobuccal root denuded almost to its apex, and necrotic granulomatous debris. *C*, Mesio-buccal root has been amputated close to trifurcation, and thorough debridement has been per-formed. *D*, Defect is filled with cultured bone–medicated surgical gelatin mixture. *E*, Final postoperative appearance three months later. Healing is complete. The gingival margin is closely adapted to the tooth, and the buccal alveolar contour is normal.

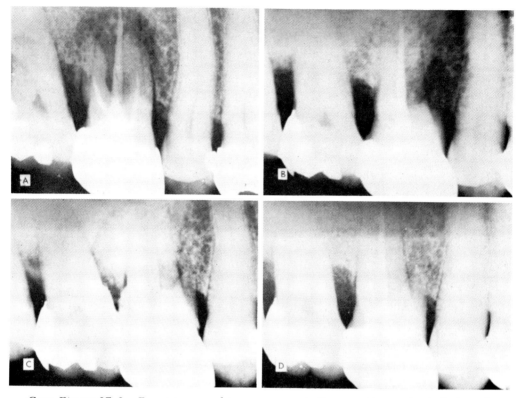

Case Figure 27–2.   Roentgenographic sequence. *A,* Preoperative periapical view shows radiolucence around mesiobuccal root and trifurcation. *B,* Immediate postoperative periapical view shows root amputation and extent of alveolar destruction. *C,* Postoperative appearance three months later. The alveolar defect is filled with partially calcified reparative bone. *D,* Final postoperative view taken six months later shows complete obliteration of radiolucent area with normal bone.

teriorly, to the third molar. The tissue was reflected from the alveolar bone and the flap was retracted, revealing a total loss of alveolar bone from the buccal surface of the mesiobuccal root and its part of the trifurcation (Case Fig. 27–1*B*).

The exposed mesiobuccal root was amputated at a point about 2 mm. above the trifurcation with a carbide fissure bur (Case Fig. 27–1*C*). Necrotic tissue present in the area was resected by electrosurgical curettage with a narrow U-shaped loop electrode. The latter was used effectively in areas usually inaccessible to conventional curets, especially in the trifurcation. Tenacious shreds that could not be resected were destroyed in situ by fulguration.

The area having been thoroughly debrided, an immediate postoperative roentgenogram was taken (Case Fig. 27–2*B*) to ascertain that all the necrotic tissue had been eliminated. The defect was then filled with cultured bone paste and medicated surgical gelatin, which were incorporated with blood in the defect (Case Fig. 27–1*D*). The flap was restored to position and sutured on the buccal aspect and interproximally. Mysteclin was prescribed and the patient was instructed in postoperative care.

She returned on the fifth postoperative day for removal of the sutures. Healing appeared to be progressing favorably. The sutures were removed and tincture of myrrh and benzoin was applied. She was seen postoperatively once a week for one month during which time healing progressed rapidly and favorably. The tooth was firmly embedded, its buccal contour was normal, and there was no evidence of alveolar depression in the amputated root space. The tissue tone remained excellent from the outset.

She was followed postoperatively for two more months. By the end of that time soft tissue healing was complete and there was no scar formation or tissue contraction. The gingival margin on the buccal aspect of the tooth extended downward toward the cemento-enamel junction farther than it had preoperatively, and appeared more normal than it had originally (Case Fig. 27–1E). A roentgenogram taken at that time (Case Fig. 27–2C) revealed regeneration of the bone in the mesial root socket and interradicularly. A final roentgenogram taken six months later shows normal calcification of the regenerated bone (Case Fig. 27–2D). The tooth has remained esthetically and functionally satisfactory in the more than 17 years since the surgery was performed.

CASE 28

This case demonstrates the fact that seemingly hopelessly involved teeth with massive periradicular bone destruction and Class III mobility can sometimes be successfully reclaimed for functional use by radical root amputations and total surgical eradication of the necrotic debris, which permits normal regeneration of the alveolar bone.

PATIENT. A 62-year-old white male.

HISTORY. A maxillary left first molar and first bicuspid, key abutments for a Chayes' bridge restoring the second bicuspid, and an edentulous span extending to the right second molar became very loose and the gingival mucosa around both teeth swelled. His dentist found evidence of massive alveolar destruction and referred the patient for amputation of the involved roots or extraction of the teeth if deemed hopeless.

CLINICAL EXAMINATION. *Extraoral.* Negative.

Intraoral. The maxillary left first bicuspid and first molar were markedly mobile: bicuspid, Class III mobility; molar, Class II mobility. The gingival mucosa around both teeth appeared edematous and hyperemic. The crowns of both teeth were restored with gold three-quarter crowns into which female attachments for a Chayes' bridge were attached. The mobility of the two teeth was not materially reduced by the presence of the bridge in the dental arch.

Roentgenographic examination revealed that the buccal root of the bicuspid was completely circumscribed by an area of radiolucence. There was also a periapical radiolucent area around the palatal root. The mesiobuccal root of the molar was surrounded by an area of marked radiolucence that involved the trifurcation. The floor of the maxillary antrum was a safe 0.5 cm. above the apices of these teeth (Case Fig. 28–2A).

TREATMENT. The patient assumed full responsibility and insisted that an attempt be made to save the two teeth despite the extremely doubtful prognosis for the successful outcome of surgery.

A fine 45-degree-angle needle electrode was selected and current output set at 3 for electrosection. *(Note: The electrosurgery was performed with a unit having silicon rectifiers which operates efficiently at a setting of 0.5 less current output than the older units require.)* A vertico-oblique incision with the activated electrode was

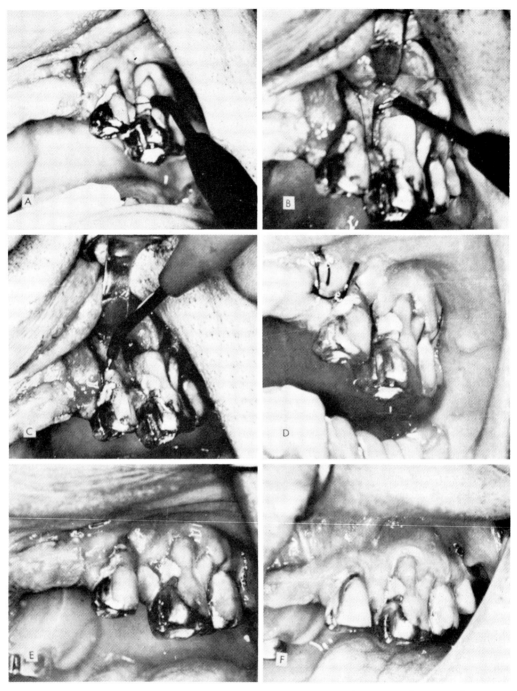

Case Figure 28–1.   Total amputation of buccal root of maxillary second bicuspid, root-end resection of palatal root of same tooth, and total amputation of mesiobuccal root of first molar close to trifurcation. *A,* Incision across interproximal papilla between the bicuspid and molar with 45-degree-angle fine needle electrode. Vertico-oblique incision anterior to the bicuspid has been performed. *B,* Incised flap has been retracted, root amputation and root-end resection of bicuspid completed, mesiobuccal root of molar resected and necrotic debris is being resected from its socket with a narrow U-shaped loop.

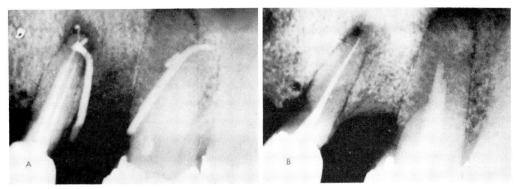

Case Figure 28-2. Roentgenographic sequence. *A,* Preoperative periapical view, with gutta-percha points inserted to determine depth of alveolar destruction around the two teeth. *B,* Immediate postoperative periapical view shows amputation of the two roots and the palatal root apex of the bicuspid.

started high in the mucobuccal fold in the cuspid area and carried downward and slightly posteriorly to the mesiogingival angle of the first bicuspid. The incision was carried across the edentulous saddle area between the two teeth; then the interproximal papilla attachment between the two molars was severed (Case Fig. 28–1*A*).

The incised tissue was undermined and retracted, exposing the alveolar bone. The buccal root of the first bicuspid was totally denuded of bone, and the mesiobuccal root of the molar was denuded about three fourths of its length. Both teeth had been devitalized many years previously.

The buccal root of the bicuspid was severed with a carbide bur immediately beyond the floor of the pulp chamber at the bifurcation. Then the mesiobuccal root of the molar was severed approximately 3 mm. beyond the trifurcation, and both roots were removed from their sockets. A huge amount of necrotic granulomatous debris was resected from the areas with surgical curets. The debris in the interradicular areas and other areas not readily accessible to curets was resected with a narrow 45-degree-angle U-shaped loop electrode (Case Fig. 28–1*B*). A few remaining adherent shreds were destroyed in situ by fulguration.

Approximately 3 mm. of the palatal root apex of the bicuspid was then resected and the necrotic periapical debris was removed. The gutta-percha root canal filling in each of the resected roots was sealed and sterilized by electrocoagulation with the small ball electrode (Case Fig. 28–1*C*). An immediate postoperative roentgenogram (Case Fig. 28–2*B*) was taken to ascertain that all the necrotic tissue had been resected.

After debridement was completed, medicated surgical gelatin powder was deposited into the defects and mixed with blood present in the two areas. The tissue flaps were restored and the margins coapted and sutured with 0000 braided silk interrupted sutures. Panalba and Kasdenol lavage were prescribed and instructions were given for postoperative home care.

The patient returned on the fifth postoperative day for removal of the sutures. The tissues were somewhat edematous but otherwise they appeared to be in reasonably good tone and healing was progressing by primary intention (Case Fig. 28–1*D*). He was seen postoperatively at weekly intervals for the next three weeks, during which time healing continued to progress favorably (Case Fig. 28–1*E*). By the end of that time there was a noteworthy decrease in mobility of the two teeth, with the bicuspid showing the greatest amount of improvement.

The patient left for a month's vacation and was not seen until the end of the second postoperative month. By that time healing was complete. The tissues were firmly reattached to the alveolar bone and readapted to the teeth (Case Fig. 28–1F). A postoperative roentgenogram taken at that time revealed evidence of regeneration of alveolar bone in the radiolucent areas.

The outcome has been highly successful and both teeth have remained functionally useful.

Maxillary Molar Palatal Roots — Subtotal Radectomy and Plastic Repair

The cases of subtotal radectomy that have just been reviewed demonstrate that it is possible with this technique to resect only the affected root or roots without need to sacrifice the corresponding coronal anatomy. The advantage is of course obvious. An abutment tooth treated in this manner continues to function as an effective abutment, undisturbed by the surgery.

It has traditionally been tacitly accepted that when the palatal root of the maxillary molar is hopelessly involved, this tooth is untreatable, regardless of technique, for two reasons; first, because the palatal root is the longest and strongest of its three roots, the all-important mainstay without which it would have difficulty withstanding the torque of function; and second, because loss of the palatal root would create a cavernous defect under the palatal aspect of the crown that would act as a food trap. Food particles trapped there would undergo decomposition. Their end-products, the amino acids, would irritate the tissues and in all probability cause tissue breakdown. Extensive decay of the crown and other roots would also be a likely aftermath.

Since the technique of subtotal radectomy results in repair of the root socket with bone and bone regeneration around the retained root stump, it prevents a cantilever effect on the crown, and eliminates the first reason cited in the preceding paragraph. By employing a simple plastic surgery procedure developed by the author, the second reason can also be effectively eliminated as a factor. The procedure consists of incising a flap of palatal tissue designed to serve as a tissue inlay that fits over and closes the root socket defect. This prevents formation of the cavernous depression under the crown and eliminates the factor of tissue irritation and decay due to trapped decomposing food debris.

The flap is contoured to fit snugly against the palatal aspect of the tooth crown, creating a surgical closure of the open root socket. The latter then proceeds to fill in with bone, like any tooth socket. Normal palatal contour is maintained partly by resting the tissue inlay flap on the 2- to 3-mm. fragment of root extending beyond the furca that is retained and partly by the sturdy texture and thickness of the flap tissue.

Most of the plastic oral surgery procedures are highly sophisticated and beyond the capabilities of the average general practitioner. The technique of plastic repair combined with subtotal radectomy developed by the author is a reasonably simple procedure that should be within the capabilities of those dentists who have had some modicum of experience and/or training in oral surgery. It is therefore being reviewed and demonstrated in this chapter instead of with the plastic oral surgery procedures that are reviewed in the following chapter.

The technique for plastic repair combined with subtotal radectomy that is about to be reviewed, and demonstrated by the following cases, overcomes the handicaps that would prevent normal repair of the bone and soft tissues and thus makes it possible to utilize the tooth for functional use as an abutment, despite the loss of this extremely important anchoring root.

CASE 29

PATIENT.   The patient in this case is the same as the one treated in Case 5 in Chapter 19.

HISTORY.   The palatal root of the isolated abutment molar that had been troublesome originally and required additional periodontal surgery several months after the initial surgery broke away from the rest of the tooth because of decay and began to cause discomfort. The isolated tooth was an invaluable abutment, since she had only the six anterior maxillary teeth remaining in addition to it. She therefore returned for the radectomy in the hope that it would succeed and permit retention of the molar to continue to serve as an abutment.

CLINICAL EXAMINATION.   The palatal root was completely separated from the rest of the tooth as a result of decay under the inferior margin of the large palatal Class V amalgam filling. The tissue around the retained root fragment appeared ulcerated (Case Fig. 29–1A). The gingivae around the remaining anterior teeth appeared to be in a normal state of health.

TREATMENT.   The tissues were prepared and a posterior superior alveolar block and palatine infiltration were administered. The palatal root was lifted out of the socket with a surgical elevator. The ulcerated palatal tissue at the root socket site was scooped out with a 45-degree-angle narrow U-shaped loop electrode with cutting current set at a power output of 5 (Case Fig. 29–1B) to create a bed for tissue inlay French sliding flap to be used for the plastic repair of the defect.

A 45-degree-angle fine needle electrode was substituted, current output was reduced to 3.5, and the activated electrode was used to incise the palatal mucosa down to, but not through, the periosteum to create a flap of mucosa that could be moved into the bed created for it, so that it would fit accurately around the palatal aspect of the molar crown and provide perfect margin coaptation with the palatal mucosa around the surgical defect (Case Fig. 29–1C).

The incised tissue was carefully elevated so as not to disturb the periosteal attachment to the bone. The tissue flap was rotated and seated into the bed that had been prepared for it, and the flap was sutured to the surrounding mucosa with which it was in perfect coaptation (Case Fig. 29–1D). A piece of Gelfoam sponge was inserted into the surgical defect created by the displacement of the tissue flap from its bed, and permitted to remain until the blood clotted with it, filling the defect. Tincture of myrrh and benzoin was applied in air-dried layers, and the denture, which had

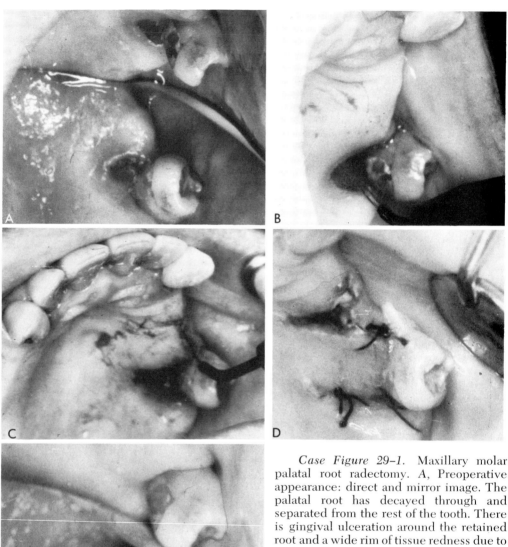

Case Figure 29–1. Maxillary molar palatal root radectomy. *A*, Preoperative appearance: direct and mirror image. The palatal root has decayed through and separated from the rest of the tooth. There is gingival ulceration around the retained root and a wide rim of tissue redness due to acute inflammation. *B*, The ulcerated tissue is being excised with a narrow U-shaped loop electrode, after the root fragment was removed from the area. The excision is being performed to create a definite bed for a tissue inlay. *C*, A mucoperiosteal flap of tissue, shaped to form a tissue inlay that will fit precisely into the bed that has been prepared to receive it is being cut with a 45-degree-angle needle electrode, with cutting current set at 4.5 on the instrument panel. *D*, The tissue inlay flap has been elevated and rotated into position to fit precisely around the palatal aspect of the tooth, and sutured into position with interrupted silk sutures, leaving a triangular surgical defect at the mesial aspect of the flap. *E*, Postoperative appearance of the tissues three weeks later, seen as a mirror image as well as directly. The distal line of incision is not visible, and the only evidence of the mesial line of incision and the surgical defect where the tissue had been shifted is a lack of fully matured keratinized epithelium which leaves the tissue surface slightly pinker in color than the almost white appearance of the heavily keratinized palatal epithelium. The tissue flap has adapted tightly around the tooth and the palatal tissue is convex, with no cavelike defect under the crown where the palatal root had been.

been sterilized, was inserted to serve as a protective surgical stent. The patient was reappointed with instructions for home postoperative care.

She returned on the fifth postoperative day for removal of the sutures. The palatal tissues showed clinical evidence of rapid, favorable repair by primary intention along the lines of incision, and the site from which the tissue flap had been removed also appeared to be progressing favorably. The sutures were removed and the patient was seen postoperatively at weekly intervals for several weeks. By the end of the third postoperative week the tissues were fully healed, and, except for a faintly pink appearance of the tissues along the original lines of incision due to incomplete maturation of the surface keratin, there was no clinical evidence of the surgery that had been performed. The palatal mucosa hugged the tooth's palatal contour tightly, and there was no cavernous or even slight depression under the crown of the tooth that could act as a food trap (Case Fig. 29–1E). The tooth continues to this day to serve as a functionally useful abutment, despite the torque to which it is being subjected from serving as an abutment for an unsurveyed half round wire clasp.

CASE 30

This case not only demonstrates the technique for the combined subtotal radectomy and plastic repair but also demonstrates how and why the procedure is successful despite what would appear to be insurmountable handicaps.

PATIENT. A 64-year-old white male.

HISTORY. He had had many maxillary teeth extracted years previously and had been wearing a very unsophisticated partial denture that was attached to the four remaining teeth in the maxilla with wrought wire clasps without rests. The palatal root of the right molar, terminal abutment for the restoration, began to cause distress, so he consulted a dentist, who found that the palatal root had decayed so badly that the root had almost separated from the rest of the tooth. He referred the patient for a root amputation, if possible, or extraction of the tooth.

CLINICAL EXAMINATION. There were four remaining maxillary teeth, all in poor condition. There was decay at the tissue level of the cuspid, and all the teeth appeared to have undergone gingival recession. The palatal root of the right molar was so badly decayed that it was obvious that it would have to be removed if the tooth were to be preserved (Case Fig. 30–1A).

TREATMENT. A posterior superior alveolar block and palatal infiltration anesthesia were administered. There was a copper cement filling on the palatal aspect of the tooth that extended almost to the level of the trifurcation. In order to remove the cement filling with the root, the latter was severed almost at the level of the furcation, leaving a stump of at most 1 mm. remaining (Case Fig. 30–1B). This was rounded as much as possible, and the gutta percha was resealed with an activated ball coagulating electrode. The bed for a tissue inlay flap was cut with a narrow U-shaped loop electrode (Case Fig. 30–2A). The incisions for the French sliding "tissue inlay" flap were made with a fine 45-degree-angle needle electrode, and cutting current output was set at 3.5 on the panel dial. The incisions were contoured to fit precisely around the palatal aspect of the crown of the tooth and into the bed that had been created for it (Case Fig. 30–2B). The tissue was elevated from the periosteum immediately after an x-ray was taken, and the freed tissue was tied with a suture to a tooth on the other

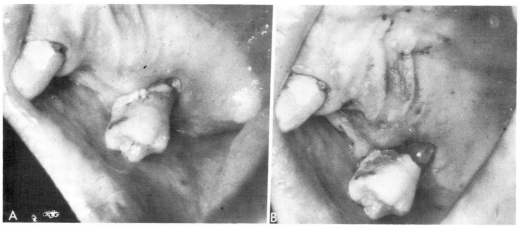

Case Figure 30–1. Radectomy of palatal and distobuccal molar roots. *A,* Preoperative appearance of maxillary right first molar. The palatal root has decayed through, is separated, and is a retained root. There is a large cement or Petralit filling between the separated root and the crown of the tooth. *B,* The palatal root is severed at the superior border of the cement filling.

side of the arch (Case Fig. 30–2C). By that time the x-ray was ready for a wet reading, and revealed a hard tumor mass on the apical two-thirds of the distobuccal root that might be a cementoma, but was also compatible with osteosarcoma (Case Fig. 30–2D).

It was imperative to remove the affected part of the root and some of the surrounding bone for differential diagnosis. The socket of the palatal root provided access to the distobuccal root, and the affected portion was severed with a fissure bur. The root fragment and some of the bone were preserved in formalin for biopsy. Another x-ray was taken to make sure that all the affected part of the root had been removed. The film verified that all that now remained was a short, slightly curved, and exostosed mesiobuccal root, and one-third of the distobuccal root (Case Fig. 30–2E).

Debridement was completed and powdered surgical gelatin was introduced into the defect and mixed with the blood present in it. The tissue flap was rotated into position in the bed prepared for it, so that it was tightly adapted around the palatal aspect of the crown of the tooth. The coapted tissue margins were perfect; they were sutured with interrupted silk sutures, and additional powdered gelatin was introduced into the surgical defect on the palate where the tissue flap had been obtained. When the blood and gelatin mixture was clotted, tincture of myrrh and benzoin was applied in air-dried layers, and the sterilized old denture was inserted to serve as a surgical stent to protect the area.

The patient returned on the fifth postoperative day for removal of the sutures. The coapted margins of tissue were almost fully healed, by primary intention, and the surgical defect on the palate showed evidence of favorable progress (Case Fig. 30–3A). Healing progressed very gratifyingly. By the end of the sixth week the palatal tissues looked quite normal and were tightly adapted around the crown of the tooth.

The patient was seen periodically for the next six months, and x-rays were taken to follow the course of bone regeneration. A final postoperative photograph taken at

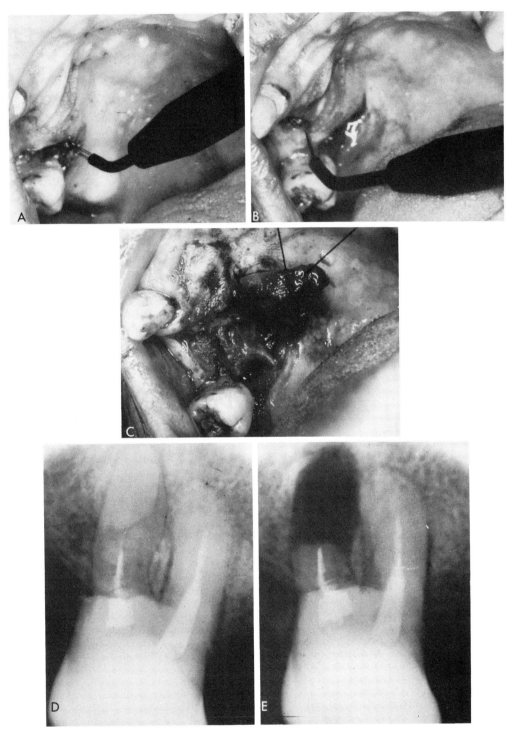

Case Figure 30–2. A, A preplanned bed for a tissue inlay is being excised with a narrow U-shaped loop electrode immediately after the root fragment has been extracted. *B*, The tissue for the "tissue inlay" is cut to fit precisely around the palatal aspect of the tooth and the bed that has been prepared for it. The mucoperiosteal flap is being incised with a 45-degree-angle needle electrode. *C*, The mucoperiosteal flap has been elevated and rotated and is tied to the two teeth on the left side to eliminate need for tissue retraction. *D*, A periapical x-ray reveals the presence of a hard tumor mass that may be malignant The apical two-thirds of the root and the mass must be removed for biopsy. *E*, The apical two-thirds and the hard mass that may be an osteoma or an osteosarcoma have been removed, as verified in the periapical x-ray film.

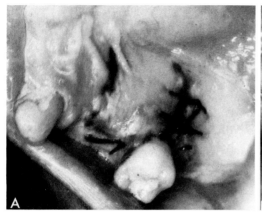
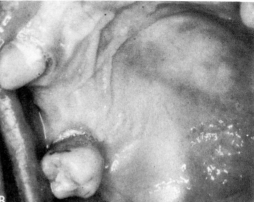
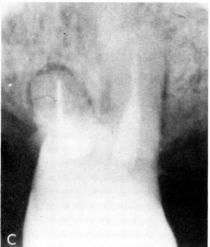

Case Figure 30–3 A, Appearance of the tissues on fifth postoperative day, before removing the sutures. There is no edema or inflammation present. B, Postoperative appearance of the tooth and tissues six months postoperatively. The healing is complete, and there is no concavitation under the crown of the tooth to act as a food trap The tooth is surprisingly firm. C, Five year postoperative x-ray shows why the tooth is so firm. There has been excellent regeneration around the remaining third of the distobuccal root and around the remaining 1 mm. of palatal root above the furcation, so that the tooth is solidly gripped by sound bone.

the end of the sixth month shows complete tissue healing, without evidence of concavitation under the crown of the molar (Case Fig. 30–3B). The tissue was firm and in excellent tone, and the tooth was the firmest of the four teeth left in the maxilla.

The patient was seen again five years postoperatively for treatment of another problem, and this made it possible to obtain a five-year postoperative x-ray of the tooth. This film revealed that the bone regeneration had filled the tooth sockets and surrounded the stump of the palatal root, so that the bone supported the crown as well as the original roots had done, and there was no cantilever effect from the loss of the roots (Case Fig. 30–3C). The bone was normal in all respects.

Results such as this present the question, when is a tooth hopeless? Apparently, only if, after having attempted to save it by surgical intervention, it fails to heal despite the effort. Such failures do not usually occur unless systemic or other unfavorable factors unrelated to the surgery are encountered, or the debridement has been incomplete, or the patient has neglected to take proper postoperative care of the wound. Otherwise, it is amazing how often apparently hopeless teeth respond favorably to electrosurgery combined with sound dental technique.

Mandibular Molar Root

CASE 31

This case offers irrefutable evidence that despite total involvement of one of the roots of a mandibular molar for which the affected root must be amputated, there is no need to perform a hemisection of the tooth in order to resect the diseased structure and retain the tooth for functional use. It offers visual evidence that there is no need to sacrifice the crown of the tooth to achieve this.

PATIENT. This was the same patient treated in Case 8 in Chapter 19.

HISTORY. The tooth being treated was the molar with the bifurcation involvement that failed to respond to periodontal therapy, perhaps owing to failure to use fulguration to assure destruction of diseased tissue fragments in the furca.

CLINICAL EXAMINATION. The infrabony pocket that communicated with the bifurcation was filled with granulomatous debris. Roentgenographic examination revealed radiolucence that enveloped the distal root entirely and also most of the mesial root (Case Fig. 31–1A).

TREATMENT. An inferior alveolar block was administered, and a molar gutta percha point was inserted into the defect to serve as a radiopaque marker for more accurate determination of the extent of bone destruction. A periapical x-ray was taken with the gutta percha point in place (Case Fig. 31–1B). This film confirmed that the destruction went to the apex of the distal root of the molar, and was just short of the apex of the mesial root.

A 45-degree-angle fine needle electrode was selected, activated with cutting current output set at 3, and used to make a vertico-oblique incision extending from the mesiogingival angle of the tooth downward and anteriorly to the mucogingival junction. The incised tissue was elevated and reflected, exposing the bifurcation and a considerable amount of denuded root. The root was severed from the tooth approximately 2 mm. beyond the furca with a fissure bur and removed from its socket. The socket was thoroughly debrided, grossly with a small surgical curet and an excavator and then with a flame-shaped loop and a narrow U-shaped loop electrode. The latter was used to debride the furca, and this was followed by fulguration, with the sparks directed into the furcation. The base of the cut root stump was then smoothed and rounded with diamond stones, and the gutta percha at the cut root end was resealed by coagulating with a ball coagulating electrode with current output set at 3 on the dial.

When it appeared that debridement was completed the surgical field was inspected with the aid of a transilluminating light and digital inspection with an inactivated 17-mm. periodontal curet electrode. This inspection confirmed that the debridement was completed, and an immediate postoperative x-ray was taken. This film revealed the huge area of radiolucence, with the 2-mm. stump of root suspended in the radiolucent void (Case Fig. 31–1C).

Powdered surgical gelatin was introduced into the defect and mixed with the blood, and the tissue flap was restored to position. The coapted margins were sutured with interrupted silk sutures. The patient was then reappointed for removal of the sutures. He returned on the fifth postoperative day, and the sutures were removed. Healing by primary intention appeared to be progressing very favorably by primary intention.

The patient was seen at regular weekly intervals for six weeks, then semimonthly

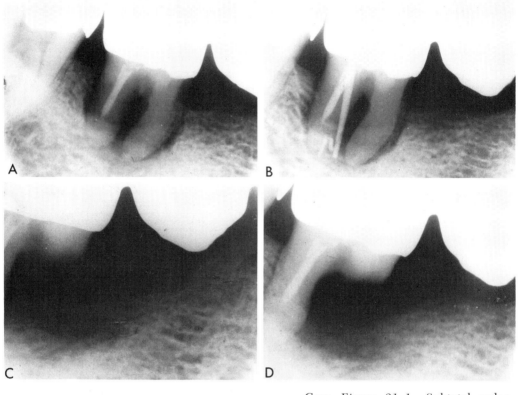

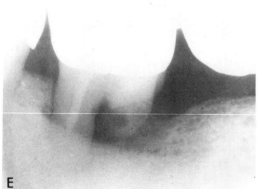

Case Figure 31–1. Subtotal radectomy of a mandibular molar root *A*, Roentgenographic appearance of the right first molar. There is an incomplete root canal filling in the mesial root and no filling in the distal root. All but the apices of the two roots appear to have had their investing alveolar bone destroyed. *B*, Roentgenogram with a molar gutta percha point inserted into the defect to serve as a radiopaque marker. The point has penetrated to the level of the apices of the tooth. The destruction appears to be slightly short of the apex of the mesial root but appears to involve the distal root apex. *C*, Roentgenographic appearance of the tooth immediately after a subtotal radectomy of the distal root had been completed and thorough debridement performed The 2-mm. stump of the distal root is suspended in a radiolucent void. *D*, Roentgenographic appearance of the tooth six weeks later. There is distinct evidence of bone regeneration filling in the void gradually from the base of the defect. *E*, Roentgenographic appearance of the tooth twelve weeks postoperatively. There is a complete fill-in of the cavity with new bone which surrounds the base of the 2-mm. root stump. The bone appears normal and normal trabeculation can be seen, although it is not yet maturely calcified. There has been equally gratifying regeneration of bone around the mesial root.

for another six weeks. By the end of that period the wound was fully healed clinically, with no visual evidence of the surgery. Roentgenograms were taken at the end of the sixth postoperative week and at the end of the twelfth week. The one taken at the end of the sixth week showed distinct evidence of bone regeneration progressing from the base of the defect upward toward the root stump (Case Fig. 31–1D). The film taken at the end of the twelfth week showed a complete fill-in of the cavity with new bone which extends to and slightly around the base of the 2-mm. root stump. The bone appeared normal, and although not yet fully calcified, normal trabeculation can be seen (Case Fig. 31–1E). The bone has regenerated completely around the mesial root. Clinically the tooth remains functionally useful without sacrifice of half of the crown.

This roentgenographic evidence of the rate and quality of bone regeneration, plus the evidence that the bone is filling into the furcation as well as the root sockets, offers visual evidence that there can be no cantilever effect on the crown of the tooth owing to the root resection, since the bone is providing the support previously provided by the roots, and that therefore there is no need whatever to sacrifice half the crown to preserve the tooth.

FOOTNOTE REFERENCES

1. Wyeth, G. A.: Surgery of Neoplastic Diseases by Electrothermic Methods. New York, Paul P. Hoeber, Inc., 1926.
2. Oringer, M. J.: Plastic oral surgery: A new term. New York J. Den., 18(11):345, Nov., 1948.
3. Archer, W. H.: A Manual of Oral Surgery. 2nd ed. Philadelphia, W. B. Saunders Co., 1956, pp. 182–222.
4. Ibid, pp. 440–448.
5. Ibid, pp. 551–556.
6. Ibid, pp. 588–613.
7. Ibid, pp. 629–668.
8. Ibid, pp. 668–720.
9. Thoma, K. H.: Oral Surgery. 3rd ed. St. Louis, C. V. Mosby Co., 1958, pp. 282–290.
10. Ibid, pp. 1388–1486.
11. Ibid, pp. 322–389.
12. Manual of Standard Practice of Plastic Maxillo-Facial Surgery. Military Surgery Manuals, National Research Council. Philadelphia, W. B. Saunders Co., 1942, pp. 253–255.
13. Color Atlas of Oral Pathology. Philadelphia, J. B. Lippincott Co., 1956.
14. Shafer, W. G., Hine, M. K., and Levy, B. M.: A Textbook of Oral Pathology. Philadelphia, W. B. Saunders Co., 1974.
15. Kruger, G. O.: Management of impactions. Symposium on Office Oral Surgery. D. Clin. North America, Nov., 1959, pp. 707–722.
16. Winter, G. B.: Exodontia. St. Louis, American Medical Book Co., 1913, pp. 137–138.
17. Ibid, pp. 179–183.
18. Ibid, pp. 283–315.
19. Winter, G. B.: Principles of Exodontia as Applied to the Impacted Mandibular Third Molar. St. Louis, American Medical Book Co., 1926.
20. Blair, V. P., and Ivy, R. H.: Essentials of Oral Surgery. St. Louis, C. V. Mosby Co., 1923, pp. 253–258.
21. Berger, A.: The Principles and Techniques of Oral Surgery. Brooklyn, N. Y., Dental Items of Interest Publishing Co., 1923, pp. 299–323.
22. Berger, A.: The Principles and Techniques of the Removal of Teeth. Brooklyn, N. Y., Dental Items of Interest Publishing Co., 1929, pp. 220–269.
23. Winter, L., Harrigan, W. F., and Winter, L. Jr.: Textbook of Exodontia. 6th ed. St. Louis, C. V. Mosby Co., 1953, pp. 173–286.
24. Pell, G. J., and Gregory, G.: Report on a ten-year study of tooth division techniques for the removal of impacted teeth. Am. J. O. & O. S., 28, Nov., 1942.
25. Oringer, M. J.: The electromagnet as an aid in the removal of a traumatically impacted metallic fragment from the body of the mandible in the vicinity of the mandibular canal. Oral Surg., Oral Med. and Oral Path., 3(2):169–178, Feb., 1950.
26. Thoma, op. cit., p. 402.
27. Blum, T.: Root amputation; a study of one hundred and fity-nine cases. J.A.D.A., 17:249–261, Feb., 1960.
28. Trice, F. B.: Periapical surgery. Symposium on Office Oral Surgery. Dent. Clin. N. Amer., Nov., 1959, pp. 735–748.

Chapter Twenty-Two

MAJOR ORAL SURGERY

Introduction

The principal difference between the electrosurgical techniques that were reviewed in the preceding chapter and those reviewed in this chapter is the greater degree of special skill and surgical training that is necessary to perform these techniques efficiently and effectively.

The cases that were reviewed in the preceding chapter dealt with surgical correction of relatively commonplace oral defects and pathologic conditions that required surgical correction. The electrosurgical techniques for effecting the corrections are more or less routine, many well within the capabilities of most general practitioners. Even the experimental techniques that were described in the first edition as imaginative and daring are now relatively commonplace, since most of them were elaborations or variations of established routine surgical procedures.

This chapter concerns itself with much more complex and sophisticated electrosurgical techniques developed by the author to treat extensive pathology,[1] unusual trauma,[2] and anatomic abnormalities and deviations.[3-8] Cases of this type usually require extensive repair or reconstruction of the damaged or destroyed anatomic structures in order to restore functional and aesthetic normalcy.

The urgent need for such restoration to normalcy will be repeatedly demonstrated in the clinical cases, which will describe a variety of techniques employed to achieve the desired results. Some of these techniques are more or less traditional and stylized; others are variations of traditional techniques. Still others are original techniques developed by the author specifically for electrosurgical instrumentation which make full use of the advantages this modality offers.

To facilitate reading and assure better continuity, the subject matter of the chapter has been subdivided into four major categories:

I. Management of extensive cysts

902

II. Plastic oral surgery techniques
III. Sialolithotomy of the submaxillary duct and gland
IV. Miscellaneous techniques

I. MANAGEMENT OF EXTENSIVE CYSTS

Oral surgeons have been using the Partsch method of marsupialization of large cysts in preference to surgical enucleation of the cystic sacs ever since this technique was introduced.

There is valid reason for their preference for marsupialization when the surgery is to be performed with a steel scalpel and curets. To marsupialize a cyst, all or only part of the covering tissue and top of the cystic sac must be excised. The resultant bleeding is superficial and can easily be controlled. If the cystic content is liquid, the fluid is evacuated through the opening which also serves as the entry for introduction of the large gauze packs that must fill the cystic cavity until the defect fills in and is obliterated. This contrasts sharply with the profuse deep bleeding that is likely to be encountered if total enucleation is attempted by steel manual instrumentation. The hemorrhagic bleeding is likely to obscure the surgical field to so great a degree that despite vigorous aspiration thorough efficient enucleation of the entire epithelium-lined sac is extremely difficult to accomplish.

That marsupialization offers distinct advantages under such conditions is undeniable, but the advantages are counterbalanced by several distinct disadvantages. It seems as though there is an immutable law of nature that a compensatory price must be paid for every advantage. The price that must be paid for the advantage of eliminating the hemorrhage and need to enucleate the entire cystic sac, with the inherent risk that failure to remove every speck of it will result in recurrence of the cyst, is the agonizingly slow rate of healing of a marsupialized defect. Not only is it necessary to devote much time to repeated repacking of the gauze until the defect has filled in, but despite the packing marsupialization usually falls short of restoring normal anatomic contours. More often than not, marsupialization results in marked concavitation that creates anatomic deformities that can seriously complicate prosthetic restoration.

With the hemostasis enjoyed with fully rectified cutting current (and the modified continuous wave current of the Ritter circuit), it is possible to surgically enucleate large cysts with meticulous thoroughness due to unimpaired visibility in the surgical field and the ability to destroy in situ by fulguration any adherent tissue shreds that cannot be removed manually.

The anatomic deformity can be averted if powdered surgical gelatin (powdered Gelfoam) is introduced into the debrided cystic cavity and mixed with blood present in the defect. The resultant spongy mass of gelatin and blood clot provides excellent support for the tissue flap when it is restored to position, thus eliminating the hazard of having the covering mucosa slough away. The gelatin also appears to accelerate the healing rate and bone regeneration.

The gelatin serves as a graft material and becomes an integral part of the repair process, thereby greatly minimizing the possibility of surgical dead spaces. It has been reported that sterile plaster of paris also can be used as the graft material, but the author has had no experience with it and therefore cannot personally recommend it. He *has* had many years of clinical experience with powdered gelatin (and the despeciated cultured calf bone products that proved superbly useful in several of the cases reported,* but regrettably are no longer available, even for experimental use). He can therefore personally testify to the beneficial usefulness of the powdered gelatin.

It is interesting to note, as was emphasized in the chapter on medication, that powdered gelatin can be used advantageously in cystic cavities that are closed by suturing, whereas the same gelatin in sponge form breaks down and liquefies when placed into closed cavities. It is, however, an excellent graft material for use in open wounds. The cystic cavity should not be overfilled with gelatin, since this would impair development of blood circulation in the repair tissue. The potential for total obliteration of the cystic cavity without anatomic deformity is greatly enhanced if, in addition to the advantages derived from use of electrosurgery and the gelatin powder graft, there is assurance that an uninterrupted postoperative blood supply to the surgical field will be attained and maintained.

Development of such a postoperative blood supply in a long-standing large cystic cavity is usually more a biomechanical problem than a biological one. The body does not discard and excrete calcium from bone that has been destroyed by a cyst except in a few isolated systemic diseases. The calcium is merely repositioned. The bone destruction is very gradual and is caused by pressure exerted against the bone by the expanding cystic sac. As the bone is being destroyed, the calcium it had contained is not carried away by the blood circulation but is displaced laterally into the immediately adjacent surrounding bone. Owing to the increase in its calcium content, this bony perimeter becomes very dense and sclerotic, and the bone surface in contact with the cyst often becomes eburnated. The nutrient foramina in the eburnated bone become sealed and obliterated. This results in cutting off the blood that circulates through the Haversian system of canals and the nutrient canals from entry into the cystic cavity.

In order to restore communication between the cystic cavity and the blood circulating in the inner spongiosum of the bone it is necessary to make a number of perforations through the eburnated layer with a small round bur. The same bur can then be used to scarify and roughen up the smooth eburnated surface of the bone to help the clotting blood to adhere as it contracts. The scarification, by preventing detachment of the blood clot from the bone surface, greatly reduces the likelihood of formation of a surgical dead space as the healing progresses. The report on treatment of a nasopalatine cyst, in which the bony surface of the cystic defect was markedly eburnated, will provide an excellent example of the advantageous use of this procedure.

---

*See Case Figure 3–2, page 914, and Case Figure 9–3, page 940.

Mandibular Cyst

Histologically, it has been accepted as factual that cysts develop from embryonal epithelial enclaves. It is true that many cysts do not develop spontaneously but are triggered by irritation and/or trauma. The first case in this series is being included because it appears to offer a direct clue to the triggering mechanism that was responsible for the cystic degeneration.

CASE 1

The tooth that was affected had been treated endodontically many years previously. Exposure of the cystic area revealed total destruction of the investing alveolar bone and physical displacement of the tooth out of the dental arch, resulting in clinical exposure of the apex of the tooth and extrusion of gutta percha beyond the apex.

When the apical end of a gutta percha root canal filling becomes extruded owing to apical resorption, the surface of the remaining root end becomes pitted and rough, with an irregular, often jagged outline. In this case the root end was smooth and normal in contour, indicating that extrusion of gutta percha had resulted from overfilling the canal originally and not from resorption.

It appears likely that detritus may have been forced through the apex of the tooth during the endodontic treatment, and chemical agents used to sterilize the canal may also have penetrated through the apical orifice and caused periapical irritation. Since development of a cyst is a slow process, continuing irritation from the protruding gutta percha appears likely to have been the major triggering mechanism.

This case also offers an interesting demonstration that the extensive destruction of investing alveolar bone and subsequent physical displacement of the tooth out of the dental arch do not necessarily make the prognosis for successful treatment hopeless.

PATIENT. A 67-year-old white female.

HISTORY. Her mandibular left cuspid had been treated endodontically several years previously. The following year the second bicuspid and first molar in that quadrant had been extracted and replaced with a fixed prosthesis. Within the past year she had begun to notice that the devitalized cuspid was moving outward toward her lip, and she was aware of discomfort in that area at mealtimes. She consulted her dentist, a roentgenogram was taken, and she was referred for either extraction or, if at all possible, treatment to retain the tooth.

CLINICAL EXAMINATION. There was a marked labial displacement of the mandibular left cuspid alveolar contour. On palpation there was no resistance but a rubbery resilience when digital pressure was applied to the bulging area. The entire tooth appeared to be displaced labially. X-ray examination revealed that the apex of the tooth was tilted labially and anteriorly, so that the root of the tooth was lying across the root of the lateral incisor. There was a huge radiolucent area between the distal surface of the displaced tooth and the mesial surface of the first bicuspid, with only a small triangle of bone remaining at the coronal end of the alveolar bone (Case Fig. 1–2A).

TREATMENT. The quadrant was prepared and an inferior alveolar block injection was administered. A 45-degree-angle fine needle electrode was selected and ac-

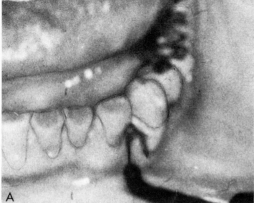

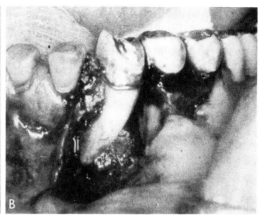

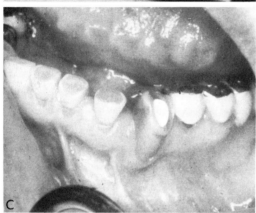

Case Figure 1–1. Surgical removal of a large mandibular cyst. *A,* The apical attachments of the interdental papillae have been severed from the lateral-cuspid embrasure posteriorly with a fine 45-degree-angle needle electrode. The activated electrode is seen being used to incise the labial mucoperiosteum in a vertico-oblique direction downward and forward from the distogingival angle of the lateral to the mesial aspect of the cuspid at its mucogingival termination. *B,* The incised mucoperiosteum has been reflected, revealing total destruction of the alveolar bone around the root of the cuspid and a large dehiscence on the mesial aspect of the first bicuspid root. A large semisolid mass of degenerative cystic tissue envelops the root of the cuspid. The latter protrudes bodily beyond the normal dental arch and could easily be removed as a finger extraction. Gutta percha can be seen extruded through the apical foramen of the tooth. Note the stainless steel ligature that has been tied to the cuspid and attached to the bicuspids to prevent accidental extraction of the tooth by displacement during debridement of the defect. *C,* Six month postoperative clinical appearance of the surgical field. The tooth is in relatively normal alignment, with very slight residual labial rotation. The gingival tissue appears firm and normal in all respects, and the tooth is nonmobile on digital palpation, without fixation to the adjacent teeth.

tivated, with cutting current set at 3, and a vertico-oblique incision was created from the marginal gingiva to the mucogingival junction. The incision was then extended to sever the apex of the lateral-cuspid interdental papilla (Case Fig. 1–1A). The mucoperiosteal flap was reflected downward and posteriorly, revealing a huge mass of cystic tissue enveloping the root except on its labial surface. About 2.5 mm. of gutta percha could be seen protruding through the apex of the tooth (Case Fig. 1–1B).

The tooth was so completely displaced from the dental arch that it was deemed impossible to attempt to treat it without some degree of immobilization to avoid displacing it irretrievably, so it was ligated to the bicuspid with a soft stainless steel ligature. The gross debridement of the cystic mass was performed with a steel curet. Fragments of cystic tissue that adhered tenaciously to the root surface and to the mesial surface of the first bicuspid, which was largely denuded of bone, and the tissue wedged between the lingual surface of the cuspid and the labial surface of the lateral root upon which it was lying were destroyed in situ by fulguration. The protruding tip of gutta percha was removed, and the apex was coagulated with a ball electrode to seal the gutta percha.

The absence of free bleeding made it possible to inspect the area meticulously to make certain that no cystic fragments had been overlooked. Debridement having been completed, bleeding was induced in the area and powdered surgical gelatin was inserted and mixed with the blood to form a spongy mass that proceeded to clot and fill the defect. Healing progressed uneventfully. On the fifth postoperative day the sutures were removed, and thereafter the patient was seen at weekly intervals and then semi-monthly for 10 weeks, during which time the periodic x-ray examinations revealed filling in of the radiolucent area. The patient was referred back to her dentist with a request that the cuspid be splinted to the first bicuspid with a pin splint.

The dentist was reluctant to drill into the veneer crown of the bicuspid, which was the anterior terminal abutment for the fixed prosthesis. He therefore permitted the ligature to remain for another month before removing it. He reported that he saw no reason for splinting the tooth, since it was now firmly embedded in the alveolar bone. The patient returned as requested at the end of 6 months for a final postoperative observation. The tooth was firm and able to withstand considerable digital pres-

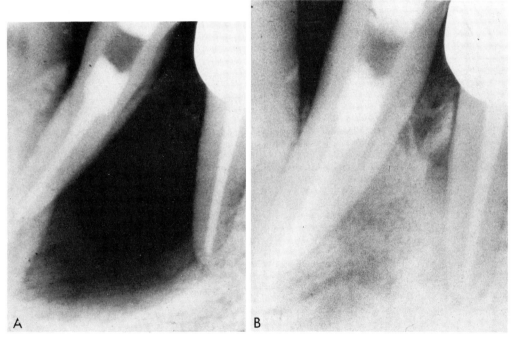

Case Figure 1–2. A, Preoperative periapical roentgenogram of the affected tooth. The left cuspid is rotated completely out of the dental arch, with a huge area of radiolucence between the cuspid and first bicuspid. The degree of radiolucence in the center of the dark area strongly suggests that both the buccal and lingual cortical plates have been perforated. The radiolucent area is circular in shape, and there is a small remnant of interseptal bone in the embrasure immediately superior to the radiolucent area, in the vicinity of the cemento-enamel junctions of the two teeth. B, Six month postoperative roentgenogram of the area shows filling in of the radiolucent area with regenerated bone, with the root of the tooth in relatively normal position in the dental arch. Evidence of bone trabeculation on the cuspid root, combined with the complete obliteration of the radiolucent area and absence of clinical labial alveolar concavitation, indicates that the labial bone as well as the interseptal bone has fully regenerated. The tooth has not been immobilized by attachment to the adjacent teeth and is therefore withstanding the torque of function solely as a result of regeneration of normal mature investing bone.

sure. The tissues around the tooth were normal in all respects, and the lines of incision were fully healed and invisible (Case Fig. 1–1C). A final roentgenogram revealed that the former radiolucent area was now filled in with bone, and there was evidence that the bond had regenerated on the labial aspect judging from the appearance of trabeculation (Case Fig. 1–2B).

Nasopalatine Cyst

According to Thoma,[9] a recognized variety of cysts form in the incisive canal of the maxilla. They may be located in the center of the bone, in which event they are incisive canal cysts, or they may develop under the papilla palatina in the incisive foramen and are cysts of the papilla palatina.

Both varieties result from persistence beyond the first year of life of embryonal epithelial tissue of the nasopalatine duct or its remnants, a middle epithelial cord or epithelial rests in the most posterior part of the papilla palatina. Both are usually referred to as a nasopalatine cyst and are reputed to occur in adults ranging from 32 to 73 years of age.[10]

The papilla palatina variety of cysts usually expand outwardly toward the buccal cavity, often destroying the thin dorsal bone plate. The cyst in the case that is about to be reviewed was somewhat atypical, since the bone destruction was not limited to the dorsal bone but also included considerable destruction of the bone base of the nasopalatine foramen, with marked eburnation of the surface of the defect.

CASE 2

PATIENT.   A 59-year-old white male in normal health. He was referred for the diagnosis and treatment of a swelling in the anterior part of the palate.

CLINICAL EXAMINATION.   There were only four teeth remaining in the maxilla: the left central and lateral incisors, cuspid, and first molar. Immediately behind the central incisor and the edentulous area of the right central incisor there was a swelling on the palate. The surface of the swelling greatly resembled enlarged rugae (Case Fig. 2–1A). On palpation the swelling was compressible, but it felt moderately firm and resilient rather than fluctuant. The swollen area appeared moderately red, in contrast to the pink color of the rest of the palate.

ROENTGENOGRAPHIC EXAMINATION.   Intraoral periapical and occlusal x-ray films were taken. They revealed a radiolucent area on the mesial aspect of the central incisor, extending beyond the apex approximately 2 cm. down toward the coronal end of the tooth. The area appeared to extend beyond the normal area of the nasopalatine foramen and seemed somewhat larger in dimension than the foramen. (See Case Fig. 2–3.)

TREATMENT.   The tissues were prepared for surgery and local anesthesia was administered. An incision for a mucoperiosteal flap was made along the edentulous

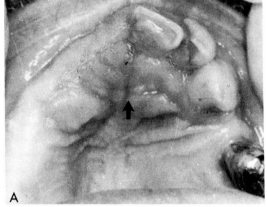
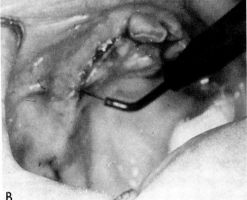
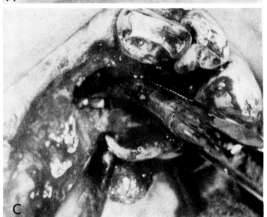

Case Figure 2–1. Elimination of a nasopalatine cyst. *A*, Preoperative appearance. A large area in the anterior part of the palate in the nasopalatine area and involving the papilla is swollen and somewhat darker in color than the surrounding tissues (arrow). There is a feeling of crepitus on digital palpation of the swelling. *B*, An incision for a mucoperiosteal flap is being made along the crest of the edentulous alveolar ridge from the distal of the left central posteriorly to the molar region. The incision is being made by electrosection with a 45-degree-angle fine needle electrode at a cutting power output of 4 on the instrument panel. Blood is present along the line of incision but there is no free bleeding. *C*, The mucoperiosteal flap has been elevated from the palate with the broad end of a periosteal elevator, which is being used to retract the tissue. A major part of the cystic sac has been enucleated. A few tenaciously adherent fragments of the sac that have torn away from the main body of the sac are being grasped with the long slender beaks of a curved mosquito hemostat and removed from the cystic crypt. Absence of free bleeding makes it possible to identify and carefully displace the nasopalatine nerve and blood vessel, so that they will not be injured by the instrumentation. (Fragments that resisted removal with the hemostat or were inaccessible to it were destroyed in situ by fulguration.)

alveolar ridge crest, from the mesial of the gingival margin to approximately the first bicuspid region (Case Fig. 2–1*B*); the apices of the interdental papillae on the palatal aspect of the central-lateral and lateral-cuspid embrasures were then incised with a 45-degree-angle fine needle electrode used with the cutting power generator knob set at 4.5 on the Coles Radiosurg unit. The incised tissue was gently but firmly pried loose from its attachment to the palate bone, with care exercised to avoid damage to the nasopalatine nerve and artery. Considerable pressure had to be exerted to pry the tissue free, and, despite precautions, the top of the cystic sac, which had coalesced to the flap at one point, tore away when the flap came free, allowing cystic fluid in the sac to escape. The remainder of the cystic sac was carefully removed from its bone crypt by blunt dissection, with care exercised to avoid injury to the nasopalatine nerve. Bleeding was minimal and readily controlled by electrocoagulation of a small bleeder vessel (Case Fig. 2–1*C*).

When all the cystic tissue appeared to have been removed, the bone cavity was packed with a strip of selvage gauze impregnated with BIP paste (bismuth, iodoform, and petrolatum), and another intraoral periapical x-ray film was taken. Being radio-paque, the pack clearly delineated the extent of the bone defect and showed that the entire cystic mass had been removed (Case Fig. 2–3B). When the pack was removed, the area was free of blood and the bone defect could be seen. The surface of the bone appeared dense and eburnated. To reduce the likelihood of a postoperative surgical dead space the sclerotic bone was perforated in several areas with a small round bur to penetrate into the underlying cancellous bone, and the surface of the bone was scarified to roughen the smooth shiny surface. When the blood that filled the bone cavity was clotted, the flap was restored to its place and sutured through the embrasures as well as along the crest of the ridge. The patient was given the usual postoperative instructions for home care and reappointed.

He was seen again on the fifth postoperative day. The tissue tone was good, there was no edema or inflammation, and the incised tissue appeared to have begun to heal by primary intention (Case Fig. 2–2A). The sutures were removed, and the patient was instructed to return in one week, at which time marked improvement was noted (Case Fig. 2–2B). He returned at weekly intervals for a month for a further post-operative follow-up. By the end of the month the area appeared fully healed and normal (Case Fig. 2–2C).

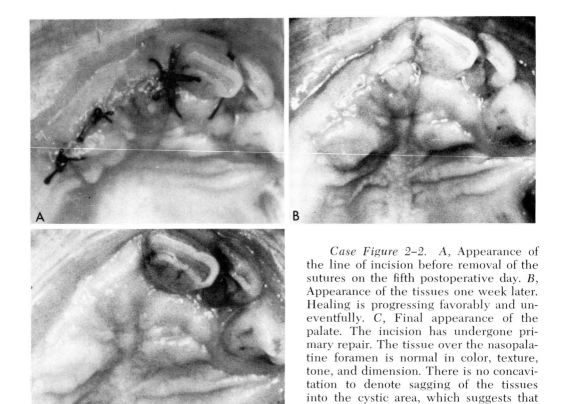

Case Figure 2–2. A, Appearance of the line of incision before removal of the sutures on the fifth postoperative day. B, Appearance of the tissues one week later. Healing is progressing favorably and un-eventfully. C, Final appearance of the palate. The incision has undergone pri-mary repair. The tissue over the nasopala-tine foramen is normal in color, texture, tone, and dimension. There is no concavi-tation to denote sagging of the tissues into the cystic area, which suggests that bone has filled in around the foramen.

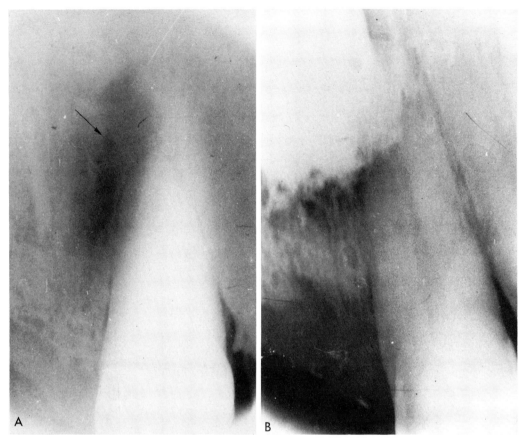

Case Figure 2–3. A, Preoperative roentgenogram. The extent of the cystic involvement is not well defined. Arrow points to what appears to be the base of the defect. *B*, Immediate postoperative roentgenogram with radiopaque gauze pack inserted into the defect to visualize its full extent and to ascertain whether complete enucleation has been achieved.

CASE 3

This case is an excellent example of the effectiveness of the combined use of electrosurgery and organic implants to produce rapid complete repair of large cystic defects by normal osteoblastic regeneration. It also demonstrates the pathologic fracture that may result from extensive bone destruction wrought by pressure from a large, progressively expanding cyst. A method of treatment is described which permits healing by primary intention without deformity or loss of normal alveolar contour.

PATIENT. A 70-year-old white male.

HISTORY. Sudden appearance of a suppurating fistulous orifice in the anterior part of the maxilla led to the roentgenographic discovery of an impacted malposed cuspid in an edentulous saddle area. His dentist planned to extract several teeth and construct partial dentures. He was referred for the removal of the impacted tooth.

CLINICAL EXAMINATION. *Extraoral.* Negative.

Intraoral. He had six teeth left in the maxilla: the left central and lateral incisors, cuspid, first bicuspid, and the right central and lateral incisors. The rest of the dental arch was clinically edentulous.

The labial alveolar bone plate bulged slightly, and there was a puffy swelling in the labial vestibule. A fistulous orifice was present close to the crest of the alveolar ridge about 1 cm. distal to the right lateral incisor. Light pressure produced a copious flow of purulent exudate from the fistulous tract.

A flexible silver probe was gently inserted into the defect. After penetrating about 1 cm. it encountered solid resistance (Case Fig. 3–1A). A roentgenogram was taken with the probe in position. This revealed the probe in contact with an impacted cuspid that was lying horizonto-obliquely parallel with the crest of the alveolar ridge. A large radiolucent area surrounded the crown of the impacted tooth and extended upward. The appearance and location of the radiolucent area suggested a follicular or dentigerous cyst.

TREATMENT. The mouth was prepared for surgery, and bilateral infraorbital and nasopalatine regional block anesthesia were administered. A heavy, long needle electrode was selected and current output set at 9 for fulguration. The orifice of the fistula was fulgurated until it was completely carbonized. The electrode was then inserted into the defect as far as it could penetrate and the tract was thoroughly desiccated.

A 45-degree-angle fine needle electrode was then selected and current output set at 3.5 for electrosection. A vertico-oblique incision was started at the mucolabial fold and extended downward to the mesiogingival angle of the left lateral (Case Fig. 3–1B). Then the crest of the alveolar ridge on the right side was incised in an antero-posterior direction to the second bicuspid area.

The incised tissue was undermined and retracted revealing a large, bulging white mass in the labial vestibule which involved the entire alveolar ridge area in the anterior region of the maxilla (Case Fig. 3–1C). The tough fibrous cystic sac was enucleated by blunt dissection and removed. Cystic pressure had destroyed the floor of the nasal fossa; when the mass was removed an aberrant blood vessel in the region of the floor, which had been attached to the mass, tore and hemorrhaged profusely.

The bleeder vessel was clamped with a mosquito hemostat and the hemorrhage was brought under control by electrocoagulation off the beaks of the hemostat. When the hemorrhage was halted, the overlying bone was removed to expose the full length of the impacted tooth (Case Fig. 3–1D). The crown of this tooth was tightly wedged between the apical third of the central and lateral roots. The labial and palatal bone around the teeth was so thin that it was evident that removal of the impacted tooth would result in pathologic fracture of the alveolar segment containing the two teeth.

Even though it was planned that these teeth would eventually be extracted, it appeared advisable to try to retain the two teeth and the maxillary fragment containing them in order to help maintain a normal ridge contour during the healing period. Otherwise, the loss of a substantial part of the anterior maxilla would cause a collapse resulting in marked deformity, particularly when superimposed on the huge bone loss due to the cystic destruction.

The impacted tooth was removed. As had been anticipated, it caused the buccal alveolar plate containing the two teeth to fracture. The fractured fragment tilted at a right angle to the alveolar ridge and the previously controlled bleeder again began to hemorrhage. It took electrocoagulation with a large ball electrode and current output set at 4 for biterminal electrocoagulation to bring it under control again (Case Fig. 3–1E).

Complete debridement of the area was then performed. Irregular bone edges, some tissue-thin, were trimmed smooth. The fracture was reduced by restoring the fragment and its teeth to normal alignment and immobilizing it with continuous-loop intramaxillary wiring. The huge defect was filled with a mixture of bone paste, bone

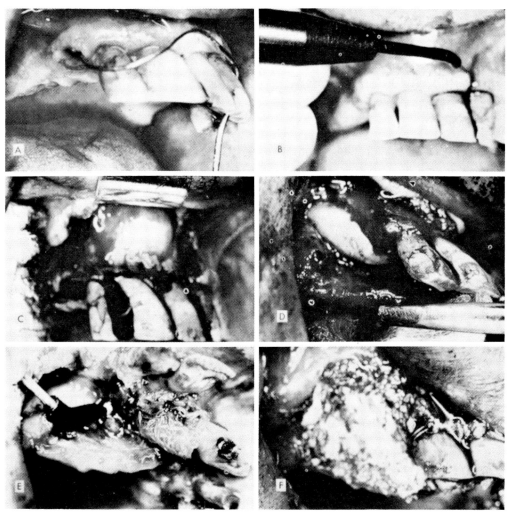

Case Figure 3-1. Removal of malposed impacted maxillary cuspid, complicated by presence of large cyst, and repair of pathologic fracture to retain normal alveolar contour. *A*, Preoperative view. Silver probe has been inserted through a labial fistulous orifice. *B*, Vertico-oblique flap incision with a fine 45-degree-angle needle electrode, extending from junction of the labiogingival mucosa to the mesiogingival angle of the lateral on the opposite side. *C*, Flap retraction exposes a huge bulging round cystic mass to view. *D*, Cyst having been enucleated, removal of overlying bone exposes the malposed ankylosed impacted cuspid to view. *E*, Hemorrhage from reinjury to an arteriole by pathologic fracture of the alveolar process with two teeth controlled by coagulation with a large ball electrode. *F*, Impacted tooth removed, fracture reduced and immobilized by intramaxillary continuous-loop wiring, the surgical defect is filled with a mixture of cultured bone paste and chips and medicated surgical powdered gelatin.

chips and surgical gelatin (Case Fig. 3–1F). The flap was restored to position; the margins were coapted and secured with 0000 braided silk interrupted sutures inserted along the lines of incision and through the papillae and their embrasures.

A roentgenogram had been taken of the fractured area. After immobilization, a BIP pack was inserted and x-rayed for visualization of the extent of defect. Another roentgenogram was taken after the defect had been filled with the bone mixture and sutured. The patient was instructed in postoperative home care and 1,000,000 units

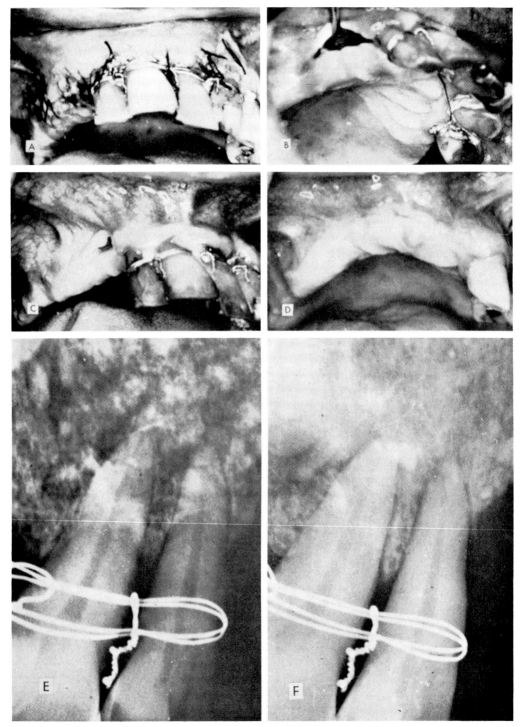

Case Figure 3–2. Postoperative sequence. *A*, Appearance on the fifth postoperative day. Healing is progressing favorably by primary intention along the lines of incision, and by granulation covered by a healthy layer of coagulum over fulgurated fistulous orifice. *B*, Appearance two weeks later. Healing has been disrupted by a fishbone embedded into the surgical site, with partial disintegration of the repair tissue. *C*, Postoperative appearance three months after surgery. All but a very shallow pit depression, seen as a small dark crescent, has of Crysticillin were administered by intramuscular injection to provide an immediate high blood level. Oral V-Cillin, Kasdenol lavage, and ascorbic acid-gelatin dietary supplement were prescribed.

He returned on the fifth postoperative day for removal of the sutures. The mouth was irrigated; then the tissues were inspected. The fulgurated fistula was granulating healthily and was covered with a thin layer of coagulum. The incisions were healing by primary union (Case Fig. 3–2A) and the maxillary alveolar contour was normal. Tincture of myrrh and benzoin was applied in air-dried layers.

The patient resented the dietary restriction to semisolid food and expressed skepticism about the need for its continuation. He said he felt quite comfortable and his mouth did not feel sore. He was cautioned about the danger of disrupting the healing process by injudicious attempts to eat solid foods and instructed to continue the postoperative home care.

He returned one week later; healing seemed to be much further advanced. The mouth was irrigated and tincture of myrrh and benzoin was applied. He was instructed to return once a week until further notice. The following week the site of the fistulous orifice which had been healing so well was badly deteriorated. The area was thoroughly irrigated. Inspection disclosed a fish bone approximately 2 cm. in length embedded into the tissues at the deteriorated site, which now was a cavelike depression about 1 cm. in diameter (Case Fig. 3–2B).

Despite repeated efforts to fill this concavitation in the alveolar ridge by scarification and insertion of surgical gelatin, the new defect filled very slowly by secondary intention. It required almost three months of semi-weekly postoperative treatments before the defect was almost fully obliterated (Case Fig. 3–2C). The defect at the end of that period was only a very shallow depression in the surface contour. A postoperative roentgenogram showed the defect uniformly filled, with no trace of surgical dead space. The bone chips which had been conspicuous in the previous postoperative film were no longer sharply delineated. The regenerating bone appeared homogenous and seemed to be undergoing normal consolidation.

The intramaxillary wiring was removed. Subsequently, the four anterior teeth were extracted and an alveoloplasty was performed. The cuspid and first bicuspid were retained. Soon thereafter he had a new set of dentures constructed. He was seen once more one year later for a final postoperative checkup. The maxillary gingival mucosa was fully healed. The tissue was firm and normal in tone and the alveolar ridge contour was highly satisfactory (Case Fig. 3–2D) and provided a stable base for the denture.

This case serves to highlight the importance of patient cooperation during the postoperative healing period. Trauma or other abnormal tissue damage incurred during the reparative stage usually does much more harm than merely

---

Case Figure 3–2   Continued.

fully repaired without loss of normal alveolar contour. D, One year postoperative checkup: The centrals and laterals have been extracted, the cuspid and first bicuspid having been retained for use as abutments. Healing is complete; the site of the defect has filled completely, and the alveolar contour is normal. E, Roentgenogram after the defect had been filled with bone mixture and sutured. F, Postoperative roentgenogram showing the defect uniformly filled, with no trace of surgical dead space.

retard the rate of healing. It can completely disrupt the healing process. As the new granulation tissue deteriorates it breaks down into basic amino acids which become an additional source of irritation. Thus, an almost endless cycle of irritation highly disruptive to the healing process results.

The supplementary postoperative treatments that must be instituted to undo the damage and reinduce tissue regeneration are usually only partially effective. The rate of renewed regeneration, therefore, is likely to be much slower than the original healing rate in spite of conscientious supplementary postoperative care.

When, in the absence of unfavorable systemic or local factors, apparently normal healing is suddenly disrupted, trauma must be suspected as the underlying cause. This is especially likely to be the case when the patient proves incapable of cooperation. Thus, when the patient is too young to be reasoned with, senile, or obstinately set in habit and behavior patterns, a traumatic basis for disrupted healing should be suspected. The precise cause should be determined and eliminated. Failure to do so may result in irreparable damage.

Traumatic Cyst

The preceding cases of this group have demonstrated the usefulness of electrosurgery for the definitive surgical management of extensive cysts. This case demonstrates that its usefulness is not limited to *treatment* of cysts, but that it can also contribute invaluably toward establishing a conclusive diagnosis where free bleeding from steel scalpel surgery could contribute to erroneous diagnosis and result in unnecessary mutilating surgery.

Although clinical appearance and roentgenographic evidence are often helpful for establishing a diagnosis, they are by no means conclusive, since they often are compatible with more than one pathologic entity. When one or more of the potential pathologic entities require radical surgery and others require comparatively innocuous surgery, the importance of being able to establish an accurate differential diagnosis is inestimable.

In the case to be reviewed, the clinical picture and roentgenographic evidence were compatible with three widely diverse pathologic entities: monostatic fibrous dysplasia, ameloblastoma, or traumatic cyst. The differential diagnosis depended on aspiration and biopsy. The hemostasis inherent in electrosection helped to facilitate both and to assure accurate results.

CASE 4

PATIENT. A 14-year-old white female.

HISTORY. The patient was a victim of grand mal since childhood and was on Dilantin therapy. She had gradually become aware of a peculiar bulging on the right cheek side of her lower jaw, and her family consulted their dentist about it. He took a

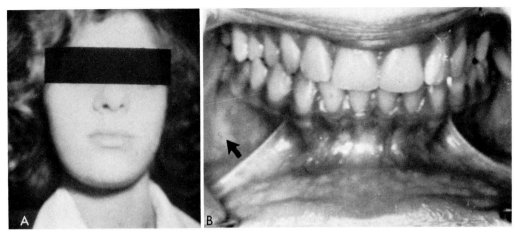

Case Figure 4–1. A, Preoperative appearance. *Extraoral:* The right side of the face is swollen from the lip level to the bottom of the jaw. The swelling has distended the right half of the lower lip slightly outward. B, *Intraoral:* The alveolar labial bone plate bulges outward from the right cuspid posteriorly to the second molar (arrow). The alveolar contour on the left side is normal. On digital pressure there is a feeling of crepitus as the swelling is palpated.

periapical x-ray and found a huge amount of radiolucence around most of the teeth in the bicuspid-molar area. He referred her to the author for diagnosis and treatment.

CLINICAL EXAMINATION. *Extraoral.* The right side of her face appeared swollen and was larger than the left side (Case Fig. 4–1A). The cheek remained asymptomatic on digital palpation.

Intraoral. The alveolar ridge on the right side of the mandible bulged convexly in sharp contrast to the left side which was concave in contour (Case Fig. 4–1B). Digital palpation elicited crepitus. The patient's temperature was normal and there was no palpable adenopathy. Intraoral and extraoral lateral jaw view roentgenograms revealed a hugh radiolucent area involving the teeth from the mesial of the second molar to the distal of the first bicuspid and extending from the crest of the ridge to the inferior border of the mandible (Case Fig. 4–3A). The cortical border of the jawbone was still intact, but it had a peculiar scalloped appearance.

TREATMENT. Before treatment could be instituted a conclusive diagnosis of the condition had to be established. Although the extraoral unilateral swelling was suggestive of monostatic fibrous dysplasia, the intraoral and roentgenographic evidence made it appear unlikely. The scalloped appearance of the remainder of the inferior border of the mandible and the large area of radiolucence was compatible with ameloblastoma, and the radiolucence and history of trauma to the face suggested the possibility of a traumatic cyst.

A traumatic cyst is not a true cyst, since it does not have an epithelium-lined sac. It is a space in the jawbone that is also known as a hemorrhagic or extravasation cyst and may be empty or filled with fluid. However, the cortical bone may be thin but is usually not expanded, as in this case. The ameloblastoma is a localized malignant lesion that rarely metastasizes and is sometimes referred to as a "benign cancer," but it tends to recur and is locally highly destructive.

Treatments for the respective conditions differ enormously. The traumatic cyst, not being a true cyst, does not require enucleation. If the bone cavity is filled with fluid, aspiration of the fluid or decomposed blood components is all that is necessary, and there follows spontaneous osteoblastic regeneration of bone. If it is an ameloblastoma, the entire lesion must be thoroughly removed and the base of the bone cauterized with chemicals or if possible by electrosurgery, to assure against recurrence. In a lesion as extensive as this one it would be necessary to eliminate it by performing a hemimandibulectomy, a disfiguringly mutilating surgical solution, particularly for a young girl.

A differential diagnosis can be established by aspiration and biopsy. Both were performed in order to assure an accurate diagnosis.

The right mandible was prepared and anesthetized by inferior alveolar block injection. A 45-degree-angle fine needle electrode was selected, cutting current was set at 3 on the power rheostat dial, and the activated electrode was used to incise the gingival mucosa covering the thin underlying bone. To assure that the incision would penetrate down to but not into the underlying bone, the thickness of the gingival tissue was established by inserting the hypodermic needle used for the injection into the labial gingiva anterior to the swollen area. The tip of the needle electrode was then allowed to penetrate precisely that far into the tissue to make the incision (Case Fig. 4–2A). The incision was made in a postero-anterior direction from the second molar anteriorly to the second bicuspid, slightly arced and angled downward as it progressed anteriorly. The lower margin of the incision was gently displaced downward with a periosteal elevator, exposing a bulge of parchment-thin alveolar bone (Case Fig. 4–2B). There was no free bleeding and the area was clearly visible.

A large Luer-type syringe with 20-gauge needle was inserted through the parchment-thin bone as easily as through soft tissue, and aspiration was performed. Since there was a total absence of free bleeding it was not possible to accidentally aspirate blood into the syringe as could occur with free bleeding caused by steel scalpel incision. The absence of bleeding during aspiration is important, because aspiration of a traumatic cyst produces fluid or decomposed blood components but no bleeding, whereas aspiration of an adamantinoma or ameloblastoma usually includes blood in the aspirated contents. A clear serous type of fluid was aspirated (Case Fig. 4–2C), suggesting strongly that this was indeed a traumatic cyst. A small specimen of the thinned out bone was removed and sent for biopsy evaluation. The biopsy confirmed that it was a traumatic cyst.

The fluid content having been evacuated, the tissue flap was restored to position and the coapted margins were sutured with interrupted silk sutures. The patient returned on the fifth postoperative day for removal of the sutures. The incision appeared to be healing satisfactorily by primary intention, except for a small vesicle that resembled a blood blister at the anterior end of the incision (Case Fig. 4–2D), which was destroyed by spot coagulation with a small ball electrode. Healing progressed rapidly and uneventfully, and three months postoperatively the intraoral appearance of the alveolar ridges in both the mandibular quadrants was identical (Case Fig. 4–2E).

The course of the healing was followed roentgenographically as it progressed, Case Figure 4–3B shows the bone repair 8 weeks postoperatively, Case Figure 4–3C shows the repair 12 weeks postoperatively, and Case Figure 4–3D shows the normal appearance of the bone 6 months postoperatively.

The pulp vitality improved comparably with the healing progress. At the time of surgery, the possibility of the lesion being an ameloblastoma appeared to be increased by the bulging of the buccal bone plate and by the fact that the teeth in the involved area, while not nonvital, responded much differently than the other teeth in the arch, suggesting a gradual death of the pulp. As the healing of the bone pro-

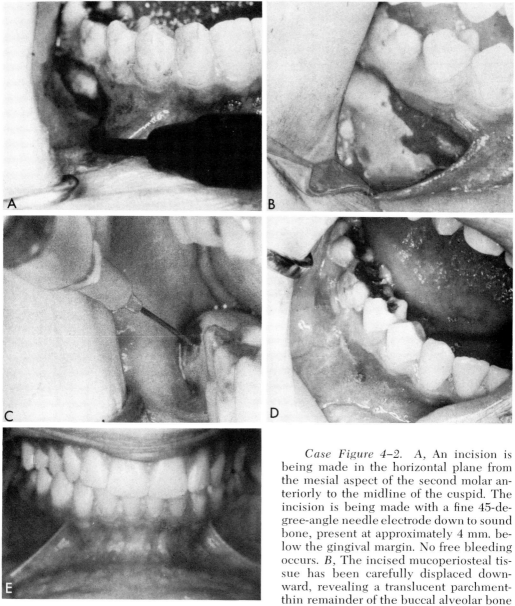

Case Figure 4–2. A, An incision is being made in the horizontal plane from the mesial aspect of the second molar anteriorly to the midline of the cuspid. The incision is being made with a fine 45-degree-angle needle electrode down to sound bone, present at approximately 4 mm. below the gingival margin. No free bleeding occurs. B, The incised mucoperiosteal tissue has been carefully displaced downward, revealing a translucent parchment-thin remainder of the buccal alveolar bone plate. C, Aspiration is being performed by puncturing into the distended area with a 20-gauge Luer-type needle attached to a Luer syringe. Air and a small amount of clear serous fluid are being aspirated. D, Appearance of the incised tissue on the tenth postoperative day. Primary healing has occurred, and the tissue appears to be healing favorably, despite a tiny red blister at the anterior terminal end, which was destroyed by superficial spot coagulation. E, Final postoperative intraoral appearance. The buccal contour of the alveolar bone is identical on both sides. The bone on the right side is rigidly firm and unyielding under maximal finger pressure.

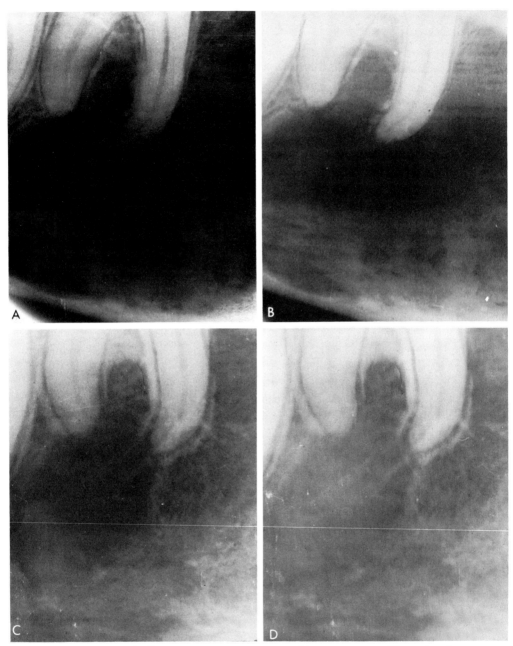

Case Figure 4–3. A, Preoperative roentgenographic appearance. There is a huge area of radiolucence in the right side of the mandible, extending from the anterior aspect of the second molar anteriorly to the distal of the cuspid. Very little bone remains intraradicularly in the first molar area, and the apices of the molar and bicuspid roots project downward into the radiolucent zone. All that remains along the inferior border of the mandible is the cortex of the inferior edge of the mandible, and even this appears thinned out under the mesial first molar root. The remaining bone presents a peculiar scalloped appearance that resembles the x-ray appearance often seen in cases of ameloblastoma. *B,* Appearance 8 weeks after aspiration. There has been a great amount of bone regeneration. The area around the roots of the first molar remains as the residual site of the radiolucence. *C,* Appearance 12 weeks postoperatively. The remaining radiolucent area is filling in with new bone. Trabeculation in the area can be seen to be forming. *D,* Final x-ray appearance, 6 months postoperatively. The bone has filled the area completely with normal bone.

gressed, the pulp vitality improved, and by the sixth month the teeth in this area responded to pulp testing exactly as the other teeth. Owing to the hemostasis with electrosurgery, a favorable result was achieved with a minimum of surgical intervention.

II. PLASTIC ORAL SURGERY

Plastic oral surgery, in common with plastic surgery procedures in other parts of the body, depends to a large extent on the use of tissue flaps and grafts. Thus, the techniques used for repair or reconstruction of oral structures often have a *basic* similarity to those used for performing plastic surgery in other parts of the body.

"Plastic surgery" is a very loose term, coined to differentiate reconstructive and cosmetic surgery from pathologic surgery. To provide more definitive terminology plastic surgery has been subclassified according to the anatomic areas involved. For example, *rhinoplasty* is the term used to describe plastic surgery of the nose. The term *plastic oral surgery* therefore properly describes comparable surgery performed on the oral structures.[10] Moreover, many oral plastic surgery procedures require more difficult and extensive surgical intervention than is involved in such typical plastic surgery procedures as rhinoplasty and mammary gland paraffin injection.

Although similar types of flaps, grafts, and implants are used in plastic oral surgery and in plastic surgery performed in other parts of the body,[11-23] there are two important differences.

1. *Difference in Purpose.* Plastic oral surgery is used primarily for functional improvement. Even when bilateral ostectomies are performed, functional improvement rivals cosmetic benefits as a motivating factor. The other forms of plastic surgery are usually utilized primarily for cosmetic improvement.

2. *Difference in Control of the Operative Field.* It is in this realm that the greatest difference exists. Plastic surgery in other areas of the body is usually performed under aseptic conditions, and it is possible to provide ample postoperative protection against contamination or irritation.

In plastic oral surgery it is impossible to provide a sterile operative field. Moreover, it is equally impossible to afford adequate local postoperative protection from contamination. Even protection of the operative field from irritation may be difficult or impossible. Thus, in plastic oral surgery the postoperative challenge is in many respects comparable to that of the surgery itself.

The inability to provide ample local protection increases the importance of using other protective measures. Beneficial indirect protection can often be provided by prophylactic use of supportive therapy. Judicious use of antibiotics, vitamins, antiseptic or bactericidal lavages, and high protein diets with ascorbic acid supplements helps greatly to mitigate the handicaps.

A universal prerequisite for the successful outcome of any form of plastic surgery is the need for a healthy host bed for the flap, graft, or implant that is employed. Failure to eradicate surgically all the diseased tissue dooms any plastic procedure to failure. Thus, when reconstructive oral surgery is performed, total eradication of all existing diseased tissue must be meticulously effected in order to insure a reasonable chance for a successful outcome. In many instances, particularly when the pathologic condition encroaches into relatively inaccessible areas, the judicious, skillful use of electrosurgery may spell the difference between success and failure of the surgical procedure.

Tissue Grafts

CASE 5

This case is an example of the usefulness of electrosurgery and tissue grafts, combined, to effect permanent repair of old soft tissue defects that fail to respond to routine treatment.

PATIENT.   A 49-year-old white female.

HISTORY.   A palatally impacted maxillary left cuspid had been surgically removed three years previously. The tooth had apparently been malposed in an oblique position and following its removal the surgeon found an oronasal perforation of the hard palate. Despite lengthy postoperative care the oronasal perforation persisted.

Eventually a palatal fistula appeared and the patient began to suffer neuralgic pains in the left side of her face and head. She also suffered frequent severe headaches. All her symptoms appeared to increase in severity as time passed. She was referred for plastic closure of the oronasal defect which was suspected to be the triggering mechanism.

CLINICAL EXAMINATION

Intraoral.   A round, bulbous defect approximately 3 mm. in diameter was visible on the left side of the hard palate. The defect was located midway between the gingival margins of the teeth and the midline approximately 1.5 cm. beyond the lingual aspect of the left central and lateral incisors. A minute dimpled depression was visible in the center of the elevation and the entire area was surrounded by an irregular, reddish areola (Case Fig. 5–1A).

An occlusal view roentgenogram taken with an intraoral cassette revealed considerable radiolucence in the palatal region on the affected side. Because of the superimposition of structures and the normal radiolucent areas found in this region this was not diagnostically conclusive.

A flexible silver probe was inserted into the dimpled orifice. After initial contact with the palatal bone, lateral manipulation located a perforation leading into the deeper structures. This provided clinical confirmation of the existence of an oronasal communication.

TREATMENT.   The mouth was prepared for surgery and the area anesthetized by a combination of circumferential infiltration plus nasopalatine regional block. A long, slender 90-degree-angle needle electrode was selected and current output set at 8 for fulguration. The fistulous orifice was thoroughly carbonized (Case Fig. 5–1B). Then the electrode was advanced into the perforation about 0.5 cm. and the epithelized tract desiccated for three seconds.

The carbonized fistulous orifice was debrided by gentle curettage to freshen the surface; the palatal bone defect was freshened in a similar manner. The nasal fossa was irrigated through the defect, then aspirated. Sulfathiazole crystals were incorporated with a small amount of cultured despeciated bone paste which was rolled into a tiny pellet. The medicated bone pellet was inserted into the defect and gently tamped down to the palatal bone base in order to seal over the perforation.

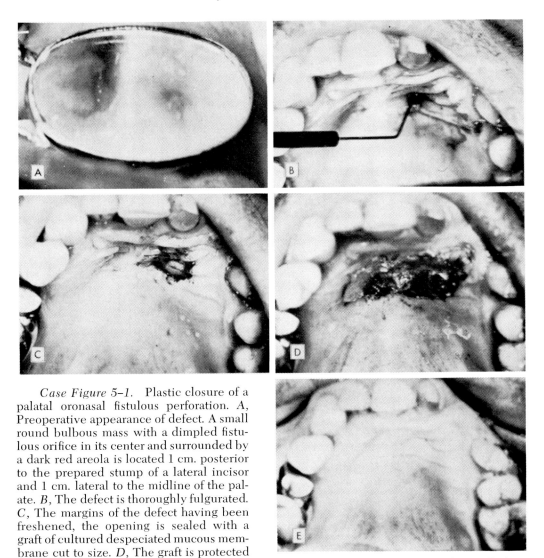

Case Figure 5–1. Plastic closure of a palatal oronasal fistulous perforation. *A*, Preoperative appearance of defect. A small round bulbous mass with a dimpled fistulous orifice in its center and surrounded by a dark red areola is located 1 cm. posterior to the prepared stump of a lateral incisor and 1 cm. lateral to the midline of the palate. *B*, The defect is thoroughly fulgurated. *C*, The margins of the defect having been freshened, the opening is sealed with a graft of cultured despeciated mucous membrane cut to size. *D*, The graft is protected with a dressing of dryfoil adapted over the area and sealed to the tissues with clear collodion. *E*, Appearance eight weeks postoperatively. The graft has "taken," and the palatal mucosa is intact and normal in tone and texture.

A small piece of cultured despeciated mucous membrane was cut to fit exactly into the palatal defect. After it was trimmed to proper shape and thickness it was soaked in soluble Terramycin solution and inserted into position in the palatal defect (Case Fig. 5–1*C*). A piece of adhesive dryfoil was cut to size, adapted over the graft, and sealed to the palatal mucosa with several air-dried layers of clear collodion (Case Fig. 5–1*D*).

The patient was given instructions in postoperative care and Terramycin was prescribed for four days. She was seen again one week later. The dryfoil dressing was still firmly attached to the palatal mucosa. It was carefully removed. The graft was found to be "taking" satisfactorily; it was beginning to assume a healthy pink color and was firmly attached to the surrounding mucosa. The area was irrigated and tincture of myrrh and benzoin was applied in air-dried layers.

When she was seen again one week later the patient reported that for the first 10 postoperative days her neuralgic symptoms had worsened but that after this initial exacerbation all her symptoms had suddenly disappeared. She was seen once a week for the next six weeks. During that period, healing progressed without incident, and by the end of that time the palatal mucosa was fully healed. The new tissue in the former defect area was firm and a healthy pink (Case Fig. 5–1E).

This patient reported semiannually for postoperative observation for the next five years. During that period the tissue remained normal and there was no recurrence of her neuralgic symptoms. The gratifying result obtained could not have been achieved if any pathology had remained in the host bed. Use of electrosurgery assured total eradication of the degenerative tissue without sbustantially increasing the size of the defect, as occurs when the resection is performed by cold-steel scalpel.

Tissue Flaps

Tissue flaps used alone or in combination with grafts or implants are basic ingredients in plastic oral surgery. Rotating palatal pedicle flaps, buccal butterfly flaps, and French sliding flaps tend to be dramatic as well as useful. Probably the simplest, least dramatic, yet often a highly successful type is the slit incision flap. It is created simply by making slit incisions in tissue in order to increase its capacity to be stretched so that it will cover the widest possible area.

If the slit is made in thin gingival mucosa it usually penetrates through the full thickness of the tissue down to the underlying bone. When working with thick, soft tissue such as buccal mucosa of the cheek, however, the slit is made just deep enough to provide the required amount of "give" to the tissue to serve efficiently.

CASE 6

This case is an unusual example of the usefulness of a simple slit incision tissue flap to effectively repair a serious traumatic oral defect.

The maxillary buccal alveolar cortex is very thin. When a maxillary molar is solidly ankylosed to its investing alveolar process, use of force in the attempt to extract the tooth may result in a fracture of the entire posterior portion of the alveolar ridge containing the tuberosity, and the embedded molar teeth.

When such an accidental traumatic fracture occurs it usually communicates with the maxillary antrum and creates a huge cleft-like defect. Unless normal anatomic contour can be adequately restored and the antral opening sealed, construction of an obturator-like prosthesis becomes the only alternative. Such prostheses are at best makeshift substitutes. Infinitely more satisfactory results are likely to be achieved through plastic repair of the defect. Plastic surgery is usually based upon formalized and standardized techniques, but occasionally situations arise for which there are no specific treatment patterns. In such instances ingenuity must provide the solution.

PATIENT.   A 19-year-old white male.

HISTORY.   While home on a brief school holiday he went to his family dentist for extraction of a painful maxillary molar. The tooth proved to be solidly embedded and immobile. The entire posterior maxillary alveolar process containing the first, second and third molars and the tuberosity fractured with a loud snap when pressure was applied injudiciously in an attempt to luxate the ankylosed tooth. As the fractured fragment tore loose it badly lacerated the mucosa of the soft palate immediately beyond its junction with the mucosa of the hard palate. The patient was immediately advised of the accident and referred for repair of the traumatic defect.

CLINICAL EXAMINATION. *Extraoral.* Negative.

Intraoral. The maxillary right molar area was still anesthetized. Immediate thorough examination and surgical repair was therefore instituted. The first molar socket was intact except at its distal margin which had been fused to the tooth and had been torn away with the fractured fragment. From the first molar posteriorly to the soft palate the alveolar ridge and tuberosity were missing, and the palatal mucosa beyond the junction of the hard and soft palate was lacerated to the pillar of the fauces and hanging into the oropharynx. In the second molar area the bony floor of the antrum was missing. The ciliated lining membrane of the sinus (Schneiderian membrane) was intact and clearly visible (Case Fig. 6–1A). With each respiration of the patient it could be seen moving rhythmically.

This type of traumatic defect can be repaired surgically or by prosthetic restoration. One surgical method consists of use of a pedicle tube graft to fill the defect and restore the alveolar ridge to normal contour. Another method involves use of autogenous or homogenous bone grafts and/or rotated pedicle palatal flaps. The disabling surgery and other handicaps inherent in these methods have been reviewed previously.

Another method consists of prosthetic restoration of the defect with obturator-like partial prosthesis. This method results in permanent maxillary defects that are almost as extensive and disabling as the congenital cleft palate, and leave the antrum permanently vulnerable to infection via the oral route.

A third surgical procedure offered an attractive alternative. The alveolar defect could be filled with cultured bone or medicated surgical gelatin, with a sliding flap created to cover the graft and simultaneously restore the alveolar ridge to a reasonable degree of normal, convex contour. The sliding flap in this instance would have to be created by making an acute-angle slit incision into the buccal mucosa of the inner aspect of the cheek in order to form a vestibular pouch. The slit would have to be made at an acute angle paralleling the alveolar ridge in order to avoid injury to the parotid (Stensen) duct. If the integrity of the vestibular pouch space could be maintained with a stent, the resulting repair should prove functionally satisfactory, although it might not recreate an anatomically or cosmetically perfect ridge and tuberosity. Electrosection is ideally suited for this type of incision.

TREATMENT. The traumatized area was irrigated and prepared for surgery. Although the area was still anesthetized, supplementary anesthesia was considered essential. This was administered by infiltration with Xylocaine (1:50,000) and also by decanting some of the solution directly into the defect.

The loose strip of torn soft palate mucosa was restored to position with two interrupted silk sutures. A strip of Gelfoam was moistened with growth inductor material and inserted to rest on top of the ciliated lining membrane that formed the floor of the antrum deep in the defect (Case Fig. 6–1B). A mixture of medicated surgical gelatin was deposited on top of the Gelfoam and mixed with the blood present, partially filling the defect.

A 45-degree-angle fine needle electrode was selected and current output set at

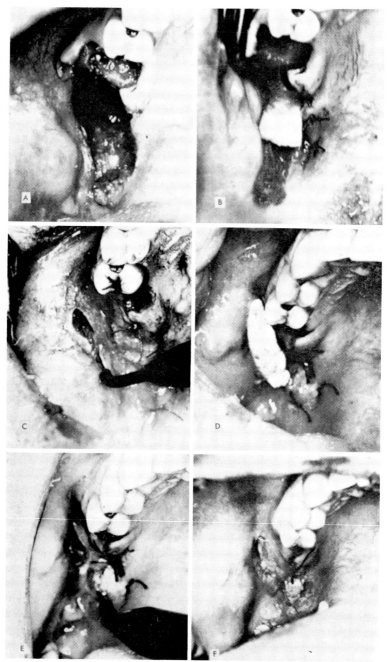

Case Figure 6–1.   Repair of traumatically fractured and displaced tuberosity. *A*, Preoperative view. The mesial half of the bony socket of the maxillary first molar still present is all that remains of the tuberosity and its alveolar ridge. The floor of the antrum has been lost, exposing to view the ciliated (Schneiderian) lining membrane of the antrum, which is intact. Immediately posterior, the mucosa of the alveolar ridge and soft palate is lacerated and hanging down into the oropharynx. *B*, The torn tissue is restored and sutured into normal position. A strip of Gelfoam sponge moistened with growth inductor material is placed into the defect to bridge over the ciliated lining membrane and provide a temporary floor for the antrum. *C*, Suturing completed, an incision is made into the buccal mucosa at an acute angle with a fine 45-degree-angle needle electrode to form a vestibular pouch and to provide tissue slack to eliminate

3.5 for electrosection. An acute-angle slit incision into the buccal mucosa paralleling the defect was made with the activated electrode. The incision was extended the full length of the defect at a 20 degree angle to the tissue surface and 1 cm. deep (Case Fig. 6–1C). Great care was taken to avoid injury to the parotid duct.

After the slit incision was made a second strip of Gelfoam was moistened with the growth inductor material and placed over the gelatin mixture previously deposited in the defect. The slit incision created enough "give" to permit the buccal and palatal margins of the defect to be brought into normal coaptation without tension and provide protective cover for the graft insert. The coapted margins were sutured with 0000 braided silk interrupted sutures. A few slightly bulging tissue puckers were created by the suturing. These were eliminated by superficial spot coagulation with a small ball electrode so that contour irregularities would be eliminated.

A stiff mix of surgical cement into which sulfathiazole and benzocaine powders had been incorporated was rolled into cigar shape, inserted into the pouch created by the buccal slit incision and sutured into position for retention (Case Fig. 6–1D). This cement pack would have to serve as a surgical stent to maintain the vestibular space created by the pouch.

Antibiotic therapy and lavage were prescribed and detailed instructions given for postoperative home care. The patient was due to return to school in another state in four days. He was therefore instructed to return daily for postoperative treatment until his departure. Each day the area was irrigated, small irregular bulging tissue tabs were lightly coagulated (Case Fig. 6–1E) and tincture of myrrh and benzoin was applied.

On the third postoperative day there was some evidence of favorable healing. The restored convexity of the alveolar ridge was still well defined. The stent-retaining sutures were removed and the stent discarded. The surface of the incised buccal pouch appeared to be granulating normally. Tincture of myrrh and benzoin was applied in air-dried layers and the patient was asked to return the following morning for a final inspection and treatment before departing on his return trip.

At the final visit the sutures were removed from the defect area. The coapted tissue margins appeared to be healing by primary union and the surface coagulum was almost completely gone from the buccal pouch (Case Fig. 6–1F). Tincture of myrrh and benzoin was applied and the patient was instructed to continue the regimen of postoperative care. His case history was forwarded to an oral surgeon near his school so that his postoperative progress could be observed and supervised.

Periodically, both the patient and the surgeon reported uneventful progress which terminated in complete healing after six weeks. The repaired alveolar ridge and tuberosity were described as resembling an alveolar ridge and tuberosity that has undergone moderately marked resorption due to advanced periodontoclasia. They remained well defined, there was a distinct buccal vestibule, and their contour was reasonably normal. The maxillary antrum has remained asymptomatic.

Case Figure 6–1 Continued.

tension against the sutures. Note that the incision is practically bloodless. *D*, Surgical cement pack inserted into the slit pouch to serve as a surgical stent and maintain the vestibular space. *E*, Forty-eight hours postoperatively. Cement pack removed, vestibular space has been maintained. Irregular tissue tabs are reduced by coagulation with a small ball electrode. *F*, Appearance last time seen, 96 hours postoperatively. The buccal pouch incision is healing well, and the vestibular space is well defined with a distinct alveolar ridge present.

Bone Grafts

Bone grafts play an important role in many plastic surgery procedures. Their role in reparative plastic surgery of the oral structures is especially important.

One of the more important uses for bone grafts is in the repair of surgical or traumatic perforations through the dense buccal cortical plate of the mandible. Such perforations are usually responsible for distressing adhesions due to invagination of gingival mucosa into the body of the mandible. If the perforations happen to communicate with the mandibular canal, fibers of the inferior alveolar nerve may emerge through the perforation to form amputation neuromas that cause acute pain.

Since obliteration of such perforations by spontaneous regeneration is highly unlikely, the most effective way to seal and obliterate such defects permanently is to plug them with bone graft inserts after all aberrant tissue has been removed.

CASE 7

This case is an example of the usefulness of bone grafts for repair of surgical perforations into the body of the mandible and of electrosurgery for total eradication of the aberrant tissue in and around such defects.

This case also illustrates the damage that can be inflicted by injudicious attempts at empirical, blind surgical correction of disorders that are relatively minor pathologically.

PATIENT. A 52-year-old white female.

HISTORY. Eight years previously she began to suffer severe pain in her lower jaw. During the next five years she had five teeth extracted in an attempt to eliminate the source of what appeared to be reflex neuralgic pains in her left mandible. Three years previously the pain seemed to localize in her mandibular left second molar.

By that time the bicuspids and first molar had been extracted, and the second molar was a valuable abutment for a partial denture. In order to retain the tooth she was referred to an endodontist for root canal therapy. The canal in the distal root was filled with vital pulp tissue and presented no problem. After it was filled the mesial canal was opened and the pulp tissue was found to have undergone liquefaction necrosis. Despite regular treatment, profuse purulent drainage persisted for 10 months. Although some improvement was noted after this canal was filled, some neuralgic pain persisted and gradually increased in severity; so one year later she consulted another dentist. He decided that the second molar was the likely offender. He removed the old canal fillings, resterilized and refilled them. This afforded a measure of relief for a few weeks but then the pain resumed with renewed intensity.

Since he had slightly overfilled the mesial canal he removed the filling and refilled it under careful measurement control. The pain persisted, however, and after a few weeks roentgenographic examination revealed a slight radiolucence developing around the mesial root apex, suggesting an early stage of periapical abscess. The patient was referred to another endodontist for resection of the mesial root end.

The root-end resection, which proved abortive, had been attempted about three months previously. Although he removed a section of buccal cortex to create a bone window he could not see the operative area. While trying to cut off the apex of the tooth his instrument suddenly gave and sank into an excruciatingly painful nonresistant area. Even direct injection of Xylocaine (1:50,000) into the bone cavity failed to produce satisfactory anesthesia. He therefore had to discontinue the surgical procedure, restore the flap, and secure it with sutures without sealing over the bone window.

Almost immediately thereafter the pain became more excruciating than ever. It radiated up the side of her face and head to the auriculotemporal region, downward into the neck in the cervical region and submaxillary triangle and into the ramus and body of the mandible. She was referred for diagnosis and treatment.

CLINICAL EXAMINATION. *Extraoral.* There was a slight amount of swelling in the lower part of the left cheek and considerable tenderness to palpation in the submaxillary and cervical regions.

Intraoral. The mucosa on the buccal aspect of the alveolar ridge in the second molar area was lumpy, fibrous, contractile and tender to pressure. The molar was somewhat sensitive to percussion and buccolingual pressure.

The patient described two simultaneous but separate types of pain. One, the original pain, was a pounding sensation in the body of the mandible, radiating postero-anteriorly. The second, more recent manifestation, was a burning sensation radiating upward toward the temple and down into the neck.

Roentgenographic examination revealed that the alveolar cortex immediately anterior to the second molar appeared radiolucent with wide trabeculations. Comparison with roentgenograms taken two years previously showed that this radiolucence had not been present at that time.

Lateral jaw views revealed two irregular radiolucent areas in the left body of the mandible that looked punched out. A small area was located near and slightly below the apex of the cuspid. The second, larger area was below and about 1.5 cm. anterior to the second molar.

The patient's physician and orthopedic surgeon were consulted about her systemic condition. The orthopedic surgeon reported she had been receiving treatment for osteoarthritis of the cervical spine for several years and that calcium had been administered a number of years earlier for treatment of osteoporotic decalcifications believed to be attributable to dietary deficiencies during the two world wars.

Biopsy of the local lesions seemed indicated in order to discount such factors as ameloblastoma, eosinophilic granuloma or amputation neuroma. If the biopsy should prove negative it was decided that bone dysplasias would have to be ruled out by laboratory tests.

TREATMENT. The mouth was prepared for surgery and inferior alveolar block anesthesia administered. A 45-degree-angle fine needle electrode was selected and current output set at 3.5 for electrosection. An incision was started with the activated electrode on the crest of the edentulous alveolar ridge posterior to the molar. It was carried to the distal of the molar, then continued along the crest of the ridge anteriorly from the mesial aspect of the tooth to within 1 cm. of the cuspid. At that point the incision was curved downward slightly for 0.5 cm. (Case Fig. 7–1A).

The incised tissue was undermined and reflected from the alveolar bone. An oval-shaped perforation in the buccal cortical plate measuring approximately 5 mm. in width and 1 cm. in length was exposed to view. A fibrous cord-like mass of scar tissue tied the buccal gingival mucosa to the bone defect. A second, softer, less fibrous cord-like mass emerged from deeper in[24] (Case Fig. 7–1B and C). It was impossible to

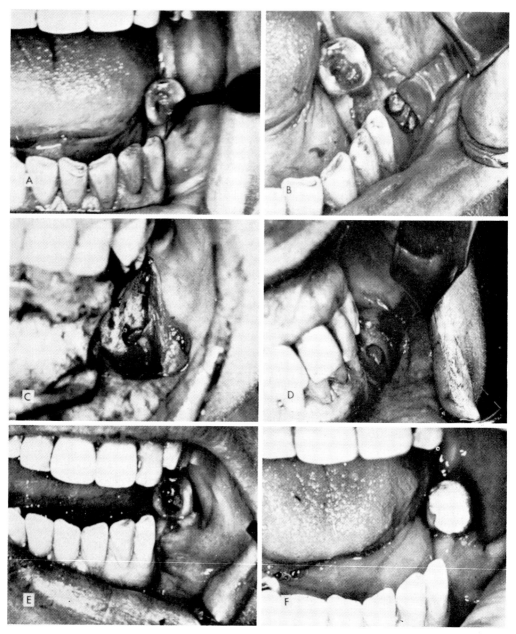

Case Figure 7–1. Repair of a mandibular traumatic cortical bone defect with a bone graft after resection of an amputation neuroma and fibrous adhesions. *A*, Incision along crest of alveolar ridge directed posteroanteriorly across edentulous area, extending from the molar to within 1 cm. of the distal of the cuspid. (Initial incision extending 1.5 cm. distal to the molar on crest of alveolar ridge can also be seen.) *B*, Flap is reflected, exposing to view two cord-like masses emerging from the defect to blend with the buccal mucosa, granulomatous debris inside the defect, and an oval perforation in the buccal alveolar cortex. *C*, Close-up view of the cord-like masses after the granulomatous tissue was resected and one fibrous attachment to the buccal mucosa severed. *D*, Cord-like masses having been resected and debridement completed, a graft of despeciated cultured fetal calf mandible is inserted to seal the perforation. *E*, Appearance on fifth postoperative day immediately after the sutures were removed. Some edema is present, and primary union has been disrupted immediately anterior to the molar where a suture had been lost. *F*, Appearance six weeks postoperatively. Soft tissue healing is complete. The tissue tone is normal, and the alveolar contour is normal. The intense local sensitivity is no longer in evidence.

930

determine whether the buccal mucosa flowed into the defect; whether these tissues emerged from deep in the body of the mandible to blend with the mucosa; or, as appeared most likely, a combination of both.

The scar-like tissue was resected from the inner aspect of the defect and then from the buccal mucosa by electrosection with the needle electrode and a narrow U-shaped loop electrode. The resected tissue was preserved in formalin solution for biopsy. Additional scar tissue and what appeared to be granulation tissue was resected from deep in the bone defect with a long, slender U-shaped loop electrode and preserved with the other tissue specimen.

Despite good anesthesia the tissue in the internal defect proved extremely sensitive to instrumentation.[24] Additional solution was injected directly into the defect — was even decanted into it — but the pain persisted until a mental foramen block was administered.

Debridement of granulomatous tissue from the bone defect was continued. When completed it was quite apparent that unless the defect were to be permanently sealed, the scar tissue adhesions or amputation neuroma would recur. The bone margin of the defect appeared eburnated; so it was freshened with a bone bur. A piece of cultured despeciated fetal calf mandible was cut to fit accurately, like a cork, into the defect. The bone graft was impregnated with sulfadiazine and Albamycin powders and wedged into the defect over a mixture of bone paste and medicated powdered surgical gelatin which was deposited into the bone cavity. The surface of the fetal calf mandible graft was trimmed level with the surrounding cortical plate with a bone file so that the continuity was unbroken (Case Fig. 7–1D).

A 2 mm. opening was made in the alveolar bone immediately anterior to the molar in order to obtain a specimen of tissue for biopsy evaluation from the radiolucent area noted on the roentgenogram. Tissue that looked granulomatous was scooped out of this area with a small curet and preserved in a second specimen bottle. This opening was effectively sealed with a small amount of bone paste. The tissue flap was restored to position and secured with interrupted silk sutures. Cosa-Tetrastatin and Kasdenol were prescribed and she was given instructions in postoperative home care.

She returned on the fifth postoperative day and reported considerable extra- and intraoral swelling and moderately severe pain. The tissues appeared to be healing satisfactorily but were being disturbed by tension from several prominent muscle attachments. Two of them were relaxed by lightly nicking them with the needle electrode activated with coagulating current. The sutures were removed (Case Fig. 7–1E) and tincture of myrrh and benzoin was applied. Healing progressed more rapidly thereafter. By the end of the sixth postoperative week the tissue healing was complete and the gingival mucosa appeared normal in color and tissue tone (Case Fig. 7–1F).

For two weeks postoperatively there was a severe exacerbation of her neuralgic symptoms; then most of the pain diminished greatly. Although the biopsy report indicated some resemblance of the resected tissue to an amputation neuroma, it was inconclusive diagnostically. Laboratory tests for possible bone dysplasia proved equally inconclusive since *all* the test results were reported to be within the *high normal* range. The only abnormal finding reported after a complete roentgenographic skeletal survey was the presence of a supernumerary cervical rib on the left side of her neck which could have been a pain factor.

Plastic closure of the mandibular perforation had produced marked local improvement in the mandible, but she still experienced some discomfort in the second molar region. The bone graft appeared to have "taken" successfully and become integrated with the surrounding bone, but the roentgenograms still suggested the periapical pathology around the second molar. Consequently, two months after the bone graft was performed this tooth was extracted and thorough curettage performed. Immediately thereafter the remaining local symptoms of discomfort in the mandible and ramus disappeared, but she continued to be troubled by symptoms in the left side of her neck and in the submaxillary gland.

Since these remaining symptoms may have been related to traumatic pressure of the supernumerary cervical rib against cervical branches of the facial nerve, the patient was referred, after consultation, to an osteopathic physician for manipulatory treatment, which is still being administered.

Despite the fact that a final diagnosis has not yet been established, this case has been reported for a number of reasons. It provides an excellent demonstration of the usefulness of bone grafts in repair of mandibular cortical perforations. It also affords an excellent example of the usefulness of electrosurgery for total eradication of aberrant tissue so that a healthy host bed can be provided for the bone graft. Finally, it is a reminder of the danger inherent in creating perforations into the mandibular cortex for endodontic or other therapeutic purposes without making adequate provision for their accurate closure.

Combined Tissue Flaps and Bone Grafts in Repair of Oro-Antral Perforations and Fistulae

Thus far we have considered surgical techniques whose success is totally dependent upon use of either a tissue flap or bone graft. There are many instances, however, where neither tissue flap nor bone graft alone may suffice, but where use of both is necessary for the success of the procedure. One of the conditions where this is very likely is in plastic closure of oro-antral perforations.

Oro-antral perforations rarely heal by primary intention. The ciliated epithelial lining membrane of the antrum cannot bridge the gap of a perforation in the floor of the antrum unless there is a bed of connective tissue or bone upon which it can grow. The lining membrane tends to grow down along the inner walls of a perforated tooth socket or other antral perforation when such a bed is not present, thereby creating an epithelized fistulous tract that prevents spontaneous healing of the defect.

A number of methods have been devised to effect satisfactory closure of antral cavities that have been perforated by oro-antral fistulas but very few are completely satisfactory.[25-27] One successful technique was described by the author in 1950.[27] This technique utilizes a palatal pedicle flap rotated into a prepared seating to form a tissue inlay that obliterates the fistulous opening and provides the necessary bed for ultimate regeneration of the ciliated lining membrane [28] (Fig. 22–1).

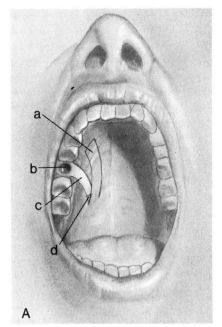
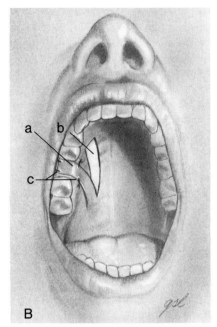

Figure 22–1. Schematic diagram for plastic closure of oro-antral fistulas or perforations with rotated palatal pedicle flaps. *A,* Diagram for incision and preparation of "tissue inlay" seating of flap. *a,* Flap incised. *b,* Oro-antral perforation freshened. *c,* Mucosa excised from area to be filled with the flap in order to prepare an accurate seating for it. *d,* Triangle of tissue excised to eliminate tissue bulge or pucker when the flap is rotated. *B,* Diagram showing flap elevated, rotated, seated and secured in its seating, by suturing to the surrounding mucosa. *a,* Pedicle flap rotated and secured into its seating. *b,* Palatal surgical defect formed by bed from which the flap was elevated, which fills in with reparative granulation tissue. *c,* Sutures retaining the flap in position.

CASE 8*

Both this case and the following one describe repair of antral perforations with the technique just mentioned.

This case offers a typical example of use of the tissue inlay technique performed with palatal flap incision and preparation of the seating area with a cold-steel scalpel. It is included for comparative purposes.

PATIENT. A 51-year-old white female.

HISTORY. The patient had had a number of teeth extracted to prepare her mouth for full denture construction. The roots of the maxillary left second molar extended up into a very low-dipping antrum. Part of the very thin bony floor of the antrum was fused to the roots of this tooth and came away with it when the tooth was extracted.

The dentist filled the socket with Gelfoam and then attempted immediate closure with parallel buccal and palatal slit incisions in order to create slack in the tissues. The respective margins were brought into coaptation and sutured with interrupted sutures. Lacking bony support, the margins sagged down into the defect, causing the sutures to tear through the tissues, thereby reopening the oro-antral communication.

The patient returned to the clinic complaining of headaches and drainage of fluids through her nose. She was referred to the author for oro-antral closure with a

---

*This case is presented to provide a clinical comparison of tissue repair following cold steel surgery and that following electrosurgery.

pedicle palatal flap. Since the dental clinic did not have electrosurgical equipment, the closure was performed with incisions made with a cold-steel scalpel.

CLINICAL EXAMINATION. *Extraoral.* Negative.

Intraoral. The alveolar ridge in the left maxillary molar area was badly resorbed. There was a pit-like depression present on the buccal aspect of the ridge, from which a discolored bluish area radiated (Case Fig. 8–1*A*).

Roentgenographic examination substantiated the loss of bone resulting in oro-antral communication.

TREATMENT. A study model of the maxilla was prepared on which the defect was reproduced. The surgical procedure was outlined on the model and a strip of rubber dam was cut to size to serve as a pattern for the preparation of the flap and for the prepared seat.

The mouth was prepared for surgery and posterior superior alveolar block anesthesia administered. The palate was incised with a No. 15 Bard-Parker scalpel blade along a line running parallel to the alveolar ridge, extending almost halfway to the incisive papilla. The base of the flap was made to extend almost into the soft palate, which assures that the pedicle flap will have a rich blood supply after it is elevated and rotated.

These palatal incisions created considerable bleeding which increased notably when the flap was undermined and reflected from the underlying periosteum and bone. The tissue on the ridge at the site of the defect was incised and excised to create a square base on sound bone for the seating of the flap. When this tissue was excised a large oro-antral perforation measuring approximately 6 mm. in diameter was exposed to view (Case Fig. 8–1*B*).

The bone at the edge of the perforation was very thin but it was freshened carefully with a bone file. Some medicated cultured bone paste was carefully inserted over the prepared base and defect by shaping it into a wafer and carefully tamping it down along the outer bony margin around the perforation. After it was seated firmly against the surrounding bone it served as a bone graft to seal the opening (Case Fig. 8–1*C*) so that the tissue flap could not sag down into the perforation. The flap was then rotated into position and sutured to the gingival mucosa around the prepared seating (Case Fig. 8–1*D*).

After the rotated flap was secured in its new position, the palatal defect created by the removal of the flap tissue filled with blood. When the blood clotted, a piece of adhesive dry-foil was placed over the entire operative field and the patient's old denture (which had been sterilized) was inserted and used as a surgical stent. Achromycin was prescribed and she was instructed to leave the denture in undisturbed for 24 hours.

She returned for postoperative treatment four days later. Inspection of the maxilla showed progress of normal healing. The flap was united to the surrounding mucosa by primary union and the palatal defect marking the flap site was filled with healthy granulation tissue (Case Fig. 8–1*E*). The sutures were removed and the area painted with tincture of myrrh and benzoin applied in air-dried layers.

She was seen postoperatively thereafter at regular weekly intervals. Healing progressed uneventfully and by the end of the eighth week the operative field was completely healed. The palatal site from which the flap had been elevated was filled with normal firm mucosa. The flap itself was contiguous with the surrounding tissue and filled the area over the original fistulous defect solidly with firm tissue (Case Fig. 8–1*F*). The only abnormality observed was a constriction of the palatal tissue along the border of its junction with the rotated flap. There, as a result of cicatricial contrac-

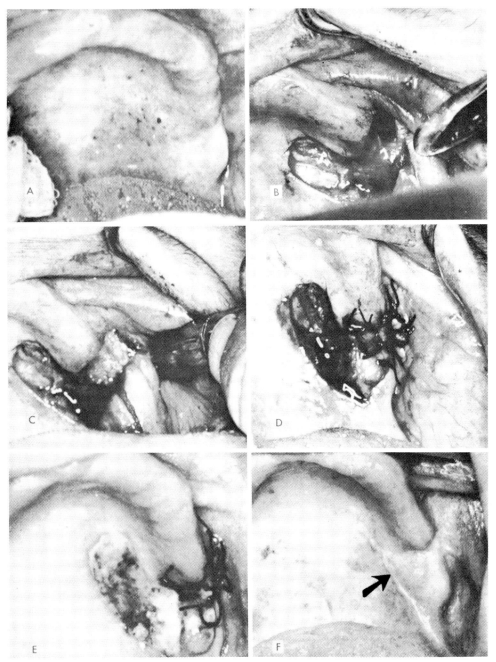

Case Figure 8–1. Closure of an oro-antral perforation with a palatal pedicle flap prepared by incision with cold-steel scalpels. *A,* Preoperative appearance of maxilla. A bluish discoloration is present near a slightly concave portion of the edentulous left molar region at the junction of the buccal and gingival mucosa. A pin-point opening in the area of discoloration permits insertion of a flexible silver probe into the maxillary antrum. *B,* Incised flap is reflected from the palate; a buccal seating has been prepared, exposing a large oval oro-antral perforation. *C,* Perforation sealed by adapting cultured bone paste to the bony base of the prepared seating area to bridge across the opening and prevent inward collapse of the flap from lack of support. *D,* Flap has been rotated, seated and sutured to surrounding mucosa. *E,* Appearance on the fourth postoperative day. The flap appears to be "taking," and the palatal surgical defect is filled with granulation tissue lightly covered with healthy coagulum. *F,* Appearance two months postoperatively. The flap now is homogeneous with the surrounding mucosa. The tissue is healthy and fully healed. The perforation is completely sealed, but an elevated, fibrous, cord-like welt of scar connective tissue is present on the palate which parallels the distal margin of the bed from which the flap was lifted (arrow).

935

tion of the tissues along the side of the base of the flap, a raised welt of cord-like scar tissue extended posteroanteriorly from the soft palate to the flap inset. The flap tissue also was slightly contracted so that it was depressed slightly beneath the level of the surrounding palatal mucosa. Neither of these contractions impaired the functional capabilities of the tissues.

CASE 9

This case is an example of the dual repair that may become necessary when a root is accidentally displaced into the maxillary antrum leaving an oro-antral perforation and a retained root fragment in the sinus cavity. An excellent contrast is afforded in this case between the quality of tissue repair achieved by cold-steel incision and by electrosection.

In this type of case, recovery of the displaced root fragment must precede repair of the perforating defect. Unlike most other traumatic injuries, where treatment often is largely improvised and empirical, the modified Caldwell-Luc procedure for recovery of roots or other foreign bodies from the antrum is a standardized, classic technique.

PATIENT.   A 43-year-old white female.

HISTORY.   During extraction of a maxillary molar the apical third of its mesial root fractured. As soon as the dentist touched it with an elevator the root disappeared from view. An apical elevator inserted into the socket penetrated upward without encountering bony resistance. Suspecting that the root had become displaced into the antrum, he made a small incision and reflected the tissues for a better view. He found an oro-antral perforation extending beyond the root socket. The patient was immediately informed of the accident and referred for removal of the displaced root and closure of the oro-antral defect.

CLINICAL EXAMINATION.   *Extraoral.*   Negative.

Intraoral.   The right molar area was still anesthetized, and blood oozed from the lacerated tissues. After the mouth was cleansed by irrigation, inspection showed that the tissue in the right maxillary first molar area was mutilated and that there probably was an oro-antral perforation in the mesiobuccal socket of the first molar. The perforation was verified by inserting a flexible silver probe into the socket. The probe penetrated into the antrum without resistance.

Roentgenographic examination revealed the presence of the root fragment in the antrum close to and immediately superior to the apex of the mesiobuccal root of the second molar. The antrum appeared to be subdivided by a number of thin bony septa.

TREATMENT.   The patient was badly shaken, apprehensive, and in no condition for further extensive surgery at the time. Treatment was limited to an attempt to locate the root clinically and if possible to recover it by irrigating the antrum and aspirating the fluid vigorously.

As anticipated, this proved unsuccessful. It was evident that it would be necessary to perform a modified Caldwell-Luc procedure to recover the root and plastic closure of the perforation. The defect was closed temporarily with two sutures and the patient was reappointed for definitive surgery after initial healing of the local tissues. In the interim, Cosa-Tetrastatin and Kasdenol lavage was prescribed prophylactically.

Three weeks later the patient returned for definitive surgery. By that time the gingival tissues were firm and healthy despite the presence of a fistulous tract leading

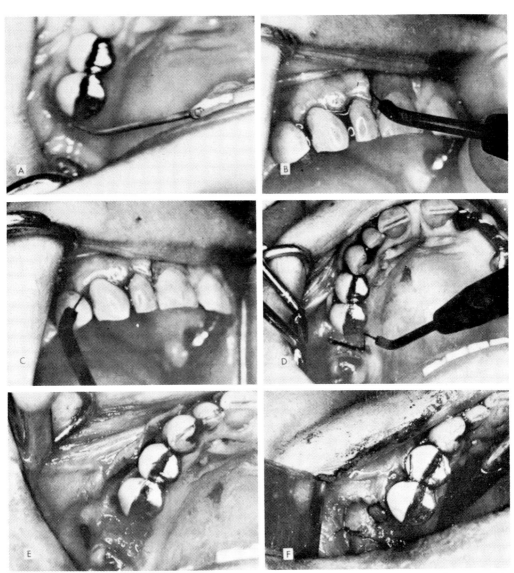

Case Figure 9–1. Removal of a root fragment displaced into the antrum, and repair of the traumatic oro-antral perforation. Stage I. Modified Caldwell-Luc procedure for removal of displaced root. *A,* Clinical appearance with silver probe inserted into the antrum through the oro-antral perforation (mesiobuccal socket of extracted first molar). *B,* Anterior incision for modified Caldwell-Luc procedure made with 45-degree-angle fine needle electrode. Incision, started in mucolabial vestibule, is extended downward obliquely 10 degrees to the mesiogingival angle of the lateral. *C,* Attachments of the interproximal papillae severed posteriorly to the second molar with the same electrode. *D,* Granulation tissue in the socket of the recently extracted molar is incised and excised to prepare a seating for the palatal pedicle flap. *E,* Buccal flap for Caldwell-Luc procedure elevated, opening for removal of displaced root fragment made high on lateral wall of the tuberosity, and walls of oro-antral perforation freshened. *F,* Graft of medicated cultured despeciated fetal calf mandible inserted into mesiobuccal socket to seal oro-antral perforation.

into the antrum. The flexible silver probe was inserted through the fistula on the crest of the alveolar ridge, communicating with the antrum (Case Fig. 9–1A). The displaced root fragment was not in evidence roentgenographically. A second view was filmed more posteriorly in order to fully include the tuberosity. This film revealed that the shifted root was now lying at the furthermost posterior portion of the tuberosity.

Stage 1. Removal of Displaced Root from Antrum.   The mouth was prepared for surgery and infraorbital, posterior superior alveolar, nasopalatine, and anterior palatine block anesthesia was administered to anesthetize the entire right half of the maxilla. A 45-degree-angle fine needle electrode was selected and current output set at 3.5 for electrosection.

A vertico-oblique incision was started in the mucolabial fold near the midline and carried downward and slightly backward to the mesiogingival margin of the right lateral incisor (Case Fig. 9–1B). All the attachments of the interproximal papillae on the right side were then severed in their respective embrasures (Case Fig. 9–1C). The incision was then extended posteriorly across the crest of the alveolar ridge to the distal aspect of the tuberosity.

As preplanned on a study model of the maxilla which had been prepared the previous week, the mucosa in the edentulous first molar area was incised with the electrode and excised (Case Fig. 9–1D) to create an accurately prepared seating for a palatal rotated pedicle flap. The incised labial and buccal gingival mucosa was then undermined and retracted, exposing the buccal aspect of the entire tuberosity. The thin buccal cortex high on the ridge was easily pierced with a Crane pick. The opening was enlarged with a rongeur forceps to create a window 8 mm. in diameter, slightly larger than the length of the root fragment (Case Fig. 9–1E).

The original oro-antral perforation's marginal wall was freshened, and through this defect the antrum was irrigated while the fluid was aspirated from the posterior window in the tuberosity. After some shaking and tilting of the patient's head, and manipulation, the root finally reached the posterior perforation and was removed.

Stage 2. Plastic Closure of Oro-Antral Perforation.   A piece of cultured fetal calf mandible was cut and trimmed to proper size and shape to fit into the old anterior perforation on the alveolar ridge. The graft was medicated with sulfathiazole powder and Albamycin, inserted into the oro-antral defect and tightly wedged into place (Case Fig. 9–1F). A few small crevices between the bone graft and the alveolar bone were sealed with medicated bone paste; then the buccal gingiva was restored to position and sutured.

The patient now was ready for the second phase: protection of the bone graft with a palatal rotated pedicle flap. The exact pattern for this flap had been designed on the study model, with strips of rubber dam used as the pattern material.

A perfect replica of the preplanned flap was painted on the patient's palate with acriviolet (Case Fig. 9–2A). The flap was then incised down to the periosteum with the needle electrode (current output increased to 5) following the flap outline exactly (Case Fig. 9–2B). When the incisions were completed—bloodlessly—the flap was undermined and reflected from the underlying periosteum and bone with a periosteal elevator. A small blood vessel was torn in the process of lifting the flap. The spurting bleeder was quickly brought under control by clamping with a mosquito hemostat. A biterminal electrocoagulating current output of 2 was applied with a small ball electrode (Case Fig. 9–2C).

The flap was then rotated to fit into the prepared seating, coapted to the surrounding palatal and gingival mucosa and secured to them with 0000 braided silk interrupted sutures. A mixture of medicated surgical gelatin was inserted into the new

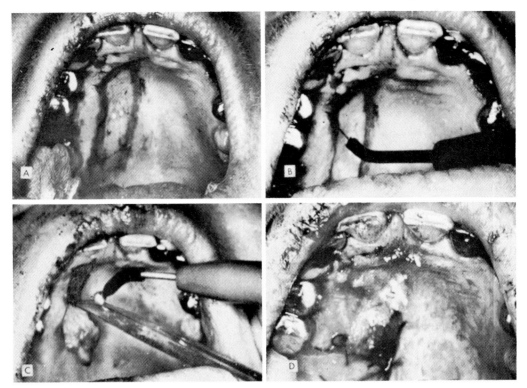

Case Figure 9–2. Stage II. Plastic closure of oro-antral defect with bone graft and rotated palatal pedicle flap. *A*, Palatal flap outlined with acriviolet, following exactly a prepared pattern. *B*, Flap incised with 45-degree-angle fine needle electrode, following precisely the outline. *C*, Flap undermined and elevated from its bed. Bleeding from a small vessel torn in lifting the flap is brought under control by coagulating off the beaks of a mosquito hemostat with a large ball electrode. *D*, Flap has been rotated, seated and sutured to the surrounding mucosa. The bed of the flap, now a surgical defect on the palate, is filled with medicated surgical gelatin. Note accurate coaptation of the flap with the surrounding mucosa.

palatal surgical defect (Case Fig. 9–2*D*). The gelatin was mixed with the blood and soon a firm clot formed. The posterior gingival incision was closed with interrupted silk sutures and the interproximal papillae were secured into their respective embrasures. A specially prepared full-palate clear acrylic spint was inserted to serve as a protective surgical stent.

The patient was instructed to leave the stent in undisturbed and to return for postoperative observation in 24 hours. The following day she reported that she had had remarkably little pain or even discomfort. Postoperative edema also was so minimal that it was practically unnoticeable.

The stent was removed and the mouth gently irrigated. A firm, healthy looking blood clot filled the palatal defect (Case Fig. 9–3*A*); the flap was perfectly adapted, firm and healthy. Tincture of myrrh and benzoin was applied and the stent replaced. The patient was instructed to remove the stent every two hours for lavage and to continue the antibiotic therapy for three more days.

She returned on the fifth postoperative day. The lines of incision and the flap were healing rapidly by primary intention and the palatal defect was beginning to form normal granulation tissue (Case Fig. 9–3*B*). The sutures were removed and tinc-

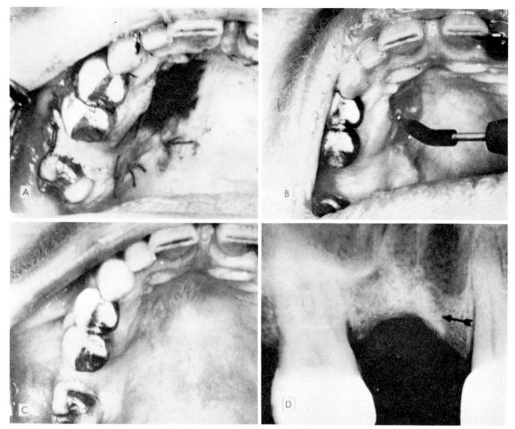

Case Figure 9–3. Postoperative sequence. *A*, Appearance of the tissues 24 hours post-operatively. The palatal defect is filled with a firm, healthy blood clot. The flap tissue is normal and beginning to show signs of primary union. *B*, Healing progress controlled and accelerated by superficial spot coagulation of irregular tissue tabs or retarded areas. Note perfect marginal coaptation and primary union of flap to surrounding mucosa. *C*, Appearance two months post-operatively. Healing is complete. The contour of the palate, the ridge and the mucobuccal fold is normal. The tissue tone is excellent and the flap tissue is indistinguishable from the surrounding mucosa. There is no scar tissue or contraction. *D*, Roentgenographic appearance four months postoperatively. Healing is complete. Arrow points to fetal calf mandible graft which appears to have formed a perfect union with the surrounding host bone. Only a difference in trabeculation differentiates it from the normal host bone.

ture of myrrh and benzoin was applied in air-dried layers. She was instructed to continue to use the stent and frequent lavage until further notice.

During the following month she returned twice a week for postoperative treatment. During this period it became obvious that the flap had taken perfectly; the palatal defect was almost fully healed by the end of the third week. The new tissue was maturing rapidly except for a few tiny dot-like spots on the surface which were superficially coagulated with a small ball electrode, with current output of 0.5, to hasten maturation (Case Fig. 9–3*B*).

She continued to be seen once a week for another month. Healing continued favorably and required only occasional spot coagulation in isolated tiny areas to assure uniformity. By the end of the sixth week the stent was discarded, and by the end of the eighth week the maxilla was fully healed.

The flap was firmly seated and the interproximal papillae tightly reattached. Both the flap and regenerated palatal mucosa were uniform in color, texture and appearance with the rest of the palatal tissue. The repair tissue was so soft and supple that it was virtually impossible to identify where the flap had united with the areolar tissue of the cheek. The palatal mucosa presented a comparably harmonious appearance. There was no visible evidence of either scar tissue or cicatricial contraction (Case Fig. 9–3C).

A follow-up roentgenogram taken two months later showed equally successful repair of the oro-antral perforation, with unmistakable evidence of harmonious consolidation of the bone graft with the surrounding alveolar bone (Case Fig. 9–3D). The patient returned for postoperative observation for the next two years. The oral tissues have remained normal and the antrum has remained asymptomatic.

III. SIALOLITHIASIS OF SUBMAXILLARY DUCT AND GLAND

Calcareous deposits are a commonplace occurrence in many parts of the body. Renal calculi are calcareous accretions that form in the kidneys or bladder. Gallstones are calcareous accretions that form in the bile duct or the common duct. Sialoliths are calcareous accretions that form in the salivary glands or ducts.

Although the sialoliths may occur in any of the salivary glands or ducts, the submaxillary *duct* is by far the most common site of sialolith formation. Submaxillary *gland* sialoliths are much more uncommon. Sialolithiasis of the sublingual glands and ducts is even more uncommon. Sialolithiasis of the parotid gland and duct is relatively rare.

Sialolithotomy of the Submaxillary Duct

Sialolithotomy, the surgical removal of the sialoliths from the submaxillary duct, has traditionally been performed via the intraoral route, by direct incision into the duct through the tissues forming the floor of the mouth.

Two factors influence the efficiency of this surgical procedure:
1. The character of the tissues that are involved.
2. The location of the calcareous mass in the duct.

TISSUE CHARACTER

The tissues forming the floor of the mouth are very delicate, highly mobile, and very vascular. It is necessary to cut through these delicate, mobile tissues to incise into the submaxillary duct. When the incision is made by "conventional" steel scalpel instrumentation, the mobility of the tissues greatly increases the difficulty of cutting through them cleanly and precisely to the duct even when they are pulled taut or have been made taut by distention, since it is necessary to exert manual pressure to force the blade into the tissue to cleave through to the duct.

The pressure that must be applied to cut with a steel scalpel blade is difficult to control when it meets variable, shifting resistance. This creates the danger of accidentally cutting through the duct or severing it and thereby creating a surgical defect that is very difficult to repair. Steel scalpel incisions are accompanied by bleeding that obscures the surgical field and increases this hazard. The profuse, usually persistent bleeding also adds to the difficulty of locating and removing the sialolith atraumatically.

When the incision is made by electrosection with the proper current, there is no need to use pressure to cut through the overlying tissues and into the duct. Thus, when the precise site for the incision has been determined, the fine needle electrode will cut through the overlying tissue down to the calcareous mass effortlessly, if an adequate amount of cutting current is employed to disintegrate and volatilize all the tissue cells in the line of cleavage efficiently. It is usually necessary to use more cutting current output than is used for cutting normal gingival tissues, owing to the vascularity of the tissues of the floor of the mouth; more current is necessary especially when there is an increase of the intracellular and extracellular fluid content of the tissues as a result of edema, engorgement, or inflammation.

In the absence of inflammation and engorgement, the incision into the duct does not cause hemorrhagic free bleeding. The resultant unobscured surgical field greatly facilitates removal of the sialolith from the duct. Inasmuch as no pressure is required to cut electrosurgically, the surgeon can control the depth of penetration of the electrode, thereby greatly minimizing the hazard of accidentally severing the duct.

LOCATION OF THE SIALOLITH IN THE DUCT

The submaxillary duct is medial to and parallel with the alveolar ridge of the mandible, with the orifice of the duct on the surface of the tissues of the anterior floor of the mouth. As the duct courses posteriorly toward the hilus of the gland, it runs deeper. Thus, the more anteriorly the sialolith is located, the more easily it can be palpated and visualized clinically.

If the sialolith is large and located anteriorly in the duct, it is easily palpated and the exact site for the incision to free the calcareous mass can be determined without guesswork. If it is slender and cylindrical and located near the orifice of the duct, it is sometimes even possible to remove it from the duct without resorting to surgery by "milking" the duct, that is, by applying gentle massage to the duct in a postero-anterior direction toward the orifice of the duct. If milking will not displace the sialolith from the duct, and an incision must be made, insertion of a suture through the duct orifice helps to pull the tissue taut and facilitates the incision.

When the sialolith is located about midway between the duct orifice and the hilus of the gland, it may or may not be clinically visible and palpable, but it can easily be located roentgenographically with an occlusal film view of the mandible (Case Fig. 12–1).

When the sialolith is located in the posterior part of the duct it is lodged so deep in the submaxillary triangle that it usually cannot be palpated even when the gland is displaced superiorly toward the floor of the mouth by extraorally applied pressure. The diagnosis and location of the calcareous mass are dependent upon the occlusal view roentgenographic visualization rather than on clinical evidence. Under such conditions determination of the precise site for the incision to release the mass from the duct presents a distinct clinical and surgical challenge. Needless to say, an attempt to incise deeply through the intervening tissues of the floor of the mouth in the hope of incising into the duct would be sheer guesswork, and such an imprecise incision would be fraught with the danger of injury to the important anatomic structures present in this area.

The author utilizes a technique that eliminates the element of guesswork. The technique consists of inserting a flexible silver lachrymal probe into the duct and advancing it *slowly* and *gently* until it encounters a slight resistance from the calcareous mas that arrests its further progress. Patience and careful instrumentation are essential, to avoid accidentally displacing the sialolith through the hilus into the gland.

Since the mass is located immediately posterior to the tip of the probe, the site for the incision is pinpointed. The incision site is then accurately visualized by lifting the probe in the duct to delineate its outline. Elevation of the probe also lifts the tissues of the floor of the mouth and pulls them taut, so that they can easily be incised downward to the duct by following the outline of the tissue elevated posterior to the probe and directing the incision in a postero-anterior direction along the elevated tissue toward the tip of the probe.

The needle electrode floats through the intervening tissues and penetrates effortlessly down to the superior surface of the calcareous mass. When the proper cutting current is used and the tissues of the floor of the mouth are normal in tone, there is almost total absence of bleeding, and vision in the surgical field remains unimpaired.

After the tissue has been incised the mass can sometimes be displaced upward into the floor of the mouth by grasping the external end of the silver probe with a mosquito hemostat and gently wiggling it. When this succeeds in displacing the mass into the mouth, need to remove it with a curet is eliminated. Even when the sialolith cannot be displaced in this manner and must be removed by curettage, the instrumentation is greatly facilitated and the efficiency of the instrumentation is greatly enhanced by the absence of hemorrhagic bleeding.

COMPLICATIONS AND HOW TO AVOID THEM

Sialolithiasis often is complicated by secondary infection. When secondary infection is present it is necessary to treat and eliminate the infection before surgical intervention is instituted. If there is purulent exudation the duct should be irrigated gently, in addition to the other local and systemic therapy that is administered and prescribed.

Failure to eliminate the infection before the surgery may result in development of a phlegmon, and the infection may spread along the fascial planes to the anterior or posterior mediastinum, with calamitous results.

**TECHNIQUE FOR REMOVAL OF
SIALOLITHS LOCATED NEAR THE
DUCT ORIFICE**

CASE 10

This case is a typical example of an uncomplicated sialolithiasis of the submaxillary duct. A simple technique for bloodless electrosurgical sialolithotomy is presented.

PATIENT. A 66-year-old white female.

HISTORY. A hard lump suddenly appeared in the floor of the mouth. Fearing cancer, she consulted her physician. In the absence of current or previous significant symptoms he suspected ranula or a mucocele. She was referred for diagnosis and treatment.

CLINICAL EXAMINATION. *Extraoral.* Negative.

Intraoral. The anterior part of the mandible was edentulous. Near the middle of the left half of the floor of the mouth there was a hard round elevation approximately 0.5 cm. in diameter. It was surrounded by a zone of moderate engorgement (Case Fig. 10–1A). On palpation the mass felt like a separate unattached body. Its location in the region of the submaxillary duct and its clinical features suggested a sialolith in the left submaxillary duct.

Roentgenographic examination with an occlusal view film confirmed the clinical diagnosis of sialolithiasis. A single, solid radiopaque mass was located opposite and about 1 cm. medial to the left bicuspids.

TREATMENT. The mouth was prepared for surgery and circumferential infiltration anesthesia was administered. A 45-degree-angle fine needle electrode was selected and current output set at 3 for electrosection. A silk suture was inserted through the orifice of the duct and used to pull the tissues of the floor of the mouth forward tautly. The tissue over the elevated mass was incised down to the calculus with a wiping motion. The incision, approximately 1 cm. in length, was made in a posteroanterior direction (Case Fig. 10–1B and C).

The margins of the incision were spread with a periosteal elevator. This exposed a round, yellowish, calcareous mass which was engaged with a small cup curet and removed through the incision (Case Fig. 10–1D). The duct was irrigated with saline solution; then the suture was removed. The entire procedure was bloodless and did not require suturing or a drain.

The patient returned 24 hours later. The engorgement was subsiding, and there was no edema. The incision was healing rapidly (Case Fig. 10–1E). She was seen again one week later. This time the incision was fully healed without visible scar or cicatricial contraction. The tissues of the floor of the mouth were normal in color and tone (Case Fig. 10–1F).

**TECHNIQUE FOR REMOVAL OF
SIALOLITHS MIDWAY BETWEEN
THE DUCT ORIFICE AND GLAND**

This type of sialolith is relatively simple to locate by digital palpation unless it is accompanied by acute or subacute infection which may produce

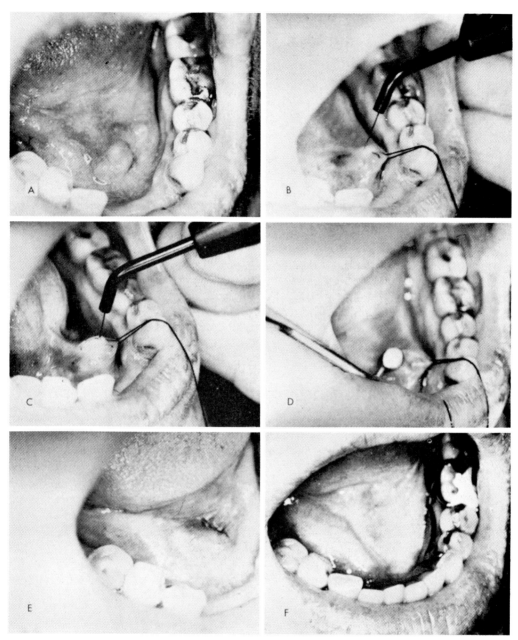

Case Figure 10–1. Sialolithotomy of the submaxillary duct. *A*, Preoperative appearance. A small, hard round mass is visible (and palpable) in the region of the left submaxillary duct. *B*, Incision of duct over the mass with a fine 45-degree-angle needle electrode started. *C*, Incision, directed anteriorly, is completed. Note complete lack of bleeding and unimpaired visibility. *D*, Calculus removed from the duct through the incision with a cup curet. *E*, Appearance 24 hours postoperatively. Healing is progressing. There is moderate engorgement but no edema or seepage of saliva. *F*, Appearance one week postoperatively. Healing is complete. There is no scar tissue or cicatricial contraction, and no edema. The tissues are completely normal except for a slightly deeper pink color along the line of incision. The patient is again able to wear her lingual bar denture.

inflammatory induration that would greatly increase the difficulty of determining its precise location in the duct.

In the absence of infection, introduction of a flexible silver lachrymal
probe into the duct until it encounters resistance from the calcareous mass is
the best way to locate the site and to make the tissues taut so that a precise incision can be made down to the mass.

CASE 11

In this case the sialolith was large and bulbous and had irritated the tissues sufficiently to cause distention and induration of the tissues of the floor of the mouth in
the vicinity of the mass. Its location was, as a result, self-evident and there was no
need to cannulize the duct with the silver probe to locate the site for the incision or to
pull the tissue taut to facilitate precise incision down to the duct.

PATIENT.   A 56-year-old white female.

HISTORY.   The patient was a victim of grand mal and had been maintained on
Dilantin medication for many years, but apparently had never developed Dilantin
hypertrophy. She suddenly developed a swelling in the floor of the mouth that caused
her discomfort from a feeling of fullness. She consulted her brother, a dentist, and he
diagnosed her condition as sialolithiasis of the submaxillary duct or gland. An intraoral occlusal view roentgenogram confirmed the presence of a sialolith in the duct,
and he referred her to the author for the surgery to remove it.

CLINICAL EXAMINATION.   The tissue over the left submaxillary duct was dark
red in color, swollen, and distended superiorly (Case Fig. 11–1A). The swelling
created a marked imbalance in the clinical appearance of the tissues of the floor of the
mouth. Despite the obvious evidence of irritation there was no evidence of infection
or purulent exudation. Palpation of the swollen tissue was not acutely painful; it
revealed the presence of a hard mass in the duct at a point parallel with the bicuspid
teeth. A slightly angulated occlusal view x-ray showed the mass to be approximately 1
cm. long and toothlike in shape, with an ovoid shape at its anterior end and tapering
conically toward its posterior end.

TREATMENT.   Despite the absence of clinical evidence of infection, Erythrocin
was prescribed 24 hours preoperatively, to be continued for a total of four days, to assure maximum precaution against complications. The following day the tissues were
prepared for anesthesia and an inferior alveolar-lingual block injection was administered. A 45-degree-angle fine needle electrode was selected, and cutting current was
set at 4 on the power output dial to assure adequate cutting power despite the
engorgement and edema of the tissue to be incised.

Since the exact site for the incision was visible and the tissues were taut from the
distention and slight induration, it was not necessary to use a silver probe insertion
into the duct for this procedure. The activated electrode was used with a wiping motion to make an incision into the duct by following the outline of the elevated tissue
(Case Fig. 11–1B). The incision was directed postero-anteriorly and extended from a
point parallel with the first molar to the lateral incisor. Some blood was released as
the tissue was incised, but there was no free bleeding, and the top of the sialolith
bulged upward into the floor of the mouth as the overlying tissue was cut (Case Fig.
11–1C). Since the top of the sialolith was widest in diameter, it spread the incision
open (Case Fig. 11–1D). Normally these incisions are not sutured, but owing to the

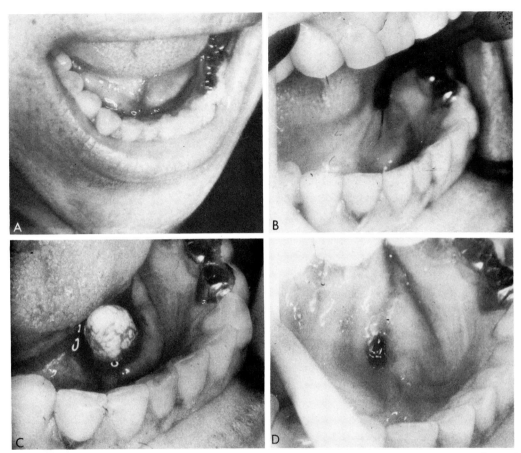

Case Figure 11–1. A, Preoperative appearance. The tissues in the left half of the floor of the mouth are engorged and swollen. The fringe tissue is distended and elevated and indurated and dark red in color. The tissue of the right half of the floor of the mouth is normal in appearance. B, An incision is being made through the left submaxillary duct with a fine 45-degree-angle needle electrode. The incision site has been predetermined by digital palpation and by inserting a flexible silver lachrymal probe into the duct until it met resistance to further penetration by a sialolith in the duct, to create an incision into the duct through which the sialolith can be expelled or removed. C, A large oval calcareous mass has been expelled from the duct into the mouth through the incision. D, The incised exit site immediately after the removal of the sialolith. The margins of the incision have been spread so wide by the expulsion of the large mass that a suture will be required to bring them into proper coaptation. Although there is no coagulation of the marginal tissue, there is no free bleeding.

width of the opening that had been spread apart by the emergence of the sialolith, the tissues were coapted with a silk suture and the patient was given dietary and lavage instructions and reappointed.

    She returned on the fifth postoperative day and reported that she had had no pain or even marked discomfort. The edema and engorgement of the tissues of the floor of the mouth were no longer in evidence, and the wound appeared to be healing by primary intention (Case Fig. 11–2A). The suture was removed and the patient was instructed to return in a week for further postoperative observation (Case Fig. 11–2B). Healing progressed uneventfully and by the end of the third postoperative week the tissues in the surgical field had returned to normal in all respects (Case Fig. 11–2C).

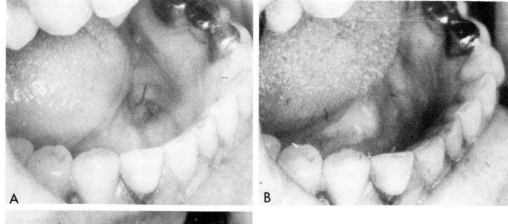

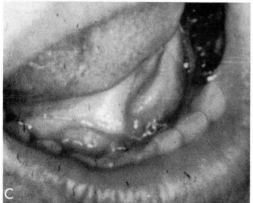

Case Figure 11–2. A, Postoperative appearance. On the fifth postoperative day, before the suture is removed, the tissues in the left half of the floor of the mouth appear greatly improved. The swelling has subsided almost completely, as has the engorgement. The coapted tissue margins appear to have begun to undergo primary repair. *B,* Appearance immediately after removal of the suture. The beginning of primary repair is confirmed. *C.* Final postoperative appearance. The incision site is not clinically visible. The tissues of the floor of the mouth are identical in appearance and dimension on both the right and left sides. Saliva flows unimpeded from the left submaxillary duct, indicating that there has been no perforation into the floor of the mouth or blockage by adhesions. This has been established by closing the orifice of the duct by finger pressure for 2 minutes and then releasing the pressure. Immediately thereafter a copious flow of saliva can be seen emerging through the orifice. No sign of saliva escaping into the floor of the mouth was manifested while the duct was sealed off.

TECHNIQUE FOR REMOVAL OF
SIALOLITHS LOCATED AT OR NEAR
POSTERIOR END OF DUCT

CASE 12

This case demonstrates the technique for removal of sialoliths located in the posterior part of the submaxillary duct, deep in the submaxillary triangle, that are clinically nonpalpable.

PATIENT. A 39-year-old white female.

HISTORY. She suddenly noticed that after eating tart or spicy foods, or smelling acrid spicy odors, a swelling developed in the floor of her mouth. The swellings subsided slowly but spontaneously, but caused her considerable discomfort while they lasted. She described this to her husband, a physician, who suspected sialolithiasis and referred her to the author for diagnosis and treatment.

CLINICAL EXAMINATION. The tissues of the floor of the mouth appeared normal at the time of the examination. There was no inflammation, redness, or other evidence of irritation of the duct or its orifice. Digital palpation of the accessible part of the duct, even with the submaxillary gland displaced superiorly toward the floor of the mouth by external pressure, was negative. An occlusal view x-ray revealed part of a sialolith at the posterior end of the film, but the mass was located so far posteriorly that only the anterior half of it was included in the intraoral film. An inferior alveolar-lingual nerve block was administered, and a flexible silver lachrymal probe was introduced into the duct and advanced carefully until it encountered resistance. The probe stopped at a point parallel with the second molar tooth, thereby indicating the precise location of the sialolith and confirming that it was in the duct (Case Fig. 12–1).

TREATMENT.   A 45-degree-angle fine needle electrode with a 2 cm. cutting filament was selected, and cutting current was set at 3.5 on the power setting dial. The silver probe was elevated forcefully (Case Fig. 12–2A and B). This pulled the tissue over the length of the probe taut and sharply delineated the duct to the end of the probe and somewhat posteriorly beyond it. The electrode was activated and used to incise along the duct outline in a postero-anterior direction from a point parallel with the distal of the third molar anteriorly to the end of the probe, terminating at a point approximately parallel with the first molar. The incision was relatively bloodless, and as the tissue was incised the dark line of the probe became visible. The free external end of the probe was grasped with a mosquito hemostat and gently wiggled until the sialolith was expelled from the duct and displaced into the oral cavity (Case Fig. 12–2C).

The sialolith was a golden yellow-colored solid mass, and there was no evidence of amorphous gravel or other calcareous fragments in the duct. The margins of the in-

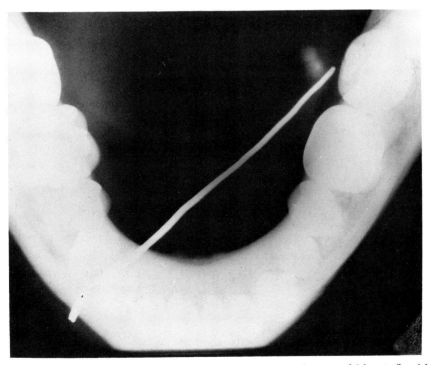

Case Figure 12–1.   Preoperative occlusal view x-ray of the mandible. A flexible silver lachrymal probe is present in the left submaxillary duct. The tip of the probe is in contact with a cylindrical salivary calculus in the posterior part of the mandible.

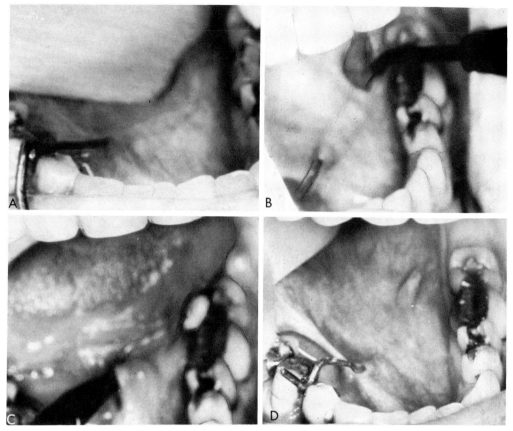

Case Figure 12–2. A, Preoperative appearance, intraoral. A flexible silver lachrymal probe has been inserted into the left submaxillary duct and advanced posteriorly until it met resistance. Approximately 5 cm. of the probe has not penetrated into the duct. B, The silver probe has been lifted to pull the tissues of the floor of the mouth taut, clearly delineating the submaxillary duct. An incision is being made along the outlined duct at the posterior end of the probe with a fine 45-degree-angle needle electrode by electrosection. The incision, approximately 3 cm. in length, starts just anterior to the pharynx and extends anteriorly to the mesial aspect of the second molar and downward to and into, but not through, the duct. Despite the vascularity of the tissues of the floor of the mouth the incision has not caused hemorrhage. C, The external end of the silver probe has been grasped with a mosquito hemostat and has been wiggled in the duct to displace the sialolith. The calcareous mass has been ejected into the floor of the mouth without need to use a curet to remove it. D, Appearance of the tissues of the floor of the mouth one week later. The tissues appear normal in tone, color, and texture. The silver probe has been reinserted into the duct and advanced posteriorly, without meeting resistance, until about 2 cm. of the probe remains externally. The reinsertion proves that the duct is patent and that the incision into the duct has healed.

cised tissue were being coapted by pressure from the tongue so that there was no need to suture the wound. Tincture of myrrh and benzoin was applied in air-dried layers, the patient was instructed in postoperative home care and reappointed for postoperative evaluation.

She returned one week later and reported an uneventful experience. The tissues along the line of incision were clinically undistinguishable from the surrounding tissues. It was now necessary to establish two things: first, whether the duct was patent or had become sealed by adhesions, and second, whether the wound in the mouth was fully healed. The silver probe was therefore reinserted into the duct, and this time it advanced unimpeded its full length, penetrating beyond the duct into the gland (Case Fig. 12–2D), thereby providing the evidence that the duct was patent and the wound in the floor of the mouth fully healed.

Sialolithotomy of the Submaxillary Gland

Prior to the development of the intraoral submaxillary gland electrosurgical sialolithotomy technique by the author, it had been considered impossible to remove calculi from the body of the submaxillary gland via the intraoral route, and sialolithectomy, or surgical extirpation of the gland, was accepted as the only realistic feasible treatment for this condition, despite numerous hazards that are inherent to this procedure.[29-32]

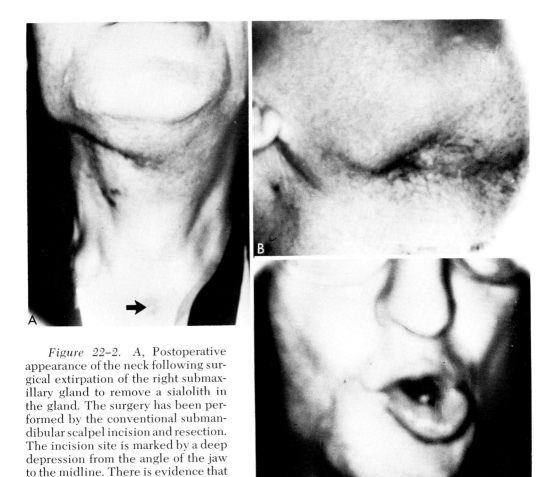

Figure 22–2. *A,* Postoperative appearance of the neck following surgical extirpation of the right submaxillary gland to remove a sialolith in the gland. The surgery has been performed by the conventional submandibular scalpel incision and resection. The incision site is marked by a deep depression from the angle of the jaw to the midline. There is evidence that a tracheostomy (arrow) had also been performed for this patient. *B,* A close-up view of the disfiguring wound healing, which is characterized by marked tissue contraction. *C,* The most damaging postoperative effect, however, is not the scar but the paralysis of the facial muscles of expression due to injury to some of the facial nerve plexus during the surgical removal, which creates a disfiguring distortion of the lips while speaking or smiling.

The extraoral incision for access to the gland is a submandibular incision that parallels the contour of the inferior border of the mandible. Although the incision is made in the tissue of the neck well beyond the body of the mandible in a caudal direction, there is an ever-constant hazard associated with it of severing some of the branches of the facial nerve plexus that ramify throughout this area, with paralysis of some of the muscles of facial expression a likely prolonged aftermath. Figure 22–2 is a typical rather than an unusual aftermath of sialolitectomy of the submaxillary gland. (The partial facial paralysis that af-

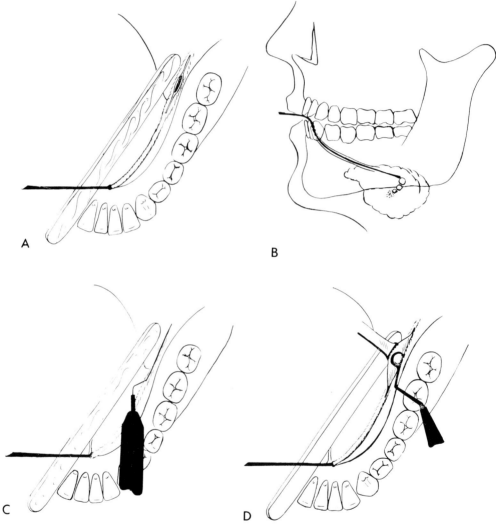

Figure 22–3. Schematic drawings of the techinque for electronic intraoral incision into the body of the submaxillary gland for intraoral sialolithotomy. *A,* Position of flexible silver probe inserted through the submaxillary duct into the submaxillary gland. *B,* A lateral jaw view shows the probe in contact with the sialoliths in the body of the gland. *C,* Incision of the floor of the mouth with a fine 45-degree-angle needle electrode following the outline of the duct along the elevated probe. The incision extends from the pillar of the fauces anteriorly to the second molar, approximately 3.5 to 4 centimeters. A clear bloodless field, essential for accuracy, is achieved. *D,* The medial incised margin is retracted, appropriate-sized cup curet inserted into body of the gland, calculus engaged and removed.

fected this patient persisted for more than two years.) The proximity of the lingual and hypoglossal nerves, the external maxillary artery, and the anterior facial vein add materially to the hazard potential of surgical extirpation of this gland.

When the sialoliths are small and scattered throughout the acini of the gland or if the calcarous mass forms in the large inferior lobe of the gland, despite the aforementioned hazards extirpation is the only feasible solution. But if the sialolith or sialoliths are located in the small superior lobe of the gland in a concentrated area it is possible to incise into the gland down to the sialoliths in a manner similar to that described for removal of sialoliths from the posterior part of the duct.

Use of a flexible silver lachrymal probe long enough to pass through the full length of the duct and penetrate through the hilus into the body of the gland is essential. Since the gland is deep in the submaxillary triangle it is necessary to use a 45-degree-angle fine needle electrode with a wire filament that is at least 2 cm. long to assure that the incision will penetrate down to the sialolith(s) with a single cutting stroke (Fig. 22–3).[33]

The end results of a successful intraoral sialolithotomy of the submaxillary gland are a normal functioning organ, a total absence of the telltale disfiguring scars that are typical of extraoral extirpative surgery, elimination of need for hospitalization to perform the surgery, elimination of the possible need for tracheostomy, and elimination of the hazard of nerve injury and postoperative functional handicap and aesthetic disfigurement due to paralysis of some of the muscles of facial expression.

The following cases of sialolithotomy of the submaxillary gland via the intraoral route demonstrate the technique and the advantages that inhere in the electrosurgical conservative procedure.

CASE 13

This case is an example of sialolithiasis of the submaxillary gland successfully treated by sialolithotomy performed via the intraoral route by electrosection.

PATIENT. A 66-year-old white male.

HISTORY. The patient was a physician. His chief complaint was severe pain in the left submandibular region, moderate extraoral swelling, tenderness in the submaxillary triangle and pain on swallowing so severe that he had to refrain from eating.

He had a history of sialolithiasis of three years duration. Recurrent episodes of pain and swelling in the past had subsided spontaneously in hours or a few days. The current episode was the most agonizing and prolonged. He was a controlled diabetic.

CLINICAL EXAMINATION. *Extraoral.* In the right submaxillary tirangle a moderate amount of swelling was visible despite the normally heavy, full jowls of an obese individual (CAse Fig. 13–1A). Light palpation in this area produced a severe pain response. No other adenopathy was present.

Intraoral. The floor of the mouth appeared normal except for a slight redness at the orifice of the right submaxillary duct and slight elevation of the duct and overlying tissues. These tissues were not tender to palpation, but intraoral palpation in the posterior part of the right side of the floor of the mouth elicited a very painful response.

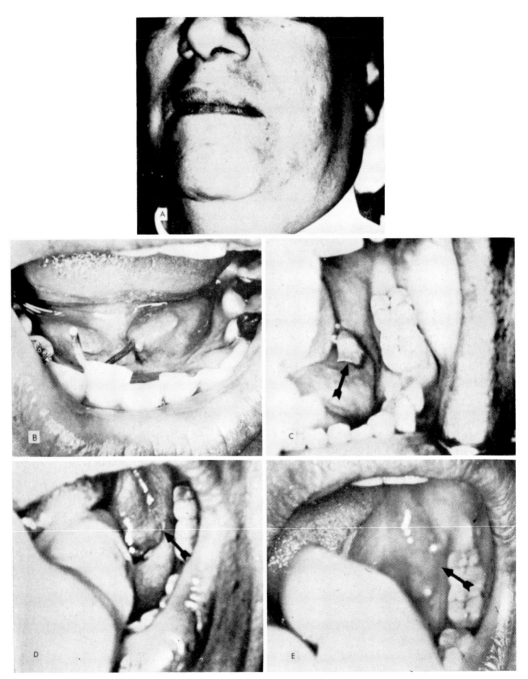

Case Figure 13–1.   Sialolithotomy of calculi embedded deep in the body of the submaxillary gland performed by intraoral electrosection. *A,* Preoperative extraoral appearance. There is typical swelling in the submaxillary triangle. *B,* Preoperative intraoral appearance of the mouth with a flexible silver probe inserted through the duct into the gland. Note the lack of involvement of the tissues of the floor of the mouth. *C,* After the sialoliths were removed intraorally, a centipede rubber dam drain was inserted through the incision into the gland, with 2 to 3 mm. projecting into the mouth. *D,* Appearance on the third postoperative day. The drain has been discarded and primary union of the incision has begun. There is very slight engorgement present in the area. *E,* Appearance on the fifth postoperative day. There is no evidence of engorgement or edema. Primary union is complete, and the intraoral and extraoral appearance is normal.

Roentgenographic examination with an occlusal view film was negative. A flexible silver probe was then introduced into the duct. It penetrated the full length of the duct without encountering resistance, but after it entered the gland it encountered hard resistance that gave off a grating sound on contact (Case Fig. 13–1B). A lateral jaw view was taken with the probe in position. This film revealed the presence of three round radiopaque masses, graduated in size, lying superimposed upon one another in a crescentic pattern. The tip of the probe was in contact with the largest mass, which was uppermost. A slightly radiopaque area between the lowest and middle calculi suggested presence of amorphous sludge or gravel in addition to the three solid masses (Case Fig. 13–2A).

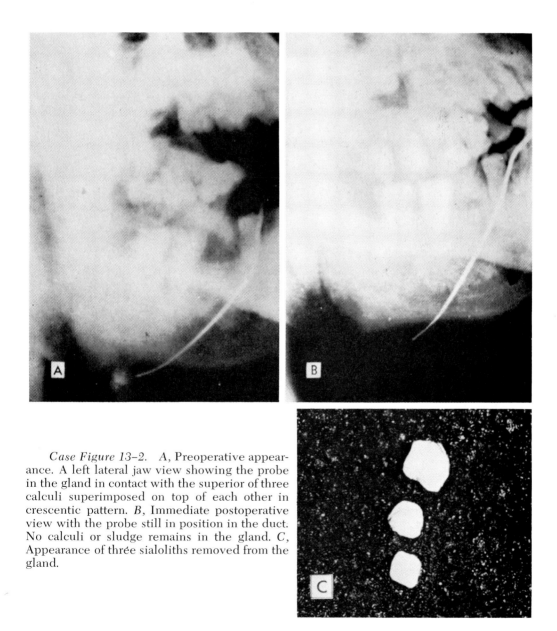

Case Figure 13–2. A, Preoperative appearance. A left lateral jaw view showing the probe in the gland in contact with the superior of three calculi superimposed on top of each other in crescentic pattern. B, Immediate postoperative view with the probe still in position in the duct. No calculi or sludge remains in the gland. C, Appearance of three sialoliths removed from the gland.

TREATMENT. Due to the acuteness of his symptoms, surgery was deferred for one day. On the first day he was premedicated with 600,000 units of Crysticillin, intramuscularly, and palliative sedation and lavage were prescribed. The following day, immediately preceding surgery, a second injection of Crysticillin was administered.

The mouth was prepared for surgery and inferior alveolar-lingual regional block anesthesia administered. A flexible silver probe was inserted into the duct and directed posteriorly until it made contact with the uppermost calculus. The probe was kept in the duct throughout the surgical procedure, being maintained in an elevated position to lift the tissues of the floor of the mouth and delineate the duct clearly.[34]

The tongue was firmly retracted toward the left side with a wooden tongue depressor, and the gland itself was displaced superiorly toward the floor of the mouth by firm extraoral pressure. With external pressure directed upward and intraoral digital pressure directed downward, the uppermost calculus could be slightly felt.

A long 45-degree-angle fine needle electrode was selected and current output was set at 3.5 for electrosection. An incision was made from the anterior pillar of the fauces anteriorly to the first molar region along the outline of the silver probe in the duct. The electrode was permitted to float downward through the tissues so that it severed the tissues of the floor of the mouth and the capsule of the gland; it penetrated into the body of the small, deep upper lobe of the gland until the electrode made contact with the top calculus, which was located in the center of the 3 cm. incision.

The incision was practically bloodless, so visibility was unimpaired. The lips of the wound were spread with the beaks of a curved mosquito hemostat and the margins were firmly retracted with Allis tissue forceps. A cup curet measuring 6 mm. in diameter was carefully inserted into the incised gland and gently manipulated until the uppermost calculus was engaged and removed. The remaining two calculi were removed in the same manner, as was a small amount of amorphous sludge. Then a blunt spoon-shaped curet was introduced and gently manipulated to break up the remaining sludge in the gland.

A Luer-type glass syringe filled with warm isotonic saline solution was attached to a flexible silver lachrymal irrigating needle. The latter was inserted through the incision and the gland was vigorously irrigated and simultaneously aspirated. A considerable amount of calcareous debris was observed (through a glass tube inserted into the aspirator rubber tubings) as it was evacuated. After a few minutes there was no further trace of debris. An immediate postoperative lateral jaw roentgenogram was taken with the silver probe still in position (Case Fig. 13–2B). This film showed that all the calcareous deposits had been removed from the gland.

In all, three calculi were removed (Case Fig. 13–2C), as well as a considerable amount of amorphous gravel. The largest calculus measured 5 mm. in diameter; the middle one, 3.5 mm.; and the smallest, most inferior one, 3 mm. A sterile centipede rubber dam drain 4 cm. long was inserted into the gland. Two millimeters of the end of the drain was permitted to project through the incision upward into the mouth (Case Fig. 13–1C). The patient was given postoperative instructions and told to return in 24 hours.

Next day the drain was removed and the gland was again irrigated with saline solution. Aspiration failed to reveal any calcareous debris. The patient was much more comfortable than preoperatively, and there was very little edema in the tissues of the floor of the mouth. A fresh drain was inserted and another dose of Crysticillin was administered.

By the third postoperative day the extraoral swelling had greatly subsided (Case Fig. 13–1D). The penicillin therapy was discontinued and the drain was discarded.

By the fifth day the intraoral swelling had completely subsided (Case Fig. 13–1E), and by the sixth postoperative day he felt sufficiently recovered to return to his home in Central America. He has written periodically and reported that the tissues of the floor of the mouth are completely normal and that there has been no recurrence of his symptoms.

CASE 14*

This case differs from the preceding cases in several important respects. Calcareous matter may be in the form of calcified masses, as gravel, or as amorphous sludge. Calcareous accretions typically are solid masses such as were removed in the preceding cases.

In this case the sialolith was a hollow shell, similar to an empty egg shell, instead of a solid mass. In this case the acute infection of the gland resulted in extraoral visible and palpable adenopathy and swelling of the submaxillary gland.

The frail texture of this hollow shell created a number of unique, atypical problems. Because of its lack of physical solid bulk it offered very little resistance to the x-rays and, as a result, produced only a faintly radiopaque image on the lateral jaw x-rays that were taken.

The frail texture also made the precise location of the mass somewhat hazardous. The flexible silver lachrymal probe usually is advanced through the duct until it meets resistance from the foreign body. A poke from the probe against this hollow shell could easily fracture it. Thus, extreme caution had to be exercised to advance the probe very gently and desist as soon as it met slight resistance.

The frailty also greatly increased the problem of removing the mass from the gland after access to it was achieved by direct incision into the gland, and there was danger that manipulation of the curet as it groped around to engage and lift out the mass could easily crush and pulverize it. In this case the latter difficulty was compounded by the fact that the surgery was being performed as one of the cases of a teaching motion picture film being made by the author.

PATIENT. A 47-year-old white female.

HISTORY. As a youngster about 33 years previously she had had submaxillary calculi removed from the duct surgically. There had been no recurrence until two weeks ago, when she suddenly felt sharp pain in the sublingual region of the mouth while eating. She continued to have acute pain from eating and even from sudden movements of the head. She also noticed a hard swelling in her neck and a peculiar taste in her mouth. She consulted her dentist and was referred to the author for treatment. She gave a history of hemorrhage after one of many extractions.

CLINICAL EXAMINATION. *Extraoral.* There was a large round hard swelling on the left side of her neck, below the inferior border of the mandible and under the bulge of the submaxillary triangle (Case Fig. 14–1A). There was palpable and visible adenopathy, but no induration, and the hard lump could be moved a little by digital palpation.

---

*This case was filmed as one sequence in a motion picture film; thus, many of the photos are enlargements from 16 mm. film instead of from 35 mm. Kodachrome transparencies. The enlargement resulted in a slight loss of sharpness and depth of field. The anatomic location of the surgery, deep in the oropharynx, has also contributed to some loss of focal sharpness. Nevertheless, considering these factors, the case figures fulfill the function of visualizing this procedure satisfactorily.

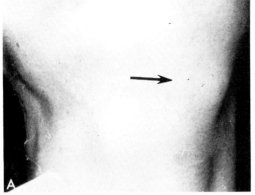
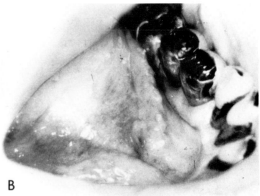
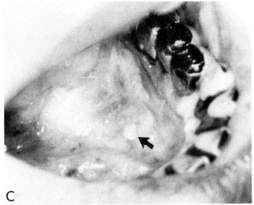

Case Figure 14–1. The author's technique for removing sialoliths from the body of the submaxillary gland via the intraoral route, thereby eliminating need for extraoral extirpation of the gland with its concomitant postoperative complications. *A,* Extraoral appearance of submandibular areas and neck. A large hard nodular swelling can be seen in the left submaxillary triangle, with the head tilted sharply upward. *B,* Intraoral appearance. There is some swelling and redness in the left side of the floor of the mouth, elevating the fringe tissue. The orifice of the submaxillary duct is red and enlarged. *C,* Light finger pressure against the swollen tissue near the orifice of the duct produces purulent exudation (arrow).

Intraoral. The floor of the mouth was elevated on the left side, the same side as the extraoral swelling. The orifice of the submaxillary duct appeared to be dilated (Case Fig. 14–1B), and light digital pressure on the tissues of the floor of the mouth on the left side produced a flow of viscous purulent exudate (Case Fig. 14–1C).

Lateral jaw x-rays revealed a thin hollow elliptical mass and two small fragments adjacent to it, in the anterior body of the small upper lobe, near the hilus of the gland. Intraoral occlusal views, with the film placed much farther posteriorly than most patients can tolerate, made possible a somewhat better visualization of the sialolith. This film, as well as the lateral jaw views, were taken with a flexible silver lachrymal probe in position against the sialolith immediately beyond the hilus of the gland (Case Fig. 14–2A). The patient had a temperature of 100.8° F. and complained of slight nausea and chills.

TREATMENT. The duct was irrigated gently with a solution of Kasdenol at body temperature (Case Fig. 14–2B), and Erythrocin was prescribed, 500 mg. stat, 250 mg. every 6 hours around the clock. She was seen again on the following day. Her temperature was almost normal, and she no longer had the chills or nausea. The duct was again irrigated, and she was instructed to return the next day.

The following day the fever was gone and the hard mass in the neck was slightly softer. She was now deemed ready for the surgery. An inferior alveolar-lingual regional block injection was administered, and the duct was cannulized with the flexible silver lachrymal probe, advanced very gently until it met a slight resistance. A special 45-degree-angle fine needle electrode with a 3 cm. wire filament was inserted

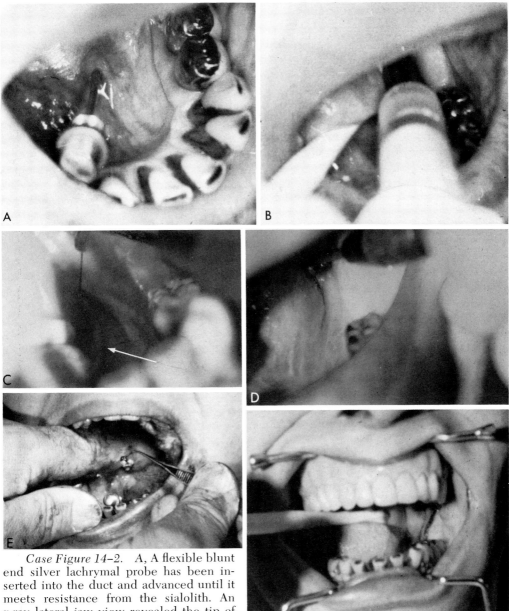

Case Figure 14-2. *A,* A flexible blunt end silver lachrymal probe has been inserted into the duct and advanced until it meets resistance from the sialolith. An x-ray lateral jaw view revealed the tip of the probe in contact with a frail, hollow-looking calcareous mass that resembled an empty eggshell. (The lack of density of the mass made it impossible to reproduce it in a black and white photograph for illustration.) *B,* The silver probe has been replaced with a flexible blunt silver lachrymal irrigating needle attached to a Luer syringe. The irrigating needle has been inserted into the duct and advanced toward the gland, and the latter is being gently irrigated with a solution of Kasdenol at body temperature. *C,* An incision is being made into the gland precisely along the line outlined by the silver probe in the duct (arrow) that has been elevated firmly while the gland is displaced superiorly toward the floor of the mouth by external pressure, so that a precise incision will be made into the gland without danger of severing any of the important anatomic structures in the area. The incision extends approximately 5 cm. postero-anteriorly, from a paint parallel with the pharyngeal tonsil to the distal of the first molar, using a long slender fine 45-degree-angle needle electrode to perform the electrosection. *D,* The incision is being extended posteriorly beyond the site of contact of the silver probe with the calcareous mass. The incision runs parallel to the pharyngeal tonsil. *E,* The sialolith, a hollow, eggshell-like mass, has been removed from the gland with a cup curet and is seen being lifted out of the mouth with ophthalmic tissue forceps. *F,* The surgery and irrigation having been completed, a centipede type of rubber dam drain has been inserted to keep the wound open for further postoperative drainage.

into the handpiece, and cutting current power was set at 4, owing to the length of the electrode and the need for hemostasis.

The gland was displaced superiorly toward the floor of the mouth by extraoral pressure upward, the probe was elevated to pull the tissues taut, and the incision was started with the activated electrode about 1 cm. beyond the tip of the probe, at a level approximately parallel with the pharyngeal tonsil (Case Figs. 14–2C and D). The tissue was incised downward until it met slight resistance. There was virtually no bleeding from the incision. A small cup curet was inserted and manipulated very gingerly until it engaged the frail mass (Case Fig. 14–2E). Fortunately only a small fragment broke away as the mass was removed, despite the blind probing to engage the mass. This fragment and two other small irregular fragments that had been adjacent to the large mass were evacuated from the gland by irrigation and aspiration. When it appeared definite that no more foreign debris was in the gland, the probe was reinserted to the same depth of penetration it had reached before, and an immediate postoperative x-ray was again taken. This film revealed the area was free of debris (Case Fig.

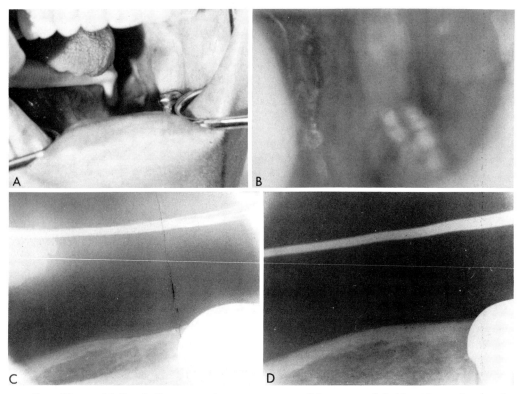

Case Figure 14–3. A, Postoperative appearance of the surgical field 24 hours later. The rubber dam drain is still in place and there is no evidence of postoperative edema or redness. B, Postoperative appearance of the wound 48 hours later. The drain having been discarded at the previous visit, the incised tissues have been healing by primary intention for 24 hours. Healing appears to be progressing so well that the patient saw no need to return for further postoperative observation, but reported complete healing without incidence or recurrence of the submaxillary swelling. C, Preoperative x-ray with flexible silver probe in contact with the sialolith in the submaxillary gland. Note the appearance of the large calcareous mass which is revealed to be hollow instead of solid. D, Postoperative x-ray with same probe inserted through the duct into the gland. The successful sialolithotomy of the submaxillary gland via an intraoral surgical route is confirmed.

14–3D). A centipede rubber dam drain was inserted, and the patient was instructed to return the following day (Case Fig. 14–2F).

When she returned, the drain was removed and the gland was irrigated and aspirated, without producing further evidence of calcareous debris. The drain was discontinued, and the wound proceeded to heal rapidly and uneventfully (Case Fig. 14–3A and B). The lump in the side of the neck disappeared after two weeks and has not recurred.

CASE 15

This case is an example of sialolithiasis of both the submaxillary duct and the gland proper treated by intraoral electrosurgical sialolithotomy.

PATIENT. A 29-year-old white female.

HISTORY. Normally healthy, she suddenly developed severe pain and swelling in the mouth and throat, causing difficulty in swallowing. These symptoms were accompanied by chills and fever, generalized malaise, a malodorous, foul-tasting oral discharge, and recurrent intraoral and extraoral swellings.

Her physician tentatively diagnosed these symptoms as sialolithiasis of the submaxillary duct. She was referred for conclusive diagnosis and treatment.

CLINICAL EXAMINATION. *Extraoral.* There was marked swelling in the left submaxillary triangle. Previous similar episodes had subsided spontaneously after a few hours, but this time it had persisted unabated for five days with increasing induration.

Intraoral. The tongue had been elevated and pushed over toward the right side by swelling and massive edema of the tissues of the floor of the mouth. The orifice of the left submaxillary duct was enlarged and ulcerated, and a thick malodorous mucopurulent exudate oozed from it. Movements of the tongue or slight pressure against the floor of the mouth increased the discharge. Swelling and induration had partially immobilized the tongue.

A flexible silver probe was inserted into the duct. It encountered grating resistance after advancing about 2.5 cm. but its progress was not completely impeded (Case Fig. 15–1A). An intraoral occlusal view roentgenogram of the mandible revealed three irregular radiopaque masses in the vicinity of the right submaxillary duct. The masses were located parallel and medial to the bicuspids.

These calculi did not appear either large or dense enough to be blocking the lumen of the duct enough to be solely responsible for the acute clinical symptoms. A lateral jaw roentgenogram was therefore taken to check on the submaxillary gland itself. This film showed two round, densely radiopaque masses, each about 0.5 cm. in diameter, located beneath the inferior border of the mandible immediately anterior to the angle of the jaw. The two calculi were superimposed upon one another vertically (Case Fig. 15–1B). A diagnosis of simultaneous sialolithiasis of the submaxillary duct and gland complicated by secondary infection was clearly established.

TREATMENT. Because of the acute infection, immediate sialolithotomy appeared contraindicated. Preliminary parenteral and palliative treatment was instituted. The first of six consecutive daily intramuscular injections of 600,000 units of Crysticillin was administered. Then the duct was gently milked to express as much of the purulent exudate as possible. One small calcareous fragment was expelled by the manipulation. When the flow of exudate stopped, a flexible blunt silver lachrymal irrigating needle was inserted approximately 2 cm. into the duct; then a 5 ml. Luer-type

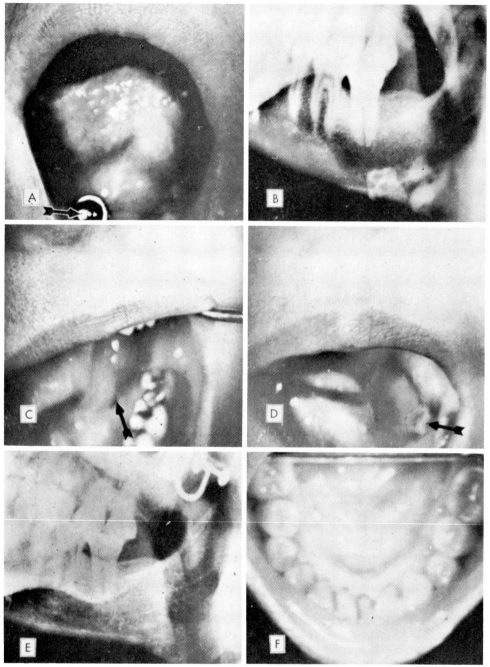

Case Figure 15–1. Sialolithotomy of the submaxillary duct and gland by intraoral electro-section. *A,* A flexible silver probe has been inserted into the duct prior to roentgenographic examination. Arrow points to head of two-piece flexible silver probe. *B,* Preoperative lateral jaw view shows two large calculi in the body of the gland. *C,* Arrow points to a curved incision of the floor of the mouth 3 cm. long, extending downward into the gland. (Curved appearance of the line of incision is due to retraction of the tongue for visibility.) *D,* Arrow points to centi-pede rubber dam drain inserted into the gland, with 2 to 3 mm. projecting upward through the incision into the mouth. *E,* Postoperative appearance. Lateral jaw view shows calculi to have been removed from the gland. No calcareous material visible. *F,* Final postoperative appear-ance of the mouth (mirror image) shows the tissues of the floor of the mouth returned to normal. There is no scar tissue or contraction present.

glass syringe filled with aqueous solution of benzalkonium chloride (1:1,000) was attached to the needle. The warm solution was instilled into the duct slowly. Irrigation was frequently alternated with aspiration performed by disengaging the syringe from the needle and attaching the latter to the aspirating tip for suction.

When the irrigation was stopped, further milking of the duct proved productive and some amorphous gravel-like sludge was expressed. Irrigation and aspiration was resumed. After the aspirated fluid viewed through the glass tube had remained free of foreign debris for several minutes, the lachrymal needle was disengaged and an occlusal view roentgenogram of the mandible was taken. This film showed the duct to be free of calcareous deposits.

When the patient returned on the following day most of the acute systemic symptoms had disappeared. The extraoral swelling was unchanged but the intraoral condition was greatly improved. The tongue was much less swollen and more mobile, and the orifice of the duct was almost normal again. Milking the duct proved unproductive. The orifice of the duct was too small to admit the lachrymal needle until it was first dilated with a flexible probe. Irrigation of the duct was somewhat more productive, and a small amount of amorphous sludge was aspirated.

When she returned on the third day her systemic and local condition appeared quite normal. Irrigating and milking the duct was totally unproductive and there was no trace of malodorous exudate. The patient was deemed ready for surgical removal of the calculi from the gland.

The mouth was prepared for surgery and inferior alveolar and lingual regional block anesthesia administered. The flexible silver probe was inserted the full length of the duct without encountering resistance, but almost immediately after entry into the gland it encountered hard resistance which produced a grating sound. A lateral jaw roentgenogram was taken with the probe in situ. This film showed the tip of the probe in direct contact with the top calculus at a point immediately beyond the duct origin.

The probe was kept in the duct throughout the surgery to serve as a guide line, and the gland was displaced upward toward the floor of the mouth by external pressure. The exact site for the incision was determined by elevating the probe to outline the duct and measuring the length of the probe along the floor of the mouth.

A long 45-degree-angle fine needle electrode was selected and current output set at 3.5 for electrosection. The incision was started at the oropharyngeal junction and carried anteriorly 3 cm. to a point equidistant to the distal aspect of the first molar (Case Fig. 15–1C). The incision ran parallel to the body of the mandible and about 1 cm. medial to it along the line outlined by the elevated probe. The electrode was permitted to float downward through the tissues toward the probe, cutting effortlessly through the capsule and body of the small upper lobe of the gland down to the top calculus.[34]

The incision was practically bloodless, even after the incision was spread wide with the beaks of a curved mosquito hemostat. A large, round, cup-shaped curet 7 mm. in diameter was inserted through the incision, and after a minimal amount of careful manipulation the uppermost calculus was engaged, elevated toward the floor of the mouth, grasped with an Allis forceps and removed.

The curet was reintroduced and the second, more deeply embedded calculus was engaged and removed in the same manner. A blunt, spoon-shaped curet was then introduced and gently manipulated in an exploratory manner. It soon encountered resistance from a substance that disintegrated readily. The curet was removed and the gland was irrigated with warm isotonic saline solution which was simultaneously aspirated. A number of small calcareous fragments and mucinous sludge were observed passing through the glass tube. After a few minutes only clear water free of debris was aspirated. The curet was reintroduced but did not encounter any resistance; again, irrigation and aspiration were unproductive.

A postoperative lateral jaw view roentgenogram was taken. This film showed that all the calculi and debris had been removed (Case Fig. 15–1E). A centipede rubber dam drain 4 cm. in length was inserted into the gland, with 2 mm. of it projecting upward into the floor of the mouth to facilitate drainage (Case Fig. 15–1D). The incision into the gland did not require suturing, but a suture was inserted at each end of the projecting drain to help keep it in position and reduce the likelihood of its displacement.

The patient returned 24 hours later for postoperative treatment. The drain was removed and the gland gently irrigated with warm saline solution. Three small calcareous fragments were aspirated. A fresh drain was inserted and she was instructed to return in 24 hours. Next day, almost all the extraoral swelling and tenderness were gone, and by the third day there was neither swelling nor tenderness. On the fourth postoperative day the two sutures were removed and the drain discarded; oral lavage was substituted for the gland irrigations. Complete healing without scar contraction ensued without incident (Case Fig. 15–1F).

In all, a total of two large and six small calculi and many minute fragments and

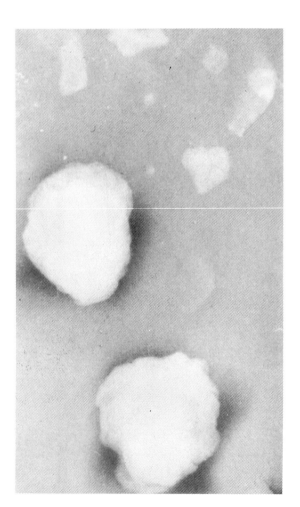

Case Figure 15–2. Appearance of the two large and numerous smaller calculi recovered from the submaxillary gland.

amorphous sludge were removed from the gland (Case Fig. 15–2). A final lateral jaw roentgenogram taken four months after she was discharged from active treatment was negative. Almost eight years have elapsed without any recurrence since this surgery was performed.

Four interrelated factors contribute to the success of this technique for intraoral sialolithotomy.

1. *Accessibility.* In order to perform an incision into the gland with a cold-steel scalpel, most of the hand would have to be inserted into the mouth to manipulate and maintain control of the instrument. With electrosurgery the long slender electrode and electrode handle easily reach the operative field without most of the hand being involved within the oral cavity, thereby leaving the site unblocked and instrumentation maneuverability unimpaired.

2. *Visibility.* Hemostasis obtained with electrosurgery greatly reduces the hazard of profuse hemorrhage such as usually results when incisions are made with cold steel into the vascular areolar tissues of the floor of the mouth. Good visibility in the operative field can therefore be maintained.

3. *Effortless Incisions.* Since the electrode can be floated downward through the tissues without pressure, the incision can be carried down through the capsule and into the gland to the calculus by electrosection without displacement or mutilation of the tissues.

4. *Safety.* Use of the silver probe as a guide for the incision assures immunity from accidental injury to nerves or blood vessels in the operative fluid, and thereby eliminates the dangers inherent in extraoral sialoadenectomy.

IV. MISCELLANEOUS PROCEDURES

There are many procedures other than those already reviewed that require special skills and therefore belong in the category of major oral surgery. The specific techniques for efficient treatment of a number of the most important of these are therefore also included in this review.

Leukoplakia

It has been estimated by students of cancer that only about 15 per cent of all leukoplakic lesions become malignant. Nevertheless, the tendency persists among many dentists and physicians to refer to all white mucous lesions as "leukoplakia."

Bernier and most other oral pathologists recommend that the term leukoplakia be applied only to those white mucous lesions that present definite histologic evidence of specific cellular alterations in content and/or arrangement, indicating that they are premalignant, with a potential for malignant degeneration.

In view of the difficulty of establishing an accurate conclusive diagnosis of leukoplakia on the basis of its clinical appearance alone and its potential for degenerating into true malignancy, the author not only concurs with their opinion but also recommends that all white mucous lesions be biopsied before treatment is instituted.

Since biopsy will be reviewed comprehensively in the next two chapters, it will not be discussed further here. But the clinical physical characteristics of the lesion that can influence treatment, the therapeutic considerations, the available methods of treatment, and the treatment of choice will be reviewed here.

After biopsy has established that the white mucous lesion is in fact leukoplakia, what is the treatment of choice for elimination of the neoplasm? Should it be removed by surgical resection? If so, should the resection be performed with a cold-steel scalpel, or with an electrode by electrosection? Or should it be destroyed in situ by coagulation? If so, should the coagulation be performed electrosurgically or chemically with potent caustics or escharotics, such as trichloracetic acid?

Leukoplakic lesions have two things in common: their malignant potential, and the fact that they, as neoplasms, are foreign bodies superimposed on the surface of normal mucosa. In other respects, however, there may be great variances that strongly influence the choice of modality and method of treatment.

The neoplasm varies greatly in clinical appearance, ranging from the thick parboiled-looking white surface of palatal mucosa to a much thinner yet well-defined whitish appearing lesion on the inner aspect of the cheek, or to a very thin, faintly whitish, lacy surface of the vermilion border of the lip that may resemble a mild lichen planus. Each presents treatment problems that influence choice of therapy. The very thin lesion would be far more difficult to resect with a steel scalpel or an electrode than the thicker variety. The location of the lesion also influences treatment, since it would be much more difficult to resect precisely a thin layer of tissue from a highly mobile surface than from tissue attached to a fixed base.

The characteristics of the various modalities are also factors that influence the choice of treatment. When the cold-steel scalpel is used, it is extremely difficult to resect the neoplastic tissue accurately and precisely from highly mobile surfaces such as the tissues of the floor of the mouth, the inner aspect of the cheek, or the vermilion border of the lip. In addition, the profuse bleeding that would accompany the dissection would make precise dissection even more difficult. The raw, denuded surface would be highly vulnerable to secondary infection. Also, the fibrous scar tissue repair creates a hazard of contractile adhesions that could produce functional and aesthetic disadvantages. This therefore appears to be the least desirable method of treatment.

Chemical coagulation presents comparable hazards and undesirable factors. Since chemical coagulation is not self-limiting in its destructiveness, it is virtually impossible for the operator to control the depth of destruction precisely. Since the liquid tends to flow beyond the perimeter of the tissue to be treated by capillary attraction and thereby to destroy adjacent normal tissue, the depth of penetration of the white coagulating effect into the underlying normal pink mucosa cannot be controlled. It may not penetrate deeply enough to destroy the basement membrane of the neoplasm, or it may penetrate much too deeply into the underlying tissue. Tissue repair with this modality, as with the steel-scalpel dissection, is characterized by cicatricial fibrous scar tissue formation, with the dangers of aesthetic and functional impairment.

Resection of the lesion by needle or loop electrode resection also presents disadvantages, despite the hemostasis that eliminates the problem of hemorrhage and the lack of pressure that eliminates much of the problem with resection from mobile tissue. It is difficult to dissect all the diseased tissue so uniformly that its complete removal is assured. It is equally difficult to avoid dissecting away much normal tissue with that which is diseased. In addition, it would leave a raw surface of tissue vulnerable to secondary infection.

The treatment of choice therefore narrows down to destruction of the tissue in situ by electrocoagulation, which offers a number of advantageous factors. When the lesion is treated by carefully applied electrocoagulation, that is, by spot coagulation rather than by scraping the electrode over the tissue surface, and the applications are made one immediately adjacent to the next, it is possible to see and determine accurately the precise depth of penetration as the coagulating effect penetrates. The depth of penetration is determined in part by the amount of electrocoagulating energy being used and in part by the period of time that the electrode is permitted to remain in contact with the tissues. As the coagulating ball electrode is applied to the tissues at the margin of the lesion it is possible to see just how deeply beyond the level of the white neoplastic tissue the coagulating effect is penetrating. The same amount of energy and time of application are allowed for each electrode contact, following the perimeter of the lesion and then continuing with the spot contacts until the entire neoplastic tissue surface has been treated, with a minimum of overlapping.

After the application has been completed, the patient must exercise reasonable postoperative care not to disturb or displace the coagulum, so that the healing will be uneventful, with a minimum of postoperative sequelae, and the coagulum can act as a protective cover, reducing the danger of secondary infection. Once healing has taken place, the coagulum peels off spontaneously, leaving a normal tissue surface that is soft, supple, and totally devoid of contractile fibrous scar tissue adhesions.

Electrocoagulation appears to offer another tremendous advantage that has been utilized for definitive treatment of "inoperable" oral cancer with remarkable results, which are reported in detail in Chapter 25. According to the reports of a number of respected research investigators, electrocoagulation initiates an antigen-antibody reaction that helps to destroy abnormal tissue cells without affecting the normal cells. It is therefore possible, if not probable, that any neoplastic cells that might not have been destroyed by the electrocoagulation would be destroyed by the antigen-antibody reaction it induces.

The following case report demonstrates the advantages of electrosurgical treatment by leukoplakia by biterminal electrocoagulation, despite the unfavorable locale the of lesion and its extensiveness.

CASE 16

This case involved leukoplakia that covered most of the floor of the mouth from the ventral attachment of the tongue anteriorly to the orifices of the submaxillary and submental salivary ducts. The fact that this was a true neoplasm and not one of many white mucous lesions was determined by biopsy.

PATIENT. A 56-year-old white female.

HISTORY. She was a chain cigarette smoker. During a periodic dental examination the presence of a thick white appearance of the tissues of the floor of the mouth was noted, and she was referred to the author for diagnosis and treatment.

TREATMENT. The mandible was anesthetized by bilateral inferior alveolar-lingual nerve blocks. A medium-width round loop electrode was selected, cutting current was set at 7, and two tissue specimens were resected for biopsy from the fringe tissue in the left side of the floor of the mouth (Case Fig. 16–1).

A large ball coagulating electrode was selected and coagulating current output was set at 3. With this electrode the white tissue, diagnosed as a true leukoplakia fulfilling Bernier's definition of this premalignancy, was destroyed by meticulously careful spot coagulation (Case Fig. 16–2A and B). The electrode was kept in contact with the tissue at each spot until the tissue immediate beneath the white layer turned white; the spot immediately adjacent was then treated, until the entire neoplastic surface was coagulated.

The patient was cautioned to avoid eating solid foods or otherwise disturbing the coagulum, which acts as a protective coating under which the tissue repair proceeds. She returned on the fifth postoperative day for postoperative observation. There was some edema present, mostly of the orifices of the submaxillary ducts, but the tongue was mobile (Case Fig. 16–2C). By the end of the third postoperative week the tissues of the floor of the mouth were fully healed with no evidence of recurrence of white tissue surface. The tissues appeared normal except that the tissue surface in the area where the biopsy tissue had been resected was not yet maturely keratinized (Case Fig. 16–2D).

The patient did not smoke for 6 months. Then, despite warnings of the potential malignant character of leukoplakia, she resumed chain smoking, and in less than 2 months there was a recurrence of the leukoplakia.

Papillary Hyperplasia

Papillary hyperplasia is one of the most perplexing pathologic entities encountered in the human mouth. We can identify it by its clinical appearance and verify the clinical diagnosis by its histologic appearance under the microscope. But we still do not know just how or why it develops. It is also one of

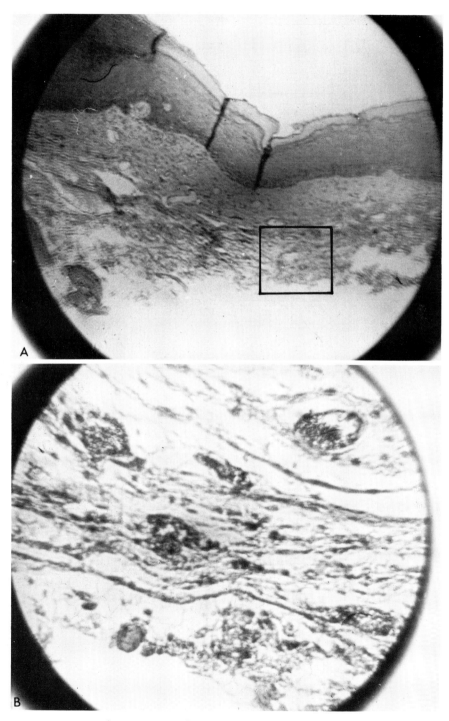

Case Figure 16–1. Photomicrographs of the loop-resected biopsy tissue. *A,* Appearance of the fringe tissue under ×100 (low power) magnification, showing the massive keratinized layer. Inset designates area of tissue that will be examined under higher magnification. *B,* Inset tissue under ×450 (medium power) magnification shows absence of coagulation of the frail areolar tissue along the cut surface.

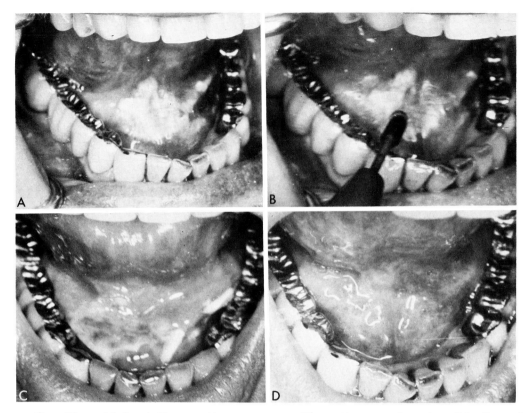

Case Figure 16–2. A, Preoperative appearance. The entire central portion of the floor of the mouth, from the junction with the tongue to the orifices of the submaxillary and sublingual ducts, and the fringe tissue on the left side were covered with a thick white surface layer that appeared superimposed over the surface of the normal mucosa. The white neoplasm extended about 1 cm. along the center of the ventral surface of the tongue at its junction with the tissues of the floor of the mouth. A dark red surgical defect is present along the left fringe tissue, where tissue had been removed with a loop electrode for biopsy evaluation. *B,* The white mass is being coagulated by meticulously careful spot coagulation with a large round, slightly flattened ball coagulating electrode. Note that each spot of coagulation is immediately adjacent to the previous one and that the electrode is not being scraped over the tissue surface. *C,* Appearance one week postoperatively. There is a surface layer of coagulum along the fringe tissue where the biopsy specimen had been removed, and a very thin film of coagulum over the field where the neoplasm had been coagulated. There is no induration, the tongue is supple, and there is relatively little edema, except of the tissue containing the orifices of the salivary ducts. *D,* Appearance of the floor of the mouth three weeks postoperatively. The tissue is normal in all respects. There is no trace of the white mucous lesion, which biopsy has confirmed was true leukoplakia.

the most frustrating conditions to treat, especially when its treatment is attempted with a steel scalpel. If the tissue is excised down to its basement membrane, the fibrous scar tissue repair results in a mutilated palatal mucosa that resembles that of a victim of cleft palate for whom a pharyngeal repair has been attempted. If the excision is not extended down far enough, the tissue promptly regenerates, with the disease recurring usually more extensively than originally.

When the excision is performed by electrosection with a loop electrode, the result is dramatically different. It is infinitely easier to resect the pathologic tissue by shaving it in layers with a loop electrode instead of trying to dissect it out with a scalpel or macerate it with a diamond stone. Since there is no bleeding and no pressure is required to resect the tissue, it is possible to plane it down to its corium without damaging the underlying periosteum. Since tissue repair from electrosection results in soft, supple tissue identical in all respects to the surrounding tissues, the mutilating effect of scar tissue repair is avoided. Also, because of the totally atraumatic nature of the surgical procedure, there is no postoperative pain. Within a matter of two to three weeks the tissue repair is complete and the palate shows no evidence of extensive surgery.

CASE 17

Since the best way to establish a conclusive diagnosis of a pathologic condition is through biopsy, the first step in treatment of this condition should be, in the opinion of the author, resection of a representative segment of tissue for histopathologic interpretation. This case demonstrates this as well as the treatment itself.

PATIENT. A 67-year-old white male.

HISTORY. He had been edentulous for more than a decade. He recently began to feel an irritation, or, as he put it, a mild burning sensation, in his palate under the denture. He consulted his dentist, who found a verrucous lesion in the center of the palate and referred him for its resection.

CLINICAL EXAMINATION. A verrucous type of irregular mass was present in the center of the palate. It measured approximately 2.5 cm. in width and 3.5 cm. in length (Case Fig. 17–1A). The clinical impression was that this was a papillary hyperplasia, but this could be confirmed only through biopsy.

TREATMENT. The area was anesthetized by nasopalatine and anterior palatine block injections reinforced with circumferential infiltration anesthesia. A 45-degree-angle fine needle electrode was selected and cutting current was set at 4 on the dial. The activated electrode was used to incise and resect a triangular segment of tissue (Case Fig. 17–1B).

The biopsy specimen having been preserved in a 10 per cent formalin solution, a medium-width round loop electrode was selected and used to resect the papillary tissue by shaving it in layers (Case Fig. 17–1C). The mass was resected down to the periosteum, with great care exercised to avoid removal of the periosteum in the process. Shaving the tissue in thin layers as the periosteum was approached controlled the resection and made it possible to avoid including the periosteum. The patient's old denture, which had been sterilized in cold sterilizing solution, was used as a surgical stent, with a very hard mix of surgical cement packed into the area that would cover the surgical field, so that it would act as a pressure bandage.

The patient returned for postoperative care on the fifth postoperative day. The surgical field was healing well; it was covered with a healthy-looking layer of coagulum (Case Fig. 17–1D). The depth to which the resection had been carried was now apparent. The patient was seen at weekly intervals, and by the end of the third week the palate was fully healed and covered with maturely keratinized epithelium except where the biopsy had been performed. The keratinization was not fully matured and the area appeared slightly pinker in color than the surrounding mucosa (Case Fig. 17–1E).

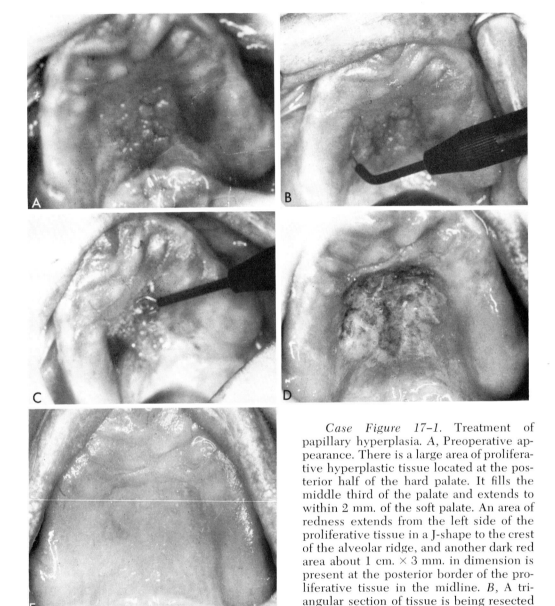

Case Figure 17–1. Treatment of papillary hyperplasia. *A,* Preoperative appearance. There is a large area of proliferative hyperplastic tissue located at the posterior half of the hard palate. It fills the middle third of the palate and extends to within 2 mm. of the soft palate. An area of redness extends from the left side of the proliferative tissue in a J-shape to the crest of the alveolar ridge, and another dark red area about 1 cm. × 3 mm. in dimension is present at the posterior border of the proliferative tissue in the midline. *B,* A triangular section of tissue is being resected from the right side of the mass with a 45-degree-angle fine needle electrode for biopsy evaluation. *C,* The proliferative tissue is being resected by loop planing with a round loop electrode down to its basement membrane. *D,* Appearance of the palate on fifth postoperative day. A surgical cement pack had been placed in the old denture to serve as a stent. The tissues are healing well, and the granulating repair is covered with a thin layer of coagulum. Note the depth to which the tissue had been resected. Also note the absence of the redness noted earlier. *E,* Appearance of the palate three weeks postoperatively. The palate is completely healed by granulation repair and is normal in appearance, except that the site of biopsy excision is still discernible as slightly redder than the surrounding tissue, because the surface epithelium has not yet fully matured and become covered with packed layers of dead cells that form the keratinized surface of mature epithelium. The biopsy report has confirmed that this was a case of papillary hyperplasia.

Ranula and Tumors of the Floor of the Mouth

Ranula and deeply penetrative pathologic conditions located in the floor of the mouth usually are considered to be inoperable by incisional excision with the cold-steel scalpel owing to the extreme mobility and vascularity of the tissues involved. These help to make such surgery too hazardous for three reasons: first, because the mobility of these tissues makes it virtually impossible to incise them precisely with the steel scalpel; second, because of the difficulty of controlling the depth of the incision precisely when the incision through the frail tissue is being made with pressure; and third, and by far most important, because the incision is accompanied by profuse hemorrhage that obscures the operative field and makes it virtually impossible to locate, identify, and preserve from harm the numerous important anatomic structures, such as the salivary ducts and lingual artery and nerve, that are located there and often are physically involved with the disease.

Because of these hazards inherent in cold-steel surgery, the ranula and tumors of the floor of the mouth are deemed inoperable by incisional excision, and marsupialization by the Partsch technique is considered the treatment of choice.

For the ranula, being a retention cyst, marsupialization usually is eminently suitable for two reasons: first, because the cystic sac is very thin and tends to adhere to the surrounding tissues, often making it virtually impossible to enucleate it and second, because it usually contains fluid that can easily be evacuated after the top of the sac and overlying mucosa have been removed.

The overlying tissue can be resected with the steel scalpel, but removal by loop resection using electrosection is infinitely superior, since it minimizes the handicap imposed by tissue mobility and eliminates the handicap of impaired visibility due to hemorrhage in the operative field. The mobility is overcome by engaging the mucosa with a tissue hook or ophthalmic tissue forceps that have been inserted through the eye of a round loop electrode.

The engaged tissue is elevated to pull it taut, and the mucosa and top of the cystic sac is resected with a single wiping stroke of the activated loop. The fluid content is evacuated, the cystic cut margin is sutured to the surrounding cut tissue margin, and the cavity is packed until the defect is obliterated.

When the ranula is atypical and contains semi-solid and solid tissue as well as fluid, or whenever the lesion resembles the ranula clinically but proves to be a solid tumor mass instead of a retention cyst, marsupialization is ineffectual, and the mass must be removed by dissection. Either type of lesion is likely to grow around and envelop the salivary ducts and other structures in the area, such as the lingual artery or nerve, which greatly magnifies the surgical hazards. If visibility in the operative field becomes impaired because of hemorrhage, the danger of injury to these structures is, of course, greatly increased.

The advantages inherent in the ability to incise the mobile tissue precisely and effortlessly without pressure and in the hemostasis that assures unimpaired visibility in the operative field make it possible to remove these lesions safely and efficiently by electrosurgical incision and excision and/or enucleation, even when the disease envelops some of the important anatomic structures in the area.

The following case report admirably demonstrates these advantages of electrosection that make it possible to resect such diseased tissue from the floor of the mouth.

CASE 18

This case offers an exceptional opportunity to see the enormous advantage of the inherent hemostasis of electrosection in performing surgery in the deep tissues of the floor of the mouth. When the surgery involves resection of a ranula-like mass enveloping the submaxillary duct and adherent to the sheath of the lingual nerve, as occurred in this case, the hemostasis made removal of the mass possible by blunt and sharp dissection without injury to any of the vital structures.

PATIENT. A 54-year-old white female.

HISTORY. She had become aware of a mass in the floor of the mouth that involved the entire right side and appeared to be gradually increasing in size. Since the lesion did not appear to be of dental origin she consulted her physician, and he referred her to an EENT specialist, who diagnosed it as a ranula. She was hospitalized, and the surface mucosa was resected in an attempt to perform a Partsch procedure to marsupialize the cyst. Unfortunately, the contents of the mass were not liquid, as usually occurs in the retention cyst called a ranula, but proved to consist of an almost gelatinous mass of soft tissue, and the area where the mucosa had been resected for the Partsch procedure was re-epithelialized.

Discouraged by the treatment failure, the patient consulted her dentist, and he referred her to the author.

CLINICAL EXAMINATION. The entire right side of the floor of the mouth was elevated almost 1 cm. above the level of the left side. There was a bluish, oval-shaped area in the anterior part of the mass which obviously was the area from which the surface mucosa had been resected so as to be able to suture the "cyst" membrane to the outer mucosa for the marsupialization attempt (Case 18–1A). The mass felt moderately firm and resilient on palpation.

TREATMENT. Inferior alveolar and lingual block anesthesia using Xylocaine (1:50,000) was administered. The oval-shaped translucent area of re-epithelialization was resected with a needle electrode by electrosection, with current output set at 3 on the cutting power knob. The mucosa of the floor of the mouth was then incised parallel to the fringe tissue (Case Fig. 18–1B). The orifice of the submaxillary duct was grasped with curved ophthalmic tissue forceps, and in the total absence of bleeding the submaxillary duct was readily visualized and preserved, while the contents of the mass closest to the floor of the mouth were resected by blunt dissection (Case Fig. 18–1C). The superior portion of the mass was then resected in a similar manner, approximately half-way posteriorly. At that point the tissue resisted enucleation by blunt dissection. A strip of selvage gauze was gently tamped into the defect to dry it, and a transilluminating light was directed into the defect. A slender, beige-yellow, cordlike structure was seen, with the tissue firmly adherent at one minute point. As the mass was gently tugged, the attachment of the tumor tissue to the cordlike structure became apparent. Borrowing an identifying procedure from the neurosurgeon to de-

(Text continued on page 982)

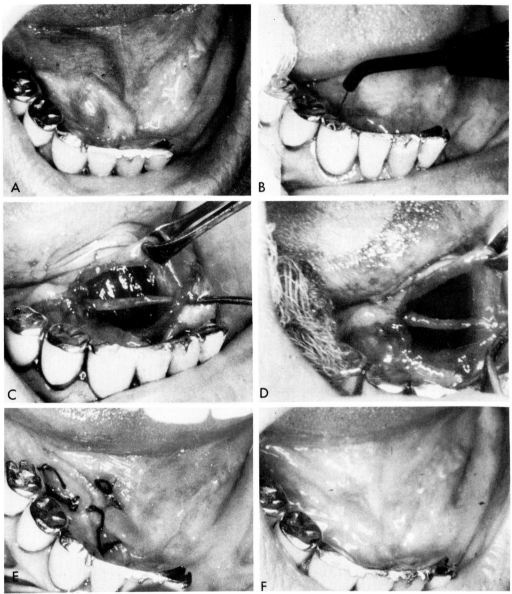

Case Figure 18–1. Surgical removal of a ranula. *A,* Preoperative appearance. The mandible is edentulous except for the left central, right central, lateral, cuspid and two bicuspids. The entire right half of the floor of the mouth is elevated several millimeters higher than the left side and is somewhat darker in color. There is an area approximately 2 cm. long and 1 cm. wide, oval-shaped, located opposite the cuspid and first bicuspid and between the fringe tissue and the alveolar ridge that is dark red in color and appears to be covered with a thin transparent membrane instead of normal surface mucosa, and bulges domelike above the level of the surrounding tissues. *B,* An incision is being made shallowly around the oval area with a fine 45-degree-angle needle electrode. *C,* There is no free bleeding. The orifice of the submaxillary duct is being grasped with ophthalmic tissue forceps, and the distal tissue of the floor of the mouth is being grasped with Allis forceps and rotated posteriorly. The traction against the tissue of the duct orifice has pulled the submaxillary duct taut, and, since the anterior portion of the mass has been removed by blunt dissection, the duct is plainly visible. *D,* The remainder of the mass has been removed by blunt dissection, leaving a clean surgical field free of any cystic tissue fragments. *E,* Appearance of the tissues of the floor of the mouth on the fifth postoperative day, before removal of the sutures. Primary healing is well advanced. *F,* Postoperative appearance of the floor of the mouth three weeks postoperatively. The entire floor of the mouth appears normal, with no evidence of where the surgery had been performed. The tissues are normal in color and uniformly level, and the submaxillary duct is functioning normally.

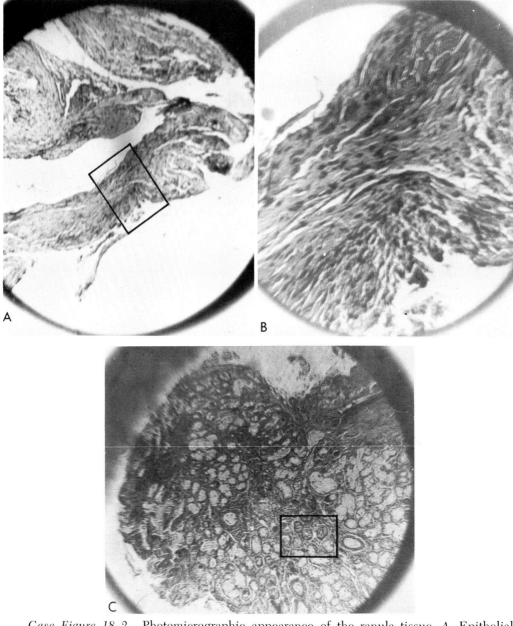

Case Figure 18–2. Photomicrographic appearance of the ranula tissue. *A,* Epithelial cystic tissue lining of the ranula as seen under 10× magnification. The box inset indicates the area that will be seen under higher magnification. *B,* Higher magnification (45×) of the inset area. *C.* Typical glandular type of tumor tissue seen under 10× magnification. The box inset indicates the area for higher magnification.

Illustration continued on opposite page.

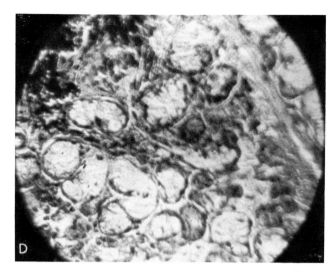

*Case Figure 18–2.
Continued. D.* Higher magnification (45×) of the inset area. Note the mucin
strands in the acini. *E.* Another view of the tumor tissue, seen under 10× magnification. The box inset
indicates the area that will
be examined under higher
magnification. *F.* Higher
magnification (45×) of the
inset area. Note how tightly
the mucin strands fill the
acini, and make the tissue
appear very dark in color.

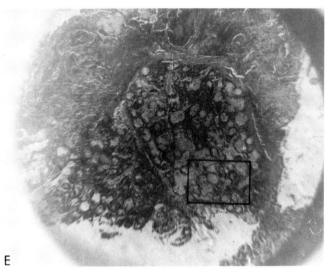

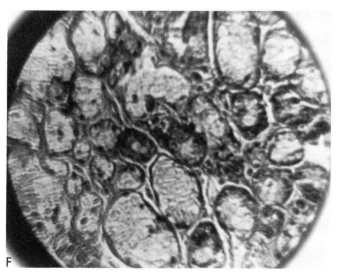

termine whether a structure is a nerve, the cordlike structure was very gently pinched with an ophthalmic forceps with serrated beaks instead of the rat-tooth beaks, such as had been used to grasp the duct orifice. The tongue twitched in response to the gentle pinch, identifying the structure as the lingual nerve. Using the very fine needle electrode such as is used for depilation procedures, the tumor tissue was pulled taut and resected from its tiny attachment to the sheath of the nerve. The remainder of the mass was enucleated by blunt dissection without further incidence (Case Fig. 18–1D). The incised margins were coapted, as were the margins of the area where the surface epithelium had been removed, and were sutured with interrupted silk sutures. Healing progressed uneventfully, and three weeks later the floor of the mouth was fully healed and in excellent tone (Case Fig. 18–1E and F).

Case Figure 18–2 shows the photomicrographic appearance at the ranular tissue.

Mental Nerve Evulsion

A number of advantages electrosection offers the oral surgeon, as well as the advantages to the patient, are dramatically demonstrated when intractable pain makes evulsion of the mental nerve necessary.

One of the advantages to the surgeon is the excellent visibility in an operative field free of bleeding. This makes location of the nerve and its meticulous resection much easier. In the absence of free bleeding it is possible to note when the nerve has been located and is elevated under traction when the maximum portion of the nerve has been elevated from the foramen. For the patient, the advantages are the reduced likelihood that the stump of the severed nerve might develop an amputation neuroma, a painful nerve tumor, and the fact that paresthesia along the distribution of the inferior alveolar nerve is far more transitory following electrosection, a totally atraumatic severing of the nerve, than it is following the traumatic severing of the nerve by sectioning with a scalpel or cutting with a scissors.

CASE 19

This case is an excellent example of the remarkable advantages electrosurgery offers in performing mental nerve evulsion.

PATIENT. A 69-year-old white female.

HISTORY. She had been edentulous for many years and wore a set of ill-fitting dentures for much of that time. As a result the mandibular alveolar ridge was completely resorbed, with concave saddle areas from the first bicuspid regions posteriorly, and the foramina of the mental nerves were palpable near the buccal margins of the saddles. Constant movement of the unstable denture and its crushing effect on the portion of the mental nerve that emerges from the canal and fans out under the periosteum in a postero-anterior direction caused such intractable pain that the author injected absolute alcohol into the right mental nerve. When absolute alcohol is injected into the Gasserian ganglion to bring relief from the pain of trifacial neuralgia the total anesthesia of the branch of the trifacial nerve involved lasts for about two years. Because of the constant traumatization of the anesthetized nerve, the effects of the alcohol block lasted less than two months. The pain was so intolerable that the patient threatened suicide unless she could obtain relief, and welcomed the evulsion of the mental nerve, despite the explanation that it would cause permanent loss of sensation along the normal distribution of the nerve.

CLINICAL EXAMINATION. The mandibular alveolar ridge was completely resorbed, with the tissues of the floor of the mouth, the crest of where the ridge had been, and the mucosa of the inner aspect of the lip forming a straight horizontal line when the lip was pulled out labially. The orifice of the mental nerve foramen could be felt on fingertip palpation.

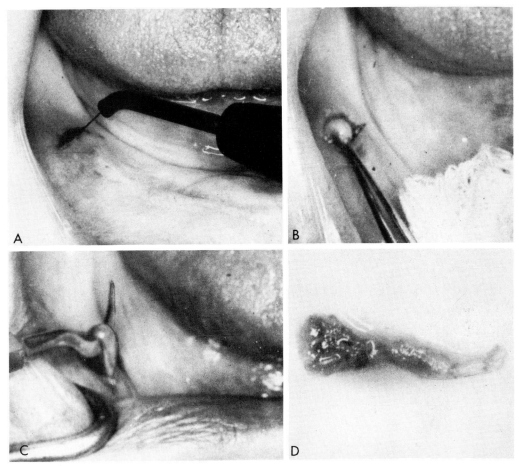

Case Figure 19–1. Evulsion of the mental nerve. *A,* Precise controlled incision being made through the thickness of the mandibular alveolar mucosa with a fine 45-degree-angle needle electrode. There is blood present at the site of incision but no free bleeding. *B,* The mental nerve, easily distinguishable in the absence of bleeding, has been identified and is being elevated with the ophthalmic tissue forceps. The beaks of the forceps have been slipped under the nerve to lift it; it is not grasping or pinching it. *C,* The ophthalmic tissue forceps has been replaced with another hand instrument that has been slipped under the nerve and is lifting it gently but forcefully upward to permit severing the distal end as close to the inferior alveolar nerve trunk as possible, without damaging the latter. *D,* The evulsed nerve. The left hand third of the nerve is the portion that fans out under the periosteum as it emerges from the foramen. The middle third is the portion that usually is resected when performing an evulsion. The right hand third of the nerve is the portion that usually remains in the foramen and often degenerates into an amputation neuroma when the nerve is severed traumatically with a scalpel, scissors, or other steel cutting instrument.

TREATMENT. Inferior alveolar and mental block anesthesia with lidocaine (1:50,000) was administered. A fine, 45-degree-angle needle electrode was selected, and an incision was made in a buccolingual direction over the nerve where it emerges from the foramen (Case Fig. 19–1A). With electrosection, since no pressure is required to cut the tissue, there is no danger of accidentally severing the nerve by exertion of too much hand pressure. But it is necessary for the surgeon to control the depth to which he permits the electrode to penetrate into the tissues, since, if left to its own devices, it will cut through the full thickness of tissue. Therefore the exact thickness of the overlying mucosa was determined by inserting the hypodermic needle used for the anesthesia and measuring the precise depth to which the needle penetrated in mucosa at a little distance from the nerve. Electrosection was then performed using cutting current set at 3 on the power output dial of the Coles Radiosurg, and the electrode was permitted to penetrate the depth of the thickness of the overlying mucosa with a rapid wiping stroke.

Since there was no bleeding once the blood that escaped from the tissue was sponged away, the nerve was easily visualized and engaged by a half-round explorer to begin elevating it enough to slide under it a thicker instrument (Case Fig. 19–1B). A curved instrument tip was then inserted under the nerve and lifted gently but forcefully until the inferior alveolar nerve was lifted toward the internal orifice of the foramen (Case Fig. 19–1C). The distal end of the elevated nerve was severed cleanly with a wiping stroke of the needle electrode, with cutting energy increased to a setting of 4 on the dial, as deep in the canal as possible.

The anterior part of the nerve that fans outward under the periosteum was dissected, with some of its overlying mucosa attached to it (Case Fig. 19–1D). The bulbous portion on the right end is the part of the nerve with its mucosa at the anteriormost end of the nerve. The middle section is the part that lies in the canal and under the periosteum for a short distance after emerging from the canal. The distal or left third is the portion that often remains behind in the canal and, when traumatized, may degenerate into an amputation neuroma.

The postoperative sequence was completely uneventful. The paresthesia of the distribution of the inferior alveolar nerve was considerable for a little more than one week. It then became a tingling sensation for about 10 days, after which the inferior alveolar nerve innervation returned to normal. The distribution of the mental nerve, of course, remained totally anesthetized, but the pain was completely eliminated.

REFERENCES

1. Oringer, M. J.: Significant recent trends in plastic oral surgery. Lecture before American Dental Association, 100th Annual Session, 1959.
2. Boyer, H. E.: Surgical repair of a severed parotid duct. J. Oral Surg., Anes. & Hosp. D. Svc., 18(3):248–251, May, 1961.
3. Calhoun, N. R.: Surgical correction of macrocheilia. J. Oral Surg., Anes. & Hosp. D. Svc., 19(1):70–71, Jan., 1961.
4. Caldwell, J. B., and Letterman, G. S.: Vertical osteotomy in the mandibular rami for correction of prognathism. J. Oral Surg., 12:185, July, 1954.
5. Caldwell, J. B., and Amaral, W. J.: Mandibular micrognathia corrected by vertical osteotomy in the rami and iliac bone graft. J. Oral Surg., Anes. & Hosp. D. Svc., 18(1):3–15, Jan., 1960.
6. Youmans, R. D.: Etiology and management of micrognathia. J. Oral Surg., Anes. & Hosp. D. Svc., 18(1):25–31, Jan., 1960.
7. Limberg, A.: Treatment of open-bite by means of plastic oblique osteotomy of the ascending rami of the mandible. D. Cosmos, 67:1191, Dec., 1925.
8. Shira, R. B.: Surgical correction of open bite deformities by oblique sliding osteotomy. J. Oral Surg., Anes. & Hosp. D. Svc., 19(4):275–289, July, 1961.

9. Thoma, K. H.: Oral Pathology. 2nd ed. St. Louis, C. V. Mosby Co., 1944, pp. 875–876.

10. Oringer, M. J.: Plastic oral surgery: A new term. New York, J. Den., 18(2):345, Nov., 1948.

11. Cooksey, D. E.: Clinical and animal experiments to investigate the healing properties of freeze-dried bone materials in the cysts of the jaws. Thesis. Graduate School of Georgetown University, 1954.

12. Boyne, P. J., and Losee, F. L.: Use of anorganic bone implants in oral surgery. J. Oral Surg., 16:53, Jan., 1958.

13. Boyne, P. J., and Lyon, H. W.: Long term histologic response to implants of anorganic heterogenous bone in man. (Abstr.) J. D. Res., 38:699, July-Aug., 1959.

14. Clayton, I.: Cultured calf bone: A new bone grafting material. Illust. Med. J., 110:49, Aug., 1956.

15. Tucker, E. J.: Studies on the use of cultured calf bone in human bone grafts. Clin. Orthoped., No. 7, 171, 1956.

16. Fischer, W. B., and Clayton, I.: Surgical bone grafting with cultured calf bone. Qtr. Bul. Northwestern Med. School, 29(4):342, 1955.

17. Fischer, W. B.: Clinical use of cultured calf bone grafts. Transplantation Bul., 4:10, Jan., 1957.

18. Tuoti, F., and Kutscher, A. H.: Relief of atypical head pain following removal of maxillary pathosis. Third Clinico-Pathologic Conference, New York D. J., 24:410, Nov., 1958.

19. Hinds, E. C., and Arnim, S. S.: Use of cultured calf bone paste in oral surgery. J. Oral Surg., 15:80, Jan., 1957.

20. Seifert, D. M., and Swanson, L. T.: Histological evaluation of bone grafts made with cultured calf bone paste: Harvard D. Alumni Bul., 19:121–128, Oct., 1959.

21. Grindlay, J. H., and Waugh, J. M.: Plastic sponge which acts as a framework for living tissue. A.M.A. Arch. Surg., 63:288–297, Sept., 1951.

22. Gale, J. W., Curreri, A. R., Young, W. P., and Dickie, H. A.: Plastic Sponge prosthesis following resection in pulmonary tuberculosis. J. Thoracic Surg., 24(6):587–610, Dec., 1952.

23. Lewin-Epstein, J.: Use of polyvinyl alcohol sponge in alveoloplasty: A preliminary report. J. Oral Surg., Anes. and Hosp. D. Svc., 18(6):453–460, Nov., 1960.

24. Oringer, M. J.: Neuroma of the mandible. Oral Surg., Oral Med. & Oral Path., 1(12):1135–1136, Dec., 1948.

25. Archer, W. H.: A Manual of Oral Surgery. 2nd ed., Philadelphia, W. B. Saunders Co., 1956, pp. 440–449.

26. Thoma, K. H.: Oral Surgery. 3rd ed. St. Louis, C. V. Mosby Co., 1958, pp. 765–773.

27. Steiner, M.: Oroantral closure with gold plate; Report of a case. J. Oral Surg., Anes. & Hosp. D. Svc., 18(6):514–515, Nov., 1960.

28. Oringer, M. J.: Plastic closure of alveolar antral traumatic perforations and chronic fistulae, presenting an improved technique. Oral Surg., Oral Med. & Oral Path., 3(4):410–420, Apr., 1950.

29. Barnhill, J. F., and Mellinger, W. J.: Surgical Anatomy of the Head and Neck. 2nd ed. Baltimore, Williams & Wilkins Co., 1940, p. 593.

30. Thoma, K. H., and Goldman, H. M.: Oral Pathology. 5th ed. St. Louis, C. V. Mosby Co., 1960, pp. 1149–1154.

31. Hayes, L. V.: Clinical Diagnosis of Diseases of the Mouth. Brooklyn, N. Y., Dental Items of Interest Publishing Co., 1935, pp. 170–174.

32. Burch, R. J., and Woodward, H. W.: Differential diagnosis and surgery of the submaxillary gland. J. Oral Surg., Anes. & Hosp. D. Svc., 18(6):470–485, Nov., 1960.

33. Burch, R. J.: Removal of sialoliths from the hilus and adjacent duct of the submaxillary gland. J. Oral Surg., Anes. & Hosp. D. Svc., 19(4):319–322, July, 1961.

34. Oringer, M. J.: Removal of submaxillary gland sialoliths by intraoral incision with electrosection. J. Oral Surg., Anes. & Hosp. D. Svc., 17:17–26, May, 1959.

Section Six

ELECTROSURGICAL BIOPSY FOR DIAGNOSIS OF ORAL PATHOLOGY

Chapter Twenty-Three

FUNDAMENTALS OF BIOPSY PROCEDURES

The electrosurgical techniques reviewed in the preceding chapters offer very tangible evidence of the innumerable invaluable services our profession can render to improve the health, comfort, and aesthetic needs of our patients. As important as these services undeniably are, they fail to fully discharge our professional responsibility to our patients.

With all due respect to the importance of those services, in the final analysis by far the most important service any member of the health professions can render his patients is the preservation of life itself. Thus, one further service of paramount importance to our patient remains—the early detection and diagnosis of oral pathology, particularly the potentially life-saving service of early diagnosis of oral malignancy.

Cancer of the oral cavity is one of the least prevalent among the important cancer sites, but it is by no means rare, and it is extremely deadly. Statistics released by the American Cancer Society reveal that only 3.9 per cent of all malignant lesions originate in the oropharynx, but that oropharyngeal cancers are responsible for 9.7 per cent of the total deaths from cancer—the highest morbidity rate ratio among all the cancer sites.

When cancer develops in a remote internal organ such as the pituitary gland, the pancreas, or the adrenal glands, fatal termination of the disease is understandable and excusable. These sites are totally inaccessible to clinical examination, and the disease remains unsuspected and progresses until the victim develops the clinical symptoms that eventually lead to a diagnosis. By the time the diagnosis is made the lesion has most likely metastasized, and fatal termination is virtually inevitable.

The oral cavity, on the other hand, is one of the most accessible and visible parts of the human body and is readily amenable to frequent visual and digital inspections. A comprehensive life-saving clinical examination can be made in substantially less than five minutes. Thus, no comparable excuse exists for the death of victims of oropharyngeal cancers.

Examination of the oral cavity for oral pathology should be as integral a part of the oral examination as the charting of caries and of periodontal lesions. Oral neoplasms are relatively commonplace and frequently encountered, as can be readily ascertained by scanning the contents of typical oral pathology texts.[1, 2, 3] Although oral malignancy is not commonplace, it is by no means rare, 'and is one of the major cancer sites of the body. Nevertheless, many busy practitioners are skeptical about oral cancer, because they have never *knowingly* encountered a single case in many years of clinical practice.

The frequency of incidence of oral cancer has varied very little over the years, from Ewing's estimate of a 4.3 per cent incidence,[4] and Boyd's estimate of 4 per cent,[5] to the current statistical 3.9 per cent. Surprisingly, the morbidity rate has been equally consistent, despite the huge increase in the number of people who undergo regular periodic recall examination and treatment. Whereas gynecologists' use of the Papanicolaou smear has greatly reduced the morbidity rate from cervical and vaginal cancers, the oral cytology smears have failed to attain comparable usefulness or achieve comparable results. Thus the huge increase in routine recall dental examinations has not produced a comparable reduction in the morbidity rate from oropharyngeal cancers. The failure to reduce the morbidity rate and the very considerable number of people who die each year from oral cancer despite its accessibility to examination must be attributed primarily to the failure to detect and clinically diagnose the malignant lesions early enough to permit effective cures.[6]

Ariel, in his review of the statistics, confirmed the importance of early diagnosis and treatment. "In 1951, 4,800 deaths from cancer of the buccal cavity and pharynx were reported. Although the lips are the most frequent site of oral cancer, 1,177 of the deaths were from cancer of the tongue, while only 392 resulted from cancer of the lips."[7] Ewing also has pointed out that, although cancer of the tongue is one of the most accessible of cancers, and readily recognizable in its early stages, it is still one of the most fatal of malignant diseases, with a mortality rate of 75 to 90 per cent.[8]

Inasmuch as both lip and tongue cancers are squamous cell carcinomas, and both have identical pathways for metastasis, the tremendous difference in their respective mortality rates must be attributed primarily to the difference in the likelihood of diagnosis. Lip cancer, being external, is so obvious that it is not likely to be overlooked and neglected, and diagnosis and treatment usually are established early enough to effect a cure. Tongue lesions are not easily recognized and must be discovered by examination. This is due to the fact that the tongue cancer is located either in the posterior part or the ventral surface of the tongue, where the patient is not likely to see it. Since the cancer remains asymptomatic until the late stages, it remains unsuspected until it has reached the terminal stage, unless it is discovered by means of a clinical examination.

It is interesting to note that, although the frequency of incidence and the morbidity rate of oral cancers have remained relatively unchanged, one intriguing significant change has occurred. In preparing the chapter on biopsy for the first edition, the author reviewed the most authoritative oncological texts available at the time, compiled and edited by the foremost students of cancer of the period. At that time the foremost authorities in the field of cancer research appeared to be in full accord that oral cancer was predominantly a disease of males. Ewing estimated (in the earliest statistical study) that the ratio of frequency of incidence was 20 times as great in the male as in the female, and that it therefore was essentially a disease of males. A subsequent similar statistical survey reported the frequency to be 12 times as great in males as in females. The latest study available at that time reported the frequency of incidence to be 8 times as great in the male. The consensus among the experts was that oral cancer occurred 12 times as often in males, and therefore it was predominantly a disease of males.[22, 24]

Just a decade later, the 1970 statistics and projections released by the Statistical Section of the American Cancer Society in 1971 belied the former statistics and conclusions. The 1972 survey reported that oral cancer now occurs with approximately *equal frequency in both sexes.*

The tremendous difference between the former statistics and the current ones of 14,000 cases of oral cancer and 7,000 deaths, occurring in *both* sexes, leads the author to speculate about whether smoking may be responsible for the statistical reversal and be as significant a carcinogenic factor in the development of oral cancer as it is reputed to be in the development of lung cancer.

It appears significant that Ewing's estimated frequency of incidence of oral cancer was based on the earliest statistical survey, and his study showed the highest sex differential estimate. The subsequent statistical surveys that were used as references for the first edition also depended on statistics gathered several years previously as the basis for their conclusions. Thus, most of the statistics dated back at least 25 years, and some as much as 45 years.

There has been a tremendous increase in the number of female smokers in that span of time. Moreover, there has been an enormous increase among women in the total consumption of cigarettes per smoker. During the same period there has been no comparable increase among males; there is a distinct likelihood that, if anything, there has been a slight reduction in the number of male smokers. The trend toward reduction in smoking by males appears to have become significant in recent years, owing to the vigorous educational campaign being waged to alert the public to the dangers of smoking as the primary carcinogenic factor in development of lung cancer and the relation of smoking to coronary episodes, Buerger's disease, and other cardiac and cardiovascular diseases that have affected males primarily.

The New York Times in a 1968 issue published a statistical table released by the American Cancer Society of morbidity from cancer and cardiovascular diseases. According to that statistical table 9.7 per cent of all deaths from the combined sources resulted from cancer of the mouth and pharynx. The high morbidity rate from these sites must be attributed largely to the extremely short pathway for metastasis from the oral cavity to the portals of entry into the main blood stream — literally a mere half a handspan in distance from the mouth to the left thoracic duct and right subclavian vein, both located in the hollow of the neck at the level of the clavicle.

Since most oral cancers are primary lesions, it must be conceded that most of the deaths are preventable; hence, the importance of early detection and diagnosis can scarcely be overemphasized. Dentistry's responsibility in the early detection cannot be evaded. Ewing, in his chapter "The Prevention of Cancer" in Pack and Livingston's *Treatment of Cancer and Allied Diseases*, underlined this when he stated: "Dentistry carries a heavy responsibility for prevention of cancer of the mouth, esophagus and stomach."[9] Most students of cancer concur with his opinion. The dental profession must accept the responsibility and include clinical visual and digital examination for oral pathology as an integral part of the dental examination.

Early detection of cancer is predicated upon thorough examination of the oral cavity and its environs. Cursory examination of just the teeth and perhaps the gingivae in a so-called "routine dental examination" is diagnostically superficial and totally unjustifiable. After the presence of pathology is discovered, clinical diagnosis can be initiated by integration of the physical factors revealed by the clinical examination with other pertinent data. Biopsy provides *conclusive* microscopic confirmation.

Many dentists do not feel qualified to perform biopsies. That they do not does not absolve them of their responsibility for the early detection and diagnosis of oral pathology. All dentists — general practitioners and specialists alike — are able at least to *detect* the presence of oral pathology clinically. Once the presence of a pathologic process has been detected the dentist should either attempt to establish a conclusive diagnosis, if qualified to do so, or promptly refer the patient to a qualified individual for conclusive diagnosis.[10, 11]

The reasons for including this chapter and the following one are threefold:

1. To alert the reader to the importance of making a thorough clinical examination of *all* the oral structures (*e.g.*, the base of the tongue, floor of the mouth, palate, lips, soft palate and oropharynx, and buccal mucosa) an integral part of every dental examination.

2. To facilitate identification of important clinical symptoms of oral malignancy, and of significant clinical indications for biopsy of oral lesions.

3. To present a number of safe, practical, clinical electrosurgical techniques for performing "properly conducted" biopsy of oral neoplasms and lesions.[12, 13]

Diagnosis of a lesion or neoplasm may be established clinically, histopathologically and/or by other laboratory examinations. Clinical diagnosis is established on collective findings gleaned from the following factors:

1. Clinical appearance of the lesion
2. Case history
3. Family history of predispositions
4. Subjective symptoms
5. Hematological and other laboratory tests

Oral cancer is essentially a disease of middle age, particularly of the fourth to sixth decades of life, although it may occur at any age.

Chemical and mechanical occupational irritants may be initiating factors. Syphilis and chronic alcoholism appear to be major predisposing factors. Solar and climatic irritation may also predispose to cancer; thus, persons with out-door occupations such as seamen, farmers or policemen are prone to develop the disease. Statistics indicate that people from warm and cold climates develop skin and lip cancers more frequently than do people from temperate regions.

INDICATIONS FOR PERFORMING BIOPSY

Malignancy should be suspected when any or all of the following symptoms are manifest:

1. Rapid, fungating growth of a new neoplasm.

2. Sudden marked alteration in the size, color, or texture of an old, presumably benign lesion.

3. Sudden unaccountable loss of body weight in the presence of existing presumably benign neoplasia.

4. Fissuring and bleeding in a white mucous lesion.

5. Any ulceration that persists despite routine care for more than 10 to 14 days.

6. Adenopathy, with fixation of the lymph nodes. When visible and palpable adenopathy occurs, as in the case of infectious mononucleosis or other infectious origin, the nodes move freely as they are palpated. But when the nodes remain frozen solidly to the underlying and/or adjacent tissues, it is diagnostic of malignancy.

The criteria for performing a biopsy do not vary, regardless of the method of instrumentation used to obtain the tissue specimen. The size of the lesion should never be considered an important factor with regard to urgency of the biopsy. Indeed, the smallest, most innocuous-looking lesions may well prove to be the most deadly.

Diagnostic Characteristics of Cancer

Cancers are new growths.

Cancers follow three typical growth patterns:

1. *The Exophytic Type.* This is the large fungating, rapidly growing lesion. There is little likelihood that this lesion will be overlooked. The large size and fearsome appearance of this type of lesion help to assure early diagnosis and treatment. This lesion therefore offers the best prognosis (Fig. 23–1A and B).

2. *The Verrucous Type.* This is a much less conspicuous lesion. It is usually a flat lesion with a rough corrugated or papillomatous surface. There is greater likelihood that this lesion might be ignored or overlooked and the prognosis actually is not quite as favorable as for the exophytic type. Nevertheless, since it is a rough-surfaced foreign mass

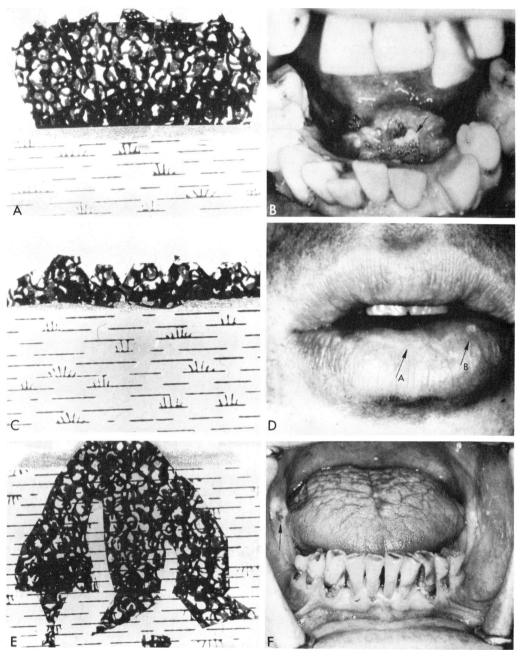

Figure 23–1. A, Schema of the exophytic type of oral cancer. This is the type of cancer that appears suddenly, mushrooms to large size almost overnight, and often is ulcerated in the center. B, A clinical example of the exophytic type of oral cancer. Note the characteristic ulceration in the center of the mass (arrow). C, Schema of the verrucous type of oral cancer. This type is characteristically a surface lesion. D, A clinical example of this type of cancer. Note the white mucous patch superimposed on the surface of the vermilion tissue of the lip; extensive leukoplakia (arrow) and verrucous lesion (arrow). E, Schema of the infiltrative or endophytic type of oral cancer. Very little of the lesion appears clinically, but it is deeply invasive and metastasizes rapidly by extension into the deeper structures, including the mandible and maxilla. F, A clinical example of the infiltrative type of oral cancer. The customary innocuous appearance of this type of lesion (arrow), frequently resembling an aphthous ulcer, often is so misleading that it is ignored.

superimposed on the normal mucosa it is likely that the patient will become aware of it and seek a diagnosis early enough to assure successful treatment (Fig. 23–1C and D).

3. *The Infiltrative or "Endophytic" Type.* Clinically this lesion all too often resembles a harmless ulceration and may be mistaken for an aphthous ulcer. Unlike the true ulcer, it persists despite normal care and medication. This type of lesion is by far the deadliest of the oral malignancies because of its deceptively innocous clinical appearance. It grows like an iceberg, mostly subsurface, penetrating inward deeply and invasively, and is likely to perforate periosteum and invade the underlying bone long before it becomes suspect. Because of its small size and harmless appearance clinically, it is very likely to metastasize into the main bloodstream before a diagnostic biopsy is performed, with fatal consequences (Fig. 23–1E and F).

Cancers show marked tendency to develop resistant ulcerations. Ninety-five per cent of all cancers are reputed to be composed of epithelial cells. Epithelial tissue has no independent blood supply. Rapid growth of the tumor mass therefore outdistances its source of nourishment. When the irritations of functional use, thermal and chemical irritations from food, bacteria and their by-products, plus lowered resistance of the local tissues are superimposed, nonhealing ulceration becomes almost inevitable.

Cancers almost invariably are accompanied by local induration. As the cancerous mass invades the adjacent tissues and destroys them it produces inflammatory responses from the surrounding tissues. The mass becomes well anchored and immobilized by the swelling of the inflammatory response, producing fixed rigidity of the entire mass.

Cancers usually are also accompanied by indurated adenopathy with fixation. When infection is present, lymph nodes often become palpable but remain mobile. When cancer is present, lymph nodes usually become enlarged and palpable, but firmly fixed to the surrounding tissues and immobilized by the induration.

Diagnostic characteristics contributed by conformations of the oral anatomic structures include the following:

1. Paresthesia of the lower lip. When considerable destruction of mandibular bone is caused by slow growth of large benign masses, the gradual pressure pushes the mandibular canal and its contents to one side without injury. Paresthesia of the lower lip therefore is not manifested.

When a comparable amount of bone is destroyed by cancer the mandibular canal and its contents are attacked by the destructive process along with the rest of the bone. Paresthesia of the lower lip on the affected side usually ensues[14] owing to damage to the inferior alveolar nerve.

2. Swelling of cheek, exophthalmos, and discharge of blood or muco-purulent exudate from the antrum through the nostrils.[15, 16] When the maxillary sinus becomes occluded by infection, cysts or benign polyps, the clinical symptoms usually consist of moderate to severe pressure, dizziness, malaise and post-nasal drip. The bony walls of the antrum remain intact and

occluding masses remain confined within the antral cavity. The osteum is located high on the intact medial antral wall and prevents drainage into the nose. Thus, facial swelling and nasal discharge of blood or pus are highly unlikely.

When the maxillary sinus is invaded by cancer the walls of the antrum are usually rapidly destroyed. The malignant mass often bulges unimpeded upward and outward into the orbit and cheek, producing visible facial swelling. If the cancer undergoes partial liquefaction necrosis, drainage of blood or mucopurulent exudate from the antrum into the nose usually produces continuous discharge through the nostrils.

3. Facial pain and muscle dysfunction emanating from the parotid gland. When acute parotitis, sialolithiasis, Sjögren's syndrome, Mikulicz's disease or benign tumors affect the parotid gland, the facial nerve plexus which ramifies through the gland remains undamaged. Neither severe pain nor functional impairment of the facial muscles is manifested.

When the parotid gland is invaded by cancer the destructive process attacks and damages or destroys facial nerve tissue in the gland. Intense facial pain and functional impairment of the muscles of facial expression on the affected side usually ensue.

Diagnostic Significance of Cancer Site

Oral malignancies show definite predilection for favored sites, while other specific areas of the oral cavity characteristically are almost immune to cancer. The area midway between the midline and commissures of the lower lip is the classic site for lip cancer. It occurs much less frequently at the angles of the lips and very rarely on the upper lip (despite infrequent reports of adenocarcinoma,[17] basal cell epithelioma or other malignant neoplasms). When cancer does occur in the upper lip it usually is much more malignant.[18,19] Further evidence of cancer selectivity is the fact that black persons seem immune to cancer of the lips.

Cancer also occurs most frequently on the lateral aspect and base of the tongue, while the dorsum of the tongue is rarely affected. Hauser estimates that 7 to 10 per cent of all intraoral cancers occur in the floor of the mouth and that the majority of them are located around the openings of the salivary ducts.[20] All suspicious lesions should be evaluated, but lesions found in favored sites must logically be more suspect than lesions with similar clinical characteristics located at uncommon sites.

The fact that cancers tend to show selectivity in sex and site of lesion does not by any means imply that when lesions of the buccal cavity occur at atypical sites or in the female sex they can be arbitrarily dismissed as nonmalignant with impunity. Nor does the presence of pre-existing precanceroses justify unsubstantiated diagnosis. A recent case which was characterized by conflicting clinical considerations demonstrates this very well. The patient, a 52-year-old white female, suddenly developed a large indurated lesion at the mucocutaneous junction of her upper lip (Fig. 23–2). Despite the

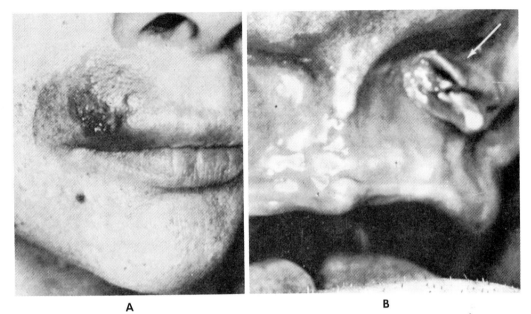

Figure 23–2. A, Basal cell epithelioma of the upper lip in a woman, an atypical cancer at an atypical site. Note presence of numerous neurofibromas of von Recklinghausen's disease on the patient's face and neck. B, Large, fungating lesions such as this one often prove benign. Size of the lesion should never be a determining factor.

atypical location of the lesion, absence of adenopathy, significant history or sudden weight loss, and the sex of the patient, the lesion created a distinct clinical impression of malignancy. To further confuse the clinical picture, the patient was a victim of von Recklinghausen's disease, which is characterized by a tendency for sarcomatous degeneration of the neurofibromas. Biopsy confirmed the clinical impression but proved the lesion to be a basal cell epithelioma, a variety of carcinoma reputed to be rarely encountered in lip cancers. Cases of this type serve to demonstrate that there are no immutable laws for cancer and that no diagnosis can be safely taken for granted. An interesting feature of this case is that on the basis of the biopsy findings x-ray therapy was instituted. The early indications suggest a successful cure without disfigurement.

Rationale for Biopsy

Identification of cancer characteristics, and related factors such as have been described, contributes greatly toward establishing a clinical diagnosis. Students of cancer are agreed, however, that while clinical diagnosis is important in order to focus suspicion on a lesion, clinical diagnosis alone is not infallible. Ariel states: "The premise is accepted that a clinical diagnosis is often misleading. Hence it cannot be utilized as a criterion for therapy. In every instance a histologic diagnosis is obtained."[18]

Benign lesions, precancerous lesions, cancer in situ and infiltrative carcinoma often present similar clinical appearance,[21] and can be accurately differentiated only by microscopic evaluation of the histologic appearance of the diseased tissue under consideration.[22] Boyd defines the precancerous state as one in which there are transitional stages between the original normal histologic picture and a definite picture of cancer in situ. He defines cancer in situ as a condition in which the epithelium shows definite evidence of malignancy, such as irregularity in size and shape of the cells, nuclear changes, anaplasia and loss of cellular polarity — but in which definite invasion of the surrounding tissue has not occurred.[23] Infiltrative carcinoma presents unmistakable evidence of marked invasion of the surrounding tissues.

Boyd states: "Precancerous lesions of the mouth may be observed to precede the onset of cancer," and regards leukoplakia, irritation from badly fitting dentures and vitamin B avitaminosis as the most important precanceroses.[24] According to Lederer and Skolnik, leukoplakia, papillomas, fissures and ulcerations are the precanceroses most likely to undergo malignant change.[25]

Need for histologic differentiation is by no means limited to lesions that are difficult to diagnose clinically. Large fulminating masses that appear to present unmistakable clinical evidence of malignancy are often misleading. To quote Haagensen: "The most experienced clinician can mistake tuberculosis or syphilis for epithelioma in the mouth. Biopsy is therefore a necessity."[26]

The biopsy also provides information that conclusively determines the nature and extent of treatment that is required. The biopsy not only tells us that the lesion is benign or malignant, but it also tells us the precise nature of the malignant cells, and whether the lesion is localized and circumscribed or is in an active state of metastasis, either by direct invasion into the adjacent tissues or via the blood or lymphatic circulation. Thus it tells us how radical the therapy should be.

Biopsy also determines the kind of treatment to institute. Some malignant cells are highly radiosensitive; others are highly radioresistant. This dictates whether radiation therapy will suffice or whether surgery is the only course of treatment. For instance, if the lesion proves to be a cylindroma or a chondrosarcoma, both of which are highly radioresistant, it would be pointless to subject the patient to radiotherapy. But if the lesion proves to be radiosensitive, such as a Ewing's sarcoma, cobalt, x-ray, or radium irradiation would usually suffice. However, if the biopsy shows that the lesion is actively invading the adjacent tissues, then surgery followed by irradiation would be indicated. If the lesion proves to be a squamous cell carcinoma, which is amenable to either surgery or irradiation, and the lesion is circumscribed and localized, surgery would be indicated; however, if the lesion showed evidence of active invasion into the adjacent tissues, surgery followed by irradiation would be indicated.

Cancer therapy must of necessity be ruthlessly thorough to be effective. It must disregard all consequences but the survival of the patient. Hence, cancer surgery invariably entails sacrifice of tissue, often accompanied by disfigurement and even functional impairment. Even so-called conservative treatment of cancer with x-ray, radium or radioactivated isotopes frequently results in osteoradionecrosis or similar damage.[27-32] When dealing with malignancy, such damage is a secondary consideration; but should postoperative evaluation prove the lesion to have been nonmalignant, such tissue destruction would be unpardonable. Haagensen asserted: "Biopsy safeguards patients from the mistake of having a benign lesion treated as a malignancy and vice versa. It also informs the surgeon of the type of malignancy he has to deal with, and enables him to select the most appropriate treatment."[33] It is therefore doubly imperative that conclusive diagnosis of cancer be established before treatment is instituted.

FACTORS THAT INFLUENCE PROPER CONDUCT OF BIOPSY

Since 1930 the procedure of removing a biopsy has been firmly established and unanimously accepted as essential for conclusive diagnosis of malignancy.[34-41] Boyd has asserted: "Biopsy should be used more, not less,[42] and Ewing advocates: "Biopsy should be made mandatory."[43] Byars agrees that microscopic confirmation is necessary, but cautions that: "Conversely, an improperly performed biopsy may cause great confusion and deny the patient an early diagnosis."[44] Cancer experts concede that removal of tissue for histopathologic interpretation can activate a premalignancy to malignant degeneration or stimulate an existing malignancy to greater malignancy. There is virtually universal agreement among them, however, that when the biopsy is "properly conducted," it can be performed safely even on actively malignant lesions.[45-48]

In a recent article, Frazell and Martin commented that: "The relative merits of surgery versus irradiation have often been expounded by enthusiasts of one school or another. . . . Rigid adherence to a strictly partisan attitude may compromise the welfare of the individual cancer patient."[49] Rigid adherence to a strictly partisan attitude regarding biopsy can be equally disadvantageous. Scientific progress and the welfare of the cancer patient dictate that an unprejudiced, sober and responsible evaluation of the respective merits of biopsy via cold-steel instrumentation versus electronic biopsy resection[12, 13, 22, 23, 46, 50-52] is long overdue.

There appears to be overwhelming evidence that the act of taking a tissue specimen is not in itself a dangerous procedure, but that two associated factors can make it dangerous. These are:

1. Traumatization of malignant tissues during biopsy. Blady specifies: "The biopsy should be cleanly cut in order to avoid trauma of the tissues, thereby preventing possible spread of cancer cells, and also to avoid crushing and distorting cells in the specimen. . . . The operator must take care not to squeeze the small fragments of tissue. . . . Squeezing may alter the histologic structure and sometimes renders the tissue useless for study."[53]

Tissue trauma resulting in mechanical dissemination of tumor emboli to distant parts of the body is usually caused by:
- a. Faulty biopsy technique
- b. Inexperienced manipulation of the tissues
- c. Traumatic instrumentation of the tissues

2. Surgical opening into lymphatic and blood circulation. Lymph channels and capillaries are incised when tissue is excised or resected for biopsy evaluation. Surgical metastasis of tumor emboli to distant parts of the body may result.[54]

Safeguards Against Biopsy-Induced Metastasis

Boyd lists the pathways and means by which tumors spread as:
1. Infiltration of tissue spaces
2. Lymph spread
3. Blood spread
4. Spread through natural passages such as bowel or bronchi
5. Spread through serous cavities (known as transcelomic spread)
6. Inoculation by surgery. The transfer of tumor cells by inoculation into surrounding tissue in the course of an operation for (or biopsy of) cancer.[55]

Our concern is with spread by lymph, blood or inoculation during surgery, producing mechanical or surgical metastasis during biopsy. There are two sure safeguards against mechanical or surgical metastasis resulting from biopsy.
1. To safeguard against mechanical metastasis:
    - a. The palpation and manipulation of neoplasia should always be very gentle and discreet. Totally inexperienced personnel should refrain from attempting to obtain biopsy specimens of suspicious lesions or masses.
    - b. In excising the biopsy specimen the tissue should be engaged with a tissue hook or ophthalmic tissue forceps and *pulled* taut to facilitate the cutting. The tissue should never be pinched or tightly bunched to make it taut.
2. To safeguard against surgical metastasis:
    - a. The biopsy should be performed by electrosection with fully rectified or modified continuous wave currents, to seal off the capillaries and lymphatics as the tissue is being incised and excised, to avert surgical entry of tumor emboli into the cut vessels and metastasis via the hematogenous and lymphatic routes.
    - b. The incisional or loop excision should be performed in normal tissue several millimeters beyond the clinical margins of the mass or lesion.

Mayo described the paths by which malignant cells reach locations beyond the primary focus thus:

"Normally only particles of molecular size such as sugars, the amino-acids, and other crystalloids, are absorbed directly through the vascular capillaries of the body, while colloids and large particles are picked up by the lymphatics. Bacteria and malignant cells do not pass directly into the capillaries, but are carried by phagocytes into the lymphatics which are a closed system of vessels."[56]

Thus, the danger inherent in surgical dissemination stems from severance of the blood vessels and the lymphatics in a malignant region by the cold-steel scalpel. To quote Wyeth, "The incomparable advantage inherent in the employment of electrosurgery which seals off these channels in the cutting should be self-evident."[57]

Ochsner expressed these conclusions when he wrote: "Later, metastases are formed by the transportation of infected cells from the original growth to distant parts of the body through the lymph channels or the blood vessels. For a time these infected cells may be interrupted in their journey by intervening lymph nodes. The removal of the original growth together with all of the infected lymph nodes may still result in a permanent cure. This can be accomplished with greater certainty if the removal is carried out with electrosurgery instead of the knife, because electrosurgery will destroy in its course any cells which may contain cancer infection. If the growth is removed with the knife and the incision is not made far beyond the infected area, the cancer is likely to spread rapidly because the lymph spaces will be opened through which infection will be carried beyond the reach of future operation. For the same reason, portions for microscopic examination should always be removed with electrosurgery before operation."[58]

Criteria for Performing Biopsy

It is advisable at this point to define biopsy. To the surgeon, biopsy represents the removal of all or part of a mass or lesion or other material from the living body for histopathologic evaluation for diagnostic purposes.[59] To the pathologist, biopsy represents preparation of the tissue specimen, mounting it for microscopic examination, and a histopathologic interpretation of the tissue cells. To the patient, biopsy suggests possible malignancy and represents hope for reassurance or for early, accurate diagnosis and a chance for survival.

Many surgeons and pathologists (including the author) are of the opinion that abnormal tissue should be submitted for biopsy examination *even when malignancy is not suspected.* The basis of this conviction is that microscopic histologic evaluation reveals the specific cellular structures involved, their characteristics, deviations from normal and degrees of abnormality. This offers valuable clues to the likelihood of recurrence, and acts as a guide to help determine the nature and extent of surgical intervention that is required.

The size of a mass or lesion is not a reliable criterion of its pathologic significance; biopsy should never hinge upon the size of the lesion. Some large fulminating masses are unmistakably malignant. Some small, insignificant-looking lesions frequently prove highly malignant, while large, unsightly ones often prove benign (Fig. 23–2B).

It is the author's firm conviction that abnormal tissue should never be arbitrarily discarded. When such tissue is removed it should be preserved in a 10 per cent formalin solution and either be submitted immediately for biopsy evaluation or at least stored during the healing period. If healing is normal, rapid and devoid of postoperative complications, the tissue can then be discarded. But if the postoperative sequence is unfavorable, the abnormal tissue is still available for biopsy evaluation.

LYMPHATIC DRAINAGE OF THE HEAD AND NECK[60]

The lymphatic circulation plays the most important role in the metastatic dissemination of tumor emboli to distant parts. The anatomic proximity of oral cancer to one of the most prolific and direct pathways of lymphatic drainage heightens the need for early accurate detection and diagnosis. For this reason the lymphatic circulation of the head and neck shall be reviewed before proceeding to consideration of surgical biopsy techniques.

The upper half of the face, the scalp, the maxillary sinuses, the maxillary posterior teeth and their gingival mucosa, and the parotid gland are drained by afferent lymph vessels that run to the parotid gland.

The maxillary anterior teeth and their investing structures, the buccal mucosa, the structures forming the floor of the mouth, the chin, sublingual and submaxillary glands, and the anterior two thirds of the tongue are drained by afferent lymph vessels leading to the submental and submandibular lymph nodes located on either side of the anterior facial vein and the external maxillary artery, which lie immediately beneath the inferior border of the mandible (Fig. 23–3A and B). The posterior third of the tongue, the soft palate and the superior part of the pharynx are drained by afferent lymph vessels leading to the "principal node" of the tongue.[61]

Efferent lymph vessels from these various lymph nodes in turn drain into the superficial and deep cervical chains of nodes which lie respectively on the superficial sheath of the sternomastoid muscle and, deep to the muscle, along the carotid sheath. The lymphatic drainage is well demonstrated in the anatomic wet specimen (Fig. 23–3A), which was specially tinted for clear visualization. Ninety per cent of these efferent vessels drain into the left thoracic duct, which drains into the blood circulation. The remaining ten per cent drain directly into the right subclavian vein.

Shafer, Hine and Levy[57] list the regional lymphatic system of the head and neck as shown in Figure 23–4. Sicher gives a much more detailed but essentially similar description.[62]

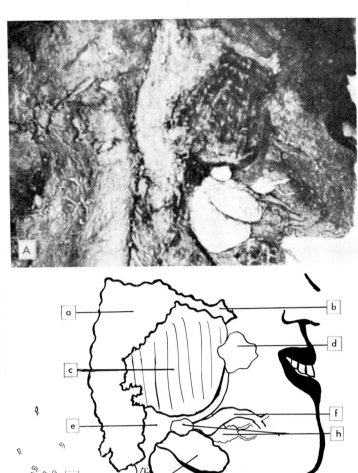

Figure 23–3. Lymphatic circulation of the head and neck. A. Illustrative anatomic wet specimen. *B*, Schematic overlay of the dissection: *a*, Parotid gland. *b*, Parotid (Stensen's) duct. *c*, Masseter muscle. *d*, Buccal pad of fat. *e*, Anterior facial vein. *f*, External maxillary artery. *g*, Submaxillary gland. *h*, Submandibular lymph nodes. *i*, Superficial chain of cervical lymph nodes. *j*, Plexus of afferent lymph vessels.

ADVANTAGES OF ELECTROSURGICAL BIOPSY

The question is often raised, "Wouldn't it be dangerous to cut into a malignant lesion to obtain a biopsy tissue specimen?" It warrants repetition that although the foremost students of cancer concede that biopsy can stimulate an existing malignancy to greater activity or activate a premalignancy to malignant degeneration, they are of the opinion that the biopsy per se is not inherently dangerous or responsible for unfavorable sequelae. Rather, they feel that the danger inheres in faulty traumatizing technique, which can, by indiscreet manipulation of the lesion, cause clumps of tumor cells to break off and invade into the adjacent tissues by extension, creating mechanical metastasis, or by surgically severing blood and lymph vessels in the process of

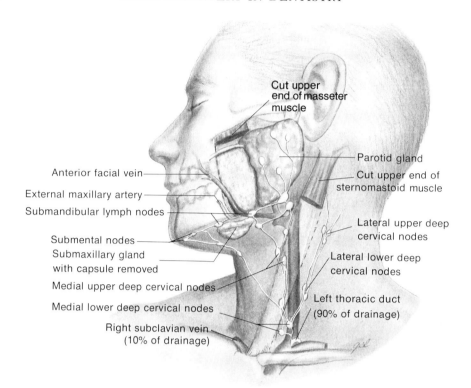

Figure 23–4. Schematic visualization of the lymph node groups involved in the efferent lymphatic drainage from the oral cavity and its environs and their relation to other major anatomic structures in the area. The appalling shortness of the pathway for metastasis along this lymphatic drainage into the main blood stream (90 per cent into the left thoracic duct, the remaining 10 per cent into the right subclavian vein, both located in the supraclavicular region) emphasizes the critical importance of early diagnosis and its relation to the prognosis of treatment of malignant lesions in this area.

cutting the biopsy tissue specimen can permit tumor cells to enter the severed vessels, thereby causing surgical metastasis.[20, 22, 62]

These cancer experts are virtually unanimous in their opinion that a *"properly conducted"* biopsy is not dangerous. The inherent characteristics of fully rectified electrosection, properly utilized with sound surgical technique, make it possible to achieve "properly conducted" biopsy. There is no need to apply pressure to cut the tissue, thus there is no need to maul or manhandle the tissues in the process of cutting them. The tissues can easily be engaged with a tissue hook or ophthalmic tissue forceps and removed atraumatically by needle or loop electrode excision. This eliminates the danger of mechanical metastasis. And since hemostasis is inherent in electrosection, the blood and lymph vessels of normal dimension are sealed off as they are severed, presumably by deposition of the atomic carbon released as the tissue cells are disintegrated and volatilized. This eliminates or tremendously reduces the danger of surgical metastasis, and thus the electrosurgical biopsy fulfills the experts' formula for "properly conducted" biopsy.

The essential diagnostic role of biopsy and safeguarding advantages of performing it electrosurgically having been established, the next step is review of biopsy techniques.

FOOTNOTE REFERENCES

1. Bernier, J. L.: The Management of Oral Diseases. 2nd ed., St. Louis, C. V. Mosby Co., 1959.
2. Shafer, W. G., Hine, M. K., and Levy, B. M.: A Textbook of Oral Pathology. Philadelphia, W. B. Saunders Co., 1958.
3. Thoma, K. H., and Goldman, H. M.: Oral Pathology. 5th ed., St. Louis, C. V. Mosby Co., 1960.
4. Ewing, J.: The Prevention of Cancer, in Pack, G. T., and Livingston, E. M.: Treatment of Cancer and Allied Diseases. Vol. I. New York, Paul B. Hoeber, Inc., 1940, p. 5.
5. Boyd, W.: Textbook of Pathology. 6th ed. Philadelphia, Lea & Febiger, 1953, p. 244.
6. Dalitsch, W. W.: Oral cancer: The role and responsibility of the dentist. J. Oral Surg., Anes. & Hosp. S. Svc., 18(3):183–193, May, 1960.
7. Ariel, I. M.: Principles in the Treatment of Lip Cancer, in Pack, G. T., and Ariel, I. M.: Treatment of Cancer and Allied Diseases. Vol. II, 2nd ed. New York, Paul B. Hoeber, Inc., 1959, p. 53.
8. Ewing, J.: Neoplastic Diseases: A Treatise on Tumors. 2nd ed. Philadelphia, W. B. Saunders Co., 1922, p. 840.
9. Ewing, op. cit., 1940.
10. The dentist mans the front lines in the fight against cancer. Editorial, J.A.D.A., 50:462, Apr., 1955.
11. The dentist takes a biopsy. Editorial, New York J.D., 26:261, Aug.-Sept., 1956.
12. Oringer, M.J.: Safeguarding biopsy by use of electronic electrosurgery. J. Oral Surg., 15:129–137, Apr., 1957.
13. Darlington, C. G.: Laboratory Diagnosis Available to the Dentist, in Miller, S. C.: Oral Diagnosis and Treatment. 3rd ed. New York, Blakiston Division, McGraw-Hill Book Co., 1957, p. 888.
14. McCall, J. O., and Wald, S. S.: Clinical Dental Roentgenology. 4th ed., Philadelphia, W. B. Saunders Co., 1957, p. 374.
15. Ewing, op. cit., 1922, p. 723.
16. Blair, V. P., Moore, S., and Byars, L. T.: Cancer of the Face and Mouth. St. Louis, C. V. Mosby Co., 1941, pp. 218, 242.
17. Meyer, I.: Current therapy of oral cancer. J. Oral Surg., Anes. & Hosp. D. Svc., 18(3):194–202, May, 1960.
18. Ariel, op. cit., p. 58.
19. Boyd, W.: Textbook of Pathology. 7th ed. Philadelphia, Lea & Febiger, 1961, p. 201.
20. Hauser, H.: Treatment of Cancer of the Floor of the Mouth, in Pack, G. T., and Ariel, I. M.: Treatment of Cancer and Allied Diseases. Vol. III, 2nd ed. New York, Paul B. Hoeber, Inc., 1959, p. 147.
21. Cruickshank, A. H.: Lips, Tongue, Mouth and Jaws, in Raven, R. W., ed.: Cancer. Vol. II, Part 2. Pathology of Malignant Tumors. London, Butterworth & Co., 1958, pp. 60–61.
22. Richards, G. E., and Ash, C. L.: Radiation Therapy of Cancer of the Buccal Mucosa, in Pack, G. T., and Ariel, I. M.: Treatment of Cancer and Allied Diseases. Vol. III, 2nd ed. New York, Paul B. Hoeber, Inc., 1959, p. 75.
23. Boyd, op. cit., 1953, pp. 226, 242.
24. Boyd, W.: Pathology for the Surgeon. 7th ed. Philadelphia, Lea & Febiger, 1955, p. 103.
25. Lederer, F. L., and Skolnik, E. M.: Precancerous Lesions of the Oral Cavity, in Pack, G. T., and Ariel, I. M.: Treatment of Cancer and Allied Diseases. Vol. III. 2nd ed. New York, Paul B. Hoeber, Inc., 1959, p. 45.
26. Haagensen, C. D.: Surgical Biopsy, in Pack, G. T., and Livingston, E. M.: Treatment of Cancer and Allied Diseases. Vol. I. New York, Paul B. Hoeber, Inc., 1940, p. 51.
27. Stafne, E. C.: Oral Roentgenographic Diagnosis. Philadelphia, W. B. Saunders Co., 1958, pp. 222–223.
28. Blum, T.: Osteomyelitis of the mandible and maxilla. J.A.D.A., 11:802–805, Sept., 1924.
29. Cook, T. J.: Late radiation necrosis of jaw bones. J. Oral Surg., 10:118–137, Apr., 1952.
30. Deschaume, M., Canhepe, J., and Goudaert, M.: Action de la radiothérapie sur le développement des maxillaires, des germes dentaires, et des glandes salivaires. (Abstr.) Oral Surg., Oral Med. & Oral Path., 4:922, 1951.
31. Lawrence, E. A.: Osteoradionecrosis of mandible. Am. J. Roentgenol., 55:733–742, June, 1946.
32. Thoma, K. H.: Oral Pathology. 4th ed. St. Louis, C. V. Mosby Co., 1954, p. 762.
33. Haagensen, op cit., 1940, p. 47.
34. McKee, G. M., and Cipollaro, A. C.: Cutaneous cancer and precancer: A practical monograph. Am. J. Cançer, 1937, p. 196.
35. Wood, F. C.: Diagnosis of cancer. J.A.M.A., 95:1141, Oct., 1930.
36. Hellwig, C. A.: Biopsy in tumors. Arch. Pathol., 13:607, Apr., 1932.
37. Donnelly, A. J.: Symposium on cancer: biopsy. Clinics, 4:97, June, 1945.
38. McGraw, A. B., and Hartman, F. W.: Present status of the biopsy. J.A.M.A., 101(16):1208, Oct., 1933.
39. Stout, A. P.: Human Cancer. Philadelphia, Lea & Febiger, 1932, p. 42.
40. Thoma, K. H.: Clinical Pathology of the Jaws. Springfield, Ill., Charles C Thomas, 1934, p. 578.
41. Bernier, J. L., and Tiecke, R. W.: Biopsy. J. Oral Surg., 8:342, 1950.
42. Boyd, W.: Textbook of Pathology. 4th ed. Philadelphia, Lea & Febiger, 1943, p. 313.
43. Ewing, J.: Neoplastic Diseases: A Treatise on Tumors. 4th ed. Philadelphia, W. B. Saunders Co., 1940, p. 110.

44. Byars, L. T.: Surgical Treatment of Cancer of the Buccal Mucosa (Cheek), in Pack, G. T., and Ariel, I. M.: Treatment of Cancer and Allied Diseases. Vol. III. 2nd ed. New York, Paul B. Hoeber, Inc., 1959, p. 88.
45. Sachs, W., *et al.*: Junction nevus-nevocarcinoma. J.A.M.A., *135*:216, Sept., 1947.
46. Barnhill, J. F., and Mellinger, W. M.: Surgical Anatomy of the Head and Neck. 2nd ed. Baltimore, Williams & Wilkins Co., 1940, p. 567.
47. Thoma, K. H., and Robinson, H. B. G.: Oral Diagnosis. 5th ed. Philadelphia, W. B. Saunders Co., 1960, p. 74.
48. Winkler, E. G.: Personal communication.
49. Frazell, E. L., and Martin, H. E.: Cancer of the head and neck. World-Wide Abst. Gen. Med., *4*(3):34–36, Mar., 1961.
50. Ariel, *op. cit.*, p. 57.
51. Darlington, *op cit.*, p. 80.
52. Hauser, *op. cit.*
53. Blady, J. V.: Biopsy in Tumor Diagnosis, in Pack, G. T., and Ariel, I. M.: Treatment of Cancer and Allied Diseases. Vol. I. 2nd ed. New York, Paul B. Hoeber, Inc., 1959, p. 76.
54. Thoma, K. H.: Oral Surgery. 3rd ed. St. Louis, C. V. Mosby Co., 1958, p. 1274.
55. Boyd, *op. cit.*, 1961, p. 702.
56. Mayo, W. J.: Relative values of surgery and radiotherapy. Minnesota Med., 8:7, Jan., 1925.
57. Shafer, et al., *op. cit.*
58. Ochsner, A. J.: Cancer infection. Surg., Gynecol. & Obstet., *40*:336, Mar., 1925.
59. Dorland's Illustrated Medical Dictionary. 23rd ed. Philadelphia, W. B. Saunders Co., 1959, p. 181.
60. deVere, C. A.: Personal communication.
61. Barnhill and Mellinger, *op. cit.*, p. 39.
62. Sicher, H.: Oral Anatomy. 3rd ed. St. Louis, C. V. Mosby Co., 1960, pp. 346–351.

Chapter Twenty-Four

CLINICAL ELECTROSURGICAL BIOPSY TECHNIQUES

MECHANICS OF RESECTION

Lesions that are less than 1 cm. in diameter invariably are resected in toto as the biopsy specimen, with a 2- to 3-mm. perimeter of normal tissue. Lesions that are more than 1 cm. in diameter usually are not removed in toto. Instead, a representative segment is removed, usually in the form of a pie-shaped wedge, with the apex of the triangle at the center of the mass and the base extending 2 to 3 mm. into the adjacent normal tissue.

There are a number of important reasons for inclusion of the perimeter or collar of normal tissue as part of the biopsy. The junction of malignant and normal tissue shows whether the lesion is circumscribed and limited or is extending into the adjacent normal tissue, which would indicate active metastasis. As has been mentioned earlier, this influences the nature and extent of the treatment to be instituted to a considerable degree. Similarly, it is desirable to extend the tissue resection 3 or more mm. beyond the base of the lesion, since presence of tumor cells in the lumen of blood or lymph vessels in the normal basal tissue would also indicate an active state of metastasis.

Resection of tissue specimens for biopsy can be performed with either needle or loop electrodes. Needle electrodes can be bent to desirable angles for greater accessibility and adaptability. Loop electrodes can be bent or shaped to meet special needs. The round, triangular, square and U-shaped loops are most useful.

To resect a small mass in toto with a needle electrode it is best to incise the area around the mass in the shape of a circumscribed ellipse (Fig. 24–1). The elliptical incision offers two advantages: it permits inclusion of the desired perimeter of normal tissue and subsequent accurate coaptation of the margins of the resultant defect without any puckering, distortion or undue tension. Small masses also can easily be resected in toto with round loop electrodes slightly greater in diameter than the masses so that the necessary perimeter of normal tissue may be included in the biopsy (Fig. 24–2).

The best method for biopsy of a large mass with a needle electrode is to incise and excise a pie-shaped triangular wedge of tissue. The apex of the triangle should be at the center of the mass, and a 3 mm. margin of normal tissue should be included at the base of the triangular segment (Fig. 24–3). Triangular, square and U-shaped loops are also useful for resecting segments of large masses for biopsy (Fig. 24–4).

Biopsy tissue should not be washed or air-dried. It should immediately be preserved in tissue fixative such as 10 per cent formalin solution.

The following case reports are presented for three reasons:

1. To describe safe, practical electrosurgical biopsy techniques.

2. To demonstrate typical quality and rate of healing after biopsy by electrosection of various types of oral tissue.

3. To demonstrate that biopsy specimens obtained by electrosection with fully rectified electronic current are comparable in all respects to the best obtainable by other surgical methods for histopathologic interpretation.

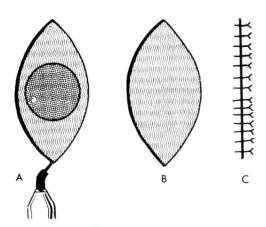

Figure 24–1. Schematic diagram for incisional biopsy of small masses. *A,* Circumferential incision with needle electrode. *B,* Incised segment resected. *C,* Cross section view of biopsy specimen. *D* and *E,* Clinical versions of this procedure.

A   B   C

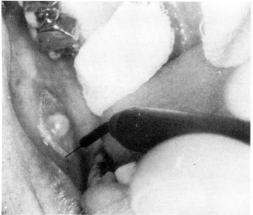

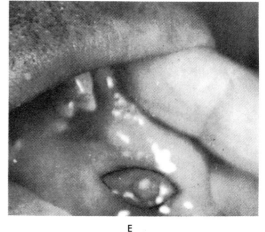

D   E

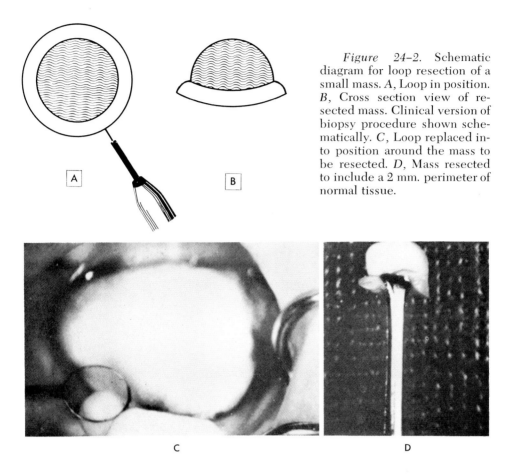

Figure 24–2. Schematic diagram for loop resection of a small mass. *A,* Loop in position. *B,* Cross section view of resected mass. Clinical version of biopsy procedure shown schematically. *C,* Loop replaced into position around the mass to be resected. *D,* Mass resected to include a 2 mm. perimeter of normal tissue.

In order to conclusively demonstrate the latter, photomicrographs of the biopsy specimens will be included with a number of case reports. These afford conclusive visual evidence that tissue properly resected by electrosection does not undergo mass coagulation necrosis, alteration of cellular contents or other deterioration that might destroy the usefulness of the tissue specimen for histopathologic evaluation. Where possible, the reports will be grouped for maximum coordination according to anatomic source or type of tissue. Since biopsy technique rather than specific pathology of the lesions is our primary concern here, the pathologists' detailed histopathologic descriptions of the biopsy tissue will be omitted.

Although all the oral biopsies involve either needle or loop resection, the techniques vary according to conditions created by their anatomic locale. The techniques shall therefore be reviewed in anatomic sequence, starting with biopsy of the lesions of the lip and progressing inward into the oral cavity to lesions of the buccal mucosa, the maxillary gingivae, the mandibular gingivae, the palate, the floor of the mouth, and the tongue. All but the latter are located in mucous membrane, and the cases reviewed in the preceding chapters have demonstrated the remarkable effectiveness of electrosection in mucous tissues. Biopsy of the tongue provides an excellent example of the comparable

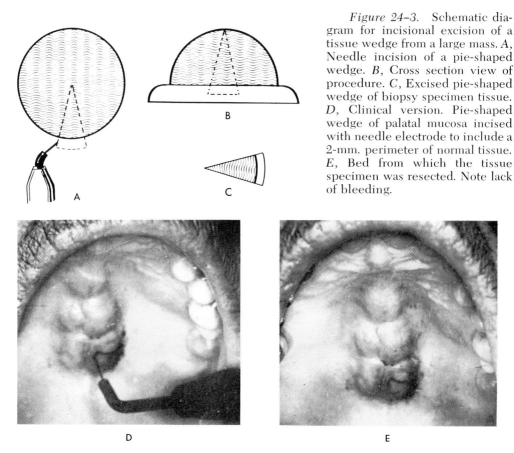

Figure 24–3. Schematic diagram for incisional excision of a tissue wedge from a large mass. *A*, Needle incision of a pie-shaped wedge. *B*, Cross section view of procedure. *C*, Excised pie-shaped wedge of biopsy specimen tissue. *D*, Clinical version. Pie-shaped wedge of palatal mucosa incised with needle electrode to include a 2-mm. perimeter of normal tissue. *E*, Bed from which the tissue specimen was resected. Note lack of bleeding.

effectiveness of electrosection in muscle tissue. Electrosection is equally effective for incising cutaneous tissue. The skin is a distinctly atypical site for oral biopsy, but special conditions may make it necessary to perform extraoral biopsy. A case that demonstrates such a procedure will also be reviewed.

BIOPSY OF LIP (AREOLAR TISSUE) LESIONS

The lip is a classic example of areolar tissue that is highly vascular. Since it is not attached to periosteum and bone it is easily displaced by pressure. Both of these characteristics constitute handicaps to biopsy by cold-steel instrumentation. As a result of the vascularity, cold-steel biopsy of these tissues is usually accompanied by profuse hemorrhage. Displacement is a handicap to precise incisional surgery.

When biopsy is performed by electrosection—particularly loop resection—these handicaps are neutralized. Since lymph channels and small capillaries are sealed by the electrosurgery, bleeding is minimized or eliminated; and, since incision or resection can be performed accurately without exerting pressure against the tissues, there is no displacement of tissues to inter-

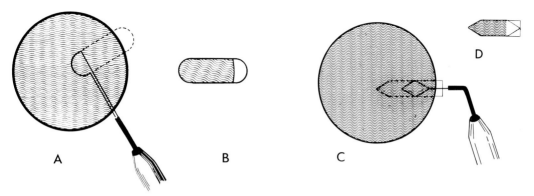

Figure 24–4. Schematic diagram for loop excision of a specimen segment of tissue. *A*, Segment of large mass resected with appropriate loop electrode. *B*, Excised segment of tissue, the biopsy specimen. *C*, Resection performed with diamond loop electrode. *D*, Excised segment of tissue, the biopsy specimen.

fere with precision. Electrosection therefore is especially advantageous for performing biopsy of areolar tissues, as the following case reports demonstrate.

Incisional Excision

CASE 1

This case demonstrates biopsy of a traumatic lesion of the lower lip by incisional electrosection and the therapeutic use of fulguration.

PATIENT. A 33-year-old white male.

HISTORY. The patient accidentally bit his lower lip three weeks previously, lacerating the surface mucosa. Being a physician, he applied antiseptic and dressed the wound. Instead of healing, the lip swelled and became indurated; a bulging round mass formed near the surface. The symptoms progressively worsened, so he came in for diagnosis and treatment.

CLINICAL EXAMINATION. *Extraoral.* The midline of the lower lip was well defined. The central third of the right half of the lip was indurated, swollen and discolored. The upper part of the swollen area projected up beyond the surface and was capped with a white circular area that appeared to consist partly of keratin and partly of coagulum (Case Fig. 1–1A). There was no adenopathy. Histories: negative.

Intraoral. Negative.

Clinical diagnosis. Soft fibroma.

TREATMENT. The lip was prepared and anesthetized by circumferential infiltration. A 45-degree-angle fine needle electrode was selected and current output set at 3 for electrosection. The lip was everted and the mass plus 2 mm. of normal tissue was incised circumferentially in an oval shape.[1] The initial incision was made about 1 mm. deep to define the biopsy area (Case Fig. 1–1B). When the entire mass was circumscribed, the incision was extended to a depth of about 5 mm. and directed at an approximate 45 degree slant toward the center (Case Fig. 1–1C). The incised mass was then grasped with an Allis forceps, pulled taut and resected with the needle electrode.

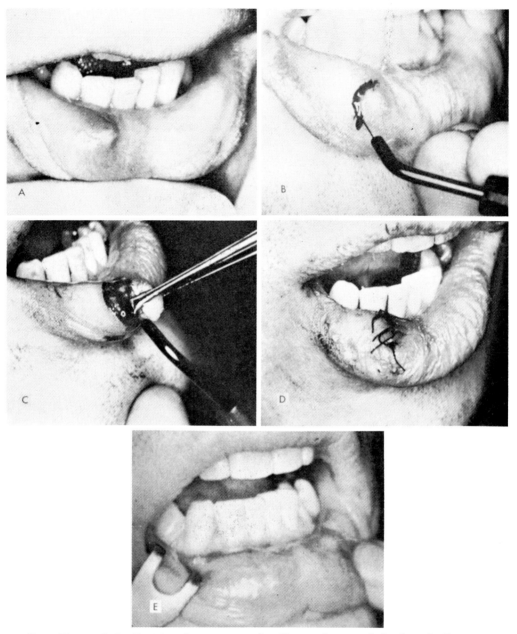

Case Figure 1–1. Incisional resection of a fibrotic lesion of the lip. *A*, Preoperative appearance of the lesion. *B*, Initial incision, elliptical in shape and shallow, is performed with a 45-degree-angle fine needle electrode. Note mere trickle of blood. *C*, The circumscribed shallow incision is then extended downward on each side at a 45-degree angle toward the midline to complete the excision with the smallest possible surgical defect. *D*, The margins of the wound are accurately coapted and sutured with interrupted silk sutures. *E*, Appearance two weeks postoperatively. The surgical defect appears almost fully healed.

The entire procedure produced only a light trickle of blood, and this was stopped by light compression. The tissue was preserved in formalin. The lip was then pulled in an anteroposterior direction so that the oval incision formed a straight line. The incised margins were coapted and sutured with interrupted silk sutures (Case Fig. 1–1D). Tincture of myrrh and benzoin was applied in air-dried layers; then clear collodion was applied over the area.

He returned on the fifth postoperative day and reported that he had removed the partially detached collodion dressing on the third day. Thereafter he had protected the area with a steroid ointment and frequent lavage and compresses. The lip was still slightly edematous and discolored, but there was no induration. Healing was progressing by primary union except where one of the sutures had exfoliated. There, healing was progressing by secondary granulation which was covered with coagulum.

The sutures were removed and tincture of myrrh and benzoin was applied. He was instructed not to apply any more ointments, but to apply tincture of myrrh and benzoin daily. He returned one week later. Healing was much further advanced. There was no more edema or discoloration; the suture line appeared almost completely healed except for the site of the exfoliated suture, which appeared slightly laggard (Case Fig. 1–1E). Tincture of myrrh and benzoin was applied and he was instructed to return in two weeks for further observation.

When he returned he reported that a new lesion had formed in the suture line, which he had noted for the first time two days previously. The lesion, a small mass about 3 mm. in diameter, spherical, resilient, and yellowish in color, projected upward 2 mm. beyond the lip surface. It seemed to contain fluid, and occupied the exact site of the exfoliated suture (Case Fig. 1–2A). Clinically this appeared to be either a dilated, blocked mucous gland or a mucocele.

The lip was prepared and topical anesthetic was applied for two minutes. A 45-degree-angle fine needle electrode was used with current output of 3 to incise the very thin distended surface tissue over the bulbous mass. The incised margins were retracted, exposing a round globule, vesicular in appearance. As it was being enucleated, it tore from its basal attachment to the lip. Additional topical anesthetic was sprayed into the defect; then the basal tissue was curetted with a sharp spoon curet. The procedure was completely bloodless. Tincture of myrrh and benzoin applied in air-dried layers substituted satisfactorily as a dry dressing.

He returned the following week. The lip appeared to be healing satisfactorily. Two weeks later, however, a similar mass appeared. This time the lip was prepared and anesthetized by infiltrating a few minims of solution. The mass was then destroyed in situ by fulguration until the site was thoroughly carbonized (Case Fig. 1–2B). Tincture of myrrh and benzoin was applied and Kenalog in Orabase was used as a protective dressing. One week later the lip was almost fully healed (Case Fig. 1–2C) and the following week it appeared completely healed (Case Fig. 1–2D).

Three weeks later another similar lesion suddenly appeared in the same area. On examination it became apparent that this lesion was almost 2 mm. to the right of the site of the previous lesions in the suture line, which, although fully healed, was just barely visible when the lip was stretched taut by eversion. The new lesion was also destroyed in situ by fulguration. Healing progressed without further incident, although a few of the surface mucous glands showed evidence of dilation. Within three weeks the lip was fully healed (Case Fig. 1–2E).

BIOPSY REPORT. Traumatic fibrosis with keratinization and ulceration (Case Fig. 1–2F).

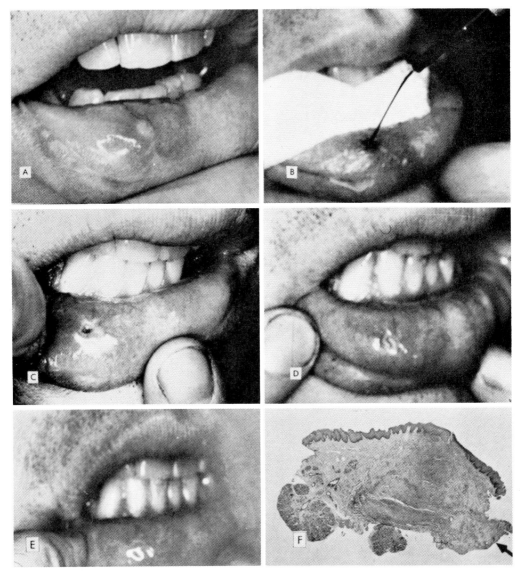

Case Figure 1–2. About three weeks later, a vesicular lesion suddenly appears in the line of incision. *A,* Clinical appearance of the new lesion. It is a vesicular mass, round and slightly elevated, surrounded by a broad areola of engorgement. A secretion of mucinous fluid is sometimes spontaneously discharged and easily milked from probable mucocele. *B,* Enucleation by curettage failed and the mucocele recurred. It is fulgurated to destroy the mass in situ, creating a carbonized crater. *C,* Appearance of the lip one week later. A fairly shallow crater remains in the fulgurated area. There is no induration or hemorrhagic extravasation into the lip. *D,* Appearance of the lip the following week. Granulation repair has almost completely obliterated the surgical defect. A number of small, superficially located mucous glands are present in the lip. *E,* Appearance of the lip approximately ten weeks after the original biopsy surgery. The lip appears normal in all respects. It is free of induration or scar tissue formation. *F,* Photomicrograph of tissue resected. Arrow points to single layer of cells destroyed by the electrosection.

The lesions have not recurred to date. This case demonstrates how easily appearance of a new lesion of similar appearance and anatomic structure in the immediate vicinity of previous lesions can simulate recurrence and be misleading if it is not subjected to thorough examination. Snap diagnoses based upon casual observation may lead to unnecessarily radical surgery.

Biopsy of the Lower Lip

CASE 2

Unlike the previous case, in which the lesion was the result of superficial trauma, this lesion involves the deep inner structures of the lip as well as the surface tissue. It also offers an excellent example of the unreliability of clinical appearances in establishing a differential diagnosis.

PATIENT. A 33-year-old white male.

HISTORY. The patient, a dentist, became aware that he was developing a habit of nibbling on a small rough spot on the vermilion surface of his lower lip. He therefore wanted to have the lesion examined and removed.

CLINICAL EXAMINATION. There was a small round verrucous lesion, approximately 0.4 cm. in diameter, surrounded by a bright red aureola that was accentuated by the presence of a very thin translucent milky white membraneous-looking surface on the vermilion surface of the lower lip (Case Fig. 2–1A).

At first glance this lesion resembled one described by Shira as an "erosive lichen planus." However, palpation revealed the subsurface presence of a firm, round mass, measuring approximately 1.5 cm. in diameter. The mass appeared to be circumscribed and suggested an encapsulated mass such as a mixed tumor. Palpation of the lip, face, and neck failed to reveal adenopathy or induration.

TREATMENT. The lip was prepared for surgery and a topical anesthetic was applied for two minutes; circumferential infiltration anesthesia was then administered. A fine 45-degree-angle needle electrode was selected and power output on the cutting rheostat dial was set at 4.5 to assure hemostasis. Circumscribing incisions were made 3 mm. beyond the clinical outline of the lesion. The lesion was excised without free bleeding, and the entire mass was preserved in a fixative solution as the biopsy specimen (Case Fig. 2–1B). The cut surface of both the biopsy specimen and the bed from which the specimen had been resected were totally free of coagulation. Blood was present on the surface of the surgical defect, but there was no free bleeding. When the surface was sponged lightly it remained dry, with no evidence of oozing. The raw tissue surface was then fulgurated (Case Fig. 2–1C).

Despite its preoperative clinical appearance, there was no evidence that the subsurface mass was encapsulated. The incised tissue margins were then coapted and wound closure was effected with 4-0 braided silk interrupted sutures (Case Fig. 2–1D). Healing appeared to be progressing without incidence, and the sutures were removed on the fifth postoperative day (Case Fig. 2–1E). However, later that day a biopsy report of squamous cell carcinoma, with the tumor tissue extending *to the line of cleavage* and a number of partially sheared tumor cells in the cleavage line, was received. The translucent thin white surface membrane was reported as leukoplakia, a premalignant lesion, according to the standards established by Bernier.[2]

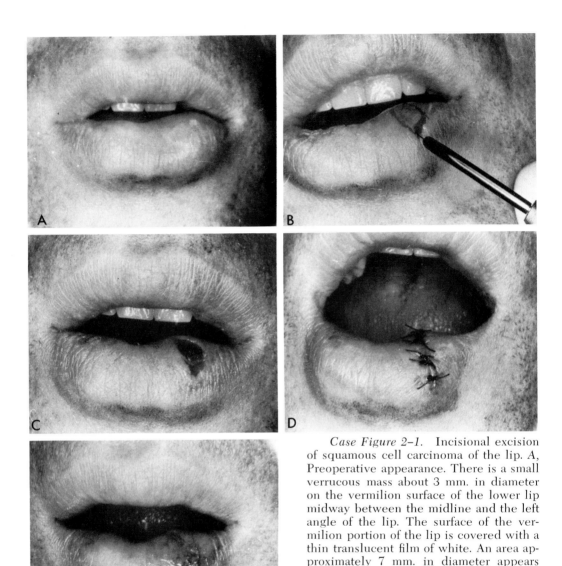

Case Figure 2–1. Incisional excision of squamous cell carcinoma of the lip. *A,* Preoperative appearance. There is a small verrucous mass about 3 mm. in diameter on the vermilion surface of the lower lip midway between the midline and the left angle of the lip. The surface of the vermilion portion of the lip is covered with a thin translucent film of white. An area approximately 7 mm. in diameter appears indurated and feels like a foreign body in the lip when palpated. *B,* Two incisions are made deep into the lip to circumscribe the mass and a 3- to 4-mm. perimeter around it. Despite the vascularity of the lip there is blood present but no free bleeding. *C,* The mass having been excised, the base of the bed from which it was removed has been fulgurated prior to closure of the wound. *D,* The incised margins are coapted and sutured with interrupted silk sutures. *E,* Appearance of the lip on fifth postoperative day immediately after the sutures were removed. The tissue appears to be healing very well, and without deformity, but the biopsy report shows the cancerous mass had extended beyond the outer perimeter of normal tissue that had been included, and several cells in the line of cleavage have been partially sheared off. The extension into the adjacent tissues necessitates further surgery.

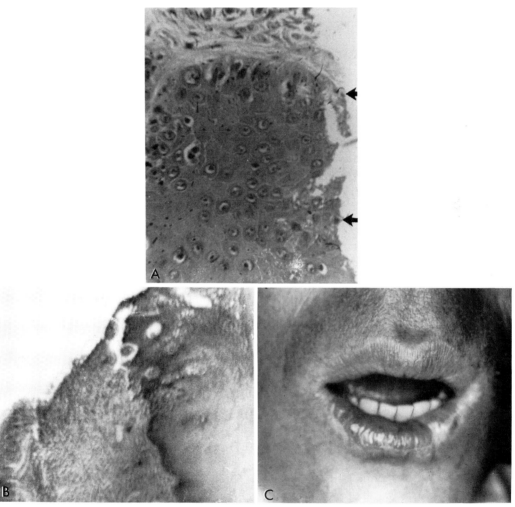

Case Figure 2–2.   *A*, Original tissue removed from the lip—a squamous cell carcinoma. A number of intact single cells and cells that have had part of their cell walls sheared off are in the line of cleavage. The contents of even the sheared cells appear intact and normal (arrows). *B*, Tissue removed by block dissection with steel scalpel 8 days after original surgery. Note almost total repair of excision site that had been treated by electrosection. *C*, Appearance of the lip one year after the block dissection with a steel scalpel and stripping of the vermilion border of the lip had been performed. Note the shortening of the left side of the lip creating a deformity owing to the contractile nature of the scar tissue repair following steel scalpel surgery.

The fact that the malignant mass extended beyond its apparent clinical delineation into the adjacent "normal" tissue suggested the possibility of an active state of metastasis by extension. This, plus the fact that the line of cleavage was apparently in malignant tissue and not in the normal perimeter tissue, created a distinct possibility that a radical neck commando dissection might be required. The author therefore consulted with Hollen Farr, M.D., of the Memorial Hospital in New York, a fellow member of the consultant staff of the St. Francis Hospital Oral Cancer Detection and Prevention Center, and decided to do a wide wedge-block dissection of the lip to evaluate the tissue on either side of the original excision site and to do a stripping of the vermilion surface of the lip.

The wedge-block dissection and vermilion stripping were performed by Dr. Farr at the Memorial Hospital with a steel scalpel on the eighth postoperative day. A serial section of the entire wedge of tissue proved to be completely free of tumor cells, despite the fact that the malignant tissue had extended to the line of cleavage, and no further treatment was required. This tissue wedge provided histologic evidence of the rate and quality of repair of the original electrosurgical excision site, which is rarely possible to determine following the usual biopsy. There was no evidence of excessive vacuolation or lymphocyte concentration in the deeper structures, and the surface repair showed a bridging of the incision site with normal epithelium (Case Fig. 2–2A). Repair of the steel scalpel excision site and the resection of the vermilion border is seen clinically as characteristic scar tissue. The contractual nature of the scar tissue repair necessitated two subsequent plastic surgery procedures to evert the vermilion tissue from the internal surface of the lip to improve the aesthetics (Case Fig. 2–2B).

Loop Resection

CASE 3

This case demonstrates resection of a lesion from the lip by loop electrosection.

PATIENT.   A 49-year-old white female in normal health.

HISTORY.   The patient had suddenly become aware of a small mass on the inner surface of her lower lip. Its presence alarmed her and made her fearful of traumatizing it, so that she avoided chewing solid foods. She was referred for diagnosis and treatment.

CLINICAL EXAMINATION.   A small round mass, measuring approximately 3 mm. in diameter, on a sessile base and slightly elevated, was located on the internal surface of the right side of her lower lip, midway between the midline and angle of the lip (Case Fig. 3–1A). There was no induration or adenopathy.

TREATMENT.   The tissue was prepared for surgery and circumferential infiltration anesthesia was administered. A round loop electrode large enough to permit resection of 2 mm. of normal tissue along with the lesion was selected and cutting current on the Coles unit was set at 5. The beaks of an ophthalmic tissue forcep were inserted through the eye of the loop and used to grasp the tissue and pull it taut, so that the lesion along with its perimeter of normal mucosa was resected with a single wiping stroke, leaving a surgical defect that was equally free of bleeding and coagulation (Case Fig. 3–1B and C). In the absence of either blood or coagulation necrosis to ob-

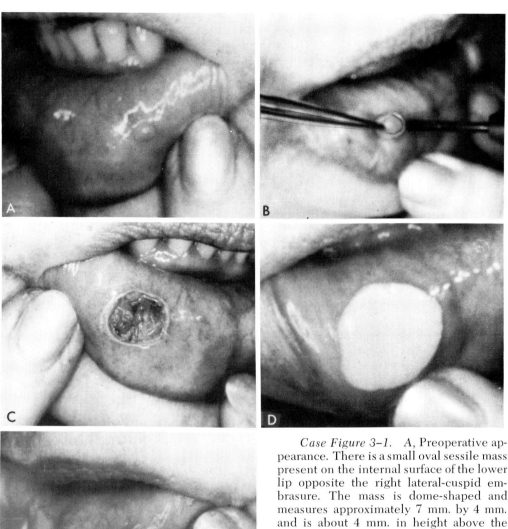

Case Figure 3–1. *A*, Preoperative appearance. There is a small oval sessile mass present on the internal surface of the lower lip opposite the right lateral-cuspid embrasure. The mass is dome-shaped and measures approximately 7 mm. by 4 mm. and is about 4 mm. in height above the level of the surrounding tissue. *B*, The edge of the mass is being grasped with a curved ophthalmic tissue forcep that has been passed through the eye of a 12-mm. round loop electrode and elevated to pull it taut, to allow resection in toto by electrosection. The electrode has cut through halfway as the photo is being taken. *C*, Immediate postoperative appearance of the lip. The internal lip structure of the bed from which the tissue was resected is intact and in the absence of bleeding is plainly identifiable. The round smooth contour of the excision is unmistakable; it cannot be duplicated by other methods of instrumentation, and there is no evidence of tissue coagulation. *D*, A bandage of Squibb Orahesive has been applied to the lip to cover the surgical field. Instead of the wound being sutured, it is being permitted to repair by granulation. *E*, Appearance of the lip on tenth postoperative day. The granulation repair is almost complete. The wound is covered with almost fully matured tissue. There is no evidence of scar contraction, and the repairing tissue is normal in all respects.

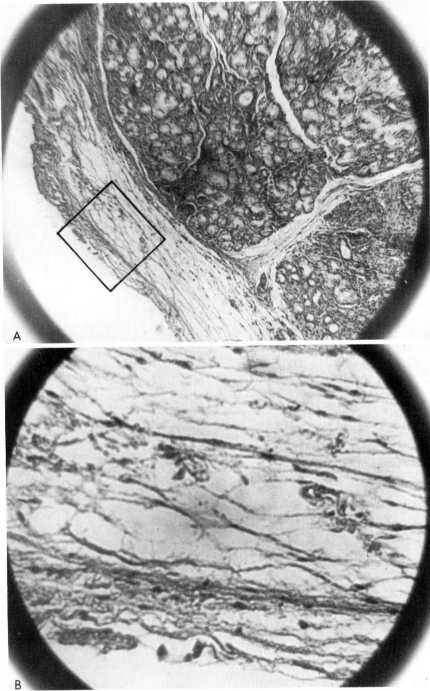

Case Figure 3–2. Photomicrographs of the biopsy tissue. *A,* Appearance of the tissue at one end of the specimen under 10× magnification. Note the areolar nature of the tissues along the line of cleavage. The tissue in the boxed area will be examined under higher magnification. *B,* Histologic appearance of the tissue in the inset area under 45× magnification. Note the intact condition of the delicate cell membranes in the areolar tissue at the line of cleavage, and the intact condition of the nuclei. *C,* Appearance of the tissue at the other end of the specimen,

Illustration continued on opposite page.

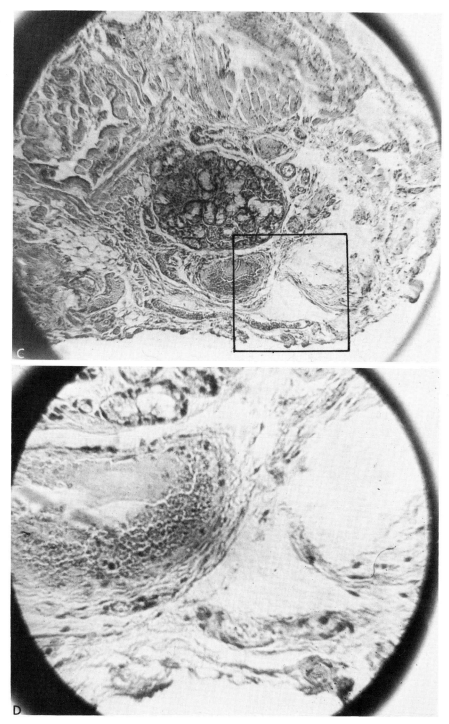

as seen under 10× magnification. Note the round contour of the tissue, characteristic of tissue resected by loop electrosection. The tissue in the boxed area will be examined under higher magnification. *D*, Histologic appearance of the tissue in the inset area at 45× magnification. Here too we see the intact cell membranes and nuclei and total absence of coagulation or cellular alteration despite the frail texture of the delicate cell membranes in this areolar tissue.

scure vision, the glandular tissue of the internal lip structure was clearly visible. The resection was so shallow that there appeared to be no need to suture the wound. A round section of Squibb's Oradhesive oral bandage was cut to size and applied to the surgical field (Case Fig. 3–1D). Although the lip is highly mobile and this bandage material adheres best to an immobile solid surface, the author has found that if it is carefully applied so that the edges of the material are held to the tissue until it adheres, in the absence of blood it not only adheres but adheres firmly enough that if the patient is careful not to displace it while eating or to hasten its disintegration by eating hot foods or performing lavage, it serves just as well on mobile mucosa as on a solid, immobile surface for approximately 12 to 18 hours. The thin bandage material is better suited for such mobile areas than is the thicker material.

The patient returned on the fifth postoperative day and reported she had been completely free of discomfort. The area was healing by secondary intention and was free of edema or inflammation. Healing progressed uneventfully, and by the end of the second week healing was complete (Case Fig. 3–1E).

See Case Figure 3–2 for photomicrographs of the biopsy tissue.

Biopsy of Lip and Buccal Mucosa (Multiple Neoplasia)

CASE 4

This case demonstrates biopsy resection of multiple neoplasia by electrosection. This patient also required a frenotomy of the mandibular lingual frenum to correct an ankyloglossia that impaired his speech.

PATIENT.   A 9-year-old white male.

HISTORY.   The largest mass, an elevated, firm, round mass 1 cm. in diameter, suddenly formed on the buccal mucosa of the right cheek about 1.5 cm. posterior to the corner of his mouth (Case Fig. 4–1A). The mass was injured several times during chewing. Two small round masses protruded from the ventral surface of the lip. A fourth slightly larger mass was submerged under the surface (Case Fig. 4–2A). He was referred for removal of the neoplasia.

CLINICAL EXAMINATION.   The large buccal mass was elevated to the same dimension as its diameter. The surface appeared keratinized and slightly grayish in color. There was a slightly redder shallow groove on the surface of the mass, where the tissue had been traumatized by the opposing teeth. This created a slight peaking of an otherwise domelike round mass on a sessile base.

TREATMENT.   The tissue was prepared for surgery, and circumferential infiltration anesthesia was administered. A round loop large enough to permit resection of 2 mm. of normal tissue around and including the lesion was selected and cutting current was set at 6 on the power output dial of the Coles unit. The beaks of a curved ophthalmic tissue forceps were inserted through the eye of the loop to grasp the tissue and lift it to pull it taut (Case Fig. 4–1B). The entire mass with its collar of normal mucosa was resected with a wiping stroke. The surgical defect created by the resection was totally free of coagulation. The glandular tissue and musculature of the internal lip structure was visible; there was just a trace of blood present, but no free bleeding (Case Fig. 4–1D). The membraneous sac of the subsurface mass, a mucocele, was

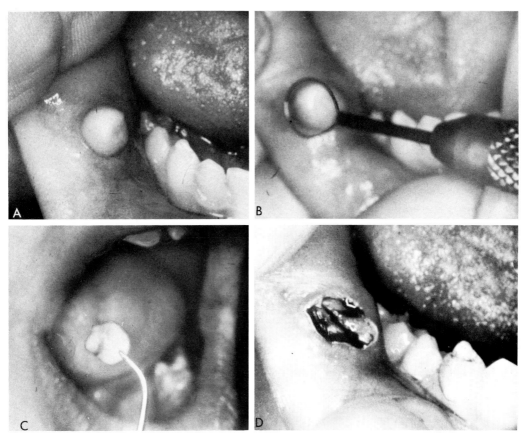

Case Figure 4–1. Multiple neoplasia and ankyloglossia. *A*, Preoperative appearance. There is a large hard white mass projecting outward from the surface of the mucosa that resembles a tooth in shape and density. *B*, The mass is being excised in toto using a large round loop electrode with a wiping, scooping motion. The electrode is seen as it has cut halfway through the tissue to resect the mass. *C*, The resected mass, grasped with an ophthalmic tissue forcep, is about to be placed into the formalin fixing solution. *D*, The bed from which the tissue has been resected shows no evidence of coagulation, but there is no free bleeding. A small amount of blood, which was released as the tissue was severed, is present on the tissue surface.

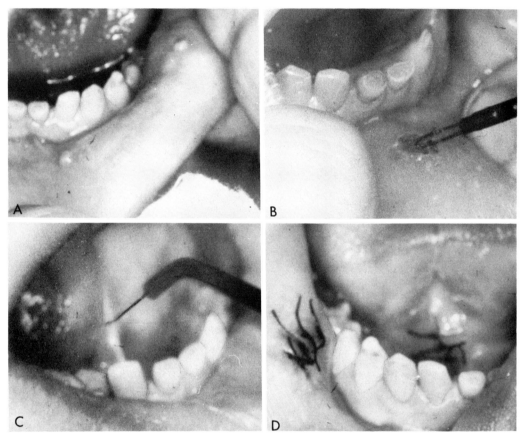

Case Figure 4–2. A, Preoperative appearance. Two nodular hard masses are present on the inner mucosa of the lip and left cheek. Both bulge upward above the tissue surface about 2 mm. A third mass immediately anterior to the one in the left cheek creates a very slight bulge above the tissue surface. This somewhat larger mass is resilient and compressible and feels slightly mobile on palpation. B, The mucocele, too frail to be enucleated, is being resected with a medium-width U-shaped loop electrode used with a scooping motion. C, The lingual frenum is being incised horizontally to sever the fibers and release the ankyloglossia. The incision is being performed with a 45-degree-angle fine needle electrode and is causing no free bleeding. D, The various wounds are closed with interrupted silk sutures.

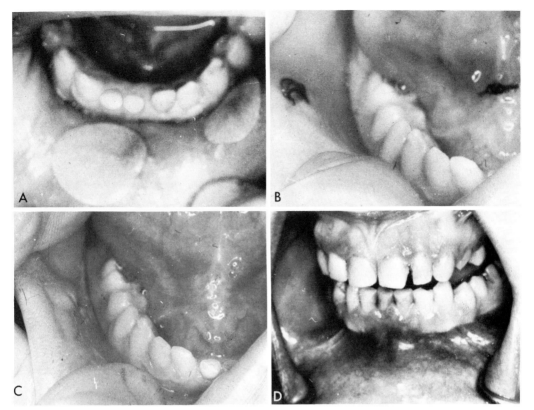

Case Figure 4–3. *A,* Squibb Orahesive bandages are placed over the wounds to provide protection for the first 12 to 18 hours. *B,* Appearance of the wounds on the fifth postoperative day. Note the absence of edema, inflammation or engorgement. *C,* Appearance of the wounds immediately after removal of the sutures. The healthy normal character of the repair process is confirmed. *D,* Final postoperative appearance. The absence of scar tissue and the complete normal tissue repair make it visually impossible to identify the surgery sites.

too thin and frail to withstand enucleation. It was scooped out by loop resection with a U-shaped loop (Case Fig. 4–2*B*). The two remaining external masses were resected with a medium-size round loop electrode and cutting power output was set at 6 on the dial.

Since the boy's speech was impaired by the mandibular lingual frenum a 45-degree-angle fine needle electrode was substituted for the loop electrode, cutting current was set at 3 on the power output dial, and the frenotomy was performed with a wiping stroke (Case Fig. 4–2*C*). The tissue around the buccal biopsy site was undermined to permit drawing the tissues together into a straight line without puckering, and the coapted margins were sutured with interrupted silk sutures; the incised frenal tissue was then sutured by drawing the incision into the vertical plane and suturing it in that position (Case Fig. 4–2*D*).

Healing progressed uneventfully. The patient returned on the fifth postoperative day and reported that he had had no pain, only the inconvenience of not being able to chew solid food. The tissues appeared to have undergone primary healing and there was no edema or inflammation present. The sutures were removed, and within 10 days thereafter the healing was complete (Case Fig. 4–3).

Photomicrographs of the loop resected biopsy tissue appear in Case Figure 4–4.

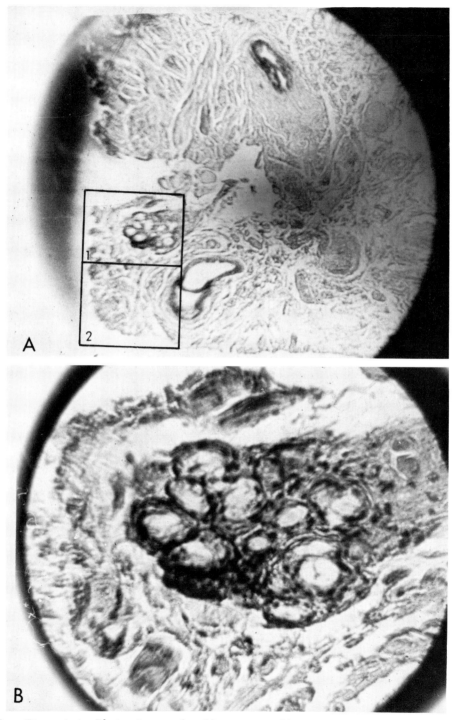

Case Figure 4–4. Photomicrographs of loop-resected biopsy tissue. *A,* Appearance of the tissue at one end of the field, under 10× magnification. Note the smooth outline and curved contour of the line of tissue cleavage. Boxed areas 1 and 2 are to be examined under higher magnification. *B,* Histologic appearance of the tissue in inset 1, seen under 45× magnification.

Illustration continued on opposite page.

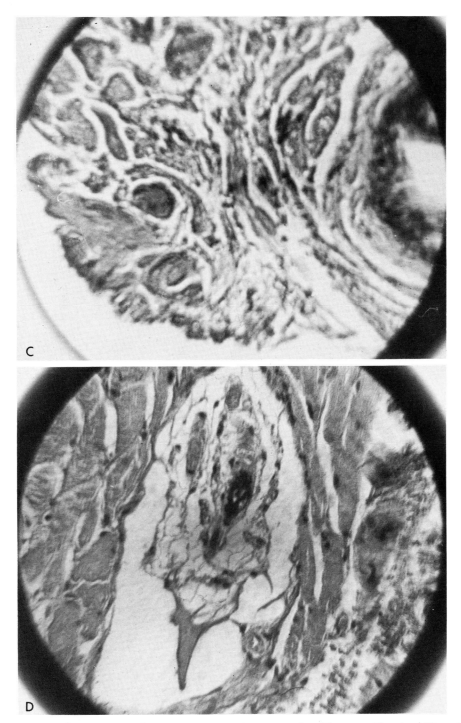

C, Histologic appearance of the tissue in inset 2, seen under 45× magnification. (Note intact nuclei along the line of cleavage.) *D*, Histologic appearance of tissue from another area of the specimen, also seen at 45× magnification.

BIOPSY OF THE BUCCAL MUCOSA

Incisional Excision of Fibroma

CASE 5

This case offers an excellent example of the total absence of fibrous scar tissue repair when tissue is properly cut by electrosection and is then not subjected to post-operative trauma. It also demonstrates well the technique of biopsy of a small lesion that includes the 2- to 3-mm. perimeter of normal tissue with the pathologic specimen, and the advantageous use of electrocoagulation to control bleeding without need to tie-off the bleeder.

PATIENT.   A 37-year-old white male.

HISTORY.   His medical history was negative. He was referred for removal of a lump on the inner aspect of the right cheek.

CLINICAL EXAMINATION.   A round, bulbous mass was present on the inner surface of the right cheek at a level parallel with the occlusal surfaces of the teeth. The mass measured approximately 7 mm. in diameter and projected about 7 mm. beyond the level of the surrounding mucosa. It was resiliently firm on palpation.

Clinical Diagnosis.   A soft fibroma, to be verified by biopsy.

TREATMENT.   Local anesthesia was administered by circumferential infiltration. A fine 45-degree-angle needle electrode was selected and cutting current power was set at 3. The mass was incised circumferentially with the activated electrode to provide an elliptical excision that included a 2 mm. perimeter of normal tissue along with the pathologic specimen (Case Fig. 5–1A and B). A bleeder in the internal incised margin was coagulated by applying a small ball coagulating electrode to a mosquito hemostat that was used to clamp the vessel (Case Fig. 5–1C).

The tissue was undermined slightly to allow slack in order to coapt the cut margins without tension, and the coapted margins were sutured with interrupted silk sutures. Tincture of myrrh and benzoin was applied in air-dried layers, and the patient was reappointed for removal of sutures on the fifth postoperative day. When he returned at that time, the line of incision appeared to have undergone primary healing. The sutures were removed and tincture of myrrh and benzoin was again applied in air-dried layers. The patient was instructed to return in six weeks for further postoperative observation. When seen at that time the tissues were fully healed and maturely keratinized, and the healed line of excision was totally indistinguishable from the surrounding tissue in color, texture, and function. Case Figure 5–2 shows photomicrographs of the biopsy specimen.

There is one interesting footnote: Two other lesions almost identical in all respects to this fibroma (one also on the inner aspect of the cheek, the other on the inner aspect of the lower lip) proved to be cavernous hemangiomas instead of soft fibromas. The undependability of clinical appearance in establishing a diagnosis of oral disease is exemplified by these cases. The textbooks describe the cavernous hemangioma as a flattened or elevated lesion, blue to red or bluish red in color[2, 3]; on pressure the blood is forced out of the lesion and on release it refills it. Neither lesion even remotely resembled the textbook descriptions but resembled the fibroma seen in this case enough to be mirror images; however, the microscope showed them to be cavernous

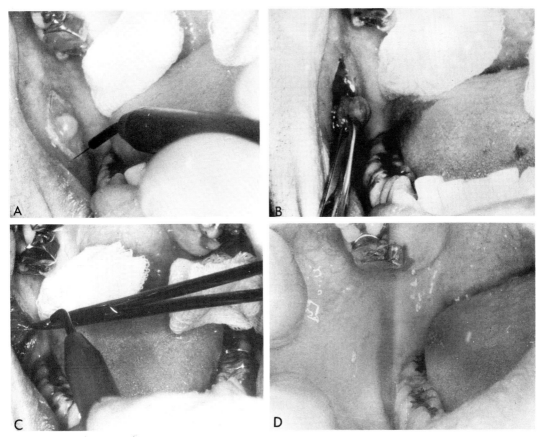

Case Figure 5–1. Fibroma on buccal surface of cheek. *A,* The neoplasm, measuring approximately 7 mm. in diameter and in height as it projects above the surface of the cheek, is being incised by electrosection for excision as a biopsy specimen and also definitive treatment. A fine 45-degree-angle needle electrode is being used to create an elliptical circumscribing incision around the lesion. Note the absence of bleeding despite the vascularity of the cheek. *B,* The mass, with its 2 mm. perimeter of normal tissue, is being removed with an Allis forceps, which had been used to grasp the incised mass as it was being resected from the internal tissues of the cheek. *C,* A bleeder in the internal incised margin has been clamped with a curved mosquito hemostat and it is being coagulated by applying the small ball coagulating current to the hemostat for 1 to 2 seconds. When the bleeding is stopped, the margins of the wound are coapted into a straight line without puckering and sutured. *D,* Postoperative appearance of the mouth seven weeks later. The tissues of the cheek are completely normal in appearance, color, texture, and function, and there is no scar tissue present to indicate where the incisions had been made. The only means for verifying that this is the patient who had had the surgery performed is by the appearance of the restorations in his teeth.

hemangiomas despite their atypical appearance. The one on the lower lip hemorrhaged so severely when it was incised for resection in a manner similar to this case that it became necessary to apply potent electrocoagulation to arrest the bleeding without doing a carotid tie-off. The full thickness of the lip had to be coagulated at the bleeding point, resulting in a permanent, tiny, brownish scar on the external surface of the lip. Had the clinical diagnosis of cavernous hemangioma been made preoperatively, it would have been a simple matter to obliterate it by electrodesiccation, but since it had inadvertently been incised it became necessary to use electrocoagulation.

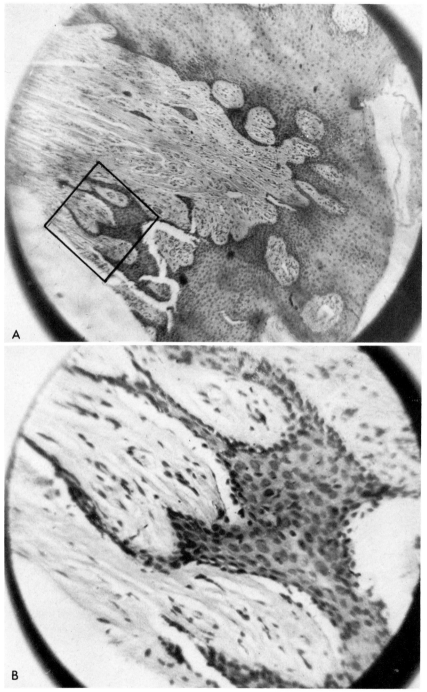

Case Figure 5–2. Fibroma of the buccal mucosa. Photomicrographs of the tissue. *A*, Appearance of the tissue under 10× magnification. Note the smooth clean line of cleavage resulting from the excisional incisions with the needle electrode. This is a typical appearance where the tissues are not torn or distorted in the process of cutting with the microtome and/or mounting on the specimen slide. The boxed area indicates the tissue that will be examined under higher magnification. *B*, Histologic appearance of the tissue under 45× magnification. The line of cleavage is smooth and sharp, there is a total absence of cellular coagulation, and many intact cell nuclei are present along the line of cleavage.

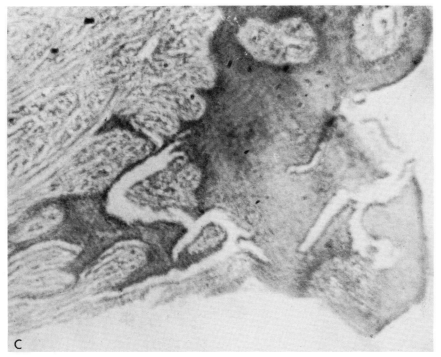

Case Figure 5–2 (continued).   C, A higher power magnification of *A* which shows the portion of the surface epithelium and cut tissue edge that is missing in the latter low power photomicrograph. Note the clean, sharp edges of the tissue specimen.

Loop Excision of Fibroma

Resection of a large lesion by steel scalpel excision on the buccal mucosa creates a particularly perplexing problem if the mass is in the center of the cheek because of contractile scar tissue repair. If excision is in the horizontal plane, the scar, being in the line of occlusion, is likely to be traumatized. If excision is in the vertical plane, the wound contracture causes facial disfigurement. Loop resection, without scar repair, avoids both hazards.

CASE 6

This case is an example of use of electrosection for loop resection of a pedunculated mass for biopsy examination.

HISTORY.   The patient was a 49-year-old white female. Her chief complaint was a large mass of tissue on the inner aspect of her left cheek. She had first become aware of it about one year previously, shortly after having accidentally bitten her cheek badly while eating. The lump persisted, so she consulted her dentist. She was reassured that it was benign, but in the intervening year it grew much larger and interfered with eating. Her brother-in-law, a dentist with whom she was visiting, referred her for its removal.

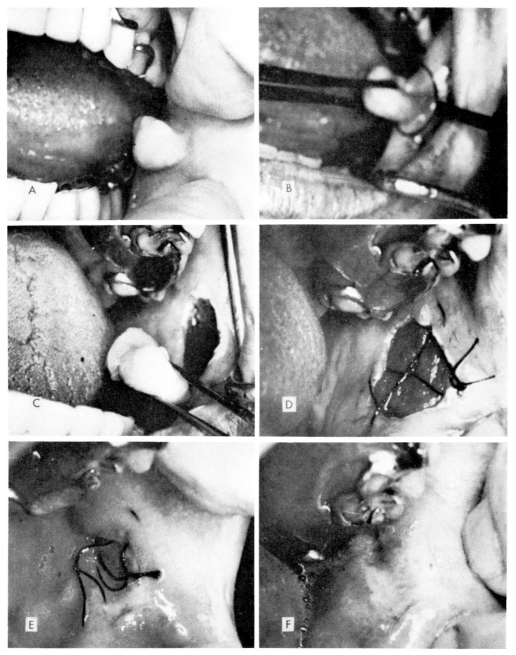

Case Figure 6–1. Loop resection of a large fibromatous mass from the buccal mucosa.
A, Preoperative appearance of the mass which lies in the occlusal line. *B,* The mass is grasped
with an Allis forceps, which has been passed through the eye of a large round electrode, and
resected with a wiping stroke of the electrode. *C,* Immediate postoperative appearance of the
buccal surgical defect. *D,* A piece of Gelfoam sponge moistened with growth indicator material
is inserted into the surgical defect, which is round and smooth, with little bleeding. Light criss-
cross suturing is utilized to help keep the graft material from being too readily displaced.
E, Appearance of the surgical defect on the fifth postoperative day. The sutures still are in the
cheek. The surgical defect is filled flush with the surrounding normal tissue and the new tissue
has a healthy pink color. *F,* Appearance of the tissues after the sutures were removed. The wide
gap created by the resection has been bridged with normal-looking tissue that is completely
free of cicatricial scar tissue formation.

CLINICAL EXAMINATION.   *Extraoral.*   Negative. Medical and family histories: negative.

Intraoral.   There was a large, firm, pedunculated, irregular-shaped resilient mass on the inner aspect of the left cheek. The neoplasm measured 1 cm. in diameter at its surface and was constricted to 0.5 cm. at the base. It was located about 1 cm. distal to the commissure of the left lip and at the level of the occlusal plane of the teeth on that side (Case Fig. 6–1*A*).

Clinical Diagnosis.   Soft fibroma or papilloma.

TREATMENT.   The area was prepared for surgery and anesthetized by circumferential infiltration. A large round loop electrode measuring 1 cm. in diameter was selected and current output set at 9 for electrosection. An Allis forceps was inserted through the eye of the loop and used to grasp the mushroom-shaped top of the neoplasm and pull it outward from the cheek (Case Fig. 6–1*B*). The entire mass with a 3 mm. perimeter of normal tissue was resected with a wiping stroke of the loop (Case Fig. 6–1*C*). The biopsy specimen was preserved in formalin.

Removal of the neoplasm left a crater in the surface of the buccal mucosa about 4 mm. deep. There was no active bleeding in this area but there was surface oozing. To prevent contraction and puckering of the buccal tissue, a piece of Gelfoam sponge moistened with medicated growth inductor material was inserted into the surgical defect; it became saturated with the blood. To help retain it in position a very superficial criss-cross suture was inserted over the defect area (Case Fig. 6–1*D*). When the blood clotted, Kenalog in Orabase was applied over it as a protective coating.

She returned on the fifth postoperative day and reported a completely uneventful postoperative sequence. The surgical defect was filled with healthy, normal-looking granulation tissue (Case Fig. 6–1*E*). After the sutures were removed, areas of normal pink coloration were seen in the repair tissue (Case Fig. 6–1*F*). The new tissue was

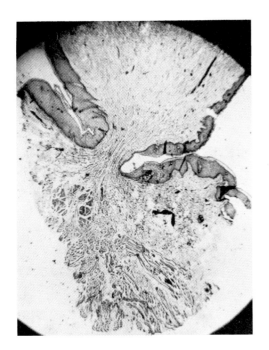

Case Figure 6–2.   Histologic section of fibroma.

completely free of cicatricial contraction; as a result there was no distortion of the angle of the lip.

The healing progressed rapidly and uneventfully. One week after the surgery was performed, the patient returned to her home in Florida. She has not been seen postoperatively since, but she has reported that there has been complete healing without recurrence or scar tissue contraction.

BIOPSY REPORT. Fibroma (Case Fig. 6–2).

BIOPSY OF ALVEOLAR MUCOSA

Maxillary Anterior Mucosa

CASE 7

This case is an example of excisional biopsy of a mass by electrosection combined with fulguration to avoid sacrifice of two teeth and their investing alveolar bone.

PATIENT. A 26-year-old white male.

HISTORY. A large mass suddenly proliferated from his maxillary left central-lateral embrasure. He was referred for diagnosis and treatment.

CLINICAL EXAMINATION. *Extraoral.* Negative. Medical and family histories: negative.

Intraoral. A firm, resilient mass measuring approximately 0.5 cm. in diameter and roughly triangular in shape was present in the left central-lateral embrasure. It extended halfway down to the incisal edges of the two teeth, was engorged and had an area of surface ulceration (Case Fig. 7–1A). When the mass was lifted with a tissue retractor it was seen to be firmly attached to the underlying periosteum and/or periodontal membrane by a sessile base (Case Fig. 7–1B).

Clinical Diagnosis. Soft fibroma or fibroid epulis.

TREATMENT. The mouth was prepared for surgery and infiltration anesthesia administered. A 45-degree-angle fine needle electrode was selected and current output set at 3.5 for electrosection. The mass plus a 2 mm. wide strip of marginal gingiva was resected (Case Fig. 7–1C) and preserved in formalin solution for biopsy. The base of the surgical defect was then fulgurated with a heavy needle electrode to destroy any invaginating fibers (Case Fig. 7–1D). Medicated surgical gelatin was inserted into the defect and mixed with the blood present in order to reconstruct a normal gingival contour (Case Fig. 7–1E). When the blood clotted, the operative field was protected with a thick coating of collodion and he was given postoperative instructions.

He returned on the fifth postoperative day and reported that the collodion had peeled off on the third day. The mucosa appeared to be healing normally. A few minute surface irregularities were reduced by superficial spot coagulation and tincture of myrrh and benzoin was applied. He returned at weekly intervals and for the first three weeks healing progressed rather slowly. By the end of the fourth week, however, the tissue appeared fully healed and the interproximal papilla was almost fully regenerated to its normal level. By the end of the sixth week the gingival tissue was normal (Case Fig. 7–1F) and he was discharged from treatment.

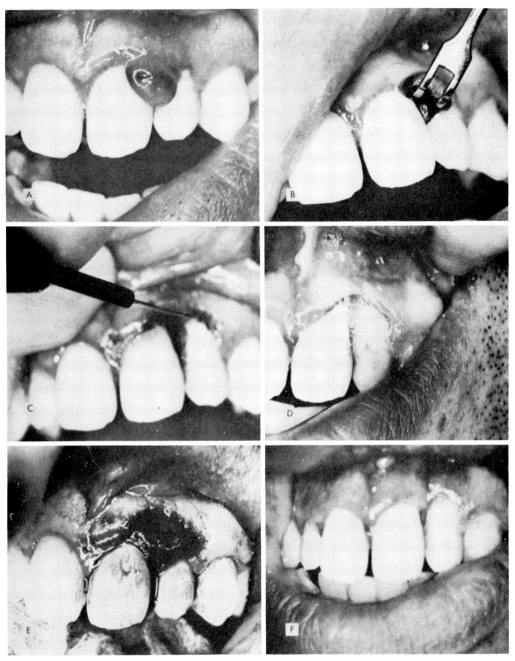

Case Figure 7–1.   Incisional resection of a fibrous bulging mass emerging from the gingival mucosa and the subgingival tissues. *A*, Preoperative labial appearance of mass, which is superimposed upon and partially covers the central and lateral. *B*, Elevation of mass with tissue retractor reveals sessile base invaginating into periosteum and/or periodontal attachment. *C*, Base and area of invaginating attachment to subgingival tissues thoroughly fulgurated after resection by incisional excision with a 45-degree-angle fine needle electrode. *D*, Appearance on the fifth postoperative day. Healing satisfactory, area covered with light layer of healthy coagulum. *E*, Graft of Gelfoam sponge saturated with growth inductor material inserted after freshening margins in order to encourage regeneration of the gingival tissue to its normal level. *F*, Appearance of the tissues six weeks postoperatively. The gingival margin is almost completely normal and the tissue tone is good.

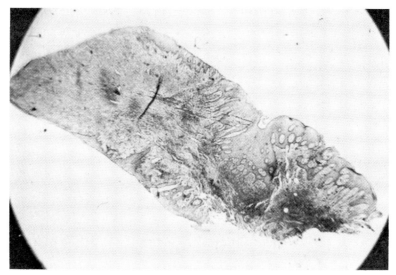

Case Figure 7–2.   Photomicrograph of the mass. Biopsy report: Ulcerated fibrous epulis with bone formation.

He was seen postoperatively six months later and at the end of the year. During that period the tissues remained normal with no sign of recurrence. He was seen again two years postoperatively and the tissues were found to be unchanged.

Biopsy report.   Ulcerated fibrous epulis with bone formation (Case Fig. 7–2).

Peripheral giant cell tumor
CASE 8

This case offers an excellent example of one of the many invaluable uses of fulguration to destroy undesirable tissue in situ in areas inaccessible using other methods of instrumentation and thereby to eliminate need to extract teeth or remove alveolar bone to do so. It also demonstrates the importance of careful treatment plan and how judicious recontouring of the marginal gingiva of a contralateral tooth can compensate for loss of gingival contour and minimize the aesthetic effects of necessary tissue resection.

Patient.   A 48-year-old white female.

History.   Medical history was negative. She was referred for diagnosis and treatment of an elevated mass on the marginal gingiva over a maxillary central incisor.

Clinical examination.   A round mass with sessile base measuring approximately 7 mm. in diameter with a convex contour projected approximately 4 mm. beyond the level of the marginal gingiva adjacent to the left central incisor. The mass appeared firm, and its color was slightly deeper red than the surrounding normal mucosa.

Roentgenographic examination.   An intraoral periapical x-ray taken of the affected area showed no pathology. However, since the lesion was on the labial aspect of the tooth, this merely indicated that no bone destruction had occurred beyond the mesiodistal dimension of the tooth.

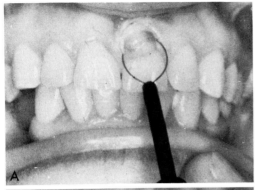
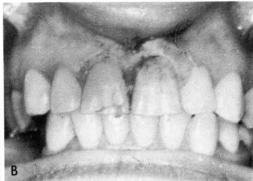
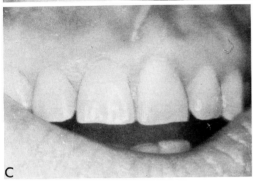

Case Figure 8–1. Peripheral giant cell tumor. *A,* A 1 cm. round mass is being resected from the labial gingiva of the maxillary left central incisor with a 14 mm. round loop electrode. *B,* The neoplasm having been resected, fulguration has been applied subgingivally to destroy any of the tumor mass that may have invaginated to the periosteum, and the gingival level of the contralateral central incisor has been raised to create better gingival harmony in the anterior part of the mouth. *C,* Appearance of the tissues by the third postoperative week. The new gingival marginal tissue over the two centrals appears moderately advanced in healing. The tissues are relatively normal in tone; there is no edema or inflammation, although the tissue over the left central lacks a maturely keratinized epithelial surface. The aesthetics are excellent, and it is difficult to realize that surgery had recently been performed on these tissues.

Clinical Diagnosis. The clinical diagnosis to be confirmed by biopsy was that this mass was a peripheral giant cell tumor—the so-called epulis.

TREATMENT. The labial gingival mucosa was anesthetized after preparation by subperiosteal infiltration anesthesia injected from the right lateral to the left lateral incisor. In order to obtain a 2- to 3-mm. margin of normal tissue along with the diseased tissue, it was necessary to use a round loop electrode measuring 12 mm. in diameter. The cutting current was set at 7; the electrode was activated and applied to the tissues approximately 2 mm. superior to the mass, and the entire mass was resected with a single wiping stroke (Case Fig. 8–1).

The tissues were recontoured to create a normal marginal gingival contour and interdental papillae by slight gingivoplasty with a flame-shaped loop electrode. Fulguration was then applied to the marginal edge of the gingiva to destroy any fibers that might be invaginating toward the periosteum or the peridental membrane. Since the removal of the mass had created a considerable discrepancy in gingival level with the adjacent gingival margins, the clinical crown of the right central was elongated and recontoured to create reasonable gingival harmony with the left central. Tincture of myrrh and benzoin was applied to the cut tissues in air-dried layers, instructions for postoperative home care were given, and the patient was reappointed. When she returned on the fifth postoperative day, healing appeared to be progressing very satisfactorily. She was reappointed to return in two weeks. When she returned, on the nineteenth postoperative day, the tissues were fully healed except for the absence of the packed layers of dead cells that make up the normal keratinized surface of mature epithelium, giving the tissue over the left central a slightly darker pink color along the edge of the marginal gingiva.

The lesion has not recurred in the seven years since it was removed.

CASE 9

This case is an example of electrosurgical incisional resection of a labio-alveolar gingival mass for biopsy, and carbonization of the surgical defect by fulguration to destroy invaginating cells. A technique for plastic repair of the surgical defect is described.

PATIENT.   A 68-year-old white female.

HISTORY.   Her upper and lower full dentures, more than 20 years old, were very unstable. The alveolar ridges had undergone marked resorption. When she consulted a dentist for construction of a new set of dentures he replaced the upper but was reluctant to undertake construction of a new lower denture unless the alveolar ridge could be improved. She was referred specifically for consultation regarding improvement of the mandibular ridge by pushback or bone graft.

CLINICAL EXAMINATION.   *Extraoral.*   Negative. Medical and family histories: negative. Her major complaint was a burning sensation in the tongue which had lasted for the past two years, painful pressure of the denture against the mandibular ridge and slight discomfort under the nose from pressure of the new upper denture.

Intraoral.   The entire mandibular ridge was resorbed down to a knife-edged crest 2 mm. high. The body of the mandible was 1 cm. in height (verified by measurements on lateral jaw plate). Palpation on the crest of the ridge revealed two slight depressions in the respective bicuspid regions, the mental foramina. These were the sore spots the patient had complained of. She was advised that very little could be done to improve the mandible except by autogenous iliac bone graft; the patient rejected this treatment. Magnet implants, or use of repellent magnetized dentures lined with velum soft acrylic was recommended as a likely alternative.

Although she had been referred for mandibular consultation, the rest of her mouth was examined prior to dismissal. Examination of the tongue and buccal mucosa was negative. But in the exact midline of the maxilla where the labial frenum normally is located, a large, spherical, avascular, white, fibrotic, indurated mass with a deep ulcerated crater in its center bulged prominently (Case Fig. 9–1A).

The maxillary alveolar ridge was almost totally resorbed from the midline to the bicuspid area on the right side and to the cuspid area on the left side. In this area the labial vestibule was nonexistent, and in addition to the bulging mass the adjacent tissue was hyperemic and hypertrophied, lying in folds. The patient stated that she was troubled by soreness in her gums and nose, especially during and immediately after eating. Her denture fitted over the round bulging mass and appeared to compress it tightly.

Immediate biopsy of the maxillary neoplasm was recommended. The patient, her daughters who had accompanied her and her dentist were consulted: all concurred.

Clinical Diagnosis.   This mass was distinctly atypical. It resembled fibroma durum in texture and avascularity, but no clinical diagnosis was established.

TREATMENT.   The mouth was prepared for surgery and bilateral infraorbital block and palatal infiltration anesthesia was administered. A 45-degree-angle fine needle electrode was selected and current output set at 4 for electrosection. A wireframe cheek-lip retractor was inserted for maximum retraction. The entire mass plus a 3 mm. perimeter of normal tissue was incised circumferentially down to underlying bone (Case Fig. 9–1B).

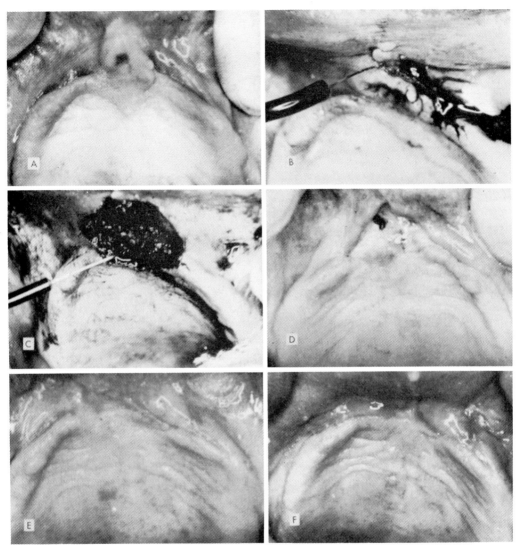

Case Figure 9–1. Incisional resection of an ulcerated mass in the median line of the maxilla which communicated with the nasal fossa. *A,* Preoperative appearance of the lesion. It is a large, bulging, fibrous mass with a large round ulcer in the center, which is attached to both the labial mucosa of the lip and the palatal mucosa including the nasopalatine papilla. Most of the anterior half of the maxillary alveolar ridge has been resorbed, with almost total loss of the labial vestibule. *B,* The mass is resected with a 45-degree-angle fine needle electrode. *C,* Following resection of the mass the basal layer is thoroughly fulgurated to destroy any aberrant cells in the substratum. *D,* Appearance of the defect on the fifth postoperative day. The area is healing well and is covered with a healthy layer of coagulum. A perforation into the nasal fossa observed when bone and cartilage fragments were removed from the fulgurated bed of the lesion still remains open despite attempted closure with 20-day chromic gut sutures. *E,* Postoperative appearance ten days after plastic closure of the oronasal perforation. Healing is progressing very well by primary union. *F,* Postoperative appearance at the end of the sixth week. Healing is complete. The perforation is sealed, and there is considerable improvement in the depth of the labial vestibule. The tissue tone is excellent, and there is no contraction of the lip.

The incised tissue was lifted taut with an Allis forceps and resected from the underlying structures with the needle electrode. A heavy needle electrode was then used with monoterminal current output set at 9 to fulgurate the entire base of the surgical defect until it was uniformly carbonized (Case Fig. 9–1C). Five bone-hard irregular-shaped fragments were found in the basal layer. They were removed and added to the biopsy specimen which had been preserved in formalin solution. The soft tissue mass measured 1 by 2 cm., by 0.8 cm. in thickness. The largest of the hard structures measured 4 by 8 by 3 mm.

When the largest hard fragment was removed by simply lifting it out, a perforation into the nasal fossa was exposed to view. When the area was irrigated during debridement, fluid passed through the perforation into the fossa and escaped through the nostrils. The perforation was sutured with 20-day chromic gut to attempt primary closure. A mixture of medicated surgical gelatin was deposited into the defect and mixed with the blood present. The sterilized denture was built up with a stiff mix of surgical cement to serve as a surgical stent. After the blood clotted in the defect area, adhesive dryfoil was adapted over it and the denture was inserted. Mysteclin and antiseptic lavage were prescribed, and ascorbic acid and Knox clear gelatin were recommended as dietary supplements.

She returned on the fifth postoperative day and reported that she had been relatively comfortable. There was no edema, and the defect was filled almost to the level of the normal adjacent mucosa with granulation tissue covered with a surface layer of healthy looking coagulum. The sutured oronasal defect was the only area not filled with repair tissue, and here the chromic gut suture was clearly visible (Case Fig. 9–1D). The mouth was irrigated and tincture of myrrh and benzoin applied in air-dried layers.

She returned at regular weekly intervals. By the third visit the chromic gut had disintegrated but its site was marked by a small residual perforation. Scarification plus cultured bone–surgical gelatin implant was attempted but failed to seal the defect. Plastic closure of the defect was planned, and performed the following week.

The mouth was prepared and bilateral infraorbital block and palatal infiltration anesthesia were administered. A 45-degree-angle fine needle electrode was selected and current output set at 3.5 for electrosection. Two parallel vertical incisions were created, one on each side of the defect. The incision on the right side was made at a point 2 cm. distal to the perforation and the one on the left side, about 1.5 cm. distal to the defect. Each incision was made 0.5 cm. deep. A thin-blade periosteal elevator was inserted through each incision and passed under the mucosa toward the central defect to undermine the tissue. This created enough tissue slack to permit use of the loosened tissue as French sliding flaps.

The surface of the defect was curetted lightly to remove the surface epithelium. The sliding flaps were accurately coapted along a line about 3 mm. to the left of the perforation which was about 3 mm. to the right of midline. The coapted margins were sutured with 0000 braided silk interrupted sutures. Two pieces of Gelfoam sponge were cut to size and moistened with medicated growth inductor solution. These were inserted into the open spaces created at the respective terminal ends of the sliding flaps. The Gelfoam was secured into position with loosely tied cross-sutures. The entire operative field was covered with a strip of adhesive dryfoil. The denture, with a fresh cement pack, was inserted to serve as a retaining surgical stent. The patient was instructed not to disturb the denture for 24 hours and then to resume regular lavage.

She returned five days later and reported uneventful postoperative recovery. The mouth was irrigated, the sutures removed and tincture of myrrh and benzoin applied.

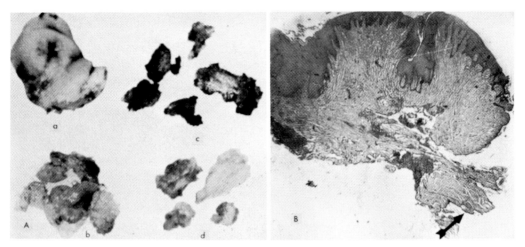

Case Figure 9–2. Gross specimens and prepared biopsy specimen. A, Gross tissue specimens. *a,* Resected tissue mass, labial view. *b,* Tissue mass, ventral surface. *c,* Bone fragments discovered in the basal area. *d,* Fragments of cartilage discovered in the basal area. The oronasal perforation was observed when the upper left fragment was removed. B, Photomicrograph of the tissue specimen obtained. Arrow points to a layer of cells that have been destroyed by the electrode.

The anterior suture line formed by the coapted flaps was healing by primary union and the posterior surgical defects were filled with healthy granulation tissue (Case Fig. 9–1E). Healing progressed without incident. By the end of the sixth week healing was complete and the tissue tone was normal (Case Fig. 9–1F).

BIOPSY REPORT. Hard tissue: Cartilage with considerable cellular alteration — but within normal limits. Soft tissue: Fibrotic tissue with ulceration perforating through its full thickness (Case Fig. 9–2).

Initially, a preliminary report of possible chondrosarcoma had been made, subject to substantiation by pathologists expert in bone and cartilage pathology. Subsequent examination by several experts led to the conclusion that the cellular alterations in the fragments of nasal cartilage were still within normal limits, but continued postoperative observation for signs of recurrence or degeneration was recommended.

The patient has been observed for five years and there has been no untoward reaction. The oronasal perforation has remained effectively sealed. An additional benefit of the plastic surgery has been improved denture stability and peripheral seal. This case highlights the importance of thorough oral examination.

Maxillary Posterior Mucosa

CASE 10

This case demonstrates a technique for electrosurgical biopsy and repair of the surgical defect.

PATIENT. A 34-year-old white female.

HISTORY. The patient was ten weeks postpartum. In the fourth month of her pregnancy she had developed marked gingival hyperemia and hypertrophy. Shortly thereafter, a large proliferative mass of tissue appeared on the buccal aspect of her maxillary right bicuspid-molar region. Her dentist diagnosed it as a pregnancy tumor and excised it with a cold-steel scalpel. A few weeks later the mass regenerated and rapidly grew larger. This time she was advised to leave it alone and wait until after delivery, at which time it should disappear spontaneously. The mass became progressively more fibrotic and persisted after childbirth. She was referred for biopsy and treatment.

CLINICAL EXAMINATION. *Extraoral.*   Negative. Medical and family histories: negative.

Intraoral.   A large irregular mass of red tissue was superimposed on the gingival mucosa in the maxillary right bicuspid-molar region. The mass extended from the interproximal embrasure between the bicuspids to the embrasure between the two molars and from the mucobuccal fold downward to the occlusal surface of the first molar. The buccal surface of the second bicuspid was partly covered and the first molar completely covered by the mass. The mass was lobulated and magenta in hue (Case Fig. 10–1A). It was firm and resilient in texture, and when elevated with a tissue retractor it was seen to be firmly attached to the alveolar bone and about 0.5 cm. thick (Case Fig. 10–1B).

Clinical Diagnosis.   Fibromatous pregnancy tumor.

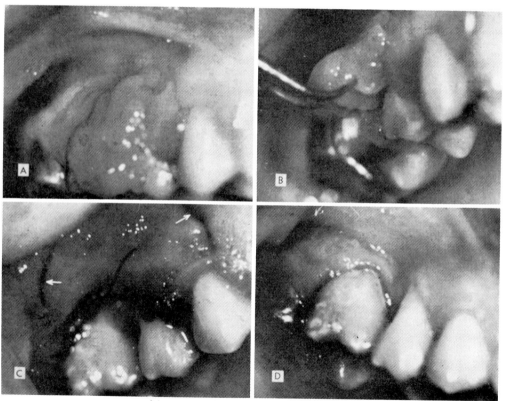

Case Figure 10–1.   Resection of large tissue-mass superimposed on the gingiva and invaginating into or emerging from the subgingival structures. A, Preoperative appearance of the mass, which covers most of the second bicuspid and first molar teeth. B, Mass, elevated, is seen firmly attached to the subgingival structures. C, Immediate postoperative appearance of the tissues after the mass was resected by electrosection and the basal layer fulgurated. Note vertical incisions for creating slack in the tissues to permit partial primary closure. (Arrow points to incisions; dark line in middle is suture.) D, Postoperative appearance of the tissues six weeks later.

TREATMENT.   The mouth was prepared for surgery and circumferential infiltration anesthesia administered. A 45-degree-angle fine needle electrode was selected and current output set at 3.5 for electrosection. The gingival mucosa 3 mm. beyond the entire mass was incised down to the alveolar bone. The incised mass was undermined with a periosteal elevator and elevated with an Allis forceps. Its basal attachment to the alveolar bone was then dissected with short brushing strokes of the electrode. The alveolar margin was thoroughly fulgurated, with current output set at 9, to destroy all invaginating fibers.

The surgical defect was approximately 2 cm. wide and almost 2 cm. in height. To facilitate rapid repair of this defect, French sliding flaps were created to cover much of this area. To do this, vertical incisions were made at each terminal end of the defect. Each incision, about 1 cm. in length, was made about 1 cm. beyond the margin of the defect and extended down to the alveolar bone. A flat periosteal elevator was inserted through each incision and used to undermine the intervening tissue between the incision and the defect in order to create tissue slack. The slack tissue became slide-flaps, which were pulled together as much as possible and secured with two silk sutures, closing the gap substantially (Case Fig. 10–1C). Medicated surgical gelatin powder was deposited into the remainder of the defect and into the two lateral defects just created and mixed with the blood in these areas. When the blood clotted, a piece of adhesive dryfoil was adapted over the operative field and covered with a surgical cement pack. Aureomycin was prescribed and the patient was given instructions in postoperative care.

She returned on the sixth postoperative day for removal of the sutures. The cement pack was removed and the area irrigated. The tissue appeared to be healing well; the vertical incisions and central defect were filled with normal granulation tissue which was covered with a very thin layer of healthy looking coagulum. Tissue repair progressed rapidly, and by the end of the fourth postoperative week healing was complete. She was seen once more two weeks later. The gingival contour around the affected teeth was normal and the tissue tone was excellent (Case Fig. 10–1D).

The patient returned one year later for final postoperative observation. The condition of her gingivae was unchanged.

BIOPSY REPORT.   Angioma.

Either of the following alternatives may account for this neoplasm:

1. It is possible that this was a true neoplasm from the outset, and was mistakenly diagnosed as a pregnancy tumor because of circumstances such as timing and similarity in appearance; or,

2. This may have started as a pregnancy tumor but degenerated into a true neoplasm as a result of untimely traumatizing surgical intervention.

This case is an excellent example of the need for biopsy when malignancy is not suspected, in order to establish an accurate differential diagnosis of the pathology.

The Buccal Vestibule

Tissue proliferations due to denture irritation are quite commonplace, and in most instances such a redundant mass, called a granuloma fissuratum, is benign. In many instances if the pressure from the denture is relieved soon after the granuloma fissuratum develops, the mass undergoes spontaneous resorption. It is not possible to make a conclusive diagnosis, however, without histopathologic interpretation of the biopsy tissue; many innocuous-looking proliferations prove to be carcinomas.[4] Even though the lesion is benign, if it is ulcerated, and especially if the ulcer is one that perforates, the biopsy surgery combined with submucous dissection becomes a definitive treatment as well as a diagnostic procedure.

The following case is an excellent example of the perforating type of lesion that requires surgical excision. It also affords an excellent example of what happens to an atraumatic electrosurgical wound if it is traumatized postoperatively.

CASE 11

PATIENT. A 61-year-old white male.

HISTORY. He had been wearing full upper and lower dentures for about 10 years. At first the dentures had fitted so well that he was able to eat almost any kind of food. For the past year or more the dentures had begun to feel loose and became displaced frequently while eating. He had noticed an irregular mass had formed in the upper jaw immediately above the upper edge of the upper denture. It began to bother him enough to consult his dentist, who referred him for diagnosis and treatment.

CLINICAL EXAMINATION. With the upper denture in place there was a bulge of proliferative tissue present at the superior edge of the labial flange in the first molar area on the left side. When the denture was removed a large elliptical mass measuring approximately 2.5 cm. in its longest dimension and 1.5 cm. in width was revealed. The tissue fungated outward about 1 cm., and there was necrotic slough in the center which proved to be covering a perforating ulcer. There was no palpable adenopathy and no induration present.

Clinical Diagnosis. Granuloma fissuratum, with necrosis and ulceration.

TREATMENT. The area was anesthetized by circumferential infiltration anesthesia. A 45-degree-angle fine needle electrode was selected, cutting current was set at 3.5, and the entire mass was resected by incisional excision(Case Fig. 11–1A). The needle electrode was replaced with a 17-mm. periodontal loop electrode and a submucous dissection was performed to create the slack needed to permit coaptation of the margins without loss of vestibular height, such as was used in many of the cases in the chapter on preprosthodontics. The margins of the wound were then coapted and sutured with interrupted silk sutures (Case Fig. 11–1B). The old denture which had been sterilized in cold sterilizing solution was built up with a roll of hard surgical cement to serve as a surgical stent to keep the vestibular tissue displaced as needed. A strip of adhesive dryfoil was placed over the sutures to prevent them from becoming imbedded into the cement, and the denture-stent was inserted and carefully contoured to the area. The patient was cautioned to avoid eating solid foods until the tissues were healed. He was instructed in home postoperative care and told to return on the fifth postoperative day for removal of the sutures.

When he returned on the fifth day and the denture was removed, the tissues were gaping wide open. The sutures were missing, and the wound was raw and angry looking (Case Fig. 11–1C). In response to questioning as to what had happened, he related that when he returned to his home he was hungry. He had no pain, no swelling, and no bleeding, and because the wound was covered with his denture he

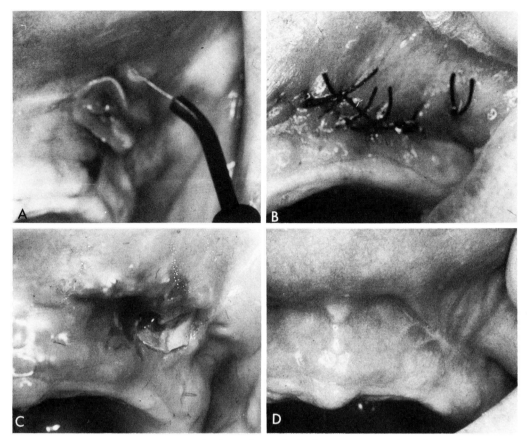

Case Figure 11-1. Biopsy in the buccal vestibule demonstrating the effects of postoperative trauma on the rate and quality of tissue repair. *A,* The mass is being incised circumferentially for biopsy excision. There is a perforating ulcer in the center of the fungating mass. *B,* The biopsy excision and the submucous dissection to permit repositioning of the sutured tissues to maintain normal vestibular height have been completed, and the coapted margins of the wound have been sutured. *C,* Appearance of the tissues on the fifth postoperative day. The sutures have been torn out and there is a wide gaping wound with much swelling and sloughing. *D,* Appearance of the fully healed wound. Note the cicatricial fibrous scar repair that is identical in all respects with the typical repair of a steel scalpel incision and totally atypical of the repair of electrosurgical wounds that have not been traumatized postoperatively.

thought it would do no harm to eat something solid. He had a delicatessen sandwich and was not aware of any damage, even though he felt a twinge of pain while chewing. When he removed the denture that evening to use the salt water lavage he became aware that the tissue had torn apart.

The tissues were too traumatized to permit resuturing for primary repair, and the wound proceeded to heal slowly by secondary intention. When healing was complete, the vestibular height was noticeably reduced, and there was a hard raised cicatricial scar line identical to the type of scar tissue repair seen when steel scalpel wounds heal (Case Fig. 11–1D).

The classic cicatricial scar tissue repair that is associated with steel scalpel surgery is not seen with wounds properly created by electrosurgery that are not subsequently subjected to trauma. The fact that the fibrous scar tissue repair occurred in this wound offers irrefutable evidence that such healing is a response to tissue trauma.

CASE 12

This case is an example of electrosurgical incisional biopsy technique for resection of maxillary alveolar mucosa.

HISTORY. The patient was a 60-year-old white male. His chief complaint was an irritated white patch on the edentulous saddle area of his maxillary right alveolar ridge. The lesion was asymptomatic; he had been unaware of it until it was discovered by his dentist. It failed to respond to routine treatment. He was referred for its diagnosis and treatment.

CLINICAL EXAMINATION. *Extraoral.* Negative. Medical history: He was frequently under treatment at the Johns Hopkins Hospital for minor arthritic and vascular ailments, and gave the impression of being a hypochondriac.

Intraoral. The maxilla was edentulous from the right cuspid posteriorly and from the left first bicuspid posteriorly. In the right second molar region near the crest of the buccal aspect of the alveolar ridge there was a thick, round, white, plaque-like patch superimposed on the mucosa.[5] This area was surrounded by a narrow red band which clearly demarcated the lesion. An irregular area of white extended beyond the circumscribed plaque. This part was not surrounded by the red areola. The white extension and a number of other small irregular areas in the mouth were covered with lacy patches of thin white film (Case Fig. 12–1A).

Clinical Diagnosis. Lichen planus.

TREATMENT. The mouth was prepared and infiltration anesthesia administered. A 45-degree-angle fine needle electrode was selected and current output set at 4 for electrosection. The circumscribed area was incised at a point 2 mm. beyond the red areolar margin, undermined with a periosteal elevator and removed (Case Fig. 12–1B and C). The tissue was preserved in formalin solution; then a piece of Gelfoam sponge was moistened with medicated bone growth inductor solution and inserted into the surgical defect where it quickly became saturated with blood present in the area. When the blood clotted, the Gelfoam was covered with a patch of adhesive dryfoil. The patient's sterilized denture was inserted to protect the area.

He was instructed to leave his denture undisturbed for 24 hours, then to follow the customary postoperative instructions. He returned on the fifth postoperative day. Inspection revealed that the surgical defect was almost completely filled with normal-looking granulation tissue, but the mucosa throughout the maxilla was spotted with numerous lacy white patches.

Fearful of malignancy, the patient persisted in anticipating the worst from the biopsy report despite repeated reassurances. Tincture of myrrh and benzoin was applied, and use of ascorbic acid and Knox clear gelatin as dietary supplements was prescribed.

BIOPSY REPORT. Lichen planus (Case Fig. 12–1F).

The report was received on the seventh postoperative day, and the patient was immediately notified that it confirmed the benign nature of his lesion. When he re-

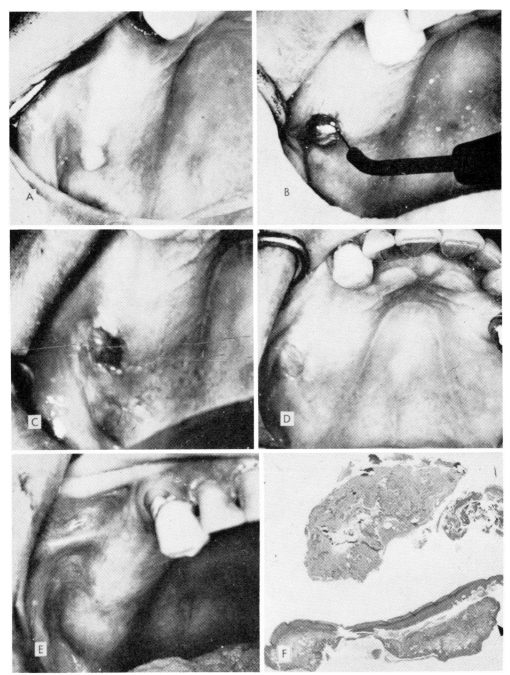

Case Figure 12–1. Incisional excision of a lesion (lichen planus) on the gingival mucosa of an edentulous maxillary alveolar ridge. *A*, Preoperative appearance of the lesion, which consists of a moderately heavy layer of white keratinization extending about 3 cm. along the buccal aspect of the ridge near the crest, and a round, densely keratinized lesion approximately 1 cm. in diameter surrounded by an areola of red discoloration. *B*, Incision performed with a 45-degree-angle fine needle electrode. *C*, Appearance of the surgical defect following excision of the biopsy. *D*, Appearance on the tenth postoperative day. The area is filled to the level of the surrounding tissue with healthy granulation tissue. It is surrounded by a very shallow depression a fraction of a millimeter deep. *E*, Appearance two months postoperatively. The area is fully healed. The evidence of lichen planus that had been scattered throughout the mouth has disappeared since the biopsy reported a benign lesion. *F*, Photomicrograph of the tissue specimen obtained. Arrow points to a layer of cells that have been destroyed by the electrode.

1043

turned on the tenth day he was buoyant and relaxed. His mouth was almost completely free of the lacy white patchwork which had been so prevalent a few days previously. Healing was well advanced in the surgical defect area (Case Fig. 12–1D) but the surface epithelium was not yet fully keratinized.

The patient remained relaxed and free of apprehension. When he returned one week later none of the white patches were present. He was seen again two weeks later, and the oral mucosa throughout the mouth appeared normal (Case Fig. 12–1E). He returned six months later for another postoperative observation and reported that he had had a brief recurrence while on a trip to Europe. It had apparently been triggered by emotional tensions relating to business transactions; the patches had undergone spontaneous remission within one week.

It is interesting to note that from the moment he had been convinced of the benign nature of his mouth lesions, the clinical manifestations of lichen planus had abated almost overnight. This affords dramatic evidence of the influence of emotional stress on this condition.

Mandibular Anterior Labial Mucosa

CASE 13

This case demonstrates use of large loop electrodes for biopsy resections and use of electrosurgery for eliminating pathology. It also presented an unusual diagnostic problem.

PATIENT. A 49-year-old white male.

HISTORY. The patient had one tooth left in the mandible and the maxilla was edentulous. He wore a full upper and partial lower denture attached to the remaining cuspid. The lower denture was very unstable and caused numerous sore spots to develop from time to time. These had healed spontaneously. A few weeks previously he had noticed a sore spot in the center of the mandibular ridge. This spot persisted and increased in size, and the surrounding tissue swelled. Neither the sore spot nor the swelling subsided, so he consulted his dentist. Roentgenographic examination showed extensive radiolucence in the area. He was referred for diagnosis and treatment.

CLINICAL EXAMINATION. *Extraoral.* Negative. Medical history: He had undergone treatment for primary lues many years previously. Serology tests had been negative since the treatment. Family history: negative. There was palpable cervical adenopathy.

Intraoral. There was a deep groove in the labiobuccal fold in the median line, with marked hypertrophy of its upper border. The groove was ulcerated and partially covered with a grayish layer of necrotic tissue. Slightly to the right of the median line and in the vertical center of the alveolar mucosa there was a fistulous orifice from which a mucopurulent exudate could readily be expressed. The alveolar mucosa from cuspid to cuspid was hyperemic, hypertrophied and somewhat indurated (Case Fig. 13–1A).

Roentgenographic examination revealed marked radiolucence in the right median region with islands of moth-eaten-appearing bone visible in the area.

The roentgenographic appearance was compatible with osteomyelitis and

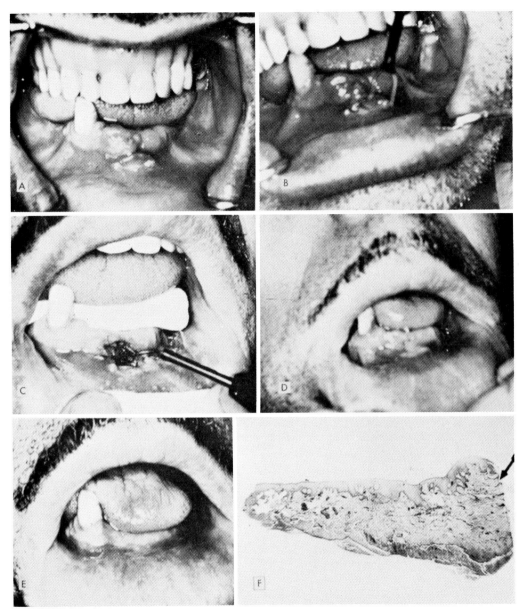

Case Figure 13–1. Granuloma fissuratum superimposed on localized osteomyelitis. *A,* Preoperative appearance of the soft tissue lesion. Note round tissue bulge near crest of the ridge with fistulous orifice from which purulent exudate could be expressed. Also note ulceration and keratinization of the groove in the granuloma fissuratum. *B,* Ulcerated, keratinized lesion resected with large U-shaped loop electrode. *C,* Basal layer thoroughly fulgurated before removing bone sequestra. The fistulous orifice also is fulgurated at this time. *D,* Appearance on the fifth postoperative day. Healing is progressing very well. The area is filled to normal level and covered with a healthy layer of coagulum. *E,* Area completely healed by the end of the sixth postoperative week. There has been no loss of vestibular space or scar tissue contraction. The alveolar ridge is well defined and normal in contour. *F,* Photomicrograph of the tissue resected. Arrow points to single layer of cells that have been destroyed by the electrosection.

sequestrum formation. The gingival lesion was clinically compatible with granuloma fissuratum with fistula. Both the clinical appearance and roentgenographic findings were compatible with invasive destruction by a malignant neoplasm. The clinical history of malaise, fever and sudden loss of body weight, and medical history of lues, was equally compatible with malignancy or osteomyelitis.

Clinical Diagnosis. Localized osteomyelitis or carcinoma.

TREATMENT. To eliminate the fever and infection, preliminary medication was instituted 24 hours prior to surgery. Accordingly, 600,000 units of Crysticillin, the first of four successive daily doses, was administered intramuscularly, and forced fluids and saline laxative were prescribed.

In view of the possibility of this being a malignancy, the treatment plan was to remove the tissue mass by electrosection for biopsy evaluation, thoroughly fulgurate and carbonize the base of the surgical defect, then remove the bone sequestra and coagulate or desiccate the affected internal bone surface after all the necrotic debris was removed.

When he returned the next day he received his second penicillin injection. Then his mouth was prepared for surgery; bilateral mental block and lingual infiltration anesthesia was administered. A large guillotine-type loop electrode was selected and current output set at 9 for electrosection. The entire ulcerated mass plus a perimeter of normal tissue was resected with a single wiping stroke of the loop (Case Fig. 13–1*B*).

The resected tissue was preserved in formalin solution. Then the entire base of the surgical defect was fulgurated with a heavy needle electrode and current output set at 10, until the surface of the defect was uniformly carbonized (Case Fig. 13–1*C*). A spoon curet was introduced through the fistulous opening into the bone defect. One large and two small bone sequestra were removed together with considerable necrotic debris. The sequestra were added to the specimen bottle for biopsy.

The bone defect was irrigated with a solution of tyrothricin followed by isotonic saline solution; both were aspirated. With current output set at 2, a large ball electrode was inserted into the bone defect and used to coagulate the entire inner surface of the bone cavity. The electrode was used with constant rotary motion until the walls were lightly coagulated. It was withdrawn and a curet inserted to remove coagulated debris. Only sound bone was contacted. Some bleeding was induced with the curettage. A mixture of medicated surgical gelatin was introduced into the defect and mixed with the blood. When the blood clotted, a piece of dryfoil was adapted to the inner surface of the sterilized denture which was then inserted as a protective surgical stent. He was given postoperative instructions and told to return daily for postoperative treatment and penicillin injections.

He received the injections for the next four days, as well as tyrothricin and saline irrigations followed by topical applications of tincture of myrrh and benzoin and acriviolet. By the fifth postoperative day the operative field was covered with a healthy looking layer of coagulum. By the tenth day only a thin layer of coagulum remained on the surface; the rest of the alveolar mucosa looked firm and healthy (Case Fig. 13–1*D*). Healing progressed rapidly thereafter. By the end of the sixth week the external appearance of the area was completely normal (Case Fig. 13–1*E*).

BIOPSY REPORT. Soft Tissue: Granuloma fissuratum with ulceration and hyperkeratosis (Case Fig. 13–1*F*). Bone: Osteomyelitis.

The patient was seen once more, three months later for roentgenographic followup. The film showed normal bone, with complete obliteration of the bone defect.

Mandibular Anterior Lingual Mucosa

CASE 14

This is the first of a series of cases involving biopsy tissue emanating from gingival crevices. This case demonstrates the usefulness of slender angulated loop electrodes for resecting small epuli or epuloid masses emanating from gingival crevices in areas that are normally awkward to get at and difficult to resect cleanly with cold-steel instrumentation.

HISTORY. The patient was a 39-year-old white male. He suddenly began to lose weight rapidly. A number of soft tissue masses simultaneously began to bulge up from under the gums of several teeth in various parts of his mouth, and his gums began to bleed profusely when he brushed his teeth. Apprehensive of cancer or leukemia, he consulted his physician. He was referred for diagnosis and treatment of the oral lesions.

CLINICAL EXAMINATION. *Extraoral.* He was slender, pallid and obviously underweight. There was no adenopathy. His eyelids and sclera appeared normal. There was no known history of trauma, alteration of dietary habits or other significant changes. Medical and family histories: negative.

Intraoral. He had a full complement of teeth. The maxillary and mandibular gingivae appeared pallid. Bulging, dark red masses of proliferative, hyperemic, friable tissue extruded from the gingival crevices of several teeth. The marginal gingivae in other areas were hypertrophic and showed surface ulceration.

An intact round globule of somewhat firmer-looking tissue extruding from the lingual aspect of the mandibular left lateral incisor appeared suitable for histopathologic evaluation. Most of the masses bled profusely upon even gentle manipulation.

Provisional Clinical Diagnosis. This case did not lend itself to specific clinical diagnosis. There was a distinct impression, however, that these oral lesions had a systemic cause, possibly being of endocrine, metabolic or hematologic origin.

TREATMENT. The mouth was prepared and lingual infiltration anesthesia administered at the mandibular right lateral and left first bicuspid. A slender right-angle U-shaped loop electrode large enough to permit intact resection of the anterior lesion was selected and current output set at 6 for electrosection. The loop was applied to the area (Case Fig. 14–1A), activated and used with a lifting motion to resect the mass in toto, plus a 2 mm. strip of marginal gingiva at its base. The biopsy specimen was preserved in formalin solution. Moderately profuse bleeding ensued. It was controlled by electrocoagulation with a small ball electrode applied with current output set at 2 (Case Fig. 14–1B). Activation was for 2-second intervals followed by a 2-second pause, repeated five times. This proved adequate for effective hemostasis (Case Fig. 14–1C).

The mass at the lingual of the bicuspid—smaller, irregular, and much more friable—was then resected in the same manner and added to the specimen in the formalin solution. The basal areas of both surgical defects were fulgurated. Surgical cement packs into which tannic acid had been incorporated were then inserted over both operative areas. Terramycin was prescribed prophylactically for three days.

The patient returned one week later for postoperative observation. The gingivae in both areas showed some evidence of healing but appeared hyperemic and desquamated. An astringent salt-alum mouthwash was prescribed; ascorbic acid (250 mg.) and Knox clear gelatin were prescribed as dietary supplements. After two weeks of

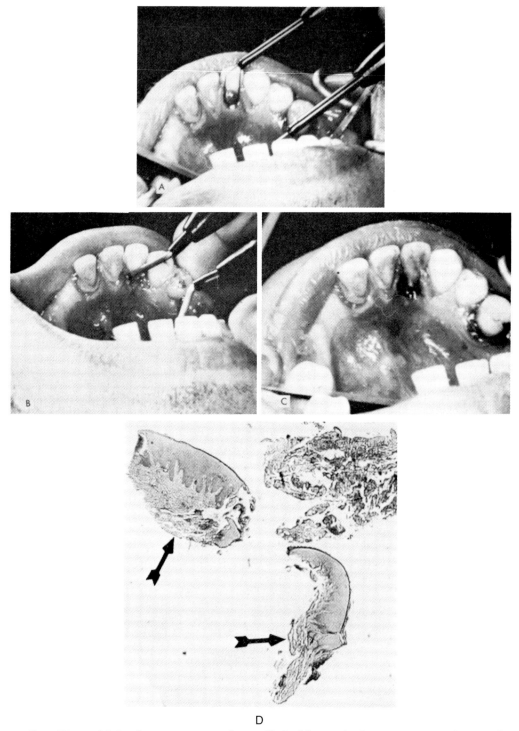

D

Case Figure 14–1.   Loop resection of a small, friable, epuloid mass emerging from under the gingival free margin. *A*, A right-angle, medium-sized U-shaped loop electrode placed in position to resect the mass with a wiping upward stroke atraumatically and bloodlessly. *B*, Basal layer of the defect thoroughly coagulated. *C*, Immediate postoperative appearance. Note lack of free bleeding after site was coagulated. *D*, Photomicrograph of the biopsy specimen. Arrows point to single layers of cells which have been destroyed by the electrosection.

this regimen some improvement was noted, but the general condition of the gingivae remained subnormal.

BIOPSY REPORT.   Nonspecific inflammatory tissue. Since the biopsy showed an absence of specific pathology and since there was a strong clinical impression that the lesions were a local manifestation of systemic factors, he was referred back to his physician for a complete medical evaluation. Laboratory work-up for incipient Hand-Schüller-Christian disease, hyperparathyroidism, scurvy or anemias were especially recommended. Roentgenographic evidence of slight radiolucence and loss of lamina dura around the roots of the affected teeth, superimposed on the clinical picture, made these diseases likely suspects.

All the laboratory tests, including calcium retention, proved either negative or inconclusive and failed to provide a diagnosis. Shortly thereafter his oral symptoms suddenly underwent spontaneous remission. For the next eight months his oral mucosa remained normal, his general well-being was improved and his weight remained constant. Then there was a sudden regression, and he experienced a second acute episode of weight loss accompanied by renewed proliferation of epuloid tissue in both the maxilla and mandible.

One of the new lesions was resected electrosurgically as described. Another of the epuloid masses was resected with a cold-steel scalpel and curet. Both tissue specimens were preserved in fixative and submitted for biopsy evaluation. The report on these was identical to the previous one. Slides of the biopsy tissue were submitted to a number of pathologists and to the Armed Forces Institute of Pathology for evaluation. All concurred with the original diagnosis (Case Fig. 14–1D).

Since no specific diagnosis had been achieved, empirical therapy was instituted. The patient was put on a high protein diet. Ten weekly therapeutic doses of vitamins B_{12} and B complex were administered intramuscularly. He also resumed the ascorbic acid, Knox gelatin and astringent lavage. His oral condition began to improve soon thereafter, and by the end of six weeks the gingivae appeared relatively normal. His condition has remained satisfactory for the past six years; there has been no further regression.

The biopsies ruled out specific pathology, thereby relieving the patient of mental anguish from fear of cancer. They also ruled out the need for extensive corrective surgery. Either of these is ample justification for performing biopsy in such cases.

Mandibular Central Mucosa

CASE 15

This case is an example of incisional resection of a mass for biopsy, combined with therapeutic electrocoagulation of a similar smaller area of mandibular alveolar mucosa.

PATIENT.   A 68-year-old white female.

HISTORY.   The patient consulted a dentist about having an ill-fitting denture replaced. He found extensive areas of dense white tissue superimposed on the alveolar mucosa. She was referred for diagnosis and treatment preliminary to multiple extractions and prosthetic restoration. (The dentist planned to extract the teeth himself.)

CLINICAL EXAMINATION. *Extraoral.* Negative. Medical history: negative. Family history: mother and one sister had died of carcinoma.

Intraoral. A slight macroglossia and small pursed lips made examination and treatment somewhat trying. Several anterior teeth and a retained right cuspid root were still present in the mandible. The gingival mucosa along the edentulous saddle areas were coated with white layers of tissue superimposed upon the normal tissue surfaces. On the right side the white mass of superimposed tissue was rough-surfaced, very thick and dense, and extended from the distal of the terminal tooth to the second molar area. There were a few additional small, thin, lacy white areas on that side. On the left side the corresponding edentulous saddle area was coated with a much thinner white layer (Case Fig. 15–1A).

The gingival areas that were not coated with white appeared hyperemic and hypertrophic. The mouth hygiene was very poor.

Clinical Diagnosis. Hyperkeratosis or parakeratosis.

TREATMENT. The mouth was prepared and inferior alveolar block anesthesia was administered on the right side. A 45-degree-angle fine needle electrode was

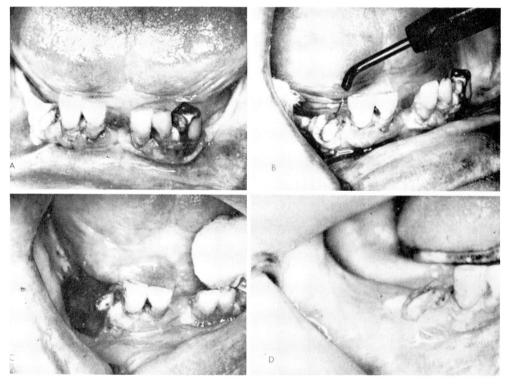

Case Figure 15–1. Incisional resection of parakeratosis from an edentulous mandibular saddle area that had been subjected to severe denture irritation. *A,* Preoperative appearance of the lesion, which consists of a dense, thick layer of tissue superimposed on the surface of the gingival mucosa. A retained root, remnant of an abutment tooth, remains in the area. *B,* Incisional resection performed with a 45-degree-angle fine needle electrode. *C,* Twenty-four hour postoperative appearance of the surgical defect. The bleeding encountered during surgery has been effectively controlled by coagulating the bleeder off the beaks of a mosquito hemostat, and the surgical defect is filled with a normal blood clot. *D,* Appearance of the tissues six weeks postoperatively. Healing is complete, without contraction. A small amount of regeneration of the hyperkeratosis has occurred around the retained root.

selected and current output set at 3 for electrosection. The entire mass, with a perimeter of normal tissue 2 mm. wide, was incised down to the periosteum (Case Fig. 15–1B). The incised tissue was undermined, resected and preserved in formalin solution. A spurting blood vessel was clamped with a curved mosquito hemostat and hemostasis effected by electrocoagulation off the beaks of the hemostat. The entire basal layer of the surgical defect was lightly fulgurated. Topical anesthesia was applied to the left saddle area and the thin white surface layer was treated by superficial electrocoagulation with a large ball electrode.

A stiff mixture of surgical cement was inserted into the right saddle area of the sterilized denture, which was utilized as a surgical stent. Because of the poor hygiene, Panalba and Kasdenol were prescribed prophylactically to reduce danger of secondary infection. The patient was instructed to leave the denture in undisturbed until seen again.

She returned in 24 hours and reported minimal discomfort and edema. The denture was removed and the mouth was irrigated. Inspection of the tissues showed the blood clot beginning to undergo organization, and the left saddle area looked almost normal (Case Fig. 15–1C). Tincture of myrrh and benzoin was applied.

She was seen at weekly intervals for the next six weeks. During that period healing progressed slowly but uneventfully. The other scattered white areas were treated with superficial electrocoagulation, and spot coagulation was applied to the regenerating tissue to control healing. By the end of the sixth week healing in the biopsy site was complete (Case Fig. 15–1D). The white areas were not entirely eliminated until her new denture was inserted. A triangular parakeratotic patch regenerated at the distobuccal angle of the retained root.

BIOPSY REPORT.   Very extensive parakeratosis and moderately severe inflammatory reaction.

Mandibular Posterior Mucosa

CASE 16

This case is an example of incisional resection of mandibular alveolar mucosa by electrosection plus use of a loop electrode to complete the biopsy.

PATIENT.   A 63-year-old white male.

HISTORY.   The patient had been wearing a lingual bar restoration for seven years. A few weeks previous to referral a sore spot suddenly developed on the posterior part of his left alveolar ridge, making eating very painful. He consulted his dentist and was referred for diagnosis and treatment.

CLINICAL EXAMINATION.   *Extraoral.*   Negative. Medical and family histories: negative.

Intraoral.   The alveolar mucosa appeared normal except for a pigmented area in the mandibular left second-third molar edentulous saddle area just anterior to the retromolar pad. In the center of the area there was an upward projecting small bulb of firm tissue. There was also a patch of white keratinized tissue located at the posterior border of the area and a small ulcerated groove on the crest of the ridge at its anterior border (Case Fig. 16–1A).

Clinical Diagnosis.   Leukoplakia with traumatic ulceration.

TREATMENT.   The mouth was prepared for surgery and inferior alveolar block

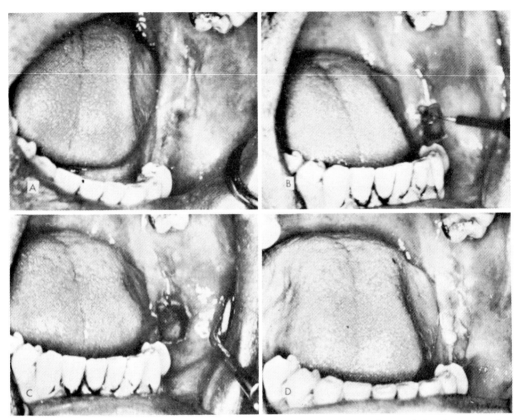

Case Figure 16–1.   Incisional resection of an ulcerated area of leukoplakia from an edentulous mandibular saddle area. *A,* Preoperative appearance of the lesion. There is ulceration, a patch of white superimposed on the epithelial surface, and an apparent hemorrhagic extravasation in the local tissues. *B,* After the mass was resected with a fine needle electrode, shreds adhering to the periosteum were resected with a flame-shaped loop electrode. *C,* Immediate postoperative appearance of the surgical defect. *D,* Appearance on the fifth postoperative day. Healing is progressing rapidly, and the defect is almost fully filled with healthy looking granulation tissue.

anesthesia administered. A 45-degree-angle fine needle electrode was selected and current output set at 4 for electrosection. The entire square of tissue in which the keratosis, ulceration and pigmentation were located, plus a 2 mm. perimeter of normal tissue, was incised down to the alveolar bone. The incised tissue was undermined, removed and preserved for biopsy evaluation. The periosteum was included with the tissue specimen, leaving a completely denuded area of alveolar bone. Marginal portions of periosteum were resected with a flame-shaped loop electrode (Case Fig. 16–1*B*).

The denuded bone appeared normal and was unaffected by the overlying gingival lesion (Case Fig. 16–1*C*). Medicated surgical gelatin was deposited into the defect and mixed with the blood. When the blood clotted it was covered with a strip of adhesive dryfoil. The patient's sterilized denture was then used as a surgical stent.

The patient returned on the fifth postoperative day and reported that he had not been troubled by pain or swelling. The surgical defect, which had measured approximately 7 mm. in width and 12 mm. in length, was almost completely filled to the level of the adjacent mucosa with healthy looking granulation tissue, and more than half of the surface area was beginning to undergo epithelization (Case Fig. 16–1*D*).

He was seen again one week later and further healing progress was noted. He was instructed to return for weekly postoperative observation and was informed of the biopsy findings.

BIOPSY REPORT.   Leukoplakia with ulceration; benign.

After the patient was informed that the lesion was benign he neglected to return for further treatment. He phoned to explain that since there was no danger and his mouth felt fully healed he saw no reason to take time off from work to come back for further observation.

BIOPSY OF THE PALATAL MUCOSA

Incisional Excision

CASE 17

This case is an example of incisional biopsy excision of wedge-shaped segments from large lesions by electrosection.

PATIENT.   A 65-year-old white male.

HISTORY.   His chief complaint was constant burning soreness of the roof of his mouth. In the 10 years he had been edentulous, he had had several dentures made, without much improvement. Patch tests for allergy to the denture acrylic were negative. He was referred for diagnosis.

CLINICAL EXAMINATION. *Extraoral.*   Negative. Medical and family histories: negative.

Intraoral.   Almost one third of his total palate was desquamated and bright red. There were many macules present in the square hemorrhagic-looking area. The labial alveolar gingiva was hypertrophic and contained several ulcerated areas (Case Fig. 17–1A and B). These appeared to be due to denture irritation.

Clinical Diagnosis.   Palate: Chronic inflammation; probably a denture sore, monilial or allergic in origin.[6] Labial: Submucous hypertrophy.

TREATMENT.   The mouth was prepared for surgery and the posterior left quadrant of the lesion was anesthetized by infiltration. A 45-degree-angle fine needle electrode was selected and current output set at 6 for electrosection. The anesthetized area was incised down to the palatal bone in the shape of a triangle, with the apex pointed inward toward the center of the lesion and the base extending 3 mm. beyond the base into normal tissue (Case Fig. 17–1C). The incised tissue was undermined, excised and preserved in formalin.

A piece of Gelfoam sponge moistened with growth inductor material was inserted into the surgical defect. The medicated Gelfoam soon became saturated with blood (Case Fig. 17–1D). An ulcerated area on the left labial alveolar ridge was anesthetized by infiltration and a flame-shaped loop electrode was substituted for the needle. Current output was reduced to 5 and a segment of the anesthetized tissue was excised with a scooping motion of the loop. This tissue was added to the palatal biopsy. The patch of hypertrophic mucosa on the right side was also resected.

By that time the blood in the palatal defect was clotted. The area was covered with a piece of adhesive dryfoil. The patient's sterilized denture was inserted over it as the surgical stent. Mysteclin was prescribed and he was given postoperative instructions. He returned the following day for observation. The defects were filled

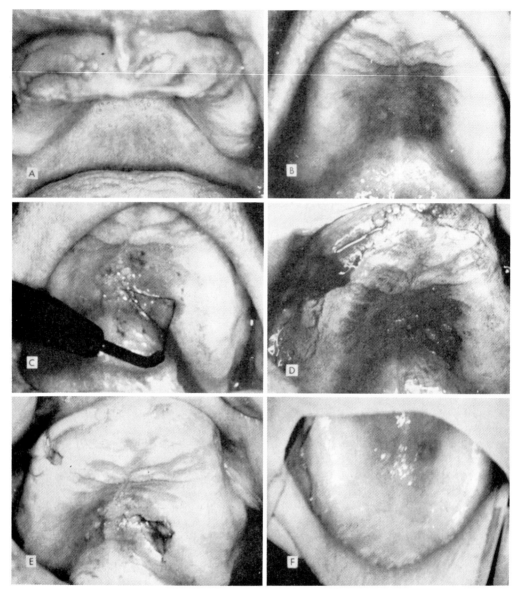

Case Figure 17–1. Incisional excision of a segment of a large palatal lesion (and loop resection of anterior hypertrophic tissue mass). *A,* Preoperative view, labial aspect, shows an ulcerated patch on the left side of the alveolar ridge and a long slender mass of hypertrophic tissue on the right side that appears to be superimposed on the gingival mucosa. *B,* Palatal view reveals a large square area in the center of the palate, dark red in color and largely desquamated of its surface keratinization. *C,* A triangular wedge of tissue is resected from the palatal defect for biopsy evaluation. The apex of the triangle is in the center of the lesion, and the base includes 3 mm. of normal tissue. Note the bloodless incisions despite the massive engorgement of the palatal lesion area. *D,* Bird's-eye view of the surgical defects after the palatal and labial tissue specimens were resected. Both surgical defects have been filled with medicated surgical gelatin and have become saturated with blood present in the defects. *E,* Appearance on the fifth postoperative day. Both defects are filled almost flush with the surrounding mucosa with healthy granulation tissue. The massive engorgement in the center of the palate is greatly reduced. *F,* Appearance of the palate seven weeks postoperatively, as seen in a mirror image. The surgical defects are fully healed, with no visible scar remaining. The engorgement has begun to manifest itself again to some extent, but to a considerably lesser degree in the vicinity of the biopsy section.

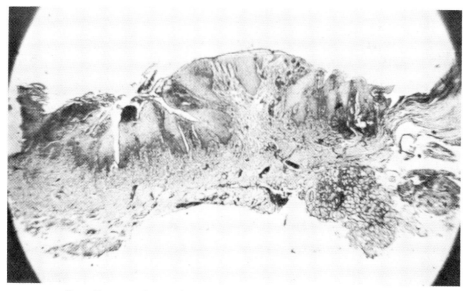

Case Figure 17–2. Photomicrograph of palatal tissue resected.

with firm blood clots which were undergoing organization. The mouth was irrigated and tincture of myrrh and benzoin applied. He was seen again four days later. All the defects were filled with normal granulation tissue (Case Fig. 17–1E). The large square area of engorgement was much improved; it was now much lighter in color, did not look as desquamated and raw, and no longer was painful. Tincture of myrrh and benzoin was applied in air-dried layers and he was instructed to continue the regimen of postoperative care.

He returned thereafter at regular weekly intervals for the next six weeks. By the end of that time the surgical defects were completely healed, but the entire palate, including the newly regenerated tissue, looked exactly as it had originally (Case Fig. 17–1F).

BIOPSY REPORT. Nonspecific inflammation with desquamation of surface epithelium (Case Fig. 17–2).

In view of the return of the palatal tissues to their former appearance, it appears likely that the immediate postoperative improvement in color was related to bleeding during surgery, which reduced the palatal engorgement temporarily.

CASE 18

This case is an example of electrosurgical biopsy by incisional and loop resections plus therapeutic electrocoagulation.

PATIENT. A 70-year-old white female.

HISTORY. Her chief complaint was pain and difficulty in swallowing due to a sore in the back part of her mouth where her full upper denture terminated.

Her dentist found a mass along the posterior border of the denture postdam. She was referred for diagnosis and treatment.

CLINICAL EXAMINATION. *Extraoral.* The patient looked pallid and emaciated.

Several lymph nodes along the plane of the sternomastoid muscle were palpable. Medical and family histories: negative.

Intraoral. hypertrophic ridge of tissue was present at the posterior end of the palate. It extended from the heel of the tuberosity toward the midline, along a plane parallel with the junction of the hard and soft palates. The mass was firm and fibrous, measured approximately 3 mm. in width by 15 mm. in length, and was elevated about 3 mm. beyond the level of the surrounding mucosa. A small ulcerated bulb of tissue was present on the soft palate, at the median termination of the fibrous ridge. There was also an ulcerated area about 6 mm. in length in the posterior part of the left buccal vestibule, which was covered with necrotic surface slough. A hypertrophic mass was present in the right central-lateral region of the mucolabial fold (Case Fig. 18–1A).

Clinical Diagnosis. Traumatic fibrous hyperplasia with ulceration.

TREATMENT. The mouth was prepared and the three lesions anesthetized by infiltration. A 45-degree-angle fine needle electrode was selected and current output set at 5 for electrosection. The palatal lesion was incised circumferentially to a depth of 3 mm., with its 2 mm. perimeter of normal mucosa included in the biopsy (Case Fig. 18–1B).

Current density was increased to 9, and an 8 mm. round loop electrode was substituted for the needle. An Allis tissue forceps was inserted through the eye of the loop and clamped to the incised tissue. The tissue was lifted in order to pull it taut; then it was resected with a wiping motion of the activated electrode. The biopsy specimen was preserved in formalin solution. A strip of Gelfoam was cut to fit the surgical defect, medicated and inserted into it. The sponge immediately became saturated with blood in the defect.

A large ball electrode was selected and current output set at 2 for electrocoagulation. The posterior vestibular lesion was coagulated by applying the ball to the tissue surface for two-second periods followed by two-second pauses until the entire surface of the lesion was coagulated to a depth of one-half millimeter. Finally, the large loop was replaced, current density set at 7, and the hypertrophic mass in the anterior vestibule was resected with a scooping motion. Medicated Gelfoam sponge was also inserted into this defect (Case Fig. 18–1C).

The patient's denture was then built up with surgical cement and dryfoil so that it would cover the posterior surgical defect and serve as an emergency surgical stent (Case Fig. 18–1D . The denture was built up with cement in the areas corresponding to the buccal and labial defects so that it would maintain the integrity of these vestibular areas. Cosa-Tetrastatin was prescribed for three days.

The patient returned on the fifth postoperative day and reported uneventful postoperative recovery. The denture was removed, the mouth irrigated and the tissues inspected. The healing was progressing splendidly. The coagulated posterior vestibule area was covered with a layer of healthy thin coagulum, and the anterior and palatal defects were filled with normal granulation tissue (Case Fig. 18–1E).

The posterior border of the palatal defect projected slightly above the level of the surrounding mucosa. A small area of tissue immediately anterior to the defect, which had not been involved in the surgery, appeared slightly irritated. Topical anesthesia was applied to both areas for two minutes. Biterminal coagulating current output was set at 0.5, and these areas were treated by superficial spot coagulation with a small ball electrode. The three operative fields were then painted with tincture of myrrh and benzoin.

The patient was seen thereafter at regular weekly intervals. At her next visit the anterior and posterior vestibular areas were completely healed, and the palatal defect

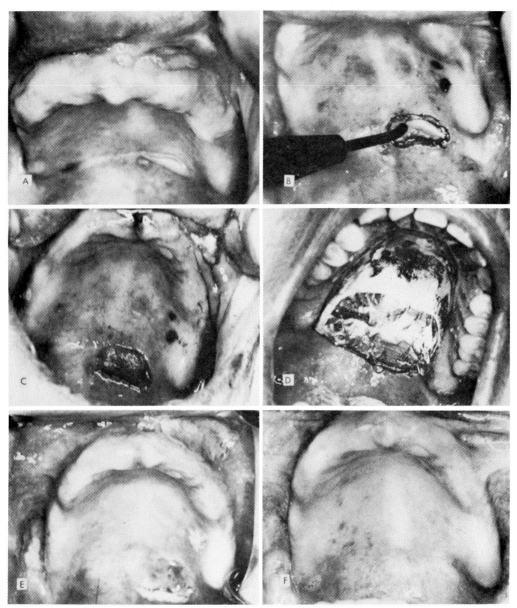

Case Figure 18–1. Incisional resection of a lesion at the junction of the hard and soft palate extending largely into the soft palate area. *A*, Preoperative view. There is a large fibrotic mass, probably granuloma fissuratum, in the left labial vestibule. There is a dense fibrotic elevated ridge of tissue with a deep groove on its anterior aspect, and a round papular lesion with an ulcerated central crater near the midline, extending along the junction of the hard and soft palates on the left side. There is also some superficial slough in the buccal vestibule on the right side. *B*, The palatal lesion is resected by circumferential incision with a 45-degree-angle fine needle electrode. *C*, Both the palatal surgical defect and labial defect (resulting when the lesion was resected with a large loop electrode) are filled with medicated surgical gelatin. *D*, The denture has been built out with surgical cement and dryfoil to extend over the palatal defect as a surgical stent. *E*, Appearance of the maxilla on the fifth postoperative day. The anterior defect is filled with granulation tissue and covered with a moderately heavy layer of healthy coagulum. The palatal defect is filled with healthy granulation tissue and covered with a light layer of coagulum. The distal margin, slightly elevated, has been reduced to normal level by superficial spot coagulation. The right buccal vestibule is covered with a moderately thick layer of coagulum where the sloughed tissue surface had been coagulated. *F*, Appearance of the maxilla three weeks later. All the lesions are fully healed with normal tissue. There is no visible evidence of the surgery, and no cicatricial contraction of the tissues of the soft palate.

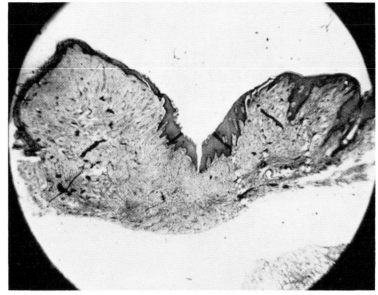

Case Figure 18–2. Photomicrograph of the palatal tissue resected.

was filled with normal tissue which had not yet undergone epithelial keratinization. Maturation progressed rapidly thereafter without incident. By the end of three weeks, the three areas were indistinguishable from the mucosa of the rest of the maxilla (Case Fig. 18–1F). The tissues were normal in tone and completely free of cicatricial scar repair.

BIOPSY REPORT. Inflammatory hyperplasia with fibrosis (Case Fig. 18–2).

The patient had a new set of dentures constructed shortly thereafter. She returned for postoperative follow-up six months later. The maxillary tissues were normal in all respects.

Loop Resection of the Hard Palate

CASE 19

This case demonstrates resection of a biopsy specimen from the mucosa of the hard palate by loop electrosection.

PATIENT. A 54-year-old white male in normal health.

HISTORY. During a regular six-month routine check-up examination his dentist found a small round mass on the mucosa of the hard palate and suggested its removal to avoid irritation resulting from normal functional use.

CLINICAL EXAMINATION. The palatal mucosa appeared normal except for a small round mass measuring approximately 3 mm. and elevated, domelike, that was present opposite and approximately 1.5 cm. medial to the right first bicuspid. The mass had a sessile base. No induration was noted.

TREATMENT. A round loop large enough to resect a 2-mm. perimeter of normal tissue along with the lesion was selected and bent to form a slight curve (Case Fig. 19–1A). The tissue was prepared for surgery and circumferential infiltration anesthe-

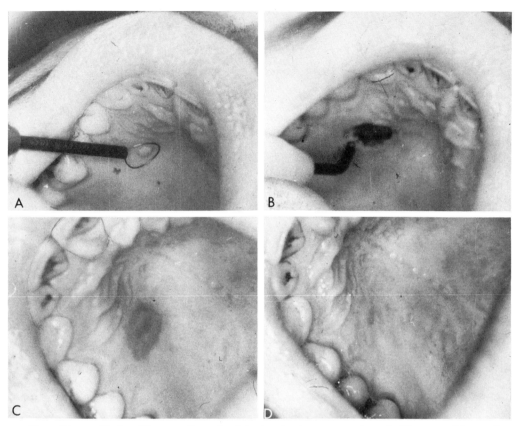

Case Figure 19–1.   Biopsy of a palatal lesion by loop resection. *A,* The round loop electrode, which has been bent to form a slight arc that will facilitate scooping out the tissue section, is about to make contact with the tissue. *B,* The tissue has been resected and a small bleeder in the cut tissue margin is being coagulated to control the bleeding. *C,* Appearance of the palate two weeks postoperatively. The defect has filled to the same level as the surrounding tissue and except for lack of surface keratin appears well healed. *D,* Appearance of the palate six weeks postoperatively. The palate is fully healed. A small elliptical area appears slightly pinker in color than the surrounding tissue owing to incomplete keratinization.

sia was administered. Cutting current was set at 6 on the power output dial, the electrode was activated, and the resection was performed with a single wiping stroke. There was no bleeding from the underlying palatal tissue, but there was some free bleeding from the medial margin of the wound, which was immediately controlled by spot coagulation with a small ball electrode and coagulating current set at 3 on the power output dial (Case Fig. 19–1*B*). The tissue in the surgical defect was totally free of coagulation. A bandage of Squibb Orahesive was cut to size and placed over the surgical defect. The patient was instructed to avoid hot liquids for the first day and to avoid chewing solid food until his return. He was seen again on the fifth postoperative day, and healing by secondary intention appeared to be progressing favorably. By the tenth postoperative day the defect was healed except for surface keratinization (Case Fig. 19–1*C*). By the twenty-first day healing was complete with all but a tiny 1 mm. area completely keratinized (Case Fig. 19–1*D*).

The preceding case involved the relatively routine electrosurgical biopsy of a small, and by all clinical indications benign, lesion by loop resection from

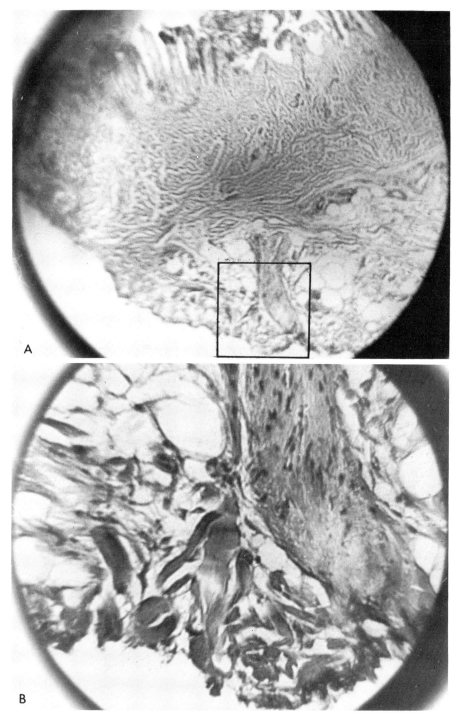

Case Figure 19–2. Photomicrographs of the biopsy specimen. *A,* Appearance of tissue removed from the hard palate by loop resection as seen under 10× magnification. Boxed area indicates the tissue that will be examined under higher magnification. *B,* Histologic appearance of the tissue in the inset area under 45× magnification. Note that the dark areas seen in *A* are not due to coagulation necrosis but to the nature of the cells and cell nuclei that are intact along the line of tissue cleavage.

the palate. This case not only involved removal of a much larger lesion by loop resection but also presented two clinical features that often are associated with malignant pathology that made the biopsy much more important and urgent from a pathologic as well as an electrosurgical standpoint.

CASE 20

The lesion in this case was about as large as could possibly be removed in toto by loop resection. It was necessary to use the largest (for dentistry) loop electrode to do so. Claims have been made that tissue cannot be removed by resection with large loop electrodes without causing notable coagulation of the biopsy specimen and the tissue of the bed from which it was removed. This case provides excellent histologic evidence that when it is properly used, tissue resection can be performed safely and efficiently even from the palatal mucosa with large loop electrodes without causing cellular coagulation or impairment of tissue repair.

PATIENT. A 58-year-old white female.

HISTORY. She had been wearing a maxillary partial denture to replace the bicuspid and molar teeth for approximately 10 years. The denture fitted well, and until recently had been trouble-free. About six weeks ago she began to feel pressure discomfort under the denture on the left side of the palate. The discomfort increased progressively into moderately severe pain, and she noticed that, although she was not dieting, she began to lose weight. She consulted her dentist, who found a large palatal lesion and referred her to the author for diagnosis and definitive treatment.

CLINICAL EXAMINATION. The edentulous alveolar ridges and their covering mucosa were normal. On the palate, in the left tuberosity area near the junction of the hard and soft palates, there was a round, firm, nonfluctuant mass with an ulcerated crater in the center. The mass was elevated convexly 0.5 cm. above the level of the surrounding mucosa at its highest point and measured 1 cm. in diameter (Case Fig. 20–1A). The rest of the palatal mucosa was normal. There was no palpable adenopathy in the submaxillary and cervical areas, and an intraoral roentgenogram of the affected area proved negative for bone disease.

TREATMENT. The adjacent palatal mucosa was prepared, and anesthesia was administered by circumferential infiltration with Xylocaine (1:100,000 solution). A round loop electrode 1.5 cm. in diameter was selected and cutting current output was set at 8 on the instrument panel rheostat dial. The electrode was activated and used with a single brushing motion to resect the mass including a perimeter of 2 mm. of normal tissue (Case Fig. 20–1B). The resected tissue was placed in formalin fixative solution and sent for biopsy evaluation.

The loop excision had been performed deeply enough to assure that the base of the excised tissue was in normal tissue, without disturbing the periosteum and denuding the palatal bone. Since the hemostasis resulted in very little bleeding, bleeding was induced by pricking the tissue in the surgical bed with the point of an explorer. Powdered Gelfoam was deposited in the defect and mixed with the blood to form a clot. A piece of adhesive dryfoil was placed over and adapted to the adjacent tissue and was sealed to the tissue by painting clear collodion over the foil and surrounding tissue, creating a firmly attached dressing over the surgical field. The dressing was level with the surrounding mucosa and did not cause any interference when the denture was inserted to serve as a surgical stent. The patient was then given instructions for postoperative care, including a regimen of semi-liquid diet, and was told to return on the fifth postoperative day.

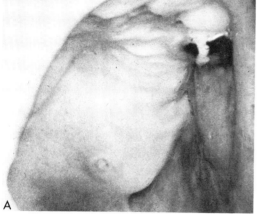

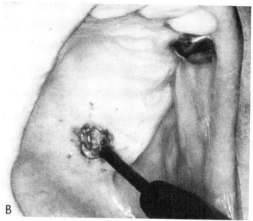

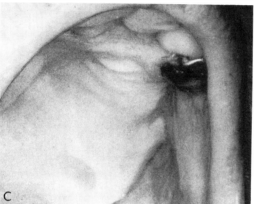

Case Figure 20–1.   Loop resection of a large posterior palatal lesion. *A,* Preoperative appearance of the lesion. It is a large round convexly elevated mass with a round ulcerated crater in the center, located near the junction of the hard and soft palates in the region of the left tuberosity. *B,* The entire pathologic mass plus a 2-mm. perimeter of normal tissue is being resected by electrosection with a large round loop electrode for biopsy evaluation. *C,* Postoperative appearance of the area less than one month later. The tissue has regenerated fully and is normal in all respects except for the incomplete keratinization of the surface epithelium.

She returned as instructed; the dressing was removed, and the surgical field was inspected. Tissue repair was progressing very favorably and the dressing was discontinued. Tincture of myrrh and benzoin was applied to the area in air-dried layers, and the patient was told to continue the postoperative care, to avoid irritating the tissue, and to return at weekly intervals until further notice for postoperative observation and supervision.

At the third of these weekly visits inspection revealed that the tissue was fully regenerated in the surgical field. The regenerated tissue appeared to be normal in all respects but was slightly darker red in color than the rest of the palatal mucosa, owing to incomplete keratinization of the surface epithelium. With the exception of this slight difference in coloration the regenerated tissue was indistinguishable in all respects from the surrounding tissues (Case Fig. 20–1C).

The biopsy report confirmed that the lesion was benign, despite the central ulceration and history of weight loss. In retrospect, the latter had probably resulted from reduced consumption of food because of the pain induced during eating. The histologic appearance of the tissue in this case as seen under 10× magnification (Case Fig. 20–2A) and under 45× magnification (Case Fig. 20–2B) proves that even when a very large loop electrode is employed for the excision, and the tissue is thick and dense, electrosection can be performed safely and efficiently without causing discernible cellular destruction or alteration, and without impairing the ability of the tissues to regenerate normally.

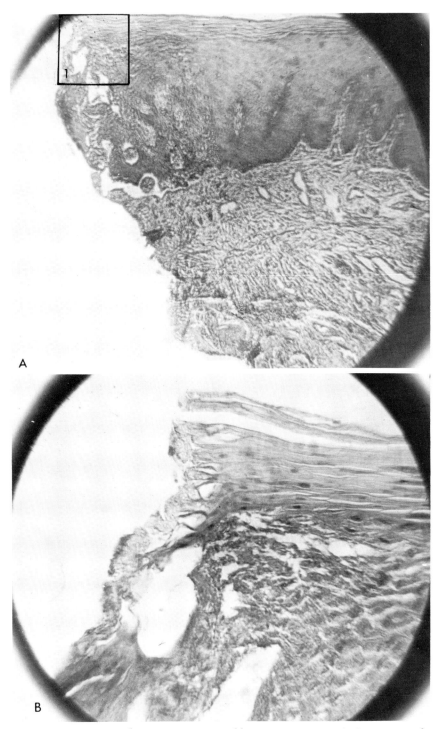

Case Figure 20–2. Histologic appearance of biopsy specimen. *A*, Specimen of tissue resected with large loop electrode at 10× magnification. *B*, Inset 1 from *A* at 45× magnification.

CASE 21

This case is an example of electrosurgical biopsy loop resection of both palatal mucosa and areolar mucosa. A rate and quality of tissue repair of thick dense palatal mucosa that is fully comparable with repair of similar defects in tissue resections where the electrode does not contact underlying bone is well demonstrated.

PATIENT. A 38-year-old white male.

HISTORY. A sore spot on the roof of his mouth was his chief complaint. Mouthwashes failed to relieve it, so he consulted his dentist, who found the palate coated with opaque white surface and ulcerations. He was referred for diagnosis and treatment.

CLINICAL EXAMINATION. *Extraoral.* Negative. Medical and family histories: negative, but he seemed to be a very tense individual and was a chain smoker. When not smoking cigars or cigarettes he chewed on cigars. There was palpable adenopathy in the left submaxillary triangle and tenderness to palpation.

Intraoral. His dentition was normal. The entire palate was covered with a thick white surface which appeared verrucose. A papular lesion measuring 2.5 mm. in diameter was located 0.5 cm. to the right of midline opposite the first molar. The papule had a punched out, crater-like ulceration in its center. Two smaller, similar lesions, each measuring 1 mm. in diameter, were located slightly to the left of midline. Posterior to this tier of papules, there were a number of similar tiny dot-like lesions. An irregular patch of verrucose keratinized mucosa also was present on the buccal aspect slightly above and posterior to the second molar (Case Fig. 21–1A).

Clinical Diagnosis. Palate: Stomatitis nicotinae. Buccal: Leukoplakia.

TREATMENT. The mouth was prepared and the buccal and largest palatal lesions were anesthetized by infiltration. A large flame-shaped loop electrode was selected and current output set at 8 for electrosection. The largest papule with a 2 mm. wide perimeter of normal tissue was resected with a single wiping stroke of the loop used with a scooping motion down to the underlying bone. A medium-sized round loop electrode was substituted and current density was reduced to 6 for resection of the buccal tissue specimen.

An ophthalmic tissue forceps was inserted through the eye of the loop, the buccal tissue was pulled taut and the buccal lesion with its perimeter of normal tissue was resected with a wiping stroke of this loop to a depth of 4 mm. Both biopsy tissue specimens were immediately preserved in formalin solution. Medicated surgical gelatin was inserted into the two surgical defects and mixed with the blood. When the blood clotted, the palatal defect was covered with adhesive dryfoil which was sealed to the tissues with a clear collodion dressing. The collodion would not adhere to the buccal tissues; this area was therefore left exposed. The patient was instructed to use oral lavage frequently.

He was too tense to permit the usual operative clinical photography so that it was not possible to obtain operative photographs of the instrumentation. When he returned postoperatively, however, he was quite relaxed and readily permitted the postoperative photography.

He returned on the first postoperative day and reported that he had had no adverse effects. The collodion dressing was removed. The palatal mucosa was normal in color and free of edema; the surgical defect was filled with a blood clot which was beginning to undergo organization. The buccal defect was also doing well but was not quite filled flush with the surrounding mucosa; the periphery was somewhat edema-

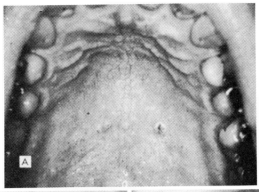

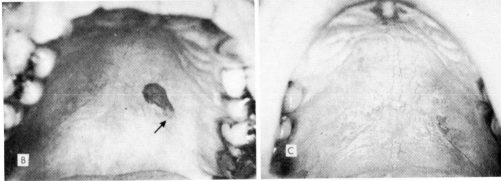

Case Figure 21-1.   Total loop resection of small ulcerated papular lesion on the palate (stomatitis nicotinae). *A*, Preoperative appearance of the lesion. The palate is covered with a heavy layer of keratinization and some fissuring. There are numerous papular lesions with punched out craters in their centers scattered over the posterior third of the palate. The papules vary in size from smaller than a pin head to almost 3 mm. in diameter. Note absence of fissuring and keratotic appearance of the tissues and the myriad papules. This temporary improvement, also displayed in Case Figure 17-1, appears to be characteristic and suggests that electrosection as well as electrocoagulation induces antibody reactions (reported in Chapter 25), although to a much lesser degree, since the improvement lasts only until repair is complete and then regresses to its preoperative condition. *B*, Appearance of the surgical defect on the fifth postoperative day. Note the smooth round outline of the defect resulting from resection with oval loop electrode. The defect is filled with healthy granulation tissue. Note the "comet-tail" effect often produced by the loop electrode as it is being lifted away from the tissue (arrow). There is no edema or engorgement present. *C*, Postoperative appearance one year later. The area where the biopsy was performed is fully healed and indistinguishable from the rest of the palatal mucosa except that, although surrounded by numerous papules, no papular lesions have developed in it.

tous, creating a raised, rolled marginal outline around the defect. Tincture of myrrh and benzoin was applied in air-dried layers to both areas.

He returned on the fifth postoperative day, at which time the healing was considerably further advanced. The palatal mucosa was intact and the defect was filled to the surface with healthy looking granulation tissue (Case Fig. 21-1*B*). The buccal defect was also filled with granulation tissue, which was covered with a thin layer of coagulum. Two weeks postoperatively the palatal defect was fully healed but the surface epithelium was not yet maturely keratinized. The buccal defect, also, was almost fully healed, but healing here was not as advanced as on the palate.

BIOPSY REPORT. Palate: Nicotine stomatitis. Buccal: Leukoplakia (Case Fig. 21-2).

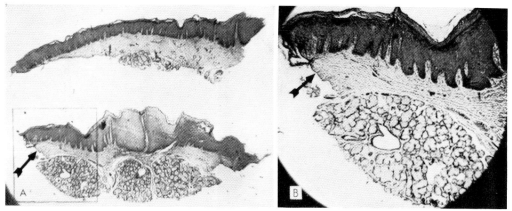

Case Figure 21–2. Photomicrographs of tissue obtained. *A*, Low power photomicrographs. Section enclosed in the square corresponds to section reproduced under higher magnification. Arrow points to single layer of cells destroyed by electrosection. Note smooth, even, round contour of tissue specimen resected with a loop electrode. This offers a favorable contrast to the irregular, often ragged margins of tissue resected with cold steel scalpels. *B*, Tissue in squared area as seen under higher magnification. Arrow points to where a few microns of adipose tissue melted, owing to greater susceptibility of fatty tissue cells to the heat.

The patient was seen again one year later for postoperative observation. The palatal biopsy site was fully healed and no visible evidence remained of the defect, but numerous papules were present on the palate (Case Fig. 21–1C). The buccal mucosa was fully healed but the site of the defect could be identified.

It is interesting to note that the site protected with dryfoil and collodion initially healed at a more accelerated rate than the totally unprotected area, although the electrode made contact with underlying bone in the former area and did not come into contact with bone in the latter area.

Incisional and Loop Resection

CASE 22

This case demonstrates a technique for incisional biopsy of thick, dense palatal mucosa by electrosection.

PATIENT. A 39-year-old white male.

HISTORY. A sore spot on his palate persisted for three weeks despite lavage with antiseptic mouthwashes and treatment by his dentist for the preceding two weeks. Topical medication and sodium perborate lavage had proved ineffectual. He was referred for diagnosis and treatment.

CLINICAL EXAMINATION. *Extraoral.* Negative. Medical history: successful treatment of primary lues in his teens, with negative serology since.

Intraoral. The entire palatal mucosa was covered with an opaque white surface, giving it a parboiled appearance. On the right side midway between the midline and the marginal gingivae there was an annular ulcerated lesion. It was oval in shape and extended from the distal of the first bicuspid to the middle of the first molar (Case Fig. 22–1A). Anterior and somewhat medial to this lesion there was a small dot-

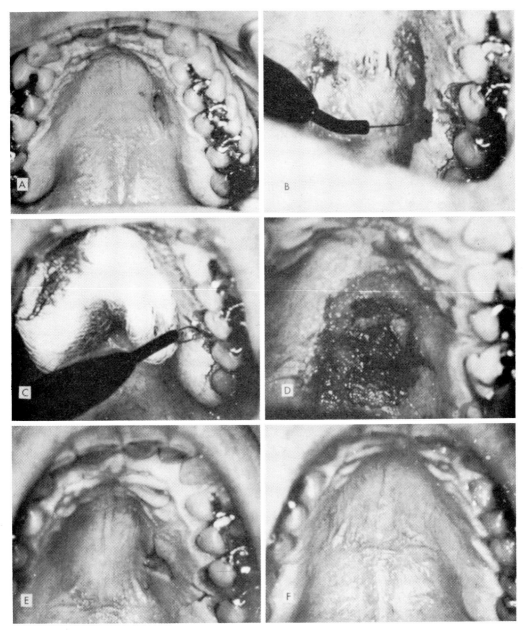

Case Figure 22–1.   Resection in toto by incisional biopsy of a small palatal lesion (leuko-plakia with ulceration) and loop resection of gingival mucosa (palatal aspect). *A*, Preoperative appearance of the annular lesion. Note thick, pearly white keratinized surface of the palatal mucosa. *B*, Incisional resection of the palatal lesion for biopsy. Note blanching of the palatal tissue as activated electrode makes contact with the underlying bone. A moderate amount of bleeding, easily staunched by pressure, occurred when the incised biopsy specimen was de-tached and elevated from the palatal bone. *C*, A small segment of keratinized tissue is resected for biopsy with a flame-shaped loop electrode. *D*, The defect is filled with mediated powdered surgical gelatin, which is mixed with the blood in the defect. Note areola of engorgement around the surgical defect. *E*, Appearance on the fifth postoperative day. There is virtually no edema, no ecchymosis. The surgical defects are almost completely filled with healthy granula-tion tissue. *F*, Postoperative appearance after one month. Healing is complete, with no cica-tricial contraction or visible scar. The epithelial surface is fully keratinized.

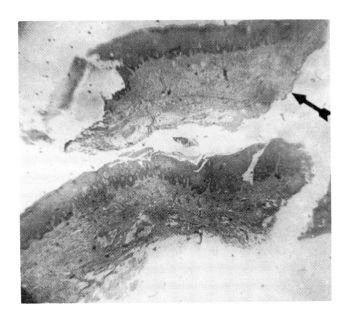

Case Figure 22–2. Photomicrograph of the palatal lesion. Arrow points to single layer of cells destroyed by electrosection at margin of specimen.

like ulcerated lesion, and extending beyond the oval area was a groove 3 mm. long shaped like a kite tail.

Clinical Diagnosis. Leukoplakia or hyperkeratosis, with ulceration; also possibly herpes simplex.

TREATMENT. The mouth was prepared for surgery and circumferential infiltration anesthesia administered. A 45-degree-angle fine needle electrode was selected and current output set at 5 for electrosection. (Note increased current density necessary to incise the thick dense palatal mucosa cleanly.) A circumscribing incision down to the palatal bone was made around the annular lesion and its 3 mm. perimeter of normal tissue (Case Fig. 22–1*B*).

The incised tissue was undermined, removed and preserved in formalin solution. The incision had been practically bloodless. When the tissue was detached from the bone, light bleeding was staunched by pressure with a sterile sponge. Some medicated powdered gelatin was introduced into the surgical defect and mixed with the blood (Case Fig. 22-1*D*). When the blood clotted, the area was covered with a protective coating of clear collodion applied thickly.

The palatal mucosa near the molars had also been anesthetized by infiltration. A flame-shaped loop electrode was substituted, current output increased to 7, and with a single scooping motion of the electrode an oval segment of mucosa was resected where the keratosis appeared thickest (Case Fig. 22–1*C*). The patient was advised to refrain from smoking and to stay on a bland diet.

He returned on the fifth postoperative day and reported that the collodion dressing had peeled away on the third day. Both surgical defects were almost fully filled with healthy granulation tissue and were showing signs of epithelization (Case Fig. 22–1*E*). The area was irrigated and tincture of myrrh and benzoin applied. Healing progressed rapidly; by the end of the first postoperative month both defects were fully healed. The tissue was normal in color, texture and density, and defied detection (Case Fig. 22–1*F*).

BIOPSY REPORT. Leukoplakia with surface ulceration (Case Fig. 22–2).

CASE 23

This case differs from the preceding cases in two respects. First, unlike the others (which involved thick, dense palatal tissue), this case involved very thin, atrophic tissue closely adherent to the underlying palatal bone. Second, whereas the previous cases involved resection or excision with either the fine needle or loop electrode, this case involved combined use of both to perform the biopsy.

PATIENT.   A 61-year-old white female.

HISTORY.   The patient had been wearing a full upper denture for more than 10 years. Two painful sore spots developed on the palate. Relieving the denture did not help. A new denture was constructed which was adequately relieved in the sore areas, but the pain persisted and the sore spots failed to respond to topical medication. She was referred for diagnosis and treatment.

CLINICAL EXAMINATION.   *Extraoral.*   Negative. Medical and family histories: negative.

Intraoral.   The palatal arch was broad with a very shallow vault. A hard bony ridge in the midline extended from the nasopalatine papilla to within 1 cm. of the junction with the soft palate and terminated in a round, slightly bulbous, lobulated mass. Midway between the alveolar ridge and the soft palate junction, just to the left of the bony ridge, there was a desquamated, red oval area measuring 4 mm. in width and 1 cm. in length. A second, smaller desquamated lesion was located at the posterior terminus of the bony ridge (Case Fig. 23–1A). The larger lesion appeared to have been ulcerated for some time. Both areas were very sensitive.

Clinical Diagnosis.   Chronic nonspecific inflammation.

TREATMENT.   The mouth was prepared for surgery and both lesions were anesthetized by circumferential infiltration. A 45-degree-angle fine needle electrode was selected and current output set at 5 for electrosection. The entire posterior lesion with a 2 mm. perimeter of normal tissue was incised circumferentially down to the underlying bone. The incised tissue was undermined, resected and preserved in formalin solution. The larger anterior lesion was also incised to include a 2 mm. perimeter of normal tissue (Case Fig. 23–1B). This tissue was undermined with a periosteal elevator but it adhered very tenaciously to the palatal bone. A 7 mm.-wide, round loop electrode was substituted and current density increased to 9; then the tissue was grasped with an ophthalmic forceps inserted through the eye of the loop and the biopsy tissue was resected from its basal attachment with a wiping stroke (Case Fig. 23–1C). Bleeding produced by undermining the segment was quickly brought under control by pressure with a sterile sponge.

Two pieces of Gelfoam were cut to size, moistened with fresh growth inductor material, medicated with sulfathiazole crystals and Albamycin powder, and inserted into the two surgical defects. Both Gelfoam grafts quickly became saturated with blood present in the defects. When the blood clotted, the areas were covered with adhesive dryfoil and the sterilized denture was inserted as a stent. Albamycin was prescribed systemically for three days and ascorbic acid and clear gelatin were prescribed as dietary supplements.

She returned on the fifth postoperative day and reported that there had been no pain, edema or difficulty in swallowing. Both areas were filled with repair granulation tissue which was beginning to look normal. The palate was irrigated and tincture of myrrh and benzoin was applied. When she was seen again one week later, the palatal defects were almost completely healed. The new tissue filled the two areas, but there

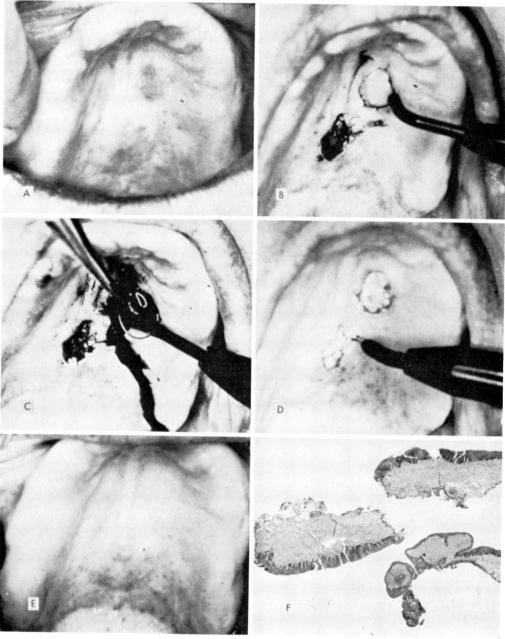

Case Figure 23–1. Combined incisional and loop resection of thin palatal mucosa overlying bony ridge of shallow palatal torus in the midline. *A*, Preoperative appearance of the
palate. There are two areas of inflammation and slight hypertrophy present: one, near the
midline in the approximate center of the palate, and the second in the midline at the junction of
the hard and soft palate on the crest of the midline torus, or sclerotic median suture line. *B*, The
posterior lesion has been incised and resected with little free bleeding. The anterior lesion is
now being incised circumferentially with a 45-degree-angle fine needle electrode. *C*, The incised tissue has been undermined and then grasped with an ophthalmic tissue forceps which
was inserted through the eye of the loop. This tissue is now being resected with the loop electrode. A considerably greater amount of bleeding has resulted with this incision. *D*, Appearance on the twelfth postoperative day. Both defects are well filled with healthy granulation

was a slight difference in the level of the marginal junction of the old and new tissues, creating a slight ledge.

A small ball electrode was selected, current output set at 0.5 for electrocoagulation, and the ledges were reduced by superficial spot coagulation (Case Fig. 23–1D). Tincture of myrrh and benzoin was applied, and use of an astringent salt-alum mouthwash starting three days hence was recommended. She returned one week later. The palatal mucosa was reasonably normal in appearance, and the tissue in the defect areas was harmoniously level with the surrounding mucosa. She was seen at regular weekly intervals for the next six weeks. By the end of that time the palate was so well healed that it was impossible to distinguish the reparative tissue from the surrounding old mucosa in color, texture or tissue tone (Case Fig. 23–1E).

BIOPSY REPORT. Inflammatory tissue with extensive desquamation of surface epithelium (Case Fig. 23–1F).

BIOPSY OF THE FLOOR OF THE MOUTH

CASE 24

This case is an example of loop resection biopsy by electrosection of a lesion in the floor of the mouth.

PATIENT. A 72-year-old white female.

HISTORY. An ulcerated lesion in the floor of the mouth near the mylohyoid ridge had been resistant to routine treatment for one month. She was referred for diagnosis and treatment.

CLINICAL EXAMINATION. *Extraoral.* The patient looked pale, frail and gaunt. There was moderate tenderness and induration in her right submaxillary triangle. Medical history: negative; family history of malignancy.

Intraoral. There was an ulcerated lesion in the floor of the mouth in the right cuspid region. The lesion, approximately 3 mm. wide and 6 mm. long, was located near the lingual aspect of the mandibular alveolar ridge (Case Fig. 24–1A). The mucosa around the lesion was hyperemic, indurated and sore.

Clinical Diagnosis. Granuloma fissuratum (denture sore).

TREATMENT. This type of lesion is one of the most common encountered in the oral cavity. Nevertheless, when accompanied by induration and adenopathy the clinical appearance of this lesion is not incompatible with that of a moderately fungating squamous cell carcinoma. It therefore should not be arbitrarily dismissed and ignored or the tissues discarded. The resected tissue should always be biopsied.

Case Figure 23–1 Continued.
tissue flush to the level of the surrounding mucosa, but both are surrounded by a shallow depressed trench, with the margin of normal surrounding mucosa slightly elevated to form a sharp-line edge. This is reduced by spot coagulation with a small ball electrode. E, Appearance of the palate two months postoperatively. Healing is complete. The palatal tissue is uniformly normal, and there is no visible evidence of the sites of biopsy resection. F, Photomicrograph of segment of the taut thin mucosa resected from over the midline torus.

PLATE VIII

Biopsy

Figure 1a. Biopsy of a small lesion on the vermilion surface of the lower lip by circumferential incisional excision by electrosection with a fine 45-degree-angle needle electrode. Note absence of free hemorrhagic bleeding despite the great vascularity of this tissue.

Figure 1b. The incised mass with its perimeter of normal tissue is being grasped with Allis forceps and is being resected from the underlying tissue with the activated electrode. Note the absence of hemorrhage even at this stage, despite the vascularity and absence of tissue coagulation.

Figure 1c. Postoperative appearance of the lip. The tissue is fully healed, and, owing to the absence of scar tissue contraction, is identical in color, texture, and function to the surrounding tissues. It is also identical in lip contour.

Figure 3a. Removal of two lesions on the hard palate by incisional excision with a fine 45-degree-angle needle electrode. Note the dense sclerotic median torus from which the thin mucosa of the posterior lesion had been removed and the absence of free bleeding from that site as well as the area being incised.

Figure 2a. Biopsy of a lesion from the tongue by loop electrosection. The tongue tissue has been grasped with ophthalmic tissue forceps that have been passed through the eye of the 12-mm. loop to pull it taut to facilitate the resection of the tissue with a single wiping motion.

Figure 2b. Appearance of the tongue immediately after the biopsy resection. Note the absence of bleeding and of tissue coagulation.

Figure 2c. Dorsal and ventral appearance of the biopsy specimen before it was preserved in a formalin fixative solution. Note the absence of any clinical evidence of coagulation even at the periphery of this tissue where it is translucently thin.

Figure 3b. Postoperative appearance of the palate eight weeks later. The palate is fully healed, and the soft, supple repair tissue is so completely normal in all respects that it is impossible to detect the surgical sites.

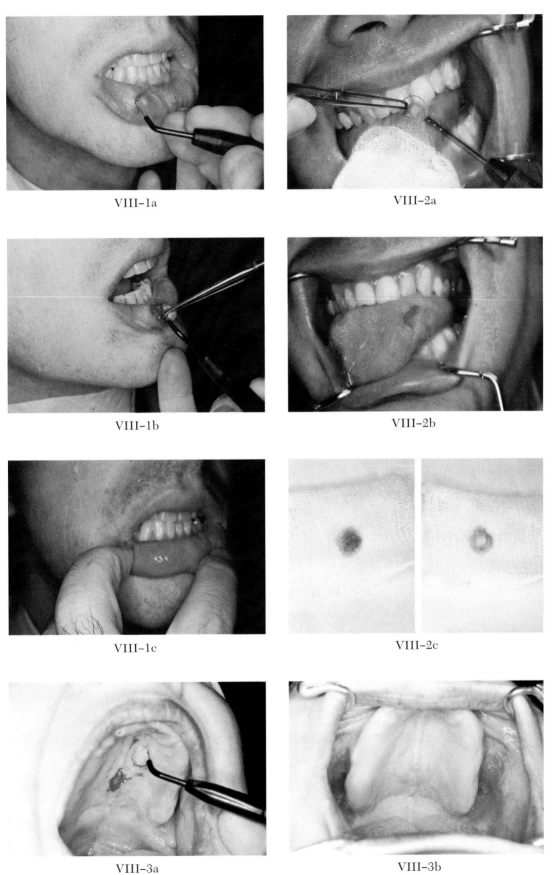

VIII–1a

VIII–2a

VIII–1b

VIII–2b

VIII–1c

VIII–2c

VIII–3a

VIII–3b

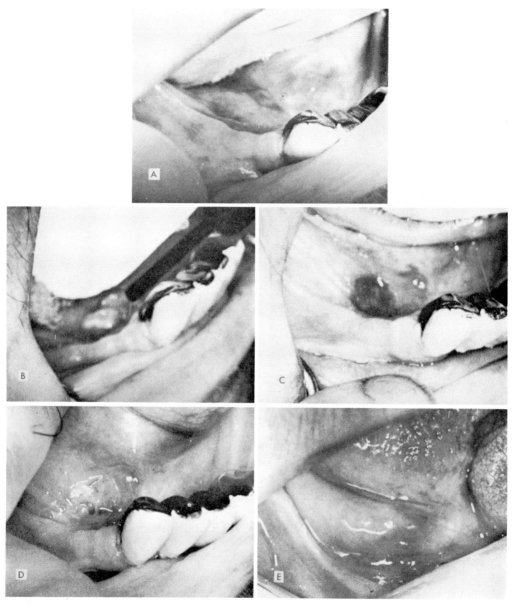

Case Figure 24–1.   Loop resection of a lesion in the floor of the mouth. *A*, Preoperative appearance of the lesion. It is an oval, elevated mass with an ulceration in its center, and is surrounded by an areola of engorgement. *B*, Entire mass is resected with a wiping stroke of a round loop electrode. *C*, Appearance of the surgical defect following resection. There is practically no bleeding, just a slight amount of surface ooze. *D*, Appearance of the tissues on the fifth postoperative day. The surgical defect is filled with healthy granulation tissue and has a surface covering of light coagulum. *E*, Appearance of the surgical defect three weeks postoperatively. The area is completely healed with normal tissue and is virtually indistinguishable from the surrounding normal tissue. There is no cicatricial contraction or other untoward effect.

The mouth was prepared for surgery and circumferential infiltration anesthesia administered. A 7 mm. round loop electrode was selected and current output set at 8 for electrosection. The tissue to be resected was grasped with an ophthalmic tissue forceps that had been inserted through the eye of the loop, and elevated to pull it taut. (Elevation also decreases danger of accidental trauma to salivary ducts in the area.) The lesion with a 2 mm. perimeter of normal tissue was then resected with a wiping stroke of the loop (Case Fig. 24–1*B*). The resected tissue was preserved in formalin. Despite the vascularity of the areolar tissue in the floor of the mouth the procedure was virtually bloodless; only a slight surface ooze of blood resulted (Case Fig. 24–1*C*). The tissue was dried and tincture of myrrh and benzoin applied.

She returned on the fifth postoperative day and reported an uneventful postoperative sequence. The surgical defect was healing very well and the resection site was covered with a healthy thin layer of coagulum (Case Fig. 24–1*D*). Healing progressed rapidly without incident. Within three weeks the area was fully healed, with no cicatricial contraction (Case Fig. 24–1*E*).

BIOPSY REPORT. Granuloma fissuratum.

It is noteworthy how often resection for biopsy serves as the cure at the same time that it provides the tissue for examination.

The next case appeared, on superficial visual oral examination, to resemble closely the clinical appearance of Case 24. However, further examination revealed a significant difference; the local lesion as well as the lymph nodes in the neck was indurated, clinically conclusive evidence of malignancy.

CASE 25

PATIENT.   A 62-year-old white male.

HISTORY: He had been losing weight unaccountably for some time. Recently he noticed a tight lumpy feeling in the floor of the mouth. He consulted a dentist and was referred for diagnosis and treatment.

CLINICAL EXAMINATION. *Extraoral.*   There was visible and palpable indurated adenopathy on the left side of his neck near the submaxillary triangle, and the submaxillary lymph gland also appeared to be enlarged and indurated.

Intraoral.   The oral hygiene of the mouth left much to be desired. A lesion was present on the left side of the floor of the mouth, opposite the bicuspids and first molar. The mass was visible but elevated very slightly. It measured about 1.2 cm. in length, 7 mm. in width, and about 1 mm. in height, but appeared to infiltrate downward. The surface of the mass was slightly ulcerated toward the anterior end. On digital palpation the intraoral mass and the lymph nodes in the neck appeared to be indurated and fixed to the surrounding tissues.

TREATMENT.   All the clinical symptoms suggested that this was a malignant lesion. The cutting current, which usually is set at 3 on the instrument panel for cutting areolar tissue with a fine needle electrode, was increased to 6 to help assure effective hemostasis.

The tissues were prepared, and a regional block inferior alveolar-lingual nerve block injection was administered. The electrode was activated and used to incise and excise a biopsy specimen, which was immediately preserved in a formalin fixative.

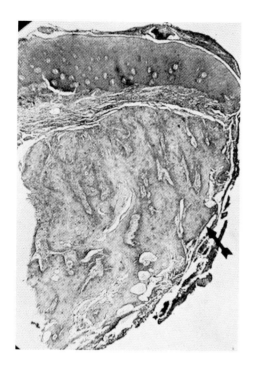

Case Figure 25–1. Photomicrograph of a grade II squamous cell carcinoma of the floor of the mouth. The current output was sharply increased for resection of this tissue, which was clinically diagnosed as a carcinoma. The arrow points to the layer of cells destroyed in the process of resection, an indication that the amount of current in excess of need is not nearly as important as the manner in which the instrumentation is performed.

The tissue in the bed from which the tissue was taken was sprayed thoroughly with sparks from fulgurating current to destroy any malignant cells that might be present there and thus to prevent surgical metastasis.

The biopsy report confirmed the clinical diagnosis; the tissue was described as squamous cell carcinoma, grade II. The patient's physician was advised of this and he concurred that cobalt irradiation might prove more effective at this stage than a commando procedure.

The patient was referred to a radiotherapist for the cobalt therapy, and at the latter's request the clinical photographs and biopsy specimen slide were sent to him. Unfortunately, he died several months later, and neither the photos nor biopsy specimen was recovered. Fortunately, the author had received two biopsy tissue slides from the Institute of Clinical Oral Pathology, and thus at least a photomicrograph of the tissue specimen was available for illustration here (Case Fig. 25–1).

The patient survived for slightly more than two years after completion of the cobalt irradiation.

BIOPSY OF THE TONGUE

Of the many advantages electrosurgery offers the therapist performing biopsy, by far the most important is the hemostasis that inherently accompanies electrosection without causing cellular coagulation necrosis or cellular alteration or distortion.

This advantage takes on added significance when the biopsy is to be performed on a highly vascular structure such as the lip or tongue for two reasons:

First, it eliminates, or at the very least, drastically reduces the hazard of encountering profound hemorrhage that would require a carotid tie-off to control. Second, and more important, it eliminates or greatly minimizes the danger of causing surgical metastasis of malignant tumor cells directly into the severed blood and lymph vessels in the surgical field.

When the biopsy is performed with a large round loop electrode there occasionally appears to be a split-second time lag between the initial contact of the activated electrode with the tissue and full output of the cutting energy. In the infrequent instances when this momentary time lag occurs, it merely causes coagulation of the top two or three layers of cells at the site of initial tissue contact. This should not be confused with coagulation necrosis of a substantial portion of the tissue, such as occurs when the electrosurgery is performed improperly or when an unsuitable current has been used. The remainder of the tissue specimen and the surface tissue in the surgical defect created by the removal are as free of coagulation or cellular alteration as is tissue removed with steel scalpel or biopsy punch.

In the vast majority of cases when the biopsy is properly performed with suitable cutting energy, regardless of the kind of electrode used, there is no histologic evidence of cellular damage, even when part of the cell wall has been sheared off from individual cells in the line of cleavage.

CASE 26

PATIENT.   A 34-year-old white male.

HISTORY.   The patient was a dentist. He suddenly became aware of a hard mass on the edge of the left side of his tongue. Aware that this is a common site for cancer of the tongue, he immediately arranged for diagnosis and treatment.

CLINICAL EXAMINATION.   On the lateral border of the left side of the tongue, approximately two-thirds posteriorly from the tip, there was a round pink-white, firm, elevated mass about 0.5 cm. in diameter, on a sessile base (Case Fig. 26–1A). Palpation for adenopathy or induration was negative.

TREATMENT.   The tongue was grasped with a sterile sponge and pulled taut. The biopsy site was prepared for surgery; topical anesthetic was applied and followed with circumferential infiltration anesthesia. A round loop electrode 1.2 cm. in diameter, large enough to permit resection of the lesion and a 3 mm. perimeter of normal tissue, was selected, and the cutting current power output dial was set at 8 on the Coles Radiosurg Scalpel IV. The fine rat-tooth tips of an ophthalmic tissue forcep were inserted through the eye of the loop and used to grasp the normal tissue immediately adjacent to the lesion to lift the tissue and pull it taut. The entire mass with its perimeter of normal tissue was resected with one wiping stroke of the activated loop (Case Fig. 26–1B).

The external margin and ventral surface of the tissue specimen were completely free of coagulation, and except for the distinguishing contour and symmetry of the tissue, it was indistinguishable from tissue cut with a steel scalpel (Case Fig. 26–2A). The surface of the surgical defect also was totally free of coagulation and was covered with blood, but there was no free bleeding (Case Fig. 26–1C).

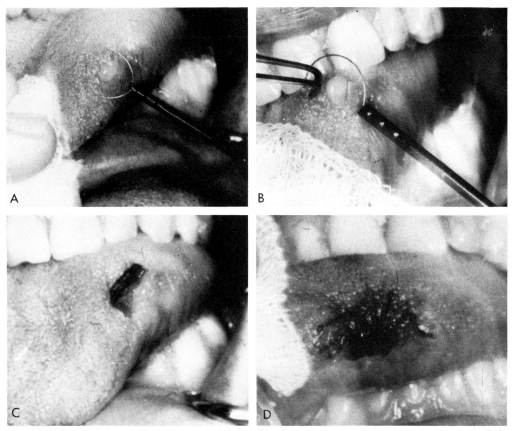

Case Figure 26–1.   Loop resection from the tongue. *A*, Preoperative appearance of the lesion. A hard sessile mass is present on the dorsal surface of the tongue near the lateral border about halfway from the tip to the base of the organ. A 14 mm. round loop electrode is being placed over the mass to determine whether it is large enough to enable resection of a 2- to 3-mm. perimeter of normal tissue with the mass. *B*, The beaks of a 90-degree curved ophthalmic tissue forceps have been inserted through the eye of the loop electrode and are grasping the perimeter tissue to pull it taut as the activated electrode is cutting into the tongue. Despite the tremendous vascularity of the tongue, there is no bleeding. *C*, Immediate postoperative appearance of the tongue. As the traction on the tongue with the finger grasp on the organ with a sterile sponge has been released, the tongue has contracted somewhat, pulling the round excision wound into an elliptical shape. Note that despite the total absence of free bleeding the tissue in the bed from which the mass was removed is normal in color, and there is no evidence of tissue coagulation. *D*, The margins of the wound have been coapted into a straight line and sutured with interrupted silk sutures. As the tongue tissue is pierced by the suture needle it begins to bleed.

The biopsy tissue having been placed in a fixative solution, the marginal tissue of the surgical defect was undermined slightly to facilitate coaptation. The coapted tissue was sutured with 4-0 braided silk interrupted sutures. Although there had been no free bleeding from removal of the tissue specimen, there was free bleeding from the suture needle puncture sites (Case Fig. 26–1*D*).

Healing progressed uneventfully, and the sutures were removed on the fifth postoperative day. Within two weeks there was no visible evidence of the surgery that had been performed.

BIOPSY REPORT.   Fibroma of the tongue (Case Fig. 26–3).

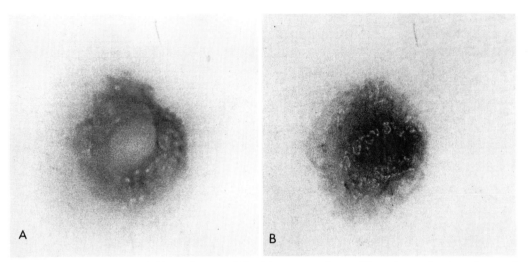

Case Figure 26–2.   A, Dorsal view of the biopsy specimen. Note the perimeter of normal tissue around the mass. B, Ventral view of the biopsy specimen. Note the total absence of clinical evidence of coagulation of the tissue, even along the very thin outer margin.

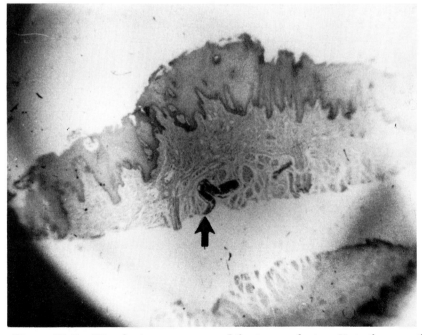

Case Figure 26–3.   Histologic appearance of the tongue lesion. Note the smooth line of cleavage and absence of coagulation along the incised edge. Note the sealed capillary (arrow), proving that hemostasis accompanies the cutting.

EXTRAORAL INCISIONAL EXCISION AND LOOP BIOPSY BY ELECTROSECTION

In dentistry, electrosurgical incisions usually involve mucous membranes. There are isolated instances where extraoral incisions through the skin are required.

CASE 27

This case is included to demonstrate the efficacy of electrosection for cutaneous incisions and extraoral biopsy.

PATIENT. A 79-year-old white male.

HISTORY. The patient was actively engaged in dental practice until a few weeks previously. Sudden rapid physical deterioration with sharp loss of weight compelled him to "temporarily" retire and go to a nursing home. While there he developed severe abdominal pains which he blamed on change of diet. Three days later a huge mass suddenly appeared on the lower left side of his face. He returned home. Since he was a colleague and personal acquaintance he consulted the author about his "abscess."

CLINICAL EXAMINATION. *Extraoral.* He looked cachectic and was very feeble. A mass approximately 7 cm. long and roughly oval in shape bulged out on the left side of his face. It extended about one half the full length of the left body of the mandible, and from 1 cm. above the inferior border of the mandible downward to the submaxillary area, involving the entire submaxillary triangle (Case Fig. 27–1A).

The mass was rubbery in consistency and markedly indurated. There were many large palpable lymph nodes in the left side of his neck and side of the face. These were all immovably fixed to the surrounding structures. He complained of weakness and malaise.

Clinical Diagnosis. Metastatic carcinoma or lymphosarcoma of the submaxillary gland.

TREATMENT. The patient, a very headstrong individual, insisted the lesion was of dental origin and refused to be hospitalized; he did consent to have it treated at the author's office. Two nephews, his only living relatives, requested that he be humored so that a biopsy could be obtained.

The skin was shaved and prepared for surgery and the head draped; then circumferential infiltration anesthesia was administered. A 45-degree-angle moderately fine needle electrode was selected and current output set at 5.5 for electrosection.

The skin, superficial fascia, deep fascia and platysma muscle were incised with a wiping motion of the activated electrode. The incision was extended 5 cm., and as larger blood vessels were traversed they were clamped with mosquito hemostats. Bleeding from all but two of the severed vessels was stopped by electrocoagulation off the beaks of the hemostats with a large ball electrode and current density set at 3 for biterminal application.

The two larger vessels had to be tied off with chromic gut. When bleeding was brought under complete control the margins of the incisions were spread wide, exposing a large mass which was encapsulated in a grayish white, fibrous-looking capsule.

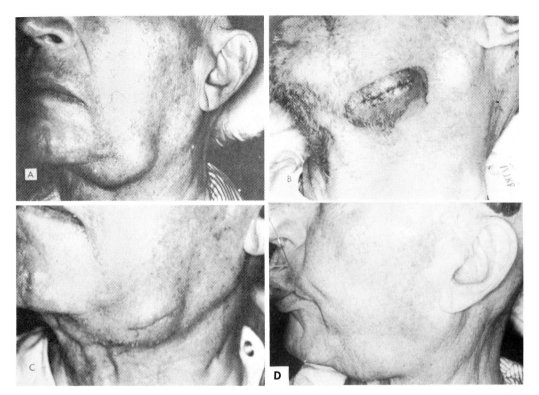

Case Figure 27-1. Extraoral cutaneous incision with fine needle electrode for biopsy of submandibular lymph nodes (reticulum cell sarcoma). *A,* Preoperative appearance of submandibular lesion. There are palpable lymph nodes in the pre-auricular region, at the angle of the jaw and on the lateral aspect of the neck. *B,* Postoperative appearance on fifth day with sutures still in position. Dark brown discoloration is tincture of myrrh and benzoin applied in air-dried layers. *C,* Appearance on tenth postoperative day. Healing is by primary intention. The darker pink color of the repair tissue and slight indentation along the original incision line make this line appear darker. *D,* Appearance by the end of the fifth week. The incision is completely healed and no longer visible. Adenopathy is greatly reduced in response to chemotherapy.

The capsule was incised and its cut margins retracted, exposing a resilient solid mass of cream-white tissue like latex.

A large U-shaped loop electrode was substituted and current density increased to 8 for electrosection. Two segments of this tissue were resected with scooping strokes of the electrode, one segment from the anterior third of the mass and the other from the posterior third. These were preserved in formalin. The neoplasm was avascular and there was no bleeding from it. The wound was closed in layers, each respective deep layer being sutured with chromic gut; then the surface skin incision was closed with interrupted silk sutures. The operative field was painted with tincture of myrrh and benzoin; then a sulfathiazole-impregnated petroleum jelly gauze dressing was applied as a pressure bandage and heavily taped to the face with adhesive tape.

BIOPSY REPORT. Reticulum cell sarcoma (Case Fig. 27–2A).

The patient was immediately hospitalized at the Mount Sinai Hospital, New York, and placed under the care of a hematologist and an internist. Blood transfusions and nitrogen mustard therapy produced immediate but temporary improvement. By the fifth day post-biopsy, healing by primary union was sufficiently advanced to permit removal of the skin sutures (Case Fig. 27–1B). The submandibular mass was getting noticeably smaller but many additional lymph nodes were plainly visible, widely distributed on the left side of his body.

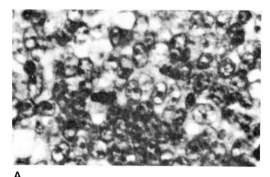

A

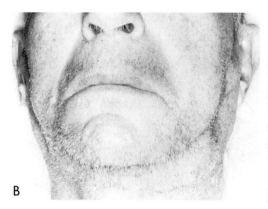

B

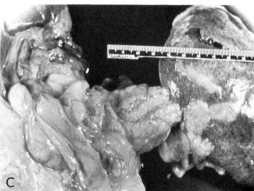

C

Case Figure 27–2. A, Photomicrograph (high power) of the resected tissue. Note the bizarre disarray of the cellular arrangement and contents that characterizes reticulum cell sarcoma. (Special staining by the late Dr. Otani of Mt. Sinai Hospital, New York.) *B,* Appearance of the facial wound one day before the demise of the patient. The wound is completely healed despite the terminal state of the patient. *C,* Autopsy specimens show massive invasion of the vital organs. The fact that the facial wound was able to heal gives eloquent testimony to the remarkable healing qualities of electrosurgical wounds.

Shortly after systemic therapy was initiated he rallied dramatically. By the tenth day the incision was fully healed and inconspicuous except for the pink color of the line of incision (Case Fig. 27–1C). By the end of the second week his adenopathy was almost fully subsided. He continued to react favorably for the next three weeks, at which time the blood transfusions were discontinued. Suddenly the adenopathy recurred more extensively than ever, with massive nodes in the preauricular, cervical, axillary and inguinal regions of his left side. He deteriorated very rapidly thereafter and died at the end of the seventh week of hospitalization. Case Figure 27–2C shows two autopsy specimens of his vital organs. Both gross specimens show massive invasion that has replaced about two-thirds of the normal tissue with malignant cells. That normal healing occurred in this patient is an indication of the favorable tissue response to electrosurgery.

Two features of this case are noteworthy. One is the fact that the huge mass from which the biopsy was obtained consisted of the submaxillary and submandibular lymph nodes, apparently fused by their enlargement, and did not involve the submaxillary gland at all. The other feature is that the skin and underlying tissues incised by electrosection healed rapidly and favorably despite the patient's weakened state.

A representative number of cases have been reported in this chapter to describe a variety of biopsy techniques, anatomic sites and types of pathology. (Figures 24–5 and 24–6 have been included as typical examples of biopsies obtained by incisional excision with a fine needle electrode, and loop resection of a small mass.) Many other excellent examples had to be omitted for

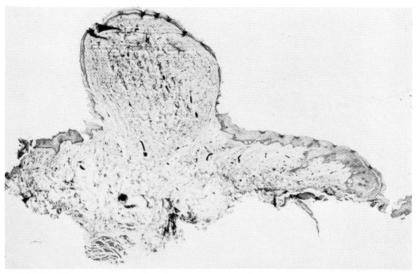

Figure 24–5. Photomicrograph of tissue resected in Figure 24–1. Note almost total lack of cellular destruction along lines of electrosurgical incision.

lack of suitable operative photographs and lack of space. The electrosurgical and histopathologic characteristics of some are too significant and interrelated to be ignored. They shall be reviewed briefly and their photomicrographs included for evaluation.

The first of these is a case of a papilloma overlying a mucous cyst.[7] In this case, although the electrode passed within a few microns of the extremely thin cyst wall, neither this tissue nor the mucous threads trapped in the cystic cavity were affected (Fig. 24–7).

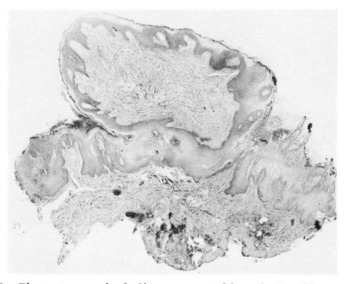

Figure 24–6. Photomicrograph of a fibroma resected from the tip of the tongue with a loop electrode. Note that only a single layer of cells along the base of the biopsy specimen was destroyed by the activated electrode.

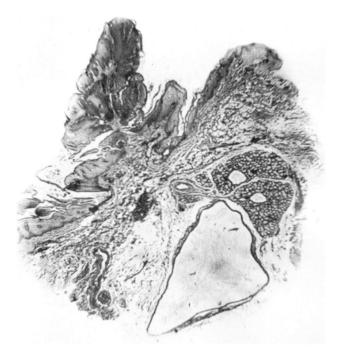

Figure 24–7. Photomicrograph of a papilloma overlying a mucous cyst. Note that neither the extremely thin membranous sac nor the mucinous contents of the cyst were affected by passage of the activated loop electrode just microns away. Note regular contour of tissue specimen.

Another is a case of cystic adenoma of the buccal mucosa. Ability to incise tissue with sharp, clean-cut edges free of coagulation and without affecting the thin cystic wall or contents of the cyst is well demonstrated in Figure 24–8.

Another case involved biopsy resection of a mixed tumor of the retromo-

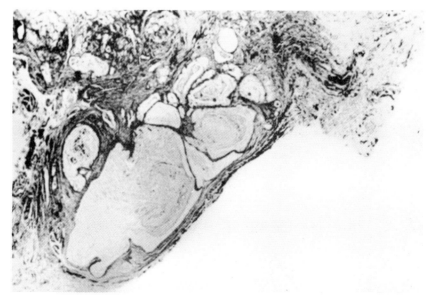

Figure 24–8. Photomicrograph of an adenomatous cyst of the buccal mucosa. Note the sharp-line angles of the tissue achieved by incisional resection with fine needle electrode.

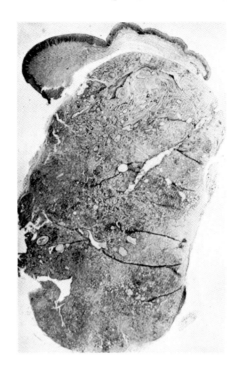

Figure 24-9. Photomicrograph of a mixed tumor of the retromolar pad. The tissue was resected with a loop electrode. Note intact capsule around the tumor.

lar pad. This case demonstrates the ability to loop resect a mass without damage to the thin capsule of the tumor (Fig. 24-9).

The next case is interesting as a rather rare oral lesion,[8] but it is especially interesting for its vivid demonstration of the value of including a perimeter of normal tissue with the biopsy specimen. The case was a Ewing's sarcoma of the mandible. The dramatic contrast created by tumor tissue contiguous to normal tissue is admirably demonstrated in Figure 24-10. The photomicro-

Figure 24-10. Photomicrograph of a Ewing's sarcoma of the mandibular gingival mucosa (soft tissue extension from alveolar sarcoma). This photomicrograph vividly demonstrates the advantage of inclusion of a perimeter of normal tissue with the neoplasm. In addition to offering a basis of contrast between the normal and pathologic cells, it also affords an opportunity to determine whether metastasis has actively begun. Arrows point to malignant nidi, indicating metastasis by direct extension.

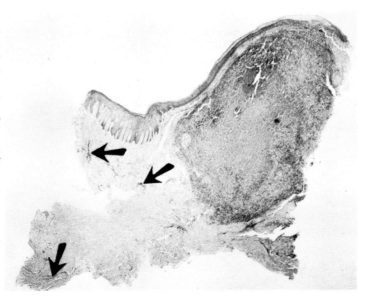

graph offers further evidence of the ability to cut tissue atraumatically by electrosection with sharp clean lines of cleavage that are free of coagulation.

FOOTNOTE REFERENCES

1. Brown, J. B., and Frayer, M. P.: Surgical Treatment of Cancer of the Lip. In Pack, G. T., and Ariel, I. M.: Treatment of Cancer and Allied Diseases. Vol. III. 2nd ed. New York, Paul B. Hoeber, Inc., 1959, p. 65.
2. Bernier, J. L.: The Management of Oral Diseases. 2nd ed., St. Louis, C. V. Mosby Co., 1959.
3. Shafer, W. G., Hine, M. K., and Levy, B. M.: A Textbook of Oral Pathology. Philadelphia, W. B. Saunders Co., 1958.
4. Color Atlas of Oral Pathology: Squamous cell carcinoma of alveolar ridge. Philadelphia, J. B. Lippincott Company, 1956, p. 151.
5. Shira, R. B.: Diagnosis of common lesions of the oral cavity. J. Oral Surg., *15*(2):95–119, Apr., 1957.
6. Zegarelli, E. V., Kutscher, A. H., Herlands, R. E., Lucca, J. J., and Silvers, H. F.: Oral lesions of interest to the prosthodontist. Part I. Denture stomatitis. J. Prosthet. Den., *2*(4):617–620, July-Aug., 1961.
7. Oringer, M. J.: Safeguarding biopsy by use of electronic electrosurgery. J. Oral Surg., *15*:129–137, April, 1957.
8. Conley, J. J.: The Treatment of Tumors of the Mandible, in Pack, G. T., and Ariel, I. M.: Treatment of Cancer and Allied Diseases. Vol. III. 2nd ed. New York, Paul B. Hoeber, Inc., 1959, p. 263.

ADVANCED ORAL CANCER

Chapter Twenty-Five

TREATMENT OF ADVANCED ORAL CANCER BY ELECTROCOAGULATION

Although the frequency of incidence of oral and pharyngeal cancer is low in comparison with the major cancer sites of the body, the incidence of morbidity from the cancers in this area is one of the highest despite the accessibility and visibility of the oral cavity. This abnormally high morbidity rate is largely due to the appallingly short pathway for metastasis from the oral cavity directly to two major portals of entry into the main bloodstream.

In the early years of this century electrocoagulation was used extensively for definitive treatment of malignant lesions. Electrocoagulation was referred to at that time as cauterization, or surgical diathermy.[1-4] In the oral cavity this method was used mostly to treat early lesions in the anterior part of the mouth.

In time surgery, particularly the introduction and subsequent advancing scope of the radical composite resection referred to as the heroic "commando" procedure, combined with postoperative use of radiation therapy, became the accepted method of treatment, and electrocoagulation fell into disuse.

RATIONALE OF TREATMENT

If oral cancer, despite being in an active state of metastasis, is considered operable, the combination of composite radical surgery followed by postoperative x-ray or cobalt irradiation therapy is usually employed.

The composite surgery, the heroic commando procedure, consists of dissection through the midline of the lower lip and chin, down the lateral midline of the neck and along the inferior border of the mandible, so that these tissues can be reflected to provide access to the contents of the digastric

1089

triangle and the sternomastoid muscle (see Case Fig. 1–1A). This makes possible resection of the submental and submaxillary lymph nodes, contents of the digastric triangle, the sternomastoid muscle, and the superficial and deep cervical chains of lymph nodes and, if involved, half of the mandible or tongue on the affected side, in the all too often vain attempt to prevent metastatic tumor cells from reaching the main bloodstream via the left thoracic duct or right subclavian vein.

Despite the radical thoroughness of this mutilating surgical procedure cancer statistics reveal that only 16 per cent of these patients achieve the 5 year survival rate that is considered optimal. This discouragingly low survival rate emphasizes dramatically the importance of early diagnosis and treatment.

It also adds greatly to the significance of a scholarly report by Drs. Merrill and Hoar, two M.D.–D.D.S. staff members of a Veterans Administration Hospital. Published in *Surgery* (November, 1962), the report describes their success in treatment of advanced oral cancer *with an extraordinarily high survival rate*.[5] Their paper reported their use of electrocoagulation to treat cases, many of which were deemed inoperable by other methods owing to advanced metastasis and extensive anatomic involvement. They found this method of treatment advantageous for a variety of reasons, most notably because it provides excellent control of the primary lesion, a lower rate of morbidity, and minimal disfigurement.

They reported successful treatment of an impressive number of advanced "inoperable" cases by partial destruction of the malignant tissue by electrocoagulation followed by irradiation similar to the dosage administered following surgery. Although anatomic limitations often limited the destruction to only two-thirds to three-quarters of the malignant masses by electrocoagulation, they found that the remaining untreated portions and metastatic lymph nodes subsequently underwent spontaneous regression, with no recurrences or need for renewed treatment over as long a period of postoperative observation as 12 years. Their results present a dramatic, hopeful contrast to the extremely poor survival prognosis for treatment of cancers, often less advanced, by the mutilating commando surgical resections.

The same issue of this journal featured a guest editorial commenting on the paper by Merrill and Hoar. This rarity in medical literature is indicative of the importance attributed to the report by the journal's editorial board. Dr. Alton Ochsner, Director of the famous Ochsner Clinic of New Orleans, was the guest editorialist.[6] He related the remarkable success that his late father, founder of the clinic that bears his name, and his father's colleagues had enjoyed with treatment of advanced cancer of the breast and other body sites by electrocoagulation. He deplored the fact that electrocoagulation has to a great extent become "a lost art" in medical surgery and stressed that the Merrill-Hoar use of electrocoagulation is not a new concept or technique, although it had been referred to earlier as cauterization, or surgical diathermy.

Dr. Ochsner concluded his editorial with a report of the results of a number of independent research investigations of the phenomenon of spontaneous regression of the untreated portions of metastatic malignancies.[7-10] Each of these investigators had arrived at the same conclusion — the regressions appeared to be attributable to an antigen-antibody reaction induced by the electrocoagulation, and this antigen-antibody reaction destroys the abnormal cells without ill effects on the normal cells of the body.

As early as 1929, Kolischer postulated that "destruction of carcinomas with cautery antibodies and the presence of the destroyed malignant cells result in development of antibodies which tend to control lesions not affected by the cautery and even metastatic ones."[7] Two years later, Henscher suggested the same theory because he had observed that the lymph nodes were destroyed after cautery of the original tumor and that the original tumor, although not completely destroyed by the cauterization, frequently disappeared. He too attributed this to development of the antibody which controls the remaining malignant cells.[8]

Alfred A. Strauss, who was reputed to have done more than anyone else to emphasize the importance of destruction of malignant tumors, particularly of the rectum, by electrocoagulation, reported as early as 1933, and in subsequent reports emphasized the value of electric cautery (electrocoagulation) for destruction of malignant tumors of the rectum.[10-12] He observed that, "although the tumor may not be completely destroyed, regression occurs, the tumor subsequently disappears, and metastatic lymph nodes become sterile."

In 1935, he reported two occasions when, several years after surgical diathermy (electrocoagulation), patients were subjected to laparotomy because of a bladder disturbance. Several large lymph nodes which were removed from the pelvis contained what appeared to be poorly staining dead carcinoma cells. He stated that he thought this indicated at least the possibility that the macrophage and reticuloendothelial reaction produced by the diathermy had destroyed the cancer cells in the regional lymph glands or rendered them inactive. The following year he and his associates reported that in a study of 73 patients with cancer of the rectum and colon treated by surgical diathermy, 52 did not require colostomy.

In addition to this purely clinical evidence there is also some supportive experimental evidence that antibodies are developed as a result of electrocoagulation of malignant tumors. In 1956, Strauss injected the Brown-Pearce carcinoma into both testicles of mongrel rabbits and Belgian hares, and at the same time pushed one testicle through the inguinal canal into the abdomen. Tumors developed in both testicles, one in the abdomen, and one in the scrotum. Upon opening the abdomen between the 14th and 21st days, he found bloody fluid and large miliary abscesses. After coagulating two-thirds of the intra-abdominal tumors, the testicular tumor in the scrotum disappeared within 3 to 6 weeks, and when the abdomen was reopened no evidence of metastasis was found. Sixty of 400 animals treated in this manner survived more than two years and were reinoculated every few months with tumors, but no tumors developed subsequently. In 1959, using white rats, he coagulated spontaneous breast cancers in the center, similar to the core of an apple, and closed the skin. After 10 to 14 days, the tumors became soft and gradually absorbed. Of the animals that lived for almost a year, none had recurrence of carcinoma of the breast.

Lewis and his colleagues observed immunity with rat sarcoma after interference with the blood supply to the sarcoma.[9] The tumor disappeared after the blood supply was ligated. The same sarcoma was reimplanted into the animals; of the 50 rats so treated, no tumors grew in 44. In the other six animals the tumor sloughed off completely, so that there was none left behind from which antibodies might presumably be produced.

Anyone who has had experience with treatment of suppuration in extremely ill patients with malignant disease by electrocoagulation of the tumors cannot help feeling greatly impressed by the well-being of the patient immediately after treatment. Elderly patients in particular withstand destruction of malignant tumors by electrocoagulation much better than they tolerate the surgery necessary to eradicate the disease by means of sharp scalpel dissection.[6]

In view of these advantages and the advantages described by Merrill and Hoar that electrocoagulation provides excellent control of the primary lesion, a lower morbidity rate, minimal disfigurement, and minimal functional impairment in contrast to the mutilating disfigurement and the very low cure rate from radical commando surgery, electrocoagulation would normally not have been replaced by the composite surgery procedure had it not been for two unfavorable factors. One is the essential need for technical skill and know-how for proper effective clinical use of electrocoagulation. The other is the grave hazard of severe postoperative hemorrhage that it entailed.

Merrill and Hoar pinpointed the reason for the first of these two factors: "This method [electrocoagulation] is so simple and direct that surgeons are tempted to use it without previous experience. Understandably poor results make them critically outspoken against this method."

The second factor relates to the methodology or technique of the electrocoagulation. The latter usually is performed with high density coagulating current provided by the very powerful hospital-size electrosurgical units, and the potent current is applied to the tissues with a Francine disc electrode. This application produces rapid, deeply penetrating electrocoagulation that quickly and very effectively destroys the malignant tissue. All the blood vessels in the area, large and small, are destroyed in the process, and there is no bleeding to indicate their destruction, so they are not tied off. The tissues subsequently heal under the coagulum, and when healing is complete, the coagulum sloughs out spontaneously.

As the healing progresses under the coagulum, blood vessels that have been destroyed also repair, but the new repair tissue often is too frail to withstand the pressure of the blood as it flows through and is likely to rupture, causing spontaneous hemorrhage. If a large blood vessel is involved, and if a carotid tie-off cannot be performed in time, hemorrhagic exsanguination may occur.

Both these factors can be effectively eliminated, the first by acquiring the training to develop the special skill and know-how that are essential for electrosurgery, including electrocoagulation, to be used efficiently and effectively, and the second by utilizing a technique refinement developed by the author for destroying the malignant tissue in layers instead of in depth. This can be easily accomplished by use of the much less powerful and thus less penetrating coagulating current provided by one of the efficient smaller "dental" types of electrosurgical units. An efficient circuit can provide ample coagulating current for effective controlled use. Owing to the more reduced potency and more limited penetration, this coagulating current permits the therapist to control the depth of penetration and thus to become aware instantly when a large blood vessel has been involved in the coagulation.

MODIFIED ELECTROCOAGULATING TECHNIQUE

The larger dental round ball coagulating electrode is best suited for this procedure. This electrode requires approximately twice the amount of current output required for coagulation with the small ball electrode. The electrode is applied to the tissues for 2 to 3 seconds at a time and then is moved to the immediately adjacent tissue rather than scraping back and forth over the entire area. The spot by spot application of the current permits the surgeon to control the depth of penetration at a uniform level and is repeated until the entire surface of the affected area has been treated. A loop electrode, either the medium-diameter round loop or medium-width 45-degree-angle U-shaped loop, is then used with a light brushing motion to shave off most of the coagulum in thin layers. The electrode may be activated with cutting current, but it is best to use the cutting electrode with the *coagulating* current and the same amount of coagulating current power output as would be used for electrosection.

The alternate spot coagulation and shaving off of coagulum in layers are continued until as much of the malignant mass as is deemed feasible has been destroyed and removed. If any large blood vessels are affected by the coagulation they can be readily located when the major portion of the coagulum is sheared off with the loop. The clinical evidence of bleeding alerts the operator and the bleeder can be immediately tied off to avert postoperative hemorrhage. If the electrocoagulation has been performed in this manner there is no spontaneous hemorrhage to be feared from blood vessels in the area when the coagulum sloughs out after the underlying tissue has healed, and healing can progress uneventfully.

The efficacy of this method is demonstrated admirably by the following case report of a patient treated at the St. Francis Hospital Oral Cancer Detection and Prevention Center of Poughkeepsie, New York, by Wallace Bedell, M.D., Melvin Engelman, D.D.S., and S. Joel Schackner, D.D.S., and their staff.[13]

CASE 1

PATIENT. A 54-year-old white female.

HISTORY. A commando procedure with hemimandilectomy had been performed for the patient about 6 months previously by Dr. Bedell to remove an actively metastasizing squamous cell carcinoma from the right mandible (Case Figs. 1–1A and B). Two weeks previously a new mass suddenly appeared on the lingual gingiva around the cuspid tooth on the opposite side (Case Figs. 1–1C and D).

CLINICAL EXAMINATION. Biopsy proved the new mass also was a squamous cell carcinoma similar to the earlier lesion. Malignant lesions are thought to be unilateral and not likely to cross the midline of the body. In this case it appeared likely, however, in view of the subsequent findings, that this was a metastatic lesion rather than a second primary lesion in the same mouth. Since in addition to the external disfigurement it would have been necessary to resect the remaining half of the mandible, and considering that the previous commando procedure apparently had been unsuccessful, it was decided to treat the new mass by the more conservative method of electrocoagulation followed by irradiation rather than to subject the patient to a second commando procedure.

TREATMENT. The patient was prepared, anesthetized, and draped in the operatory, and electrocoagulation was begun with a large dental ball electrode and current provided by a Coles Radiosurg Scalpel IV electrosurgical unit (Case Fig. 1–2A).

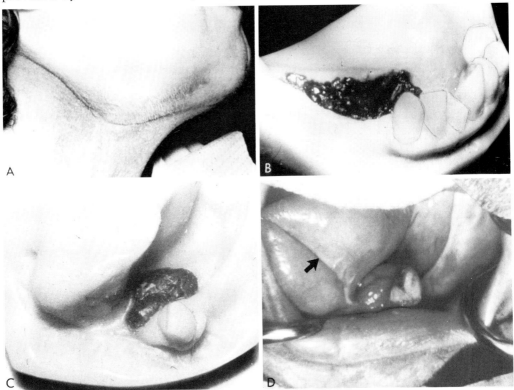

Case Figure 1–1. A, Preoperative: External, lateral view. Scar extends from midline of lower lip posteriorly along submandibular region along the inferior border of the jaw and terminates posteriorly slightly behind the neck; a second, joining scar extends downward from the angle of the jaw to the clavicle, along the line created by the sternomastoid muscle—classic scars of the heroic "commando" procedure. *B*, A model depicting appearance and site of the original carcinoma on the opposite (right) side of the jaw. *C*, Preoperative study model of new mass. *D*, Intraoral. The left cuspid is the sole remaining tooth in the mandible. There is a large bulging friable looking mass on the lingual aspect of the tooth, extending around to and beyond the distal of the tooth. The right side of the tongue is tied down to the floor of the mouth by scar adhesions from the previous commando surgery (arrow).

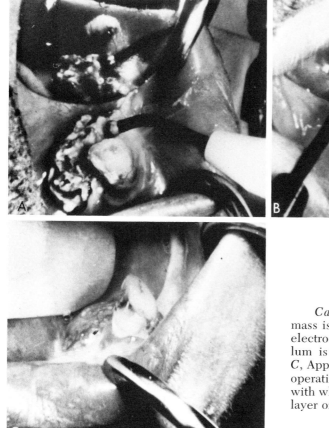
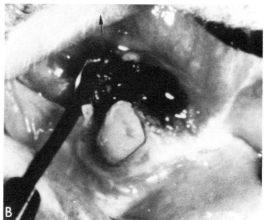

Case Figure 1–2. A, Operative: The mass is being coagulated with a large ball electrode. *B,* The major part of the coagulum is being removed by electrosection. *C,* Appearance of the tissue on tenth postoperative day. The surgical field is covered with what appears to be a moderately thick layer of reparative coagulation.

When all the tissue had been coagulated to a depth of approximately 3 mm., all but the basal portion of the coagulum was resected with a round loop electrode by electrosection (Case Fig. 1–2*B*).

The alternate procedures of coagulation and resection in layers were repeated until the entire mass was destroyed and removed, and the surface of the mandible was then also treated by superficial electrocoagulation. The patient suffered only mild postoperative discomfort, and healing progressed uneventfully (Case Fig. 1–2*C*).

About three months later the patient's condition began to deteriorate rapidly and one month later she expired at Memorial Hospital, New York. An autopsy performed at that institution revealed that metastasis from the original cancerous lesion had invaded and involved most of her vital organs, but the area that had been treated by electrocoagulation was found to be completely free of malignant cells.[14]

Although this case did not require only partial destruction of the malignant mass, the technique involved was the same as it would be for such cases. In view of the research reports that an antigen-antibody reaction appears to be induced by electrocoagulation, similar treatment of a major portion of a large carcinomatous mass and leaving the inoperable remainder untreated appears to offer far better prognosis for successful cure than the mutilating heroic commando surgery, and performing it by the author's combined coagulation-excision technique as described virtually eliminates the hazard of dangerous postoperative hemorrhage.

The author recently had an opportunity to employ the alternate coagulation-excision technique, while in Montreal, Canada, conducting an electrosurgery course.

This case demonstrates the incredible advantages of this technique when the anatomic location of a lesion makes its surgical excision not only difficult but extremely hazardous and would result at best in extensive functional and aesthetic impairment, when conservative treatment by irradiation therapy alone would be of highly questionable efficacy and when massive uncontrolled electrocoagulation would be very likely to result in severe spontaneous postoperative hemorrhage.

(This case report differs in one important respect from other reports in this text. The author did not have photographic equipment with him when he was unexpectedly invited to treat this patient. With the exception of the photomicrographs of the biopsy specimen removed by the author by loop electrosection immediately before definitive treatment was instituted, the report is entirely verbal and without the benefit of the step by step operative illustrations that are normally included in the reports. However, the photomicrographs of the biopsy specimens do provide histologic evidence of the totally self-limiting destruction that makes possible superbly efficient electronic biopsy.)

CASE 2

PATIENT.   A 39-year-old white female.

HISTORY.   While hospitalized for medical reasons, a routine oral examination was performed on her by the oral surgery resident. He found a small ulcerated somewhat fungating lesion on the crest of the maxillary right tuberosity. He also noted that her tongue appeared somewhat limited in mobility, and on palpation detected a slight amount of induration at the posterior right lateral border of the tongue but found no clinically visible lesion to account for it. The patient was totally asymptomatic with regard to pain or even discomfort.

One week earlier the attending oral surgeon removed the maxillary lesion by steel scalpel excision for biopsy evaluation. He also found a small lesion at the right lateral extreme posterior border of the tongue by grasping the organ and extending it forcefully as far forward as he could pull it with his fingers.

Since there were multiple lesions, and on the basis of their clinical appearance, he suspected the possibility that these might be metastatic, with a primary lesion in the lung. He therefore ordered a bronchoscopic examination to rule out the possibility of pulmonary carcinoma, and planned to perform a biopsy on the tongue lesion while she was under nasopharyngeal general anesthesia for the bronchoscopy. The attending oral surgeon was one of the course participants, and, although personally untrained in electrosurgery, recognized its potential value in this case. He therefore invited the author to perform the biopsy and, if indicated, definitive treatment by the electrocoagulation technique that had been described to the class by the author.

CLINICAL EXAMINATION.   The patient was on the operating table under intravenous anesthesia with nasopharyngeal intubation, and the bronchoscopic examination was in progress. The bronchoscopist reported that the lungs were clear, with no evidence of any primary or secondary lesions present there. He had clamped the tongue with a sterile towel clamp to pull it forward forcefully, and when the tongue was being pulled forward to its fullest extent to remove the bronchoscope, a round ulcerated lesion measuring approximately 2 cm. in diameter came into view at the extreme base of the tongue on the right side, deep in the throat. On examination the mass was indurated and appeared to be approximately 7 mm. deep, and the surrounding tissue was somewhat swollen. The left side was normal in all respects.

TREATMENT.   A Coles Radiosurg Electronic Scalpel IV on loan from the dental department was present in the operating room, with a supply of electrodes. The unit was activated, cutting current was set at 7, and a round loop electrode 1 cm. in diameter made of very fine gauge wire was selected. The activated loop was used to resect three tissue specimens from three areas. Each biopsy specimen was removed with a single rapid wiping motion of the electrode to slice off the tissue.

A large round ball coagulating electrode was selected and used with coagulating current power output set at 4 to spot coagulate the entire surface of the mass. When the coagulation had penetrated about 3 mm., most of the coagulum was resected by shaving it with a planing motion of the loop electrode that had been activated with the cutting current, with power output set at 8.*

The coagulation was then repeated and followed by resection of most of the coagulum until approximately 75 per cent of the mass had been coagulated and resected. This method of removal would have revealed destruction of large blood vessels that would have to be tied off, which would eliminate the hazard of postoperative hemorrhage when the coagulum sloughed off. Since no evidence of bleeding was manifested during the procedure, there was no need to tie off any blood vessels.

Because of the anatomic location of the mass and its contiguity to the lateral wall of the throat, it was decided that the remainder of the mass would be left untreated rather than to have the electrocoagulation penetrate deeper. Hopefully the antigen-antibody reaction attributed to the electrocoagulation, plus postoperative irradiation, would destroy the remaining diseased tissue.

Although the author has not seen the patient since the surgery, he has been kept informed about the progress of the case by the attending oral surgeon[15] and received a slide of the biopsy tissue from the pathologist with the diagnosis, which confirmed the clinical diagnosis of squamous cell carcinoma[16] (Case Fig. 2–1).

The patient appears to have responded very favorably to the therapy, and the indications are that she will have a total, permanent cure rather than the usually optimal 5 year cure. Moreover, not only do the prospects appear excellent for her complete recovery, but she will not undergo the functional impairment and aesthetic facial disfigurement that would have resulted from treatment by means of the commando procedure.

The attending oral surgeon's report of her postoperative progress is very revealing and significant in view of the fact that the anatomic site of the squamous cell carcinoma, at the base of the tongue, is usually associated with an exceedingly high morbidity rate and consequently makes the prognosis after the commando procedure extremely poor. He also reported that the patient had had no postoperative pain or complications and remarkably little physical discomfort. Her sole complaint was soreness in the tip of her tongue, which had been punctured with the towel clamp to fully extrude her tongue.

This patient's experience bears out previous observations that when electrosurgery is performed properly there is a remarkable absence of pain and the other unfavorable customary postoperative sequelae. The fact that the patient did not require narcotics for relief of pain despite the extensiveness of the treatment and the unfavorable surgical site bears out the observation very gratifyingly.

---

*If the lesion does not permit coagulation to a depth of 3 to 5 mm., the coagulum can be sheared off with the loop activated by coagulating current instead of cutting to minimize the risk of surgical metastasis.

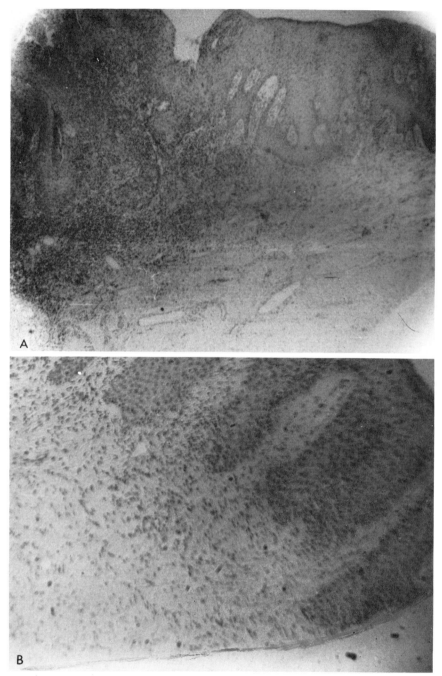

Case Figure 2–1. Photomicrographs of biopsy taken from an oral carcinoma by loop electrosection from the lateral base of the tongue. *A,* Low power photomicrograph, showing the disarray of the rete pegs and the cellular arrangement. *B,* A slightly higher magnification showing a cut edge of the tissue that had been resected with the loop electrode. Note the sharp clean tissue edge, with no evidence of charring or coagulation.

Illustration continued on opposite page.

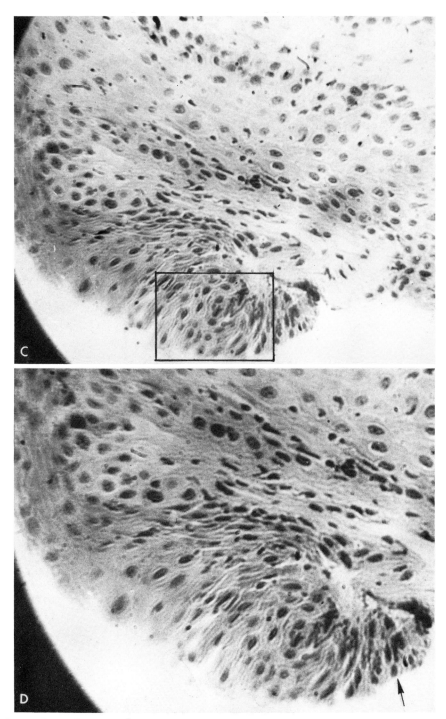

Case Figure 2–1   Continued.

C, Photomicrograph (10×) of the cut edge of the tissue. We see the characteristic curved contour of the cut tissue edge and the absence of coagulation or charring. *D*, Inset of *C* at 45×. Many intact cells are seen along the line of cleavage, and one cell appears to have had the outer edge of its cell wall sheared off (arrow).

Illustration continued on following page.

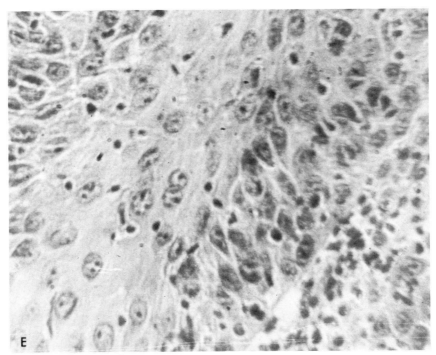

Case Figure 2-1 Continued.

E, High power photomicrograph (45×) of the bizarre cellular disarray that is indicative of malignancy. Many multinucleated cells are present, and some cells appear to be undergoing mitosis. It is obvious from the appearance of the cells that not only has there been no coagulation or charring despite the high output of cutting power used for the biopsy but there has been no alteration of the cellular components by the heat generated by the RF current.

The cumulative clinical, histologic, and research evidence of the efficiency, safety, and diversified usefulness of electrosurgery in modern dentistry that have been presented lead to an inescapable conclusion: it is timely and eminently fitting, in this electronic age, with the current refinements it has produced, that our profession should universally avail itself fully of the innumerable clinical advantages that are mutually beneficial to the patient and the therapist, as well as the potential for financial benefits that accrue from elimination of unproductive chair operating time loss. The safety features incorporated into the new equipment combined with sound dental and electrosurgical technique eliminate completely the potential hazards that have in the past been the main reason for failure to utilize this remarkable modality.

This concludes the instructional part of the text. The text that follows is a convenience feature.

FOOTNOTE REFERENCES

1. Cade, S.: Carcinoma of the floor of the mouth. Brit. J. Surg., *41*:225, 1953.
2. Gardham, A. J.: Carcinoma of the floor of the mouth. Brit. J. Surg., *41*:241, 1953.
3. Hoover, W. B., and King, G. D.: The present status of intraoral cancer. Surg. Clin. N. Amer., *34*:663, 1954.
4. Kelly, H. A., and Ward, G. E.: Electrosurgery. Philadelphia, W. B. Saunders Co., 1932, p. 305.

5. Merrill, K., Jr., and Hoar, C. S., Jr.: Electrocoagulation for local treatment of advanced oral carcinoma. Surgery, 52:5, 699–708; Nov. 1962.
6. Ochsner, A.: Editorial—Treatment of malignant disease by cauterization. Surgery, 52:5, 1962.
7. Kolischer, G.: Surgical diathermy in malignancy. Amer. J. Surg., 7:249, 1929.
8. Henscher, C.: Die Behandlung des Karzinoms in der Chirurgie. Schweiz. Med. Wchnschr., 61:441, 1931.
9. Lewis, M. R., Maxwell, D. B., and Aptekman, P. M.: Atrophy of sarcoma in rats followed by tumor immunity. Surgery, 30:689, 1951.
10. Strauss, A. A.: Surgical diathermy of carcinoma in the rectum and its clinical end results. Arch. Phys. Ther., 14:212, 1933.
11. Strauss, A. A., Strauss, S. F., Crawford, R. A., and Strauss, H. A.: Surgical diathermy of carcinoma of the rectum. JAMA, 104:1480, 1935.
12. Strauss, A. A., Strauss, S. F., and Strauss, H. A.: A new method and end results in the treatment of carcinoma of the stomach and rectum by surgical diathermy. S. Surgeon, 5:348, 1936.
13. Bedell, W., Engelman, M., and Schackner, J.: Oral Cancer Detection and Prevention Center, St. Francis Hosp., N.Y. Personal communication to the author.
14. Autopsy report, Memorial Hospital, N.Y.
15. Mercier, P.: Oral Surgeon, St. Mary's Hosp., Montreal, Quebec, Canada. Personal communication to the author.
16. Kahn, D. S.: Pathologist, St. Mary's Hosp., Montreal, Quebec, Canada. Personal communication, biopsy report, and histologic specimen.

Chapter Twenty-Six

MEDICAMENTS AND INSTRUMENTS MENTIONED IN THE TEXT

This appendix has been prepared to facilitate location of specific items by the reader.

To facilitate immediate identification of *potentially life-saving emergency drugs and instruments* with a minimal loss of time when anesthetic, surgical, or other clinical emergencies arise in the dental office, these items are listed separately immediately below. All are so critically important that, wherever applicable, the preferred methods of administration are also included. It would be highly advisable that every dental office include these items in its armamentarium, to assure their availability for immediate use in the event of an emergency.

EMERGENCY ARMAMENTARIUM

The most important and universal single emergency item is **oxygen,** administered by manual or automatic positive pressure.

ITEM	CHAPTER	SOURCE
Oxygen (from inhalation anesthesia and analgesia units)	10, 11	S.S. White; Carbide Reduction Co.
Oxygen Resuscitator Cylinders	10, 11	McKesson Co. and others

1102

Emergency Drugs

FOR ANAPHYLAXIS AND PROFOUND SHOCK

ITEM	CHAPTER	SOURCE
Hydrocortisone Hemisuccinate (IV administration)	10	Parke-Davis Co.
Solu-Cortef (IV administration)	10	Upjohn & Co.
Solu-Medrol (Sodium Succinate) (IV administration)	10	Upjohn & Co.

FOR ANGIONEUROTIC EDEMA

ITEM	CHAPTER	SOURCE
Benadryl Steri-Vials (IV or IM administration)	10	Ciba Pharmaceutical Co.
Chlor-Trimetron (subcutaneous administration)	10	Schering Co.

FOR CARDIAC AND RESPIRATORY STIMULATION

ITEM	CHAPTER	SOURCE
Coramine (IV or IM administration)	10, 11	Ciba Pharmaceutical Co.

FOR CIRCULATORY AND RESPIRATORY STIMULATION

ITEM	CHAPTER	SOURCE
Metrazol (IV administration)	10, 11	Knoll Pharmaceutical Co.

FOR CARDIAC MANAGEMENT (ANGINA PECTORIS)

ITEM	CHAPTER	SOURCE
Nitroglycerin USP (oral—sublingual administration)	10	Eli Lilly & Co.
Nitroglyn (Long-Acting) (oral—sublingual administration)	10	Key Pharmaceuticals, Inc.

Emergency Instruments

RESPIRATORY

ITEM	CHAPTER	SOURCE
Disposable Plastic Endo-tracheal Airways (Fig. 26–1)	11	Foregger Co.

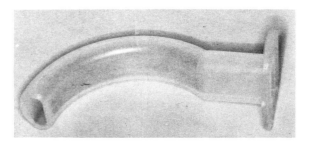

Figure 26–1 Disposable plastic airway, which is light in weight, smooth, and nonirritating.

Monoject Emergency Tracheal Catheter (Fig. 26–2)	11	Sherwood Medical Industries

CARDIAC – CIRCULATORY

ITEM	CHAPTER	SOURCE
Stethoscope (Bowles or Ford Type)	11	Medical Supply Companies
Sphygmomanometer (Mercury Manometer)	11	Medical Supply Companies

Drugs for Minor to Moderate Emergencies

FOR SYNCOPE AND MILD SHOCK

ITEM	CHAPTER	SOURCE
Amyl Nitrite (Inhalation)	10	Burroughs-Welcome; Eli Lilly & Co.
Aromatic Spirits of Ammonia	10	Burroughs-Welcome; Eli Lilly & Co.; Johnson & Johnson;
Novocol Emergency Therapules	10	Novocol Chemical Co.

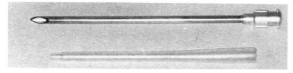

Figure 26–2. Emergency tracheal catheter. *Top,* Tracheal stylus with cutting tip. *Bottom,* Catheter tube.

GENERAL ARMAMENTARIUM*

Anesthetic Agents

LOCAL ANESTHETICS

ITEM	CHAPTER	SOURCE
Carbocaine	10, 11	Cook-Waite Co.
Citanest	10, 11	Astra Pharmaceutical Co.
Lidocaine	10, 11	Graham Chemical Co.
Octocaine	10, 11	Novocol Chemical Co.
Procaine	10, 11	Winthrop Chemical Co.
Xylocaine	10, 11	Astra Pharmaceutical Co.

TOPICAL ANESTHETICS

ITEM	CHAPTER	SOURCE
Graham's Topical	10, 11	Graham Chemical Co.
Novol Benzocaine-Tetracaine	10, 11	Novocol Chemical Co.
Xylocaine Topical	10, 11	Astra Pharmaceutical Co.

GENERAL — INHALATION

ITEM	CHAPTER	SOURCE
Fluothane	11	Ayerst Laboratories
Nitrous Oxide–Oxygen USP	3, 11	S.S. White; Carbide Reduction Co.

GENERAL — INTRAVENOUS

ITEM	CHAPTER	SOURCE
Brevital Sodium	10, 11	Eli Lilly & Co.
Pentothal Sodium	10, 11	Abbott Laboratories
Seconal Sodium	10, 11	Eli Lilly & Co.

---

*Items mentioned in this listing represent those which are referred to by brand or generic name in the text and which are familiar to the author. In many instances other manufacturers have marketed similar products, but it is neither practical nor possible to include all such products here.

Anesthetic Instruments

HYPODERMIC SYRINGES

ITEM	CHAPTER	SOURCE
Metal – Aspirating	11	Cook-Waite Co.;
Metal – Aspirating	11	Graham Chemical Co.;
Metal – Aspirating	11	Astra Pharmaceutical Co.
Plastic, Disposable – Aspirating	11	Astra Pharmaceutical Co.;
Monoject Dental Injector #418	11	Sherwood Medical Industries

HYPODERMIC NEEDLES

ITEM	CHAPTER	SOURCE
Disposable Needles	11	Astra Pharmaceutical Co.; Bard-Parker Co.; Getz Dental Product; Hypo Corp.; Sherwood Medical Industries

JET SYRINGES

ITEM	CHAPTER	SOURCE
Syriject, Mark II	11	Mizzy, Inc.

Antibiotics

ITEM	CHAPTER	SOURCE
Cleomycin	10	Whitehall Laboratories
Declomycin HCL	10	Lederle Laboratories
Erythromycin Products	10	
Ilosone	10	Eli Lilly & Co.
Ilotycin	10	Eli Lilly & Co.
Erythrocin	10	Abbott Laboratories
Lincocin	10	Whitehall Laboratories
Penicillin Products	10	
Oral:		
Biosulfa	10	Upjohn & Co.
Pentids	10	E. R. Squibb & Sons
Pen-Vee K	10	Wyeth Laboratories
Resistopen	10	E. R. Squibb & Sons
V-Cillin	10	Eli Lilly & Co.

Parenteral Systemic:

Item	Chapter	Source
Abbocillin	10	Abbott Laboratories
Bicillin	10	Wyeth Laboratories
Crysticillin	10	E. R. Squibb & Sons
Depo-Penicillin (fortified)	10	Upjohn & Co.
Duracillin Products	10	Eli Lilly & Co.
Terramycin (Oxytetracycline)	10	Pfizer Laboratories
Tetracycline Products	10	Lederle Laboratories

Antisialogogues

Item	Chapter	Source
Artane	10	Lederle Laboratories
Banthine	10	Searle Laboratories
Probanthine	10	Searle Laboratories
Pamine	10	Upjohn & Co.

Ataraxics — Tranquilizers

Item	Chapter	Source
Compazine	10	Smith, Kline & French
Equanil	10	Wyeth Laboratories
Librium	10	Roche Laboratories
Miltown	10	Wallace Products
Thorazine	10	Smith, Kline & French
Trilafon	10	Schering Co.
Ultran	10	Eli Lilly & Co.
Valium	10	Roche Laboratories

Coagulants — Hemostatics

Local

Item	Chapter	Source
Adrenalin Chloride Solution (1:1,000)	10, 18	Parke-Davis Co.
Adrenosem Salicylate	10	S. E. Massengill Co.
Menadione	10	Merck & Co.
Oxycel	10, 21	Parke-Davis Co.
Surgicel	10, 21	Johnson & Johnson
Synkayvite (Vitamin K Analog)	10, 21	Roche Products
Tannic Acid USP	10, 19, 21	Pharmacy Item

Thrombin Topical	10, 20, 22	Parke-Davis Co.
Thromboplastin	10	Cutter Laboratories

PARENTERAL

ITEM	CHAPTER	SOURCE
Adrestat	10, 21	Organon, Inc.
Bivam	10	U.S. Vitamin & Pharmaceutical
Ceanothyn	10	Flint, Eaton & Co.
CVP Products	10	U.S. Vitamin & Pharmaceutical
Koagamin	10	Chatham Pharmaceuticals
Rutascorb	10	U.S. Vitamin & Pharmaceutical
Rutorbin	10	E. R. Squibb & Sons

Dietary Supportives and Vitamins

ITEM	CHAPTER	SOURCE
Ascorbic Acid USP	10, 18	Pharmacy Item
Gelatin (clear, unflavored)	10, 18, 21, 22	Grocery Item (Knox, etc.)
Meritene	10	Doyle Pharmaceutical Co.
Nutriment	10, 21	Mead Johnson Co.
Sustagen	10	Mead Johnson Co.
Multiple Vitamins, USP	10, 18	Pharmacy Item
Vitamin B Complex (therapeutic)		
Becotin Products	10	Eli Lilly & Co.
Stresscaps	10	Lederle Laboratories
Theragren Products	10	E. R. Squibb & Sons

Dressings, Periodontal and Surgical Packs

ITEM	CHAPTER	SOURCE
B.I.P. Formula	10, 21, 22	Prescription Item
Burlew Adhesive Dryfoil	10, 22	J. F. Jelenko & Co., Inc.
Cavit	10, 14	Premiere Dental Co.
Coepac	10, 14, 18	Coe Laboratories, Inc.
Flexible Collodion USP	10, 22	Pharmacy Item
Gelfoam Powder	10, 22	Upjohn & Co.

Gelfoam Sponge	10, 22	Upjohn & Co.
Kenalog In Orabase	10	E. R. Squibb & Sons
Orabase	10	E. R. Squibb & Sons
Orahesive Bandage	10, 20	E. R. Squibb & Sons
Periodontal Pack Formula	10, 19	Prescription Item
Peripak	10, 19	deTrey Co.
Tincture of Myrrh and Benzoin Formula	10, 19 to 22	Prescription Item
Quickseal	10, 14	Interstate Dental Co.

Lavages

ITEM	CHAPTER	SOURCE
Chloraseptic	10	Eaton Laboratories
Glyoxide	10	International Pharma- ceutical Corp.
Kasdenol	10, 19, 22	Kasdenol Corp.
Salt and Alum Formula (Alum USP, powdered)	10, 19	Pharmacy Item

Narcotics

ITEM	CHAPTER	SOURCE
Demerol HCL (IV or IM administration)	10	Breon Laboratories; Winthrop Laboratories
Numorphan (IM or rectal administration)	10	Endo Laboratories
Percodan (Synthetic Codeine)	10	Endo Laboratories

Sedatives — Analgesics

ITEM	CHAPTER	SOURCE
Anacin	10	Whitehall Laboratories
APC with Codeine	10	Prescription Item
Aspirin	10	Bayer, Squibb, etc.
Bufferin	10	Bristol-Myers Co.
Darvon Products	10	Eli Lilly & Co.
Empirin Compound	10	Burroughs-Welcome Co.
Excedrin	10	Bristol-Myers Co.
Talwin (Pentazocaine)	10	Winthrop Laboratories

Miscellaneous

Cold Sterilizing Solution

ITEM	CHAPTER	SOURCE
Alcohol-Formaldehyde Formula	10, 18, 21	Prescription Item
Cidex	10	Johnson & Johnson

Hygroscopic Deodorizing Agent

ITEM	CHAPTER	SOURCE
Ozium (Fig. 26–3)	10, 18	Woodlets, Inc.

Neuromuscular Relaxant

ITEM	CHAPTER	SOURCE
Tolseram (Mephenasen)*	10	E. R. Squibb & Sons

Radiopaque Visualizer

ITEM	CHAPTER	SOURCE
Lipiodol Lafay	10, 22	E. Fougera & Co., Inc.

---

*Discontinued owing to inadequate sales volume.

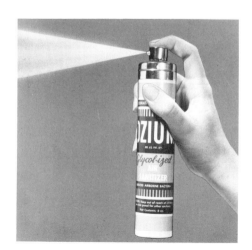

Figure 26–3. Hygroscopic deodorizing agent.

INSTRUMENTS

Electrosurgical Equipment

CONTINUOUS WAVE—FULLY RECTIFIED UNITS

ITEM	CHAPTER	SOURCE
Coles TR-1; TR-2	2	Cavitron Corp.
Dento-Surg 90 FFP	2	Ellman Dental Manu-facturing Co.
L.A.S.E.R.	2	LASER Co. (Milan, Italy)
Strobex	2	Whaledent

FULLY RECTIFIED UNITS

ITEM	CHAPTER	SOURCE
Cameron-Miller #26-230-R; 26-240-R; 26-250-R; 26-255-R	2	Cameron-Miller Surgical Instruments Co.
Coles Radiosurg Scalpel IV	2	Cavitron Corp.
Electrosurg	2	Hampton Research
Elektrotom 70D	2	Gebrueder Martin (W. Germany)
Parkell 25; 255	2	Parkell Electronics Division
"Sirotom" (35W)	2	Siemens AG (W. Germany)

PARTIALLY RECTIFIED UNITS

ITEM	CHAPTER	SOURCE
Cameron-Miller #250; 265	2	Cameron-Miller Surgical Instruments Co.
Joulisator	2	Joulisator Co. (Denmark)
Siemens Units	2	Siemens AG (W. Germany)

SPARK-GAP GENERATORS

ITEM	CHAPTER	SOURCE
Hyfrecator	2	Birtcher Corp.
Bantam Bovie	2	Leibel-Flarscheim Co.
Electricator	2	National Electric Co.

Electrosurgical Accessories

SURGICAL ELECTRODES

ITEM	CHAPTER	SOURCE
Basic and Special Electrodes	1	Coles-Cavitron Corp.
Basic and Special Electrodes	1	Cameron-Miller Surgical
Basic and Special Electrodes	1	Instruments Co.
		Gebrueder Martin

SURGICAL ELECTRODE HANDPIECES

ITEM	CHAPTER	SOURCE
Chuck Type #26 Universal Handpiece	1	Cameron-Miller Surgical Instrument Co.
Coles Barbed Broach Electrode Handpiece	1	Coles-Cavitron Corp.
Coles Handpiece Adapter for TR-1, TR-2	1	Coles-Cavitron Corp.

SUCTION—COAGULATING HANDPIECE AND ELECTRODE

ITEM	CHAPTER	SOURCE
Handpiece (Anthony–Fischer #26-1106-A) Electrode (Anthony-Fischer #26-1104-A)	1	Cameron-Miller Surgical Instruments Co.

COAGULATING FORCEPS

ITEM	CHAPTER	SOURCE
Oringer Coagulating Forceps	1	Euram Instrument Co.

INDIFFERENT SEAT ELECTRODE

ITEM	CHAPTER	SOURCE
Oringer Internal Indifferent Seat Assembly	1	Euram Instrument Co.

Ancillary Surgical Instruments

HEMOSTATS

ITEM	CHAPTER	SOURCE
Mosquito Hemostats (curved, straight)	5, 22	Hu-Friedy; Gebrueder Martin; Friedman; Sklar Surgical Instrument Co.

SUTURE AND SUTURE NEEDLES

ITEM	CHAPTER	SOURCE
Ethicon 3-0 Silk, Black Braided, X-8	19, 20, 22, 24	Johnson & Johnson Dental Division
Ethicon 4-0 Silk, Black Braided, FS-2	19, 20, 22, 24	Johnson & Johnson Dental Division
Ethicon 5-0 Silk, Braided, FS-2	22, 24	Johnson & Johnson Dental Division
Ethicon 5-0 Ethiflex, Green Braided, V-5	22, 24	Johnson & Johnson Dental Division
Deknatel 4-0 Silk, Braided Suture	19, 20, 22, 24	J. A. Deknatel & Sons
#1821 – 16, 18, 20 Half Round Needles	19, 20, 22, 24	Anchor Brand

TISSUE FORCEPS

ITEM	CHAPTER	SOURCE
Ophthalmic (curved, straight)	5, 13, 20, 22	Gebrueder Martin; Sklar Surgical Instrument Co.

Miscellaneous Ancillary Instruments

ASPIRATING AND SALIVA EJECTOR TIPS

ITEM	CHAPTER	SOURCE
Metal, Rubber Insulated (Fig. 26–4)		Lorvic Corp.
Plastic, Disposable, Monoject		Lorvic Corp

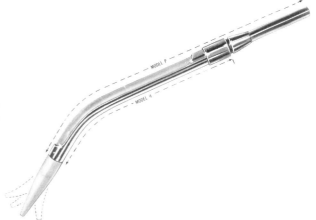

Figure 26–4. Lorvic rubber-shielded nonconductive metal aspirator tip.

Plastic, Disposable, Monoject (Fig. 26–5) Sherwood Medical Industries, Inc.

PINS: NONPARALLEL, SPLINTING

ITEM	CHAPTER	SOURCE
Splintmate, ReSeté, etc., Pin Systems	15	Whaledent Corp.

PERIODONTAL POCKET PROBES AND MARKERS

ITEM	CHAPTER	SOURCE
10-mm. Probe, Flat	3, 18, 19	Gebrueder Martin
Endodontic Silver Points	14, 19, 22	
Omnidepth Probe	19	Whaledent

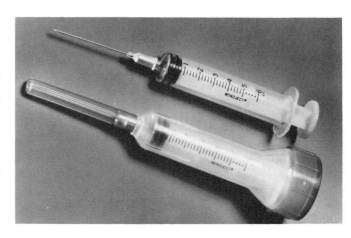

Figure 26–5. Typical aspirational biopsy syringe (monoject #502-Ed). A 16 to 18 gauge needle and 6 to 10 cubic centimeter syringe will provide enough suction to pull tissue cylinder punch-out into the lumen with enough force to detach it from the underlying tissues. *Top,* Syringe removed from its plastic shield.

PROBE — LACHRYMAL

ITEM	CHAPTER	SOURCE
Flexible Silver Probe	19, 22	S. S. White

RETRACTORS

ITEM	CHAPTER	SOURCE
Oringer Self-Retaining Cheek-Lip Retractor (Fig. 26–6)	12 to 22	Euram Instrument Co.
Fiberglass Mirrors	12 to 22	Sam Dixson Co.

SYRINGES

ITEM	CHAPTER	SOURCE
Irrigating, Monoject #412 Irrigating, Endodontic, with Needle, #502-Ed Aspirating, Monoject #135 S–R	14, 19, 22	Sherwood Medical Industries
Controlled Pressure Endodontic Syringe	14, 19	The Endovage Company

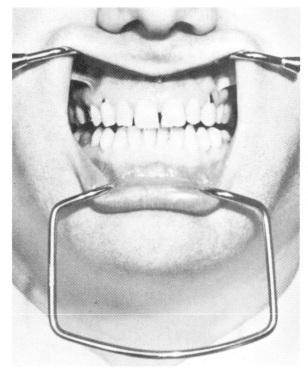

Figure 26–6. Self-retaining cheek-lip retractor (Oringer) eliminates need for manual traction and exposes the mouth fully for active treatment or photography. Its uniform distribution of traction minimizes postoperative effects of retraction and does not interfere with movement of electrodes.

STERILIZERS

ITEM	CHAPTER	SOURCE
Cold, Tray Type	10	Bard-Parker Co.
Cold, Tray Type #18/8	10	Inox Co.
Autoclave	10, 14, 22	Castle, Pelton & Crane
Dry Heat Sterilizer	10	Dri-Clave Co.

TOOTHBRUSHES — MANUAL

ITEM	CHAPTER	SOURCE
Natural Bristle, Hard, Extra-Hard	18, 19	Lactona, Pycopay
Nylon, Soft, Ultra-Soft (Fig. 26–7)	18, 19	Lactona; Pycopay; Butler; Oral-B; Anchor

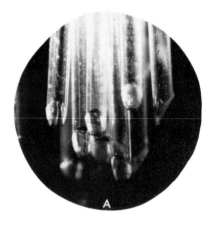

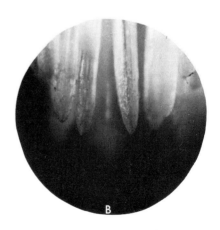

Figure 26–7. Nylon toothbrush bristles. *A,* Appearance of tips of bristles that have been cut, resulting in irregular and often razor-sharp edges. *B,* Appearance of tips of bristles that have been rounded to eliminate trauma from jagged tips such as those in *A.*

TOOTHBRUSH—ELECTRIC

ITEM	CHAPTER	SOURCE
Universal Action (Up-Down and Horizontal Strokes)	18, 19	General Electric Co.
Broxodont	18	E. R. Squibb Sons

TRANSILLUMINATING LIGHT

ITEM	CHAPTER	SOURCE
Electrosurgical Unit Transilluminator	5, 19, 22	Coles-Cavitron Corp
Disposable Pen-Type Light (Fiberoptic)	22	Kendall Corp.

ULTRASONIC PROPHYLACTIC UNIT

ITEM	CHAPTER	SOURCE
Cavitron "660" and "1010"	18, 19	Dentsply International
Sonus	18, 19	Litton Dental Products
Rittertron	18, 19	Ritter Co.

INDEX

Note: Page numbers in *italic* represent illustrations.

A

Abscess(es), alveolar, acute, drainage of, *868*
  drainage of, 816–821, *818*, *820*
    electrosurgery vs. scalpel surgery, 817
  paradontal, 592
    in trifurcation involvement, 705, *706*
Acetone, in root canal sterilization, 330
Acrylic crown forms, 439
Acrylic template, prior to denture fitting, 730
Acusection, 73–76. See also *Electrosection.*
Adenoma, cystic, of buccal mucosa, 1084, *1084*
Adenopathy, in oral cancer, 991
Aesthetics, elongation of clinical crown for, 395–397, *396*, 405–416, *406*, *407*, *409*, *411*, *413*, *414*, *415*
Alcohol-formaldehyde solutions, 259
Allergy, drugs for control of, 242, 245
Allis forceps, in suturing, 812
Alternating current. See *Current, alternating.*
Alveolar bone. See *Bone, alveolar.*
Alveolar contour, loss of, 829
Alveolar fistula, destruction of, *824*
Alveolar gingiva, 422
Alveolar mucosa, resection of, *749*
Alveolar nerve, damage to, in cancer, 991
Alveolar nerve fibers, in perforation, 928
Alveolar ridge
  atrophy of, 730
  extension of, 745
    maxillary, *782*
    vestibulotomy for, 767–783
  functional stress, and resorption, 748
  high, elongated tuberosity and, 786, *787*
  reduction of, prior to extraction, 733
  resorption of, and denture failures, 729
    implantology for, 774
    in denture wearer, 767
    total, vestibulotomy for, 780–783, *782*
  sharp, and denture instability, 730
Alveolectomy, 730, 732–736
  horizontal, to reduce vertical dimension, 786, *787*
Alveoloplasty, 730, 732–736
  for denture insertion, 739, *740*
  injudicious, correction of, 748–760
  routine, *735*
  with pushback, 778–780, *779*
Ameloblastoma, treatment of, 918

Amelogenesis imperfecta, in adolescent, elongation of clinical crown for, 416–418, *416*, *417*, *418*
Amplitude, of waveforms, 15
Amputation, root. See *Radectomy.*
Amputation neuroma, mental nerve evulsion and, 978
  resection of, 928, *930*
Analgesia, in electrosurgery, 88
Analgesics, 239–241, 1109
Anaphylaxis, drugs for, 1103
Anatomic defects, and denture failures, 729
  injudicious alveoloplasty and, 748–760
Anemia, effect on healing, 804
  periodontoclasia in, 626, 629, *630*, 631, 638, 641
Anesthesia
  balanced local and general, 235
  general, 234, 235
  hypodermic needles for, 230, *232*, *233*
  in abscess drainage, 817
  in electrosurgery, 211–235
    profundity of, 212
  jet syringes for, 231, *233*
  local, anatomic sites in, 214
    choice of, 213
    contraindications for, 233
    emergencies during, 234
    infiltration, 215
  regional block, 215, 217–234
    anterior palatal (nasopalatine), 220, *223*, *224*
    inferior alveolar-lingual, 223, *226*, *227*, *228*, *229*
    infraorbital, 218, *220*, *221*, *222*
    mental, 229, *230*
    posterior palatine, 223, *225*, *226*
    posterior superior alveolar, 217, *217*, *218*, *219*
    topical, 231, 248
Anesthetic agents, 1105
  explosive and flammable, 88
Anesthetic armamentarium, 230–233, *232*, *233*, 248
Anesthetic cartridge, blood contamination of, 216
Anesthetic drugs, local, pharmacodynamics of, 212–235
Anesthetic instruments, 1106
Anesthetic shock, prevention of, 215
Anesthetic solution, temperature of, 215
Angina pectoris, drugs for, 1103
Angioma, biopsy of, 1039

1119

Angle-edgewire orthodontic technique, 528–531, *530*
   lingual frenotomy for, 866, *867*, 1018, *1020, 1021*
Ankylosis, of roots, 834
Antibiotics, 241
   for root canal sterilization, 325–327
   in armamentarium, 1106
   in plastic surgery, 921
   vs. electrosurgery, in osteomyelitis, 825
Antiformin, 571
Antigen-antibody reaction, in electrocoagulation for oral cancer, 1092
Antiseptics, 251
Antisialogogues, 237, 1107
Antrum, maxillary. See *Maxillary antrum.*
Aphthous ulcer, nonelectrosurgical treatment of, 85
   vs. infiltrative lesion, 991
Apical cavity, sealing of, 340, *341*
Apicoectomy, 335–376, 878–901. See also *Root-end resection.*
Arc incision, in root-end resection, 366
Arch bar, stainless steel, 658, 661, *662*
   to immobilize after periodontal therapy, 576
   with acrylic, in periodontal splinting, 634
Areolar gingiva, 422
Areolar tissue, biopsy of, 1006–1023
Armamentarium, 1102–1117
   emergency, 1102–1104
      minor drugs for, 1104
   general, 1105–1110
   in oral surgery, 811–815
   instruments in, 1111–1117
Asepsis, in plastic surgery, 921
Aspirating tips, 1113, *1114*
Aspiration, in infraorbital block anesthesia, 220
   of traumatic cyst, 918, *919*
   prior to anesthetic injection, 216
   syringes for, 231, *232, 233*
Astringents, 251
   for gingival retraction, 423, 426
Ataraxics, 1107
Axial floor, of inlay preparation, exposure of, 284–290, *285, 286, 287, 289*

B

Band(s), elastic-Japanese grassline, in periodontal therapy, 577, *632, 638, 667*
   orthodontic, and interproximal papillae inflammation, 531
      and subgingival irritation, 532
      contact with electrodes, 506, 555–556, *556*
Bandages, oral, 252, *255, 256*
Barbed broach electrode handle, *328*
Basal cell epithelioma, of lip, 993
Beveling, in traumatic occlusion, 744
Bifurcation involvement, in periodontoclasia, 624
   treatment of, 691, *691*, 699–705, *701, 703*
Biopsy
   criteria for performing, 997
   dangers of, 995–998
   electrosurgical, 7, 84
      advantages of, 999–1000

Biopsy (*Continued*)
   electrosurgical, clinical techniques in, 1003–1086
      for diagnosis of oral pathology, 983–1086
   in diagnosis of cancer, 988
   incisional, *1004, 1006*
   indications for, 989–995
   inducing metastasis, 996
   loop excision, 119, *119*
      extraoral, 1080–1086
   of buccal mucosa, 1024–1030, *1026, 1027, 1028, 1029*
   of buccal vestibule, 1039–1044
   of floor of mouth, 1071–1076
   of gingival mucosa, 1030–1053
      mandibular anterior labial, 1044–1046, *1045*
      mandibular anterior lingual, 1047–1049, *1048*
      mandibular central, 1049–1051, *1050*
      mandibular posterior, 1051–1053, *1052*
      maxillary anterior, 1030–1037
      maxillary posterior, 1037–1039
   of labio-alveolar gingival mass, 1034–1037
   of lips, 1006–1023
   of lip and buccal mucosa, 1018–1023, *1019, 1020, 1021, 1022, 1023*
   of lower lip, 1011–1014, *1012, 1013*
   of maxillary alveolar mucosa, 1042–1044, *1043*
   of maxillary antrum and parotid gland, 85
   of palatal mucosa, 1053–1071
   of tongue, 1072, *1073*, 1076–1078
   procedures in, 985–1002
   properly conducted, factors influencing, 995–998
   rationale for, 993–995
   resection of specimens for, 1003–1006, *1004, 1005, 1006*
   using scalpel, disadvantages of, 1006
Biopsy specimen, preservation of, 1004
Biopsy syringe, *1114*
Bipolar electrode, definition of, 13
Birtcher Blendtome unit, *51, 52*
Biterminal currents. See *Currents, biterminal.*
Biterminal electrode, definition of, 13, *14, 27*
Bleaching, of teeth, by electrocoagulation, 301–305, *303*
Bleeding, free, in unhealthy tissue, 810
Blood dyscrasia, periodontoclasia related to, 626
Blood flow, to tissues, in periodontia, 668
   to bone, in cystic disease, 904
Bone, alveolar, atrophy of, and denture instability, 745
   destruction of, *703*
      around palatal roots, 705, *706*
      endodontic-periodontal deterioration and, 604, *605*
      in cystic disease, 905
      intraradicular, 702, *703*
      periradicular, 889, *890, 891*
      root-end resection for, "biased," 353–356, 354
   disintegration of, improper occlusion and, 744
   eburnated, 904
   edentulous, exposure of, in implantation, 469–480
   regeneration of, after bifurcation debridement, *626*
      after periodontal pocket debridement, 600, *601, 603*, 640, *663*, 704

Bone (*Continued*)
  regeneration of, after radectomy, *900*
    after treatment of endodontic-periodontal disease, 604, *605*
    and graft materials, 568
    stimulation of, 667
  removal of, to maintain crown-root ratio, 397
  resorption of, circumscribing, 576, 635, *636*, *653*
    in frenal traction, 712
  response to electrosurgical scalpel, 182–189, *183–187*, 810
  sequestration of, 301
    in osteomyelitis, 825
  trimming of, use of study model in, 730, 733, 784, *785*
  cortical, perforation of, 365
    repair of with graft, *930*
  denuded, in elongation of clinical crown, 298, *299, 300*, 301
  despeciated, 568, 904
  interseptal, destruction of, 696, 699
Bone fragments, in biopsy specimen, *1037*
Bone grafts, 928–932, *930*
Bone loss
  horizontal, 576
    circumscribing, *692*
  in furcation, 699–701
  in periodontia, 631, 652, *653*
    interdental, reduction of, 664
  uniform, 566
  vertical, 657
Bone paste, despeciated, 568, 904
Bone ramping, in periodontal therapy, 638
Bone spurs, interseptal, and denture failures, 729
Bridge, ill-fitting, and tissue proliferation, 405–406, *406*
  repair of, anterior, 388–389, *388*
    posterior, 389–391, *390*
Bruxism, elongation of crown in, 406–409, *407*, *409*
Buccal mucosa, biopsy of, 1024–1030, *1026, 1027*, *1028, 1029*
  and lip, 1018–1023
  incidence of cancer in, 986
  slit incision flap in, 924

C

Calcareous deposits. See *Calculus.*
Calcium excretion, in cystic disease, 904
Calculi, in submaxillary duct. See *Sialoliths.*
Calculus
  and gingival irritation, 582, 668
  removal of, prior to periodontal therapy, 574
  salivary, removal of, 574
  serumal, 575
    removal of, 574
Caldwell-Luc procedure, 936–941
Calf mandible, in practice of electrosurgical technique, 104
  subgingival trough preparation on, *433*
Callus formation, denture stent and, 764
Cameron-Miller units, 52, *53*, 55
Cancer
  oral
    advanced, electrocoagulation for, 1089–1100

Cancer (*Continued*)
  oral, age incidence of, 988
    biopsy for, 989–1000
    causes of, 988–989
    characteristics of, 989, *990*
    detection of, 985–986, 988
    differential diagnosis of, 994
    in male vs. female, 987
    incidence of, 985, 986
    metastasis in, 996
      routes of, 987
    significance of site of, 992–993
    symptoms of, 991–992
    treatment for, 994
      electrosurgical, 84
  oropharyngeal, 985, 986
Carbohydrate-rich diet, and periodontia, *642*, 643
Carbonization, tissue. See *Fulguration.*
Carcinoma, of submaxillary gland, 1080
  squamous cell, of floor of mouth, 1075, *1076*
  oral, 986
  of lip, 1011, *1012*
Cardiac pacemakers, use of electrosurgery with, 84
Cardiac patients, therapeutic drugs for, 245
Cardiac responses to electrosurgery, 151–153, *152*, *153*
Caries, interproximal, gingivectomy in, 290–292, *291, 293*
  removal of proliferative tissue from, 274, *276*, 277
  subgingival, and periodontal deterioration, 563, 582
  exposure of, 272–274, 277, *278, 279, 280, 281*, *302, 303*
Cartilage, nasal, in biopsy specimen, *1037*
Cauterization, for oral cancer, 1089
Cavity preparation, removal of tissue proliferation from, 274–276, *275*
Cement, surgical, in denture flange, 737, *738*
Cement pack, in orthodontic therapy, 534, 557
  in periodontal therapy, 604, *605, 656*
    proper vs. improper, *722*
  surgical, 252
Cementum, viable, retention in root planing, 575
Centrals, permanent, delayed eruption of, 316–318, *317*
Ceramic restorations, and periodontoclasia, 612, *614*
Cervical crowns, in vertico-oblique incision, 359–360, *361*
Cheek, swelling of, in cancer, 991. See also *Buccal mucosa.*
Chemical coagulation, of leukoplakia, 966
Chemical retraction of gingiva, 423, 426
Chemical solvents, in periodontal curettage, 571
Chemotherapeutics, 241
Chlorine, nascent, in root canal sterilization, 330
CIDEX, 260
Cigarette smoking, and leukoplakia, 968
  and oral cancer, 987
Circuits, fully rectified, 27, 31–35, *32, 33, 34, 35*, 48, 52–64
  partially rectified, 27, 28, *30*, 47, 50–52, *51*
  unrectified, 27, 28, *29*
Cleft, traumatic fracture and, repair of, 924, *926*
Cleft palate, elongation of clinical crown in, 410
  surgery for, 808

Cleft palate abnormalities, and denture failures, 729
  electrosurgical treatment of, 537–558
Coagulants, 1107
Coagulating electrode, in sterilization of root canal apex, 340, *341*
Coagulating forceps, 111, *112*
Coagulation, chemical, of leukoplakia, 966
  currents for, 36
  superficial spot, *306, 307*
    for tissue proliferation, after root-end resection, *358, 359*
Coles, 8, 29, 31, *33*
Coles Electrosurg TR-1, 58, *58*
Coles Radiosurg Electronic Scalpel IV, 55, *56*, 142, *143*
Collodion, flexible, 254
Commando procedure, 1094, *1095*
  for oral cancer, 1089
Constant-wave power supply, 48
Crown
  artificial, reaction of gingival tissues to, 384
  causing subgingival impingement, and periodontoclasia, 616, *620*
  cervical, in vertico-oblique incision, 359–360, *361*
  clinical, elongation of, 292–301, *295, 297–300*, 391–418
    electrosection vs. electrocoagulation for, 391–392
    for aesthetics, 395–397, *396*
    for amelogenesis imperfecta, 416–418, *416, 417, 418*
    for combined aesthetics and function, 405–416, *406, 407, 409, 411, 413, 414, 415*
    for function, 397–405, *399, 400, 401, 402, 403, 404*
    in cleft palate patient, 409–414, *411, 413, 542–547, 543, 545, 546, 551, 553*
    in orthodontics. See *Orthodontics.*
  exposure of, in cleft palate, 539–540, *539, 541*
    in delayed eruptions, 508–524, *509, 515, 517, 523*
    in fibromatosis, *671*
  full, types of restoration of, 419, *422*
  gold, in vertico-oblique incision, 359–360, *361*
  single, replacement of, 386, *387*
  unerupted, surgical exposure of, 312–314, *313, 314*
Crown and bridge prosthodontics, 378–504
  contributions of electrosurgery in, 379–383
  electrosurgical techniques, 83, 385–491
    elongation of clinical crown. See *Crown, clinical, elongation of.*
    exposure of key retained abutment roots. See *Roots, key retained abutment.*
    implants. See *Implants.*
    preparation of subgingival trough. See *Subgingival trough, preparation of.*
    processing of intermediate splint. See *Splint, intermediate.*
    reduction of redundant tissue. See *Hypertrophic tissue.*
    repairs, 385–391
      anterior, 388–389, *388*
      posterior, 389–391, *390*
      single crown, 386, *387*

Crown and bridge prosthodontics (*Continued*)
  factors influencing tissue tolerance in, 383–385
  failures in, 480–503
    extensive, 485–499
    gingival recession, 488–490, *489, 490, 491*
    improper occlusion, 480
    improper treatment plan, 494–499, *495, 497, 498*
    in diabetes, 492–494, *493*
    insufficient subgingival trough, 482, *483*, 483–485, *484*
    iatrogenic periodontoclasia, 480, 481–482, 485–488, *487*
    nonelectrosurgical, iatrogenic periodontoclasia, 499, *500, 500, 501*
      insufficient subgingival trough, 499, *500, 501, 502*
      traumatic occlusion, 502, *503*
    simple, 482–485
Crown forms, acrylic, 439
Crown-root ratio, elongation of clinical crown and, 293, *295, 297–300*, 397–414
  reversal in periodontia, 657
Curet, electrosurgical, 572, *572*
Curettage, periodontal, chemical, 571
  electrosurgical techniques for, 570–573, *572*
  manual, 571
Current(s)
  alternating, 27–35
    envelope of, 16, 28, 31
    fully rectified, 27, 31–35, *32, 33, 34, 35*, 48
    partially rectified, 27, 28, *30*, 47
    unrectified, 27, 28, *29*
  application of, monoterminal vs. biterminal, 27
  biterminal, evaluation of, 148–151
    experimental procedures with, 108–126
  damped, 28, 50
  electrosurgical, behavioral characteristics of, 141–151
    effect on gingival tissues, 154–165, *157, 158, 159, 161, 163, 164*
  flow during operation, 22–24, *23*
  "full-wave," 31, *32*, 48
  fully rectified, 8, 12
    oscilloscopic evaluation of, 143–148, *146, 147*
  "half-wave," 28, *30*, 47
  high frequency, 4, 12
  misconceptions about, 66
  monoterminal, experimental procedures with, 106–108
  Oudin, 44
  radio-frequency, 16
  regulation of, 49
  therapeutic electrosurgical, 10–41, 36–40
  undamped, 31
  waveforms of, 13
Current density, 15
  in electrocoagulation, 108
  in fully rectified circuits, 31, 32, *32, 33, 34, 35*, 48
  in medical vs. surgical diathermy, 11–12
Cuspid, malposed, exposure of, 315, *315*
  removal of, complicated by large cyst, *913*
  palatally impacted, 845, 847, *848, 849–851, 850*
CWRF current, 57
Cyst(s), adenomatous, of buccal mucosa, 1084, *1084*

Cyst(s) (*Continued*)
  and denture instability, 730
  complicating removal of malposed cuspid, *913*
  enveloping impacted molar, 841, *843*
  extensive, management of, 903–921
  follicular, treatment of, 520–521, *520*
  incisive canal, 908
  mandibular, 905–908, *906, 907*
  nasopalatine, 908–916, *910, 911, 913, 914*
  of papilla palatina, 908
  traumatic, 916–921, *917, 919, 920*

D

Damping. See *Currents, damped.*
D'Arsonval, 4, 12, 44
Dead space, surgical, avoidance of, 340
Debridement, of periodontal pockets, 568, *569.*
  See also *Periodontal pockets.*
Deciduous teeth, treatment of, 309–320
DeForest, 4, 46
Deglutition impairment, neoplasms and, 730
Dehydration, currents for, 36
  tissue. See *Electrodesiccation; Fulguration.*
Dental arch, alignment of, prior to immobilization
  of teeth, 577
Dental examination, and detection of cancer, 988
Dental school curriculum, 265
Dental student, experimental practice techniques
  for, 101–132
  prelaboratory electrosurgical exercises for, 93–
  100
Dentin, exposed, desensitization of, 266–272
Dentistry, operative. See *Operative dentistry.*
  restorative, 265–504
  classification in dental education, 265
Dentition, anterior, maxillo-mandibular relation
  in, 744
  permanent, aids to eruption of, 309–320
Denture
  acrylic template for, 730
  as surgical stent, 748, *753*, 770
  and irritation, 763
  clasp of, and enamel erosion, 271, *272*
  ill-fitting, and hypertrophic degeneration, 754,
  755
  and periodontoclasia, 607
  irritation from, and granuloma fissuratum, 764,
  765, 1039, *1041*
  and necrosis, 747
  and parakeratosis, *1050*
  poor adaptation of, 758
  seating of, impairment of, 730
Denture failures, causes of, 728–729
Denture flange, building of, 737, *738*
  labial, overextended, 762
Denture materials, old vs. new, 744
Denture sore, 1053, 1071, *1074*
Denture wearer, and trauma during mastication,
  744
Desensitization, of hypersensitive dentin, 266–272
  reaction of pulp to, 177–182, *178–182*
Desiccation, to debride necrotic tissue, 828. See
  also *Electrodesiccation.*
Desquamation, gingival, in periodontia, 629, *630*
  of surface epithelium, biopsy of, *1055*

Diabetes insipidus, and periodontal deterioration,
  564
Diastema, frenal attachment and, 710, *710*
  in Dilantin hypertrophy, 670
  in periodontoclasia, 631, *632*, 635, *636*
Diathermy, medical, 11
  surgical, 12
  for oral cancer, 1089
Diet, in plastic surgery, 921
Dietary deficiency, and periodontia, 629, *630*, 643
Dietary supplements, 249, 1108
  in periodontal therapy, 578
Dilantin, and tissue hypertrophy. See *Hypertrophy, Dilantin.*
Diode, 16, 46
Discoloration, of teeth, 301, 302, *303*
Dissection, mucous and submucous, for hyperplasia due to trauma, 745–748, *747*
  of redundant submucosa, with preservation of
  gingiva, 762
Drainage, incisions for, of acute abscess, 816–821
  lymphatic, of head and neck, 998, 999, *1000*
Dressings, surgical, 1108
Drifting. See *Migration.*
Drugs
  in emergency armamentarium, 245, 1103, 1104
  local, 237, 238–260
    anti-inflammatory, 250
    antiseptics and astringents, 251
    hemostatic, 249
    heterogenous grafts, 257
    oral bandages, 252
    physiological stimulants, 250
    sterilizing agents, for electrodes, 259
      for operative field, 258
    topical anesthetics, 248
  systemic, 236, 237–248
    for allergy and respiratory management, 245
    for cardiac management, 245
    hemostatic, 246
    preanesthetic-preoperative, 237–239
    premedication and postmedication, 239
    vitamins and dietary supplements, 248
Dryfoil, in orthodontic treatment, 557
Duct, submaxillary, "milking" of, 942
  sialoliths of. See *Sialoliths, of submaxillary
  duct.*

E

Edema, angioneurotic, drugs for, 1103
Edentulous areas, reduction of hypertrophic tissue
  in, 463–469, *464, 466, 467, 468*
Electrocardiogram (canine), during electrosurgical
  procedure, *152, 153*
Electrocautery, 3–4
  vs. electrosurgery, 10–12
Electrocoagulation, 36, 39, 73
  biterminal application of, *110*
  contraindicated in creation of subgingival
  trough, 87
  effect on tissue temperature, *159*, 160
  experimental procedures with, 108–112, *109,
  110, 112*
  for advanced oral cancer, 1089–1100

Electrocoagulation (*Continued*)
  for coronal exposure in delayed eruptions, 509–524, *510*
  for elongation of clinical crown, 391–392
  for endodontic sterilization, 208
  for experimental abortion of mandibular third molars, 205–207
  for granuloma fissuratum, *766*
  for hemangiomas, 831
  for hypertrophy in orthodontic treatment, 531–534, *533*
  for reduction of proliferative tissue, 272–274
  for root canal sterilization, 325–335, *334*
  for tooth bleaching, 301–305, *303*
  in control of granulation repair in tooth socket, 822–823, *822*
  in desensitization of exposed dentin, 267–272, *269, 271, 272*
  in pulp exposure, 306–307, *306*
  in sterilization of root canal apex, 340, *341*
  in subgingival trough preparation, 427
  of bleeder, 696–697
  of tooth socket, 736, *737*
Electrode(s)
  applications of, intermittent, 811
  coagulating, cylindrical, 271, *272*
    small ball, 268, *269*
    solid conical, 267, 269–271, *271*
  contact with orthodontic band, 555–556, *556*
  electrosurgical, placement of, 25–27
    types of, 19–25, *20, 21, 22*
  endodontic barbed broach, in root canal sterilization, 328–330, *328, 334*
  experimental techniques in use of, 105–126
  for biopsy, 1003–1006, *1004, 1005, 1006*
  indifferent, 13, *14*, 19, *22, 23, 24*
    for infant, 320
    placement of, 26
    seat, 1112
  loop, in frenectomy, *740*
    in periodontal pocket debridement, 568, *569*
    to facilitate inlay preparation, 284–290, *285, 286, 287, 289*
  needle, for gingivectomy, 290–292, *291*
    in drainage of abscess, 816–821, *818, 820*
  periodontal curet loop, in subgingival fracture, 274
  reshaping of, in operculotomy, *869*
    in treatment of endodontic-periodontal disease, 600
  surgical, 19, *20, 21*, 1112
    placement of, 25
Electrode contact points, 13
Electrode handle, barbed broach, *328*
Electrodesiccation, 36, 37, *37*, 71
  effect on tissue temperature, 156, *158, 159*
  experimental procedures with, *107*, 108
  of hemangiomas, 831
Electrolyte imbalance, 86
  effect of during anesthesia, 235
Electromagnetic waves, 17
Electromedical Systems unit, 59
Electronic scalpel, prototype, 4
Electrosection, 36, 39, 73–76
  biterminal, for infant, 320
  effect on bone, 810
  effect on tissue temperature, 160–162, *161, 162*

Electrosection (*Continued*)
  experimental procedures with, 112–126, *113–126*
  extraoral, 1080–1086
  for biopsy, 999–1000
  for coronal exposure in delayed eruption, 508–524, *509, 515, 517, 523*
  for mucoperiosteal flaps, 810. See also *Mucoperiosteal flaps.*
  for reduction of proliferative tissue, 273
  in subgingival trough preparation, 427
  in treatment of hypertrophy, 672–673
  loop, for elongation of clinical crown, 391, 392–395, *394*
    of granuloma fissuratum, *761*
  subgingival, for inlay preparation, 284–290, *285, 286, 287, 289*
  vs. steel scalpel surgery, 808
Electrosurgery
  advantages of, over caustics and escharotics, 80
    over steel scalpel, 78
  anesthesia in, 211–235
  basic physics of, 10–90
  cardiac response to, 151–153, *152, 153*
  causes of failures in, 81
  contraindications to, 84–88
    in aphthous ulcer, 85
    in biopsy of maxillary antrum and parotid gland, 85
    in creation of subgingival trough by electro-coagulation, 87
    in electrolyte imbalance, 86
    with cardiac pacemaker, 84
  dental, 42–44
  disadvantages of, 80
  explosive and flammable anesthetic agents in, 88
  for epileptic patient, 90
  historical background, 3–9
  indications for, 83–84
  medical, 42–44
  nitrous oxide-oxygen analgesia in, 88
  principles of, 18–35
  terminology in, 12–18
  vs. antibiotics, in osteomyelitis, 825
  vs. electrocautery, 10–12
  vs. steel scalpel surgery, *131*, 132, 263–264
    electron microscope histologic evaluation of, 195–200, *196–200*
    in gingivectomy for Dilantin hypertrophy, 200–205, *202, 203, 204*
    in periodontics, 561
    for subgingival curettage, 191–195, *192, 193*
Electrosurgical currents, 10–41. See also *Currents, electrosurgical.*
Electrosurgical equipment
  accessories to, 1112–1117
  dental, 42–70
    evaluation of, 65–70
  in armamentarium, 1111
  misconceptions about, 67–68
  placement of, 78
  purchasing guide for novice, 69
  qualifications of, 3, 4, 11
Electrosurgical instrumentation techniques, 70–78
  clinical. See under specific disciplines, e.g., *Crown and bridge prosthodontics; Endodontics; Orthodontics; Pedodontics; etc.*

Electrothermic endothermy, 4–8
Ellman Dento-Surg unit, 55, *55*
Embrasure tissue, removal of, for inlay preparation, 284–290
Emergency armamentarium, 245
Emergency drugs and instruments, 1102–1104
Enamel erosion, denture clasp and, 271, *272*
Endocrine imbalance, and periodontal deterioration, 564
Endodontics, 83, 321–377
Endodontic sterilization, electrocoagulation for, 208
Endodontic-periodontal disease, 582, 599–602
Endophytic lesion, *990*, 991
Endotherm knife, advantages of, 4–8
Endotracheal airway, emergency, 1103, *1104*
Envelope, of alternating current cycle, 16, *28*, 31
Epilepsy, and Dilantin hypertrophy. See *Hypertrophy, Dilantin.*
    and electrosurgery, 90
Epithelial rests, and cyst formation, 908
Epithelioma, basal cell, of lip, *993*
Epulis, loop resection of, *1048*
Epulis fibroma, biopsy of, 1030, *1031, 1032*
Epulis fissuratum, bifid, 730
    reduction of, 745
Epulis granulomatosa, 745
Equipment, electrosurgical. See *Electrosurgical equipment.*
Eruption, delayed, electrosurgical exposure for, 312–314, *313, 314*, 507–531
    partial, of malposed teeth, 518–531, *519*
    surgical exposure for, 314–316, *315*
Escharotics, and hemorrhage, 272
Estrogen deficiency, and periodontia, *647*
Excision, loop, 119, *119, 120, 121*
    of epithelial debris in socket, 621
Exodontia, 832–858
Exophthalmos, in oral cancer, 991
Exophytic lesion, 989, *990*
Experimental practice techniques, for practitioner and student, 101–132

F

Facial nerve plexus, in anesthesia administration, 226–228, *226*
Facial pain, in oral cancer, 992
Facial paralysis, in extraoral sialolithotomy, 952
Fail-safe switch, on unit, 78, *79*
Fiberglass mirror, in retraction, 813
Fiberoptics, in transillumination, 814–815, *815*
Fibroma, destruction of, by fulguration, *830*
    elongating tuberosity, 789
    gingival, biopsy of, 1030, *1031, 1032*
    incisional excision of, 1024–1026, *1026, 1027*
    loop excision of, 1027–1030, *1028, 1029*
    of tongue, 1077, *1078, 1093*
Fibromatosis, generalized gingival, 670, *671*
    in alveolar portion of arch, excision of, *860*, 861
Fibromatous pregnancy tumor, biopsy of, 1037–1039, *1038*
Fibrosis, complicating root-end resection, 346–348, *347*
    traumatic, of lip, 1009
Fistula(s), alveolo-gingival, complicating root-end resection, 342–345, *343, 345*

Fistula(s) (*Continued*)
    destruction of by fulguration, 823–825, *824*
    oro-antral, 372, 376
        repair of, 932–941
    palatal, plastic closure of, 922–924, *923*
Fixation, of tissue, after electrocoagulation, 267–268, 269, 271
Flame-shaped electrode, in elongation of clinical crown, 298, *298*
Flap(s). See also *Mucoperiosteal flap.*
    apically repositioned, for ridge extension, 771–774
        mandibular, in iatrogenic periodontoclasia, 717–721
    palatal, for root socket defect, 892, *933*
    palatal pedicle, 932, *933*
    slit incision, in gingival vs. buccal mucosa, 924
    tissue, 924–927, *926*
        in removal of impacted teeth, 835
        with bone grafts, in repair of oro-antral perforations, 932–941
    tissue inlay, 893, *894, 895, 897, 898*
Floor of mouth, biopsy of, 1071–1076
    tissues of, 941
    tumors of, 973–978
Foramen(ina), nasopalatine, destruction of, 908
    nutrient, sealed, 904
Forceps, Allis, 812
    coagulating, 1112
    in suturing, 812–813
    ophthalmic, in electrosurgery, 813
    tissue, 1113
Formalin, combined with electrocoagulation, 267–268, 269, 271
Fracture, pathologic, from extensive bone destruction, 911, *913*
    pulp exposure in, 305–306, *306*
    subgingival, electrosection for rubber dam isolation, 322, *322, 323*, 324, *324, 325*
    surgical removal of impacted teeth and, 834
    transverse, of maxilla, correction of, 795–806, *799, 800*
    traumatic, tissue flap for, 924, *926*
    vertical, infrabony pocket in, 695
Fracture site, subgingival, 278, 281, *282–283*
    exposure of, 272, *274*
Frenectomy
    electrosurgical, 534–536, *535*, 739–741, *740*
        in Dilantin hypertrophy, 672, *673*
    steel scalpel, 506, 534, 738, *739*
    to correct injudicious alveoloplasty, *749*, 750
    with vestibulotomy, 775
Frenectomy-frenotomy, 709–712
    experimental, 122, *123*
    for orthodontic purposes, 534–536, *535*
    in child, for aesthetics, 318–320, *319*
        for eruption of permanent centrals, 316–318, *317*
    of maxillary labial frenum, 861
Frenotomy, for ankyloglossia, 1018, *1020*, 1021
    lingual, 866, *867*
    of mandibular labial frenum, 862
Frenum(a), abnormal, and denture failures, 729
    and facial disharmony, 318
    deeply invaginated, resection of, 741
    elimination of. See also *Frenectomy-frenotomy.*
    in preprosthodontics, 737–743

Frenum(a) (*Continued*)
   lingual, high, and denture instability, 730
   mandibular, and traumatic traction, 712–713
   nonfibrous, resection of, by electrosurgery,
     739–741, *740*
Fulguration, 36, 37, 38, 71
   experimental procedures with, 106, *107*
   for hemostasis, in pocket debridement, *590*
   for osteomyelitis, 825
   in bleeding pulp exposure, 306, *306*
   in destruction of fistulae, 823–825, *824*
   in destruction of tumor masses, 829–831, *830*
   in necrotic tissue debridement, *828*
   in root debridement, *602*
   of bleeder, *298*
   of fistulous orifice, 922, *923*
   of follicular cyst, 843, *844*
   of muscle fibers, 717
   of necrotic tissue, in bifurcation involvement,
     703
   of pin-point pulp exposure, in child, 309–310,
     311
   of vesicular lip lesion, *1010*
   Oudin vs. simulated spark-gap current in, 141–
     142, *143*
   to treat periapical necrosis, *339*
Fully rectified circuits, 27, 31–35, *32, 33, 34, 35,*
   48
   invention of, 8, 12, *33*
   units supplying, constant-wave with coaxial
     shielding, 57–63, *58, 59, 60*
     dual-circuit, 55
     filtered, 57, *57*
     multiple-circuit, 55–57, *56*
     single circuit, 52–55, *53, 54, 55*
     oscilloscopic evaluation of, 143–148, *146, 147*

G

Gelatin, powdered surgical, 257, 903
Gelfoam, 249
Generators, spark-gap, 44, *45*
Generators, vacuum-tube, 4, 46
Geriatric patient, alveolar ridge resorption in, 770
Giant cell tumor, peripheral, biopsy of, 1032, *1033*
Gingiva, alveolar, 422
   areolar, 422
   atonal, in nutritional-hematologic deficiencies,
     629, *630*
     rekeratinization of, 721–726, *724, 725*
   cemental, in preparation of subgingival trough,
     422–423
   detachment of. See *Periodontal pockets.*
   fibromatosis of, 670, *671*
   health of, and periodontal deterioration, 563
   hyperplasia of. See *Hyperplasia, gingival.*
   invaginating into mandible, 928, *930*
   irritation of, in iatrogenic periodontoclasia, 603
   keratinized zones of, regeneration of, 721–726,
     724, 725
   marginal, debridement of, around fresh socket,
     821
     electrosection vs. scalpel cutting of, 397
     in preparation of, subgingival trough, 422,
       423, 434–438, *436, 437, 438*
     thin, gingivoplasty in, *688*
   massage of, 578

Gingiva (*Continued*)
   normal-appearing, in periodontia, 646
   recontouring of, 568, 569. See also
     Gingivoplasty.
   regeneration of after electrosection, 165–176,
     165–175
     after periodontal curettage, 573
   repositioning of, with frenectomy, 712–717
   stripping of, 566, *567*
   thin, slit incision flap in, 924
   trauma to, from frenal attachments, 709–717
Gingival harmony, elongation of clinical crown
   for, 395, *396,* 414–418
Gingival mucosa, biopsy of, 1030–1053
   histology of, 336
Gingival recession, 652, *653*
   prevention of, 434–435, *436*
   subgingival impingement and, 452
Gingival retraction, using astringents, 423, 426
Gingival tissue, effect of heat of electrosurgical
   currents on, 154–165, *157, 158, 159, 161, 163,*
    164
   postoperative inflammation of, electrosurgery
     vs. steel scalpel, 174, 174(t), *175*
   response to artificial crown, 384
Gingivectomy. See also *Subgingival trough*
   preparation.
   experimental, *120*
   full mouth, in periodontoclasia, 608
     in porcelain restorations, *614*
   of Dilantin hypertrophy, evaluation of healing
     following, 200–205, *202, 203, 204*
   of interdental papillae, to facilitate cavity prep-
     aration, 290–292, *291, 293*
   of unsupported gingiva, 398, *399*
   to elongate clinical crown, 401–403, *401, 402,*
    403
   with infrabony pocket eradication, 588
Gingivectoplasty, 654, *655, 659, 660*
   experimental, 122, *124, 125*
   for elongation of clinical crown, 293
   in periodontoclasia, 637
   loop planing for, 393, *394*
   tissue regeneration after, despite blood dys-
     crasia, 626, *627*
   to expose partially erupted teeth, 314–316, *315*
Gingivitis, necrotizing, and periodontal deterioration, 563
Gingivoplasty, 122, *124, 125,* 568, *569,* 573
   full mouth, 588, *589*
   in handicapped patient, *688, 690*
   in periodontoclasia, 604, *605, 632, 633*
   in traumatic occlusion, *596*
Gold crowns. See *Crowns, gold.*
Graft(s)
   bone, 928–932, *930*
     with tissue flaps, in repair of oro-antral perfo-
       rations, 932–941
   heterogenous, 257
     for periodontal pockets, 568
   mucous membrane, *803*
   powdered gelatin, 904
   split-thickness skin, 770
     in re-creation of vestibular space, 718
   tissue, 922–924, *923*
Granuloma fissuratum, 760–767
   biopsy of, 1039, *1041*
   electrocoagulation of, *766*

Granuloma fissuratum (*Continued*)
  from traumatic occlusion, 762, *763*
  multiple, denture irritation and, 764, *765*
  of floor of mouth, 1071, *1074*
  resection of, by loop electrosection, *761*
  superimposed on osteomyelitis, *1045*
Gutta percha, triggering mandibular cyst, 905, *906*

H

Hampton Electro Surgical unit, 57, *57*
Hawley retainer, after periodontal therapy, 634
Healing. See *Wound healing.*
Heart disease, periodontia in, 652
Heat dispersion, lateral, in electrosurgery, 562
  in periodontal curettage, 572
Hemangioma, cavernous, atypical, 1024
  obliteration of, 831
Hematologic disease, periodontia related to, 626
  with nutritional deficiency, 629, *630*
Hemimandibulectomy, 918, 1094, *1095*
Hemisection, of multirooted teeth, 878
  avoidance of, 899
Hemorrhage
  drugs to control, 246, 249
  electrocoagulation for, 110–112
  electrodesiccation for, 37–38
  escharotics and, 272
  from exposed pulp tissue, fulguration for, 306,
    306
Hemostasis, electrocoagulation for, 696–697, 810
Hemostats, mosquito, 1113
Hemostatic agents, 1107
High-frequency circuits, development of, 4, 12
High-frequency currents, 28–35, 46–49
Histologic comparison of electrosurgery and
    scalpel surgery, 195–200, *196–200*
Hormonal imbalance, and periodontia, 646
  effect on healing, 594. See also *Endocrine
    imbalance.*
Hydrocolloid impressions, of inlay preparations,
    in subgingival trough preparation, *419*
Hygroscopic deodorizing agent, 1110
Hyperemia, inflammatory, and periodontal
    deterioration, 563
Hyperkeratosis, denture irritation and, *1050*
  of palate, 1068
Hyperplasia. See also *Hypertrophy.*
  of mucosa, and denture instability, 730
  papillary, 968–971, *972*
  subgingival impingement and, 452
  trauma and, treatment of, 745–748, *747*
  traumatic fibrous, biopsy of, 1056, *1057, 1058*
Hypertrophy, Dilantin, 670, *671*, 672, 674, *675*
  electrosurgery vs. steel scalpel surgery, *677*
  gingivectomy for, evaluation of healing
    following, 200–205, *202, 203, 204*
  fibrous, resection of, 758, *759*
  ill-fitting denture and, 754, *755*
  in edentulous areas, reduction of, 463–469,
    464, 466, 467, 468
  in orthodontic treatment, electrocoagulation for,
    531–534, *533*
  in tooth socket, electrocoagulation for, 822–823,
    822
Hypodermic needles and syringes, 1106
  for oral local anesthesia, 230, *232, 233*

I

I and D. See *Drainage, incisions for.*
Iatrogenic periodontoclasia. See *Periodontoclasia,
    iatrogenic.*
Immobilization, of teeth, prior to periodontal
    therapy, 575–577, *577*
  permanent, after periodontal therapy, 657
  temporary, after periodontal therapy, 657
Impaction, preorthodontic treatment of, 507–531,
    520, 527, 530
Impedance, 17–18, 22
  evaluation of, in biterminal current application,
    149, 151
Implants, blade, 469, 470, 472, 473–480, *474, 475,
    476, 478, 479*
  mucoperiosteal flap incisions in, 469–480, *472,
    474, 475, 476, 478, 479*
  organic, to repair cystic defects, 911
Implantology, in treatment of alveolar ridge
    resorption, 774
Impression materials, old vs. new, 744
Impression-taking, electrosection to facilitate,
    284–290
Incision(s), in root-end resection, 336, 337–338
  purse-mouth, in hard palate, *793*
  semilunar, 337, *337*
  vertico-oblique, 337, *338*
Incisional biopsy, *1004, 1006*
Incisional excision, extraoral, by electrosection,
    1080–1086
  of palate, 1053–1058
Incisive canal cysts, 908
Indifferent plate, evaluation of, 148–151
Indifferent electrode, 13, *14*, 19, *22, 23, 24, 26*
Induration, local, and oral cancer, 991
Infection(s), chronic, and healing, 592, 594
  complicating removal of impacted molar,
    839, *840*
  control of, drugs for, 241
  in periodontia, 648
  mixed, therapy for, 244
  of submaxillary duct, 943
Infiltrative lesions, 990, 991
Infrabony pockets. See *Periodontal pockets.*
Infrabony pocket debridement, experimental, 122,
    124, 125
Inlay preparation, electrosection for, *276, 277*,
    284–290, *285, 286, 287, 289*
Instrument(s), broken, in root canal, 368–372
  broken fragment of, root-end resection for, 368
  emergency, circulatory and respiratory, 1103–
    1104
Instrumentation, control of, 129–132, *130, 131*
Instrumentation techniques, causes of failure of,
    81
  electrosurgical, 70–78
  experimental practice of for practitioner and
    student, 101–132
  preclinical exercises for, 91–100
  types of meat used in, 126–132, *130, 131*
Iodophors, 259

J

Jaw, impaction of metallic fragment in, 834
  pathologic fracture of, 834, 841
Jet injection anesthesia, 231, *233*

Jet syringes, 1106
J-loop electrode, in excision of subgingival tissue, 284–290, *285*, *286*, *289*

K

Kazanjian technique, 745
Kenalog in Orabase, 250, 253, 255
Keratinization, in attached gingiva, regeneration of, 721–726, *724*, *725*
    loss of, in periodontoclasia, 629, *630*, 635, *636*, 643

L

Lachrymal probe, 1115
Lavages, in armamentarium, 1109
Leukoplakia, 965–968, *990*
    biopsy of, *1052*
    biopsy specimen of, *969*
    clinical appearance of, 966
    of lip, 1011
    of tongue, 1064
    spot coagulation of, 968, *970*
    with ulceration, of palate, *1067*
Lichen planus, biopsy of, 1042–1044, *1043*
Lidocaine, pharmacodynamics of, 214
Liebel-Flarscheim Bovie unit, 59
Lip, biopsy of, 1006–1023, *1012*, *1013*, 1072, *1073*
    and buccal mucosa, 1018–1023
    cancer of, 992, *993*
        incidence of, 986
    lesion of, incisional resection of, 1007, *1008*
        loop resection of, 1014–1018, *1015*, *1016*, *1017*
    lower, paresthesia of, 991
    paresthesia of, root-end resection and, 365
Loop electrode, for elongation of clinical crown, 293, *294*, *295*, *297*, *298*
    in subgingival trough preparation, 423–426, *425*
    to expose unerupted crowns, 312–314, *313*, *314*
    uses of, 116–126, *116–126*
Loop electrosection, for gingivectoplasty, 314–316, *315*
    of exposed pulp tissue, 305–306, *306*
Loop resection, of hard palate, for biopsy, 1058–1066
    of lip lesion, 1014–1018, *1015*, *1016*, *1017*
Lymphatic drainage, of head and neck, 998, *999*, *1000*
Lymphosarcoma, of submaxillary gland, 1080

M

Malocclusion, and periodontal disease, 587
    longstanding, 583
Mandible. See also *Jaw*.
    cyst of, 905–908, *906*, *907*
    dentulous, contacting edentulous maxilla, 745, 746
    root-end resection in, 364–368
Mandibulo-maxillary relations, proper, 743–744
Manufacturers. See *Armamentarium*.
Marsupialization, of cysts, 903
    of tumors, 973
Martin Elektrotom units, 54, *54*, 55

Mastication, traumatic forces in, 744
Maxilla, cyst in, 908–916, *910*, *911*, *913*, *914*
    deformed, repair of, 544–547, *545*, *546*
    edentulous, contacting dentulous mandible, 745, 746
    ridge reduction of, 780–783, *782*
    transverse fracture of, correction of, 795–806, *799*, *800*
Maxillary antrum
    biopsy of, 85
    diseases of, electrosurgery for, 359
    projection of roots into, 834
    perforation of, accidental, 359, 365
        repair of, 932–941
    purulent exudate from, in oral cancer, 991
    root fragment in, removal of, 933–941
Maxillo-mandibular relations, proper, 743–744
Medication, 236–261. See also *Drugs*.
Menadione, 249
Menopause, and periodontal deterioration, 564, 646
Menstruation, and periodontal deterioration, 564, 646
    healing in, 592
Mental nerve, injury to, 365, 366
Mental nerve evulsion, 978–980, *979*
Metabolism, alterations in, and periodontal deterioration, 564
Metastasis, biopsy-induced, 996
    mechanical safeguards against, 996
Methemoglobin, and tooth discoloration, 301
Microglossia, 549, *550*
Micrognathia, 549, *550*
Migration, in alveolar bone loss, 631, *632*
    in periodontoclasia, pathologic, 635, *636*, 657
    loss of opposing dentition and, 786
    prevention of, after periodontal therapy, 634
Mirror, fiberglass, 813
Mobility, of teeth, in periodontoclasia, 657
Model, trimming of, prior to preprosthodontic electrosurgery, 730, 733, 784–785, *785*
Molars
    displacement of, in surgery for impacted teeth, 834
        into sphenomaxillary fossa, 844
    impacted, experimental exposure of, 122, *128*
        multiple involvement in, 841, *842*
        vertically, operculotomy for, 873, *874*
    mandibular third, complicated by pericoronitis, 839, *840*
        experimental abortion of, 205–207
        impacted, 835, *836*, *838*
        palliative exposure of, 875, *877*
    maxillary, palatal roots of, radectomy of, 892–898
    maxillary third, impacted, 844–845, *846*
Monopolar electrode, definition of, 13
Monoterminal currents. See *Currents, monoterminal*.
Monoterminal electrode, definition of, 13, *14*, 27
Mucocele, resection of, 1018–1023, *1020*
Mucoperiosteal flaps
    electrosection for, 810
    for debridement of dead cementum, 604, *605*
    for root-end resection, 302, *303*
    in bifurcation debridement, *625*
    in Dilantin periodontoclasia, *682*, *683*
    in periodontal curettage, *586*
        disadvantages of, 571

Mucoperiosteal flaps (*Continued*)
  in removal of cystic odontoma, 854, 855, 857
  in treatment of endodontic-periodontal disease, 600, *602*
  incision for, 337–338, *338*, 341, *341, 343, 347, 349, 352, 354, 357, 361,* 366, *367, 371, 375*
  in implantation, 469–480, *472, 474, 475, 476, 478, 479*
Mucosa, alveolar, resection of, *749*
Multiple sclerosis, periodontia in, 685
Muscle attachment. See also *Frenum.*
  abnormal traction of, frenectomy-frenotomy for, 709–717
  in mandible, 712–713
  low, correction of, 737
Muscle dysfunction, in oral cancer, 992

N

Narcotics, 241, 1109
Nasal spine, reduction of, 781
Nasopalatine cyst, 908–916, *910, 911, 913, 914*
Nasopalatine foramen, destruction of, 908
Necrosis, denture irritation and, *747*
  fulguration of, to restore alveolar contour, 829
  of pulp tissue, silver nitrate and, 267
  periapical, removal of, 338–339, *339*
Needles, suture, 811
Needle electrode, for elongation of clinical crown, 293
  improper use of, 113, *114, 115*
  proper use of, 113, *113, 115*
  use in subgingival trough preparation, 432–434, *433*
Neoplasms. See also *Osteofibromas; Tumors.*
  and deglutition impairment, 730
  and denture failures, 729
  leukoplakic, 965–968
  multiple, biopsy of, 1018–1023, *1020*
  oral, 985–986
  palpation of, prior to biopsy, 996
Nerve, mental, injury to, 365, 366
Nerve plexuses, in anesthesia, facial, 226–228, *226*
  pterygoid, 217
Neurofibromas, 993
Neuroma, amputation, mental nerve evulsion and, 978
  resection of, 928, *930*
Neuromuscular relaxant, 1110
Neutropenia, cyclic, and infection, 592
Nitrous oxide-oxygen analgesia, in electrosurgery, 88
Nutrient foramina, in eburnated bone, 904
  opening of, 340

O

Occlusion, disharmonies of, 563
  nonfunctional, and periodontal disease, 594, *596*
  proper maxillo-mandibular relations in, 743–744
  traumatic, and granuloma fissuratum, 762, *763*
  and periodontal deterioration, 563, 582, 583, *584,* 587, 594, *596,* 669, *669*
Odontoma, cystic, treatment of, 851, 854, 855, 856, 857.
Operative dentistry, 266–308
  electrosurgery for, 83

Operculotomy, experimental, 122, *127*
  for resection of pericoronal flaps, 866–878
  reshaping electrode in, *869*
  to eliminate pericoronitis, 871, *872*
  to expose vertically impacted molar, 873, *874*
  to facilitate tooth removal, 869, *870*
Orabase, 253, 255
Orahesive, 254, *255, 256*
Oral bandages, 252, *255, 256*
Oral cavity, lymphatic drainage of, 998, *999, 1000*
Oral surgery. See *Surgery, oral.*
Oro-antral fistula, and delayed healing, 372, 376
Oro-antral perforation, repair of, 932–941
Oronasal defect, plastic closure of, 922–924, *923*
Oropharyngeal cancer, incidence of, 985, 986
Orthodontics, 505–558
  electrosurgery for, 84
  frenectomy-frenotomy in, 534–536, *535*
  impediments to, 507–536
  pre-treatment for, electrosurgical, 507–536
  techniques in cleft palate abnormalities, 537–558
  unfavorable tissue reactions to, 531–534
Orthodontic bands, and subgingival impingement, 582
Oscillograph, 15
Oscilloscope, 15
Osteitis, heat in pulp chamber and, 301
Osteofibromas, bilateral, of hard palate, reduction of, 791–795, *792, 793, 794*
Osteofibromatous tuberosity, reduction of, 789, *789*
Osteomyelitis, biopsy of, 1044–1046, *1045*
  fulguration for, 825
Oudin, spark-gap current, 29, 44
  physical features of, 107
Oxycel, 249
Oxygen, in emergency armamentarium, 246, 1102
Ozium, *1110*

P

Pacemakers, cardiac, use of electrosurgery with, 84
Pain, facial, in oral cancer, 992
Pain response, 817, *818*
Palatal mucosa, biopsy of, 1053–1071
  reduction of, for rubber dam isolation, 322, *322, 323, 324, 324, 325*
Palatal pedicle flap, 932, *933*
Palatal vault, collapse of, 754, *755*
Palate, bilateral osteofibromas of, reduction of, 791–795, *792, 793, 794*
  fistula in, plastic closure of, 922–924, *923*
  hard, incisional and loop resection of, 1066–1071, *1067, 1068, 1070*
  loop resection of, for biopsy, 1058–1066
  infrabony pocket on, 707, *708*
Papilla(e), interdental, hypertrophic, in pocket debridement, *591*
  gingivectomy of, 290–292, *291, 293*
  reduction of, 568, 665
Papilla palatina, cyst of, 908
Papillary hyperplasia, 968–971, *972*
Papilloma, overlying mucous cyst, 1083, *1084*
Parakeratosis, biopsy of, 1049–1051, *1050*

Paralysis, of facial muscles, in extraoral sialo-
lithotomy, 952
Paresthesia, of lip, root-end resection and, 365
of lower lip, 991
Parkell Electronic Electrosurgery unit, 54, 55
Parotid gland, accidental anesthesia of, 227, 228,
229
dysfunction of, in oral cancer, 992
Partially rectified circuits, 27, 28, 30, 47
units supplying, 50–52, 51
Partsch technique of marsupialization, 903, 973
failure of, 974
Pedodontics, 309–320
electrosurgery for, 83
Pedunculated mass, loop resection of, 1027, 1028
Penicillin, 242
Perforation(s)
mandibular, repair of, 928, 930
of root canal, accidental, 368
oro-antral, traumatic, 932–941, 937
oronasal, plastic repair of, 1034
traumatic, 928, 930
Periapical defect, "biased" root-end resection for,
353–356, 354
Pericementitis, acute, 583
Pericoronitis, acute, drainage for, 819, 820
complicating removal of impacted molar, 839,
840
operculotomy for, 866, 868, 871, 872
Periodontal curettage. See Curettage, periodontal.
Periodontal degeneration, iatrogenic, 382, 383.
See also Crown and bridge prosthodontics.
Periodontal disease, and endodontic involvement,
599–602
causes of, 582
biomechanical, 599–626
mechanical, 583–599
related to blood dyscrasia, 626
related to nutritional-hematologic deficiencies,
629, 630
Periodontal packs, 1108
Periodontal pocket(s), debridement of, 573, 586,
590, 604, 605
in traumatic occlusion, 596, 597
deep infrabony, and loss of bone structure, 635,
636
cross-section of, 692
treatment of, 691–709
deep irregular, 589, 692
eradication of, 569
with gingivectomy, 588
graft materials for, 568
horizontal, 566
in presence of vertical fracture, 695
instrumentation of, 566–570
intraradicular, 699–709, 701, 703, 706
measuring depth of, 659
of difficult access, 707
of key abutment tooth, 692, 693
resection of, 572, 572
vertical, 566
Periodontal pocket probes, 1114
Periodontal structures, repair of, 560
Periodontia, complicated by unrelated systemic
disease, 685–691
electrosurgery for, 84
normal-appearing gingiva in, 646
related to cell abnormalities, 670–684

Periodontics, 559–727
clinical techniques in, 581–727
electrosurgery in, 564–570
interceptive, using electrosurgery, 197
methods of treatment in, 559–563, 570
objectives of, 559
postoperative treatment in, 577–579
preoperative treatment in, 573–577
Periodontium, deterioration of, 563–564
Periodontoclasia, 566. See also Periodontal
pocket(s).
advanced, treatment of, 604, 605
and ill-fitting dentures, 607
complicated by unrelated systemic factors, 685–
691
iatrogenic, 602–626
poor restoration and, 606
traction from marginal gingivae and, 717–721
influence of oral hygiene on, 668, 669
porcelain restorations and, 612, 614
related to nonspecific systemic factors, 657–684
related to systemic factors, 626–691
relation of abnormal traction to, 709–717
subgingival impingement and, 616, 620
traumatic occlusion and, 583, 584
Periosteum, in suturing, 812
shifting, and denture instability, 730
Peripheral seal, disruption of, 729
Pharynx, cancer of, incidence of, 986
Physics, of electrosurgery, 10–90
Physiological pen recorder, 156, 157, 178, 179
Physiotherapy, and periodontal tissues, 560
in retention of maturely keratinized gingiva, 726
oral, in periodontics, 573–574, 577
Pins, in armamentarium, 1114
Planing, of tissue, by electrosection, for inlay
preparation, 118, 284–290, 285, 286, 287, 289
Plastic surgery, for skin grafting in bone resorp-
tion, 770
oral, 921–941
reconstructive, 730
with subtotal radectomy, 893, 894, 895–898
Pocket marker, 659
Pockets, periodontal. See Periodontal pocket(s).
Pontics. See Bridge.
Porcelain pontics, repair of, 388–391, 388, 390
Porcelain restorations, and periodontoclasia, 612,
614
Postmedication, 239
Power output, adjustment guideline, 77
linear, 64
nonlinear, 65
Practitioner, experimental practice techniques for,
101–132
Premaxilla, floating, immobilization of, 410
Premedication, 239
Preprosthodontics, 728–806
criteria for surgical intervention in, 728–730
electrosurgical techniques in, 730
Probe(s), 1114, 1115
flexible silver, in location of sialolith, 952, 953,
955, 962
Procaine, pharmacodynamics of, 214
Proliferation, of tissue, impeding inlay preparation, 276, 277, 284–290, 285, 286, 287, 289
in tooth socket, 736
into cavity preparation, 274–276, 275
into interproximal caries site, 274, 276, 277

Proliferation (*Continued*)
　of tissue, prosthetic restorations and, 405–406, *406*
　subgingival, 272–274
Prosthesis(es). See also *Denture(s)*.
　ill-fitting, and iatrogenic periodontoclasia, 603
　improper, and periodontoclasia, 582
　obturator-like, in traumatic fracture, 924, 925
Prosthodontics, 84. See also *Preprosthodontics*.
Pterygoid venous plexus, in anesthesia administration, 217
Pulp, histologic reaction to dentin desensitization, 177–182, *178–182*
　hypersensitive, in treatment of infrabony pockets, 693
Pulp capping, electrosurgery in, 305–308, *306*
Pulp chamber, oxidation of, 301
Pulp exposure, pinpoint, in adult, *306*
　in child, 309–310, *311*
　pseudo-, *306*, 307
　traumatic, 305–308, *306*
Purulent exudate, from antrum, in oral cancer, 991
Pushback procedure. See also *Vestibule, pushback of; Vestibulotomy*.
　in periodontoclasia, 709–717
　to re-create vestibular space, 719

R

Radectomy, subtotal, 878–901
　of mandibular molar root, 899–901, *900*
　of maxillary molar palatal roots, 892–898
　with plastic repair, 893, *894*, 895–898
Radio-frequency current, 16
Radioknife, 4–8, 46–64
Radiopaque visualizer, 1110
Radiotherapy, for oral cancer, 994
Ranula, biopsy specimens of, *976, 977*
　incisional excision of, 973–978, *975*
　of floor of mouth, removal of, 852, 853
Research, in electrosurgery, ground rules in, 138–140
　indications and standards for, 135–140
　reports of, behavioral, 141–153
　　clinical techniques on human subjects, 191–208
　　laboratory experiments in clinical techniques, 154–190
　relation to clinical electrosurgery, 136–140
Resection, incisional, of proliferative hypertrophy, 745
　loop, 116–118, *116, 117, 118*
　of lip lesion, 1014–1018, *1015, 1016, 1017*
　of ranula, 973
　of biopsy specimens, mechanics of, 1003–1006, *1004, 1005, 1006*
　of redundant mucous tissue, 749, 750
　of redundant submucous tissue, 752, *753, 755*, 756
　root-end. See *Root-end resection*.
Resorption, of alveolar bone. See also *Bone, alveolar, resorption of*.
　senile vs. functional, 748
Respiratory emergency, control of, 245
Restoration, ill-fitting, and pericementitis, 583
Restorative dentistry, 265–504
Retraction, in oral surgery, 813–814

Retractor(s), 1115
　cheek-lip, 537, *538*, 813, *1115*
Ridge, alveolar. See *Alveolar ridge*.
Ritter Mode[4] unit, 60, *61*
Root(s), amputation of, 886, *887*, 889, *890*
　ankylosis of, 834
　buccal, apicoectomy of, 879–892, *880, 881*
　denuded, in periodontia, 658
　dilaceration of, 834, 841, *843*
　exposure of, for rubber dam isolation, 322, *322, 323, 324, 324, 325*
　key retained abutment, exposure of, 420, *421*, 456–463, *457, 460, 461, 462*
　of mandibular molar, amputation of, 899–901, *900*
　palatal, bone destruction around, 705, *706*
　projecting into maxillary antrum, 834
　retained, exposure of, for removal, 832–834, *832, 833*
　treatment of infrabony pocket in, double, 691, *691*, 699–705, *701, 703*
　　single, 691, *691*, 692–699, *693, 694, 696*
　　triple, 691, *691*, 705–709, *706, 708*
Root amputation, 335–376. See also *Root-end resection*.
Root canal, accidental perforation of, 368–372, *371*
　chronically suppurating, one-sitting treatment of, 331–335, 334
Root canal apex, sealing of, 340, *341*
Root canal filling, incomplete, and surgical dead space, *374*
Root canal sterilization, by electrocoagulation, 325–335, *334*
Root-end resection, 335–376, 878–901
　arc incision in, 366
　failures in, 336, 372–376
　for broken instrument fragments, 368–372
　in mandible, 364–368
　root retention in, 353–356, *354*
Root fragment, removal of, scalpel vs. electrosection, 936–941, *937, 939, 940*
Root planing, prior to periodontal therapy, 575
Root socket defect, palatal flap for, 892, *933*
Rubber dam drains, centipede, 818, *819*
Rubber dam isolation, 321–325, *325*

S

Saliva, viscous, in dietary deficiency, 629
Saliva ejector tips, 1113, *1114*
Salivary calculus. See *Calculus, salivary*.
Scaling. See also *Calculus, removal of*.
　in handicapped patient, 686
Scalpel
　electronic, prototype, 4
　steel, and metastasis, 7
　　and tissue trauma, 808
　　for frenectomy, 738, 739
　　for marsupialization of cysts, healing in, 903
　　for semilunar incision in root-end resection, 337, *337*
　　for vestibulotomy, 770
　　hazards of, 808
　　in exposure on unerupted tooth, *513*
　　in implantology, 469, 470, *471*
　　use in hypertrophied tissue, 672–673, *676*
　　vs. electrosurgery, 263–264
　　　in periodontics, 561

Scalpel (*Continued*)
   steel, vs. endotherm knife, 7
Scar tissue, in cold-steel semilunar incision, *337, 341*
   of lip, *1013,* 1014
Scar tissue adhesions, and denture failures, 729
   in steel scalpel frenectomy, 739
Scarification, of bone, in cystic disease, 904
Schmutzpyorrhea, 582, *582*
Scissors, suture, 813
Sclerosing solutions, for obliteration of hemangiomas, 831
Sclerosis, in long-standing cystic disease, 904
Seal, peripheral, disruption of, 729
Sealing, of root canal apex, 340, *341*
Sedatives, 240, 1109
Semilunar incision, in root-end resection, 362–364, *363, 364*
Senility, and alveolar ridge resorption, 729
Serumal calculus. See *Calculus, serumal.*
Shock, anaphylactic, during local anesthesia, 234
   drugs for, 1103
   mild, drugs for, 1104
Shoulder preparation, types of, *422, 426*
Sialoliths, *964*
   hollow, removal of, 957–961, *959, 960*
   locating in duct, 942, *949*
   of submaxillary duct, removal of, 852, *853*
   removal of, at posterior end of duct, 948, *950*
      midway between duct orifice and gland, 944, 946, *947*
      near duct orifice, 944
Sialolithiasis, of submaxillary duct and gland, 941–965, *962*
   secondary infection in, 943
Sialolithotomy, extraoral, 952
   intraoral, *952,* 953–965, *954, 959, 962*
      advantages of, 965
   of submaxillary duct, 941–965, *945*
Siemens Radiotome, 52
Silver nitrate, for desensitization of exposed dentin, 267
Sinus, maxillary, occluded, in oral cancer, 991
Slit incision flap, in gingival vs. buccal mucosa, 924
Sluiceway, creating in embrasure, experimental, 122, *126*
Smoking, and leukoplakia, 968
   and oral cancer, 987
Socket, tooth. See *Tooth socket.*
Sodium sulfite, 571
Solid-state circuitry, 16
Spark-gap circuit, *47*
Spark-gap current, 28, *29*
   Oudin vs. simulated, evaluation of, 141–142, *143*
   physical features of, 107
Spark-gap generators, 44, *45,* 1111
   development of, 4
Splint, for floating premaxilla, in cleft palate, 542–544, *543*
   in frenectomy and gingival repositioning, 715, *716*
   in periodontal therapy, 576
      causing periodontoclasia, 616, *620*
      Whaledent, 641

Splint (*Continued*)
   intermediate, processing of, 438–456, *441, 442, 443, 445, 446, 447, 449, 450, 451, 452, 453, 454, 455*
Splint bands, temporary, 439, *439*
Splinting pins, 1114
Split mucosal flap procedure, 571
Spray bandages, 254
Squamous cell carcinoma, of tongue, coagulation-excision for, 1096–1100, *1098, 1099, 1100*
Steel scalpel. See *Scalpel, steel.*
Steele's facing, replacement of, 388
Stent, surgical, after frenectomy and gingival positioning, *716*
   as denture flange, 737, *738*
Sterilization, in electrosection, 809
   inherent in electrocoagulation, 307
   of curved roots, by electrocoagulation, 328–329
   of root canal, by electrocoagulation, 325–335, *334*
   of surgical field, by electrocoagulation, in root-end resection, 356
Sterilizers, 1116
Sterilizing agents, for electrodes, 259
   for operative field, 258
Sterilizing solutions, 1110
Steroids, 250
Stimulants, circulatory and respiratory, 1103
   physiological, 250
Stomatitis, Vincent's, and periodontal deterioration, 563
Stomatitis nicotinae, 1064
Stripping, gingival, 566, *567*
Subgingival curettage, cold-steel vs. electrosurgical, 191–195, *192, 193*
Subgingival impingement in orthodontic treatment, 531–534
Subgingival trough, preparation of, 419–438, *420*
   atraumatic, 430, *431*
   by electrocoagulation, 87
   electrodes used in, 423–426, *425,* 432–434, *433*
   experimental, 119, *120, 121, 122*
   in fixed prosthodontics, 426–428
   in full crown preparation, 419–426, *419, 422, 423, 425*
   in temporary and permanent fixed restorations, 428–432
   in thin marginal gingiva, 434–438, *436, 437, 438*
   inadequate, and impingement, 444–456
   using astringents, 423, 426
   using full loop, 285, *287*
   using J-loop, 284, *286,*
Submaxillary gland, carcinoma of, 1080
Suction-coagulating handpiece, 1112
Sulfonamides, 244
Surgery. See also *Electrosurgery; Scalpel.*
   of cleft palate, 808
   of soft tissues, 858–878
   oral, 807–815
      associated unfavorable factors, 807
      electrosurgery for, 84
      major, 902–981. See also under individual procedures.

Surgery (*Continued*)
  oral, minor, 816–901. See also under individual procedures.
  plastic. See *Plastic surgery*.
Surgical gelatin, powdered, 903
Surgical stent. See *Stent, surgical*.
Surgical packs, 1108
Surgicel, 249
Sutures, 811, 1113
Suture needles, 811, 1113
Suturing, of flap in root-end resection, *341*
  of periosteum, 812
Syncope, drugs for, 1104
Syringes, 1106
  aspirational biopsy, *1114*
  irrigating, 1115
    endodontic, *332, 333*

T

Teeth, displacement of, in cystic disease, 905
  impacted, exposure of, 507–523, *520*
    in edentulous areas, 845
    malposed, and denture instability, 730
    removal of, 524–531, *527, 530*
    surgical hazards in, 834
    surgical removal of, 834–851
  key abutment, periodontal pockets of, 692, *693*
  malposed, and hyperplastic gingiva, 582
    preorthodontic exposure of, 507–531, *519*
  migration of, in alveolar bone loss, 631, *632*
  mobile, immobilization of, prior to periodontal therapy, 575–577, *577*
  multirooted, amputation of, 886, *887*
    subtotal radectomy of, 878–901
  supernumerary, removal of, 524–526, *525*, 851–858
  unerupted, exposure of, by electrosurgery, 507–536
    by steel scalpel surgery, 858–860, *859*
Thermistor probe, 156, *157*
Thrombin, topical, 249
Tinctures, aromatic, 250
Tissue(s), cell cleavage in, scalpel vs. electrosurgery, 808
  cicatricial repair of, 808
  conservation of, in periodontics, 565
  excess, excision of, determining extent of, 784–786, *785, 786*
  hypertrophic, reduction of, in edentulous areas, 463–469, *464, 466, 467, 468*
  of floor of mouth, 941
  redundant, mucous and submucous, resection of, 743–767
  regeneration of following electrosection, 165–176, *165–175*, 176(t)
  response to Dilantin therapy, atypical, 676–684, *678*
    typical, 672–676
  soft, defects of. See *Preprosthodontics*.
    surgery of, 858–878
  temperature of, effect of electrosurgical currents on, 154–165
    in periodontal electrosurgery, 562
  trauma to, in biopsy, 996
    in scalpel surgery, 808

Tissue carbonization. See *Fulguration*.
Tissue flaps, 924–927, *926*. See also *Mucoperiosteal flaps*.
Tissue grafts, 922–924, *923*
Tissue inlay technique, using scalpel, 933, *935*
Tissue planing. See *Planing, of tissue*.
Tissue proliferation. See *Proliferation, of tissue*.
Tissue reactions, to orthodontic treatment, 531–534
  undesirable, causes of, 81
Tissue resistance, 76
Tissue tabs, removal of, in preprosthodontics, 730, 732, *732*
Tissue tone, subnormal, and free bleeding, 810
Tomes' fibers, coagulation of, 266, 267
Tongue, biopsy of, 1072, *1073*, 1076–1078
  cancer of, 992
    incidence of, 986
  squamous cell carcinoma of, coagulation-excision for, 1096–1100, *1098, 1099, 1100*
Tongue blades, wooden, in retraction, 814
Tooth bud, of mandibular third molar, abortion of, 205–207
Tooth movement, in periodontia, 657
  rapid, and periodontal disease, 582
Tooth socket, debridement of, by loop excision, 821–822, *821*
  granulation repair in, control of, 822–823, *822*
  tissue proliferation in, 736
Toothbrush, electric, 578, 579, 1117
  manual, 578, 1116
Toothbrushing, in periodontal physiotherapy, 577
Topical anesthesia, 231, 248
Torus(i), bilateral, reduction of, 802–806, *803*
  palatal, and denture failures, 729
Traction, abnormal, related to periodontia, 709–717. See also *Muscle attachments*.
Tranquilizers, 238, 1107
Transillumination, 814–815, *815*
  of infrabony pockets, 646, *649, 650*
  to determine extent of debridement, 855
  to visualize calculus, 575
Transilluminator, 1117
Transistor, 16
Trauma, and cyst formation, 916–921, *917, 919, 920*
  and hyperplasia, treatment of, 745–748, *747*
  during mastication in denture patient, 744
  tissue, in biopsy, 996
Trifurcation, debridement of, *598*
  in multiple sclerosis patient, *688*
Trifurcation involvement, 691, *691*, 705–709, *706, 708*
  ill-fitting dentures and, 607, *611*
Tuberosities, abnormal, correction of, 783–791
  and denture failures, 728, 729, 730
  deformed, restoring contour of, *790*
  reduction of, predetermination of, 784–786, *785, 786*
  types of, 783
Tumors, destruction of, by fulguration, 829–831, *830*
  fibromatous pregnancy, 1037–1039, *1038*
  nerve. See *Neuroma*.

U

Ulcer, aphthous, nonelectrosurgical treatment of, 85
  nonhealing, 991
Ulceration of hypertrophied tissue, incisional excision of, 745
  vs. infiltrative lesion, 991
Ultrasonic prophylactic unit, 1117
Units, electrosurgical, 1111
Unrectified circuits, 27, 28, 29
U-shaped loop electrode, in excision of subgingival tissue, 284–290, 285, 287
  to remove necrotic periapical debris, 339

V

Vacuum tube generator, 4, 46
Valleylab units, 59
Vermilion stripping, by steel scalpel, 1013, 1014
Verrucous lesion, 989, 990
Vertico-oblique incision, for mucoperiosteal flap, in Dilantin periodontoclasia, 682, 683. See also Mucoperiosteal flap.
Vestibule, buccal, biopsy of, 1039–1044
  pushback operation for, 516, 517
  loss of, 729
  occluded, expanded tuberosities, and, 788, 789
  scar tissue and, 758
  pushback of, 547–549, 547, 548
  re-creation of, apically repositioned flap for, 717–721
Vestibulotomy, for alveolar ridge extension, 767–783
  in totally resorbed alveolar ridge, 780–783, 782
  mandibular, with submucous dissection, 771–774, 772
    without submucous dissection, 774–778, 775
  procedure for, 770
  with alveoloplasty, 778–780, 779

Vincent's stomatitis, and periodontal deterioration, 563
Vitamins, 249, 1108
  in periodontal therapy, 578
  in plastic surgery, 921
Vitamin deficiency, and periodontoclasia, 631
von Recklinghausen's disease, 993, 993
V-Y incision, 682, 683
  with electrosurgery, 742
  with steel scalpel, 738, 739

W

Water jet spray, in oral physiotherapy, 578
Watts, 17
  misconceptions about, 67
Waveform(s), 13
  modified continuous, 62, 63
  of alternating current, 27–35
    fully rectified, 27, 31–35, 32, 33, 34, 35
    partially rectified, 27, 28, 30
    unrectified, 27, 28, 29
  of fully rectified circuit, oscilloscopic comparison of, 143–148, 146, 147
"Webb" technique, 110
Whaledent Omni-Depth pocket marker, 659
Whaledent Strobex unit, 57, 57
Wound closure, suture materials in, 811
Wound healing, after electrosection, 809
  after electrosurgical root-end resection, 348–351, 349
  after periodontal electrosurgery, histologic nature of, 727
  after steel scalpel surgery, 809
  during menstrual cycle, 592, 594
  in electrosurgery vs. cold-steel surgery, in periodontics, 562

Z

Zephyr Temporary Splint Bands, 439